# Respiratory Genetics

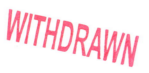

# Respiratory Genetics

**Edited by**

**Edwin K. Silverman** MD, PhD
Channing Laboratory and Division of Pulmonary and Critical Care Medicine
Brigham and Women's Hospital
Harvard Medical School
Boston, MA
USA

**Scott T. Weiss** MD, MS
Channing Laboratory
Brigham and Women's Hospital
Harvard Medical School
Boston, MA
USA

**David A. Lomas** PhD, ScD, FRCP, FMedSci
Department of Medicine
University of Cambridge
Cambridge Institute for Medical Research
Cambridge, UK

**Steven D. Shapiro** MD
Division of Pulmonary and Critical Care Medicine
Brigham and Women's Hospital
Harvard Medical School
Boston, MA
USA

# Hodder Arnold

A MEMBER OF THE HODDER HEADLINE GROUP

First published in Great Britain in 2005 by
Hodder Education, a member of the Hodder Headline Group,
338 Euston Road, London NW1 3BH

http://www.hoddereducation.com

Distributed in the United States of America by
Oxford University Press Inc.,
198 Madison Avenue, New York, NY10016
Oxford is a registered trademark of Oxford University Press

Whilst the advice and information in this book are believed to be true and
accurate at the date of going to press, neither the author[s] nor the publisher
can accept any legal responsibility or liability for any errors or omissions
that may be made. In particular, (but without limiting the generality of the
preceding disclaimer) every effort has been made to check drug dosages;
however it is still possible that errors have been missed. Furthermore,
dosage schedules are constantly being revised and new side-effects
recognized. For these reasons the reader is strongly urged to consult the
drug companies' printed instructions before administering any of the drugs
recommended in this book.

*British Library Cataloguing in Publication Data*
A catalogue record for this book is available from the British Library

*Library of Congress Cataloging-in-Publication Data*
A catalog record for this book is available from the Library of Congress

ISBN 0 340 814322

1 2 3 4 5 6 7 8 9 10

Commissioning Editor:      Joanna Koster
Project Editor:            Naomi Wilkinson
Production Controller:     Lindsay Smith
Cover Design:              Sarah Rees
Index:                     Dr Laurence Errington

Typeset in 10/12 Minion by Charon Tec Pvt. Ltd
www.charontec.com
Printed and bound in Great Britain by CPI Bath

What do you think about this book? Or any other Hodder Arnold title?
Please visit our website at **www.hoddereducation.com**

*This book is dedicated to our patients with respiratory diseases*

# Contents

# Contributors

Edwin K. Silverman MD, PhD
Channing Laboratory and Division of Pulmonary and
Critical Care Medicine
Brigham and Women's Hospital
Harvard Medical School
Boston, MA
USA

Stavros E. Anevlavis MD
Department of Pulmonology
Dimokritio University of Thrace
Medical School
University Hospital of Alexandroupolis
Alexandroupolis, Greece

Paul A. Beirne MA MSc MRCP
Interstitial Lung Disease Unit
Department of Occupational and Environmental Medicine
National Heart and Lung Institute
Imperial College of Science, Technology and Medicine
London, UK

Didier Belorgey PhD
Department of Medicine
University of Cambridge
Cambridge Institute for Medical Research
Cambridge, UK

Juan C. Celedon MD, PhD
Channing Laboratory
Brigham and Women's Hospital
Harvard Medical School
Boston, MA
USA

David C. Christiani MD, MPH, MS
Harvard Medical School
Massachusetts General Hospital
Harvard School of Public Health

Damian C. Crowther MA, PhD, BH, BCh, MRLP
Department of Medicine
Cambridge Institute for Medical Research
University of Cambridge
Cambridge, UK

Garry R. Cutting MD
Department of Pediatrics and Medicine
Johns Hopkins University School of Medicine
Baltimore, MD
USA

Timothy R. Dafforn PhD
Department of Biosciences
University of Birmingham
Edgbaston
Birmingham, UK

Elizabeth A. Davidson BSc, MSc
Department of Clinical Biochemistry
Addenbrooke's Hospital
Cambridge, UK

Dawn L. DeMeo MD, MPH
Channing Laboratory and Division of Pulmonary and
Critical Care Medicine
Brigham and Women's Hospital
Harvard Medical School
Boston, MA
USA

Roger B. Dodd PhD
Structural Medicine Unit
Department of Haematology
University of Cambridge
Cambridge Institute for Medical Research,
Cambridge, UK

Jeffrey M. Drazen MD
Division of Pulmonary and Critical Care Medicine
Brigham Women's Hospital
Harvard Medical School
Boston, MA
USA

Roland M. du Bois MA, MD, FRCP, FCCP
Interstitial Lung Disease Unit
Department of Occupational and Environmental Medicine
National Heart and Lung Institute
Imperial College of Science, Technology and Medicine
London, UK

**Natasha Y. Frank** MD
Division of Genetics
Children's Hospital
Harvard Medical School
Boston, MA
USA

**Joshua Groman** PhD
Johns Hopkins University School of Medicine
Institute of Genetic Medicine
Baltimore, MD
USA

**David J. Halsall** PhD
Department of Clinical Biochemistry
Addenbrooke's Hospital
Cambridge, UK

**Craig P. Hersh** MD, MPH
Channing Laboratory and Division of Pulmonary and
Critical Care Medicine
Brigham and Women's Hospital
Harvard Medical School
Boston, MA
USA

**Gary Hunninghake** MD
Department of Internal Medicine
University of Iowa
Iowa City, IA
USA

**Isaac Kohane** MD, PhD
Children's Hospital
Harvard Medical School
Boston, MA
USA

**Peter Kraft** PhD
Departments of Epidemiology and Biostatistics
Harvard School of Public Health
Boston, MA
USA

**Nan Laird** PhD
Department of Biostatistics
Harvard School of Public Health
Boston, MA
USA

**Christoph Lange** PhD
Department of Biostatistics
Harvard School of Public Health
Boston, MA
USA

**Ross Lazarus** MD, MBBS, MPH, MMed, GDIP CSCi
Channing Laboratory
Brigham and Women's Hospital
Harvard Medical School
Boston, MA
USA

**Augusto Litonjua** MD, MPH
Channing Laboratory
Brigham and Women's Hospital
Harvard Medical School
Boston, MA
USA

**David A. Lomas** PhD, ScD, FRCP, FMedSci
Respiratory Medicine Unit
Department of Medicine
University of Cambridge
Cambridge Institute for Medical Research
Cambridge, UK

**James Loyd** MD
Division of Allergy, Pulmonary and Critical Care Medicine
Department of Medicine
Vanderbilt University School of Medicine
Nashville, TN
USA

**Francis X. McCormack** MD
Division of Pulmonary and Critical Care Medicine
Department of Internal Medicine
University of Cincinnati
Cincinnati, OH
USA

**Nicholas W. Morrell** MD, FRCP
Division of Respiratory Medicine
Department of Medicine
University of Cambridge School of Clinical Medicine
Addenbrooke's Hospital
Cambridge, UK

**Michael F. Murray** MD
Divisions of Genetics and Infectious Diseases
Department of Medicine
Brigham and Women's Hospital
Harvard Medical School
Boston, MA
USA

**John H. Newman** MD
Division of Allergy, Pulmonary and Critical Care Medicine
Department of Medicine
Vanderbilt University School of Medicine
Nashville, TN
USA

Ralph J. Panos MD
Division of Pulmonary and Critical Care Medicine
University of Cincinnati College of Medicine
Cincinnati, OH
USA

John A. Phillips III MD
Division of Medical Genetics
Departments of Pediatrics, Medicine and Biochemistry
Vanderbilt University School of Medicine
Nashville, TN
USA

Benjamin A. Raby MD, CM, MPH
Channing Laboratory
Brigham and Women's Hospital
Harvard Medical School
Boston, MA
USA

Randy J. Read
Structural Medicine Unit
Department of Haematology
University of Cambridge
Cambridge Institute for Medical Research
Cambridge, UK

Steven D. Shapiro MD
Division of Pulmonary and Critical Care Medicine
Brigham and Women's Hospital
Harvard Medical School
Boston, MA
USA

Rebecca Suk MD
Dana-Farber/Partners Cancer Care
Harvard Medical School
Boston, MA
USA

Jody S. Sylvia
Channing Laboratory
Brigham and Women's Hospital
Boston, MA
USA

Kelan G. Tantisira MD
Channing Laboratory
Brigham and Women's Hospital
Harvard Medical School
Boston, MA
USA

Karl Thomas MD
Department of Internal Medicine
University of Iowa
Iowa City, IA
USA

Peter V. Tishler MD
Channing Laboratory
Brigham and Women's Hospital
Harvard Medical School
Boston, MA
USA

Bruce C. Trapnell MD
Pulmonary Biology
Children's Hospital Research Foundation
Cincinnati Children's Hospital Medical Center
Cincinnati, OH
USA

Paul D. Upton PhD
Division of Respiratory Medicine
Department of Medicine
University of Cambridge School of Clinical Medicine
Addenbrooke's Hospital

Kristel Van Steen PhD
Department of Biostatistics
Harvard School of Public Health
Boston, MA
USA

Scott T. Weiss MD, MS
Channing Laboratory
Brigham and Women's Hospital
Harvard Medical School
Boston, MA
USA

Lisa R. Young MD
Divisions of Pulmonary and Critical Care Medicine and
Pulmonary Medicine
Departments of Internal Medicine and Pediatrics
University of Cincinnati and Cincinnati Children's Hospital
Medical Center
Cincinnati, OH
USA

# Preface

The impressive success of the Human Genome Project and the identification of the genetic basis for many monogenic disorders have generated a great deal of interest in genetic research among scientists and clinicians. However, we are at the beginning of the application of new genetic technology to pulmonary disease. New tools, methods and resources are needed to bring the full potential of genetics to the point of clinical relevance for complex traits. An additional issue is that the multidisciplinary nature of genetic research, which includes molecular biology, epidemiology, statistical genetics, and bioinformatics, has limited the accessibility of genetic approaches to many pulmonary researchers and physicians. Even among genetic researchers, no single investigator can have complete mastery of clinical phenotyping, molecular characterization, and statistical genetic approaches.

Our goals in this book are to provide an introduction to the major fields and genetic approaches to respiratory disorders (Chapters 1 to 8), and to provide an integrated discussion of progress in genetics of both common and rare respiratory diseases in a comprehensive fashion (Chapters 9 to 18). We have used a broad definition of "genetics." One might ask: Why are animal models discussed so prominently? What does X-ray crystallography have to do with genetics? We contend that genetics is not limited to the study of rare monogenic disorders, and that genetic investigation does not end with the identification of significant genetic association. Essentially every pulmonary disease has some degree of genetic determination and many have significant interaction with key environmental factors. We wish to show how genetic methods will change the research practices of pulmonologists and demonstrate that genetic research can and should lead to the understanding of molecular mechanisms of disease and functional effects of genetic variation. This requires both genomic physiology in animals (Chapter 7) and functional genomic studies of in vitro systems (Chapter 6).

We have attempted to demonstrate the links between rare monogenic disorders and more common complex diseases by including discussions of epidemiology, natural history, monogenic syndromes, complex disease components, and animal models within each of our disease-specific chapters. Genetic nomenclature is often not standardized, but we have tried to refer to the HUGO symbols for human genes that are discussed in each chapter. Other aspects of nomenclature remain non-uniform; for example, although many geneticists prefer "Marfan syndrome" to "Marfan's syndrome," the possessive form remains in widespread use for genetic syndromes in the medical literature, and we have left these decisions to the authors of each chapter.

We hope that this book will be useful for pulmonary researchers, both students at the beginning of their careers and experienced investigators who are well established. We are particularly hopeful that those at the beginning of their investigative careers will turn to genetics as a way forward to understanding respiratory diseases and that this book will help them in this task. We also hope that clinicians, both pulmonologists and medical geneticists, will find useful reference information as well; although genetics does not yet influence treatment of most of the conditions discussed, it often does influence our understanding of disease pathophysiology. As progress continues, we expect that genetic insights will lead to additional treatment options and pharmacogenetic insights into treatment responses and adverse events. This is already beginning in asthma (Chapter 8).

As in any multi-author book, the success of the endeavor relates to the commitment and creativity of the collaborating authors; we are extremely thankful for the hard and careful work of each of our contributors. They represent an important resource as we enter the genetic and genomic era of pulmonary medicine. We would also like to thank our colleagues at Hodder Arnold who provided outstanding support for this project, including Joanna Koster, Naomi Wilkinson, Sarah Burrows, Carole Goodall, Heather Smith, and Alyson Thomas. Finally, we must thank our families for their support, their patience, and their love during this long and arduous project: Rachel, Anna, and Andrew; Nicole, Calli, Tess, and Skylar; Judith, Tim, James, and Ben; and Debby, Ben, and Matthew.

Edwin K. Silverman, Steven D. Shapiro,
David A. Lomas, and Scott T. Weiss

# Acknowledgements

We would like to thank Dr James Huntington from the University of Cambridge for providing the Alpha 1 molecule image for the cover.

# List of abbreviations used

A2M        alpha 2-macroglobulin
AAT        alpha 1-antitrypsin
AAV        adeno-associated virus
ABC        ATP-binding cassette
ACD        acid citrate dextrose
ACE        angiotensin converting enzyme
ACRN       Asthma Clinical Research Network
ADR        adverse drug reaction
AIDS       acquired immunodeficiency syndrome
AIP        acute interstitial pneumonia
ALS        amyotrophic lateral sclerosis
APTI       airway pressure time index
APTT       activated partial thromboplastin time
ARDS       acute respiratory distress syndrome
ARPKD      autosomal recessive polycystic kidney disease
ATP        adenosine triphosphate
ATS        American Thoracic Society
AV         atrioventricular
AVM        arteriovenous malformations
AWUV       alveolar wall per unit volume
BAL        bronchoalveolar lavage
BCG        Bacillus Calmette–Guerin
BeS        beryllium sensitization
BHD        Birt–Hogg–Dube syndrome
BHL        bilateral hilar lymphadenopathy
BiPAP      bilateral positive airway pressure
BMP        bone morphogenetic proteins
BUP        beta upstream regulator
CASP       critical assessment of structure prediction
CASR       calcium-sensing receptor gene
CBAVD      congenital bilateral absence of the vas deferens
CBD        chronic beryllium disease
CBP        CREB-binding protein
CBS        cystathione beta-synthase
CC10       Clara Cell Protein 10
CCHS       congenital central hypoventilation syndrome
CD         circular dichroism
CDH        congenital diaphragmatic hernia
CEPH       Centre d'Etude du Polymorphisme Humain
CF         cystic fibrosis
CFTR       cystic fibrosis transmembrane conductance regulator
CGH        comparative genomic hybridization
CHO        Chinese hamster ovary
CIE        crossed immunoelectrophoresis
CNS        central nervous system
CO         cardiac output
COGA       Collaborative Study on the Genetics of Alcoholism

COP        cryptogenic organizing pneumonia
COPD       chronic obstructive pulmonary disease
CR1        complement receptor 1
CREB       cAMP-responsive element binding protein
CSF        colony-stimulating factor
CSGA       Collaborative Study on the Genetics of Asthma
CSGE       conformation-sensitive gel electrophoresis
CSS        Churg–Strauss syndrome
CT         computed tomography
CTEPH      chronic thromboembolic pulmonary hypertension
CYP        cytochrome P450
ddF        dideoxy fingerprinting
DHPLC      denaturing high-performance liquid chromatography
DIOS       distal intestinal obstructive syndrome
DIP        desquamative interstitial pneumonia
DLD        Division of Lung Diseases
DNA        deoxyribonucleic acid
DRC        DNA repair capacity
DZ         dizygous
EBC        exhaled breath condensate
EBV        Epstein–Barr virus
ECM        extracellular matrix
ECP        eosinophil cationic protein
EDN        eosinophil derived neurotoxin
EDP        extreme discordant phenotype
EDS        Ehlers–Danlos syndrome
EGFR       epidermal growth factor receptor
ELISA      enzyme linked immunosorbent assays
EN         erythema nodosum
EPO        eosinophil peroxidase
ER         endoplasmic reticulum
ERS        European Respiratory Society
ES         embryonic stem
ESR        erythrocyte sedimentation rate
EST        expressed sequence tag
ETS        environmental tobacco smoke
FBAT       family-based association test
$FEV_1$    forced expiratory volume at one second
FHS        Family Heart Study
FISH       fluorescence in situ hybridization
FPF        familial pulmonary fibrosis
FPPH       familial primary pulmonary hypertension
FRET       fluorescence resonance energy transfer
FTQ        Fagerstrom tolerance questionnaire
FVC        forced vital capacity
G6PD       glucose-6-phosphate dehydrogenase deficiency

| | | | | |
|---|---|---|---|---|
| GEE | generalized estimating equation | | MHC | major histocompatibility antigen |
| GFP | green fluorescent protein | | MI | meconium ileus |
| GO | gene ontology | | MIP | macrophage inflammatory protein |
| GPCR | G-protein coupled receptors | | MM | mismatch |
| GSEC | gene susceptibility to environmental carcinogenesis | | MMP | matrix metalloproteinase |
| GST | glutathione S-transferase | | MnSOD | manganese superoxide dismutase |
| H&E | hematoxylin and eosin | | MPI | mucus proteinase inhibitor |
| HD | Huntington disease | | MPO | myeloperoxidase |
| HES | hypereosinophilic syndrome | | MPS | mucopolysaccharidoses |
| hGH | human growth hormone | | MRI | magnetic resonance imaging |
| HHRR | haplotype-based haplotype relative risk | | MSI | microsatellite instability |
| HHT | hereditary hemorrhagic telangiectasia | | MZ | monozygous |
| HHV | human herpes virus | | NETT | National Emphysema Treatment Trial |
| HIES | hyperimmunoglobulin E syndrome | | NHLBI | National Heart Lung and Blood Institute |
| HIPAA | Health Insurance Portability and Accountability Act | | NMR | nuclear magnetic resonance |
| HIV | human immunodeficiency virus | | NO | nitric oxide |
| HLA | human leukocyte antigen | | NOTT | Nocturnal Oxygen Therapy Trial |
| HMOX1 | heme oxygenase-1 | | NPD | nasal potential difference |
| HNE | human neutrophil elastase | | NSIP | nonspecific interstitial pneumonia |
| HPS | Hermansky–Pudlak syndrome | | nt | nucleotides |
| HRCT | high-resolution computed tomography | | OI | osteogenesis imperfecta |
| HRR | haplotype relative risk | | OMIM | Online Mendelian Inheritance in Man |
| HU | Hounsfield units | | OVA | ovalbumin |
| HUV | hypocomplementemic urticarial vasculitis | | OVW | optimal ventilation waveform |
| HWE | Hardy Weinberg equilibrium | | PAGE | polyacrylamide gel electrophoresis |
| I/D | insertion/deletion | | PAI | plasminogen activator inhibitor |
| IATA | International Air Transport Association | | PAP | pulmonary alveolar proteinosis |
| ID | identification | | PAS | periodic acid Schiff |
| IDS | iduronate sulfatase | | PASP | pulmonary artery systolic pressure |
| IEF | isoelectric focusing | | PCD | primary ciliary dyskinesia |
| IFN | interferon | | PCR | polymerase chain reaction |
| IFNG | interferon gamma | | PDGF | platelet-derived growth factor |
| IHC | immunohistochemistry | | PDGFRA | platelet-derived growth factor receptor alpha |
| IL13 | interleukin-13 | | PDI | prolyl disulfide isomerase |
| ILD | interstitial lung disease | | PEF | peak expiratory flow |
| INR | international normalized ratio | | PEFR | peak expiratory flow rate |
| IPAH | idiopathic pulmonary arterial hypertension | | PET | positron emission tomography |
| IPF | idiopathic pulmonary fibrosis | | PFT | pulmonary function test |
| IRB | institutional review board | | PGK | phosphoglycerate kinase |
| IRT | immunoreactive trypsinogen | | PHA | phytohemagglutinin; Pulmonary Hypertension Association |
| ISAAC | International Society of Asthma and Allergy in Childhood | | PI | protease inhibitor |
| KS | Kveim–Siltzbach | | PM | perfect match |
| LAM | lymphangioleiomyomatosis | | poly-A | poly-adenine |
| LD | linkage disequilibrium | | PPE | porcine pancreatic elastase |
| LHS | Lung Health Study | | PPH | Primary pulmonary hypertension |
| LIP | lymphocytic interstitial pneumonia | | PVOD | pulmonary veno-occlusive disease |
| LOH | loss of heterozygosity | | PVR | pulmonary vascular resistance |
| LTA | lymphotoxin alpha | | PWS | Prader–Willi syndrome |
| LTF | lactoferrin | | QTL | quantitative trait locus |
| LVRS | lung volume reduction surgery | | RAMP | receptor activity-modulating proteins |
| MAD | multiple-wavelength anomalous dispersion | | RANTES | regulated on activation, normal T lymphocyte expressed and secreted |
| MAPK | mitogen activated protein kinases | | | |
| MBL | mannose binding lectin | | RAST | radioallergosorbent test |
| MBP | major basic protein | | RBC | red blood cells |
| MDA | malondialdehyde | | RB-ILD | respiratory bronchiolitis-interstitial lung disease |

| | | | | |
|---|---|---|---|---|
| RF | radiofrequency | | TCR | T-cell receptor |
| RFLP | restriction fragment length polymorphism | | TDT | transmission disequilibrium test |
| RIA | radioimmunoassay | | TEM | transmission electron microscopy |
| ROS | reactive oxygen species | | TGF | transforming growth factor |
| rtTA | reverse tetracycline transactivator | | Th | T helper |
| SAGE | serial analysis of gene expression | | TIMP | tissue inhibitor of metalloproteinases |
| SDS–PAGE | sodium dodecyl sulfate polyacrylamide gel electrophoresis | | TK | thymidine kinase |
| | | | TLC | total lung capacity |
| SEA | soluble egg antigen | | TNF | tumor necrosis factor |
| SIR | standardized incidence ratio | | TRE | trinucleotide repeat expansion |
| SLPI | secretory leukoproteinase inhibitor | | TSC | tuberous sclerosis complex |
| SMCD | systemic mast cell disease | | TUG | transverse urea gradient |
| SNP | single nucleotide polymorphism | | UIP | usual interstitial pneumonitis |
| SP-C | surfactant protein | | VDR | vitamin D receptor |
| SSCP | single-stranded mobility methods | | VEGF | vascular endothelial growth factor |
| STR | short tandem repeat | | VTE | venous thrombosis complicated by pulmonary embolism |
| SVC | superior vena cava | | WASOG | World Association of Sarcoidosis and Other Granulomatous Disorders |
| TAP | transporter associated with antigen processing | | | |

# Reference annotation

The reference lists are annotated, where appropriate, to guide readers to primary articles, key review papers, and management guidelines, as follows:

● Seminal primary article
◆ Key review paper
❊ First formal publication of a management guideline

We hope that this feature will render extensive lists of references more useful to the reader and will help to encourage self-directed learning among both trainees and practicing physicians.

# Key concepts in respiratory genetics

# Overview of human genetics

EDWIN K. SILVERMAN AND SCOTT T. WEISS

## REVIEW OF BASIC GENETICS CONCEPTS

We will provide a very brief review of key genetics concepts that will be relevant throughout the book. For a more thorough discussion of molecular or population genetics, a series of references is provided at the end of this chapter.[1–6] For definitions of common genetic terms, a glossary has been included at the end of the book.

### Structure and function of DNA

The genetic alphabet consists of four different types of biochemical 'letters,' which are nucleotide bases. Our genetic material, which is made of deoxyribonucleic acid (DNA), consists of a linear sequence of these four different nucleotide bases. The four nucleotide bases in DNA include two purines (adenine and guanine) and two pyrimidines (cytosine and thymidine). The human DNA sequence comprises approximately 3 billion of these nucleotide bases. DNA is located within the cell nucleus and is packaged into chromosomes. Genes are located at specific locations along each of the 22 autosomal and two sex chromosomes that humans normally inherit. These genes provide coding instructions for the proteins that perform the functions of the cell; the DNA sequence is copied into messenger RNA (mRNA) – a process called transcription, and the mRNA sequence is used to direct the addition of amino acids into proteins – a process called translation. We inherit one set of chromosomes from each parent, so we have two copies of most genes. The exact number of genes in the human genome is unknown but is thought to be approximately 30 000.[7]

## Types of genetic variation

Every person except identical twins has a unique DNA sequence. There are at least 10 million locations in the genome where the DNA sequence commonly varies between people. These locations are referred to as polymorphisms when there are at least two variants (also known as alleles) that occur with greater than 1 percent frequency. Variations at some of these polymorphic sites lead to common genetic diseases such as different inherited forms of alpha 1-antitrypsin (HUGO symbol SERPINA1) and the cystic fibrosis transmembrane conductance regulator (CFTR) delta F508 allele. However, most genetic variants do not have a major functional effect.

The most commonly studied polymorphisms in human genetics are short tandem repeat (STR) markers, also known as microsatellites, and single nucleotide polymorphisms (SNPs), these types of variants are discussed in detail in Chapter 4B. STR markers are repeats of two, three, or four bases, which are reasonably frequent in the genome. They tend to have multiple common alleles, and therefore frequently allow the transmission of chromosomal regions to be tracked accurately through a pedigree. Although they are extremely useful as markers of different chromosomal regions, STR markers are usually not disease susceptibility variants themselves. Huntington disease and some other rare disorders are exceptions to this general rule.

SNPs are much more frequent in the genome than STR polymorphisms. A SNP typically occurs approximately every 500 base pairs. There are many methods used to genotype SNPs, which will be reviewed in Chapter 4B. SNPs are commonly used in genetic association studies, and many

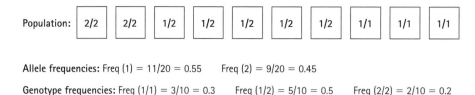

Population: 2/2 2/2 1/2 1/2 1/2 1/2 1/2 1/1 1/1 1/1

Allele frequencies: Freq (1) = 11/20 = 0.55    Freq (2) = 9/20 = 0.45

Genotype frequencies: Freq (1/1) = 3/10 = 0.3    Freq (1/2) = 5/10 = 0.5    Freq (2/2) = 2/10 = 0.2

**Figure 1.1** *Calculation of allele frequencies and genotype frequencies: A hypothetical population of 10 individuals is shown at the top of the figure, with the genotype at a two allele SNP specified within the symbol for each individual.*

disease susceptibility gene variants are likely SNPs. In addition to SNPs and STRs, short insertion or deletion variants (indels) occur commonly in the genome.

## KEY POPULATION GENETICS CONCEPTS

### Allele and genotype frequencies

If all of the alleles at a particular genetic locus in a population are tabulated, the percentage of the total number of alleles represented by each variant is known as the allele frequency. The genotype of an individual is the set of alleles (two for autosomal loci) that are inherited at a particular genetic locus. If the assumptions of random mating within a population are met, including the absence of inbreeding, population stratification, migration, selection, and mutation, the genotype frequencies can be estimated accurately from the allele frequencies, and Hardy–Weinberg equilibrium is present for this genetic locus. Under Hardy–Weinberg equilibrium, the genotype frequency of a homozygous genotype is estimated as the (allele frequency)$^2$ for the allele present in that genotype; for a heterozygous genotype, the genotype frequency is estimated as $2 \times$ (allele frequency 1) $\times$ (allele frequency 2) for the two alleles in that genotype. The calculation of allele and genotype frequencies directly from the observed genotypes is shown in Fig. 1.1.

The assessment of Hardy–Weinberg equilibrium can be performed using a chi square goodness-of-fit test, where the expected number of genotypes calculated from the allele frequencies is compared to the observed number of genotypes. The chi square statistic is calculated by summing the following quantity over all genotypes:

$$\frac{\left(\begin{array}{c}\text{Expected number} \\ \text{of genotypes}\end{array} - \begin{array}{c}\text{Observed number} \\ \text{of genotypes}\end{array}\right)^2}{(\text{Expected number of genotypes})} \quad (1.1)$$

If there are small sample sizes and/or rare allele frequencies leading to small expected numbers of any genotype, the asymptotic assumptions of the chi square statistic will not be met. As a rule of thumb, the expected number of individuals in all genotypic classes should be greater than five for the chi square goodness-of-fit test to be valid. If these criteria are not met, exact tests of Hardy–Weinberg proportions, such as

the method proposed by Haldane, should be performed.[8] The assessment of deviation from Hardy–Weinberg proportions for a locus with multiple alleles, such as STR markers, is more complicated, especially when the sample size and/or some of the genotype frequencies are small. However, methods to estimate the exact significance level of Hardy–Weinberg proportions for multiallelic loci have been developed.[9] Absence of Hardy–Weinberg equilibrium means that one of the assumptions of random mating has been violated, or that genotyping error is present.

### Haplotypes

Although many disease susceptibility loci are likely SNPs, there is increasing interest in the use of haplotypes of adjacent SNPs as a tool for susceptibility gene localization. A haplotype is the series of specific alleles at loci inherited from one parent; it typically refers to closely grouped loci on one chromosome. Haplotypes are gaining popularity because they are often more informative about the parental origins of a particular genomic region than an individual SNP. They also reflect evolutionary history more accurately, and they can capture the linkage disequilibrium patterns of a genomic region more completely; it is linkage disequilibrium that drives genetic association between a genetic marker and an untyped nearby disease susceptibility locus. In addition, it is possible that combinations of adjacent SNPs are required to confer a particular phenotype; haplotype analysis may allow identification of key combinations of SNPs.

### Linkage disequilibrium

The tendency of nearby genetic loci to be inherited together is the result of linkage disequilibrium. A variety of measures of linkage disequilibrium have been proposed, which are typically related to a linkage disequilibrium parameter (D) calculated from the frequencies of the four possible haplotype combinations (11, 12, 21, and 22) for two loci with two alleles each: $D = (P_{11})(P_{22}) - (P_{12})(P_{21})$. Because these haplotype frequencies are not directly observed, statistical estimates must typically be used. Commonly used measures of linkage disequilibrium based on the D parameter include D′, a standardized measure of D, and $r^2$, the square of the correlation coefficient between the alleles at two loci on a chromosome.[10]

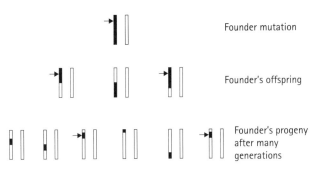

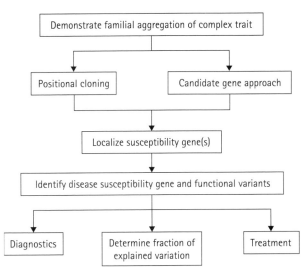

**Figure 1.2** *Reduction in linkage disequilibrium across generations. When a new disease mutation occurs in a single individual, or when a single individual with a disease mutation migrates into a population, the entire chromosome bearing that mutation in that founder individual is initially in linkage disequilibrium with the disease mutation (indicated by an arrow). With successive generations and meiotic events, the amount of the founder's DNA that tracks with that disease mutation becomes progressively smaller and the linkage disequilibrium dissipates.*

When a mutation occurs on a particular chromosome, initially there is a large shared segment of linkage disequilibrium around it. As shown in Fig. 1.2, this region of linkage disequilibrium dissipates over time with meiotic recombination – the process of crossing over between homologous chromosomes that occurs during gametogenesis. With successive generations, the region of linkage disequilibrium is reduced, and only individuals who inherited a narrow genetic region around the disease susceptibility variant will express the disease. However, this single founder mutation model is likely not valid in many cases. In general, loci that are located more closely together on a chromosome will be in stronger linkage disequilibrium than those loci that are far apart, but the actual degree of linkage disequilibrium is very difficult to predict based on physical distance alone. Some loci that are separated by 100 base pairs will not be in linkage disequilibrium, while other loci separated by many thousands of nucleotide bases will be in tight linkage disequilibrium.[11] Therefore, if one finds a significant and valid genetic association in a population of unrelated individuals, the distance from the tested marker to the disease locus may be relatively small, but the linkage disequilibrium pattern of the region will need to be examined carefully.

## APPROACHES TO FIND GENETIC DETERMINANTS OF RESPIRATORY DISEASES

### Monogenic versus complex diseases

Diseases influenced by genetic determinants can be classified as monogenic or complex. Monogenic disorders are influenced by a single major gene; they typically demonstrate a classic pattern of Mendelian inheritance (e.g., autosomal dominant, X-linked recessive). Complex disorders are presumably influenced by multiple genetic determinants and

**Figure 1.3** *Schematic overview of the steps involved in identifying a genetic determinant for a complex disorder. After familial aggregation has been shown, either positional cloning or candidate gene approaches can be used to find the general location of a disease susceptibility gene. Identification of the key susceptibility gene and its functional variants can be performed by systematic fine mapping or by candidate gene approaches. If a new susceptibility gene is found, new diagnostic tests can be designed, the fraction of cases related to the variant can be determined, and new pathways for treatment may result.*

environmental factors, as well as gene-by-gene and gene-by-environment interactions. They do not follow a pattern of simple Mendelian inheritance. However, the distinction between monogenic and complex disorders is becoming increasingly blurred, as many classic monogenic disorders demonstrate features of complexity. For example, as discussed in Chapter 10, the development of chronic obstructive pulmonary disease (COPD) in severe alpha 1-antitrypsin deficiency, which results from mutations in a single major gene (SERPINA1), is strongly influenced by cigarette smoking, an environmental factor, and likely by genetic modifiers as well.

Finding the genetic determinants of complex traits is a challenging task. As shown in Fig. 1.3, the first step is to determine if genetic factors are likely to be involved in a trait, by assessing for familial aggregation. Two general approaches have been used to find complex disease genes: positional cloning and candidate genes. In both cases, the goal is to localize the susceptibility gene to a genomic region. Subsequently, one would like to identify the actual causative gene in that region and to determine the important functional variants. When that has been achieved, it is conceivable to develop new diagnostic tests for the condition, to determine what fraction of disease cases are caused by a particular genetic variant, and to identify pathways that can be used as targets of new treatments.

The most popular hypothesis for the genetic basis of complex diseases is the common disease/common variant hypothesis. This hypothesis states that key genetic determinants of common diseases have relatively high allele frequencies (they are common), and they likely have modest effect sizes.[12] In complex diseases, common variants of very large effect are unlikely to exist. Thus, common complex diseases are likely influenced by common variants of modest effect and/or rare variants of modest-to-large effect. If complex respiratory diseases such as asthma and COPD are really homogeneous entities, then the common disease/common variant hypothesis seems quite reasonable. However, a key question is whether these complex disorders are really one homogeneous common entity, or a collection of rarer entities, which could include less common but greater genetic effects.

## Study design issues in complex disease genetics

In complex disease genetic studies, careful measurements of phenotype and genotype in selected populations are analyzed with appropriate statistical methods (Fig. 1.4). The integration of expertise in bioinformatics is critical to manage phenotype and genotype data for statistical analysis; epidemiology to characterize the phenotypes within populations of interest; statistical genetics to perform analysis of risk to relatives, linkage, and association; and ultimately functional genomics to determine the impact of genetic variation on pathophysiology.

The selection of phenotypes in complex disease genetic studies is challenging and important. It is intuitively appealing to use the disease diagnosis as the phenotype, because the disease is the condition of interest. However, diagnostic misclassification of something as subjective as a

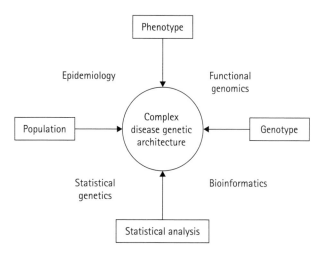

**Figure 1.4** *Designing a genetic study for a complex disease requires a multidisciplinary approach, involving the fields of epidemiology, statistical genetics, bioinformatics, and functional genomics to measure the appropriate phenotypes in a well-characterized population, and to genotype relevant genetic variants and perform statistical genetic analysis.*

disease diagnosis is not uncommon, and if it occurs can be problematic. Moreover, disease diagnosis is a qualitative rather than a quantitative phenotype, and quantitative phenotypes are often more powerful for identification of disease susceptibility loci. For these reasons, intermediate phenotypes, which are intermediate between the disease gene and the disease diagnosis, have significant utility. For example, total serum immunoglobulin E level is an intermediate phenotype commonly used in asthma genetics. Intermediate phenotypes are typically objective and quantitative. However, they are not the same as the disease, and genes influencing the intermediate phenotype may not influence the disease of interest.

The population studied is also critical in complex disease genetics. Although studies of humans involve the species of interest, controlled crosses are fortunately not permissible. Animal models offer unique opportunities for genetic studies. In studies of human populations, isolated populations, such as the Central Valley of Costa Rica, offer some significant advantages. Fewer susceptibility genes may be present in populations founded by a smaller number of founders, so there may be increased homogeneity for a complex disorder. On the other hand, most human populations are heterogeneous, and the ability to generalize to such heterogeneous populations is an important goal in complex disease genetics.

In addition, the type of individuals sampled must be considered. Study populations can include affected cases and unaffected control subjects, population-based samples which will include some affected and some unaffected individuals, or families (nuclear family units or extended pedigrees). For a case–control association study, one tries to enroll unrelated but reasonably matched case and control subjects. Parent–child trios or larger nuclear families can be used for linkage and/or association studies, while very extended pedigrees are typically used for linkage studies, although association studies may also be performed.

Complex disease genetic studies are inherently multidisciplinary, and the optimal study designs and analytical approaches are changing rapidly. The three most widely used techniques in genetic epidemiology are assessment of risk to relatives, linkage analysis, and association studies. We will briefly review each of these methods.

## Familial aggregation

Assessing for increased risk to relatives for a disease is a commonly used approach to assess for familial aggregation. The risk to relatives is calculated by comparing the risk of a disease phenotype in relatives of affected individuals compared to the general population. For example, the risk of airflow obstruction in smoking first-degree relatives (parents, siblings, and children) of severe, early-onset COPD subjects is three-fold higher than smokers from the general population.[13] Demonstrating an increased risk to relatives is consistent with a genetic influence on a disease, but it does not prove it. Shared family environment can also cause an increased risk to relatives. For quantitative phenotypes, demonstrating significant positive correlations for pairs of relatives (e.g., sib–sib, parent–offspring) also provides evidence for familial aggregation, which could be caused by genetic factors or shared family environment. The estimated percentage of phenotypic variation that is due to genetic factors is known as the heritability. Heritability can be estimated in twin studies; greater concordance between identical (monozygotic) twins than fraternal (dizygotic) twins provides evidence for significant heritability. Segregation analysis is another genetic epidemiological method to study the pattern of familial aggregation. In segregation analysis, the distribution of a phenotype within a family is assessed to determine if the pattern is consistent with a single major gene mode of inheritance.

## Linkage analysis

Linkage analysis includes a group of methods that analyze the distribution of DNA markers within families to determine if a particular region of the genome contains a gene related to the phenotype of interest. The basic approach in linkage analysis is to determine whether the alleles at two loci segregate together more often than one would expect by random assortment. This can be assessed by comparing the frequency of recombinant chromosomes, in which a crossing over event has rearranged the parental chromosomes, to the frequency of nonrecombinant chromosomes. With extended pedigrees and observed genetic loci, it is possible to determine the phase of the genetic variants (their specific arrangement on each chromosome) and to determine if a meiotic recombination event has occurred. In Fig. 1.5, the paternal grandparents are homozygous at the A and B loci, so the phase of these variants on the father's chromosomes is known with certainty (AB and ab). Thus, since the mother is homozygous in this example, we can determine that there are two recombinant and two nonrecombinant children in the third generation.

If the loci are on different chromosomes or are greatly separated on one chromosome, they will be unlinked, and recombinant and nonrecombinant chromosomes will each be observed approximately half of the time. When the loci are linked, parental chromosomes are more common than recombinant chromosomes. The strength of the linkage, expressed as the recombination fraction, is dependent on the genetic distance between loci; the more tightly linked two loci are, the less likely it is to find recombinant chromosomes. Of course, in most real pedigrees, with missing subjects and less than fully informative combinations of alleles, it is often not possible to determine recombinant and nonrecombinant subjects with certainty. Assessing linkage to a hypothesized and unobserved disease locus rather than genotyped markers creates additional complexity. In

those cases, complicated statistical genetic approaches to assess for linkage are required.[2,14]

Linkage results are often expressed as a lod score, which is the result of a statistical test to determine if genetic loci are linked. Lod scores are log to the base 10 of the odds that the loci are linked, and depending on study design, lod scores of 3.0 to 3.6 correspond to significant linkage.[15] Linkage studies are usually based on STR or SNP markers distributed throughout the genome, such that if a major disease susceptibility gene is located anywhere in the genome, one of the tested markers will be close enough to demonstrate evidence for linkage. Typically, a genome-wide linkage scan requires about 400 STR markers or 1500 SNP markers that are appropriately distributed. To adjust for the multiple statistical testing involved in genome scans, the lod score thresholds for significant linkage correspond to stringent levels of significance. Linkage analysis can be performed with one marker at a time, which is known as two point analysis because the evidence for linkage between a marker and a hypothetical disease locus is assessed. Multipoint linkage analysis is more commonly performed and uses information from adjacent markers to assess the transmission of a particular chromosomal region in a family. Linkage analysis was initially developed in a model-based or parametric framework, which required specification of a variety of model parameters including the disease allele frequency, penetrance of the various genotypic classes, and

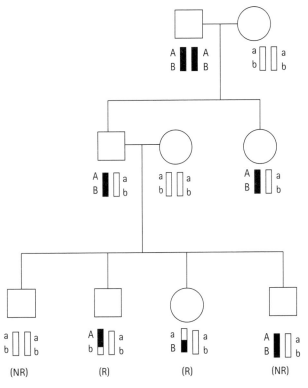

**Figure 1.5** *Hypothetical three-generation pedigree with genotypes specified for locus 1 (alleles A and a) and locus 2 (alleles B and b). In the third generation of this pedigree, recombinant (R) and nonrecombinant (NR) individuals can be determined.*

mode of inheritance. For classical monogenic disorders, this information can often be estimated with reasonable accuracy, but for complex diseases, these variables are typically unknown. Thus, nonparametric methods based on allele-sharing among affected relatives have been more widely used in complex diseases, because such model parameters do not need to be estimated. Linkage analysis can be based on qualitative (e.g., affected/unaffected) or quantitative (e.g., $FEV_1$ level) phenotypes. Some of the more commonly used linkage methods are compared in Table 1.1.

## Types of genetic association studies

Association studies, perhaps the most widely used approach in genetic epidemiology, determine if a particular allele or genotype occurs more frequently in subjects with a phenotype of interest. A genetic association can occur if the specific allele is a cause of the disease. In many cases, association occurs when the specific allele is not the true disease mutation, but is tightly linked to the true disease mutation.

As discussed in Chapter 3, association studies can be performed with unrelated individuals (case–control or population-based) or families. In the case–control design,

the distribution of alleles in case and control subjects is compared. In the hypothetical example in Fig. 1.6, there appear to be more '1' alleles in cases than in controls. If this constituted a statistically significant difference, it would support a genetic association between the '1' allele at this locus and disease. Population-based methods are similar, but the affected and unaffected individuals within the population are compared; alternatively, quantitative phenotypes can be tested for association to particular alleles or genotypes. Family-based methods use internal controls to test for genetic association. In the most widely used family-based association analysis approach, the transmission-disequilibrium test (TDT), the transmission of alleles from heterozygous parents to affected offspring is assessed. In the example shown, the '1' allele is transmitted while the '2' allele is not transmitted from the heterozygous father to the affected daughter. If statistically significant overtransmission of one particular allele from heterozygous parents is found, this constitutes evidence for genetic association in the presence of linkage.

As discussed in more detail in Chapter 3, the statistical significance of a genetic association is based on the probability of rejecting the null hypothesis of no association. However, this $P$ value does not necessarily reflect the effect

**Table 1.1** *Comparison of some commonly used linkage analysis methods*

| Method | Family units | Phenotypes | Model assumptions | Example programs |
|---|---|---|---|---|
| Parametric | Any pedigree | Qualitative or quantitative | Disease allele frequency, penetrance, dominance | LINKAGE[32] |
| Affected sibling | Nuclear families | Qualitative | None | ASPEX[33] |
| Haseman–Elston | Nuclear families[a] | Qualitative or quantitative | None | SIBPAL[34] |
| Affected relative | Pedigrees (computational limits are present) | Qualitative | None | MERLIN[35] |
| Variance component | Any pedigree | Quantitative | Multivariate normality for phenotypes | SOLAR[36] |
| Markov chain Monte Carlo | Any pedigree | Quantitative | None | LOKI[37] |

[a]Analytical theory for extended pedigrees has been developed.

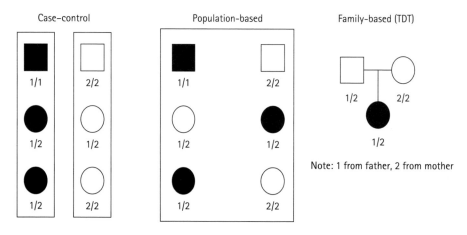

**Figure 1.6** *The major study designs in genetic epidemiology are demonstrated: case-control, population-based, and family-based. Affected individuals are denoted by filled symbols and the genotype at a two allele SNP locus is specified below each symbol.*

size of the genetic association. Effect size in case–control and population-based genetic association studies can be expressed as an odds ratio; the percentage of explained variation of the measured genotype can also be estimated.[16] For family-based association methods like the TDT, the ratio of transmissions of the alternative alleles has been suggested as an effect size estimate.[17]

## Replication of genetic association studies

One of the major challenges in complex disease genetics has been the inconsistent results of genetic association studies, which could be the result of several factors. Genetic heterogeneity, or different genetic mechanisms, in different populations could contribute to difficulty in replicating associations between studies. In addition, false positive or false negative results could contribute as in any study design. A potentially important factor is that case–control association studies are susceptible to supporting (or refuting) associations based purely on population stratification. Population stratification occurs when differences in allele frequencies between cases and controls relate to differences in ancestry rather than association of genetic variants with disease. Population stratification can cause false positive or false negative results in association analysis. Case–control and population-based association analysis methods are certainly susceptible to population stratification, but some family-based methods are also not completely immune to population stratification effects.[18] There is a great deal of controversy regarding the importance of population stratification; recent data suggest that population stratification is a bigger problem for larger studies.[19,20] Potential approaches to avoid population stratification include careful matching of cases and controls, although it is difficult to know if this has been done carefully enough. Genotyping multiple unlinked markers to test for, and potentially adjust for, population stratification is a reasonable approach,[21–23] as are the use of family-based methods that are not susceptible to population stratification effects.

Dealing with multiple comparisons is one of the major challenges in genetic association studies. Multiple statistical testing results from testing multiple phenotypes, multiple SNPs in a gene, and/or multiple genes. Adjusting the observed $P$ values using the conservative Bonferroni approach, or a variety of other somewhat less conservative approaches, is an option. Simulation to obtain empirical $P$ values is another reasonable approach. Screening for significant associations using population-based association analysis of the individuals in a set of families that are uninformative for association analysis, followed by family-based association analysis of significant association results in the screening phase, has also been proposed.[24] However, the best approach is typically to replicate the association findings in an independent population. Additional potential problems in many case–control association studies include control groups that are selected based on convenience (such as blood donors)

rather than careful matching, small sample sizes such that reclassification of a few individuals would lead to loss of statistical significance, and testing only a single SNP rather than a comprehensive set of SNPs that capture the linkage disequilibrium pattern of the candidate gene.

Several criteria have been proposed to evaluate the quality of case–control genetic association studies.[25] As shown in Table 1.2, the first criterion is the selection of the candidate gene polymorphism. Is it a biologically reasonable choice, preferably also a positional candidate in a region of linkage? Possible solutions to this issue include demonstration of a biologically functional effect of a particular polymorphism, or selection of a candidate gene within a region of linkage in man or model organisms. We previously discussed population stratification; it is important to attempt to match case and control groups appropriately. Matching on ethnicity is one approach; testing unlinked markers and showing no association can increase one's confidence that

**Table 1.2**  *Evaluation of candidate gene case–control association studies*

| Criteria | Key questions | Possible solutions |
|---|---|---|
| Selection of candidate gene and genetic variants | Is it biologically reasonable? Is it a positional candidate within a linked region? | Demonstrate functional effect Located with a linked region in man or syntenic from a linked region in an animal model |
| | Are an adequate number of genetic variants studied? | Select SNPs to capture linkage disequilibrium pattern of the gene |
| Population stratification | Are cases and controls well matched? | Matching on ethnicity Family-based association analysis Assessment/ adjustment for population stratification |
| Hardy–Weinberg equilibrium | Is the control group in Hardy–Weinberg equilibrium? | Calculation and reporting of Hardy–Weinberg proportions |
| Multiple comparisons | Number of alleles and genetic loci tested? Number of phenotypes tested? | Bonferroni correction Alternative $P$ value correction (e.g., false discovery rate). Estimation of empirical $P$ values |

Note: Adapted from Silverman and Palmer.[25]

population stratification is not an important factor in a study. Family-based association analysis approaches can avoid the problem of population stratification altogether. Third, it is important to determine if Hardy–Weinberg equilibrium is present. A variety of factors can interfere with Hardy–Weinberg equilibrium, including deviations from random mating (e.g., inbreeding, population stratification) and genotyping errors. True genetic associations can cause deviations from Hardy–Weinberg equilibrium among affected individuals, so it is important to test for Hardy–Weinberg equilibrium in control subjects. Finally, one must consider the implications of multiple statistical testing.

The differences between linkage and association analysis are highlighted in Fig. 1.7. Three families are represented in the top panel; affected individuals are denoted by solid symbols. In the first family, the '3' allele tracks with disease, while in the second family it is the '2' allele, and in the third family, it is the '1' allele. In each case, there is some evidence for linkage; however, no single allele tracks with disease across families, so there is no evidence for association. In the bottom set of families, the '1' allele tracks with disease in each pedigree. Thus, there is evidence for association as well as for linkage in these pedigrees.

In fact, linkage analysis and association analysis can be viewed as ends of a continuum of genome segment sharing.[26] Affected close relatives, like sibs, share large segments of DNA around a disease locus, because only a few meiotic steps separate them. Unrelated affected individuals, if they share the same ancestral disease mutation, are separated by many more meiotic steps, and only a small segment of DNA around a disease locus is shared by them. Intermediate numbers of meiotic steps can lead to sharing of large enough segments of DNA, as in some isolated populations, that covering the genome with a relatively sparse set of polymorphic markers can lead to the identification of shared genomic segments containing disease susceptibility genes.

## Candidate gene vs. positional cloning approaches

As mentioned earlier, the two general approaches to gene localization in complex diseases are positional cloning and the candidate gene approach. Positional cloning typically begins with genomewide linkage analysis, followed by progressive narrowing of the location of the susceptibility gene using association analysis with individual SNPs and/ or haplotypes. Although positional cloning has been extremely successful in monogenic disorders, it has only been modestly successful in complex disorders. The identification of ADAM33 as a susceptibility gene for asthma is one of the few success stories, and there is still controversy about the importance of this gene in asthma (Chapter 9).[27] Candidate gene approaches typically involve selection of candidate genes from the known pathophysiology of a disease. These approaches also have only had modest success in complex disorders; one example is the identification of Factor V Leiden as a risk factor for deep vein thrombosis. Hybrid approaches, including elements from both the positional cloning and the candidate gene approaches may have the greatest likelihood of success. Examples of such hybrid approaches include human studies of genome scan linkage analysis followed by positional candidate gene studies; this was one of the approaches that led to the identification of NOD2 as a genetic determinant of Crohn's disease.[28]

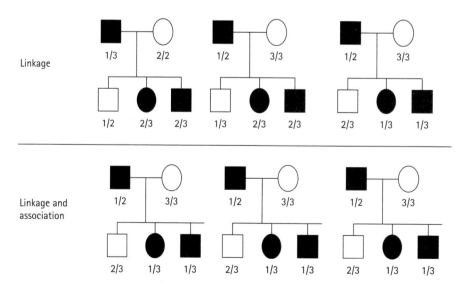

**Figure 1.7**   *The distinction between linkage without association and linkage with association is shown. Affected individuals are denoted by filled symbols. The top three pedigrees provide evidence for linkage but no association, because a different allele tracks with disease in each pedigree. The bottom three pedigrees provide evidence for linkage and association because the same allele tracks with disease in each pedigree.*

## Fine mapping of disease genes

One of the great challenges of complex disease genetics is how to perform fine mapping. Fine mapping can be defined as narrowing the genomic region that contains a susceptibility gene, with the eventual goal of identifying that susceptibility gene and its key functional variants.

Fine mapping in classical monogenic disorders is relatively straightforward. Critical recombinants can be identified in families that progressively narrow the genomic region that contains the susceptibility gene. Within such families, shared haplotypes of adjacent markers can be used to define the location of the susceptibility gene precisely.

In complex diseases, fine mapping is more challenging, because critical recombinants cannot be reliably identified. Some individuals, referred to as phenocopies, may develop a complex disease for purely environmental reasons. Genetic heterogeneity, or different genetic causes of a complex disorder, may be present; incomplete penetrance, or individuals that inherit a susceptibility gene but do not develop disease, may also complicate the identification of critical recombinants. Thus, in complex diseases, shared haplotypes define the location of the susceptibility gene probabilistically and with less certainty than single gene disorders.

A variety of approaches may help to overcome the challenges of fine mapping in complex diseases. The identification of increasing numbers of SNPs and improving genotyping technology allow testing of a dense panel of SNPs within linked regions to assist in complex disease gene localization. The integration of other genomic information, such as expression array analysis of mRNA levels in relevant tissue from affected and unaffected individuals, can assist in selecting candidate genes for further study. Finally, improvements in the measurement and statistical analysis of genotype-by-environment interactions will be required, since it may not be possible to localize some complex disease genes without including relevant environmental measurements.

Recent evidence suggests that many regions of the genome contain haplotype blocks of linkage disequilibrium.[29,30] These haplotype blocks, which are the basis for the HapMap project, may make it easier to localize regions of the genome that contain a susceptibility gene.[31] However, they may also limit the resolution at which a susceptibility gene may be identified.

## Animal models

Animal models offer unique advantages in the study of complex disease phenotypes, which are reviewed in Chapter 7. Inbred lines of essentially genetically identical individuals are often available. Crosses between such inbred strains, that differ in a quantitative phenotype of interest, can be used to determine the location of quantitative trait loci (QTL) influencing that phenotype. Although the offspring of a cross between two parental inbred strains

(known as the F1 generation) will be genetically identical, the second generation (F2) formed from crosses between F1 individuals or between F1 and parental individuals will give a range of genetic combinations as a result of chromosomal segregation and recombination that can be related to the phenotypes by linkage analysis to determine the likely locations of QTLs.

Mice have been especially useful model organisms for respiratory genetics, because they are rapidly reproducing mammals in which extensive genetic investigation has been performed. Strain-to-strain variability in a phenotype for mice exposed to the same environmental conditions strongly suggests that genetic differences influence that phenotype. After parental strains that consistently differ in a phenotype of interest have been identified, quantitative trait locus identification using crosses or bioinformatic comparisons relating known genetic variation between strains to phenotypic differences can be used. However, fine mapping and gene identification for a QTL in model organisms, as in humans, is difficult. Comparing the genetic results in model organisms to humans can assist in candidate gene selection and identification.

If a potentially susceptible gene is identified, model organism studies are especially valuable, because overexpression of the gene (transgenic), removing expression of the gene (knock-out), or introducing specific genetic variants (knock-in) can be used to demonstrate a functional effect.

## CONCLUSION

How do you know when a genetic determinant for a disease has been found? The standards have changed over time. In the 1980s and early 1990s, a new gene was named based on finding a significant linkage result, which at that time was judged to be a lod score above 3. In 1995, Lander and Kruglyak[15] published stringent significance levels for linkage and required linkage replication to have a confirmed linkage. By the late 1990s, association analysis had become more popular, and significant association results led to claims for new susceptibility genes. However, inconsistent replication was soon noted, and the requirement for replicated association became prominent. Currently, a replicated association by multiple groups, as well as compelling functional data, should be required before a new susceptibility gene is claimed.

Genetics has the potential to identify new mechanisms of disease and to identify new targets for treatment intervention. Genetics has the potential to identify clinically meaningful subgroups of patients with different pathophysiological mechanisms for their illness or differential responses to treatment. Genetics has the potential to allow the early detection of susceptible individuals at risk for disease, to allow avoidance of key environmental risk factors or preventative therapy before disease develops. However, the application of genetic insights in respiratory medicine is still in its infancy, and major scientific advances will be required to bring genetic medicine routinely to the bedside.

## Key learning points

- The identification of genetic determinants of complex diseases is challenging and evolving.

- The major methods in genetic epidemiology are familial aggregation analysis, linkage analysis, and association analysis.

- Genetic studies of complex diseases require a multidisciplinary approach, with careful consideration of the phenotypes to be measured, the genotypes to be assayed, the source population and family units to be studied, and the statistical genetic analysis to be performed.

- Both candidate gene and positional cloning approaches have been used in complex disease genetics, but the optimal approach has not yet been determined.

- Integration of genetic results from human and animal studies can provide useful insights into complex diseases.

## REFERENCES

●1 Hartl DL, Clark AG. *Principles of population genetics*, 3rd edn. Sunderland, MA: Sinauer Associates, 1997: 542.

●2 Thomas DC. *Statistical methods in genetic epidemiology*. Oxford: Oxford University Press, 2004.

●3 Rao DC, Province MA (eds) *Genetic dissection of complex traits*. San Diego, CA: Academic Press 2001.

●4 Lewin B. *Genes VIII*. Upper Saddle River, NJ: Pearson Prentice Hall, 2004.

●5 Khoury MJ, Little J, Burke W. *Human genome epidemiology*. Oxford: Oxford University Press, 2004.

●6 Cavalli-Sforza LL, Bodmer WF. *The genetics of human populations*. Mineola, NY: Dover Publications, Inc, 1999.

7 Pennisi E. Bioinformatics. Gene counters struggle to get the right answer. *Science* 2003; **301**: 1040-1.

8 Haldane JBS. An exact test for randomness of mating. *J Genet* 1954; **52**: 631-5.

9 Guo SW, Thompson EA. Performing the exact test of Hardy-Weinberg proportion for multiple alleles. *Biometrics* 1992; **48**: 361-72.

10 Devlin B, Risch N. A comparison of linkage disequilibrium measures for fine-scale mapping. *Genomics* 1995; **29**: 311-22.

◆11 Pritchard JK, Przeworski M. Linkage disequilibrium in humans: models and data. *Am J Hum Genet* 2001; **69**: 1-14.

●12 Zondervan KT, Cardon LR. The complex interplay among factors that influence allelic association. *Nat Rev Genet* 2004; **5**: 89-100.

13 Silverman EK, Chapman HA, Drazen JM et al. Genetic epidemiology of severe, early-onset chronic obstructive pulmonary disease: Risk to relatives for airflow obstruction and chronic bronchitis. *Am J Resp Crit Care Med* 1998; **157**: 1770-8.

●14 Ott J. *Analysis of human genetic linkage*. Baltimore: Johns Hopkins University Press, 1999.

15 Lander E, Kruglyak L. Genetic dissection of complex traits: Guidelines for interpreting and reporting linkage results. *Nat Genet* 1995; **11**: 241-7.

16 Boerwinkle E, Sing CF. Bias of the contribution of single-locus effects to the variance of a quantitative trait. *Am J Hum Genet* 1986; **39**: 137-44.

17 Mitchell LE. Relationship between case-control studies and the transmission/disequilibrium test. *Genet Epidemiol* 2000; **19**: 193-201.

18 Cervino AC, Hill AV. Comparison of tests for association and linkage in incomplete families. *Am J Hum Genet* 2000; **67**: 120-32.

19 Freedman ML, Reich D, Penney KL et al. Assessing the impact of population stratification on genetic association studies. *Nat Genet* 2004; **36**: 388-93.

20 Marchini J, Cardon LR, Phillips MS, Donnelly P. The effects of human population structure on large genetic association studies. *Nat Genet* 2004; **36**: 512-7.

◆21 Pritchard JK, Rosenberg NA. Use of unlinked genetic markers to detect population stratification in association studies. *Am J Hum Genet* 1999; **65**: 220-8.

22 Reich DE, Goldstein DB. Detecting association in a case-control study while correcting for population stratification. *Genet Epidemiol* 2001; **20**: 4-16.

◆23 Devlin BL, Roeder K. Genomic control for association studies. *Biometrics* 1999; **55**: 997-1004.

24 Lange C, DeMeo D, Silverman EK et al. Using the noninformative families in family-based association tests: a powerful new testing strategy. *Am J Hum Genet* 2003; **73**: 801-11.

●25 Silverman EK, Palmer LJ. Case-control association studies for the genetics of complex respiratory diseases. *Am J Respir Cell Mol Biol* 2000; **22**: 645-8.

◆26 Houwen RHJ, Baharloo S, Blankenship K et al. Genome screening by searching for shared segments: mapping a gene for benign recurrent intrahepatic cholestasis. *Nat Genet* 1994; **8**: 380-6.

27 Van Eerdewegh P, Little RD, Dupuis J et al. Association of the ADAM33 gene with asthma and bronchial hyperresponsiveness. *Nature* 2002; **418**: 426-30.

28 Ogura Y, Bonen DK, Inohara N et al. A frameshift mutation in NOD2 associated with susceptibility to Crohn's disease. *Nature* 2001; **411**: 603-6.

◆29 Daly MJ, Rioux JD, Schaffner SF et al. High-resolution haplotype structure in the human genome. *Nat Genet* 2001; **29**: 229-32.

◆30 Gabriel SB, Schaffner SF, Nguyen H et al. The structure of haplotype blocks in the human genome. *Science* 2002; **296**: 2225-9.

31 Couzin J. Human genome. HapMap launched with pledges of $100 million. *Science* 2002; **298**: 941-2.

32  Terwilliger JD, Ott J. *Handbook of human genetic linkage.*
    Baltimore: Johns Hopkins University Press, 1994.

33  Hinds DA, Risch N, The ASPEX package: Affected sib-pair
    exclusion mapping. http://aspex.sourceforge.net

34  Haseman JK, Elston RC. The investigation of linkage between a
    quantitative trait and a marker locus. *Behav Genet* 1972; **2**:
    3–19.

35  Abecasis GR, Cherny SS, Cookson WO, Cardon LR. Merlin–rapid
    analysis of dense genetic maps using sparse gene flow trees.
    *Nat Genet* 2002; **30**: 97–101.

36  Almasy L, Blangero J. Multipoint quantitative-trait linkage
    analysis in general pedigrees. *Am J Hum Genet* 1998; **62**:
    1198–211.

37  Heath SC. Markov chain Monte Carlo segregation and linkage
    analysis for oligogenic models. *Am J Hum Genet* 1997; **61**:
    748–60.

# 2

# Phenotypes for human respiratory genetics

AUGUSTO A. LITONJUA AND SCOTT T. WEISS

## INTRODUCTION

Essential to performing genetic linkage and association studies is the ability to relate phenotype to genotype. A list of the common phenotypes for respiratory genetics and how they are assessed is presented in Table 2.1. In this chapter, each of these phenotypes will be discussed in turn, detailing how they can be utilized by the respiratory geneticist, in either a family-based, case–control, or population-based cohort study design. It is important to recognize that the choice of a particular phenotype and its assessment in a respiratory genetics study is dependent on many factors. Participant burden (how much the subjects can actually tolerate), scientific research question, cost, and the specific hypothesis of interest are all important factors that influence phenotypic choice and assessment. An important area not covered in this chapter is the role of environmental exposures. Ultimately, phenotype is determined by genes interacting with other genes and environmental factors in a developmental context. As important as measuring phenotypes, respiratory geneticists must be willing to consider and assess environmental exposures such as cigarette smoking, allergen levels, diet, and infections (viral, bacterial, and parasitic) as well as clinical phenotypes and DNA markers in their genetic studies. Consideration of all of the relevant environmental exposures is beyond the scope of this chapter; however, it is very clear that any respiratory genetics study that does not assess environmental tobacco smoke exposure and/or active cigarette smoking for virtually any respiratory disease outcome is missing an important opportunity for studying a potentially highly relevant environmental exposure at relatively low cost.

Table 2.1 *Phenotypic assessment of respiratory disease*

| Phenotype | How assessed |
|---|---|
| Symptoms | Standardized questionnaires |
| Doctor's diagnosis | Subject self report of doctor's diagnosis |
| Lung function | Spirometry. Less commonly diffusing capacity (DLCO) or lung volume measurements by He dilution or body plethysmography |
| Airway responsiveness | Challenge with cold air, methacholine, histamine or AMP |
| Bronchodilator response | Spirometry before and after albuterol |
| Allergy | Skin prick test and/or total and specific IgE levels in serum |
| Radiology | Chest X-ray, chest computerized tomography (CT) |
| Inflammation | Exhaled gases, sputum, blood, or urine biomarkers |

## RESPIRATORY SYMPTOMS/QUESTIONNAIRES

Standardized respiratory questionnaires have an extremely long history. They were first used in the 1950s in Great Britain to assess subjects in epidemiologic studies with the realization that clinical assessment of such subjects was plagued by uncontrollable bias. The British Medical Research Council approved a standardized questionnaire in 1960 and it was subsequently approved by the American Thoracic Society (ATS) in 1969. In 1978, the ATS and the Division of Lung Diseases (DLD) performed a major revision of this questionnaire.[1] This standardized ATS–DLD respiratory questionnaire remains in widespread use. However, this questionnaire, which was primarily developed to assess chronic obstructive pulmonary disease (COPD), has limitations, including the assessment of children and asthma. The American Thoracic Society is developing a modular version of both the child and adult questionnaire, and the International Society of Asthma and Allergy in Childhood (ISAAC) has adapted a questionnaire originally developed by the International Union Against Tuberculosis for use in childhood asthma. These questionnaires consider standard respiratory symptoms such as cough, phlegm, wheezing, shortness of breath, and nocturnal awakenings. It is important to ascertain information about environmental exposures such as smoking, parental history of respiratory disorders or allergic diseases, and occupational information. It is impossible to utilize symptoms alone to differentiate COPD and asthma. The British Thoracic Society has defined six clinical features that separate these disorders. These clinical features are shown in Table 2.2. Bronchodilator response is not an absolute discriminator and cannot be used to definitively distinguish asthma from COPD.

Traditionally, a doctor's diagnosis of asthma or COPD is elicited from self-report of the subject of a doctor's diagnosis of these conditions. In the case of young children, it would be the self-report of the parent reporting the child's diagnosis. Self-report of a doctor's diagnosis of asthma has a very high correlation with the presence of asthmatic range airways responsiveness on methacholine or cold air challenge testing.[2] It is impossible to independently validate a doctor's diagnosis for either asthma or COPD because there is no gold standard for these airways diseases. More precise disease definitions can be obtained by using a combination of self-report of respiratory symptoms and objective abnormalities on lung function tests. For example, persistent wheezing (i.e., wheezing most days and nights apart from colds) in combination with a $PC_{20}$ methacholine $<16\,mg/mL$ is a standard objective definition of asthma.[3] Similar constructs can be made for COPD. Using these more objective definitions, potential biases in relation to reporting of a doctor's diagnosis of airways disease can be effectively eliminated from genetic studies.

## LUNG FUNCTION

The three separate types of tests utilized to measure lung function are: (1) spirometry, which is used to define whether airflow obstruction is present or absent; (2) lung volumes, which are utilized to determine lung size; and (3) diffusion capacity, which is used to determine the volume of gas and blood exchanging surface area in the lung. For practical purposes, spirometry is the only realistic test for phenotyping lung function in large-scale genetic studies in families and populations. Figure 2.1 depicts two spirograms – one in an asthmatic and the other in a normal control subject. In the spirometric maneuver, a subject takes a deep breath in

**Table 2.2** *Clinical features differentiating COPD and asthma in adults*

|  | COPD | Asthma |
| --- | --- | --- |
| Smoker or exsmoker | Nearly all | Can occur, usually lower dose |
| Symptoms under age 35 | Rare | Common |
| Chronic productive cough | Common | Uncommon in adults |
| Breathlessness | Persistent and progressive | Variable |
| Nighttime awakening with breathlessness or wheeze | Uncommon | Common |
| Significant variation or day-to-day variation of symptoms | Uncommon except in severe disease | Common |

*Thorax* 2004; **59**(suppl 1):33

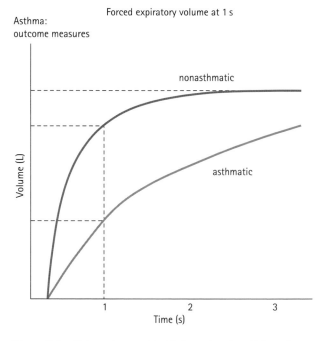

**Figure 2.1** *Spirometry: a subject takes a deep breath in and blows it out as hard and as fast as they can. Normal (non-asthmatic) subjects get all the air out of their lungs rapidly. An asthmatic has decreases in the amount of air expired in the first second of exhalation called the forced expiratory flow in 1 s (FEV$_1$).*

and blows it out as hard and as fast as he/she can. In this maneuver, one can determine the forced vital capacity (FVC), which is the maximum volume of air expired from the lung. The forced expiratory volume in 1s ($FEV_1$) is the amount of air expired in the first second of exhalation. The peak expiratory flow (PEF) is the maximum flow at the initiation of expiration. Flows at lower lung volumes can also be calculated such as the forced expiratory flow 25–75 percent ($FEF_{25-75}$), which is the flow between 25 and 75 percent of the vital capacity. The ATS has published two important documents detailing critical information for respiratory geneticists who desire to perform spirometry as a phenotype in their genetic studies. In 1994, in the Standardization of Spirometry Update, the ATS gives detailed recommendations about instruments, quality control, maneuver performance recommendations, end of test criteria, maximum number of maneuvers, the use of nose clips, and the position in which testing should be performed.[4] Also available are recommendations on reporting of results, maneuver acceptability, test result reproducibility, and reference values.[5] It is beyond the scope of this chapter to review all of these recommendations; however, there are important features of the testing that should be emphasized. First, the greatest source of error in spirometry is failure to obtain a maximum effort from the study subject. The vital capacity maneuver requires coordination and cooperation from the subject. The research technician performing the study must know how to coach the subject appropriately to achieve a maximum effort. The research technician must understand the nature and extent of unacceptable FVC maneuvers and nonreproducible tests, corrective actions to take to improve the quality and number of acceptable maneuvers, and the requirements for equipment quality control, including calibration. The machine should be checked on a daily basis for leaks as well as volume recording accuracy. Linearity of the machine should be checked for flow spirometers on a regular basis. A minimum of three acceptable FVC maneuvers should be performed. Reproducibility criteria may require that up to, but not more than, eight maneuvers be performed, and the best three of these maneuvers are retained for analysis. The exhalation time of 6 s should not be shortened unless there is an obvious plateau in the volume–time curve and is required to obtain maximal FVC results. When testing children, young adults, and some patients with restrictive lung disease, shorter exhalation times may be acceptable. Use of a nose clip is optional and subjects may be tested either sitting or standing but these testing criteria should be consistent across the whole study population. The temperature of the spirometer should be recorded and BTPS correction should be performed when necessary. The criteria of unacceptable spirometric maneuvers include: (1) an unsatisfactory start of expiration characterized by excessive hesitation; (2) false start; (3) extrapolated volume of greater than 5 percent of FVC or 0.15 L, whichever is greater; (4) coughing during the first second of the maneuver; (5) early termination; (6) glottic closure; (7) leak; or (8) obstructed mouth piece. Acceptable reproducibility should produce vital capacities within 0.2 L.

## AIRWAY RESPONSIVENESS TESTING

Airway responsiveness is the term used to describe the tendency of the airways to bronchoconstrict to a variety of nonspecific stimuli. Nonspecific airway responsiveness refers to responsiveness to nonantigenic stimuli including pharmacological agents (methacholine, histamine) and physical stimuli such as cold air and exercise. Nonspecific airway responsiveness is considered an independent host characteristic, and an important intermediate phenotype in both asthma and COPD. Methacholine, histamine, and AMP are the pharmacologic agents most widely used to assess nonspecific airway responsiveness. Methacholine is the one most commonly used. The ATS has issued a guideline statement for methacholine and exercise challenge testing that summarizes the important information needed to perform this testing.[6] It is important to recognize that there are a variety of absolute and relative contraindications to performing this testing. These contraindications are listed in Table 2.3. Safety is paramount in airway responsiveness testing and it is critical that the absolute contraindications be adhered to. A physician should perform a pretest evaluation of the patient to ensure that he/she has been evaluated for contraindications. In addition, a review of patient medications and a general health assessment should be performed by the physician to ensure that the patient understands the procedure and can reliably perform spirometric maneuvers. Short-acting bronchodilators, longer-acting bronchodilators, and foods containing caffeine, such as coffee, tea, and chocolate, should be stopped 24 h prior to testing. A variety of techniques are available to perform the tests but all follow the same basic procedure. Varying increasing doses of a bronchoconstrictive agent such as methacholine are inhaled by the study subject and forced expiratory volume maneuvers are performed. The procedure begins with baseline testing of $FEV_1$, then use of a diluent alone, followed by

Table 2.3    *Contraindications to airway responsiveness testing*

| **Absolute** |
| --- |
| Severe airflow limitation ($FEV_1$ < 50% predicted or <1.0 L)<br>Heart attack or stroke in last 3 months<br>Uncontrolled hypertension (systolic BP >200, or diastolic BP >100)<br>Known untreated aortic aneurysm |

| **Relative** |
| --- |
| Moderate airflow limitation (FEV < 60% predicted or <1.52L)<br>Inability to perform acceptable quality spirometry<br>Pregnancy<br>Nursing mothers<br>Current use of beta blocker inhibitor medication |

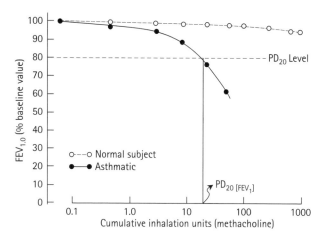

**Figure 2.2**  *Methacholine challenge testing: normal subject (open circle) and asthmatic subject (closed circle) decline in FEV$_1$ as a percentage of baseline with increasing doses of inhaled methacholine. PD$_{20}$ is the dose of methacholine associated with a 20 percent drop in FEV$_1$ from baseline.*

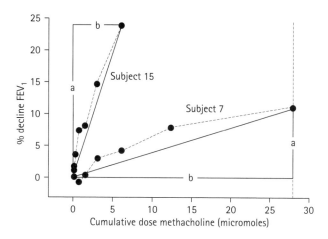

**Figure 2.3**  *Dose response slope is a continuous measurement of airway responsiveness, which is simply the slope of the line from the initial FEV$_1$ to the final FEV$_1$ after methacholine. Taken from O'Connor et al.[99]*

increasing doubling concentrations of methacholine via inhalation, and measurement of FEV$_1$ 30 and 90 s after nebulization is complete. If the FEV$_1$ falls by less than 20 percent of the baseline value, the subject moves on to the next dose. As soon as the FEV$_1$ is ≤20 percent of baseline, the test is terminated (Fig. 2.2). Standards for the use of nebulizers and monitoring nebulizer performance are provided in the ATS guidelines.[6] The guidelines summarize the methods of nebulization of methacholine or histamine. Tidal breathing for a fixed period of time from a continuous output nebulizer is often used, or the administration of a specific number of inhalations of aerosol using a dosimeter or hand-held nebulizer are the two primary methods of choice. The dosimeter method has the advantage that an inhaled dose of aerosol can be directly estimated from the number of inhalations and measurement of nebulizer output. These two methods give comparable results in terms of PC$_{20}$ FEV$_1$, which is the dose of methacholine provoking a 20 percent decline in FEV$_1$. Figure 2.3 shows the calculation of the methacholine dose response slope curve. An important problem in population studies is that the majority of study subjects fail to experience a 20 percent fall in FEV$_1$ during the bronchial challenge test. Hence, PC$_{20}$ FEV$_1$ cannot be calculated for these subjects. A variable such as dose response slope can be calculated with a line connecting the origin of the dose response curve with the final point of the curve, providing a single numerical summary of the whole dose response curve for each subject, and, thus, allowing one to assign a value to all study participants (Fig. 2.3). This may be particularly important in family genetic studies where missing data should be minimized. This approach gives some categorization of airway responsiveness by severity in all subjects. In general, individuals whose PC$_{20}$ value is >16 mg/mL are considered to be normal, values 8–16 mg/mL are considered borderline, and values

**Table 2.4**  *Categorization of severity of airway responsiveness*

| PC$_{20}$ (mg/mL) | Interpretation |
| --- | --- |
| >16 | Normal airway responsiveness |
| 16–8 | Borderline airway responsiveness |
| 8–4 | Mild AR |
| <4 | Moderate to severe AR |

below 8 are considered asthmatic range airway responsiveness, with individuals having values 4–8 having mild and individuals having values <4 having moderate to severe airway responsiveness. Airway responsiveness is clearly related to both bronchodilator responsiveness and level of FEV$_1$.[7] Individuals with lower levels of FEV$_1$ will have greater degrees of airway responsiveness. Lower levels of FEV$_1$ are criteria for nonperformance of the test because of concerns with safety. This censoring creates significant problems with missing data and is not remedied by using dose response slope as a phenotype.

## BRONCHODILATOR RESPONSIVENESS TESTING

Because of subject safety, not all individuals can undergo bronchoconstrictive challenge testing. It is also likely that genes associated with the bronchoconstrictor response may not completely overlap with the genes associated with the bronchodilator response. In any case, independent assessment of bronchodilator responsiveness is a necessary and important feature of respiratory genetic studies of airways diseases such as cystic fibrosis, asthma, and COPD. Testing is typically performed by having the subject inhale two puffs (90 μg per puff) from a metered-dose inhaler of albuterol. A spacer device can be used to improve the consistency of bronchodilator administration. Spirometry is measured before inhalation and at 15 min following the second inhalation. Bronchodilator responsiveness is usually normally distributed, and an abbreviated dose response curve may be obtained by repeating the maneuver after a second dose of four puffs of albuterol. Bronchodilator responsiveness can be expressed in many different ways; commonly used phenotypes are: (1) an absolute volume change in $FEV_1$ (post $FEV_1$ − pre $FEV_1$); (2) a percentage of the baseline $FEV_1$ [(post $FEV_1$ − pre $FEV_1$) divided by the pre $FEV_1$ as a raw value]; or (3) a percentage of predicted $FEV_1$ [(post $FEV_1$ − pre $FEV_1$) divided by the predicted $FEV_1$ value adjusting for age, height, and gender].

## ALLERGY TESTING/SKIN TESTING

IgE-mediated hypersensitivity is characterized by the presentation of antigen to dendritic cells, which then interact with $CD4^+$ T lymphocytes to elaborate a series of proinflammatory cytokines (IL4, IL5, IL9, IL13). In addition, the activation of mast cells and $CD4^+$ lymphocytes via these cytokines produces isotype switching in the production of IgE antibody, which is characteristic of this particular immediate type hypersensitivity immune response. IgE-mediated hypersensitivity is characteristic of three organs: (1) the respiratory epithelium; (2) the gastrointestinal epithelium; and (3) the skin. Respiratory geneticists assess IgE-mediated hypersensitivity utilizing either skin prick tests or the measurement of IgE levels in serum. The two principal methods of skin testing utilized in respiratory genetic studies are the prick test and the intradermal test. The prick test is utilized almost exclusively in genetic studies. A drop of antigen is applied to the skin and a skin test needle is injected through the solution pricking the superficial epidermal layer of the skin without inducing bleeding. The introduction of antigen into the skin results in raised red lesions characterized by a wheal (i.e., the size of the bump) and flare (the degree of redness) measured at 15–20 min after antigen application. There are two types of control tests required for skin testing. The first contains the aqueous vehicle without antigen to assess nonspecific reactivity unrelated to allergy. The most commonly used vehicle used in the prick methods is 50 percent glycerol. Any reaction to this negative control is routinely subtracted from that of the test reactions in recording wheal size. The second, or positive, control is histamine, usually administered as 1 mg/mL of histamine hydrochloride. A several centimeter size wheal is expected from the histamine control, reaching its peak 8–10 min following application. A negative histamine reaction indicates either lack of mast cell histamine release in the skin, the inactivation of the histamine by antihistamine preparations, or the test agent itself was misapplied. Several issues should be considered in this type of testing: (1) the choice of the area of the body; (2) the choice of antigens to be applied; and (3) interpretation of the test results. There are several body areas generally deemed to be of equal reactivity. The back is thought to be more sensitive than the forearm, and the upper back is more sensitive than the lower back. Usually, both forearms are used. The time of day of application of the antigens may also influence results. There is no absolute rule as to the number of antigens that should be applied. Different antigens may be important in different regions of the world. In general, indoor antigens are thought to be more important than outdoor antigens, though Alternaria has been shown to be a major antigen in desert regions such as Tucson, Arizona. As a general rule, the more antigens applied, the greater the reactivity prevalence rate in the population. Four or five judiciously applied antigens with a positive and negative control should be adequate in most populations. It is important to measure the size of both the wheal and flare reaction in millimeters. This can be accomplished using a marker and clear adhesive tape. A potential problem remains in the combining of antigens of different concentrations and potency to create an overall index. A simple index is the number of positive reactions simply added up and used as an index of skin test positivity.

## SERUM IGE LEVELS MEASURED BY STANDARD IMMUNOASSAY TECHNIQUES

This test is performed using a variety of enzyme linked immunosorbent assays (ELISAs) that are commercially available. Also commercially available are standard radioimmunoassay (RIAs). For measurement of specific IgE, the radioallergosorbent test (RAST) is used. This is similar to the total IgE test except that a single antigen is bound to the paper disk rather than the total IgE. Although radioactively labeled antibodies were used initially, fluorescence-based assays for specific IgE measurement are also commercially available and in widespread use. Test serum is added, specific IgE antibodies are bound to the allergen disk complex and subsequently measured by a labeled anti-IgE. Investigators routinely measure total IgE and either skin test reactivity or RAST to a specific IgE. The importance of measuring both total and specific IgE is that they appear to be under separate genetic control.[8]

## NONINVASIVE BIOMARKERS OF INFLAMMATION FOR RESPIRATORY GENETIC STUDIES

Airway inflammation is central to asthma, COPD,[9] and other lung diseases.[10,11] While the cell type and location of the inflammatory process in these disorders differ, markers of inflammation have been studied in relation to the presence of disease, disease severity, and response to treatment.

To date, there have been no estimates of heritability of markers of inflammation in respiratory genetic studies. Nevertheless, assessment of inflammation in these disorders holds promise either in helping to refine the phenotype or as an intermediate phenotype in gene identification, association, or pharmacogenetic studies.

Studies that have investigated airway and lung parenchymal tissue samples obtained by fiberoptic bronchoscopy (either bronchial biopsies or bronchoalveolar lavage) have elucidated the role that inflammation plays in lung disorders. However, bronchoscopy is invasive and unsuitable for studies of human complex genetic disorders, such as asthma and COPD, where large numbers of cases and controls, or family members, need to be phenotyped. Thus, noninvasive measures of inflammation that can be collected easily, in some cases collected multiple times on the same person, in large numbers of subjects, are necessary for these studies.

Many biomarkers have now been studied in asthma, COPD, and other lung disorders. Some of the more common biomarkers are reviewed here. Since most respiratory genetic studies have blood collection as part of their study protocols, measurement of many of these biomarkers in either serum or plasma has been utilized. Because of its ease of collection, particularly for adult subjects, urine samples have also been used to measure many of the biomarkers that are found in blood. It may be argued, however, that markers that are measured in blood and urine are reflective of systemic inflammation, or may be affected by co-morbid conditions (particularly with urinary measures), and not truly reflective of airway inflammation. To address this, there has been great interest in measurement of inflammatory biomarkers in sputum, exhaled gases, and exhaled breath condensate as more proximate measures of airway inflammation, as evidenced by several recent reviews.[12–14] Eventually, the choice of which biomarker to measure, and in which compartment to measure them, will be dependent on the particular research question being asked.

## CIRCULATING BIOMARKERS

The eosinophil is the predominant cell in the inflammatory response in asthma, and circulating levels of these cells[15–17] or their associated proteins have been used as markers of inflammation in asthma. The eosinophil contains four cationic proteins – eosinophil cationic protein (ECP, also known as RNASE3), major basic protein (MBP, also known as PRG2), eosinophil peroxidase (EPO, also known as EPX), and eosinophil derived neurotoxin (EDN, also known as RNASE2), that are released during their activation. In serum and plasma, methods of collection may affect measured levels of these proteins.[18] For example, levels of ECP in serum are higher than in EDTA-plasma. Furthermore, it appears that serum levels reflect the releasability of proteins from eosinophils whereas plasma levels reflect baseline circulating levels.[19] Thus, to ensure repeatable results, blood should be collected under tightly controlled and standardized conditions.[18–21] Eosinophil granule proteins can also be detected in urine, although fewer studies have assessed this method of collection compared to blood. As with blood, attention to proper and standardized collection is crucial.[18] Both blood and urine levels are affected by diurnal variation,[18,22] and there is evidence for genetic control of eosinophil counts.[23,24]

Neutrophil-derived proteins have also shown promise as biomarkers of airway inflammation. While less useful for asthma,[25] high levels of these proteins, such as myeloperoxidase (MPO), lactoferrin (LTF), and human neutrophil lipocalin (also known as NGAL) have been found in cystic fibrosis.[26] Processing of samples for neutrophil-derived proteins is not as demanding as for eosinophil granule proteins, however, consideration must be given to bacterial infections outside the airways, as these may increase the circulating levels of these proteins.[18]

Oxidative stress results from an imbalance between reactive oxygen species (ROS) production and antioxidant defenses, and has been implicated in many respiratory diseases. Because of their ubiquitous distribution within cell membranes and their propensity to contain double bonds, unsaturated lipids are often targets of ROS via peroxidation reactions. Isoprostanes are made by ROS-mediated peroxidation of arachidonic acid, which circulate in the plasma and can be excreted in the urine.[27] Although over 60 different isoprostanes can arise from the oxidation of arachidonic acid, 8-iso-prostaglandin $F_{2\alpha}$ is one of the most stable products and, as a consequence, has received most attention in human studies. However, measurement requires expensive instrumentation for gas chromatography/mass spectrometry, and sample processing is relatively labor intensive. While a commercial immunoassay kit is available, comparisons between the two methods have revealed significant inconsistencies.[28] Both plasma and urinary isoprostanes are elevated in many respiratory disorders.[29–31] Malondialdehyde (MDA) is an end product of the oxidation and decomposition of polyunsaturated fatty acids containing three or more double bonds, and has been found to be elevated in plasma of asthma and COPD subjects.[32] Proteins are also targets of oxidation, giving rise to protein carbonyls, and oxidized and nitrated proteins, which can all be measured in plasma.[33]

Multiple cytokines and adhesion molecules have been measured in peripheral blood of patients with asthma, cystic fibrosis, and other respiratory disorders. However, since these are also local messengers, there is debate as to the functional relevance of these measurements.[18]

## INDUCED SPUTUM

Sputum induction was introduced in the 1950s as a noninvasive method of screening for lung cancer.[34] Much later, it was recognized that studying the cellular composition and soluble constituents in sputum reflects the inflammatory processes in the airways.[35] This method entails the inhalation of hypertonic saline aerosol to induce coughing up of sputum. Afterward, two methods of sputum processing are available, one by using the whole sputum sample[36] and the other by separating the solid portion from the remainder.[37] Normal levels for sputum cell counts have been published for adults,[38] but there is not as much reliable information available for children.[39] Aside from cell counts, many of the markers that can be measured in blood samples may be measured in sputum samples.[40,41] Recent advances in the use of sputum as a reflection of airway inflammation include the measurement of cysteinyl leukotrienes, prostaglandins, thromboxanes, and interleukins.[39,42]

## EXHALED GASES

The analysis of breath constituents has received great interest, because it provides a potentially easily accessible, noninvasive method to measure airway inflammation and oxidative stress. Because the collection of exhaled gases or exhaled breath condensate is relatively noninvasive, it lends itself to repeated measurements, which may be very helpful in studies that seek to define changes in phenotypes over time (e.g., studies that investigate genetic determinants or modifiers of exacerbation of disease over time) or for determining response to an intervention (e.g., pharmacogenetic studies).

A number of volatile gases, such as nitric oxide (NO), have been measured in exhaled gases and have been shown to be elevated in a number of respiratory disorders. While the details of the sample collection, measurement, and sources of variation of each of these markers is beyond the scope of this chapter, recent detailed reviews have been published.[13,43]

Exhaled NO has been the most extensively studied biomarker, and levels have been documented to be elevated in asthma,[44–46] unstable COPD,[47] and bronchiectasis;[48] normal in stable COPD;[49,50] and decreased in pulmonary hypertension[51] and cystic fibrosis.[52,53] Recently, genetic determinants of exhaled NO levels have been suggested by genetic association studies.[54,55] Because NO levels are higher in nasal cavities and are affected by flow rate, samples are collected by exhalation against a resistance to ensure closure of the soft palate, and a constant flow rate is used. NO may be measured from exhaled breath by continuous sampling by the NO analyzer ('online measurements') or from exhaled gas previously collected in a reservoir ('offline measurements'). Extensive recommendations for these and other standardized collection procedures from the American Thoracic Society[56] and the European Respiratory Society[57] have been published, and particular recommendations for measurement in children were prepared by a joint task force from the two respiratory societies.[58]

Carbon monoxide, volatile hydrocarbons such as ethane, pentane, and isoprene, and other markers of lipid peroxidation such as malonaldehyde and aliphatic hydrocarbons have been measured in exhaled breath.[43] However, these markers have not been extensively studied, and their practical value must still be demonstrated.

## EXHALED BREATH CONDENSATE

While sputum induction is a relatively noninvasive method of obtaining samples from the respiratory tract, there is evidence that repeated induced sputum collection can provoke inflammatory responses,[59,60] which may limit the usefulness of this method in some circumstances. Collection of exhaled breath condensate (EBC) is a new method of detecting nonvolatile mediators and inflammatory markers that does not influence airway function or inflammation.[61] Collection entails passing exhaled air through a condensing apparatus, resulting in fluid that is predominantly derived from water vapor. Several methods of EBC collection have been described, with at least one commercially available method. The list of biomarkers that can be measured from EBC is long, and includes pH,[62] hydrogen peroxide,[63] cytokines,[64] aldehydes,[65] isoprostanes, and other products of oxidation.[66,67] To underscore the potential for EBC as a noninvasive and easily obtainable sample in which to measure inflammatory biomarkers, EBC has been studied in a wide variety of respiratory disorders, such as asthma,[62,65,68] COPD,[66,68] cystic fibrosis,[69] interstitial lung disease,[70] and acute lung injury/ARDS,[71] and in both children and adults. Factors that affect collection of samples include salivary contamination, contamination of exhaled breath with nasal air, and humidity and air temperature.[43] EBC collection is a promising method for collection of respiratory samples, but collection methods and techniques need to be standardized before it can be advocated as a means of phenotyping subjects for genetic studies.

## COMPUTED TOMOGRAPHY IN PHENOTYPE DEFINITION

Conventional lung function tests are excellent measures of overall level of ventilation and degree of ventilatory obstruction. However, they are limited in the amount of information they provide with regard to the regional heterogeneity of lung parenchyma or airways. Computed tomography (CT) scanning has the potential to refine our definitions of phenotypes by differentiating between subjects who have primarily parenchymal involvement from those with primarily airway pathology and by quantitative assessment of the degree and distribution of parenchymal and airway lesions.

Computed tomography provides transverse anatomical images in which the value of each picture element (pixel) corresponds to the radiographic attenuation of a defined volume of tissue (voxel).[72] The radiographic attenuation values for each set of CT slices are registered by the computer and organized in a matrix form. The radiographic attenuation, also called tissue density, is numerically expressed in Hounsfield units (HU), with the scale of values ranging from $-1000$ HU (the attenuation value of air) to 3000 HU; 0 HU corresponds to the attenuation value of water. The thousands of pixels in one CT scan make this modality the most precise method for assessing lung structure in vivo.[72,73] While CT scanning can help in the diagnosis of respiratory disorders such as interstitial lung disease and bronchiolitis,[74] probably the most promising use of this modality is in refining the subphenotypes in COPD. The presence, severity, and distribution of emphysema can be determined, and there is the potential to determine the importance of small airway obstruction as well.

The assessment of emphysema by CT scan has been conducted by both qualitative (visual assessment of the presence/absence of emphysema or the use of radiologist severity scoring[75,76]) and by quantitative (computerized image analysis[77]) methods, which rely on the detection of relatively large radiolucent areas within the lung. While the qualitative methods are easier to implement and do not require dedicated software, computerized image analysis methods have been shown to be more reproducible across institutions[78] and have greater correlation with macroscopic morphological measurements.[79] Several lung attenuation methods based on histogram analysis of the frequency distribution of the attenuation values of the lung have been developed to quantify emphysema objectively.[72] Most commonly, emphysema has been quantified on CT by examining the frequency distribution of the X-ray attenuation values within the lung, and those areas that fall below a predetermined threshold are considered emphysematous.[80–82] In an early study, Müller et al.[82] found that X-ray attenuation values lower than $-910$ HU correlated best with the extent of lesions on gross pathologic lung specimens, and as a consequence, this threshold was recommended for the identification of emphysema. More recently, a threshold of $-950$ HU was suggested to be optimal for thin (1 mm) section CT scans.[83] The second most common technique involves defining a predetermined percentile of the lung attenuation distribution curve.[84,85] The lowest fifth percentile of the HU distribution was found to correlate significantly with both the mean value of the surface area of the alveolar wall per unit volume (AWUV) and the extent of emphysema measured pathologically,[85] while the lowest 15th percentile was found to be appropriate for individuals with severe alpha-1-antitrypsin deficiency.[84] Other techniques to quantify emphysema on CT scans have been developed and involve predicting the lung surface-to-volume ratio from CT attenuation values,[86] assessing the relation between lesion size and spatial distribution (expressed as a fractal dimension),[81] and a texture-based adaptive multiple feature method.[87]

While most of the chest CT analytical techniques have dealt with quantifying parenchymal lesions, there have also been attempts to measure airway wall dimensions. Many of these methods make use of qualitative visual assessment.[88] However, several quantitative methods have recently been developed.[89,90] The most common method in use is the full width at half-maximum method ('half-max').[89,91] This method casts rays from a seed point in the airway lumen through the airway wall and measures the X-ray attenuation within the wall and back to low attenuation in the parenchyma. The advantages of this method are that it is relatively operator-independent and very fast. Another method makes use of a maximum-likelihood technique to estimate the airway inner and outer radius.[92] The main limitation, however, of all the above methods, is that accurate airway luminal area (Ai) and airway wall area (Aaw) can be measured only from airways that are oriented approximately perpendicular to the plane of scanning.[88] Wood and coworkers[93] overcame this limitation by converting the asymmetric CT voxels into cubic dimensions, allowing the images to be reconstructed in any orientation. King and colleagues[94] reported an automated CT image analysis algorithm based on the principle of score-guided erosion to measure Ai, Aaw, and airway angle of orientation. Finally, Saba and colleagues[95] have proposed a new technique of fitting ellipses to airway walls, which substantially reduces the amount of error in these measurements.

While research into the measurement of airway dimensions is continuing, the current methods have been studied in both asthma and COPD. In asthma, airway wall thickness was negatively correlated with the $PD_{20}$,[96] spirometric indices of $FEV_1$ and $FEV_1/FVC$[i], and was directly related to duration of disease.[97] Nakano and colleagues[91] developed software to measure the dimensions of the apical segmental bronchus in 94 COPD patients and 20 asymptomatic smokers. Although the upper lobe apical segmental bronchus is a large airway, they showed that the airway dimensions of this airway correlated well with the smaller airways. They also found that the COPD patients could be divided into groups with predominant loss of lung attenuation and those with predominant thickening and narrowing of the apical segmental bronchus. This finding highlights the heterogeneity that is present in subjects with COPD, whose diagnosis relies heavily on spirometric indices, and underscores the need for better characterization of subphenotypes in genetic studies of respiratory disorders.

CT scanning holds promise as a means to noninvasively assess structural characteristics of the lung that will aid in phenotyping subjects for respiratory genetics studies. Most of the studies that have investigated the use of CT scanning have focused on defining the presence, extent, and distribution of emphysematous lesions. Thus, it is likely that CT scanning will play an immediate role in dissecting genetic determinants for subtypes of emphysema (e.g., different genes influencing apical predominance versus basal predominance of emphysematous lesions). More work needs to be done with quantifying airway dimensions, and it appears that this will be important in studying airway wall remodeling in both asthma and COPD.[98]

## Key learning points

- The amount and type of phenotyping in a genetic study must be related to specific hypotheses.

- Most phenotyping in respiratory genetics follows well-established clinical protocols.

- All phenotyping involves some risk for the subject. It is important for the investigator to know the details of these risks for human subjects purposes as well as protocol design.

## REFERENCES

◆1  Ferris BG, Jr. Epidemieology standardization project. *Am Rev Respir Dis* 1978; **118**: 1–88.

2  Weiss ST, Tager IB, Weiss JW et al. Airways responsiveness in a population sample of adults and children. *Am Rev Respir Dis* 1984; **129**: 898–902.

3  Toelle BG, Peat JK, Salome CM et al. Toward a definition of asthma for epidemiology. *Am Rev Respir Dis* 1992; **146**: 633–7.

◆4  Standardization of Spirometry, 1987 Update. Statement of the American Thoracic Society. *Am Rev Respir Dis* 1987; **136**: 1285–98.

◆5  Standardization of Spirometry, 1994 Update. American Thoracic Society. *Am J Respir Crit Care Med* 1995; **152**: 1107–36.

◆6  Crapo RO, Casaburi R, Coates AL et al. Guidelines for methacholine and exercise challenge testing – 1999. This official statement of the American Thoracic Society was adopted by the ATS Board of Directors, July 1999. *Am J Respir Crit Care Med* 2000; **161**: 309–29.

7  Rijcken B, Schouten JP, Weiss ST et al. The relationship between airway responsiveness to histamine and pulmonary function level in a random population sample. *Am Rev Respir Dis* 1988; **137**: 826–32.

8  Marsh DG. Mapping the genes for IgE production and allergy. *Adv Exp Med Biol* 1996; **409**: 43–53.

9  O'Byrne PM, Postma DS. The many faces of airway inflammation: asthma and chronic obstructive pulmonary disease. *Am J Respir Crit Care Med* 1999; **159**: S41–S66.

10  Strieter RM. Mechanisms of pulmonary fibrosis: conference summary. *Chest* 2001; **120**: 77S–85S.

11  Chmiel JF, Berger M, Konstan MW. The role of inflammation in the pathophysiology of CF lung disease. *Clin Rev Allergy Immunol* 2002; **23**: 5–27.

12  Kharitonov SA, Barnes PJ. Biomarkers of some pulmonary diseases in exhaled breath. *Biomarkers* 2002; **7**: 1–32.

13  Paredi P, Kharitonov SA, Barnes PJ. Analysis of expired air for oxidation products. *Am J Respir Crit Care Med* 2002; **166**: S31–7.

14  Rahman I, Kelly F. Biomarkers in breath condensate: a promising new non-invasive technique in free radical research. *Free Radic Res* 2003; **37**: 1253–66.

15  Fujitaka M, Kawaguchi H, Kato Y et al. Significance of the eosinophil cationic protein/eosinophil count ratio in asthmatic patients: its relationship to disease severity. *Ann Allergy Asthma Immunol* 2001; **86**: 323–9.

16  Stelmach I, Majak P, Grzelewski T et al. The ECP/Eo count ratio in children with asthma. *J Asthma* 2004; **41**: 539–46.

17  Tang RB, Chen SJ. Serum levels of eosinophil cationic protein and eosinophils in asthmatic children during a course of prednisolone therapy. *Pediatr Pulmonol* 2001; **31**: 121–5.

18  Koller DY. Sampling methods: urine/blood analysis. *Am J Respir Crit Care Med* 2000; **162**: S31–3.

19  Reimert CM, Poulsen LK, Bindslev-Jensen C et al. Measurement of eosinophil cationic protein (ECP) and eosinophil protein X/eosinophil derived neurotoxin (EPX/EDN). Time and temperature dependent spontaneous release in vitro demands standardized sample processing. *J Immunol Methods* 1993; **166**: 183–90.

20  Pronk-Admiraal CJ, Bartels PC. Effect of clotting temperature and eosinophil concentration on the eosinophil cationic protein concentration in serum. *Scand J Clin Lab Invest* 1994; **54**: 185–8.

21  Wempe JB, Tammeling EP, Koeter GH et al. Blood eosinophil numbers and activity during 24 hours: effects of treatment with budesonide and bambuterol. *J Allergy Clin Immunol* 1992; **90**: 757–65.

22  Peterson CG, Enander I, Nystrand J et al. Radioimmunoassay of human eosinophil cationic protein (ECP) by an improved method. Establishment of normal levels in serum and turnover in vivo. *Clin Exp Allergy* 1991; **21**: 561–7.

23  Chae SC, Lee YC, Park YR et al. Analysis of the polymorphisms in eotaxin gene family and their association with asthma, IgE, and eosinophil. *Biochem Biophys Res Commun* 2004; **320**: 131–7.

24  Evans DM, Zhu G, Duffy DL et al. Major quantitative trait locus for eosinophil count is located on chromosome 2q. *J Allergy Clin Immunol* 2004; **114**: 826–30.

25  Tauber E, Herouy Y, Goetz M et al. Assessment of serum myeloperoxidase in children with bronchial asthma. *Allergy* 1999; **54**: 177–82.

26  Eichler I, Nilsson M, Rath R et al. Human neutrophil lipocalin, a highly specific marker for acute exacerbation in cystic fibrosis. *Eur Respir J* 1999; **14**: 1145–9.

27  Morrow JD, Roberts LJ. The isoprostanes: unique bioactive products of lipid peroxidation. *Prog Lipid Res* 1997; **36**: 1–21.

28  Proudfoot J, Barden A, Mori TA et al. Measurement of urinary F(2)-isoprostanes as markers of in vivo lipid peroxidation – A comparison of enzyme immunoassay with gas chromatography/mass spectrometry. *Anal Biochem* 1999; **272**: 209–15.

29  Dworski R, Roberts LJ, II, Murray JJ et al. Assessment of oxidant stress in allergic asthma by measurement of the major urinary metabolit of F2-isoprostane, 15-F2t-IsoP (8-iso-PGF2alpha). *Clin Exp Allergy* 2001; **31**: 387–90.

30  Pratico D, Basili S, Vieri M et al. Chronic obstructive pulmonary disease is associated with an increase in urinary levels of

isoprostane F2alpha-III, an index of oxidant stress. *Am J Respir Crit Care Med* 1998; **158**: 1709–14.

31    Wood LG, Fitzgerald DA, Gibson PG et al. Lipid peroxidation as determined by plasma isoprostanes is related to disease severity in mild asthma. *Lipids* 2000; **35**: 967–74.

32    Rahman I, Morrison D, Donaldson K, MacNee W. Systemic oxidative stress in asthma, COPD, and smokers. *Am J Respir Crit Care Med* 1996; **154**: 1055–60.

33    Boots AW, Haenen GR, Bast A. Oxidant metabolism in chronic obstructive pulmonary disease. *Eur Respir J Suppl* 2003; **46**: 14s–27s.

34    Bickerman HA, Sproul EE, Barach AL. An aerosol method of producing bronchial secretions in human subjects: a clinical technic for the detection of lung cancer. *Dis Chest* 1958; **33**: 347–62.

◆35    Pin I, Gibson PG, Kolendowicz R et al. Use of induced sputum cell counts to investigate airway inflammation in asthma. *Thorax* 1992; **47**: 25–9.

36    Fahy JV, Boushey HA, Lazarus SC et al. Safety and reproducibility of sputum induction in asthmatic subjects in a multicenter study. *Am J Respir Crit Care Med* 2001; **163**: 1470–5.

37    Jayaram L, Parameswaran K, Sears MR, Hargreave FE. Induced sputum cell counts: their usefulness in clinical practice. *Eur Respir J* 2000; **16**: 150–8.

38    Belda J, Leigh R, Parameswaran K et al. Induced sputum cell counts in healthy adults. *Am J Respir Crit Care Med* 2000; **161**: 475–8.

◆39    Wilson N. Measurement of airway inflammation in asthma. *Curr Opin Pulm Med* 2002; **8**: 25–32.

40    Nagayama Y, Odazima Y, Nakayama S et al. Eosinophils and basophilic cells in sputum and nasal smears taken from infants and young children during acute asthma. *Pediatr Allergy Immunol* 1995; **6**: 204–8.

◆41    Twaddell SH, Gibson PG, Carty K et al. Assessment of airway inflammation in children with acute asthma using induced sputum. *Eur Respir J* 1996; **9**: 2104–8.

42    Brightling CE, Ward R, Woltmann G et al. Induced sputum inflammatory mediator concentrations in eosinophilic bronchitis and asthma. *Am J Respir Crit Care Med* 2000; **162**: 878–82.

43    Kharitonov SA, Barnes PJ. Exhaled markers of pulmonary disease. *Am J Respir Crit Care Med* 2001; **163**: 1693–722.

44    Henriksen AH, Lingaas-Holmen T, Sue-Chu M, Bjermer L. Combined use of exhaled nitric oxide and airway hyperresponsiveness in characterizing asthma in a large population survey. *Eur Respir J* 2000; **15**: 849–55.

45    Kharitonov SA, Yates D, Robbins RA et al. Increased nitric oxide in exhaled air of asthmatic patients. *Lancet* 1994; **343**: 133–5.

46    Persson MG, Zetterstrom O, Agrenius V et al. Single-breath nitric oxide measurements in asthmatic patients and smokers. *Lancet* 1994; **343**: 146–7.

47    Maziak W, Loukides S, Culpitt S et al. Exhaled nitric oxide in chronic obstructive pulmonary disease. *Am J Respir Crit Care Med* 1998; **157**: 998–1002.

48    Kharitonov SA, Wells AU, O'Connor BJ et al. Elevated levels of exhaled nitric oxide in bronchiectasis. *Am J Respir Crit Care Med* 1995; **151**: 1889–93.

49    Kharitonov SA, Robbins RA, Yates D et al. Acute and chronic effects of cigarette smoking on exhaled nitric oxide. *Am J Respir Crit Care Med* 1995; **152**: 609–12.

50    Rutgers SR, van der Mark TW, Coers W et al. Markers of nitric oxide metabolism in sputum and exhaled air are not increased in chronic obstructive pulmonary disease. *Thorax* 1999; **54**: 576–80.

51    Kharitonov SA, Cailes JB, Black CM et al. Decreased nitric oxide in the exhaled air of patients with systemic sclerosis with pulmonary hypertension. *Thorax* 1997; **52**: 1051–5.

52    Balfour-Lynn IM, Laverty A, Dinwiddie R. Reduced upper airway nitric oxide in cystic fibrosis. *Arch Dis Child* 1996; **75**: 319–22.

53    Thomas SR, Kharitonov SA, Scott SF et al. Nasal and exhaled nitric oxide is reduced in adult patients with cystic fibrosis and does not correlate with cystic fibrosis genotype. *Chest* 2000; **117**: 1085–9.

54    van's Gravesande KS, Wechsler ME, Grasemann H et al. Association of a missense mutation in the NOS3 gene with exhaled nitric oxide levels. *Am J Respir Crit Care Med* 2003; **168**: 228–31.

55    Wechsler ME, Grasemann H, Deykin A et al. Exhaled nitric oxide in patients with asthma: association with NOS1 genotype. *Am J Respir Crit Care Med* 2000; **162**: 2043–7.

◆56    American Thoracic Society. Recommendations for standardized procedures for the on-line and off-line measurement of exhaled lower respiratory nitric oxide and nasal nitric oxide in adults and children-1999. This official statement of the American Thoracic Society was adopted by the ATS Board of Directors, July 1999. *Am J Respir Crit Care Med* 1999; **160**: 2104–17.

57    Kharitonov S, Alving K, Barnes PJ. Exhaled and nasal nitric oxide measurements: recommendations. The European Respiratory Society Task Force. *Eur Respir J* 1997; **10**: 1683–93.

◆58    Baraldi E, de Jongste JC, European Respiratory Society, American Thoracic Society. Measurement of exhaled nitric oxide in children, 2001. *Eur Respir J* 2002; **20**: 223–37.

59    Holz O, Richter K, Jorres RA et al. Changes in sputum composition between two inductions performed on consecutive days. *Thorax* 1998; **53**: 83–6.

60    Nightingale JA, Rogers DF, Barnes PJ. Effect of repeated sputum induction on cell counts in normal volunteers. *Thorax* 1998; **53**: 87–90.

◆61    Hunt J. Exhaled breath condensate: an evolving tool for noninvasive evaluation of lung disease. *J Allergy Clin Immunol* 2002; **110**: 28–34.

62    Hunt JF, Fang K, Malik R et al. Endogenous airway acidification. Implications for asthma pathophysiology. *Am J Respir Crit Care Med* 2000; **161**: 694–9.

63    Jobsis Q, Raatgeep HC, Schellekens SL et al. Hydrogen peroxide in exhaled air of healthy children: reference values. *Eur Respir J* 1998; **12**: 483–5.

64    Scheideler L, Manke HG, Schwulera U et al. Detection of nonvolatile macromolecules in breath. A possible diagnostic tool? *Am Rev Respir Dis* 1993; **148**: 778–84.

65    Corradi M, Folesani G, Andreoli R et al. Aldehydes and glutathione in exhaled breath condensate of children with asthma exacerbation. *Am J Respir Crit Care Med* 2003; **167**: 395–9.

66    Corradi M, Rubinstein I, Andreoli R et al. Aldehydes in exhaled breath condensate of patients with chronic obstructive pulmonary disease. *Am J Respir Crit Care Med* 2003; **167**: 1380–6.

67    Montuschi P, Collins JV, Ciabattoni G et al. Exhaled 8-isoprostane as an in vivo biomarker of lung oxidative stress in

patients with COPD and healthy smokers. *Am J Respir Crit Care Med* 2000; **162**: 1175-7.

68   Montuschi P, Corradi M, Ciabattoni G et al. Increased 8-isoprostane, a marker of oxidative stress, in exhaled condensation in asthma patients. *Am J Resp Crit Care Med* 1999; **160**: 216-20.

69   Montuschi P, Kharitonov SA, Ciabattoni G et al. Exhaled 8-isoprostane as a new non-invasive biomarker of oxidative stress in cystic fibrosis. *Thorax* 2000; **55**: 205-9.

70   Montuschi P, Ciabattoni G, Paredi P et al. 8-Isoprostane as a biomarker of oxidative stress in interstitial lung diseases. *Am J Respir Crit Care Med* 1998; **158**: 1524-7.

71   Carpenter CT, Price PV, Christman BW. Exhaled breath condensate isoprostanes are elevated in patients with acute lung injury or ARDS. *Chest* 1998; **114**: 1653-9.

◆72   Madani A, Keyzer C, Gevenois PA. Computed tomography assessment of lung structure and function in pulmonary emphysema. In: Bankier A, Gevenois PA (eds). *European Respiratory Monograph*. Vol. 30, 2004: 145-60.

◆73   Hoffman EA, McLennan G. Assessment of the pulmonary structure-function relationship and clinical outcomes measures: quantitative volumetric CT of the lung. *Acad Radiol* 1997; **4**: 758-76.

74   Ujita M, Hansell DM. Small airways diseases: detection and insights with computed tomography. In: Bankier A, Gevenois PA (eds). *European Respiratory Monograph*, Vol. 30, 2004: 166.

75   Bergin C, Muller N, Nichols DM et al. The diagnosis of emphysema. A computed tomographic–pathologic correlation. *Am Rev Respir Dis* 1986; **133**: 541-6.

76   Hruban RH, Meziane MA, Zerhouni EA et al. High resolution computed tomography of inflation-fixed lungs. Pathologic–radiologic correlation of centrilobular emphysema. *Am Rev Respir Dis* 1987; **136**: 935-40.

77   Webb WR, Stein MG, Finkbeiner WE et al. Normal and diseased isolated lungs: high-resolution CT. *Radiology* 1988; **166**: 81-7.

78   Kazerooni EA. Radiologic evaluation of emphysema for lung volume reduction surgery. *Clin Chest Med* 1999; **20**: 845-61.

79   Bankier AA, De Maertelaer V, Keyzer C, Gevenois PA. Pulmonary emphysema: subjective visual grading versus objective quantification with macroscopic morphometry and thin-section CT densitometry. *Radiology* 1999; **211**: 851-8.

80   Gevenois PA, de Maertelaer V, De Vuyst P et al. Comparison of computed density and macroscopic morphometry in pulmonary emphysema. *Am J Respir Crit Care Med* 1995; **152**: 653-7.

81   Mishima M, Hirai T, Itoh H et al. Complexity of terminal airspace geometry assessed by lung computed tomography in normal subjects and patients with chronic obstructive pulmonary disease. *Proc Natl Acad Sci USA* 1999; **96**: 8829-34.

82   Muller NL, Staples CA, Miller RR, Abboud RT. 'Density mask'. An objective method to quantitate emphysema using computed tomography. *Chest* 1988; **94**: 782-7.

83   Gevenois PA, De Vuyst P, Sy M et al. Pulmonary emphysema: quantitative CT during expiration. *Radiology* 1996; **199**: 825-9.

84   Dirksen A, Friis M, Olesen KP et al. Progress of emphysema in severe alpha-1-antitrypsin deficiency as assessed by annual CT. *Acta Radiol* 1997; **38**: 826-32.

85   Gould GA, MacNee W, McLean A et al. CT measurements of lung density in life can quantitate distal airspace enlargement – an essential defining feature of human emphysema. *Am Rev Respir Dis* 1988; **137**: 380-92.

86   Coxson HO, Rogers RM, Whittall KP et al. A quantification of the lung surface area in emphysema using computed tomography. *Am J Respir Crit Care Med* 1999; **159**: 851-6.

87   Uppaluri R, Mitsa T, Sonka M et al. Quantification of pulmonary emphysema from lung computed tomography images. *Am J Respir Crit Care Med* 1997; **156**:248-54.

88   Nakano Y, Muller NL, King GG et al. Quantitative assessment of airway remodeling using high-resolution CT. *Chest* 2002; **122**: 271S-5S.

89   Amirav I, Kramer SS, Grunstein MM, Hoffman EA. Assessment of methacholine-induced airway constriction by ultrafast high-resolution computed tomography. *J Appl Physiol* 1993; **75**: 2239-50.

90   McNitt-Gray MF, Goldin JG, Johnson TD et al. Development and testing of image-processing methods for the quantitative assessment of airway hyperresponsiveness from high-resolution CT images. *J Comput Assist Tomogr* 1997; **21**: 939-47.

91   Nakano Y, Muro S, Sakai H et al. Computed tomographic measurements of airway dimensions and emphysema in smokers. Correlation with lung function. *Am J Respir Crit Care Med* 2000; **162**: 1102-8.

92   Reinhardt JM, D'Souza ND, Hoffman EA. Accurate measurement of intrathoracic airways. *IEEE Trans Med Imaging* 1997; **16**: 820-7.

93   Wood SA, Zerhouni EA, Hoford JD et al. Measurement of three-dimensional lung tree structures by using computed tomography. *J Appl Physiol* 1995; **79**: 1687-97.

94   King GG, Muller NL, Whittall KP et al. An analysis algorithm for measuring airway lumen and wall areas from high-resolution computed tomographic data. *Am J Respir Crit Care Med* 2000; **161**: 574-80.

95   Saba OI, Hoffman EA, Reinhardt JM. Maximizing quantitative accuracy of lung airway lumen and wall measures obtained from X-ray CT imaging. *J Appl Physiol* 2003; **95**: 1063-75.

96   Boulet L, Belanger M, Carrier G. Airway responsiveness and bronchial-wall thickness in asthma with or without fixed airflow obstruction. *Am J Respir Crit Care Med* 1995; **152**: 865-71.

97   Niimi A, Matsumoto H, Amitani R et al. Airway wall thickness in asthma assessed by computed tomography. Relation to clinical indices. *Am J Respir Crit Care Med* 2000; **162**: 1518-23.

98   Brown RH, Mitzner W. Understanding airway pathophysiology with computed tomography. *J Appl Physiol* 2003; **95**: 854-62.

99   O'Connor G, Sparrow D, Taylor D et al. Analysis of dose-response curves to methacholine. An approach suitable for population studies. *Am Rev Respir Dis* 1987; **136**: 1412-7.

# 3

# Testing for association in genetic studies

NAN LAIRD, PETER KRAFT, CHRISTOPH LANGE, AND KRISTEL VAN STEEN

## BASIC CONCEPTS UNDERLYING GENETIC ASSOCIATION ANALYSIS

The goal of a genetic association analysis is to show that a disease phenotype varies in a predictable manner with a marker genotype. In some respects, testing for an association between a disease phenotype (or trait) and a genotype is no different from testing for statistical association between any two variables, whether they are genetic or not. Indeed, many of the statistical techniques used to analyze ordinary statistical association are used for genetic association as well. However, there are important differences in study design and analysis and in the interpretation of the findings. In this chapter we will describe statistical methods used for testing association between a trait and a genetic marker.

There are two basic types of study designs that are used in genetic association analysis: standard (or population-based) and family-based. Analytic methods appropriate for these two designs are quite different and will be discussed separately under sections Standard designs for association studies and Family-based designs for genetic association, respectively. In this introductory section we will provide an overview of common themes in genetic association analysis, including a detailed discussion of study design, the nature of genetic association, standard approaches to association analysis, coding of variables for analysis, and analyses of multiple and quantitative traits.

### The nature of genetic association

We define genetic association broadly to mean that the variation in the disease trait of interest is explained at least in part by an individual's genotype at a genetic marker. Association analyses are used in many settings: looking at the effects of markers in candidate genes, fine mapping under linkage peaks, and even whole genome scans. If the marker genotype being tested is a known mutation which influences the trait, values of the trait will be directly associated with presence or absence of the mutation. Typically, however, we are testing association between a disease trait and a genetic marker which is chosen because of its location in the genome and not its biological function. Even with candidate genes, there may be no known functional mutation to test. Thus, in many settings, the markers selected for testing may well have no causal relationship to the disease phenotype. Instead, an association between a marker and the trait may be present if there is allelic association between an unobserved mutation at the disease susceptibility locus and the marker being tested.

Allelic association is a population concept which implies that the alleles at one genetic locus are associated with the alleles at a second genetic locus. For two randomly selected markers in a randomly mating population, there should be no allelic association because of the genetic reshuffling that occurs during meiosis; in this case, the markers are said to be in linkage equilibrium. Many factors can create an observed allelic association in a population: mutation, selection, genetic drift, founder effects, and population admixture or stratification. Ordinarily, allelic association will dissipate over time due to meiosis, however it can continue for many generations if the two loci are tightly linked; this phenomenon is called linkage disequilibrium (LD). LD occurs when the genetic material at the two loci is inherited as a single unit, i.e., there is little or no recombination between the two loci. If one locus is a disease susceptibility locus and the other is a nearby marker, the presence of LD between the two loci provides the rationale for using association studies to locate disease susceptibility loci. LD between a disease susceptibility locus and a marker can induce an association between the marker and the disease trait.

There is currently much debate over how far LD extends to markers around a disease mutation, and mathematical and simulation models do not correspond well in practice to actual data. It is important to remember that LD depends very much on the selected population and on the allele frequencies of the marker and the hypothesized disease locus. In addition, genetic distance and LD are not highly correlated within a relatively small region and the extent of LD can vary according to type of marker, e.g. SNP, or microsatellite. All of this makes it very difficult to establish precise guidelines for spacing of markers in a genetic study.[1]

It is important to keep in mind that although LD implies association between a marker and a disease trait, association does not necessarily imply LD. Association can also be spurious; spurious association is context dependent. When studying association between a marker and a disease trait, we take spurious association to mean that there is actually no disease susceptibility locus in linkage disequilibrium with the marker even though the trait and the marker are associated. Spurious association is most plausibly related to the presence of population stratification or admixture. An early example of this is given by Knowler et al.,[2] who studied diabetes mellitus in a population of American Indians with mixed Caucasian heritage. They were able to classify all of their subjects according to the number of grandparents of Indian heritage and to show that the degree of Indian heritage was strongly related to a genotype from the GM system of human immunoglobulin G. The crude analysis, not correcting for heritage, was highly suggestive of an association between presence or absence of diabetes and the genotype, but the association disappeared when the analysis was stratified on the degree of Indian heritage. Methods for dealing with potential admixture or stratification are discussed under Standard designs for association studies.

## Study design for genetic association analysis

The defining feature of a genetic association study is whether the sampled unit consists of unrelated individuals or multiple members of a family. We refer to the former as a standard design because variants of these designs, e.g., case–control or cohort designs are commonly used for testing association in any setting. However, family-based designs are unique to genetic association studies. Designs which sample families, usually through one or more probands, are commonly called family-based association studies. We first briefly review standard designs because of their greater familiarity.

Standard designs sample independent individuals. They can be further classified as case–control or cohort depending on how subjects are selected for study. In principle, individuals can be randomly sampled from a population of interest without any regard to their trait or genotype; this would be a true population-based study. This is rare in practice because such designs are not efficient, especially if the trait is rare in the population. Although it is generally desirable from an efficiency viewpoint to select subjects into a study based on their predictor variable, this is not feasible when the predictor is a genotype. Hence, it is common to select subjects on the basis of their trait value. With dichotomous traits, this yields the standard case–control study; i.e., we select cases (or subjects who are positive for the trait of interest) into the study and choose appropriate controls. If the trait is rare, invasive, and/or expensive to determine, using trait unknown subjects as controls can be an effective strategy, although larger samples will generally be required. Case–control and cohort designs will be discussed in some detail under Standard designs for association studies. Selecting subjects on the basis of their quantitative traits is also possible, but may require screening a large population (see the discussion under Family-based designs).

With family-based designs, the sample will ideally include at least one offspring assessed for both the genotype and the trait, and the genotype data for their parents. The family-based design is attractive for many reasons. This design protects against a finding of spurious association due to population admixture or stratification. The reason for robustness is that the analysis uses parental genotypes to determine the distribution of the test statistic. As discussed under Family-based designs for genetic association, the analysis effectively compares the distribution of alleles transmitted to the affected subjects with the distribution of those alleles which are not transmitted. The analysis cannot be biased by admixture or stratification because the 'case' and 'control' alleles are drawn from the same set of parents; therefore they have the same genetic background. Although three subjects need to be genotyped, the trait has to be determined only in the offspring.

There are many variations to the simple 'trio' design with two parents and an affected offspring, for example, designs which include multiple affected offspring, or multiple offspring with at least one affected. With late onset traits, it may not be feasible to obtain parental genotypes. In this case, it is necessary to have additional family genotype data, and the best approach is to collect genotype data from siblings. In contrast to the setting where siblings are used to provide additional phenotypic information for the association analysis, here, siblings are primarily used to provide information on the unobserved parental genotypes. As a result, larger sample sizes will generally be required to compensate for the missing parental data. More information about efficient family-based designs will be given under Family-based designs for genetic association.

Another important distinction between standard and family-based designs is the null and alternative hypotheses that are tested. With a standard design, the null and alternative hypotheses are simply:

Null: no association

Alternative: association is present.

Exactly how association is defined will depend on the model used in the analysis. For example, in a regression analysis, the null hypothesis is formulated by setting the regression coefficient of the genetic predictor to zero.

With a family-based test, the null and alternative hypotheses can be phrased in terms of the underlying genetics in the population. To have any power to reject the null hypothesis, both linkage and LD must exist between the trait locus and the marker. Thus, the alternative hypothesis for a family-based test is always:

both linkage and linkage disequilibrium are present.

There are two possibilities for the null hypothesis:

no linkage and no association

linkage, but no association.

When testing candidate genes, the appropriate null hypothesis will ordinarily be

no linkage and no linkage disequilibrium.

However, if we are testing for association in a region of known linkage, then a more appropriate null hypothesis is

linkage but no linkage disequilibrium.

This distinction is not relevant when our sample consists of parents and one offspring. However, when the sample includes multiple offspring from the same family, with or without parents, the distribution of the test statistic under the null differs for the two null hypotheses. In Family-based designs for genetic association, we will show how to construct valid tests under both types of null hypotheses.

## Association analysis: an overview

This section provides a very brief overview of statistical methods that can be used in any standard association analysis and how they translate in the genetic context. Methods used to test association between two variables depend on the nature of the two variables. While phenotypes or traits can be measured, dichotomous or time-to-onset, genetic marker data are inherently categorical, although it can also be recoded as a count or as a dichotomous variable.

A general paradigm for testing association between a response variable (disease trait) and a predictor (genotype at a marker) is a regression analysis. A regression analysis (linear, logistic, or proportional hazards) can accommodate all types of outcomes and all types of predictors. When the trait is quantitative, we use linear regression; with dichotomous traits we use logistic regression, and with time-to-onset data, we use proportional hazards regression. The null hypothesis of no association can be expressed simply as the coefficient of the predictor is zero in the population. Either likelihood ratio or Wald tests can be used. One advantage

of a regression analysis is that covariates can be included as a way of adjusting for potential confounding variables and increasing efficiency. Another is that the predictors can be dichotomous, quantitative, or categorical.

Although regression analysis has many advantages and is widely used in epidemiological investigations, it does require specifying a model for how the trait depends upon the genotype. If the model is incorrect, the power may be reduced. Depending upon study design and analysis, there may be consequences for the validity as well. Some data analysts prefer simple, 'model'-free approaches. For example, the Wilcoxon rank sum (or the Kruskal–Wallis) test[3] can be used for association analysis when the response is quantitative and the predictor is dichotomous (or categorical). With dichotomous traits and categorical predictors, a chi-square analysis is commonly used to test association in the $2 \times C$ cross-classification of trait by predictor. When the predictor is quantitative, one can use modifications of the standard chi-square (e.g. Cochran–Armitage test-for-trend in a $2 \times C$ table). When the trait is a time-to-onset variable and the predictor is categorical, the log-rank test can be used.

## CODING GENOTYPES FOR ANALYSIS

By their nature, genotypes are categorical data, but how they are coded can be an important feature of the analysis. For example, consider a single nucleotide polymorphism (SNP) with two possible alleles, which we label 1 or 2; there are three possible genotypes: 11, 12, 22. It is possible to analyze association by considering the three genotypes as three separate groups (i.e., as a categorical variable), assessing variation across the three groups. This will lead to global tests of association with two degrees of freedom. We refer to this as 'genotype' coding. However, simpler codings offer the possibility of more powerful tests with reduced degrees of freedom, and may better reflect the underlying disease process. Commonly used codings are recessive, dominant, and additive. With a recessive or dominant coding, we construct a dichotomous variable which reflects the assumed gene action. Suppose we test for a recessive model in allele 1. In constructing the dichotomous predictor, the 11 genotype is coded as 1 and the 12 and 22 genotypes are both coded as 0. For the dominant coding, the 11 and the 12 genotypes are coded as 1, and the 22 genotype is coded as 0. For the additive model, the coding variable is quantitative; it counts the number of 1 alleles present in the genotype. Therefore, the coded values for the 1 allele are 0, 1, 2 for the genotypes 22, 12, 11, respectively.

If there are just two alleles at the locus, choice of allele (1 versus 2) is only important in the context of testing recessive or dominant models, since the additive coding for the 2 allele is a linear transformation of the 1 allele coding. The additive coding also has the general appeal that it has reasonably good power even when the true disease model is dominant or recessive, but the reverse does not hold. That is, if we use a dominant or recessive coding when the true gene action is not the assumed model, there can be substantial loss of power, especially with the recessive model.[4–6] Thus, the additive model serves as a useful coding when nothing can be assumed about the underlying disease process. Martin et al.[7] has shown similar results for the genotype model; that is, the genotype model gives reasonably good power when the true model is additive, recessive, or dominant, although the use of the additive versus the genotype model as a general purpose testing strategy is still debatable. Once we have narrowed our search to only a handful of putative disease mutations, the genotype coding may be helpful in trying to discriminate the mode of action.

When there are more than two marker alleles, say $C > 2$, the problem of multiple genotypes is compounded for the genotype model, but each allele can be coded to construct global tests of association with $C - 1$ degrees of freedom for the additive model, or $C$ degrees of freedom for the recessive and dominant models. See Schaid[8] for additional details on coding.

## Types of traits and multiple traits

Historically, many genetic studies used dichotomous traits, e.g., presence or absence of a disorder; simple Mendelian diseases are typically characterized by dichotomous traits. In studies of complex diseases, many quantitative traits are often recorded that either describe the severity of the disease or are disease-related phenotypes. Dichotomous traits may be based on conventional, or even arbitrary, rules for defining affection status, while many continuous traits are obtained by objective and reproducible standardized measurements. Dichotomous descriptions are often defined for the purpose of prevalence estimates and may not best reflect the underlying disease process. By their nature, quantitative traits take values in a broad range and thereby contain more information which makes them potentially more powerful in a genetic analysis than dichotomous traits.[9]

The advantages of using quantitative traits come with a few caveats. Many quantitative traits also reflect the influences of other important factors, e.g., body characteristics, environmental effects, etc. For example, the measurements for forced expiratory volume at one second measured before and after bronchodilator (PRE $FEV_1$ and POS $FEV_1$) are important disease-related phenotypes for asthma and chronic obstructive pulmonary disease (COPD). Nevertheless, their unadjusted, raw measurements do not reveal the affection status. Besides the affection status, the measurements of PRE $FEV_1$ and POS $FEV_1$ also depend upon body characteristics, e.g., height, age, and sex, upon environmental factors, e.g., smoking, etc., and upon ethnicity. Adjusting the raw $FEV_1$ measurements for all known covariates decreases the outcome variability, and thus can increase the power of an association analysis. For $FEV_1$, standard adjustment formulas based on the variable's height, age, and sex, have been established in the literature.[10] Since they have been derived for unaffected individuals and do not include other important confounding variables such as smoking, their applicability to samples obtained through an ascertainment condition for the affection status is debatable. In this setting, an alternative approach is a study-specific adjustment, for example, adjusting the raw measurements by regressing them on the confounding variables.[11,12] The adjustments by this approach may not be reproducible in other studies and require careful model building. Ideally, all environmental factors and other covariates should be known, measured, and included in the regression model used for the adjustment. For many quantitative traits, not all confounding variables are known prior to the study, and they can be difficult to measure and to model.

The affection status and the severity of complex diseases are usually manifested in many symptoms/traits. For example, groups of quantitative traits can be defined that describe similar symptoms for asthma, e.g., lung-function phenotypes, atopy phenotypes, etc. DeMeo et al.[13] called the sets of traits 'symptom groups.' By their nature, the traits in one symptom group may be correlated and it is not clear which trait is the best single choice to test for association with a selected SNP or haplotype. Hence, one usually has to test several correlated traits. For example, the phenotypes percent of predicted $FEV_1$ post-bronchodilator, percent of predicted FVC post-bronchodilator, mean of morning peak expiratory flow, mean of evening peak expiratory flow, and peak expiratory flow variability (as a function of evening minus morning peak flow to evaluate circadian changes in peak flow) constituted the symptom group 'Pulmonary function' in DeMeo et al.[13] Each single trait by itself may not capture the 'entire picture' of the symptom group very well. Looking at each trait separately and, consequently, having to adjust for multiple comparisons, may diminish the power advantages of quantitative traits.

The problem is magnified when we are interested in many measures of severity or symptoms. Genes that have an impact on one symptom group are unlikely to affect another symptom group that does not share the same biological basis. Since the underlying biological processes and their links to the phenotypes are usually not known prior to the study, their understanding is the primary goal of the study. Without knowledge about the underlying biological processes, the definition of symptom groups can be based on clinical intuition,[13] but this approach becomes difficult in situations when there is little knowledge about the joint genetic components of the phenotypes, and may not be reproducible by other investigators. In such situations, defining symptom groups with a joint genetic component is not a trivial problem. The success of the association analysis will depend upon the group definitions. Even assuming that the traits have successfully been assigned to symptom groups, the symptom group with the strongest genetic component for a particular SNP or haplotype is not known before the analysis. Testing all symptom groups for association with a particular locus causes, again a multiple comparison problem. Strategies for handling multiple traits will be discussed in detail under Family-based designs for genetic association.

The coding of traits is straightforward in standard designs; quantitative traits may be transformed to make their distribution more normal. The standard coding for dichotomous traits is 1/0. In both cases, standard regression analyses can be used to adjust for covariates.

The situation is quite different for family-based analyses. In the simple setting where all offspring have the same trait value (e.g., all diseased), the trait can be coded as 1 for every subject without loss of generality. If there are also unaffected offspring, or if the trait is quantitative, then the coding of the trait can have a substantial impact on the power. Intuitively, we would expect the pattern of transmissions to unaffected or low trait offspring to be the reverse of the pattern of transmissions seen in the affected or high trait offspring. The purpose of the coding is to ensure that the test statistic forms this contrast. Coding details will be discussed in some detail for family-based tests under Family-based designs for genetic association.

## Haplotypes

When multiple markers are sufficiently closely linked so that it is reasonable to assume no recombination has occurred between them, construction of multilocus haplotypes is a popular strategy for combining information from markers. A multilocus haplotype refers to the set of alleles, one from each marker, which are inherited from a single parent, either from the mother or the father. If a disease locus is present in the region flanked by the markers, but does not correspond exactly to any of the markers tested, it may not be in sufficiently high disequilibrium with any one marker to be detected by one-at-a-time testing of the markers. If we use enough markers to capture the haplotype diversity in the population, then the haplotypes should capture the variation directly at the disease locus. Thus, in principle, tests using haplotypes can be more powerful than those using single markers.

If we know each person's haplotype, then in principle, the set of markers forming the haplotypes can be considered as a single marker with many alleles, and methods used for multiallelic markers apply. However, constructing haplotypes can be challenging, particularly when there are no family data, because the observed data consist of pairs of alleles at each marker. For example, consider an individual who is heterozygous at two different markers: (12) and (12). Without further information, haplotypes cannot be constructed, because we do not know which alleles are inherited from which parents. Strategies for haplotype analyses will be discussed for both standard and family-based designs.

## STANDARD DESIGNS FOR ASSOCIATION STUDIES

Here, we consider standard case–control and cohort designs using unrelated subjects. The design and analysis of such studies for genetic risk factors is almost identical to those for studying nongenetic risk factors. As introduced above, the main novelty in genetic association studies is the particular form of confounding known as population stratification bias. We review some of the theoretical and empirical work on the severity of population stratification bias. We also outline proposed 'genomic control' procedures that use multiple unlinked markers to estimate and adjust for population stratification. We close with a discussion of haplotype inference using unrelated individuals.

### Case–control studies

Many excellent references review the basic principles behind the design of case–control studies.[14–16] Briefly, the study should be designed to minimize selection bias, information bias, and confounding.[17]

Selection bias occurs when the controls do not come from the appropriate study base for the cases, that is, the population which was eligible to become diseased and be enrolled in the study as cases. Say, for example, that cases are taken from clinics in Bigtown City and controls from Smallville County, 1000 miles away. Then, cases and controls may differ in ethnicity or key environmental exposures simply due to the sampling scheme. Selection bias can also arise when using hospital-based controls or controls diagnosed with diseases other than the condition being studied.[17] In those situations, a marker may be associated with a different disease that occurs only among the controls. If the majority of controls have that disease, then that marker will (falsely) appear to be associated with the condition under study. This problem can be ameliorated by choosing controls from several different disease groups.

Another drawback of convenience controls (e.g., patients at the same hospital as cases without the condition being studied or disease-free children from the same school) is that only relative risks can be estimated. To estimate absolute risks from case–control data, the sampling fractions must be known. This would be true if cases were sampled from a disease registry, and the controls were sampled at random from the underlying at-risk population (e.g., all persons living in a city or country). For convenience controls, the underlying control sampling population is unknown or difficult to specify and absolute risks cannot be calculated.

Recall bias – a form of information bias that occurs when cases are more likely to (mis)remember past exposures relative to controls – is often a concern in case–control studies. It is very unlikely that the genetic data would be affected by this kind of error, as appropriate laboratory procedures should ensure that any genotyping errors occur with equal probability among cases and controls (e.g., cases and controls should be randomly distributed across genotyping plates). However, differential recall of past environmental exposures (proximity to pollution sources, exposure to allergens) could bias analyses that look at the joint effect of genes and environment.[17]

Confounding bias can occur when a covariate is a risk factor for disease and associated with the marker under study. Clayton and McKeigue[18] have argued that genetic studies inherently minimize confounding, since genotypes at a given locus are independent of most environmental factors and genotypes at other loci. However, there are important cases where genotypes at a locus are not independent of other environmental or genetic factors. For example, if disease rates and allele frequencies vary by ethnicity, an allele can appear to be associated with disease, even though within each ethnic group it plays no causal role (population stratification bias). Age-at-onset is another potential confounder. If a gene influences either disease age-at-onset or death due to competing risks (or some other censoring process), then the genotype frequency in the source population varies with age.[19,20] Comparing younger cases to older controls (or vice versa) can lead to reduced power or spurious results. To minimize confounding, appropriate matched or stratified analyses should be performed. If ethnicity information is available, cases and controls should be matched on ethnicity. If cases' age-at-onset varies (and follow up on cases and controls also varies), controls should be matched to the cases on age and appropriate analysis methods should be used (e.g. Cox proportional hazards).

## Cohort studies

There are a number of advantages for cohort studies relative to case–control studies.[21] First, because the study base is explicitly defined and all cases can be ascertained (except where participants are lost to follow up) absolute risks can be estimated. Second, because information about environmental exposures is collected before diagnosis, cohort studies are not susceptible to recall bias. Third, multiple disease outcomes can be studied using the same cohort, while case–control studies are limited to the disease used to define cases. In the context of genetic studies, cohort studies have the additional advantage of being able to reduce possible population stratification by focusing recruitment on one population – or by explicitly seeking to recruit sufficient numbers from multiple populations.

The primary disadvantage to cohort studies is the large investment in both money and time required to recruit and measure baseline environmental data on the original cohort, which may require (hundreds of) thousands of subjects to achieve the necessary number of cases needed to detect the moderate genetic effect sizes expected in complex diseases. The size of the cohort depends on the incidence of the disease(s) being studied. For relatively common diseases – or if 'normal' phenotypic variation in the general population is the principal focus – a prohibitively large cohort may not be needed. After the initial steps of recruiting the cohort and accruing a sufficient number of cases for meaningful analysis, genetic studies can be conducted rather economically by using a nested case–control strategy: instead of genotyping all controls in the cohort, a few controls (matched where appropriate) are selected for each case.[21]

A secondary disadvantage to cohort studies is the fact that they are often restricted to a particular population, limited perhaps in terms of location, age, profession, or ethnicity. What in some respects is a strength – homogeneity alleviates concerns of population stratification and other confounding – is also a limitation, as results cannot be immediately transferred to other populations. However, a strong result in one population should be a fruitful candidate for further molecular studies and follow-up epidemiologic studies in other populations. It is better to have valid estimates and good power in one population than potentially biased or underpowered in several.

Although the majority of genetic association studies using unrelated individuals are case–control studies, there are a number of cohort studies that have begun to study genetic associations, such as the Children's Health Study[22,23] and the Boston Home Allergens and Asthma Study.[24]

## Single-marker analyses

Given a particular coding (dominant, additive, etc.) for genotypes, standard analyses for case–control and cohort studies can be used.[14–16] Table 3.1 shows a $3 \times 2$ contingency table analysis for an unmatched case–control study using genotype coding. This table presents the raw genotype data and relevant summary statistics in a simple and familiar format. The covariate-adjusted odds ratios in Table 3.1 can be calculated using a logistic regression model with two genotype 'dummy variables:' the first is 1 if a subject is heterozygous and 0 otherwise; the second is 1 if a subject is homozygous for the A allele and 0 otherwise.

Absent specific knowledge of the biologic role of the marker being tested, the temptation to present results only for the 'best fit' coding (as measured, for example, by Akaike's Information Criterion) or to present results for all genotype codings, should generally be avoided. Presenting only the 'best fit' coding ignores the model selection problem. $P$ values and confidence intervals from the 'best fit' will be overoptimistic (too small), unless they are adjusted in some way for the model selection process. As discussed above, the additive and genotype-coding models are most robust to misspecifying the genetic model; the genotype coding has the additional advantage of yielding genotype-specific odds ratios, which give some broader insight into the mode of action. One of these two codings should be chosen as the

**Table 3.1** *Association between a diallelic marker and disease*

| Genotype | Cases | Controls | OR[a] | OR[b] |
|---|---|---|---|---|
| aa | $n_{10}$ | $n_{00}$ | ref | ref |
| Aa | $n_{11}$ | $n_{01}$ | $\dfrac{n_{11}n_{00}}{n_{10}n_{01}}$ (95% CI) | $\widehat{OR}_{Aa}$ (95% CI) |
| AA | $n_{12}$ | $n_{02}$ | $\dfrac{n_{12}n_{00}}{n_{10}n_{02}}$ (95% CI) | $\widehat{OR}_{AA}$ (95% CI) |

[a] Unadjusted odds ratio.
[b] Odds ratio adjusted for known risk factors via e.g. logistic regression.

primary analysis. Given strong evidence for association from the primary analysis, other codings can be used in secondary analyses. Detecting the true mode of action from clinical or epidemiological data is quite difficult, however, both for technical reasons (the additive, recessive, and dominant models are not nested and cannot be evaluated in a likelihood-ratio testing framework) and due to a lack of power (the ability to discriminate between the additive and genotype coding models is driven by the number of homozygous individuals; for rare alleles this number will be small except in unrealistically large sample sizes).[25]

## Gene–environment interaction

Complex diseases such as asthma are, by definition, multifactorial, resulting from the interplay of several genes and environmental exposures. Phenylketonuria, for example, results when an individual has two copies of a defective *PAH* gene *and* is exposed to dietary phenylalanine. Khoury et al.[26] give several other examples of plausible patterns of disease risk across genotypes and environmental exposure. Botto and Khoury[27] argue that a saturated model should be fit for single-gene-by-single-environmental-factor analyses – that is, a simple cross-tabulation of the data by case status, genotype, and environmental exposure, with odds ratios relative to a common reference category (e.g., unexposed noncarriers). This has the advantage of efficiently presenting all of the data and emphasizing joint effect estimation instead of tests of departure from specific statistical models of interaction. Departures from such models can be tested and estimated, but the meaning of such tests and estimates depends on the specific statistical model of interaction and the scale of the effects being estimated (e.g., relative or absolute).[27,28] Which model and scale is most appropriate depends on the goal of the analysis, for example, to compare specific hypotheses about biologic mechanisms or estimate the public health impact of an exposure across different genetic subgroups. (Note that failure to depart from a particular statistical 'main effects only' model does not necessarily mean two exposures do not interact biologically, in the sense that they may be part of the same causal pathway).[28]

Logistic regression methods can be used to fit and assess gene-by-environment interaction models. The standard multiplicative odds ratio model has the form $\log(\Pr[D]/(1 - \Pr[D])) = \beta_0 + \beta_1 G + \beta_2 E$, where $G$ and $E$ are codings for the genetic and environmental factors, respectively. (For simplicity, we assume $G$ and $E$ are 0/1 codings.) Departures from this model can be assessed by fitting a model with the $G \times E$ cross product term, $\log(\Pr[D]/(1 - \Pr[D])) = \beta_0 + \beta_1 G + \beta_2 E + \beta_3 G \times E$, and calculating a Wald's test for the interaction term $\beta_3$ or a likelihood ratio test comparing the two models. Somewhat surprisingly, the additive model (on the incidence scale) can also be fit using case–control data, by exploiting the fact that under this model, $(OR_{ge} - 1) = (OR_g - 1) + (OR_e - 1)$.[28] This leads to a model where $\log(\Pr[D]/(1 - \Pr[D])) = \beta_0 + \beta_1 G$ for unexposed carriers; $\log(\Pr[D]/(1 - \Pr[D])) = \beta_0 + \beta_2 E$ for exposed noncarriers; and $\log(\Pr[D]/(1 - \Pr[D])) = \beta_0 + \log(\exp\{b_1\} + \exp\{b_2\} - 1)$ for exposed carriers. This model is no longer linear in the parameters, however, and will require specialized software for nonlinear models.

## Power

Power and sample size calculations are important in both the design and interpretation of genetic association studies, as underpowered studies are a major reason why many reported associations fail to replicate.[29,30] The program Quanto (http://hydra.usc.edu/gxe/) calculates power for a variety of genotype codings and study designs (matched and unmatched case–control studies, population-based studies of quantitative traits, as well as variety of family-based studies). Quanto also calculates power to detect departures from a multiplicative odds ratio model for gene–environment and gene–gene interaction analyses.[22,31] A limitation to Quanto is that it assumes either a dichotomous or normally distributed environmental exposure. Power depends on sample size and the size of the odds ratio to be detected, as well as the allele frequency and the assumed genetic model. For example, a study with 150 cases and 150 (unmatched) controls will have 81 percent power to detect an odds ratio of 2.0 for a dominant allele with 15 percent frequency, but only 52 percent power to detect a dominant allele with 5 percent frequency and only 6 percent power to detect a recessive allele with 5 percent frequency.

## Population stratification

The existence and magnitude of population stratification bias are somewhat controversial. For example, Wacholder et al.[32,33] have argued that the classic example presented in Knowler et al.[2] is an extreme situation involving two subpopulations with very different incidence rates and allele frequencies. In other situations, such as non-Hispanic European Americans, where there are many subpopulations with modest differences in allele frequencies and disease incidence, noticeable population stratification bias is not likely to occur.[32] They suggest following basic principles of study design and matching on ethnicity as a surrogate for genetic subpopulation. Ardlie et al.[34] found little evidence for population stratification in four case–control studies that were matched on grandparents' ethnicity. However, others have argued that such detailed information on ethnic background is rarely available, and may be a poor surrogate for genetic heritage in recently admixed populations such as African Americans and Hispanic Americans. It may also be difficult to find appropriate controls for mixed-ethnicity individuals, who are increasingly common in many parts of the United States.[35]

Furthermore, aside from confounding due to population stratification, tests of genetic association may have inflated significance levels due to 'cryptic relatedness.' Cases may be more related than controls because they share a recent ancestor who had a disease-predisposing allele (not necessarily at the marker being studied). Thus the cases' contributions to the analysis are correlated, while the usual statistics assume that they are independent. This leads the standard analyses to overestimate the effective sample size and produce overoptimistic $P$ values.[36] There are limited data on the relative magnitude of the effects of population stratification bias or cryptic relatedness, but even if modest, the large sample sizes proposed for studies of complex diseases raise the likelihood that the false positive rates for standard analyses will be inflated.[35,37]

A number of authors have proposed using multiple unlinked markers to estimate and adjust for population stratification bias or cryptic relatedness. There are two basic approaches. In the first, the markers are used to estimate population substructure and incorporate this into the analysis.[38,39] In the second, the markers are used to estimate the inflation in the test statistic due to population stratification or cryptic relatedness; the test statistic at the marker under study is then corrected for this inflation factor.[36,40] Recent empirical and simulation studies suggest that hundreds of markers may be required to detect or adequately adjust for population stratification or cryptic relatedness in large studies of modest genetic effects. However, for smaller studies aimed at detecting substantial genetic effects, only a few dozen markers may be needed to rule out population substructure as an explanation for a significant association.[37,41]

## Haplotype analysis

Analyses of haplotypes from unrelated cases and controls have been proposed in two contexts: fine-mapping under a linkage peak (which involves relatively sparsely spaced markers over long distances)[42–45] and testing candidate–gene association (which involves densely-spaced markers over short distances).[46–49] The main difference between these two approaches is that the former depends on the presence of recombination (roughly, cases should show less evidence for recombination around the causal locus than controls), while the latter depends on the absence of recombination.

Here, we focus on testing association between haplotypes in a candidate gene. There are two principal reasons researchers may be interested in haplotypes. First, the haplotypes per se may be of interest, such as when researchers wish to evaluate *cis* interaction. In this case, two alleles confer higher risk only when they lie on the same haplotype; hence phase information – knowing which chromosome each allele lies on – is essential. Second, haplotype analyses may be more powerful and cost-effective than multiple single-SNP analyses.[46,50–52] This idea is based in part on the observation that in regions of high LD (correlation among markers), there is typically limited haplotype diversity, so collecting information on all SNPs may be quite redundant (see Fig. 3.1). The assumption that the candidate gene can be divided into 'haplotype blocks' or regions of limited haplotype diversity and high LD is important and can be assessed via several different measures.[53–56] It makes little sense to test the association of disease with haplotypes over large regions of low LD: most subjects will have unique haplotype pairs, making inference unreliable if not impossible.

A key element in the design of haplotype-association analysis is marker selection. Known or putative functional

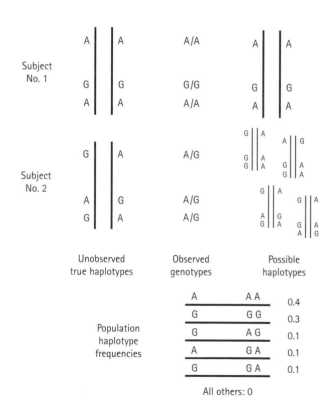

**Figure 3.1**  *Inferring phased haplotypes from unphased genotypes on unrelated individuals: an example.*

SNPs (such as non-synonymous coding SNPs) could be genotyped. However, if a previously unknown functional SNP or a variant in a non-coding region plays a causal role, it is unlikely that this approach will detect those variants. To capture information on SNPs of unknown function, one could genotype all known SNPs in the candidate gene (as well as some distance upstream and downstream, as these regions may play a role in gene regulation). Typically, this involves searching public databases such as dbSNP (www.ncbi.nlm.nih.gov/SNP) and perhaps resequencing a subsample of subjects to discover new SNPs and to verify that the public SNPs are present in the study population. As discussed above, however, genotyping all SNPs on all subjects may be redundant and prohibitively expensive.

Alternatively, a number of authors have suggested a two-stage approach.[51,57,58] In the first stage, a relatively small portion of the subjects (or an external sample from the same population), is resequenced or genotyped on a dense panel of markers. This information is then used to choose 'tag SNPs,' a subset of the SNPs that contains most (or all) of the information in the whole panel. In the second stage, these tag SNPs are genotyped and analyzed in all subjects.

A number of measures of tag SNP performance have been proposed. For example, some algorithms seek to maximize the ability of tag SNPs to predict individual untyped SNPs;[46,52,59] others ('haplotype-tagging SNPs' or htSNPs) seek to maximize the ability of tag SNPs to predict haplotypes over the panel of markers.[57,60] A key point here is that the tag-SNP-selection algorithm should correspond to the planned analysis. If researchers want to test multiple SNPs in a candidate gene one by one, they should use a method that maximizes the ability to predict individual SNPs. If they want to test haplotype-disease association, they should choose a method that maximizes the ability to predict haplotypes. Several tag-SNP selection algorithms also give estimates of the correlations ($r^2$) between the tag SNPs and unobserved variants (SNPs or haplotypes). This can be useful in the design phase, as it provides an estimate of the effective sample size, $N^* = r^2 \times N$. The power of a study using tag SNPs with sample size $N$ will roughly be the same as a study where all the relevant variants are observed with sample size $N^*$.[1,57]

This is an area of active research and many design questions remain. For example, how many subjects should be included in the first stage sample? A reasonable rule-of-thumb seems to be to resequence or genotype enough chromosomes to be able to detect a haplotype of moderately low frequency with high probability. (Approximately 60 chromosomes or 30 subjects would be needed to detect a haplotype with 5 percent frequency with 95 percent certainty.) However, this may not be enough chromosomes to give an accurate picture of the correlation structure. For further discussion, see Thompson et al.[58]

Given a set of SNPs genotyped on a set of subjects, the principal statistical problems are how to infer phased haplotypes given unphased genotypes and how to account for this inference in the association analysis. Genotypes from related individuals can be used to accurately infer haplotypes (see Schaid[8] and the discussion below for family-based association tests), but for large population-based studies (the focus of our attention here), such information is infeasible to collect. Instead, some algorithm which uses estimates of the population haplotype distribution to infer haplotypes for unrelated individuals must be used.[61–65]

Figure 3.1 illustrates how the popular expectation–maximization algorithm infers phase for two individuals: one who is homozygous at three loci, and one who is heterozygous at three loci. In the first case, phase is unambiguous. Only one pair of haplotypes is consistent with the observed genotypes. In the second case, phase is ambiguous. Four pairs of haplotypes are consistent with the observed genotypes. However, assuming this individual is drawn at random from a randomly mating population, and given estimates of the haplotype frequencies, some pairs are more likely than others. In this case, haplotypes pairs AGG–GAA and GGA–AAG are impossible, while pair AAA–GGG is $0.4 \times 0.3/(0.4 \times 0.3 + 0.1 \times 0.1) = 95$ percent likely and pair GAG–AGA is 5 percent likely.

It is common practice in association analysis to assign each individual to his or her most likely haplotype pair and then treat the inferred haplotypes as if they were multiallelic markers. There are two potential problems with this approach. First, it can induce a form of measurement error. In this example, the most likely haplotype pair for subject No. 2 is AAA–GGG, although in reality this individual carries pair GAG–AGA. This measurement error can lead to biased estimates of haplotype-association parameters. Second, this procedure does not take the added uncertainty due to the estimation of haplotype frequencies into account.

A number of procedures that account for uncertainty in haplotype estimates have been proposed. Several of these treat this as a missing data problem and jointly estimate haplotype effect parameters by summing over the unknown phase assignments.[66–69] These approaches are computationally intensive and require specialized software, for example, the haplo.stats package for R and stand-alone programs like HPLUS (http://cougar.fhcrc.org/hplus/) and Chaplin (http://server2k.genetics.emory.edu/chaplin/down-load.html). Another simpler and somewhat more flexible approach involves using expected haplotype codings (instead of the codings from the most likely haplotype pairs). This can be implemented using software that estimates haplotype frequencies in unrelated individuals and standard biostatistical packages. This 'expectation–substitution' approach can be shown to have negligible bias in case–control studies for a range of realistic relative risks.

A subtlety here is that some of these methods assume the subjects in the analysis are drawn from a single, randomly mating population.[48] This will not be true for a case–control study away from the null, that is, when one or more of the haplotypes is associated with an increased risk of disease. Tests of the null hypothesis of no association remain valid (have appropriate type I error rates) if the random-mating assumption is not met, but estimates of relative risks or odds ratios may be biased. If possible, a method that accounts for the ascertainment scheme should be used.[66]

The haplotype association methods discussed here all aim to estimate parameters from a standard epidemiologic analysis (such as logistic regression or survival analysis), while taking haplotype uncertainty into account. These standard analyses all fit models based on a haplotype coding, often chosen by the user. Just as with multiallelic markers, there are a large number of such codings. Absent a priori information on the function of particular haplotypes, an additive coding seems sensible. Here, one haplotype (e.g., the most common) is chosen as the reference, and count variables are created for the remaining H-1 haplotypes. A likelihood ratio or score test (on H-1 degrees of freedom) can be created to test general association between haplotypes and disease. The additive coding has the advantage that these tests do not depend on the choice of reference haplotype.

## FAMILY-BASED DESIGNS FOR GENETIC ASSOCIATION

Here, we describe the basic analytical principles that underlie the analysis of family-based data. The underlying approach is to derive the distribution of the observed genotype data in offspring under H0 by using Mendel's basic laws of inheritance. We begin by considering genotype data on a trio consisting of an affected individual and both parents. Every individual inherits discrete genetic information from each of his or her parents; each human carries two variants (alleles) of the same gene: one inherited from the father and one from the mother. Disentangling the transmitted and nontransmitted alleles from each parent leads to the 2 by 2 table representation for biallelic marker data (alleles 1 and 2), as shown in Table 3.2.

Each entry in the table is a parent. Thus n11 counts the number of parents who are homozygous for the '1' allele, n12 counts the number of 12 parents who transmitted the '1' allele to the offspring, etc. The benefits of organizing the data in this 2 by 2 table were described by Ott[70] and Terwilliger and Ott,[71] who proposed the haplotype-based haplotype relative risk, or HHRR, test. This test is similar to the haplotype relative risk test (HRR) proposed by Rubinstein et al.[72] and Falk and Rubinstein.[73]

Spielman et al.[74] recognized that the tabulated data in Table 3.2 can also be used to perform a test of linkage and

association. Unlike the case–control method, where the distribution of the alleles has to be estimated from the data under the null, with parental data we use Mendel's laws to assign a distribution to the cell counts, conditional on the traits, the parental genotypes, and a null hypothesis of either no association and no linkage, or linkage but no association. In this way, problems with population stratification or admixture are avoided. The transmission disequilibrium test (TDT) is based upon the idea that the expected counts, $E(n12)$ and $E(n21)$, are equal under the null hypothesis of no association (LD). Moreover, it is clear that no information with respect to allelic transmission preference can be retrieved from homozygous 11 or 22 parents when the distribution of cell counts is computed in this manner. Hence, the classical McNemar test serves the purpose of testing for equal allelic transmissions, but was renamed TDT in the context of genetic associations:

$$\text{TDT} = \frac{(n_{21} - n_{12})^2}{n_{21} + n_{12}}$$

The TDT can be viewed either as a test for linkage, or a test of association, depending upon the setting. If the null hypothesis is no linkage and no association, it is a valid test of both. It is also a valid test of association (LD) if linkage is present provided only unrelated trios are used. Although the TDT is always a valid test of linkage, there will be little power to detect linkage unless strong LD is present.

### Extensions of the TDT

Since its conception, many generalizations to the affected child (trio) setting with biallelic markers have been proposed. Extensions for multi-allelic markers are described by, for example, Sham and Curtis,[75] Bickeboller and Clerget-Darpoux,[76] Spielman and Ewens,[77] Schaid,[8] and Horvath and Laird.[78] Rice et al.[79] describe an extension to the TDT that not only allows for multi-allelic markers, but also for covariates measured on the parent or offspring as well. Ewens and Spielman[80] and Horvath and Laird[78] extended the TDT for use in sibships with at least one affected and one unaffected child. Knapp has a more general approach to missing parental information. Bias problems arising when parental information is (partially) missing are addressed by, for example, Curtis and Sham,[81] Schaid and Li,[82] and Rabinowitz and Laird.[83] A more thorough account of statistical properties of the classical TDT test and these extensions is given in Ewens and Spielman[84] and Zhao.[85]

Clayton and Jones[86] and Clayton[87] formulated a generalization of the TDT based on likelihood analysis which can handle missing parental data and haplotype data in the context of nuclear families with dichotomous outcomes. In principle, the method can be extended to handle other types of traits as well. It is similar in spirit to the approach of Rabinowitz and Laird[83] described below, but the missing

**Table 3.2** *Cross-classification of transmitted and not-transmitted alleles in parent/child trios*

| Allele not transmitted | | 1 | 2 |
| --- | --- | --- | --- |
| Transmitted allele | 1 | n11 | n12 |
| | 2 | n21 | n22 |

parental data (and the missing phase data for haplotype analysis) are handled by assigning the missing genotypes a distribution and estimating the parameters of that distribution from the data. This approach is not robust to population admixture because the approach fails to condition on founder genotypes.[88]

## A unifying framework

The large number of extensions to the TDT reflects the utility of this simple statistic, and speaks to the importance of a unifying framework. A unified approach to family-based tests of association, introduced by Rabinowitz and Laird[83] and Laird et al.,[89] builds on the original TDT method.[74] The method puts tests of different genetic models, tests with different family structures, tests involving different disease phenotypes, tests with missing parents, and tests of different null hypotheses, all in the same framework. For the rest of this chapter, we will discuss this unified approach to the construction of family-based tests. The methods we discuss have been implemented in the software packages FBAT and PBAT: http://www.biostat.harvard.edu/~fbat/default.html and http://www.biostat.harvard.edu/~change/default.htm

This framework has two basic components: the construction of the test statistic and the construction of the distribution of the test statistic under H0.

Understanding the two components of the framework enables one to construct a family-based test for virtually any setting.

## The test statistic

The general family-based association test (FBAT) statistic[89] is based on a linear combination of observed offspring genotypes and phenotypes. In particular, we define the FBAT test statistic S as

$$S = \sum_{ij} T_{ij} X_{ij},$$ (3.1)

with $X_{ij}$ denoting some function of the marker genotype of the jth offspring in family i; $X_{ij}$ will depend on the selected coding of the genotypes. It can be a vector or a scalar. The trait of the jth offspring in the ith family, $T_{ij}$, is some function of the phenotype, depending upon possibly unknown (nuisance) parameters. $T_{ij}$ can also be a vector, as described below.

The expectation of S, conditional on the traits is:

$$E(S) = \sum_{ij} T_{ij} E(X_{ij}).$$

$E(X_{ij})$, is computed with respect to the offspring genotype distribution under the null hypothesis; computation of

this distribution is discussed below. Let C be defined as $S - E(S)$, i.e.

$$C = \sum_{ij} T_{ij}(X_{ij} - E(X_{ij})).$$

By construction, C has mean zero when $H_0$ is true. In general, the trait $T_{ij}$ will be mean centered, so that C can be thought of as the covariance between the trait and the genotype taken over all offspring in all families. Except as indicated below, $V = \text{Var}(S)$ is also calculated with respect to this same distribution and used to standardize S. For an explicit formula for V, refer to the technical report by Horvath et al.[6]

If $X_{ij}$ is a scalar summary of an individual's genotype, then the large sample test statistic

$$Z = C/\sqrt{V}$$ (3.2)

is approximately $N(0,1)$. If $X_{ij}$ is a vector, then

$$x^2 = C'V^-C,$$ (3.3)

has an approximate $\chi^2$-distribution with degrees of freedom equal to the rank of V. Here, $V^-$ denotes a generalized inverse of V.

Both Z and $\chi^2$ are large sample tests, based on the number of informative families. With 10 or more informative families, these asymptotic tests are usually adequate. When very low $\alpha$ values are used, the minimum number of informative families should be higher than 10, as $\alpha$ values smaller than 0.05 tend to make the large sample tests conservative. Alternatively, Monte Carlo approximations to an exact test are available.

## Distribution of the test statistic under H0

In deriving the conditional null distribution of the genotype marker data (required in Eq. (3.1)), we need to be more specific about the null hypothesis itself. As discussed under Basic concepts underlying genetic association analysis, family-based tests have a composite alternative hypothesis and, consequently, also a composite null hypothesis: Either the null hypothesis is 'no association and no linkage' or 'no association in the presence of linkage'.[89] The null hypothesis of no linkage and no association is easiest to handle because there are no nuisance parameters to consider in the distribution.

With complete parental data, the null distribution is obtained by conditioning on the observed traits in all family members and on the parental marker genotypes. In this case, transmission to each offspring of each parental allele has a probability of ½, and all transmissions from both parents to all offspring are independent. For incomplete parental data, the null distribution is obtained, not only by conditioning on all observed traits and any observed parental marker genotypes, but also on the offspring genotype configuration. Rabinowitz and Laird[83] showed that any partially observed parental genotypes and the offspring genotype configuration are sufficient statistics for the missing parental genotypes. In summary, the expected value and the variance of the test statistic are derived using Mendel's law of segregation and conditioning on the sufficient statistics for any nuisance parameters under the null. Since conditioning eliminates all nuisance parameters, the technique avoids biases due to population admixture or stratification, misspecification of the trait distribution, and/or selection based on phenotype.[83,90]

When multiple sibs are present in a family and the null hypothesis assumes no association but linkage, the siblings genotypes are correlated, with correlation depending upon the recombination parameter. The patterns of allele sharing (identity-by-descent relationships) are the sufficient statistics for the recombination parameter and the minimal sufficient statistics used in computing the conditional distribution of S.[83] However, conditioning on the identity-by-descent relationships is very restrictive, and can cause considerable reduction in power. Thus, with multiple sibs in a family and testing for association in an area of known linkage, a valid association test in the presence of linkage is performed using the mean of the test statistic computed via the Rabinowitz–Laird algorithm under the null hypothesis of 'no association and no linkage,' and using an empirical variance–covariance estimator for V that adjusts for the correlation among sibling marker genotypes.[91]

If the data include pedigrees with more than one nuclear family, the FBAT approach is to decompose the pedigree into distinct nuclear families and use an empirical variance calculation. The PBAT approach conditions on the sufficient statistics for the founder genotypes and computes the statistic over all offspring of the pedigree, computing the distribution under the null hypothesis of no linkage and no association.

## Coding traits

While the general remarks in Basic concepts underlying genetic association analysis apply, there are several issues concerning the coding of the traits that are unique to family-based designs:

- $T_{ij}$ can be any function of the phenotype and other information in the data provided that it is not a function of the offspring marker genotype.
- Sample design and nature of the trait (e.g., trios only versus sampling unaffecteds and qualitative versus quantitative traits) influence optimal choices for $T_{ij}$.
- Coding strategies can be based on model assumptions (prior knowledge about the population prevalence) or can be purely statistically based (e.g., choose a coding that minimizes the variance of the test statistic under

the null or maximizes its variance under the alternative).
- In addition, $T_{ij}$ can be adjusted to include covariates in the association model for $Y_{ij}$.

The discussion on the use of trait information is organized separately for the case of a single dichotomous or a single continuous quantitative phenotype. Special attention is given to centering the traits. Time-to-onset traits are considered in Lange et al.[12]

### A SINGLE DICHOTOMOUS TRAIT

When a trait is dichotomous, the usual approach in family-based association testing has been to consider allele transmissions from parents to affected offspring only.[74] This can be achieved by setting $T_{ij} = 1$ for affected individuals and $T_{ij} = 0$ for all others. Subjects with $T_{ij} = 0$ contribute nothing to the statistic, but may contribute information about the distribution of $X_{ij}$ when parental genotype is missing. The classical TDT test uses the 1/0 coding for $T_{ij}$, and an additive coding for the genotype. The introduction of an offset of the form $T_{ij} = Y_{ij} - \mu$ where $\mu$ is an offset between 0 and 1, allows one to control the contribution of affecteds and unaffecteds to the test statistic. A clever choice may substantially increase the power of the test.[92] In theory, one should take the offset to be the disease prevalence or mean trait when it is continuous.[9,92,93] This may be difficult to specify in practice, especially when sampling is based on the trait, hence the offset can be chosen to minimize the variance of S[94] or maximize the power of the test under an assumed alternative.[9]

### A SINGLE QUANTITATIVE TRAIT

With a quantitative trait, the use of an offset can have a very powerful effect on the P value. A trait which is mean centered is designed to have power against an alternative which specifies that the presence of the tested allele increases trait value, while absence of the allele decreases the trait. In contrast, a trait which has not been mean centered, and consists entirely of positive or entirely negative values, mimics an affected only TDT, with the magnitude of the trait determining the 'weight' assigned to a transmission. If the sample is selected randomly from the population, the mean centered trait is preferred; if the sample is selected for extreme values on the trait, dichotomizing the trait is preferable (see Sample size and power).

Although the validity of the FBAT test does not depend on making any distributional assumptions on the trait, it will be most powerful when the trait is normally distributed. Further, the test can be sensitive to outlying values. Thus, it may desirable to consider transformations of the trait, based on ranks or normal scores.

Finally, with quantitative variables, it is often the case that much of the variability in the response can be explained by covariates unrelated to the marker under test. Using the residuals from a regression analysis that incorporates these covariates can result in large power gains. In the next section on multiple traits, we discuss adjustment techniques for both single and multiple quantitative traits.

## ADJUSTING QUANTITATIVE TRAITS FOR CONFOUNDING VARIABLES

When the confounding variables for the quantitative traits are known and have been recorded, their effects on the traits can be removed by proper statistical adjustment. For example, the trait values can be regressed on the covariates and the trait is then defined as the residuals from the regression on the covariates.

As discussed in Lunetta et al.[94] and Lange et al.[11,12] we use ordinary linear regression to estimate the effects of the covariates and compute the residuals (possibly after transforming the traits and/or the covariates). To avoid biasing the significance level of the FBAT statistic, the marker information is not used in the regression. The phenotypic mean model is given by

$$Y = \mu + \beta_1 \text{*covariate} + \cdots + \beta_m \text{*covariate}_m \quad (3.4)$$

where $\mu$ is the overall mean and $\beta_1, \ldots, \beta_m$ are the coefficients of the $m$ covariates. If there is only one trait involved, this completes the model specification. If there are multiple correlated traits, then each trait has a separate regression model with possibly different predictors. For the phenotypic variance–covariance matrix, we assume that the same phenotypes within one family are modeled by an exchangeable correlation structure and different phenotypes measured on the same person are modeled by an unstructured correlation matrix.

Using these assumptions for the phenotypic mean and variance structure, we can estimate all parameters by the generalized estimating equation (GEE) approach.[95] The GEE-methodology allows us to handle multiple correlated traits, either on the same subject or on related subjects in a single analysis. Non-normally distributed traits can easily be incorporated and the GEE estimates of the mean parameters are robust against a misspecification of the variance assumption.[11] Based on the mean parameter estimates, the phenotypic residuals are computed and coded as

$$T_{ij} = Y_{ij} - \hat{Y}_{ij} = Y_{ij} - \hat{\mu}$$
$$- \hat{\beta}_1 \text{covariate}_{1ij} - \cdots - \hat{\beta}_m \text{covariate}_{mij}$$

The residual $T_{ij}$ can then be used directly as the trait in the FBAT statistics (Eqns (3.1–3.3)).

It is important to note that the validity of the FBAT statistic, as opposed to the likelihood based methods,[96,97] does not depend upon the correctness of the regression model. The $P$ values of the FBAT-statistic are valid regardless of the user-defined coding for $T_{ij}$ and, therefore, regardless of the correctness of the mean model used for their computation.

Nevertheless, the quality of the mean model will directly influence the power of the corresponding test statistic.

When the confounding variables are either unknown or difficult to model, Lange et al.[98] suggest an alternative approach, FBAT-PC. FBAT-PC does not require any specification of a regression model for the confounding variables. Instead, multiple measurements of the quantitative trait of interest have to be recorded under the same or varying conditions. The approach is based on generalized principal component analysis. Using a mean Eqn. (3.4) without any covariates, FBAT-PC constructs an overall phenotype that has maximal locus-specific heritability. Using generalized principal component analysis, FBAT-PC calculates weights that amplify the heritability of each trait, making a covariate adjustment of the trait unnecessary.

When quantitative traits are important disease-related phenotypes in a genetic association study and the traits may be confounded by extraneous variables, it is important to consider the best way to adjust the quantitative traits for the confounding variables during the planning phase of the study. For asthma, for example, when the sample is ascertained through the affection status, $FEV_1$ measurements can be repeated inexpensively at each office visit during a study. For a large study without ascertainment conditions and only one visit, it can be more efficient to measure the confounding variables, for example, height, weight, etc., and adjust the $FEV_1$ measurements by regression.

## HAPLOTYPES

Although more can be inferred about haplotypes in the family-based setting than in population-based studies, phase cannot always be resolved. If all offspring are homozygous at all markers, or heterozygous at no more than one marker, then phase is observed in the offspring and thus in the parents. Phase is also observed if at least one parent is homozygous at all markers. In other cases, it is necessary to handle missing phase. The principle of conditioning on the sufficient statistics for missing parental genotypes extends quite straightforwardly to handle missing phase.[88] One now obtains a distribution for the phased offspring genotype. The test statistic can be computed in the same way, recognizing that the set of markers forming the haplotypes is treated as one multi-allelic marker with each haplotype forming an allele. In principle, with n SNPs, there can be $2^n$ haplotypes, but in practice the number of haplotypes observed in a family-based analysis are usually quite a bit less than $2^n$. The availability of family data enables one to eliminate many possibilities as not compatible with observed family data.

The haplotype analysis implemented in FBAT and PBAT uses the principle of conditioning on the sufficient statistics for both phase and any missing parental data, and on offspring traits, and hence is not biased by population stratification and/or admixture. Either bi-allelic or multi-allelic tests are computed in the usual way, and the empirical variance option can be used to account for the presence of linkage. The usual set of traits can be used. A feature of the implementation is that it also allows one to recover information from only partially phase known families by using weights.[88] FBAT also offers a Monte Carlo approximation to an exact $P$ value for both bi-allelic and multi-allelic tests.

## MULTIVARIATE FBATS

As discussed under Basic concepts underlying genetic association analysis, methods for handling several traits simultaneously are desirable in order to maximize power and avoid multiple comparison problems. Lange et al.[11] introduced a multivariate extension of the FBAT-approach, the FBAT-GEE statistic. FBAT-GEE, like the original FBAT statistic, is straightforward to compute, it does not require any distributional assumptions for the phenotypes, and it tests different trait types simultaneously. Assuming that we observed $m$ traits for each offspring that we want to test simultaneously by the FBAT approach, we denote the vector containing all m observations for each offspring by $Y_{ij} = (Y_{ij1}, ..., Y_{ijm})$ where $Y_{ijk}$ is the $k$th phenotype for the $j$th offspring in the $i$th family. The multivariate FBAT-GEE statistic is constructed by replacing the univariate coding variable $T_{ij}$ in $C$ by the coding vector defined by

$$T_{ij} = Y_{ij} - \hat{Y}_{ij} = \begin{pmatrix} Y_{ij1} \\ \vdots \\ Y_{ijk} \\ \vdots \\ Y_{ijm} \end{pmatrix} - \begin{pmatrix} \hat{Y}_{ij1} \\ \vdots \\ \hat{Y}_{ijk} \\ \vdots \\ \hat{Y}_{ijm} \end{pmatrix}$$

where the $\hat{Y}_{ijk}$s are either the observed sample means for the $k$th trait or the predicted trait values based on the regression model given in Eqn. (3.4), when confounding variables are given. By replacing the coding variable by the coding vector $T_{ij}$ in the FBAT-statistic, the FBAT-GEE statistic is derived,

$$T_{FBAT-GEE} = C^T V^- C.$$

Under the null-hypothesis that the marker is unlinked and not associated with any disease locus affecting any trait, the statistic $T_{FBAT-GEE}$ has a $\chi^2$ distribution with $m$ degrees of freedom. Because $T$ is a vector, $S$ is a vector and $V$ is an $m \times m$ matrix, even though $X_{ij}$ is a scalar. Although the test statistic seems to be ad hoc, it can be motivated as a score test from a multivariate normal. However, the advantage of the FBAT-GEE approach is that it can be extended to handle generalized linear models and missing data. The FBAT-GEE statistic does not depend upon the validity of any model assumptions about the generalized linear model or missingness process. In simulation studies,[92] FBAT-GEE has been shown to be very powerful.

## SCREENING ALGORITHMS FOR DETERMINING THE BEST PREDICTED TRAIT

Here, we describe an approach to screening a large number of potential traits for association with a marker (or haplotypes). In such situations, grouping the traits may not be feasible and carries the risk of misclassification. On the other hand, univariate testing is underpowered and is unlikely to find an existing association.

Lange et al.[11,12] introduced testing strategies that find the group of traits that have the strongest potential genetic effects and test that group with FBAT-GEE without having to adjust for multiple comparisons. The testing strategies take advantage of the natural decomposition of family-based data sets into informative and non-informative families. Since the non-informative families are not used in the computation of the FBAT statistic, they can be used in the first stage of the testing strategy to find the most 'promising' combination of phenotypes for a particular SNP or haplotype without biasing the significance level of any subsequently computed FBAT statistic. The first stage uses the conditional linear mean regression model (Eqn. (3.4)) which now includes both the marker genotypes and the covariates in the following form:

$$\text{Phenotype} = \mu + \alpha E(X) + \beta_1 {}^*\text{covariate}_1 + \cdots + \beta_m {}^*\text{covariate}_m. \tag{3.5}$$

Note that, as in Eqn. (3.4), this can be extended to include multivariate phenotypes. To increase the power of this approach, we also include the informative families in the first stage by replacing the proband's genotypes by their expectation based on the parental information or sufficient statistic as calculated by FBAT.[83] The screening is based on the fact that the mean model Eqn. (3.5) can be estimated without biasing the significance level of any subsequent FBAT statistic computed using the actual $X_{ij}$'s. This is because $E(X_{ij})$ does not depend upon the actual $X_{ij}$ for the informative families. For the non-informative families, $X_{ij} = E(X_{ij})$, but they are excluded from the FBAT test statistic.

The parameter estimates from Eqn. (3.5) can be used in two different ways to select the most promising traits for use in subsequent FBAT testing. The first method uses the genetic effect size estimate (based on alpha and the residual standard error) to compute the power for the observed traits (using the multivariate generalization of the power calculations described earlier). Different combinations of phenotypes are ranked on the basis of these power calculations. The second algorithm computes a Wald test for alpha in model Eqn. (3.5) and uses the $P$ values of the Wald tests to rank the different combinations of traits. In general, ranking the groups of traits based on the power is preferable. It is a yardstick that combines the effect size estimates with the number of informative families. The Wald test does not take the number of informative families into account. The power estimates seem to be also more robust against misspecification of the regression model Eqn. (3.5), when confounding variables are left out, and more efficient in the presence of population admixture and stratification. However, for large pedigrees, computing the power is not feasible and ranking based on the $P$ values of Wald tests is the only feasible method.

Both methods can be divided into six steps as described below. The first five steps of the algorithm are repeated for all possible subsets of phenotypes. In the last step, either based upon the estimated power levels or the $P$ values of the Wald tests, the subset of traits that is most promising is selected, and tested for association with the FBAT-GEE statistic. The steps of the algorithm are given by:

1 Select any subset of quantitative traits.
2 Posit a multivariate model that describes the selected phenotypes as a function of the genotypes.
3 Replace the observed offspring genotypes in the multivariate model by their expected values conditional on the parental genotypes or the sufficient statistic.[83]
4 For this adjusted multivariate model, estimate the parameters using the generalized estimating equation approach of Liang and Zeger[95] which is robust against misspecification of the environmental variance.
5 Method 1: Estimate the conditional power for the selected phenotypes and estimated model. Method 2: Compute the $P$ value of the Wald test for the genetic effect size estimates.
6 Use the multivariate FBAT-GEE on the subset of traits with maximal power (method 1) or low $P$ values of the Wald test (method 2).

Both algorithms are entirely robust against population admixture and stratification. The decision regarding a potential association is solely based on the FBAT-GEE statistic which is robust against these effects. Nevertheless, population admixture and stratification that is not accounted for in the multivariate model Eqn. (3.5) will affect the quality of the phenotype selection. In conclusion, population admixture and stratification will have an influence on the power of our testing strategy, but the strategies themselves remain robust against these effects. Since both approaches utilize the data on all available families to estimate the effect size of the tests, they are far more powerful than standard methodology, even in the presence of population admixture and stratification.

This general screening approach has been implemented in PBAT for a single marker. Extensions to include testing haplotypes or multiple markers are straightforward.

## Sample size and design issues

Several papers[99–101] have suggested that family-based studies are inefficient compared to population-based studies, for example, case–control or cohort studies. This popular opinion stems mainly from two prejudices towards family-based studies:

- Family-based studies require the genotypes of the parents who may be not available. The recruitment and the genotyping of the parents entail the need for additional resources, making family-based studies more costly than population-based studies.
- Since family-based association tests do not utilize information on all genotyped families, they lose power relative to population-based studies.

Although FBATs certainly do have these properties to some extent, their impact on the power of the study and on the required sample size can be easily compensated for by appropriate study designs. Further, many researchers have not considered the most powerful approaches to analyze family-based data. The requirements for family-based studies are known at the design stage and can be integrated in the design of the study in order to diminish their impact. In this section, we will discuss general approaches to power calculations and how they can be used to design efficient and powerful family-based association studies. We give general rules of thumb for family-based designs.

Traditionally, most authors of family-based association tests assess the power of their proposals for test statistics by simulation studies.[4,96,102] However, during the design stage of the study, the power of many potential designs has to be assessed. Simulation studies make the design phase of the study slow and cumbersome. Analytical approaches to power calculations have been discussed by Knapp,[4] Chen and Deng,[103] Lange and Laird,[92] and Lange et al.[9]

There are several types of power calculations that can be done in this setting. Because family-based tests are conditioned on offspring traits and on parental genotypes (or on the sufficient statistics for parental genotypes if they are missing) we can calculate the power conditioning on these quantities, if data are available, using the method developed in Lange and Laird.[104] One can use these conditional power calculations to determine the power of the data to detect a specific alternative hypothesis. As described under screening multivariate traits, conditional power calculations can also be used to choose a set of traits for analysis. However, in study design, we need to be able to calculate the power for a proposed design, regardless of the realized traits or parental genotypes. We refer to these as prospective power calculations; they can be done by averaging over the conditional power calculations. We now outline the basic approach.

### A UNIFYING FRAMEWORK FOR POWER CALCULATIONS

The conditional power of any FBAT statistic can be derived given the vector of observed traits and the vector of sufficient statistics for each family's parental genotype data, using the algorithm given in Lange and Laird.[104] The prospective power for the design under consideration is obtained by averaging the conditional power calculations over the distribution of parental genotype and over the offspring traits, conditional on the ascertainment condition, for example, affected offspring only. For the computation of both the conditional and the prospective power, the mode of inheritance and the disease penetrance functions have to be specified. Additionally, for the prospective power, you must specify the allele frequencies, a distribution for the trait, and the ascertainment condition. Using the formulas discussed in Lange and Laird,[104] it is straightforward to compute prospective power by numerical integration for any phenotype for which a probability density conditional upon the marker score can be defined. The design of the study influences the power calculations through the ascertainment condition.

For dichotomous and continuous traits, the PBAT software contains implementations of the approach to prospective power calculations for FBATs given by Lange and Laird.[104] The power can be calculated for families with multiple offspring and with missing parental information. PBAT is able to assess the power of designs that contain different family-types where the family-types can be sampled through a different ascertainment condition. These features of PBAT can be used to evaluate many different designs for a study and help to find a design with ascertainment conditions that are powerful and feasible at the same time.

## RULES OF THUMB FOR DESIGNS WITH DICHOTOMOUS TRAITS

Using PBAT, prospective power calculations are used to examine the effects of missing parental information, additional siblings and the ascertainment condition under the following four scenarios:

1   Common disease and common disease allele. The disease allele frequency is 0.2, the population prevalence of the disease is 0.3 and the attributable fraction of variation in the phenotype to this disease locus is 0.15.
2   Common disease and rare disease allele. The disease allele frequency is 0.05, the population prevalence of the disease is 0.3 and the attributable fraction is 0.10.
3   Rare disease and rare disease allele. The disease allele frequency is 0.05, the population prevalence of the disease is 0.05 and the attributable fraction is 0.10.
4   Rare disease and common disease allele. The disease allele frequency is 0.2, the population prevalence

of the disease is 0.3 and the attributable fraction is 0.15.

The power is computed under the following assumptions: the marker allele is the causative allele; the significance level is 5 percent; 200 families are ascertained. Two ascertainment conditions are considered in the power calculations:

**A**  At least one affected offspring in each family.
**B**  At least one affected offspring and one unaffected offspring in each family.

Table 3.3 shows prospective power calculations for the different scenarios. The results are grouped according to the number of individuals that must be genotyped per family, 2, 3, or 4.

In general, despite the small sample size of 200 families and an attributable fraction between 0.1 and 0.15, we observed reasonable power for many family types, especially for the first three scenarios. Based on the power calculations in Lange and Laird[9,92] and based on Table 3.3, the following rules of thumb are recommended:

- For common diseases (scenarios I and II), regardless of the allele frequency, the parental genotypes are not necessary to obtain powerful designs. In comparison to the trio design, higher power can be obtained by genotyping additional siblings instead of genotyping the parents. One can either ascertain two additional siblings regardless of their affection status or ascertain one additional unaffected sibling. While genotyping two additional siblings entails the same amount of genotyping as for the trio design (three individuals per family), sampling discordant sib-pairs requires genotyping only two individuals per family.
- For rare diseases, imposing ascertainment conditions for the affection status of the additional offspring increases the power of the study only mildly and is usually not worthwhile pursuing. When the parental genotypes are not known, either two or three additional siblings have to be recruited to obtain power levels that are similar to the trio design.
- When both parents are genotyped and additional siblings are available, imposing ascertainment conditions on the affection status of the additional siblings may decrease the power.

**Table 3.3**   *Power calculations for a dichotomous trait with 200 families*

| No. offspring | No. parents | No. genotypes per family | S I | | S II | | S III | | SIV | |
|---|---|---|---|---|---|---|---|---|---|---|
| | | | A | B | A | B | A | B | A | B |
| 2 | 0 | 2 | 0.40 | 0.55 | 0.65 | 0.82 | 0.46 | 0.48 | 0.30 | 0.32 |
| 1 | 2 | 3 | 0.52 | – | 0.74 | – | 0.73 | – | 0.52 | – |
| 3 | 0 | 3 | 0.65 | 0.68 | 0.92 | 0.93 | 0.61 | 0.61 | 0.42 | 0.42 |
| 2 | 2 | 4 | 0.69 | 0.59 | 0.93 | 0.82 | 0.76 | 0.73 | 0.54 | 0.52 |
| 4 | 0 | 4 | 0.79 | 0.79 | 0.98 | 0.98 | 0.70 | 0.70 | 0.48 | 0.47 |

## RULES OF THUMBS FOR DESIGNS WITH CONTINUOUS TRAITS

The results by Lange et al.[9] on power calculations for continuous traits can be summarized by the following rules of thumb:

- In general, when quantitative traits are analyzed, missing parental information can be well compensated for by additional siblings, positive correlation between the traits of the siblings and by the ascertainment condition (with greater information provided by phenotypically discordant sibs).
- For families with two siblings that are sampled from the population without any ascertainment condition, i.e., total population samples, the power calculations by Lange et al.[9] suggest the following:
  1 When parents are not genotyped and there is no correlation among sibling phenotypes, one has to recruit about twice as many families to maintain the same power level achieved as when the parents are genotyped. More resources for the screening process are then necessary, but the cost of genotyping is less affected, because only two family members must be genotyped.
  2 In the presence of moderate correlation (about 0.4), one has to recruit approximately 60 percent more families to maintain the same power level when the parents are not genotyped. The cost of the screening process is increased by approximately 60 percent, but the cost of genotyping is decreased by 20 percent.
- When the families are ascertained through discordant conditions on the traits of both siblings, for example, one sib from the upper tail of the distribution and the other from the lower, the power is dramatically increased and the benefits of genotyping the parents are further reduced.
- When a quantitative trait has been measured and no ascertainment conditions have been imposed on the trait, for example, total population sample, the trait should be analyzed as a quantitative trait. Transforming the trait to a dichotomous trait will reduce the power.
- When a quantitative trait has been measured and an ascertainment condition has been imposed on the trait, for example, sampling only trios whose offspring are from the upper 5 percent of the phenotypic distribution, the trait should be analyzed as a dichotomous trait after an appropriate transformation. Analyzing such a trait as a continuous variable can be difficult because results are highly sensitive to choice of offset.

The rules of thumb discussed in this section provide guidelines for the construction of powerful and efficient family-based designs. For the final decision about the study design, the feasibility and the costs of genotyping the parents, the general costs of genotyping and the costs of the various ascertainment conditions have to be known. Without the information about these study parameters, a decision about the most cost-effective design is not possible.

## Key learning points

- Analyzing association between disease traits and genetic markers can be an effective strategy for locating disease susceptibility loci. To be successful, the markers tested must be in high LD with the disease locus.

- There are two basic designs for association studies: standard (case–control or cohort) and family-based.

- The design and analysis of genetic association studies using unrelated individuals are very similar to the design and analysis of studies testing the association between non-genetic risk factors and disease. Two primary differences are the possibility of inflated type I error or bias due to population stratification and the specification of coding for the genetic variables.

- The effects of population stratification can be ameliorated through careful study design and novel analytic techniques that use multiple unlinked markers to measure and adjust for latent stratification.

- Family-based samples typically include offspring and their parents and/or siblings. Efficiency of different designs depends upon disease prevalence as well as ascertainment of offspring.

- Methods for the analysis of family-based designs are specialized but software for the analysis is widely available and adaptable to most settings.

## ACKNOWLEDGEMENT

The authors were supported in part by a grant from the National Institutes of Health, MH59532.

## REFERENCES

◆1 Pritchard J, Przeworski M. Linkage disequilibrium in humans: Models and data. *Am J Hum Genet* 2001; **69**: 1–14.
●2 Knowler W, Williams R, Pettitt D, Steinberg A. Gm3,5,13,14 and type 2 diabetes mellitus: an association in American Indians with genetic admixture. *Am J Hum Genet* 1988; **43**: 520–6.
3 Rosner B. *Fundamentals of biostatistics*, 5th edn. Pacific Grove, CA: Duxbury, 2000.

4   Knapp M. A note on power approximation for the transmission/disequilibrium test. *Am J Hum Genet* 1999; **64**: 1177–85.

5   Tu I-P, Whittemore AS. Power of association and linkage tests when the disease alleles are unobserved. *Am J Hum Genet* 1999; **64**: 641–9.

6   Horvath S, Xin X, Laird NM. The family-based association test method: Strategies for studying general phenotype-genotype associations. *Eur J Human Genet* 2001; **9**: 301–6.

7   Martin ER, Bass MP, Gilbert JR et al. Genotype-based association test for general pedigrees: The genotype-PDT. *Genet Epidemiol* 2003; **25**: 203–13.

8   Schaid DJ. General score tests for association of genetic markers with disease using cases and their parents. *Genet Epidemiol* 1996; **14**: 1113–18.

9   Lange C, DeMeo D, Laird NM. Power and design considerations for a general class of family-based association tests: Quantitative traits. *Am J Hum Genet* 2002; **71**: 1330–41.

10  Weiss ST, Ware JH. Overview of issues in the longitudinal analysis of respiratory data. *Am J Respir Crit Care Med* 1996; **154**(6 Pt 2):S208–11.

11  Lange C, Silverman E, Xu X et al. A multivariate family-based association test using generalized estimating equations: FBAT-GEE. *Biostatistics* 2003; **4**: 195–206.

12  Lange C, Blacker D, Laird NM. Family-based association tests for survival and times-to-onset analysis. *Stat Med* 2004; **23**: 179–89.

13  DeMeo DL, Lange C, Silverman EK et al. Univariate and multivariate family-based analysis of the arg130gln polymorphism of the IL13 gene in the Childhood Asthma Management Program. *Genet Epi* 2002; **23**: 335–48.

14  Breslow NE, Day NE. Statistical methods in cancer research: I. In: Davis W (ed.) *The analysis of case-control studies.* Lyon: IARC Scientific publications, 1980.

15  Breslow NE, Day NE. Statistical methods in cancer research: II. In: Heseltine E (ed.) *The design and analysis of cohort studies.* Lyon: IARC Scientific publications, 1987.

16  Rothman K, Greenland S. *Modern epidemiology.* Philadelphia: Lippencott-Raven, 1998.

◆17  Garcia-Closas M, Wacholder S, Caporaso N, Rothman N. Inference issues in cohort and case-control studies of genetic effects and gene-environment interactions. In: Khoury M, Little J, Burke W (eds) *Human genome epidemiology: a scientific foundation for using genetic information to improve health and prevent disease.* Oxford: Oxford University Press, 2004.

18  Clayton D, McKeigue PM. Epidemiology methods for study genes and environmental factors in complex diseases. *Lancet* 2001; **358**: 1356–60.

19  Kraft P, Thomas D. Case-sibling gene-association studies for diseases with variable age at onset. *Stat Med* 2004; **23**: 3697–712.

20  Li H, Hsu L. Effects of age at onset on the power of the affected sib pair and transmission/disequilibrium tests. *Ann Hum Genet* 2000; **64**: 239–54.

◆21  Langholz B, Rothman N, Wacholder S, Thomas D. Cohort studies for characterizing measured genes. *Monogr Natl Cancer Inst* 1999; **26**: 39–42.

22  Gauderman WJ. Sample size requirements for association studies of gene-gene interaction. *Am J Epidemiol* 2002; **155**: 478–84.

23  Peters JM, Avol E, Navidi W et al. A study of twelve Southern California communities with differing levels and types of air pollution. I. Prevalence of respiratory morbidity. *Am J Respir Crit Care Med* 1999; **159**: 760–7.

24  Gold DR, Burge HA, Carey V et al. Predictors of repeated wheeze in the first year of life: the relative roles of cockroach, birth weight, acute lower respiratory illness, and maternal smoking. *Am J Respir Crit Care Med* 1999; **160**: 227–36.

25  Thompson W. Effect modification and the limits of biological inference from epidemiologic data. *J Clin Epidemiol* 1991; **44**: 221–32.

26  Khoury MJ, Adams MJ, Jr, Flanders WD. An epidemiologic approach to ecogenetics. *Am J Hum Genet* 1988; **42**: 89–95.

◆27  Botto L, Khoury M. Facing the challenge of complex genotypes and gene-environment interaction: the basic epidemiologic units in case-control and case-only designs. In: Khoury M, Little J, Burke W (eds) *Human genome epidemiology: a scientific foundation for using genetic information to improve health and prevent disease.* Oxford: Oxford University Press, 2004.

28  Greenland S, Rothman K. Concepts of interaction. In: Rothman K, Greenland S (eds) *Modern epidemiology.* Philadelphia: Lippincott Williams & Wilkins, 1998.

29  Hirschhorn JN, Altshuler D. Once and again – issues surrounding replication in genetic association studies. *J Clin Endocrinol Metab* 2002; **87**: 4438–41.

30  Wacholder S, Chanock S, Garcia-Closas M et al. Assessing the probability that a positive report is false: an approach for molecular epidemiology studies. *J Natl Cancer Inst* 2004; **96**: 434–42.

31  Gauderman W. Sample size requirements for matched case-control studies of gene-environment interaction. *Stat Med* 2001; **15**: 35–50.

◆32  Wacholder S, Rothman N, Caporaso N. Population stratification in epidemiologic studies of common genetic variants and cancer: quantification of bias. *JNCI* 2000; **92**: 1151–8.

33  Wacholder S, Rothman N, Caporaso N. Counterpoint: Bias from population stratification is not a major threat to the validity of conclusions from epidemiological studies of common polymorphisms and cancer. *Cancer Epidemiol Prev Biomarkers* 2002; **11**: 513–20.

34  Ardlie K, Lunetta K, Seielstad M. Testing for population-subdivision and association in four case-control studies. *Am J Hum Genet* 2002; **71**: 304–11.

◆35  Thomas D, Witte J. Point: Population stratification: a problem for case-control studies of candidate gene associations? *Cancer Epidemiol Prev Biom* 2002; **11**: 505–12.

●36  Devlin B, Roeder K. Genomic control for association studies. *Biometrics* 1999; **55**: 997–1004.

37  Freedman ML, Reich D, Penney KL et al. Assessing the impact of population stratification on genetic association studies. *Nat Genet* 2004; **36**: 388–93.

38  Pritchard J, Rosenberg N. Use of unlinked genetic markers to detect population stratification in association studies. *Am J Hum Genet* 1999; **65**: 220–8.

●39  Pritchard J, Stephens M, Rosenberg N, Donnelly P. Association mapping in structured populations. *Am J Hum Genet* 2000; **67**: 170–81.

40 Reich D, Goldstein D. Detecting association in a case-control study while correcting for population stratification. *Genet Epidemiol* 2001; **20**: 4–16.

41 Marchini J, Cardon LR, Phillips MS, Donnelly P. The effects of human population structure on large genetic association studies. *Nat Genet* 2004; **36**: 512–7.

42 Liu J, Sabatti C, Teng J et al. Bayesian analysis of haplotypes for linkage disequilibrium mapping. *Genome Res* 2001; **11**: 1716–24.

43 Molitor J, Marjoram P, Thomas D. Application of Bayesian spatial statistical methods to analysis of haplotype effects and gene mapping. *Genet Epidemiol* 2003; **25**: 95–105.

44 Morris R, Kaplan N. On the advantage of haplotype analysis in the presence of multiple disease susceptibility alleles. *Genet Epidemiol* 2002; **23**: 221–33.

45 Thomas DC, Stram DO, Conti D et al. Bayesian spatial modeling of haplotype associations. *Hum Hered* 2003; **56**: 32–40.

46 Chapman JM, Cooper JD, Todd JA, Clayton DG. Detecting disease associations due to linkage disequilibrium using haplotype tags: a class of tests and the determinants of statistical power. *Hum Hered* 2003; **56**: 18–31.

47 Schaid D, Rowland C, Tines D et al. Score tests for association between traits and haplotypes when linkage phase is ambiguous. *Am J Hum Genet* 2002; **70**: 425–34.

48 Stram D, Pearce C, Bretsky P et al. Modeling and E-M estimation of haplotype-specific relative risks from genotype data for a case-control study of unrelated individuals. *Hum Hered* 2003; **55**: 179–90.

49 Zhao H, Zhang S, Merikangas K et al. Transmission/disequilibrium tests using tightly linked markers. *Am J Hum Genet* 2000; **67**: 936–46.

50 Akey J, Jin L, Xiong M. Haplotypes vs single marker linkage disequilibrium tests: what do we gain? *Eur J Hum Genet* 2001; **9**: 291–300.

51 Johnson G, Esposito L, Barratt B et al. Haplotype tagging for the identification of common disease genes. *Nature Genet* 2001; **29**: 233–7.

52 Carlson CS, Eberle MA, Rieder MJ et al. Selecting a maximally informative set of single-nucleotide polymorphisms for association analyses using linkage disequilibrium. *Am J Hum Genet* 2004; **74**: 106–20.

53 Gabriel SB, Schaffner SF, Nguyen H et al. The structure of haplotype blocks in the human genome. *Science* 2002; **296**: 2225–9.

54 Wall J, Pritchard J. Haplotype blocks and linkage disequilibrium in the human genome. *Nat Rev Genet* 2003; **4**: 587–97.

55 Wall JD, Pritchard JK. Assessing the performance of the haplotype block model of linkage disequilibrium. *Am J Hum Genet* 2003; **73**: 502–15.

56 Zhang K, Jin L. HaploBlockFinder: haplotype block analyses. *Bioinformatics* 2003; **19**: 1300–1.

57 Stram D, Haiman C, Hirschhorn J et al. Choosing haplotype-tagging SNPs based on unphased genotype data using a preliminary sample of unrelated subjects with an example from the multiethnic cohort study. *Hum Hered* 2003; **55**: 27–36.

58 Thompson D, Stram D, Goldgar D, Witte JS. Haplotype tagging single nucleotide polymorphisms and association studies. *Hum Hered* 2003; **56**: 48–55.

59 Lazarus R, Silverman E, Raby B et al. Choosing subsets of SNP for genotyping in association studies: htSNP and ldSNP. *Am J Hum Genet* 2003; **73**: A387.

60 Sebastiani P, Lazarus R, Weiss ST et al. Minimal haplotype tagging. *Proc Natl Acad Sci USA* 2003; **100**: 9900–5.

61 Chiano M, Clayton D. Fine genetic mapping using haplotype analysis and the missing data problem. *Ann Hum Genet* 1998; **62**: 55–60.

62 Clark AG. Inference of haplotypes from PCR-amplified samples of diploid populations. *Mol Biol Evol* 1990; **7**: 111–22.

63 Excoffier L, Slatkin M. Maximum-likelihood estimation of molecular haplotype frequencies in a diploid population. *Mol Biol Evol* 1995; **12**: 921–7.

64 Qin Z, Niu T, Liu J. Partition-ligation-expectation-maximization algorithm for haplotype inference with single-nucleotide polymorphisms. *Am J Hum Genet* 2002; **70**: 157.

65 Stephens M, Donnelly P. A comparison of Bayesian methods for haplotype reconstruction from population genotype data. *Am J Hum Genet* 2003; **73**: 1162–9.

66 Epstein M, Satten G. Inference on haplotype effects in case-control studies using unphased genotype data. *Am J Hum Genet* 2003; **73**: 1316–29.

67 Lake S, Lyon H, Tantisira K et al. Estimation and tests of haplotype-environment interaction when linkage phase is ambiguous. *Hum Hered* 2003; **55**: 56–65.

68 Lin DY. Haplotype-based association analysis in cohort studies of unrelated individuals. Genet *Epidemiol* 2004; **26**: 255–64.

69 Zhao L, Li S, Khalid N. A method for the assessment of disease associations with single-nucleotide polymorphism haplotypes and environmental variables in case-control studies. *Am J Hum Genet* 2003; **72**: 1231–50.

●70 Ott J. Statistical properties of the haplotype relative risk. *Genet Epidemiol 1989*; **6**: 127–30.

71 Terwilliger JD, Ott J. A haplotype-based 'haplotype relative risk' approach to detecting allelic associations. *Hum Hered* 1992; **42**: 337–46.

72 Rubinstein P, Walker M, Carpenter C et al. Genetics of HLA disease associations: The use of the haplotype relative risk (HRR) and the 'haplo-delta' (Dh) estimates in juvenile diabetes from three racial groups. *Hum Immunol* 1981; **3**: 384.

●73 Falk CT, Rubinstein P. Haplotype Relative Risks: an easy reliable way to construct a proper control sample for risk calculations. *Ann Hum Genet 1987*; **51**: 227–33.

74 Spielman RS, McGinnis RE, Ewens WJ. Transmission test for linkage disequilibrium: the insulin gene region and insulin-dependent diabetes mellitus (IDDM). *Am J Hum Genet* 1993; **65**: 578–80.

75 Sham PC, Curtis D. An extended transmission/disequilibrium test (TDT) for multi-allelic marker loci. *Ann Hum Genet* 1995; **59**: 323–336.

76 Bickeboller H, Clerget-Darpoux F. Statistical properties of the allelic and genotypic transmission/disequilibrium test for multiallelic markers. *Genet Epidemiol* 1995; **12**: 865–70.

●77 Spielman R, Ewens W. The TDT and other family-based tests for linkage disequilibrium and association. *Am J Hum Genet* 1996; **59**: 983–9.

78 Horvath S, Laird NM. Discordant sibship test for disequilibrium/ transmission: No need for parental data. *Am J Hum Gen* 1998; **63**: 1886–97.

79 Rice JP, Neuman RJ, Hoshaw SL et al. TDT with covariates and genomic screens with mod scores: their behavior on simulated data. *Genet Epidemiol* 1995; **12**: 659–64.

80    Ewens WJ, Spielman RS. Disease associations and the transmission/disequilibrium test (TDT). *Curr Protocols Hum Genet* 1997; Supplement **15**: 1.12.1–13

81    Curtis D, Sham PC. A note on the application of the transmission disequilibrium test when a parent is missing. (letters to the editor), *Am J Hum Genet* 1995; **56**: 811–12.

82    Schaid DJ, Li H.Genotype relative-risks and association tests for nuclear families with missing parental data. *Genet Epidemiol 1997*; **14**: 1113–1118.

●83    Rabinowitz D, Laird NM. A unified approach to adjusting association tests for population admixture with arbitrary pedigree structure and arbitrary missing marker information. *Hum Hered* 2000; **50**: 211–23.

84    Ewens WJ, Spielman RS. The transmission/disequilibrium test. In: *Handbook of Statistical Genetics*, 2nd edn, Chapter 18. Wiley Europe, 2003.

●85    Zhao H. Family-based association studies. *Stat Methods Med Res* 2000; **9**: 563–87.

●86    Clayton D, Jones H. Transmission/disequilibrium tests for extended marker haplotypes. *Am J Hum Genet* 1999; **65**: 1161–9.

87    Clayton D. A generalization of the transmission/ disequilibrium test for uncertain-haplotype transmission. *Am J Hum Genet* 1999; **65**: 1170–7.

88    Horvath S, Xu X, Lake SL et al. Family-based tests for associating haplotypes with general phenotype data: application to asthma genetics. *Genet Epidemiol* 2004; **26**: 61–9.

89    Laird NM, Horvath S, Xu X. Implementing a unified approach to family-based tests of association. *Genet Epi* 2000; 19(Suppl 1): S36–S42.

90    Lazzeroni L, Lange K. A conditional inference framework for extending the transmission/disequilibrium test. *Hum Hered* 2001; **48**: 67–81.

91    Lake S, Blacker D, Laird NM. Family-based tests of association in the presence of linkage. *Am J Hum Gen* 2000; **67**: 1515–25.

92    Lange C, Laird NM. Analytical sample size and power calculations for general class of family-based association tests: Dichotomous traits. *Am J Hum Genet* 2002; **71**: 575–84.

93    Whittaker JC, Lewis DM. The effect of family structure on linkage tests using allelic association. *Am J Hum Genet* 1998; **63**: 889–97.

94    Lunetta KL, Farove SV, Biederman J, Laird NM. Family-based tests of association and linkage using unaffected sibs, covariates and interaction. *Am J Hum Gen* 2000; **66**: 605–14.

95    Liang K-Y, Zeger SL. Longitudinal data analysis using generalized linear models. *Biometrika* 1986; **73**: 13–22.

96    Abecasis GR, Cardon LR, Cookson WOC. A general test of association for quantitative traits in nuclear families. *Am J Hum Genet* 2000; **66**: 279–92.

97    Gauderman WJ. Candidate gene association analysis for a quantitative trait, using parent-offspring trios. *Genet Epidemiol* 2003; **25**: 327–38.

98    Lange C, Andrew T, MacGregor AJ et al. A family-based association test for repeatedly measured quantitative traits adjusting for unknown environmental and/or polygenic effects. *Stat Appl Genet Mol Biol* 2004; **3**, Article 17.

99    Morton NE, Collins A. Tests and estimates of allelic association in complex inheritance. *Proc Natl Acad Sci USA* 1998; **95**: 11 389–93.

100    Risch N, Teng J. The relative power of family-based and case-control designs for linkage disequilibrium studies of complex human diseases I. DNA pooling. *Genome Res* 1998; **8**: 1273–88.

101    McGinnis R, Shifman S, Darvasi A. Power and efficiency of the TDT and case-control design for association scans. *Behav Genet* 2002; **32**: 135–44.

102    Monks SA, Kaplan NL. Removing the sampling restrictions from family-based tests of association for a quantitative-trait locus. *Am J Hum Genet* 2000; **66**: 576–92.

103    Chen W-M, Deng H-W. A general and accurate approach for computing the statistical power of the transmission disequilibrium test for complex disease genes. *Genet Epidemiol* 2001; **21**: 53–67.

104    Lange C, Laird NM. On a general class of conditional tests for family-based association studies in genetics: The asymptotic distribution, the conditional power and optimality considerations. *Genet Epidemiol* 2002; **23**: 165–80.

# 4

# Molecular characterization of genetic variation

# Sample collection and processing in human respiratory genetics

BENJAMIN A. RABY, JODY S. SYLVIA, AND EDWIN K. SILVERMAN

This section on subject recruitment and sample management for respiratory genetic studies will provide a brief overview of some of the important practical issues involved in performing a human genetic research study. For the non-researcher, this review will provide insight into the mechanics of performing such studies, while for researchers interested in this area, we will try to provide some useful guidelines. When performing human genetic studies, it is essential to anticipate what samples and information need to be tracked for the current project and for potential future projects within a study cohort.

## SUBJECT RECRUITMENT

### Institutional review board issues

The study design employed significantly impacts subject recruitment issues. Some of the common genetic study designs were reviewed in Chapter 1. In all cases, subject recruitment needs to be performed in accordance with local institutional review board (IRB) or ethical committee requirements, and there are major differences in the requirements between countries. In the USA, if the institution at which the genetic research is performed does not have an IRB, a federally approved external IRB may be used.

For a case–control genetic association study nested within an ongoing population cohort, subjects have already agreed to participate in a research study, and recontacting them to participate in a related genetic study may be relatively straightforward. On the other hand, use of previously collected biological samples for new genetic studies raises a variety of contentious issues,[1] and options such as obtaining a waiver of informed consent from the IRB, recontacting subjects to obtain consent, or removing links to identifying information (anonymization) may be required. For prospective studies involving the identification of new subjects, potential participants identified by a medical record review will likely not be expecting to be contacted about research studies, and consideration of the most appropriate method to contact such subjects is required. As an added element of complexity, there are marked variations between IRBs in the USA regarding requirements and reviews of genetic studies.[2]

The enactment of the Health Insurance Portability and Accountability Act (HIPAA) in April 2003 has made subject recruitment into clinical research studies in the USA much more challenging. The ability to review medical records and transfer data between collaborators in different institutions has been affected by the HIPAA. Even before the HIPAA was enacted, particular scrutiny had focused on human genetic studies due to concerns about confidentiality and stigmatization of study participants. Because genetic studies can provide information relevant not just for the study participant but also for their relatives and even for their entire racial or ethnic group, a variety of unique human studies issues are raised by genetic studies.[3] A widely publicized case at Virginia Commonwealth University, in which the parent of a research participant learned that his confidential psychiatric information had been collected without his consent, has led to increased efforts to protect family members in genetic studies.[4] An IRB review of genetic studies includes a determination of whether relatives about whom information is collected from a study participant should be considered as human subjects in that project, and if so, whether informed consent from those relatives must be obtained before such data can be collected. Concerns about the impact of genetic discrimination in maintaining employment or obtaining insurance resulting from participation in genetic studies have also been raised.

Clearly, the requirements for subject recruitment in genetic studies are rapidly changing, and uniform guidelines have not been developed. However, a few general principles can be widely applied. First, it is always preferable for the initial contact of a potential research participant to come from someone that they know (e.g., their own healthcare provider or a relative), rather than by a researcher that they have never met. Second, the subject must not be coerced into participating in a research study, for example, by linking their research participation to their standard clinical care. Third, the procedures, risks, and benefits of participating in the research study must be clearly explained to the subject, with written informed consent obtained in essentially all cases. Fourth, adequate efforts to maintain subjects' confidentiality must be taken, with secure storage of data and limited access to identifying information. A certificate of confidentiality can be obtained in the USA from the Department of Health and Human Services to provide protection against involuntary release of research information in response to a subpoena. This protection is valuable and should be considered for genetic studies, but the limited nature of such a certificate must also be understood by the research participant – voluntary disclosures are not protected. In efforts to protect the confidentiality of individual research participants, it is especially important to avoid discussing the research data or study participation of one family member with another. Finally, family studies must effectively balance the need to recruit relatives with the rights of those relatives to protection of their confidential health information.

## Data management

### FINDING STUDY PARTICIPANTS

A variety of sources can be used to identify participants in a genetic study, depending on the study design, with IRB approval. If IRB approval is obtained for review of medical records, computerized database searches based on diagnostic codes or various laboratory values (e.g., low $FEV_1$), may be appropriate if they are available. Referrals from other physicians, direct responses from potential participants to study advertising (e.g., posters, internet summaries) and mailings to disease-specific patient organizations are also potential sources of research subjects. As noted above, contacting potential research subjects that do not initiate contact with the research group directly typically requires assistance of the primary physician of that potential research subject. Initial contact is usually by mail, often with an opt-out postcard for subjects to indicate that they do not want to receive additional information or an opt-in postcard to indicate that they do wish to receive such information. For family studies, after the initial subject is enrolled in the family (proband or index case), that proband may be asked to assist in contacting relatives that might be eligible for study participation. Various methods for family enrolment have been used, including: (1) the proband obtains permission from their relatives for contact by the research team; and (2) the proband delivers a letter from the research team to their relatives.

After a potential research participant in a genetic study is identified, determination of their eligibility to participate

is performed by reviewing the inclusion and exclusion criteria for the study with the subject, and documenting their responses to these criteria in a standard fashion.

Special consideration by the IRB is typically required before enrolling members of vulnerable populations, such as prisoners or cognitively impaired individuals, into a genetic study. Although there is considerable controversy regarding the returning of clinical genetic test results to children, children can often participate in genetic research studies with parental consent. An assent form for older children can be used to indicate their willingness to participate in the study.

### ASSIGNING ID NUMBERS

A large variety of different identification (ID) code schemes has been used in genetic studies. For example, investigators can assign ID codes during recruitment in a sequential order to track biological samples that are collected in the study protocol. Using a sequential ID code provides very limited information to the laboratory staff managing the samples, however. Therefore, it can be very helpful to include some type of verification code in order to minimize sample misassignments. The local IRB typically determines what information is allowed to be included in the ID codes for genetic research studies. For family studies, including a family ID code and a subject ID code, along with a verification code (e.g., year of birth), is recommended.

### TYPES OF DATA IN GENETIC STUDIES

In terms of individual subject identifying information, there are several major categories of biological samples in genetic studies.[5] Identified samples are labeled with personal identifying information, such as the subject's name; storage of samples in this manner is not recommended. Coded samples are labeled with an identification code that the investigator can decode; this type of sample is typically used in genetic studies. De-identified samples are labeled with a code that is unknown to the investigator, but could be decoded with the appropriate key to the codes. Multicenter studies often use de-identified samples. Anonymized samples have no linkage between the sample and the identifying information; a data set for analysis is created and the links to identifiers are broken. Anonymized samples may be appropriate when previously collected samples were obtained from subjects who did not give consent for a particular genetic test. Anonymous samples were never linked to identifying information; for example, buccal swabs for DNA were collected from random subjects on the street, and identifying information was never collected.

### COMPLETION OF THE STUDY PROTOCOL

Genetic research studies may last for many years to collect the required number of trios, families, or case–control pairs to be a viable resource for the analysis of genetic influences on respiratory diseases. Samples from each subject need to be tracked and stored in a uniform format. A manual of procedures for the study that contains easy-to-follow protocols for each member of the research team is essential. An example of sample flow for the multicenter Alpha 1-Antitrypsin Genetic Modifier Study is shown in Table 4A.1. It is important to establish a chain of custody for the biological samples, which should include log forms and record sheets. Logging information into an electronic database at the point of recruitment is optimal, because it provides rapid and simple tracking information for subjects and at the same time protects the participant's confidential information.

## PEDIGREE DATA

In family studies that involve more complex units than sibling pairs or parent–child trios, it is very helpful to maintain a pedigree diagram. Standard pedigree nomenclature has been developed, as discussed by Bennett and colleagues.[6] Accurate records of pedigrees are essential for human genetic research, since they can assist in guiding additional enrollment of family members into the study as well as the interpretation of Mendelian inconsistencies observed in genotyping data. An example pedigree is shown in Fig. 4A.1. Males are denoted by squares and females by circles. Filled

**Table 4A.1**  *Sample flow in the multicenter Alpha 1-Antitrypsin Genetic Modifier Study*

| Samples collected | Initial storage | Shipment | Laboratory log-in | Initial laboratory processing | Procedure for long-term storage |
|---|---|---|---|---|---|
| Blood in EDTA (20 mL) | Label with subject ID | By overnight express mail in an IATA/DOT approved shipment box with a shipment log form | Enter sample into LIMS | Lyse red blood cells | Complete DNA extraction with Gentra Kit |
| | Store at 4°C | | Apply barcode label to each tube | Store white blood cells (one aliquot at −70°C; one aliquot in liquid nitrogen) | Quantify DNA with Pico Green<br>Store two undiluted master tubes and two 50 ng/μL tubes (one each −70°C and liquid nitrogen) |
| | | | Make blood spot card from one of the vacutubes | Send blood spot card for AAT type | |
| Blood without anticoagulant (10 ml) | Label with Subject ID | As above | As above | Aliquot serum into 200 μL aliquots | Store half of aliquots at −70°C and half in liquid nitrogen |
| | Centrifuge and place serum in polypropylene tube<br>Store at 4°C | | | | |

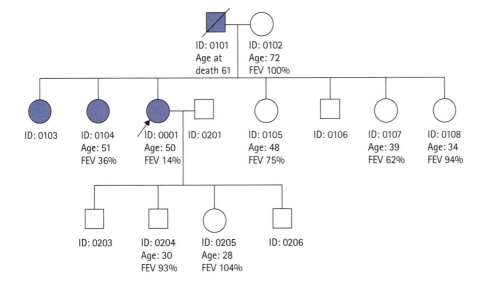

**Figure 4A.1**  *An example pedigree from the Boston Early-Onset COPD Study is provided. In this three-generation pedigree, subjects are listed with their subject ID number. The proband is indicated by an arrow, and individuals previously diagnosed with COPD are shown by filled symbols. The age and FEV$_1$ (percent predicted) values are provided for subjects that participated in the study.*

symbols indicate an affected individual, and partitions within the individual symbol can be used to record affection status for multiple conditions. An arrow below and to the left of an individual symbol identifies the proband; in clinical genetic counseling a 'P' is included to denote the first affected pedigree member who was identified, and to distinguish that individual from the subject who is seeking genetic counseling and/or testing. Deceased individuals are indicated by a diagonal slash through the individual's symbol, and pregnancies are indicated by a 'P' within the individual's symbol.

Each generation in a pedigree should be on the same horizontal plane. Relationship lines identify spousal relations with a horizontal line reaching the middle of the symbol for each of the spousal partners. A horizontal sibship line denotes individuals that are full biological siblings and individual vertical lines descend from the sibship line. Siblings are recorded from left to right in birth order, starting with the first-born. Vertical lines of descent connect the relationship line of parents to the sibship line of their offspring. The notation for a variety of pedigree complexities including twins, adoption, consanguinity, divorce, and assisted reproductive technologies are discussed by Bennett and colleagues.[6]

In pedigrees presented in publications, usually a roman numeral defines each generation, and each person in the generation is given an arabic number, from left to right in the diagram. This makes it easy to refer to family members in the pedigree by number, and thus protects family confidentiality.[7] To format information for a study database, the individuals in the pedigree are often denoted by their subject ID number (Fig. 4A.1). It is helpful if the subject ID number allows the study staff to know how the subject is related to the proband within the family, by using standard relationship codes for the subject ID numbers within a family (e.g., the proband's father is always denoted by 0101). By drawing the pedigree, it may be possible to recognize patterns of inheritance, such as X-linked recessive or autosomal dominant, for a monogenic disorder. The inheritance patterns for complex diseases are not readily determined from pedigree inspection, but the pedigree diagram provides a record of family relationships and affection status.

In addition to the identification number, supplemental information can be recorded on the pedigree diagram including names, ages, and other medical conditions. However, confidentiality issues must be respected when recording such information, especially if the pedigree is to be shown to outside investigators or family members.

### FOLLOW-UP WITH STUDY PARTICIPANTS

The genotypic information generated in genetic research studies can have important implications for research participants. If a known genetic disorder is assessed, such as alpha 1-antitrypsin deficiency, there may be proven disease risks associated with the genotype. Genetic research studies also have the potential to identify novel genetic determinants of disease. Even the act of participation in a genetic research study could have implications for genetic discrimination in employment or insurance. Whether research information will be returned to study participants should be decided before the study begins and clearly stated in the informed consent form. One complicating factor is that most research laboratories do not meet the standards for clinical laboratory testing, which are known in the USA as CLIA or Clinical Laboratory Improvement Amendments (initiated in 1988). Thus, research results typically should be repeated in a clinical laboratory, even if results are released to study participants. Another important issue to consider regarding returning research results to study participants is that research results are often of uncertain clinical utility, and thus may not be of benefit to the subjects.[8] Due to the nature of these results and the need to maintain confidentiality, genetic research results are not typically placed in the participant's medical record. If research results are returned to subjects, access to genetic counseling should be provided. Although it may not be appropriate to provide individual research results, it is often beneficial to send out newsletters to study participants, which summarize the progress made in the research project and the results in aggregate.

## SAMPLE COLLECTION AND MANAGEMENT

It is essential to establish standardized sample collection protocols within the study recruitment team and to insure open lines of communication between laboratory staff, research coordinators, and investigators. It is helpful to perform pilot studies to obtain an estimate of the time and resources needed to complete the study protocol. In addition, the locations where the study protocol will be performed should be determined. With appropriate IRB approval and study equipment, home visits can often be performed if the study procedures are safe and portable (e.g., questionnaire, spirometry, phlebotomy). In other cases, such as protocols involving chest CT scans or bronchoscopy, study visits at the medical center will typically be required. If only a blood sample is required for the study, it may be possible for the research subject to ship their blood sample, collected by a local healthcare provider and placed in an approved shipping container for diagnostic specimens. International regulations for shipping biological materials have been developed by the International Air Transport Association (IATA), and US federal regulations are enforced by the Department of Transportation.[9]

The total volume of biological samples collected is determined by the study requirements as well as the health and age of the study participants. In studies of pediatric populations, the quantity and timing of blood collection require special consideration. If blood collection for required testing, such as blood lead analysis, can be combined with study sample collection, then children can avoid a separate blood draw for the research project. It is important to determine what sample source is needed to perform the study laboratory assays most efficiently and to anticipate what samples will need to be stored, and under what conditions, for future biological assays.

## Sample types

### SOURCES OF DNA

For genetic studies, obtaining DNA is a primary goal. Any source of nucleated cells can provide DNA. Blood remains the most commonly used source of DNA in genetic studies, and guidelines for the collection of blood samples in epidemiological studies have been proposed.[10,11] DNA can be extracted directly from white blood cells, with yields of approximately 30 μg/mL of blood. Blood that is anticoagulated with EDTA is commonly used for genetic studies; heparin can interfere with some PCR-based genotyping assays and is less commonly used.[12] Alternatively, Epstein–Barr virus transformation can be performed to create lymphoblastoid cell lines and an essentially inexhaustible source of DNA; blood is typically collected in acid citrate dextrose (ACD) as an anticoagulant for lymphoblastoid cell lines.[11]

Smaller amounts of DNA can be obtained from buccal cells, which can be collected using brushes or mouthwash protocols; DNA yields are typically higher with mouthwash protocols.[13–15] A substantial portion of the DNA extracted from buccal samples is nonhuman, so it is useful to quantify the human DNA in such samples.[9] Dried blood spots, such as Guthrie cards collected from newborns, can also provide small amounts of DNA.[16] The development of whole genome amplification approaches, especially using the multiple displacement amplification approach which uses a high fidelity DNA polymerase, has allowed large quantities of DNA to be derived from small DNA samples such as buccal brushes.[17] Other tissue samples, such as lung tissue, can also serve as sources of DNA, but typically these valuable samples are used for other assays that specifically require tissue (e.g., immunohistochemistry, expression array analysis).

### OTHER SAMPLES IN RESPIRATORY GENETIC STUDIES

Depending on the goals of the study, a variety of additional samples may be useful; a discussion of phenotypes that can be measured in some of these samples is included in Chapter 2. Serum, the noncellular component of blood after clotting has occurred, and plasma, the noncellular component of blood before clotting has occurred, can be valuable samples for biomarker measurement. Plasma can be obtained from the same blood tubes used to collect

white blood cells for DNA extraction; collection of serum requires a blood collection tube without anticoagulant. RNA can be extracted from a variety of tissue types, including whole blood or purified cell populations from blood, for studies including expression array analysis and assessment of alternative splicing. Red blood cells can also be obtained from anticoagulated blood for biomarker measurement. Urine samples can be used for measurement of biomarkers including desmosine, a specific breakdown product of elastin, and leukotriene E4, a metabolite of arachidonate that is elevated in asthmatics.[18,19] Samples from proliferation assays of peripheral blood mononuclear cells in response to various allergens have been collected in a variety of asthma studies; in addition to proliferation assays, cytokine measurements are often performed from these cultured cells.[20] Measurement of some biomarkers may require specific anticoagulants, other chemical additives, or collection tubes, and should be clarified before sample collection begins.

Various samples can be collected during bronchoscopic procedures, including bronchoalveolar lavage fluid, bronchial washings, and endobronchial biopsies.[21,22] Skin biopsies can provide fibroblast cultures for molecular studies and histological analysis of elastic fibers. Exhaled breath condensate has been used to measure a range of biomarkers.[23]

## Sample processing and storage

Proper handling and shipping of biological samples between collection and storage is critical. In general, the amount of time between sample collection and processing should be minimized, but the requirements vary with the samples collected. Buccal brushings are stable at room temperature for extended periods, while blood that is collected for DNA extraction and/or other components (e.g., serum, plasma) should be refrigerated if more than several hours are to elapse between collection and processing. Although DNA yields from blood decrease with longer storage before extraction, reasonable DNA yields can be obtained in blood that has been refrigerated for up to 1 week.[24] Blood samples for DNA extraction can be shipped by overnight express mail, preferably with a cooling pack (e.g., frozen water bottle). The impact of shipping samples on serum and plasma biomarkers is variable and should be determined before sample collection begins. In addition, the recent plans for electron beam irradiation of mail in the USA to protect against bioterrorism may have a deleterious effect on DNA-containing samples shipped through the US postal service.[9]

Several methods are commonly used to extract DNA from blood.[10] Phenol/chloroform extraction was primarily used in the past, but the organic waste generated from this procedure has been one factor in a shift towards alternative approaches. High salt concentrations cause protein precipitation, and this approach followed by ethanol precipitation of DNA provides excellent DNA yields using the kit from Gentra systems.[25] Use of DNA-binding surfaces followed by elution is also a very effective DNA purification procedure, and it has been implemented commercially by Qiagen.[26] Finally, DNA binding to magnetic beads followed by elution, marketed by Roche, is a viable alternative as well. In the system marketed by Dynal, magnetic beads are also used to purify DNA; the DNA can be eluted from the magnetic beads, or the DNA-bound beads can be used directly in PCR-based genotyping.[27] Some of the widely used and commercially available DNA extraction methods are compared in Table 4A.2.

After DNA is extracted, quantification and dilution to uniform concentrations of a portion of the DNA sample is typically performed. In addition, it is advisable to store some undiluted master DNA tubes in case higher DNA concentrations are required for future assays. DNA can be quantified using a spectrophotometer by assessing the absorbance at 260 nm; the ratio of A260/A280 provides an index of DNA purity, with a ratio of approximately 1.8 indicating excellent DNA purity. Quantification using fluorescent dyes such as PicoGreen may be more accurate than spectrophotometric measurements and is gaining popularity.[28]

After extraction, DNA is diluted to the appropriate concentration; this concentration varies from laboratory to laboratory; our laboratory typically stores DNA at 50 µg/mL. Subsequently, aliquots are made and stored. Although different protocols are used in different laboratories, a few general principles are widely followed. First, more than one aliquot should be stored, preferably in more than one location. DNA samples for genetic studies are quite valuable, and storing multiple tubes in multiple locations protects against loss of the sample. Second, storing too many low volume aliquots is not efficient, since evaporation can lead to loss of sample volume. Third, although DNA is reasonably stable at 4°C, it is prudent to store at least a portion of the DNA sample in a −80°C or liquid nitrogen freezer. Repeated freeze–thaw cycles can damage DNA, but maintaining at least some of the DNA in long-term freezer storage should be strongly considered.

Optimal storage of non-DNA samples depends upon the sample types and the assays to be performed. For example, since some cytokines are easily degraded, storage conditions are critical in cytokine assays from cellular proliferation experiments.[20] Routinely, any biological samples to be used in cytokine assays should be stored at or below −80°C unless they are assayed immediately after collection. Since cytokines may be damaged by repeated freezing and thawing, the samples should be collected and stored under uniform conditions, with efforts to minimize the number of freeze–thaw cycles. RNA can be readily degraded by RNAses, so use of RNAse-free laboratory equipment, use of RNA-stabilizing reagents (e.g., beta-mercaptoethanol), and storage at or below −80°C is typically required.[9]

**Table 4A.2** *Representative commercially available DNA extraction methods*

| | Blood <1 mL manufacturer: | | | Blood >1 mL | |
| | Gentra | Qiagen | Roche | Gentra | Qiagen |
|---|---|---|---|---|---|
| Manual method | Puregene: High salt precipitation Generation: Ion binding/Column capture | QIAamp: Ion Binding/Column Capture Flexigene: High salt precipitation MagAttract: Magnetic-particle technology | N/A | Puregene: High salt precipitation | QIAamp: Ion Binding/Column capture |
| Throughput volume | 200–1000 µL | 50–200 µL | | 0.1–10 mL | 0.2–10 mL |
| Automated method | Autopure: High salt precipitation | BioRobot: QIAamp technology | MagNAPure LC: Magnetic-particle technology (automated PCR set up) | Autopure: High salt precipitation | QiaVac24 (with QIAamp Columns is semi-automated) |
| Throughput (samples; × volume) | 72 × 1 mL | 96 × 0.2 mL | 32 × 0.2 mL | 96 × 10 mL | 72 × 10 mL |
| DNA yield | 7 µg/200 µl | 6 µg/200 µl | 10 µg/200 µl | 350–500 µg/10 mL | 300–450 µg/10 mL |
| Extraction time[a] | 60 min | 45 min | 85 min | 9 h | 8 h |

[a]Approximation based on a minimum of 96 reactions and including other required steps.

## Key learning points

- Human genetic studies require careful consideration of ethical, legal, and social issues, with adherence to local institutional review board guidelines.

- Standardized protocols for data collection, record-keeping, and pedigree drawing are essential to the success of a human genetic research study.

- A variety of DNA extraction protocols are available, which vary in their cost, throughput volume, and biochemistry.

# REFERENCES

1 Dalton R. Tribe blasts 'exploitation' of blood samples. *Nature* 2002; **420**: 111.

2 McWilliams R, Hoover-Fong J, Hamosh A et al. Problematic variation in local institutional review of a multicenter genetic epidemiology study. *J Am Med Assoc* 2003; **290**: 360–6.

◆3 Ashburn TT, Wilson SK, Eisenstein BI. Human tissue research in the genomic era of medicine: balancing individual and societal interests. *Arch Intern Med* 2000; **160**: 3377–84.

4 Botkin J. Protecting the privacy of family members in survey and pedigree research. *J Am Med Assoc* 2001; **285**: 207–11.

5 Terminology for sample collection in clinical genetic studies. *Pharmacogenomics J* 2001; **1**: 101–3.

◆6 Bennett RL, Steinhaus KA, Uhrich SB et al. Recommendations for standardized human pedigree nomenclature. Pedigree Standardization Task Force of the National Society of Genetic Counselors. *Am J Hum Genet* 1995; **56**: 745–52.

7 Bennett RL. *The practical guide to the genetic family history.* New York: Wiley-Liss, 1999.

8 Fuller BP, Kahn MJ, Barr PA et al. Privacy in genetics research. *Science* 1999; **285**: 1359–61.

9 Holland NT, Smith MT, Eskenazi B, Bastaki M. Biological sample collection and processing for molecular epidemiological studies. *Mutat Res* 2003; **543**: 217–34.

10 Austin MA, Ordovas JM, Eckfeldt JH et al. Guidelines of the National Heart, Lung, and Blood Institute working group on blood drawing, processing, and storage for genetic studies. *Am J Epidemiol* 1996; **144**: 437–41.

11 Steinberg K, Beck J, Nickerson D et al. DNA banking for epidemiologic studies: a review of current practices. *Epidemiology* 2002; **13**: 246–54.

12 Beutler E, Gelbart T, Kuhl W. Interference of heparin with the polymerase chain reaction. *Biotechniques* 1990; **9**: 166.

13 Richards B, Skoletsky J, Shuber AP et al. Multiplex PCR amplification from the CFTR gene using DNA prepared from buccal brushes/swabs. *Hum Mol Genet* 1993; **2**: 159–63.

14 Lench N, Stanier P, Williamson R. Simple non-invasive method to obtain DNA for gene analysis. *Lancet* 1988; **1**: 1356–8.

15 Garcia-Closas M, Egan KM, Abruzzo J. Collection of genomic DNA from adults in epidemiological studies by buccal cytobrush and mouthwash. *Cancer Epidemiol Biomarkers Prev* 2001; **10**: 687–96.

16 Makowski GS, Davis EL, Nadeau F, Hopfer SM. Polymerase chain reaction amplification of Guthrie card deoxyribonucleic acid: extraction of nucleic acid from filter matrices. *Ann Clin Lab Sci* 1998; **28**: 254–9.

17 Hosono S, Faruqi AF, Dean FB et al. Unbiased whole-genome amplification directly from clinical samples. *Genome Res* 2003; **13**: 954–64.

18 Israel E, Fischer AR, Rosenberg MA. The pivotal role of 5-lipoxygenase products in the reaction of aspirin-sensitive asthmatics to aspirin. *Am Rev Respir Dis* 1993; **148**(6 Pt 1): 1447–51.

19 Stone PJ, Gottlieb DJ, O'Connor GT et al. Elastin and collagen degradation products in urine of smokers with and without chronic obstructive pulmonary disease. *Am J Respir Crit Care Med* 1995; **151**: 952–9.

20 House RV. Cytokine measurement techniques for assessing hypersensitivity. *Toxicology* 2001; **158**: 51–8.

◆21 Klech H, Pohl W. Technical recommendations and guidelines for bronchoalveolar lavage (BAL). Report of the European Society of Pneumology Task Group. *Eur Respir J* 1989; **2**: 561–85.

22 Jeffery P, Holgate S, Wenzel S. Methods for the assessment of endobronchial biopsies in clinical research: application to studies of pathogenesis and the effects of treatment. *Am J Respir Crit Care Med* 2003; **168**(6 Pt 2): S1–17.

23 Hunt J. Exhaled breath condensate: an evolving tool for noninvasive evaluation of lung disease. *J Allergy Clin Immunol* 2002; **110**: 28–34.

24 Schunemann HJ, Stanulla M, Trevisan M. Short-term storage of blood samples and DNA isolation in serum separator tubes for application in epidemiological studies and clinical research. *Ann Epidemiol* 2000; **10**: 538–44.

25 Miller SA, Dykes DD, Polesky HF. A simple salting out procedure for extracting DNA from human nucleated cells. *Nucleic Acids Res* 1988; **16**: 1215.

26 Scherczinger CA, Bourke MT, Ladd C, Lee HC. DNA extraction from liquid blood using QIAamp. *J Forensic Sci* 1997; **42**: 893–6.

27 Rudi K, Kroken M, Dahlberg OJ et al. Rapid, universal method to isolate PCR-ready DNA using magnetic beads. *Biotechniques* 1997; **22**: 506–11.

28 Ahn SJ, Costa J, Emanuel JR. PicoGreen quantitation of DNA: effective evaluation of samples pre- or post-PCR. *Nucl Acids Res* 1996; **24**: 2623–5.

# Genetic variation, genotyping, and sequencing

BENJAMIN A. RABY, JODY S. SYLVIA, AND EDWIN K. SILVERMAN

## INTRODUCTION

The human genome is highly polymorphic, with substantial quantitative and qualitative variation in DNA sequence distributed across all chromosomes. While much of this variation is situated in the approximately 97 percent of genomic DNA sequence that is devoid of transcribed elements and is likely of little consequence, virtually all heritable phenotypic variation is conferred by a subset of these variants that interfere with normal gene function or regulation. The primary aim of human genetic research is to identify this functional subset of variation, and correlate genetic variants with their phenotypic outcomes. A major challenge of this research is to characterize the genetic variation in populations reliably, with high accuracy and at low cost. The advent of a comprehensive physical map of the human genome, public databases to catalog identified variants, and the development of accurate high-throughput sequencing and genotyping technologies have helped to overcome many of the obstacles, usher in the post-genomic era, and accelerate the pace of genetic research to unprecedented levels. In this chapter we outline the common forms of genetic variation implicated in health and disease, and provide a survey of the contemporary technologies available for identifying and genotyping genetic variation. Due to the rapid pace of technological advancement and the virtually continuous announcement of new technologies and applications, we are unable to provide a comprehensive review of all available platforms. Rather, we hope to describe the current state-of-the-art in molecular genetic technologies, with the aim to introduce the reader to the fundamental concepts of this research.

## Chromosomal abnormalities

Gross chromosomal abnormalities are those variants that can be directly visualized through karyotyping and chromosome banding techniques. They can be broadly classified into two categories: aberrations in chromosome number and aberrations in chromosome structure. Abnormalities can also be classified as either constitutional (present in all cells, due to origins in the germline or early embryonic period) or somatic (present in only a limited number of cells, due to origins later in life). Most chromosomal abnormalities result from errors in chromosome recombination during meiosis (for germline mutations) or aberrant chromosomal migration and segregation during either meiosis or mitosis. While chromosomal abnormalities are frequently implicated in rare genetic syndromes, they have rarely been observed in common disease. Aside from lung cancer, chromosomal abnormalities have been implicated in few pulmonary disorders. A brief discussion of the types of abnormalities follows, with attention placed on those that have been implicated in pulmonary disease.

## NUMERICAL ABNORMALITIES

Polyploidy refers to abnormal copy number of the genome. Approximately 1–3 percent of pregnancies are triploidy (69XXX, XXY, or XYY), usually resulting from dispermy. Polyploidy is not compatible with life. Aneuploidy refers to an abnormal copy number of one chromosome. Aneuploidy is thought to result through two mechanisms: nondysjunction, where chromosomes paired in meiosis or mitosis fail to separate, and anaphase lag, where a chromosome does not localize to its pole in a timely manner and is not incorporated into a daughter nucleus. Trisomy is the presence of an additional chromosome (e.g., an additional copy of chromosome 21 in Down syndrome, trisomy 21), while monosomy is the absence of a chromosome (e.g., monosomy X in Turner syndrome). All autosomal monosomies involving complete chromosomes are embryonic lethal, as are most trisomies. Trisomy 13 (Patau syndrome) and 18 (Edwards syndrome) can survive to term, but rarely longer. Trisomy 21 is viable, manifesting as Down syndrome. Monosomies and trisomies of chromosomal fragments resulting from aberrant chromosomal exchange during meiosis, are often viable, several of which have associated pulmonary phenotypes (see below).

## STRUCTURAL ABNORMALITIES

Structural abnormalities arise either through improper repair of chromosomal breaks or through aberrant meiotic recombination. Chromosomal breaks can arise through exposure to radiation or other mitogenic agents, and are commonly observed in malignant clones, where cellular mechanisms responsible for identifying and correcting these breaks are often defective. These breaks are usually recognized by DNA repair systems, resulting either in break repair or the initiation of cellular apoptosis. Occasionally, the repair is faulty, resulting in structural abnormalities. The spectrum of structural errors observed in the context of abnormal break repair includes chromosomal deletions (terminal deletions at the end of chromosomes and interstitial deletions in the middle of chromosomes), gene duplication (due to unequal sister chromatid exchange), gene inversions, and ring chromosome formation. Pulmonary manifestations including pulmonary atresia and hypoplasia have been reported in several structural chromosomal syndromes, usually in association with diaphragmatic herniation.[1–5] A 4.2 kb interstitial deletion on chromosome 4q12 has been implicated in the idiopathic hypereosinophilic syndrome. This interstitial deletion results in the approximation of the FIP1L1 gene to exon 12 of platelet-derived growth factor receptor alpha (PDGFRA), and the creation of a novel fusion gene product with uninhibited tyrosine kinase activity.[6,7] Unusual chromosomal structures with abnormal centromere number (acentric or dicentric chromosomes) or two copies of one chromosome arm (isochromosomes) can also result through abnormal break repair. Gene inversions, such as those observed in Factor VIII deficiency (40 percent of hemophilia A),[8] can also result through other mechanisms likely related to abnormal chromatin folding patterns.[9]

In addition to improper repair of chromosomal breaks, structural abnormalities may also result from aberrant chromosome recombination during meiosis. These errors are either homologous (occurring between two copies of the same chromatid) or nonhomologous (occurring between two unrelated chromosomal regions). Homologous recombination errors result from improper alignment of the two chromatids, and generate novel chromatids with unequal amounts of genetic information, with the malaligned region being represented twice on one chromatid, and absent on the other. Subsequent fertilization with these gametes will result in chromosomal duplication or deletion, respectively. It should be emphasized that this mechanism of mutation results in the generation of two gametes, one with excess genetic information, the other missing that portion of the chromosome. It is the random acquisition of one of these two gametes that determines whether progeny manifest gene duplication (by inheriting the former product) or gene deletion (by inheriting the latter). There is evidence that

the unequal crossovers occur in regions of high sequence similarity, including those genomic regions containing multiple members of a gene family (including regions containing genes and their pseudogene counterparts) or those with multiple tandem repeat sequences.

Recent genome-wide surveys have demonstrated that large-scale deletion and duplication polymorphism is more common then perhaps initially considered.[10,11] Such copy number polymorphisms, spanning 25–3000 kb in length, are dispersed throughout the genome, with evidence of clustering, suggesting regions of hotspot.[10,11] In two surveys of 20 and 39 individuals, approximately 50 and 41 percent of the copy-number variants were observed in two or more individuals, with common variants of greater than 10 percent frequency observed frequently. More than 50 percent of identified copy number variants spanned genomic sequence that includes gene-coding regions, including genes known to influence heritable phenotypes, suggest-ing that this form of variation may impact phenotypic variation of common traits, in addition to their well-documented role in monogenic syndromes.

Hotspots of unequal homologous recombination have been observed in several disorders, including Duchenne's muscular dystrophy (where the largest gene duplications have been observed) and osteogenesis imperfecta.[12–14] Unequal homologous recombination has also been observed between repetitive elements such as Alu repeat sequences: 15–20 percent of patients with hereditary angioneurotic edema have deletions of complement component 1 inhibitor (C1NH, OMIM No. 606860) due to unbalanced homologous exchange at this locus.[15] Nonhomologous recombination typically occurs between differing chromosomes and results in the distribution of chromosomal segments to differing chromosomes. If both recombination products segregate together, the translocation is balanced, as no genetic information is lost. In contrast, separation of the recombination products into differing gametes results in one gamete having three copies of one chromosomal segment (partial trisomy) and only one copy of the other involved segment (partial monosomy). The alternate gamete has the complementary chromosomal components. Aside from gene deletion, unequal crossover, whether homologous or nonhomologous, can disrupt gene function in other ways. Frequently, the translocation results in the approximation of two functionally distinct genetic elements, with the generation of a new genetic unit with unique functional properties. This can include approximation of coding sequence of two genes (resulting in a gene fusion product), or coding sequence from one gene with regulatory sequence (resulting in aberrant expression of the approximated coding sequence).[6,16]

## Cytogenetics

Cytogenetics, the study of chromosome structure and function, began with the discovery that hypotonic solutions could be used to prepare chromosome spreads on glass slides for phenotypic evaluation.[17,18] Subsequent refinements in techniques of DNA isolation, chromosome staining, and the use of molecular probes have led to the widespread application of cytogenetic methods for both research and clinical uses. The basic methods of karyotyping are essential for the study of gross chromosomal abnormalities, and in conjunction with fluorescence in situ hybridization (FISH), have become the most commonly used method for identifying and characterizing gene deletions, duplications, and inversions.

Although a comprehensive discussion of cytogenetic techniques and their application is beyond the scope of this text (and is readily available in several well-referenced sources, see Ref. 19), a brief description of the basic methods follows. Chromosomes are only easily visualized during mitosis, which can be induced in cultured T lymphocytes using phytohemagglutinin (PHA). To ensure that a high proportion of cells are isolated during mitosis, cells are cotreated with colcemid, a colchicine analog that prevents cells from leaving the M phase of mitosis. High resolution FISH and chromosome banding techniques require the isolation of genomic DNA at phases during the cell cycle when the chromosomes are least contracted. While chromosomes isolated during metaphase are adequate for simple karyotyping, the longer chromosomes isolated in prophase or prometaphase are needed for high-resolution studies, such as physical mapping and complex gene rearrangement and small gene deletion detection. Prophase isolation is achieved by combining cell cycle synchronization (using colcemid) with inhibition of chromosome condensation (using ethidium bromide). The latter method is more intricate, requiring attention to precise timing of the duration of each step,[19] but results in longer, less condensed chromosomes, that can be visualized with greater detail.

While basic karyotyping permits visualization of the chromosomes, reliable identification of each chromosome and characterization of most abnormalities is only possible with the use of chromosome banding. Various banding agents are available, including chemical agents such as Giemsa (which preferentially stains GC-rich regions) and fluorescent dyes such as quinacrine or 4′, 6-diamidino-2-phenylindole (which stain AT-rich regions). Alterations of the staining protocol, including the addition of denaturing solutions or heat-denaturing steps, alters the normal banding patterns to accentuate various chromosomal regions (for instance centromeres or telomeres). Based on these banding methods, gross chromosomal abnormalities can be readily identified, including relatively precise localization of chromosomal break points. More detailed analysis, however, requires the use of molecular probes and in situ hybridization.

## FISH

Molecular probes generated from fragments of cDNA or genomic DNA can be labeled and hybridized with chromosome slide preparations to map gene segments and their arrangement. The use of fluorescent labels has greatly enhanced the resolution of in situ hybridization over radio-labeled probes, permitting precise localization and arrangement of genetic components.[20–22] The fluorescent label is either direct (incorporated in the DNA probe) or can interact indirectly through reporter molecules (digoxigenin or biotin). The chromosome preparation with the hybridized probes is then visualized using a fluorescence microscope. Double spotting of the probe denotes visualization of the probe bound to each sister chromatid. Multiple probes labeled with fluorophores of different spectra can be used to demonstrate gene order (for identification of rearrangements or translocations). The utilization of FISH for the study of lung cancer pathobiology has resulted in the identification of several targets for possible therapeutic intervention, including the epidermal growth factor receptor (EGFR).[23–26]

## COMPARATIVE GENOMIC HYBRIDIZATION

Comparative genomic hybridization (CGH) enables the evaluation of DNA sequence copy number across the genome by hybridizing differentially labeled test and control genomic DNA to fixed samples with normal karyotype.[27] Classical CGH protocols hybridized test samples to normal metaphase DNA spreads on glass slides, with high sensitivity to detect variations of approximately 1 Mb in length. Adaptations using chip-based platforms of cDNA, oligonucleotide, or BAC arrays and restriction digestion protocols have enabled higher throughput and greater sensitivity to detect smaller variants, with resolution to within 100 kb.[28–30] Initially developed to screen for sequence gains or losses in tumor cell lines,[31] this technique has been expanded to screen for similar variation in nonmalignant genomes, providing evidence of important common copy-number variation in both human and murine populations.[11,32] Given that these copy variants often involve genes, these techniques may eventually play a larger role in complex genetic mapping studies.

# Fine-scale genetic variation

While chromosomal aberrations typically have a dramatic impact on clinical phenotype and are frequently implicated in rare genetic syndromes, smaller variations, including single nucleotide substitutions and small insertion/deletions, are likely responsible for most of the genetic variance for heritable traits in general populations, as well as the majority of disease-causing variations (Table 4B.1). These variants are not discernible using the molecular methods previously described, and until recently could only be studied through examination of the abnormal prote in products which they encoded. The development of recombinant technologies in the 1980s removed this limitation, enabling direct characterization of genetic variation at any position in the genome.

**Table 4B.1** *Distribution of disease-causing genetic variation by mutation type in the human genome mutation database*

| Mutation type | Number of entries | % of total |
|---|---|---|
| Micro-lesions | | |
| Missense/nonsense | 25 266 | 57.3 |
| Splicing | 4182 | 9.5 |
| Regulatory | 483 | 1 |
| Small insertions and deletions | 10 727 | 24.3 |
| Gross lesions | | |
| Repeat variations | 91 | 0.2 |
| Gross insertions and duplications | 406 | 0.9 |
| Complex rearrangements (including inversions) | 514 | 1.2 |
| Gross deletions | 2421 | 5.5 |
| Total | 44 090 | |

Reproduced with permission from the HGMD database (http://www. hgmd.org) (accessed 13 December 2004).

As a result, the last quarter of the twentieth century witnessed the identification of the molecular causes of numerous diseases and the cloning of thousands of genes, culminating in the construction of high-resolution physical genomic maps and complete genomic sequences for humans and a range of other organisms. The advent of high-throughput sequencing and genotyping technologies now enables the comprehensive evaluation of variant loci across the genome in large cohorts, with the promise of identifying the genetic basis for most heritable traits. Among the most important milestones on this road of progress was the development of the polymerase chain reaction.

## POLYMERASE CHAIN REACTION

The major challenge for both variation discovery and genotyping is to interrogate one fraction of the genome reliably, at the exclusion of the other three billion nucleotides that comprise the human genome. Virtually all methods used to resolve genomic variation at the nucleotide level require use of the polymerase chain reaction (PCR). First described in 1985 as a method to characterize variation at the sickle cell locus in the beta-globin gene,[33] the method revolutionized the field of genetics by enabling rapid analysis of individual genomic segments without the need for use of laborious cloning systems. The reaction has been optimized to perform reliably with small amounts of DNA (often less than 10 ng) and in very small volumes (less than 5 $\mu$L), and is highly adaptable for a high-throughput environment. In addition to its role in DNA sequencing and genotyping, PCR is also central in gene expression studies (both qualitative and quantitative) and recombinant DNA applications, including in vitro mutagenesis and transgenic animal models (see Chapter 7).

PCR amplifies targeted segments of DNA by cycling through three principal reaction steps (DNA denaturation, primer annealing, and DNA synthesis) that duplicate both strands of DNA in an iterative manner (Fig. 4B.1). Double-stranded source DNA is separated to single strands (denatured) by heating to approximately 95°C. These single strands are then targeted by two short sequences of DNA (oligonucleotides) that are designed to bind specifically to the regions of DNA flanking the region of interest (annealing step). For this binding to occur reliably the reaction temperature is dropped to 50–70°C; the precise temperature is reaction-specific, and is determined by the melting temperature ($T_m$) of the reaction. Once bound, these oligonucleotides (amplimers) serve to prime the duplication reaction, whereby single deoxynucleotides present in solution are added sequentially in a 5′ to 3′ orientation to extending strands (DNA synthesis). DNA synthesis is catalyzed by heat-stable DNA polymerase, which incorporates nucleic acids that are complementary to the targeted DNA. Amplification of the targeted region results from cycling through the three reaction temperatures from 95°C (denaturing), to 50–70°C (annealing), to 73–74°C (DNA synthesis), with newly synthesized strands serving as the template for subsequent cycles. This is possible because the newly synthesized strands are complementary to the second primer. With each cycle, the number of newly synthesized strands, templates for the subsequent cycle, doubles, and the total copy number of the targeted region grows exponentially. Typically 25–30 cycles are performed, yielding more than $10^7$ copies of amplified sequence. The reaction is best suited for amplification of targets 500–2000 bases in length, although larger products can be amplified using long-range protocols.

A principal aspect of PCR setup is PCR primer design. Primer pairs suitable for robust PCR should have similar melting temperatures (ideally within 1–2° of each other, between 55–58°C), should not be self-complementary (which results in self-hybridization rather than primer–template hybridization), and should not be complementary with each other (resulting in primer pair heterodimer formation). In standard reaction buffer, the quality of the primer–template interaction is determined primarily by primer length and nucleotide sequence. Primers with high GC content (>50 percent) will hybridize at lower temperatures, but with reduced specificity. The complexity of the primer sequence is also critical – greater complexity, including avoidance of GC-rich regions and polypyrimidine tracks, is preferred to prevent nonspecific binding. Several freeware applications are available to automate primer selection (for example, Primer3.0 at http://frodo.wi.mit.edu/cgi-bin/primer3/primer3_www.cgi). To ensure that amplification is restricted to one genomic region of interest, primers should (where possible) be designed to anneal to unique genomic sequences that flank the target sequence. This is usually easily accomplished by designing primers of 18–25 nucleotides in length, which are typically represented only

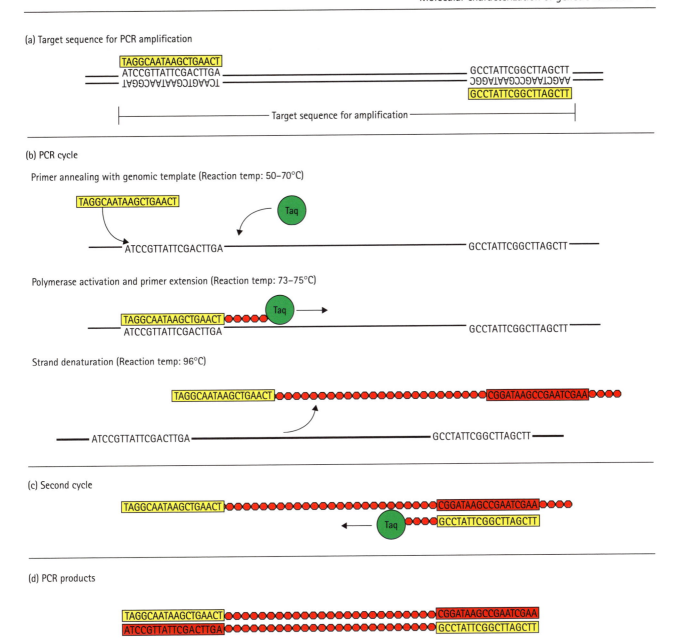

(a) Target sequence for PCR amplification

(b) PCR cycle

Primer annealing with genomic template (Reaction temp: 50–70°C)

Polymerase activation and primer extension (Reaction temp: 73–75°C)

Strand denaturation (Reaction temp: 96°C)

(c) Second cycle

(d) PCR products

**Figure 4B.1** *The polymerase chain reaction. (a) The target region of double stranded genomic DNA serving as the template for PCR reaction is bounded by forward (F) and reverse (R) oligonucleotide primers (yellow). The initial step of PCR is genomic DNA denatured at 96°C (not shown). (b) PCR cycle: In annealing step, forward primer binds to target DNA (optimal temperature depends on primer-DNA melting temperature, typically 50–70°C). DNA synthesis is initiated by activation of Taq Polymerase upon raising reaction temperature to 73–75°C. Strand synthesis proceeds 5'→3' with incorporation of deoxynucleotides (red circles). Extension continues until temperature is raised to 96°C (denaturing step). Not shown is simultaneous synthesis of complementary strand using reverse primers. (c) Second cycle using PCR product as template. Following denaturing, a second cycle of PCR is initiated by cooling reaction to annealing temperature. For this and subsequent PCR cycles, strands generated in previous rounds can serve as the template, as shown here. (d) Final targeted PCR product, bound by PCR primers.*

once in the genome. Because the reaction mandates that these primers hybridize to the target genome in a complementary orientation, it is unusual for such combinations to be seen in more than one genomic region. However, simultaneous amplification of multiple regions is observed when primers are designed to highly repetitive sequence (Alu or LINE elements), to regions of low complexity, or to pseudogenes. The latter scenario is more often seen when both primers are designed to hybridize with exonic sequence. Primer uniqueness should be evaluated by aligning their sequence with the target genome using internet-based bioinformatic tools (e.g., BLAST at http://ncbi.nih.gov/BLAST/). Many primer design programs can screen the sequence for repetitive elements prior to primer selection.

PCR is capable of amplifying extremely small quantities of DNA (only 1–2 copies of a template are needed).[34] Due to this robustness, reaction contamination by foreign DNA is a common problem, and can radically influence interpretation of results. Contamination of test samples is often difficult to appreciate, as the contaminant product may be identical in size and sequence (primarily if the contaminant is from the same organism). Positive (known standard samples) and negative (water) controls should be routinely performed with all experiments to ensure early identification of contamination. The source of foreign DNA is often difficult to identify. Contamination of PCR reagents (nucleotides, polymerases, or buffers) results in evidence of contamination in all samples, while contamination of individual samples or DNA spotting equipment may affect only subsets of samples. The latter type of contamination is more difficult to identify. A common problem in laboratories that frequently amplify the same targets is cross-contamination by the PCR product. This is also of major concern for high-throughput genotyping protocols that use uniform secondary primers for large-scale multiplexing reactions (see below). As such, PCR setup should ideally be performed in a well-ventilated area removed from the thermocycling units and post-PCR laboratory space.

The basic PCR protocol can be modified in a variety of ways that make the reaction highly adaptable for numerous applications. PCR primers or individual nucleotides can be labeled and used to generate labeled PCR products. Radioactive labeling with [33]P-labeled or [32]P-labeled nucleotide enables visualization of PCR products with autoradiography, and is used routinely for Southern blotting and dot-blot hybridization. Formerly also used for genotyping and sequencing, radiolabeling has been largely replaced by nonisotopic labels, including chemical labels (digoxitinin or biotin), and more recently, fluorescent labels. Fluorescent labeling has gained widespread popularity owing to its usefulness in high-throughput genome sequence analysis. Another modification of the basic PCR protocol is the use of dideoxynucleotides to force premature termination of strand elongation. This adaptation is the key element of dideoxy sequencing and genotyping (see DNA sequencing).

## SCREENING FOR GENETIC VARIATION

Numerous methods are available for the identification of single nucleotide variations, also known as point mutations. Unlike screening methods for gross deletions that are typically laborious and not amenable to high-throughput, these screening methods are primarily PCR-based. The major challenge in screening for point mutations is that the regions to be screened are often quite large, with the goal of identifying single base pair changes buried within kilobases of normal sequence. For single gene disorders with large effects, mutations typically (but not always) localize to coding sequence, untranslated regions, intron/exon boundaries, or known regulatory regions. For screening of genes in these conditions, targeted surveys of these high-probability areas are typically performed, reducing the amount of genomic DNA to be screened. However, the increasing evidence in both monogenic and complex disease, that regulatory or splicing variants located in deep intronic regions and remote 'gene deserts' impact phenotypic variance, also mandate the screening of these regions.[35,36] In addition, when searching for rare variants, large numbers of chromosomes need to be surveyed to achieve statistical power.[37] Therefore, methods are required to rapidly screen for polymorphisms that are not prohibitively expensive. Included here is a brief description of the more commonly used methods for point-mutation screening. These methods can be broadly classified in two groups: direct methods (sequencing based protocols) and indirect methods (which identify DNA fragments harboring variation, but typically cannot characterize the precise variation). While direct resequencing is the most informative method and is becoming more accessible in core sequencing facilities in many academic institutions, indirect methods for screening remain important tools for the rapid screening of larger regions of genome at considerably lower financial and DNA cost.

## INDIRECT MUTATION SCREENING METHODS

There are three types of indirect mutation screening: single-stranded mobility methods (SSCP), heteroduplex-based methods (mismatch screening, DDGE, and DHPLC), and DNA cleavage assays (ribonuclease protection assays, chemical cleavage, and fluorescence assisted mismatch analysis). These methods differ in their sensitivity rates for mutation detection, degree of throughput, and ease of set up and overhead cost. While no single method is ideal, SSCP and DHPLC have gained increased favor over recent years with the development of fluorescence-based high-throughput platforms.

### Single strand conformational polymorphism
DNA molecules of equal length but differing base composition demonstrate observable differences in electrophoretic migration patterns because of the differing secondary structures formed.[38] These differences are observable even when strands differ at only one nucleotide. SSCP differentiates wildtype DNA fragments from those with nucleotide variation by leveraging this property.[39] The methods can also be used to identify small insertions or deletions. In its most rudimentary form, the method is technically simple and requires no specialized laboratory equipment, consisting of PCR of the target region followed by electrophoresis of the heat-denatured PCR products through a nondenaturing gel. Migration patterns are then compared and abnormal variants identified, which can then be sequenced to characterize the variant. The protocol is technically simple to run and can rapidly screen large regions of sequence over a series of runs. However, careful attention to initial optimization of the migration patterns through the manipulation of buffer concentration, pH, and temperature is

required as the migration rates are not predictable from the known sequence data. Also, control samples known to be devoid of mutation should also be included, unless the variants being looked for are rare (so that most samples can be regarded as negative controls). While some mutations produce overt differences in migration, others are subtler and require experience to detect. One limitation of the basic protocol is that approximately 20 percent of variants do not alter electrophoretic mobility, resulting in a variation detection sensitivity of only approximately 80 percent. This is particularly true for fragments larger than 300 bases in length.[40] Other determinants of sensitivity include gel quality and sequence composition of the target region. SSCP is easily adapted for high-throughput analysis using fluorescent labeling of PCR primers and capillary electrophoresis, and the method is amenable to multiplexing.[41,42]

Where capillary electrophoresis is not available, the limitations of SSCP (namely low sensitivity and requirement of small DNA fragments) can be overcome by analyzing the migration patterns of fragmented amplicons – techniques known as fingerprinting. The fragments can be generated with one of two methods: dideoxysequencing (dideoxyfingerprinting) or digestion with restriction enzymes (restriction endonuclease fingerprinting).[43,44] These modifications improve the likelihood of detection by creating multiple products containing the polymorphism (at least one of which should demonstrate altered mobility) and by allowing interpretation of the sequencing or restriction patterns themselves. These methods greatly improve sensitivity,[45,46] but are more sensitive to errors in gel loading and atmospheric conditions in the laboratory. As in simple SSCP, these techniques can be modified to accommodate fluorescently labeled primers and analyzed with a DNA sequencer.

## Heteroduplex screening

When amplified diploid DNA differing by at least one base pair is denatured and then allowed to anneal, two types of annealing pairs are produced: pairing of perfectly complementary strands (homoduplex), and mispairing of strands that are not complementary at the site of polymorphism (heteroduplex). In theory, 50 percent of strands from an individual heterozygous for a genetic variant should form heteroduplexes. Because of the mispairing, heteroduplexes have altered tertiary structure, and can be distinguished from homoduplexes based on their altered mobility on electophoresis or by altered chromatograph patterns. Mismatched heteroduplexes migrate through nondenaturing polyacrylamide gels more slowly than their corresponding homoduplexes.[47] Varying gel composition (using vinyl polymers) enabled the use of non-radiolabeled samples in heteroduplex screening without significant loss in assay sensitivity,[48] greatly enhancing the utility of this technique. As with SSCP, mismatch heteroduplex screening is dependent on the size of the amplicons to be screened, with a conservative upper limit of good sensitivity at 500 bp. Modification of this technique, using gels with graduated

denaturing agent concentrations or temperature graduated electrophoretic units, can improve band resolution and increase sensitivity.[38,49] This method is also adaptable to capillary electrophoresis to increase throughput and resolution.[50]

## Denaturing high-performance liquid chromatography

The structural differences between heteroduplexes and homoduplexes can also be resolved using denaturing high-performance liquid chromatography (DHPLC).[51–54] This methodology is highly sensitive for amplicons as large as 1500 bp (with sensitivities approaching 100 percent for amplicons of 500 bp or smaller), and is very fast, requiring no post-PCR manipulations.[53] In addition, while each amplicon screened must be optimized to run at its individual melting temperature, the melting temperatures are predictable from the sequence, which can be ascertained using internet-based freeware (DHPLC Melt at http://insertion.stanford.edu/melt.html) greatly reducing the time required for optimization. Multiplexing is also possible, with multiplex sets arranged by similarity in melting profiles. DHPLC has been used successfully to screen hundreds of genes (Oefner P, Trebo M, 2002 http://insertion.stanford.edu/ human_genes_DHPLC.pdf). Assays for screening cystic fibrosis transmembrane conductance regulation (CFTR) for cystic fibrosis mutations have been used by many groups.[53] DHPLC was also used to screen bone morphogenetic protein receptor II (BMPR 2) in the positional candidate screening effort that identified mutations in this gene responsible for familial pulmonary hypertension.[55] The method has also been applied in studies of asthma[56–58] and bronchiolitis.[59]

In addition to its usefulness in mutation screening, DHPLC has also been successfully adapted for assessing DNA methylation,[60] gene expression,[61] and molecular fingerprinting in microorganisms, including mycobacteria.[62]

## Nucleic acid cleavage

A third set of indirect methods for polymorphism screening includes those that cleave mismatched DNA or RNA complexes. The most widely used of these methods is DNA chemical cleavage.[63] In this technique, probes complementary to wildtype sequence are hybridized with targeted amplicons. Probe–target hybrids will have mismatches at sites of variation on the target strands. Mismatched cytosine and thymine residues are recognized and oxidized by hydroxylamine and osmium tetroxide, respectively. The probes are then cleaved following addition of piperidine, and the digested products are size-separated and analyzed. Because only cytosine or thymine mismatches are recognized, assays must be designed to interrogate both strands of DNA to insure identification of all types of polymorphism. Advantages of this method include the ability to screen kilobases of DNA rather than 500–1000 bp, and the ability to determine the precise location of variation based on the cleavage patterns observed. However, the method is labor intensive, requiring multiple purification steps between reactions, and the need for protective equipment (including the use of a fume hood when working with the potent oxidizing agents). Solid-phase platforms have been developed to overcome some of these issues and improve throughput.[64] Many other cleavage-based methods have been developed, including T4 endonuclease VII cleavage, RNase cleavage assays, and fluorescence-assisted mismatch analysis, although these methods are not typically amenable for high-throughput screening.[65,66]

## DNA sequencing

DNA sequencing is the most reliable, and most commonly used, method for single-base pair variation discovery as it allows for direct comparison of multiple homologous sequences, the identification of heterozygous loci, and the precise localization of the variant alleles.[67] Modern DNA sequencing is performed using single-stranded DNA targets that serve as a template for unidirectional duplication by the chain-termination method (Fig. 4B.2).[68] The chain-termination method, first proposed by Sanger in 1977, is a modified PCR protocol, where dideoxynucleotides (ddNTPs) are included in the reaction mix. Dideoxynucleotides lack a second (di) hydroxyl group at the 3′ position of the nucleotide carbon ring, the position needed for normal phosphodiester bond formation with subsequent nucleotides. Incorporation of a ddNTP into a nascent strand results in chain termination because the addition of subsequent nucleotides is prevented. Prior to the advent of individual nucleotide labeling with distinct fluorophores, four separate reactions were required per template, each including only one type of terminating nucleotide. The amount of dideoxynucleotide relative to the amount of deoxynucleotide is optimized to insure that terminating nucleotides are incorporated randomly along each nascent strand, so that strands up to 1000 bases long can be generated. 35–40

thermal-cycled reactions (identical to PCR) are executed, resulting in the generation of millions of strands of varying length, each terminating with a dideoxynucleotide present in the reaction mix. The four separate reactions are then subjected to electrophoresis in four parallel lanes, resulting in size separation of the various fragments. Bands are then 'read' from lowest molecular weight to highest (corresponding to 5′ to 3′ sequence reads) and the sequence is determined. Radiolabeling has largely been replaced by fluorescent labeling of either the sequencing primer or the dideoxynucleotides. Primer labeling has the advantage of producing very even peak patterns but mandates four separate reactions per sequence. Using fluorophore-labeled dideoxynucleotides and automated DNA sequence analyzers, the four reactions can be condensed to one, with differentiation of the four nucleotides by their spectral output. In addition, electrophoresis using high-resolution urea-based polyacrylamide denaturing gels can be replaced with capillary-based electrophoresis in order to increase automation and throughput. Although not the sole method for DNA sequencing, and initially less accurate in earlier versions, cycle sequencing offers several important advantages over alternative methods, including its high-throughout capacity (particularly if using automated sequence analyzers), and the small amount of template needed (50–75 fmol of DNA). These properties, along with the availability of ready-made reaction mixes (sequencing kits) from many companies, have made it the sequencing protocol of choice by most investigators and core sequencing facilities.

Earlier versions of the cycle sequencing protocol were less accurate than other methods (chemical cleavage analysis, for example) due to reduced sequence quality and consistency. These limitations have been largely overcome with the development of better quality fluorophores and more sensitive

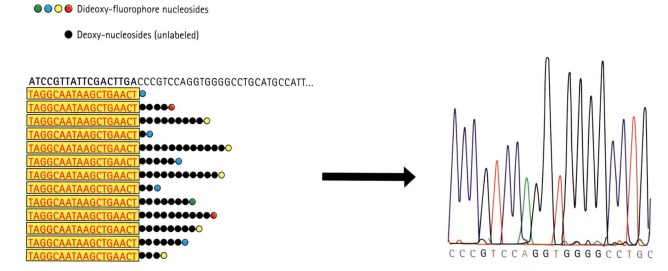

**Figure 4B.2** *Dye-terminator sequencing reaction. Fluorophore-labeled dideoxynucleotides are randomly added during single-strand synthesis reactions, thereby simultaneously terminating chain extension and labeling strands. Size separation via capillary gel electrophoresis through an Applied Biosystems 3737 DNA Sequence Analyzer permits visualization of the fluorescence sequence, as seen in the accompanying tracing.*

analyzers. The frequent problem of GC compression resulting from intraprimer self-hybridization and hairpin formation, resulting in abnormal band migration and read errors, has been largely overcome by replacement of dGTP by either dITP or 7-deaza-dGTP. Currently, the major limitation of DNA sequencing is the length of sequence that can be interrogated per reaction, typically 500–1000 bases. As a result, multiple reactions, using sets of tiled primers, are required to characterize larger regions.

Recently, additional non-gel-based methods have been developed for DNA sequencing. These methods have the advantage of avoiding electrophoresis-related artifacts such as GC compressions, and more easily differentiate insertions and deletions. Sequence variation can be determined by real-time evaluation of inorganic phosphate release during nucleotide incorporation.[69–71] This luminometric detection system avoids the need for labeled primers or nucleotides, and is quite rapid, particularly for short fragments, making it ideal for genotype characterization at a series of closely spaced variants. Longer fragments are less amenable to this platform. Because multiple enzymes and many reaction steps are required, this method cannot be used efficiently in a high-throughput environment.

Mass spectrometry permits the differentiation of oligonucleotide fragments that vary only slightly in length. This technology, commonly used for high-throughput genotyping (see below), can be applied to mutation discovery using RNase fingerprinting. Targeted regions are amplified using PCR with T7-tagged primers. The products are then transcribed to RNA by RNA polymerase bound to the T7 elements, and digested through a modified RNase I reaction. Digestion products are analyzed by mass spectrometry. Although four digestion reactions are required to identify all possible base-pair combination variations, this platform has the potential for higher throughput rates.

The main applications of DNA sequencing include characterization of novel DNA sequence, the identification of novel polymorphisms within known DNA sequence, and use as a genotyping method. The experimental approach and primer selection strategy will differ significantly depending on the goals of sequence analysis. Sequencing through previously uncharacterized DNA sequence requires some prior knowledge of at least a part of the flanking sequence for initial primer design. When such information is not available, target DNA fragments must first be amplified using specialized cloning vectors that include specific flanking sequences that can be used for the initial sequencing runs. Alternative strategies using degenerate primers have been used with some success, but are typically more laborious and prone to error. Resequencing of previously characterized regions for mutation screening or genotyping is typically more straightforward. Primers should be designed at a distance of approximately 50 bases from the beginning of the region of interest, as the first bases of sequence are difficult to resolve with nucleotide-labeled protocols. It should be emphasized that variants located

within the sequence with which the sequencing primer hybridizes will not be detected, as sequence reads will be off the primer sequence, not the template. In general, primers should not be designed over regions of known variation, as initial hybridization may not occur, and strands with variant bases may not amplify. Because of the size limitation of 500–600 bases, larger regions are often screened in multiple reactions. For regions up to 1200 bases, bidirectional sequencing can achieve one-pass coverage of the region. Larger regions must be sequenced using sets of tiled primers or sets of nested primers. Protocols for efficient primer design in the context of targeted sequencing or genotyping of known variants have been published.[72]

It is often advantageous to screen mRNA for variation, particularly for large genes with multiple short exons separated by large intronic regions. This is accomplished by first generating cDNA from mRNA using reverse transcriptase.[73] cDNA serves as a template for sequencing and can expedite sequencing of large genes. Despite the appeal, there are important limitations to cDNA mutation screening. Attention should be placed on the tissue source for mRNA – many genes demonstrate a high degree of tissue specificity. However, it is often possible to amplify small amounts of mRNA from most genes from peripheral blood lymphocytes, even those demonstrating high tissue specificity, due to the phenomenon of ectopic gene expression.[74,75] Of greater importance is the concern that mutated transcripts are often differentially expressed or maintained in cells, due to a variety of mechanisms including nonsense mediated decay. As a result, deleterious mutations easily identifiable by DNA screening may not be represented in cellular mRNA and would be completely overlooked. Moreover, this strategy only enables screening of transcript and ignores non-coding regulatory and intronic regions of the genome, which are known to harbor substantial variability.

## GENOTYPING

Genotyping is the evaluation of allelic status for individuals at known polymorphic genetic loci. While the characterization of large chromosomal abnormalities using FISH or Southern blotting certainly meets this broad definition, these types of variation represent a very small proportion of total genetic variation, and probably do not represent the bulk of pathogenic variation. Most genetic variation, and that which probably confers most heritable trait information for disease susceptibility and variation in therapeutic response, consists of smaller variants, including short tandem repeat polymorphisms, single nucleotide substitutions, and short insertions and deletions. Given the extent of both phenotypic and genetic heterogeneity, genetic epistasis (gene–gene interaction), and the important effects of the environment, it is likely that the magnitude of risk conferred by a given polymorphism influencing a complex respiratory disease will be small (i.e., relative risks of 1.5–2.0). As a result, population- or family-based genetic studies designed to identify these variants require large numbers of subjects to achieve sufficient statistical power (see Chapter 3). A major challenge facing gene hunters today is to develop inexpensive and accurate high-throughput genotyping technologies that will permit screening of large numbers of variants (i.e., thousands) in large study populations. Numerous genotyping platforms are currently available, each with inherent strengths and limitations. The following is a brief overview of the current technologies available for moderate- to high-throughput genotyping. Due to the rapid pace of technology development and the wide array of technologies already in use, this presentation cannot specifically address all of the technologies available. Rather, we will attempt to: (1) provide an introduction to the basic concepts in genotyping technologies; (2) highlight the strengths and limitations for the most commonly used genotyping platforms currently available; and (3) discuss the practical considerations that investigators should bear in mind when performing large-scale genotyping studies.

## Short tandem repeat markers

Short tandem repeat markers (STRs), also known as microsatellite markers, are sequences of tandemly repeated 2–4 base pair sequences flanked by non-repetitive sequence amenable to PCR amplification. The genetic variation is the length of the sequence due to variable number of tandem repeats present. Typical tandem motifs are [CA]n, [GATA]n, and [CAG]n, but other combinations have been observed. Such polymorphism is generated by slip-mispairing during DNA replication, with formation of DNA loops and back priming of the leading strand.[76,77] Longer STRs are more susceptible to slip-mispairing and mutation rates for STRs are substantially higher than for point mutations (see below). As a result, STRs are highly polymorphic, with many markers demonstrating heterozygosity greater than approximately 0.70. Moreover, microsatellites are relatively widely and evenly distributed across eukaryotic genomes. Dinucleotide CA repeats are most common, occurring approximately once per 0.4 cM.[78] Tri- and tetranucleotide repeats are less abundant than dinucleotide repeats, but alleles are more easily differentiated compared to dinucleotide repeats due to larger length difference and less PCR-related stutter.[79] These features, along with their ease of amplification and length scoring, have made STRs an extremely useful class of genetic markers for genome mapping, physical map construction, and linkage studies. However, because of the high rates of mutation and the relatively low density across the genome compared to single nucleotide polymorphisms (SNPs), STRs are less suited for association mapping, although they have also been used with some success in this context. For example, Cookson and colleagues demonstrated

strong genetic association with asthma and related phenotypes in a family-based association analysis to STR markers in asthma-linked regions on chromosomes 13q14 and 2q14.[80,81] Linkage disequilibrium patterns surrounding these loci extended no more than 100 kb, focusing attention to candidate genes in these regions, and eventually resulting in the identification of two asthma-related genes, PHF11 and DPP10.

In addition to their usefulness in genome mapping, pathologic expansion of tandem repeat sequences has been described in several neurogenetic conditions. While most STRs are relatively stable, with mutation rates as high as $8 \times 10^{-3}$,[82,83] several tandem repeats have been described with greater tendency to massive expansion and that have pathologic consequences. The most notable of these include Fragile X (which results from expansion of a CGG repeat sequence in the 5′UTR of the FMR1 gene), myotonic dystrophy (due to an expansion of a CTG repeat in the 3′UTR of the DMPK gene),[84–86] and Huntington disease (due to CAG expansion within the coding region of huntington (HD).[87] Disease-causing expansions of tandem repeat sequence in coding regions of genes, intronic sequence, and 5′ genomic sequence have also been described.[87–89] Diseases resulting from STR-based mutations typically have several unique clinical features that can be correlated with the molecular defect, including anticipation, variable penetrance, and parent of origin effects. Anticipation is the clinical phenomenon whereby disease severity (including age of symptom onset) worsens in subsequent generations. Mild forms of the disease in elderly patients that have gone unrecognized until late age are frequently brought to medical attention as a result of the diagnosis in a severely affected grandchild. This phenomenon, typically seen in myotonic dystrophy, reflects worsening expansion of the repeat copy number with each generation. The converse phenomenon of repeat length contraction has also been observed, and may explain variable penetrance observed in myotonic dystrophy.[90] Parent of origin biases have also been observed in several of these conditions, probably due to gender-related differences in repeat expansion rates.

### GENOTYPING STRs

The three main steps of STR genotyping are: (1) PCR amplification; (2) product separation; and (3) product detection and allele calling.[91,92] As in most PCR-based methods, early applications of STR genotyping required the use of radiolabeled primers or nucleotides for product detection, followed by Southern blotting and manual allele calling. The advent of fluorophores and automated DNA sequencing platforms (particularly those implementing capillary electrophoresis) greatly enhanced the throughput and ease of STR genotyping (see Fig. 4B.3). DNA sequencers and capillary electrophoresis eliminate the need for gel loading and manual allele calling – two steps that introduce the potential for sample loss and genotype error. DNA sequencers

(a)

**ATCCGTTATTCGACTTGA**CAGCAG[CAG]$_n$CAGCAG**GCCTATTCGGCTTAGCTT**

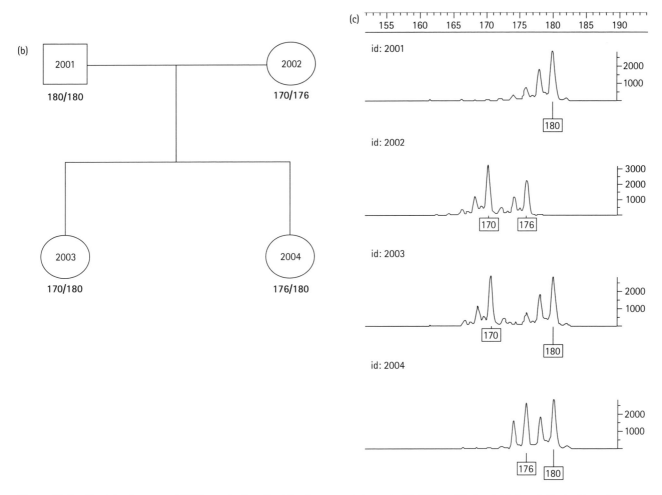

**Figure 4B.3** *Short tandem repeat (STR) genotyping. Short tandem repeat element with CAG motif of variable length flanked by unique genomic sequences (in bold) can be used as polymorphic marker for familial studies (a). Amplification of this region from related DNA samples (b) with fluorophore-labeled primers complementary to the unique flanking sequences generates products of variable length that can be visualized with capillary-gel electrophoresis and a fluorimeter (c). Amplicon size is determined by comparison to size standard (not shown). Stutter bands due to in vitro slip-mispairing can be seen. Automated genotype calls confirm allelic transmission compatible with Mendelian inheritance.*

have greater resolution than solid-phase denaturing gels (to the nucleotide level), enabling more accurate allele calling and binning. Primer labeling with fluorescent probes of differing spectral output allows for multiplexing of two or more markers of similar length. Standard reference sets of variable marker density (typically between 5 and 20 cM sets) are available for both the human and mouse genomes, and are commercially available from several distributors. Additional sequence information for thousands of validated and mapped STRs is available through internet-based services (for example, UniSTS at www.ncbi.nlm.nih. gov). Genetic maps including many of these markers have been generated to facilitate accurate linkage analysis, including maps generated with more than 1000 meiotic events.[93–95]

Most commercially available linkage marker panels group STRs into sets of three or four of similar length, label each marker within the group with differing fluorophores, and combine 3–4 non-overlapping sets of markers into one multiplex reaction. This allows for 12–16 markers to be run simultaneously, reducing the number of reactions per individual in a typical 10 cM genome-wide screen from approximately 380 to less than 30. When fluorescent labeling approaches are used, there are two stages at which point multiplexing can be implemented, with either the PCR performed separately for each marker, with products then pooled and analyzed simultaneously, or multiplex PCR. The former method has the advantage of eliminating the possibility of cross-marker primer interactions, and maximizes amplification of each marker. The latter approach is typically higher throughput (once the multiplex reaction is optimized) and less expensive, primarily due to the smaller amount of Taq polymerase used, but more prone to genotyping error. Time should be invested in the optimization of PCR reactions for STR genotyping outside of a standard panel, with particular focus on the effects of multiplexing on genotype quality. Each marker should be amplified in single plex on a subset of individuals, including control samples, to ensure robust amplification and reproducible genotype calls. Once optimized, multiplex PCR or pooling of PCR products should be performed on the same samples to confirm assay stability. This two-stage approach minimizes the likelihood of genotyping error due to unrecognized interactions between primers from different assays in one multiplex. Tracings should also be examined for evidence of spectral pull-up from markers of a different hue, which can complicate allele calling. Dinucleotide markers are prone to PCR stutter, whereby multiple non-allelic bands are observed and hamper correct allele calling. This phenomenon is due to in vitro slip-mispairing during PCR, reminiscent of the in vivo mutation-generating effect. Stutter effects are less common and less problematic in tri- and tetranucleotide repeat markers, and can be substantially reduced by modifying one of the PCR primers by the addition of neutral oligomers or poly-A tails that stabilize the reactions.

STR genotyping quality control is of critical importance, particularly for large studies requiring multiple plates. Between plate and within plate standards are required to ensure that allele binning is consistent. The former is achieved by including replicate samples across all plates and verifying consistent genotype calling. The latter is achieved by the addition of fluorescently labeled size standard. In addition, water controls should be included on all plates to screen for contaminant, a common source of error. Automated allele calling and high-capacity bioinformatic interfaces are essential to avoid human error in data handling, but a protocol for manual inspection and verification of genotype calls should be implemented in most settings.

## SINGLE NUCLEOTIDE POLYMORPHISMS

Single nucleotide polymorphisms represent the most abundant form of genetic variation in mammals. Estimates of the degree of polymorphism have reported differences between haploid genomes of unrelated humans averaging every 185–2000 nucleotides.[96–99] Differences in these estimates likely relate to the number of genomes evaluated (depth of screening) and the number and characteristics of the genomic regions screened. The rate of polymorphism is highly variable across the genome, with some regions (for instance, the HLA complex and olfactory gene complexes) demonstrating very high heterozygosity, while others display restricted variation.[98,99] This variability is

likely due to the effects of selective pressures that either promote or restrict genetic variability. In addition to the variability between genomic regions, within gene heterozygosity rates also differ substantially. A survey of nucleotide variation among 313 genes revealed much lower rates of base substitution in coding regions of genes (average of 3.4 substitutions per 1000 bases) compared to untranslated regions, upstream promoter sequence, or exon–intron boundaries (5.3–7.0, 5.9, and 6.5 substitutions per kb, respectively).[98]

## Mechanisms of mutation

Genetic variation is introduced into a population through germline mutation and transmission to offspring. It is estimated that each nucleotide in the human genome undergoes mutation at an average rate of $1.8–2.5 \times 10^{-8}$ mutations per nucleotide per generation.[100–102] Although the vast majority of these mutations occur in nonfunctional genome and are of no consequence, these estimated rates of germline mutation suggest that between one and three new deleterious mutations are passed from parent to offspring. The eventual population frequency of a given variant so introduced depends largely on the effects of selective forces, random genetic drift, and migration patterns. For convention, in the context of both population genetics and complex trait mapping, single-base pair changes that achieve a population frequency of at least 0.01 are referred to as SNPs, while less frequent substitutions are labeled as mutations. This convention is not universally accepted, particularly among medical geneticists, who reserve the term mutation for those variants that have clinically deleterious functional consequences. The argument is semantic and contextual: regardless of nomenclature, single base substitutions should be considered as one form of genetic variation that arises through shared mechanisms, whose frequency distribution and functional significance are determined by genomic location and population genetic effects.

Single nucleotide substitutions probably arise through several distinct mechanisms, of which CpG-mediated cytosine deamination and single-base slip mispairing are the two most important. 5-methylated cytosine is susceptible to demethylation and tautomeric shift with subsequent transformation to thymine.[103] Cytosine positioned 5′ to guanine (CpG) is commonly methylated and as a result is frequently observed as the site of single-base substitution, and is a major source of variation (representing approximately one third of all variation).[98,104,105] This phenomenon provides a partial explanation for the substantial overrepresentation of transition substitutions (pyrimidine to pyrimidine and purine to purine) compared to transversions (pyrimidine–purine changes). While cytosine deamination is an important source of these biases, it is probable that additional mechanisms are also responsible given that transition substitutions are also more frequent at non-CpG sites.

A second common mechanism for substitution is replicative misincorportation of nucleotides by DNA polymerase.[106,107] The major mechanism for nucleotide misincorporation is thought to be single-base slip-mispairing, similar to that observed with short tandem repeat variability.[107–109] Support for this mechanism comes from the observation that there is an overrepresentation of substitutions by nucleotide complementary to the adjacent base position.[105] This mechanism probably also explains insertion/deletion creation. Although these two mechanisms are most common, others are probably also important, including errors in DNA repair machinery, and direct isotopic and chemical mutagenesis.

### INSERTION/DELETION POLYMORPHISM

A subset of common small-scale variation is the indel – a polymorphic site of insertion or deletion of one or more nucleotides. Indels are distributed throughout the genome and represent approximately 18–20 percent of human DNA variation.[110] As in single base substitutions, most indels (particularly insertions) arise through slip-mispairing.[111,112] Based on sequence comparisons with non-human primates, it is estimated that most indels result from deletional mutation, with an observed insertion:deletion ratio of 1:4.[110] Moreover, it appears that the vast majority of human indels arose following human divergence from other primates, as most (>99 percent) indel loci are monomorphic in apes.[110] Most indels range in length between one and four nucleotides, of which the vast majority are one nucleotide. Unless situated at the most 3′ end of a gene, indels situated in coding regions typically result in frameshift mutations, often with radical alterations in protein structure (typically truncation) and function. That these variants more greatly impair gene function than SNPs can be inferred by their over-representation (30 percent) in the Human Gene Mutation Database.[113] While most of these pathogenic indels result in frameshift mutations, 3 and 6 nt repeats can have pathogenic consequences despite maintaining normal reading frames. The most common mutation in cystic fibrosis, a 3 nucleotide (CTT) deletion at codon 508 of the CFTR gene, results in deletion of phenylalanine residue 508, situated in one of the two nucleotide-binding folds, and results in improper trafficking of mature CFTR to the cell surface.[114–116] This mutation has a carrier frequency of 1 in 25 European Caucasians, and is responsible for 70 percent of cystic fibrosis cases in people of this ancestry. Substantially larger indels have been implicated in human disease, including a 32 base pair deletion in the coding region of chemokine-receptor 5 (CCR5), a T-cell surface receptor which serves as a co-receptor for HIV transfection. The delta32 CCR5 deletion is observed in 16 percent of Caucasians. By impairing normal CCR5 function, this variant substantially impairs HIV infection of T cells,

protecting delta32 homozygotes from HIV infection, and slowing the rate of disease progression among heterozygote carriers.[117–119]

## SNP genotyping

A wide choice of genotyping methodologies is available to investigators. Many of these are well suited for small-scale projects, where a limited number of samples and loci are evaluated. However, for larger-scale studies that are required in complex disease gene mapping, high-throughput systems are needed that minimize DNA and time requirements, as well as cost. Several approaches have been used to achieve these goals. PCR reaction volumes have been reduced to 0.5–5 µL, significantly reducing Taq polymerase amounts (the most expensive reaction component). Sample processing and genotyping-reaction time requirements can be shortened at three stages: (1) assay optimization (by reducing the stringency of reaction conditions); (2) assay reaction time (by reducing the number of reaction steps and assay manipulations); and (3) data extraction and analysis (by developing automated assay detection systems with bioinformatic interfaces). One approach to achieve all of these goals is the development of large-scale multiplex reactions, whereby multiple loci are simultaneously evaluated in one reaction, in one tube or well. As a result, the amount of DNA expended, reagent costs, and time costs are reduced proportional to the number of assays plexed together. Maximizing plex size is a major focus of ongoing research and development. In general, the critical limitation in maximizing plex size is not in increasing the number of PCR reactions that can be pooled (now numbering more than 2000 with some platforms), but rather in the subsequent separation and differentiation of the individual assays. Two approaches to assay separation are currently available: (1) length-based discrimination and (2) solid-phase separation. In length-polymorphism based methods, assays are separated based on the length of oligonucleotides generated. PCR primers are tagged with oligonucleotides of varying length (with each SNP-specific assay assigned a different length tag), which can then be separated either with electrophoresis or mass spectrometry (see below). Using this technique, up to 50-plex reactions have been reported, with 4–7 plex reactions now routinely being performed. In solid phase separation, assays are separated via secondary hybridization of assay products to short oligonucleotides (or antibodies) fixed to predetermined sites on a solid matrix (typically chips, slides, or beads).[120,121] Alternatively, the assay-specific oligonucleotides are embedded on the solid array, and the allele-discriminating reactions take place locally. Platforms using this approach (AffiCHIP, Orchid, Illumina) are capable of separating thousands of assays, with the promise of increasing throughput by several orders of magnitude. Methods using a solid-phase approach are becoming increasingly flexible and affordable, and are among the methods preferred for large-scale high-resolution fine-mapping projects.[122]

## GENOTYPING ASSAYS AND PLATFORMS

Unlike the limited number of well-accepted, robust methods for genotyping STR polymorphisms, there are numerous platforms commercially available for SNP genotyping. These platforms differ in the type of assay used and their methods of assay detection, which translate into important differences in their capacity for reliable assay development and reaction optimization, capacity for multiplexing, and efficient automation and bioinformatic interface. Despite their differences, virtually all assays are PCR-based, and can generally be grouped into one of five types: (a) enzymatic digestion/cleavage reactions; (b) probe hybridization; (c) primer hybridization; (d) primer extension/minisequencing

reactions; and (e) ligation reactions. Each method has unique advantages and limitations, relating to equipment requirements, flexibility, and capacity for high-throughput applications. While all have been successfully adapted for large-scale projects, primer extension-based methods have been more amenable for multiplexing, as have new methods that combine primer extension reactions with DNA ligation (e.g., Perlegen and Illumina).

## ENZYMATIC DIGESTION AND RESTRICTION FRAGMENT LENGTH POLYMORPHISM

Restriction digest enzymes are proteins of typically bacterial origin that recognize and cut specific DNA sequences. The recognized sequences are typically 4–8 bases long, and are often palindromic (i.e., GGTCC – see Fig. 4B.4). The distribution of these sites along the genome is random and

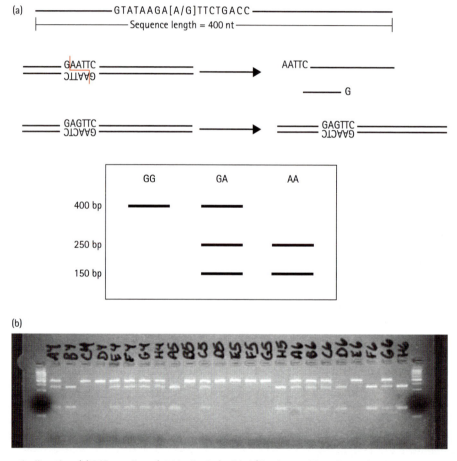

**Figure 4B.4** *Enzymatic digestion. (a) PCR amplicon (400 bp in size) with A/G polymorphism situated at base pair position 250. The variant is situated within the 6-base palindrome GAATTC. Presence of the A allele results in sequence recognition and cleavage by restriction enzyme EcoRI into two fragments of 250 and 150 bp. Presence of the G allele alters the palindrome, thereby preventing digestion. Digestion patterns are then evaluated by electrophoresis, with banding patterns corresponding to fragments. (b) RFLP analysis of CD14 promoter polymorphism with AvaII restriction enzyme. PCR amplicons were treated with AvaII restriction enzyme, which recognizes the palindrome sequence GGTCC, present only on − 159 T chromosomes. PCR products were incubated for 2 h at 37°C and run on a 3.5 percent agarose gel at 120 volts for 1.5 h. Undigested amplicons bearing the C allele migrate to 497 bp (for example, lanes C4 and D4, homozygotes CC), while digested amplicons bearing the T allele show bands at 144 and 353 bp (for example, lanes B4 and A5, TT homozygotes). CT heterozygotes display three bands (for example, lanes F4 and G4), at 144, 353, and 497 bp.*

directly proportional to the power of sequence length. For example, a 4-base sequence will on average be represented once every 256 nucleotides ($4^4$), and a six-base cutter every 4096 bases ($4^6$). Nucleotide variations present within these recognition sites typically alter the restriction enzyme's ability to cleave the sequence, thereby altering the digestion patterns of fragments separated on electrophoretic gel. Restriction fragment length polymorphism (RFLP) quickly gained widespread use with the availability of numerous restriction enzymes and the realization that polymorphic cleavage sites are widely dispersed across the genome.[123] The major advantage of RLFP over all other methods is the lack of sophisticated equipment for the platform, requiring only a thermocycler for PCR and enzyme incubation and an electrophoresis apparatus, and the availability of relatively inexpensive restriction enzymes. The technique requires minimal technical expertise and difficulties in assay optimization are unusual. There are, however, several important disadvantages to RFLP that make it undesirable for large-scale genotyping, including the need for manual allele calling, lack of bioinformatic interface, and long digestion reaction times to avoid incomplete enzymatic digestion. It is also not possible to interrogate sequence variants that do not reside within recognized restriction sites. Nevertheless, RFLP remains an important tool for small-scale genotyping projects. In addition, enzymatic digestion remains one of the few methods readily available for molecular haplotyping.

## ALLELE-SPECIFIC OLIGONUCLEOTIDE PROBE HYBRIDIZATION

In probe hybridization methods, two oligonucleotides are designed that are each complementary to one of the two alleles and the flanking sequence at a polymorphic site. The probes compete for hybridization to target DNA under stringent reaction conditions, whereby only one of the probes binds its corresponding polymorphic amplicon. Hybridization has been adapted to both solid- and liquid-phase formats. In solid phase, probes representing thousands of loci are arrayed in fixed positions on glass slides, and labeled target DNA binds to their allele-specific sites (Fig. 4B.5). Because noncomplementary targets do not bind, allelic discrimination can be reliably determined for thousands of loci simultaneously by knowing the precise location of each probe.[124] The major advantage of the solid phase method is the high throughput capacity. When a more limited number of loci are to be evaluated, liquid-phase homogenous assays are more appropriate.[125,126] In the most popular application of this technology (the 3′ exonuclease assay – TaqMAN), probes are modified to carry two fluorophores: a reporter and a quencher (Fig. 4B.5). Upon laser excitation, the reporter fluorophore emits fluorescence that can be measured quantitatively to distinguish the allele-specific probes. In contrast, the quencher fluorophore is modified to capture the fluorescent energy from the reporter through fluorescence resonance energy transfer (FRET). When in close proximity (i.e., on the same oligonucleotide probe), the fluorescence emitted by the reporter element is transferred to the quencher, thereby preventing detection of fluorescence when analyzed using a fluorimeter. These probes are included in the PCR reaction mix, and hybridize competitively to the amplified targets during the PCR annealing step. During the PCR primer extension, the probe is digested (its component nucleotides are liberated into solution) by the 3′ exonuclease function of Taq polymerase. As a result of this digestion, the reporter and quencher are separated, preventing FRET-mediated inhibition of the reporter fluorescence, and the allele-specific fluorescent spectrum is detectable in solution. Only hybridized probe is digested, allowing for discrimination of SNP allele status. Unlike most other genotyping platforms available, the 3′ exonuclease assay is a homogenous single-step system (one 3 h reaction), making it highly amenable high-throughput typing. Accuracy of allelic discrimination can also be enhanced using fluorescence polarization.[127] The relatively low start-up costs for the fluorescence-detection systems, recent advances in reducing reaction volumes and enhancing hybridization using minor groove binders, and the ease of performing a single-step closed-tube reaction have made this platform one of the most commonly used by moderate-size genotyping laboratories. A similar platform also employing a closed-tube system has been developed using probes with complex stem-loop structures.[126] Unfortunately, due to the cost of individual probe design, per-SNP reagent costs remain relatively high (approximately 30 cents per genotype) for both platforms, limiting their use in very large-scale projects. In addition, assay set-up can require significant optimization time to ensure good separation of the three-genotype spectral outputs.

## ALLELE-SPECIFIC PRIMER HYBRIDIZATION

In this method, allelic discrimination is determined by the formation of allele-specific PCR products. In this reaction, three PCR primers are designed: two forward primers with the most 3′ nucleotide complementary to each of the two SNP alleles, and a third common reverse primer. Because of the specificity of each forward primer for only one of the two SNP alleles, only the allele-specific primer can successfully be extended, resulting in allele-specific PCR product formation. Several methods for distinguishing the allele-specific PCR products have been devised, including fluorescent tagging, ligation techniques or melting curve profile analysis.[128–131] As in the probe-hybridization platforms, the requirement for relatively stringent reaction conditions mandates significant set-up time for assay-specific optimization, reducing its usefulness as a principal high-throughput platform. Adaptation of this technique, incorporating a secondary ligase reaction, has been developed with promising results.[132]

(a)    Target single nucleotide polymorphism

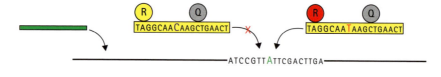

Primer annealing and competitive hybridization of complementary molecular probes

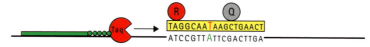

PCR extension reaction with Taq polymerase 3' exonuclease activity

Probe digestion and reporter fluorophore liberation

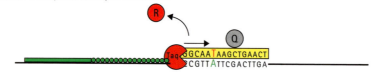

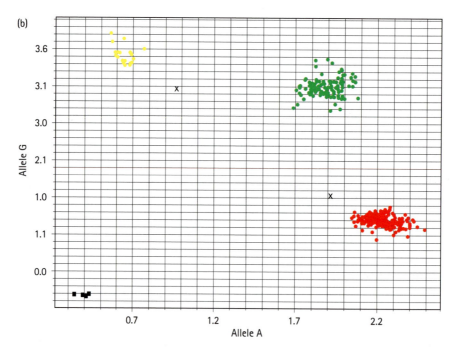

**Figure 4B.5**    *Probe-hybridization genotyping. (a) 2-probe set targeting A/G polymorphism designed to be complementary to allelic forms of locus. Probes are modified with reporter (yellow for G-complement probe, red for A-complement probe) and quencher (grey) fluorophores. While approximated, quencher absorbs reporter fluorescence by FRET. Repetitive PCR cycles result in probe-target hybridization and subsequent probe digestion by the 3' exonuclease function of Taq Polymerase. Only bound (i.e., complementary) probe is digested, resulting in liberation of reporter fluorophore into reaction solution. Upon stimulation, liberated reporter molecules emit fluorescence. Samples carrying G alleles would demonstrate digestion of 'G' probes (not shown). (b) Genotype scatter plot. VIC and FAM fluorescence intensities plotted on X and Y axes, respectively. AA homozygotes (red) localize to right lower quadrant, corresponding to high VIC and low FAM fluorescence. GG homozygotes (yellow) localize to left upper quadrant, corresponding to high FAM and low VIC fluorescence. Heterozygotes (green), manifesting equal amounts of VIC and FAM fluorescence, localize to right upper quadrant. Negative control water samples, exhibiting little or no amplification, localize to left lower quadrant (black squares). Poorly segregating samples (X) plotted between genotype clusters are not called.*

## PRIMER EXTENSION/MINISEQUENCING REACTIONS

Primer extension reactions are widely used in a variety of allele detection platforms owing to their flexibility and adaptability. In these reactions, PCR-generated amplicons that include the target locus serve as a template for an internal primer that binds 5' adjacent to the SNP location. The extension reactions can be allele-specific, where two internal primers that are complementary at their most 3' position with the variant allele extend only when they bind to their corresponding allele, similar to the allele-specific PCR-based methods above.[133] More typically, however, only one internal primer is designed that binds to the target sequence immediately 5' to the variant allele, with primer extension beginning by incorporation of the variant allele. The reaction mix is modified to contain dideoxynucleotides, which result in chain-termination when incorporated in the growing oligonucleotide chain. A variety of detection systems have been developed, including those that can identify labeled terminating nucleotides by fluorescent labels,[134] fluorescence polarization,[135] or hapten labels,[136] or those that differentiate nucleotide mass by mass spectrometry.[137,138] Mini-sequencing reactions have several important advantages over the other methodologies previously described. Typically, they do not require significant modification of the synthetic oligonucleotides, reducing assay-design costs. Because the reactions are not competitive, stringent assay-specific conditions are not required, typically resulting in less optimization time. In addition, minisequencing reactions are highly amenable to multiplexing; reactions performed in multiplex can be distinguished from each other by modifying the 5' end of the internal minisequencing primer with assay-specific tags that can either be separated by hybridization to solid phase or by size-separation using length-tagging. Microarray-based single base extension has also been developed, which can simultaneously differentiate thousands of loci.[139,140] These newer methods are significantly more accurate than their solid-phase probe hybridization counterparts.[140] As a result, minisequencing has been the most widely applied biochemical reaction in currently available platforms.

## LIGATION ASSAYS

Oligonucleotides hybridized to adjacent sites on target DNA can be joined together to form one contiguous strand by DNA ligase. The ligase enzyme is highly specific, and sensitive to mispriming.[141,142] Moreover, ligation can be performed using unamplified genomic DNA as a template using a variety of complex molecular probes, including padlock probes[143] and circularized molecules.[142] These features make ligase-based assays attractive for multiplexing. Ligation products can be separated either by electrophoresis or on solid media. An interesting adaptation has been the combination of ligation and single-base extension, as implemented in several genotyping platforms such as the Illumina Bead-Array and Parallele MegAllele

platforms.[144,145] The high multiplex capacity of these platforms (1500 to 20 000 assays in parallel) with resultant reduction in genotyping cost and dramatic increase in throughput capacity lends these platforms to large-scale SNP surveys.

## DNA POOLING

In case–control genetic association studies, allele frequencies are compared across populations of affected individuals (cases) and unaffected controls, with the expectation that disease-susceptibility variants will be over-represented among cases. Despite advances in SNP genotyping technology, and the availability of high throughput genotyping methods at relatively low cost (10–20 cents per SNP), large-scale projects of thousands of SNPs in thousands of individual samples remain quite expensive. An alternative approach to individual sample genotyping that is gaining increasing acceptance involves the use of DNA pooling.[146] In this approach, equimolar amounts of DNA from individual samples contribute to large DNA pools, from which allele frequency estimates across samples can then be performed. Because each individual should in theory contribute equal numbers of chromosomes to the pool, the relative proportion of each allele in the pooled samples should reflect the allele frequency in the individual samples from which the pools were generated. In simple case–control association study designs, only two pools (cases and controls) are constructed and evaluated. The cost savings (financial, DNA loss, and time) are directly proportional to the original sample size and inversely related to the number of pools generated. For example, using a pooling approach with two pools, each composed of 1000 individual samples (1000 cases and 1000 healthy controls) and each sampled once per SNP tested, 1000 SNPs could be screened at the cost of typing only one of the SNPs in all 2000 individual samples. More complex designs, using multiple pools stratified by gender, ethnicity, age, or environmental exposures have also been described,[147] as have family-based pooling methods.[148,149]

Numerous genotyping platforms have been adapted for DNA pooling, including methods for typing either microsatellite or SNP markers. The critical requirement for any platform is that it is quantitative; that is, it has the capability of accurately quantifying the relative contribution of each allele within pools. In general, methods that are purely qualitative (allele is present or absent) are not suitable for use in evaluating pools. This quantitative nature of the platform deems that all three stages of the genotyping protocol (initial PCR, allelic interrogation, and signal detection) are stable and reproducible across specimens. Although many systems have been adapted for quantitative fluorescence-based assays, mass spectroscopy and array-based methods appear to have greatest accuracy and throughput capacity, and more integrated bioinformatics support.[150–152]

The earliest applications of pooling-based genotyping centered on screening for regional homozygosity in Mendelian traits exhibiting autosomal recessive patterns of inheritance. This method is most powerful in consanguineous pedigrees or genetic isolates, where homozygosity at the disease locus is highly probable given the increased probability that disease alleles are identical by descent. Because pooling strategies make feasible the evaluation of thousands of SNPs, there is increasing use of this methodology to perform regional fine-mapping association studies[153] as well as genome-wide association studies in complex traits.[154,155] As an illustration of the potential for pool genotyping in complex trait mapping, Herbon and colleagues generated pools from individuals with Crohn's disease, schizophrenia, type 1 diabetes, and asthma, as well as healthy controls, and genotyped 534 SNPs across a 25-Mb region on chromosome 6p21 that has been linked to all four diseases.[156] Ten polymorphisms demonstrated significant differences ($P$ values $10^{-4}$–$10^{-9}$) in allele frequency in the disease pools compared to the control pool, including several for asthma.

Despite the potential cost savings and the rapidity with which pooling experiments can be performed, there are several important caveats in the use of pooling. The major reservation to adopting pooling as a primary gene finding strategy has been the loss of power associated with using indirect estimates of allele frequency rather than typing individual samples. Although genotyping errors are also a source of both false discovery rate inflation and loss of power in individual genotyping studies, the impact of measurement error in pooling experiments appears to be much greater, and is dependent on the underlying genetic model. Experimental error can be introduced at two levels: pool construction and allelic measurement.[157] Ensuring precise allele frequency estimation requires careful attention to pool construction, including accurate quantification of individual sample DNA concentration prior to pooling, and the use of large volumes from each sample to avoid pipetting error. Generation of multiple replicate pools consisting of the same individuals, or generating multiple smaller pools (each with a unique set of individuals), are two additional means for reducing and assessing pool construction error. Measurement error inherent to the platform used can also reduce statistical power. The standard measurement error varies across platforms and laboratories, and should be estimated using calibration pools prior to initiating large-scale projects. Small increases in this measurement error can radically diminish statistical power. Several technologies appear to have smaller inherent error, and are probably more robust for large-scale pooling projects. One method to reduce pool measurement error (and to continuously monitor the accuracy of the platform) is to genotype multiple replicates of each pool. Although adding cost, it is suggested that at least 4–16

replicates be performed per pool, so as to reduce measurement error sufficiently. Despite this, it is clear that in most laboratories there remains a significant loss of efficiency from pooling, particularly for genetic variants with relatively low minor allele frequencies ($<0.10$). In this range, statistical power is dramatically reduced when using a pooling strategy, even when measurement error is relatively low.[146,150] An additional consideration is that some assays exhibit differential amplification of alleles during PCR due to regional sequence-specific conformational changes, hybridization affinities, and nucleotide incorporation rates. Failure to adjust for this differential amplification, which can be observed by genotyping individual heterozygotes, can result in biased estimates of allele frequency differences. To obtain unbiased allele frequency estimates, the degree of differential amplification should be included as a correction factor (see Le Hellard et al.[150]). Screening of a random sample of individuals to identify heterozygotes adds additional genotyping cost.

The second major limitation of DNA pooling is that the loss of information at the level of the individual makes analysis of haplotypic association, gene-by-environment interactions, and quantitative trait locus mapping significantly more challenging. Haplotype-based association studies in very large pools are not possible because allelic-phase is not discernible. Methods have been proposed to address this concern by using mini-pools of 5–10 individuals,[158–160] but this greatly reduces the time and cost savings of pooling-based strategies. Evaluation of quantitative trait loci is also problematic for similar reasons. Strategies to evaluate quantitative trait loci (QTLs) in pools include using pools of individuals at the extremes of the trait distribution, or generating multiple pools of incremental trait values.[161] Adjustment for known covariates and evaluation for gene-by-environment interactions is also not feasible without increasing the number of pools considerably. As a result, investigators must determine which, if any, of these design issues is most important, as high-order combinations are not realistic. Finally, it is clear that because of the potential sources of error, DNA pooling should be used primarily as a screening technique, whereby positive results are then confirmed both by individual genotyping, adjusting for covariates, and by replicating results in additional populations. Published reports of significant disease association based solely on pooling studies should be interpreted with caution.

## QUALITY CONTROL

Genotyping error is a critical obstacle that must be carefully addressed in genetic linkage and association studies. The quality and completeness of the genotyping data can impact studies in several ways, and genotyping error may be an underappreciated cause of false-positive and false-negative claims of genetic association. The two broad types of genotyping error include missing data and incorrect genotype call (miscalls). Missing data directly impact statistical power, by reducing the effective sample size. Missing data also impact haplotype analysis, particularly as the number of loci analyzed increases. Miscalled genotypes are also quite deleterious. In linkage analysis, unrecognized errors will inflate marker recombination rates, weakening evidence for linkage and broadening linkage support intervals. In case–control genetic association studies, miscalling error will typically bias towards the null. False-positive association in family-based studies can occur due to miscalling errors, which often provides evidence of overtransmission of the common allele from parents to affected offspring.[162]

Although newer methodologies have greatly improved genotyping completion rates and miscalling error rates, such errors remain an important consideration in all laboratories. Assessing genotype quality is often difficult, and systematic errors can often go unrecognized, particularly in the high-throughput setting. Whereas in small samples, repeat typing of the cohort with secondary methods (such as RFLP) are easily performed to insure reproducibility, repeat typing of multiple SNPs in large-scale studies is often not feasible. As a result, great care should be placed on assay optimization, with emphasis placed on reliable separation of genotypes. Rigorous protocols for quality assurance should be implemented in each laboratory, with only those markers and DNA samples with the highest quality included in subsequent analysis. Negative and positive control samples should be included on all plates to assess for evidence of contamination, assay stability, and correct plate orientation. The latter is achieved by spotting the negative and positive controls in predetermined locations on all plates, and confirming the correct location on subsequent analysis. By using two negative controls placed in different locations on each plate, plate signatures can be established to avoid sample mix up. Standard features of adequate assay performance include high genotype completion rates and low between-run discordances of repeated samples. In our laboratory, we routinely repeat genotyping on a random subset of the cohort (approximately 10 percent). Ideally, this should be performed with

**Table 4B.2** *Methods for evaluating genotyping quality control*

| Characteristic | Method of assessment | Comments |
| --- | --- | --- |
| Plate orientation and identification | Confirm well positions of both negative and positive controls | Pattern of well distribution for negative and positive controls should uniquely identify each plate in study and its orientation |
| Well contamination | Negative water controls | Genotype data in negative control suggest cross-contamination of plates |
| Genotype completion rates | Percent missing data | Minimum 95% completion, particularly for haplotype-based analysis |
| | Distribution of missing data | Assess missingness in context of DNA plate layout, family structure, and genotype at surrounding loci to assess for patterns of nonrandom missing data |
| Reproducibility | Repeat genotyping of sample subset to assess concordancy. Ideally use alternate genotyping platform | Even low levels of discordancy (i.e., less than 1%) may indicate important genotype errors. To ensure adequate power for detection of low discordancy rates repeat sample should be of sufficient size |
| Genotype distribution | Hardy–Weinberg equilibrium | Most suitable for control population in case–control studies. May be inappropriate in family-based analysis depending on method of ascertainment |
| Allelic transmission inconsistent with Mendelian inheritance | PEDCHECK[163] | Genotype error detection rates using patterns of inheritance estimated at 51–77% for multiallelic markers and 13–75% for biallelic markers[166] |
| Familial relationships | RELPAIR,[167] PREST,[168] GRR[169] | Non-paternity and misspecified familial relationships are frequently observed in large family-based studies. Power increases with number of markers tested and decays with more distant relative pair comparisons |

a different genotyping platform, although that may not always be practical. Assays that demonstrate a high degree of discordance should be considered unreliable and not analyzed. For very large projects, where hundreds or thousands of SNPs are screened simultaneously, it is advisable to select a subset for repeat genotyping on the entire cohort (ideally using a different genotyping platform), particularly those demonstrating positive results. For platforms with quantitative properties, plots of genotype data should form distinct clusters that can be easily distinguished from each other (see Fig. 4B.5). Once assay stability has been assured, secondary quality control analysis should be performed (Table 4B.2). This includes assessing for evidence of Hardy–Weinberg equilibrium (HWE), particularly in the control group, for case–control designs. HWE should be observed at most loci in outbred populations. Although deviations from random mating assumptions can also lead to the absence of HWE, significant evidence of HW disequilibrium also raises concerns about biased assay performance. Even in the face of good assay performance, evidence of HW disequilibrium among controls may represent undetected population substructure or biased control population ascertainment, and complicate genetic association analyses. Analysis of HWE among samples ascertained on disease status (i.e., case populations) is less helpful, as deviation from HWE may represent true disease-marker associations rather than systematic errors in marker typing. It must be emphasized that the usefulness of HWE as a screen for genotyping error is limited, particularly in small samples that are underpowered to detect significant within-sample deviations from HWE. Similarly, the usefulness of HWE among parental genotypes as a screen for genotyping error in family-based studies is also of limited value, as families ascertained on disease status may demonstrate disequilibrium at or near disease loci. For family-based studies, unrecognized genotyping error can be detected by examining for pedigree inconsistencies in allelic transmission. Several algorithms are available for this type of analysis, usually providing reports of problematic pedigrees.[163] Other analytical packages are available to verify familial relationships from available genetic data, so as to identify unreported non-paternity, adoption, data entry errors, or in-house sample mix up.[164,165]

## CONCLUSIONS

There are a variety of genotyping platforms now available for moderate-to large-scale projects, and studies using this technology are now commonplace. Although many of the more advanced platforms require significant infrastructure support (both with respect to spatial considerations, technical support, and financial investments), many universities are now developing core high-throughput genotyping facilities, available for investigators to use. Alternatively, many companies now offer off-site genotyping services for large-scale projects. Because the primary investigators who use these services are often disengaged from the actual genotyping, it is of utmost importance that they familiarize themselves with the pitfalls of the platform being used for their studies, and make a concerted effort to assess for systematic genotyping errors and incomplete data collection. Laudable and certainly foreseeable, the focus of much research and development is to create tools that permit individual genome-wide resequencing and genotyping at very low cost.

## Key learning points

- Virtually all heritable phenotypic variation results from the subset of genetic polymorphism that interferes with normal gene function or regulation. The primary aim of human genetic research is to identify this functional subset, and correlate genetic variants with their phenotypic outcomes.

- Large size chromosomal abnormalities, including trisomy, monosomy, chromosomal translocations and inversions, and interstitial deletions, result either from errors in chromosome recombination or aberrant chromosomal migration and segregation, and are frequently implicated in rare genetic syndromes. These abnormalities can be detected by karyotyping and fluorescence in situ hybridization (FISH). Common large-scale segmental duplications and deletions have recently been recognized as a potential cause of common disease, and can be evaluated using comparative genomic hybridization (CGH) arrays.

- Single nucleotide variation is the most common type of human polymorphism and is responsible for most heritable variation. The majority of disease-related variants identified to date are coding polymorphisms, particularly for monogenic disorders. It is anticipated that non-coding regulatory variation represents a substantially larger proportion of pathogenic variation in complex disease, although the difficulties in recognizing such regulatory variation have limited their identification.

- The polymerase chain reaction (PCR) is the cornerstone of all current polymorphism discovery and genotyping technologies, as it enables the amplification and evaluation of targeted genomic regions at the exclusion of non-target genome. The reaction is robust, but sensitive to contamination.

- Methods for point variation discovery can be classified as either indirect or direct. Indirect methods including SSCP, DDGE, DHPLC, and DNA cleavage assays are used to screen for variation, but rarely can be used to identify precise nucleotide changes. Direct screening using fluorescence-based sequencing chemistry permits direct visualization of polymorphic variation. These methods have been adapted for high-throughput screening. Sample sizes for SNP discovery should be sufficiently large to ensure statistical power to detect variation at lower frequency.

- Highly polymorphic short tandem repeat (STR) marker genotyping using labeled PCR primers provide high information content and is therefore favored for family-based linkage studies. Rarely, these markers are pathogenic, particularly in disease states exhibiting genetic anticipation (i.e., myotonic dystrophy).

- Numerous platforms are available for single nucleotide polymorphism genotyping. Most are well suited for small-scale projects, while a limited (but ever growing) number of platforms is available for larger-scale studies, as required for complex disease gene mapping. High-throughput systems should minimize DNA and time requirements, reduce per-genotype costs, and have automated allele calling and strong bioinformatics support.

- DNA pooling is gaining increasing acceptance for comparing allele frequencies in large case-control studies. While reducing per-locus genotyping costs, results from such studies should be validated by individual genotyping due to inaccuracies in DNA quantitation and allele frequency estimation errors. Pooling is less efficient for studies of quantitative traits.

- Quality control measures are essential to reduce the impact of genotyping error in genetic studies. High completion rates, evidence of genotype reproducibility, and the use of negative and positive controls are very useful for identifying poorly performing assays. Deviations from Hardy–Weinberg equilibrium among control subjects or evidence of non-Mendelian patterns of inheritance suggest poor marker performance. Non-paternity and misclassification of familial relationships are common in genetic studies and can be identified using genotype data from markers distributed throughout the genome.

# REFERENCES

1 Kristoffersson U, Heim S, Mandahl N et al. Monosomy and trisomy of 15q24–qter in a family with a translocation t(6;15)(p25;q24). Clin Genet 1987; 32: 169–71.
2 Tachdjian G, Fondacci C, Tapia S et al. The Wolf–Hirschhorn syndrome in fetuses. Clin Genet 1992; 42: 281–7.
3 Hofbeck M, Leipold G, Rauch A et al. Clinical relevance of monosomy 22q11.2 in children with pulmonary atresia and ventricular septal defect. Eur J Pediatr 1999; 158: 302–7.
4 Puvabanditsin S, Garrow E, Zia-Ullah MO et al. Monosomy 11Q: report of new phenotypic manifestations. Genet Couns 2001; 12: 283–6.
5 Kramer BW, Martin T, Henn W et al. Lung hypoplasia in a patient with del(2)(q33–q35) demonstrated by chromosome microdissection. Am J Med Genet 2000; 94: 184–8.
6 Cools J, DeAngelo DJ, Gotlib J et al. A tyrosine kinase created by fusion of the PDGFRA and FIP1L1 genes as a therapeutic target of imatinib in idiopathic hypereosinophilic syndrome. N Engl J Med 2003; 348: 1201–14.
7 Griffin JH, Leung J, Bruner RJ et al. Discovery of a fusion kinase in EOL-1 cells and idiopathic hypereosinophilic syndrome. Proc Natl Acad Sci USA 2003; 100: 7830–5.
8 Higuchi M, Kazazian HH Jr, Kasch L et al. Molecular characterization of severe hemophilia A suggests that about half the mutations are not within the coding regions and splice junctions of the factor VIII gene. Proc Natl Acad Sci USA 1991; 88: 7405–9.
9 Jennings MW, Jones RW, Wood WG, Weatherall DJ. Analysis of an inversion within the human beta globin gene cluster. Nucleic Acids Res 1985; 13: 2897–906.
10 Sebat J, Lakshmi B, Troge J et al. Large-scale copy number polymorphism in the human genome. Science 2004; 305: 525–8.
11 Iafrate AJ, Feuk L, Rivera MN et al. Detection of large-scale variation in the human genome. Nat Genet 2004; 36: 949–51.
12 Hu XY, Ray PN, Worton RG. Mechanisms of tandem duplication in the Duchenne muscular dystrophy gene include both homologous and nonhomologous intrachromosomal recombination. EMBO J 1991; 10: 2471–7.
13 Lau YL, Srivastava G, Wong V et al. Deletions, duplications and novel restriction fragment length polymorphism in Duchenne and Becker muscular dystrophies. Clin Genet 1992; 41: 252–8.
14 Cohn DH, Zhang X, Byers PH. Homology-mediated recombination between type I collagen gene exons results in an internal tandem duplication and lethal osteogenesis imperfecta. Hum Mutat 1993; 2: 21–7.
15 Stoppa-Lyonnet D, Duponchel C, Meo T et al. Recombinational biases in the rearranged C1-inhibitor genes of hereditary angioedema patients. Am J Hum Genet 1991; 49: 1055–62.
16 Van den Berghe H. Letter: The Ph1-chromosome: translocation to chromosome 9. Lancet 1973; 2: 1030–1.
17 Tijo JH, Levan A. The chromosome number of man. Hereditas 1956; 42: 1–6.
18 Hsu T. Mammalian chromosomes in vitro I. J Heredity 1952; 43: 167–72.
19 Morton CC. Cytogenetics. In: Dracopoli NC, Haines JL, Korf BR et al. (eds), Current protocols in human genetics, Vol. 1. New York: John Wiley & Sons, 2003, 4.1.1–17.
20 van Ommen GJ, Breuning MH, Raap AK. FISH in genome research and molecular diagnostics. Curr Opin Genet Dev 1995; 5: 304–8.
21 Trask BJ. Gene mapping by in situ hybridization. Curr Opin Genet Dev 1991; 1: 82–7.
22 Trask BJ. Fluorescence in situ hybridization: applications in cytogenetics and gene mapping. Trends Genet 1991; 7: 149–54.
23 Hirsch FR, Varella-Garcia M, Bunn PA Jr et al. Epidermal growth factor receptor in non-small-cell lung carcinomas: correlation between gene copy number and protein expression and impact on prognosis. J Clin Oncol 2003; 21: 3798–807.
24 Berrieman HK, Ashman JN, Cowen ME et al. Chromosomal analysis of non-small-cell lung cancer by multicolour fluorescent in situ hybridisation. Br J Cancer 2004; 90: 900–5.

25  Nakamura H, Saji H, Idiris A et al. Chromosomal instability detected by fluorescence in situ hybridization in surgical specimens of non-small cell lung cancer is associated with poor survival. *Clin Cancer Res* 2003; **9**: 2294–9.

26  Buys CH, Osinga J, van der Veen AY et al. Genome analysis of small cell lung cancer (SCLC) and clinical significance. *Eur J Respir Dis Suppl* 1987; **149**: 29–36.

27  Kallioniemi OP, Kallioniemi A, Sudar D et al. Comparative genomic hybridization: a rapid new method for detecting and mapping DNA amplification in tumors. *Semin Cancer Biol* 1993; **4**: 41–6.

28  Snijders AM, Nowak N, Segraves R et al. Assembly of microarrays for genome-wide measurement of DNA copy number. *Nat Genet* 2001; **29**: 263–4.

29  Pollack JR, Perou CM, Alizadeh AA et al. Genome-wide analysis of DNA copy-number changes using cDNA microarrays. *Nat Genet* 1999; **23**: 41–6.

30  Lucito R, Healy J, Alexander J et al. Representational oligonucleotide microarray analysis: a high-resolution method to detect genome copy number variation. *Genome Res* 2003; **13**: 2291–305.

31  Taguchi T, Cheng GZ, Bell DW et al. Combined chromosome microdissection and comparative genomic hybridization detect multiple sites of amplification DNA in a human lung carcinoma cell line. *Genes Chromosomes Cancer* 1997; **20**: 208–12.

32  Li J, Jiang T, Mao JH et al. Genomic segmental polymorphisms in inbred mouse strains. *Nat Genet* 2004; **36**: 952–4.

33  Saiki RK, Scharf S, Faloona F et al. Enzymatic amplification of beta-globin genomic sequences and restriction site analysis for diagnosis of sickle cell anemia. *Science* 1985; **230**: 1350–4.

34  Li HH, Gyllensten UB, Cui XF et al. Amplification and analysis of DNA sequences in single human sperm and diploid cells. *Nature* 1988; **335**: 414–17.

35  Cimbora DM, Schubeler D, Reik A et al. Long-distance control of origin choice and replication timing in the human beta-globin locus are independent of the locus control region. *Mol Cell Biol* 2000; **20**: 5581–91.

36  Horikawa Y, Oda N, Cox N et al. Genetic variation in the gene encoding calpain-10 is associated with type 2 diabetes mellitus. *Nat Genet* 2000; **26**: 163–75.

37  Kruglyak L, Nickerson DA. Variation is the spice of life. *Nat Genet* 2001; **27**: 234–6.

38  Fischer SG, Lerman LS. DNA fragments differing by single base-pair substitutions are separated in denaturing gradient gels: correspondence with melting theory. *Proc Natl Acad Sci USA* 1983; **80**: 1579–83.

39  Orita M, Suzuki Y, Sekiya T, Hayashi K. Rapid and sensitive detection of point mutations and DNA polymorphisms using the polymerase chain reaction. *Genomics* 1989; **5**: 874–9.

40  Sheffield VC, Beck JS, Kwitek AE et al. The sensitivity of single-strand conformation polymorphism analysis for the detection of single base substitutions. *Genomics* 1993; **16**: 325–32.

41  Inazuka M, Wenz HM, Sakabe M et al. A streamlined mutation detection system: multicolor post-PCR fluorescence labeling and single-strand conformational polymorphism analysis by capillary electrophoresis. *Genome Res* 1997; **7**: 1094–103.

42  Kuypers AW, Willems PM, van der Schans MJ et al. Detection of point mutations in DNA using capillary electrophoresis in a polymer network. *J Chromatogr* 1993; **621**: 149–56.

43  Liu Q, Sommer SS. Restriction endonuclease fingerprinting (REF): a sensitive method for screening mutations in long, contiguous segments of DNA. *Biotechniques* 1995; **18**: 470–7.

44  Liu Q, Feng J, Sommer SS. Bi-directional dideoxy fingerprinting (Bi-ddF): a rapid method for quantitative detection of mutations in genomic regions of 300-600 bp. *Hum Mol Genet* 1996; **5**: 107–14.

45  Liu Q, Feng J, Sommer SS. In a blinded analysis, restriction endonuclease fingerprinting detects all the mutations in a 1.9-kb segment. *Biotechniques* 1997; **23**: 836–9.

46  Felmlee TA, Liu Q, Whelen AC et al. Genotypic detection of *Mycobacterium tuberculosis* rifampin resistance: comparison of single-strand conformation polymorphism and dideoxy fingerprinting. *J Clin Microbiol* 1995; **33**: 1617–23.

47  White MB, Carvalho M, Derse D et al. Detecting single base substitutions as heteroduplex polymorphisms. *Genomics* 1992; **12**: 301–6.

48  Keen J, Lester D, Inglehearn C et al. Rapid detection of single base mismatches as heteroduplexes on Hydrolink gels. *Trends Genet* 1991; **7**: 5.

49  Fischer SG, Lerman LS. Two-dimensional electrophoretic separation of restriction enzyme fragments of DNA. *Methods Enzymol* 1979; **68**: 183–91.

50  Gelfi C, Cremonesi L, Ferrari M, Righetti PG. Temperature-programmed capillary electrophoresis for detection of DNA point mutations. *Biotechniques* 1996; **21**: 926–8, 930, 932.

51  Oefner PJ, Bonn GK, Huber CG, Nathakarnkitkool S. Comparative study of capillary zone electrophoresis and high-performance liquid chromatography in the analysis of oligonucleotides and DNA. *J Chromatogr* 1992; **625**: 331–40.

52  Xiao W, Oefner PJ. Denaturing high-performance liquid chromatography: A review. *Hum Mutat* 2001; **17**: 439–74.

53  Underhill PA, Jin L, Lin AA et al. Detection of numerous Y chromosome biallelic polymorphisms by denaturing high-performance liquid chromatography. *Genome Res* 1997; **7**: 996–1005.

54  O'Donovan MC, Oefner PJ, Roberts SC et al. Blind analysis of denaturing high-performance liquid chromatography as a tool for mutation detection. *Genomics* 1998; **52**: 44–9.

55  Deng Z, Morse JH, Slager SL et al. Familial primary pulmonary hypertension (gene PPH1) is caused by mutations in the bone morphogenetic protein receptor-II gene. *Am J Hum Genet* 2000; **67**: 737–44.

56  Yoshida N, Nishimaki Y, Sugiyama M et al. SNP genotyping in the beta(2)-adrenergic receptor by electronic microchip assay, DHPLC, and direct sequencing. *J Hum Genet* 2002; **47**: 500–3.

57  Kabesch M, Tzotcheva I, Carr D et al. A complete screening of the IL4 gene: novel polymorphisms and their association with asthma and IgE in childhood. *J Allergy Clin Immunol* 2003; **112**: 893–8.

58  Graves PE, Kabesch M, Halonen M et al. A cluster of seven tightly linked polymorphisms in the IL-13 gene is associated with total serum IgE levels in three populations of white children. *J Allergy Clin Immunol* 2000; **105**: 506–13.

59  Hull J, Ackerman H, Isles K et al. Unusual haplotypic structure of IL8, a susceptibility locus for a common respiratory virus. *Am J Hum Genet* 2001; **69**: 413–19.

60  Baumer A, Wiedemann U, Hergersberg M, Schinzel A. A novel MSP/DHPLC method for the investigation of the methylation

status of imprinted genes enables the molecular detection of low cell mosaicisms. *Hum Mutat* 2001; **17**: 423–30.

61 Hayward-Lester A, Oefner PJ, Sabatini S, Doris PA. Accurate and absolute quantitative measurement of gene expression by single-tube RT-PCR and HPLC. *Genome Res* 1995; **5**: 494–9.

62 Cooksey RC, Morlock GP, Holloway BP et al. Temperature-mediated heteroduplex analysis performed by using denaturing high-performance liquid chromatography to identify sequence polymorphisms in *Mycobacterium tuberculosis* complex organisms. *J Clin Microbiol* 2002; **40**: 1610–16.

63 Cotton RG, Rodrigues NR, Campbell RD. Reactivity of cytosine and thymine in single-base-pair mismatches with hydroxylamine and osmium tetroxide and its application to the study of mutations. *Proc Natl Acad Sci USA* 1988; **85**: 4397–401.

64 Bui CT, Lambrinakos A, Babon JJ, Cotton RG. Chemical cleavage reactions of DNA on solid support: application in mutation detection. *BMC Chem Biol* 2003; **3**: 1.

65 Youil R, Kemper BW, Cotton RG. Screening for mutations by enzyme mismatch cleavage with T4 endonuclease VII. *Proc Natl Acad Sci USA* 1995; **92**: 87–91.

66 Myers RM, Larin Z, Maniatis T. Detection of single base substitutions by ribonuclease cleavage at mismatches in RNA:DNA duplexes. *Science* 1985; **230**: 1242–6.

67 Kwok PY, Carlson C, Yager TD et al. Comparative analysis of human DNA variations by fluorescence-based sequencing of PCR products. *Genomics* 1994; **23**: 138–44.

68 Sanger F, Nicklen S, Coulson AR. DNA sequencing with chain-terminating inhibitors. *Proc Natl Acad Sci USA* 1977; **74**: 5463–7.

69 Nordstrom T, Ronaghi M, Forsberg L et al. Direct analysis of single-nucleotide polymorphism on double-stranded DNA by pyrosequencing. *Biotechnol Appl Biochem* 2000; **31**(Pt 2): 107–12.

70 Ronaghi M, Uhlen M, Nyren P. A sequencing method based on real-time pyrophosphate. *Science* 1998; **281**: 363, 365.

71 Alderborn A, Kristofferson A, Hammerling U. Determination of single-nucleotide polymorphisms by real-time pyrophosphate DNA sequencing. *Genome Res* 2000; **10**: 1249–58.

72 Vieux EF, Kwok PY, Miller RD. Primer design for PCR and sequencing in high-throughput analysis of SNPs. *Biotechniques,* 2002; **Suppl**: 28–30, 32.

73 Poon R, Paddock GV, Heindell H et al. Nucleotide sequence analysis of RNA synthesized from rabbit globin complementary DNA. *Proc Natl Acad Sci USA* 1974; **71**: 3502–6.

74 Chelly J, Kaplan JC, Maire P et al. Transcription of the dystrophin gene in human muscle and non-muscle tissue. *Nature* 1988; **333**: 858–60.

75 Sarkar G, Sommer SS. Access to a messenger RNA sequence or its protein product is not limited by tissue or species specificity. *Science* 1989; **244**: 331–4.

76 Schlotterer C. Evolutionary dynamics of microsatellite DNA. *Chromosoma* 2000; **109**: 365–71.

77 Ellegren H. Microsatellite mutations in the germline: implications for evolutionary inference. *Trends Genet* 2000; **16**: 551–8.

78 Weber JL. Informativeness of human (dC-dA)n.(dG-dT)n polymorphisms. *Genomics* 1990; **7**: 524–30.

79 Edwards A, Civitello A, Hammond HA, Caskey CT. DNA typing and genetic mapping with trimeric and tetrameric tandem repeats. *Am J Hum Genet* 1991; **49**: 746–56.

80 Zhang Y, Leaves NI, Anderson GG et al. Positional cloning of a quantitative trait locus on chromosome 13q14 that influences immunoglobulin E levels and asthma. *Nat Genet* 2003; **34**: 181–6.

81 Allen M, Heinzmann A, Noguchi E et al. Positional cloning of a novel gene influencing asthma from chromosome 2q14. *Nat Genet* 2003; **35**: 258–63.

82 Mahtani MM, Willard HF. A polymorphic X-linked tetranucleotide repeat locus displaying a high rate of new mutation: implications for mechanisms of mutation at short tandem repeat loci. *Hum Mol Genet* 1993; **2**: 431–7.

83 Weber JL, Wong C. Mutation of human short tandem repeats. *Hum Mol Genet* 1993; **2**: 1123–8.

84 Verkerk AJ, Pieretti M, Sutcliffe JS et al. Identification of a gene (FMR-1) containing a CGG repeat coincident with a breakpoint cluster region exhibiting length variation in fragile X syndrome. *Cell* 1991; **65**: 905–14.

85 Buxton J, Shelbourne P, Davies J et al. Detection of an unstable fragment of DNA specific to individuals with myotonic dystrophy. *Nature* 1992; **355**: 547–8.

86 Harley HG, Brook JD, Rundle SA et al. Expansion of an unstable DNA region and phenotypic variation in myotonic dystrophy. *Nature* 1992; **355**: 545–6.

87 The Huntington's Disease Collaborative Research Group. A novel gene containing a trinucleotide repeat that is expanded and unstable on Huntington's disease chromosomes. *Cell* 1993; **72**: 971–83.

88 Lalioti MD, Scott HS, Buresi C et al. Dodecamer repeat expansion in cystatin B gene in progressive myoclonus epilepsy. *Nature* 1997; **386**: 847–51.

89 Muragaki Y, Mundlos S, Upton J, Olsen BR. Altered growth and branching patterns in synpolydactyly caused by mutations in HOXD13. *Science* 1996; **272**: 548–51.

90 Shelbourne P, Winqvist R, Kunert E et al. Unstable DNA may be responsible for the incomplete penetrance of the myotonic dystrophy phenotype. *Hum Mol Genet* 1992; **1**: 467–73.

91 Weber JL, May PE. Abundant class of human DNA polymorphisms which can be typed using the polymerase chain reaction. *Am J Hum Genet* 1989; **44**: 388–96.

92 Litt M, Luty JA. A hypervariable microsatellite revealed by in vitro amplification of a dinucleotide repeat within the cardiac muscle actin gene. *Am J Hum Genet* 1989; **44**: 397–401.

93 Murray JC, Buetow KH, Weber JL et al. A comprehensive human linkage map with centimorgan density. Cooperative Human Linkage Center (CHLC). *Science* 1994; **265**: 2049–54.

94 Broman KW, Murray JC, Sheffield VC et al. Comprehensive human genetic maps: individual and sex-specific variation in recombination. *Am J Hum Genet* 1998; **63**: 861–9.

95 Kong A, Gudbjartsson DF, Sainz J et al. A high-resolution recombination map of the human genome. *Nat Genet* 2002; **31**: 241–7.

96 Chakravarti A. It's raining SNPs, hallelujah? *Nat Genet* 1998; **19**: 216–17.

97 Li WH, Sadler LA. Low nucleotide diversity in man. *Genetics* 1991; **129**: 513–23.

98 Stephens JC, Schneider JA, Tanguay DA et al. Haplotype variation and linkage disequilibrium in 313 human genes. *Science* 2001; **293**: 489–93.

99 Halushka MK, Fan JB, Bentley K et al. Patterns of single-nucleotide polymorphisms in candidate genes for blood-pressure homeostasis. *Nat Genet* 1999; **22**: 239–47.

100 Kondrashov AS. Direct estimates of human per nucleotide mutation rates at 20 loci causing Mendelian diseases. *Hum Mutat* 2003; **21**: 12–27.

101 Nachman MW, Crowell SL. Estimate of the mutation rate per nucleotide in humans. *Genetics* 2000; **156**: 297–304.

102 Giannelli F, Anagnostopoulos T, Green PM. Mutation rates in humans. II. Sporadic mutation-specific rates and rate of detrimental human mutations inferred from hemophilia B. *Am J Hum Genet* 1999; **65**: 1580–7.

103 Rideout WM 3rd, Coetzee GA, Olumi AF, Jones PA. 5-Methylcytosine as an endogenous mutagen in the human LDL receptor and p53 genes. *Science* 1990; **249**: 1288–90.

104 Cargill M, Altshuler D, Ireland J et al. Characterization of single-nucleotide polymorphisms in coding regions of human genes. *Nat Genet* 1999; **22**: 231–8.

105 Krawczak M, Ball EV, Cooper DN. Neighboring-nucleotide effects on the rates of germ-line single-base-pair substitution in human genes. *Am J Hum Genet* 1998; **63**: 474–88.

106 Kunkel TA, Alexander PS. The base substitution fidelity of eucaryotic DNA polymerases. Mispairing frequencies, site preferences, insertion preferences, and base substitution by dislocation. *J Biol Chem* 1986; **261**: 160–6.

107 Kunkel TA. The mutational specificity of DNA polymerase-beta during in vitro DNA synthesis. Production of frameshift, base substitution, and deletion mutations. *J Biol Chem* 1985; **260**: 5787–96.

108 Dover G. Slippery DNA runs on and on and on. *Nat Genet* 1995; **10**: 254–6.

109 Levinson G, Gutman GA. Slipped-strand mispairing: a major mechanism for DNA sequence evolution. *Mol Biol Evol* 1987; **4**: 203–21.

110 Weber JL, David D, Heil J et al. Human diallelic insertion/deletion polymorphisms. *Am J Hum Genet* 2002; **71**: 854–62.

111 Krawczak M, Cooper DN. Gene deletions causing human genetic disease: mechanisms of mutagenesis and the role of the local DNA sequence environment. *Hum Genet* 1991; **86**: 425–41.

112 Taylor MS, Ponting CP, Copley RR. Occurrence and consequences of coding sequence insertions and deletions in mammalian genomes. *Genome Res* 2004; **14**: 555–66.

113 Antonarakis SE, Krawczak M, Cooper DN. Disease-causing mutations in the human genome. *Eur J Pediatr* 2000; **159**(Suppl 3): S173–8.

114 Kerem B, Rommens JM, Buchanan JA et al. Identification of the cystic fibrosis gene: genetic analysis. *Science* 1989; **245**: 1073–80.

115 Riordan JR, Rommens JM, Kerem B et al. Identification of the cystic fibrosis gene: cloning and characterization of complementary DNA. *Science* 1989; **245**: 1066–73.

116 Rommens JM, Zengerling S, Burns J et al. Identification and regional localization of DNA markers on chromosome 7 for the cloning of the cystic fibrosis gene. *Am J Hum Genet* 1988; **43**: 645–63.

117 Liu R, Paxton WA, Choe S et al. Homozygous defect in HIV-1 coreceptor accounts for resistance of some multiply-exposed individuals to HIV-1 infection. *Cell* 1996; **86**: 367–77.

118 Samson M, Libert F, Doranz BJ et al. Resistance to HIV-1 infection in Caucasian individuals bearing mutant alleles of the CCR-5 chemokine receptor gene. *Nature* 1996; **382**: 722–5.

119 Eugen-Olsen J, Iversen AK, Garred P et al. Heterozygosity for a deletion in the CKR-5 gene leads to prolonged AIDS-free survival and slower CD4 T-cell decline in a cohort of HIV-seropositive individuals. *AIDS* 1997; **11**: 305–10.

120 Fan JB, Chen X, Halushka MK et al. Parallel genotyping of human SNPs using generic high-density oligonucleotide tag arrays. *Genome Res* 2000; **10**: 853–60.

121 Chen J, Iannone MA, Li MS et al. A microsphere-based assay for multiplexed single nucleotide polymorphism analysis using single base chain extension. *Genome Res* 2000; **10**: 549–57.

122 The International HapMap Consortium. The International HapMap Project. *Nature* 2003; **426**: 789–96.

123 Botstein D, White RL, Skolnick M, Davis RW. Construction of a genetic linkage map in man using restriction fragment length polymorphisms. *Am J Hum Genet* 1980; **32**: 314–31.

124 Wang DG, Fan JB, Siao CJ et al. Large-scale identification, mapping, and genotyping of single-nucleotide polymorphisms in the human genome. *Science* 1998; **280**: 1077–82.

125 Livak KJ. Allelic discrimination using fluorogenic probes and the 5′ nuclease assay. *Genet Anal* 1999; **14**: 143–9.

126 Kostrikis LG, Tyagi S, Mhlanga MM et al. Spectral genotyping of human alleles. *Science* 1998; **279**: 1228–9.

127 Latif S, Bauer-Sardina I, Ranade K et al. Fluorescence polarization in homogeneous nucleic acid analysis II: 5′-nuclease assay. *Genome Res* 2001; **11**: 436–40.

128 Nazarenko IA, Bhatnagar SK, Hohman RJ. A closed tube format for amplification and detection of DNA based on energy transfer. *Nucleic Acids Res* 1997; **25**: 2516–21.

129 Myakishev MV, Khripin Y, Hu S, Hamer DH. High-throughput SNP genotyping by allele-specific PCR with universal energy-transfer-labeled primers. *Genome Res* 2001; **11**: 163–9.

130 Ye S, Dhillon S, Ke X et al. An efficient procedure for genotyping single nucleotide polymorphisms. *Nucleic Acids Res* 2001; **29**: E88–88.

131 Germer S, Higuchi R. Single-tube genotyping without oligonucleotide probes. *Genome Res* 1999; **9**: 72–78.

132 Mein CA, Barratt BJ, Dunn MG et al. Evaluation of single nucleotide polymorphism typing with invader on PCR amplicons and its automation. *Genome Res* 2000; **10**: 330–43.

133 Pastinen T, Raitio M, Lindroos K et al. A system for specific, high-throughput genotyping by allele-specific primer extension on microarrays. *Genome Res* 2000; **10**: 1031–42.

134 Vanden Haesevelde MM, Peeters M, Jannes G et al. Sequence analysis of a highly divergent HIV-1-related lentivirus isolated from a wild captured chimpanzee. *Virology* 1996; **221**: 346–50.

135 Chen X, Levine L, Kwok PY. Fluorescence polarization in homogeneous nucleic acid analysis. *Genome Res* 1999; **9**: 492–8.

136 Nikiforov TT, Rendle RB, Goelet P et al. Genetic bit analysis: a solid phase method for typing single nucleotide polymorphisms. *Nucleic Acids Res* 1994; **22**: 4167–75.

137 Ross P, Hall L, Smirnov I, Haff L. High level multiplex genotyping by MALDI-TOF mass spectrometry. *Nat Biotechnol* 1998; **16**: 1347–51.

138 Buetow KH, Edmonson M, MacDonald R et al. High-throughput development and characterization of a genomewide collection of gene-based single nucleotide polymorphism markers by chip-based matrix-assisted laser desorption/ionization time-of-flight mass spectrometry. *Proc Natl Acad Sci USA* 2001; **98**: 581–4.

139   Shumaker JM, Metspalu A, Caskey CT. Mutation detection by solid phase primer extension. *Hum Mutat* 1996; **7**: 346–54.

140   Pastinen T, Kurg A, Metspalu A et al. Minisequencing: a specific tool for DNA analysis and diagnostics on oligonucleotide arrays. *Genome Res* 1997; **7**: 606–14.

141   Barany F. Genetic disease detection and DNA amplification using cloned thermostable ligase. *Proc Natl Acad Sci USA* 1991; **88**: 189–93.

142   Lizardi PM, Huang X, Zhu Z et al. Mutation detection and single-molecule counting using isothermal rolling-circle amplification. *Nat Genet* 1998; **19**: 225–32.

143   Nilsson M, Malmgren H, Samiotaki M et al. Padlock probes: circularizing oligonucleotides for localized DNA detection. *Science* 1994; **265**: 2085–8.

144   Oliphant A, Barker DL, Stuelpnagel JR, Chee MS. BeadArray technology: enabling an accurate, cost-effective approach to high-throughput genotyping. *Biotechniques* 2002; **Suppl**: 56–58, 60–61.

145   Hardenbol P, Baner J, Jain M et al. Multiplexed genotyping with sequence-tagged molecular inversion probes. *Nat Biotechnol* 2003; **21**: 673–8.

146   Sham P, Bader JS, Craig I et al. DNA pooling: a tool for large-scale association studies. *Nat Rev Genet* 2002; **3**: 862–71.

147   Weinberg CR, Umbach DM. Using pooled exposure assessment to improve efficiency in case–control studies. *Biometrics* 1999; **55**: 718–26.

148   Risch N, Teng J. The relative power of family-based and case-control designs for linkage disequilibrium studies of complex human diseases I. DNA pooling. *Genome Res* 1998; **8**: 1273–88.

149   Kirov G, Williams N, Sham P et al. Pooled genotyping of microsatellite markers in parent-offspring trios. *Genome Res* 2000; **10**: 105–15.

150   Le Hellard S, Ballereau SJ, Visscher PM et al. SNP genotyping on pooled DNAs: comparison of genotyping technologies and a semi automated method for data storage and analysis. *Nucleic Acids Res* 2002; **30**: e74.

151   Ross P, Hall L, Haff LA. Quantitative approach to single-nucleotide polymorphism analysis using MALDI-TOF mass spectrometry. *Biotechniques* 2000; **29**: 620–6, 628–9.

152   Uhl GR, Liu QR, Walther D et al. Polysubstance abuse-vulnerability genes: genome scans for association, using 1004 subjects and 1494 single-nucleotide polymorphisms. *Am J Hum Genet* 2001; **69**: 1290–300.

153   Arnheim N, Strange C, Erlich H. Use of pooled DNA samples to detect linkage disequilibrium of polymorphic restriction fragments and human disease: studies of the HLA class II loci. *Proc Natl Acad Sci USA* 1985; **82**: 6970–4.

154   Liguori M, Sawcer S, Setakis E et al. A whole genome screen for linkage disequilibrium in multiple sclerosis performed in a continental Italian population. *J Neuroimmunol* 2003; **143**: 97–100.

155   Coraddu F, Lai M, Mancosu C et al. A genome-wide screen for linkage disequilibrium in Sardinian multiple sclerosis. *J Neuroimmunol* 2003; **143**: 120–3.

156   Herbon N, Werner M, Braig C et al. High-resolution SNP scan of chromosome 6p21 in pooled samples from patients with complex diseases. *Genomics* 2003; **81**: 510–18.

157   Barratt BJ, Payne F, Rance HE et al. Identification of the sources of error in allele frequency estimations from pooled DNA indicates an optimal experimental design. *Ann Hum Genet* 2002; **66**: 393–405.

158   Pfeiffer RM, Rutter JL, Gail MH et al. Efficiency of DNA pooling to estimate joint allele frequencies and measure linkage disequilibrium. *Genet Epidemiol* 2002; **22**: 94–102.

159   Chae SC, Yoon KH, Chung HT. Identification of novel polymorphisms in the Adam33 gene. *J Hum Genet* 2003; **48**: 278–81.

160   Yang Y, Zhang J, Hoh J et al. Efficiency of single-nucleotide polymorphism haplotype estimation from pooled DNA. *Proc Natl Acad Sci USA* 2003; **100**: 7225–30.

161   Jawaid A, Bader JS, Purcell S et al. Optimal selection strategies for QTL mapping using pooled DNA samples. *Eur J Hum Genet* 2002; **10**: 125–32.

162   Mitchell AA, Cutler DJ, Chakravarti A. Undetected genotyping errors cause apparent overtransmission of common alleles in the transmission/disequilibrium test. *Am J Hum Genet* 2003; **72**: 598–610.

163   O'Connell JR, Weeks DE. PedCheck: a program for identification of genotype incompatibilities in linkage analysis. *Am J Hum Genet* 1998; **63**: 259–66.

164   Boehnke M, Cox NJ. Accurate inference of relationships in sib-pair linkage studies. *Am J Hum Genet* 1997; **61**: 423–9.

165   Broman KW, Weber JL. Estimation of pairwise relationships in the presence of genotyping errors. *Am J Hum Genet* 1998; **63**: 1563–4.

166   Douglas JA, Skol AD, Boehnke M. Probability of detection of genotyping errors and mutations as inheritance inconsistencies in nuclear-family data. *Am J Hum Genet* 2002; **70**: 487–95.

167   Epstein MP, Duren WL, Boehnke M. Improved inference of relationship for pairs of individuals. *Am J Hum Genet* 2000; **67**: 1219–31.

168   Sun L, Wilder K, McPeek MS. Enhanced pedigree error detection. *Hum Hered* 2002; **54**: 99–110.

169   Abecasis GR, Cherny SS, Cookson WO, Cardon LR. GRR: graphical representation of relationship errors. *Bioinformatics* 2001; **17**: 742–3.

# 5

# Bioinformatics

# Public databases and SNPs

ROSS LAZARUS

## INTRODUCTION

### Opportunities and challenges

Researchers studying the association between genetic variation and respiratory diseases face both new opportunities and new challenges. Opportunities arise from a wide range of resources offering ready access to the virtual flood of data, including genomic data from an increasingly wide range of organisms. Challenges include learning how to make the most efficient use of these rich, new resources, without being overwhelmed by complexity.

Although many of these resources are freely available and readily accessible using the internet, uptake and use does not seem to be keeping up with the prodigious rate at which data are being generated, suggesting that there are practical barriers to its application in research and clinical practice. These barriers are gradually being overcome by the development of integrative bioinformatics applications and by educational efforts for potential consumers, many of which are freely available, even if not yet as widely appreciated as they might be.

This chapter introduces basic nomenclature for describing genomic data, together with some readily available tools and resources which can be accessed to harvest genetic and genomic data and to assist in the design, execution, and interpretation of respiratory disease genetic research. In order to make the chapter as practical as possible, typical uses of some of these resources are illustrated with some simple 'walk through' examples drawn from the range of tasks a researcher may need to perform.

The remainder of this section outlines the discipline of bioinformatics, the browser metaphor for accessing genomic data, the scope, assumptions, and limitations of the rest of this chapter, and provides a brief introduction to common nomenclature for genomic bioinformatic resources.

### Bioinformatics – techniques and tools for managing data

The term 'bioinformatics' is applied to a wide range of activities and is difficult to define in a universally agreed way, partly because the field is evolving so rapidly, and partly because it relies and builds upon so many disciplines. One simple and inclusive definition is that *Bioinformatics is the evolving, multidisciplinary art and science of transforming biological data into information using automated methods.* Although biologists were early adopters of modern computing developments, bioinformatics emerged as a formal discipline relatively recently, largely in the context of developing methods to support modern genome science. The scope of bioinformatics now extends much more widely to supporting data transformation over the entire range of biological research. The boundaries between bioinformatics, information science, and computational biology are indistinct and a source of ongoing debate among academics. In practice, the distinctions are of little or no importance to most users of bioinformatic resources.

Note that this definition does not mention computers. Bioinformatics practitioners nearly always use computers to implement their ideas, so there are elements of computer science necessarily underlying all practical bioinformatic implementations and the user invariably uses a computer to access the resource. While the computer is an obvious and visible component, it is nothing more or less than a means to an end – a tool which makes it feasible to implement techniques for making biological data more easily understood. To paraphrase the great computer scientist E.W. Dijkstra, bioinformatics is no more about computers than astronomy is about telescopes.

Bioinformatics is multidisciplinary because in practice, it is nearly always necessary to integrate theoretical and practical developments from a wide range of disciplines in order to solve interesting and important biological problems. Ideas from mathematics, statistics, information sciences, epidemiology, genetics, and genomics are often used in theoretical and applied bioinformatic developments. Managing and transforming biological data is at the root of the most useful and practical bioinformatic applications because, at heart, applied bioinformatics is driven by challenges arising in the study of biology.

Formal training in bioinformatics is important for scientists involved in actually designing and implementing tools, but it is not needed to use well-designed bioinformatic resources. While each individual resource discussed below requires specific instruction (nearly always available from the resource itself) for efficient and effective use, in nearly all cases, content knowledge in the specific biological problem domain which drives the researcher is the only other prerequisite.

## The browser metaphor

Many of the major genomic and related bioinformatic resources have interactive, internet-accessible interfaces which provide flexible and powerful means of finding important features and other information. These interfaces are very general and sometimes referred to as 'genome browsers' because the user can navigate the resource using one of the commonly used 'web browsers' available on nearly all modern personal computers. The browser metaphor is simple, easy to understand, powerful, and widely employed. For example, while browsing a section of a chromosomal region of interest, the user can typically move the browser view linearly along the chromosome using forward and back arrow buttons. Similarly, 'zoom' buttons are usually available which change the size of the genomic region displayed, allowing the user to see more detail around features of interest, or zoom out to see less local detail, but more of the regional context including potentially important nearby features.

Despite the simplicity of the browser interface, the underlying data which they expose is complex. For many new users, even the best designed interfaces may appear complicated and intimidating at first glance. However, once some of the basic navigational and other interface conventions are understood, these resources become much more useful and easy to access. In addition, most of the resources described in this chapter have extensive support material and documentation, which allow users to learn at their own pace as needed. Learning to find and use the documentation is a valuable skill. Finally, many of the larger resources offer email or other help desk support services when specific questions cannot be answered using available on-line documentation.

## Scope of this chapter

This chapter is intended to provide a practical introduction to some important bioinformatic resources for the busy scientist who needs to perform some of the more common research planning and data interpretation tasks in respiratory genetics. The main focus is on a small selection of freely available internet-accessible 'user-friendly' interfaces to public repositories of genetic and genomic data and information. Many of these interfaces are integrative, combining data from multiple primary collections in ways which make each of the individual data collections easier to use. In addition, some freely accessible tools which can transform raw genotypic data into more accessible forms such as images or summaries are briefly touched upon. The chapter presents this information firstly as a brief overview of some major web sites and then as specific tasks which the reader may need to perform.

This chapter is not meant to cover the field of bioinformatics as such. Rather, it is about bioinformatic resources and tools which allow scientists to make efficient use of readily available genomic and genetic data, with an emphasis on single nucleotide polymorphisms (SNPs), sequences, and disease association resources. There are many excellent resources available for learning about bioinformatics. Some of these are briefly touched upon in the final section of this chapter. The somewhat indistinct boundaries between 'pure' bioinformatics and more general information sciences is completely ignored in this chapter, because there is no obvious benefit to the reader in distinguishing between them in getting research done.

## Assumptions

The reader is assumed to have both access to and experience using a computer connected to the internet, using a reasonably recent version of any one of the common web browsers. Some introductory hints on how to use a web browser are provided, but it is assumed that the reader has already discovered the basic principles or can obtain help with the commonest tasks like navigating to a specific web address and exploring a web browser screen full of interesting hyperlinks. These basic skills can provide access to a vast store of data and knowledge through judicious use of the internet.

## Caveats

Bioinformatics is an evolving discipline, characterized by extremely rapid change. Bioinformatic resources and tools for accessing genomic data are constantly being modified and improved. By the time the ink is dry on this chapter, some of the contents may be out of date. New tools and resources spring up regularly. Sometimes old resources fall into disrepair or simply disappear from the bioinformatic landscape due to the vagaries of funding or because newer resources make them redundant. These considerations lead to two major caveats for the reader. The first is that any map or guide to such a constantly evolving landscape is quickly dated, so only the larger and more stable resources are mentioned here. The second caveat is that it is almost impossible for any individual to claim to know everything about the field, so material covered here is, of necessity, biased by the authors' experience and personal interests.

Readers should be aware that the material of this chapter is not meant to be a complete catalog of useful bioinformatic resources. Only a small fraction of all potentially important resources are mentioned, and for each of these, only a tiny part of the entire available depth is described. It is hoped that this very simple and brief introduction will enable, and encourage, the reader to dive into the resources and explore them more fully. In nearly all cases, the resources have their own in-depth tutorials or other support material for users.

Finally, readers should be aware that all of these resources are, by design, extremely robust. As a user, you are unlikely to cause any damage to either the resource or yourself by trying things out on your web browser. A willingness to experiment is an important element in learning to make the best use of the wide range of bioinformatic resources which can help support respiratory genetics research.

## Bioinformatic nomenclature for genomic architecture

Genomic architecture describes the physical layout of genomes and their features. In this section, some basic terms and frameworks are briefly reviewed. These are all described in more detail elsewhere in this book, but they are briefly summarized and reviewed here because they are useful for many bioinformatic tools.

The term 'sequence' is used to describe the linear arrangement of nucleotides, one after the other, as might be found on one strand of a chromosome. A worldwide consortium (described below) collaborates to assemble the sequence of the entire genomes of many organisms and to make the resulting data freely available. Although the complete sequences of many genomes, including the human genome, are available, the process by which sequence fragments are joined into each completed chromosome is far from straightforward. Technical challenges remain, particularly in genomic regions where it is difficult to obtain high quality sequence reads such as near the centromere, or where joining sequences into longer completed fragments is made difficult by the presence of long runs of repetitive patterns of nucleotides or large duplicated segments. In practice, each new version of the finished assembly of the human genome produces a more complete result, but some ambiguity and uncertainty remains. Each sequence assembly of each organism is given a revision number and it is important to understand that even for the human sequence, for which a first draft was published in 2001, the process of refinement and revision of the finished sequence will continue for some time to come.[1]

One fundamental framework for bioinformatic nomenclature is to number the individual nucleotides along each chromosome. The linear arrangement of nucleotide bases along a chromosome leads naturally to the idea of a linear coordinate system, counting nucleotides from one end of the chromosome (conventionally, the distal end or telomere of the short arm) to the other. Given these 'chromosome absolute' coordinates, any genomic feature such as a polymorphism or a gene can be unambiguously mapped to a specific place on a specific chromosome.

The term 'feature' is often used to refer to more sequence which functions as a more complex genomic structure such as a gene or an evolutionarily conserved sequence. The process of uniquely identifying the location of genomic features is often referred to as 'mapping'. Unambiguous mapping can only be accomplished when a counting scheme is in place for the basic linear scaffolding – the sequence. For example, the notation chr4:38598801 refers to the nucleotide 38 598 801 bases from the start of chromosome 4. Positions may change between revised genome assemblies, so this notation should be used in the context of one specific assembly, such as the 35th NCBI revision of the sequence of the human genome.

Historically, some genes have acquired more than one name in the literature, and this can lead to confusion. For example, CARD4 and NOD1 refer to the same gene. Many bioinformatic resources allow gene symbols assigned by the international HUGO gene naming committee as text search terms and these are generally referred to as HUGO symbols or HUGO gene names (www.gene.ucl.ac.uk/nomenclature). For example, *TLR10* is the HUGO symbol for the gene encoding the Toll-like receptor 10 protein. Genes have a complex substructure of important genomic features. The genomic region containing a gene contains features such as a promoter region, a 3′ untranslated region, exons, and introns. Exons contain nucleotide sequences which encode the amino acids of the final protein product of the gene. Most genes have multiple exons, separated by introns – genomic sequences which are not represented in the final protein product. As a result, there is generally no simple correspondence between linear genomic sequence and final gene protein product, so any scheme for describing genomic architecture must allow for complex biological transformation and for the wide range of interests and needs of biologists.

The chromosomal coordinates of a gene may be guessed by looking for features typical of genes 'in silico,' using bioinformatic resources. Truly functional genes are identified and located by the position of the appropriate sequence of nucleotides encoding a sequence of messenger RNA (mRNA) observed to be an intermediate step in the production of the gene's protein product. For nearly all proteins, the transcripts representing the exons are spliced together in a complex post-transcriptional process. Many genes have more than one possible pattern of splicing, resulting in distinct isoforms of the final protein product – for example, Toll-like receptor 4 (*TLR4*) is known to produce four distinct isoforms referred to as isoforms A through D. Since each of these isoforms consists of a different selection of exons, the relative positions of amino acids may vary, making nomenclature more complex.

Once the structure of a gene is identified, it is possible to locate features within or near a gene, using 'gene relative' coordinates. The first nucleotide in coding sequence is generally counted as 1. Nucleotides upstream of this position are generally designated as negative numbers, counting back from −1 so there is no nucleotide zero. In this framework, chr4:38598801 is the 977th nucleotide in the translated sequence of the human gene which encodes Toll-like receptor 10 (*TLR10*), where it is the second base of the three base codons translated into the 326th amino acid of the protein product of the gene. For a protein with multiple isoforms, it is necessary to specify a position and an isoform to avoid ambiguity.

While the vast majority of the bases in the genomic sequence are invariant between individuals, as discussed in Chapters 1 and 4B, sites where individuals may each have different nucleotides are termed polymorphic sites or polymorphisms. The most abundant of these polymorphisms are single base substitutions, which when present at 1 percent or greater in a population are termed single nucleotide polymorphisms or SNPs. A catalog of SNPs is maintained by an international consortium described in more detail below. As SNPs are discovered, they are submitted to the consortium and after careful checking, given a unique identifier (a reference SNP or rs number). Knowing an SNP rs number, it is possible to use an SNP catalog (such as dbSNP) to find the chromosomal absolute (and where relevant, the gene relative) coordinates of the SNP, and to identify some of the basic properties such as whether it is located in a coding region (a coding SNP), and whether it induces a change in the protein product (termed a nonsynonymous SNP) or not (termed a synonymous SNP). The human genome location chr4:38598801 is the site of a single nucleotide polymorphism (known as rs11466653 in the dbSNP database). At this nucleotide position, most humans have a thymine base, but approximately 4 percent have a cytosine. This is a nonsynonymous SNP, because it is the 977th position in the coding sequence, and the substitution of a cytosine changes the 326th amino acid of the TLR10 protein from the usual methionine to a threonine.

## AN OVERVIEW OF THREE MAJOR INTERNET-BASED RESOURCES

The three data resources introduced here are only a small fraction of all bioinformatic resources available through the internet. Many important sites have been left out, but the sites described here were chosen as being immediately useful in the study of respiratory genetics as evidenced by the fact that these are resources used regularly by authors of this book. In this section, resources are grouped by individual web site. They are briefly introduced here, and followed below with detailed examples illustrating how these and other web sites can be used in common research tasks.

## NCBI – www.ncbi.nlm.nih.gov

An extensive collection of important resources, conveniently accessible through a common searchable interface, the National Center for Biotechnology Information (NCBI) web site integrates a vast and wide range of individual databases, many of which have their own specialized web sites, within the framework of a consistent design and user interface.

### INTERFACE

Entrez is the name given to the interface or gateway through which all major NCBI bioinformatic resources can be conveniently accessed. The main NCBI page is itself an Entrez page which includes a search facility that operates on all of the databases in the NCBI site. This allows less experienced visitors to find their way with a simple text search, while more experienced users can quickly access specific information using far more sophisticated search strategies and techniques. Exact match text searches are performed by typing a word or phrase into the search bar illustrated in Fig. 5A.1 and described in more detail below. The Entrez search and results pages also offer lists of potentially useful and important links (including help and tutorials) on the navigation bar on the left side of the browser screen. Links to major NCBI resources are arranged horizontally, near the top of the page where the search bar is located.

The default NCBI page has the word Entrez showing in the resource selector to the left of the text term entry box. This resource selector is a drop down list which enables the search to be targeted at individual NCBI resources when necessary. If the search is run with Entrez as the target resource, all major NCBI resources are searched. Otherwise, the search is run on the specific selected resource only. For Entrez searches, a summary of the matching text 'hits' is presented in a neatly organized results page. This is all viewed through a web browser, so the result page offers direct links to each resource with the appropriate result set displayed. The volume of material which is searched through the single Entrez interface is hard to comprehend. A brief outline and some current statistics for major components are presented below.

### SEQUENCE

GenBank is a collaborator in a worldwide consortium which creates and maintains a shared database of nucleotide sequences. Material from more than 130 000 organisms

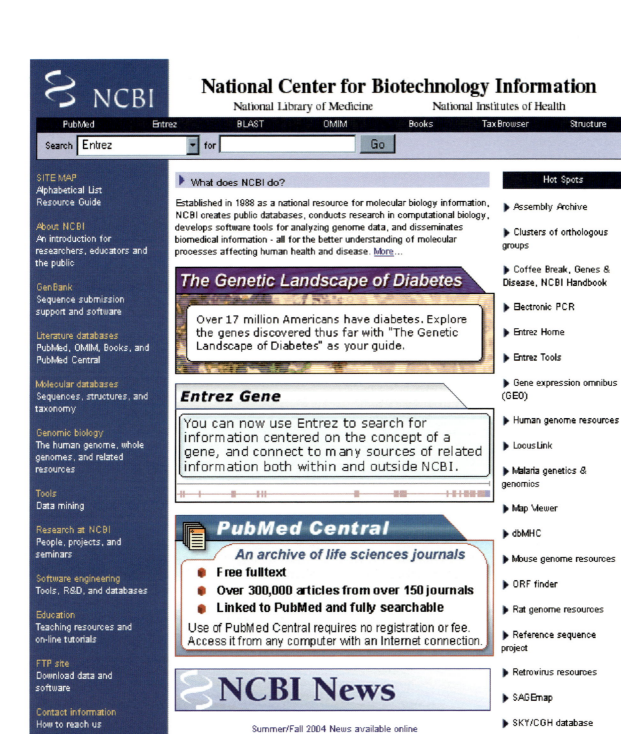

**Figure 5A.1** *NCBI web site home page. Note search bar below double helix logo with search scope set to the default 'Entrez' – a text search will return results from all NCBI database resources – 28 at the time of writing.*

is currently available. Many genomes have been completely assembled, and many sequences have been annotated with the position and layout of genes, and other features of potential interest. The June 2004 release offered 35 532 003 individual sequences totaling 40 325 321 348 nucleotides. All of these data are freely downloadable, requiring 160 gB of storage for the sequence and annotation. This is twice the size of the June 2002 release[2] and the count of nucleotides in GenBank appears to be growing exponentially.[3]

## LITERATURE

PubMed is a web-accessible gateway which offers a searchable database of more than 11 million bibliographic citations[4] from the biomedical literature. It is a very busy resource, providing an average of 22 bibliographic searches a second or more than 60 million searches each month. The NCBI web site is also an entry point for other important and useful literature-related databases. These include MeSH which is a controlled vocabulary for medical subject classification, and OMIM which is a manually curated database currently containing 15 582 records (www.ncbi.nlm. nih.gov/Omim/mimstats.html August 14 2004), each record summarizing published information about genes and the genetics of a human disease.

## MOLECULAR INFORMATION

A wide variety of resources are available including proteins, gene expression data, and variations including *dbSNP*,

a searchable SNP database currently containing detailed information on nearly 10 million SNPs.[5]

## TOOLS AND VIEWERS

The NCBI offers genome map viewers, specialized protein structure viewers, and many specialized search methods. As other resources, these are all accessible through the single, integrated Entrez interface.

## UCSC Bioinformatics (GoldenPath) – http://genome.ucsc.edu

The Genome Bioinformatics Group of University of California, Santa Cruz maintain the UCSC genome and annotation browser, integrated with a search engine optimized for relatively short sequences (Blat) and a variety of other valuable tools. These all operate consistently on assemblies of the whole genomes of a variety of organisms – 15 at the time of writing. Opening a browser screen at a specific feature or genomic location is very easy, for example, it is possible to navigate directly to a gene by typing the HUGO symbol for the gene (e.g., *TLR10*) into a text box, and opening a genome browser page illustrated in Fig. 5A.2. Help, in the form of an on-line user guide and frequently asked questions, is available from links near the top of each page as seen in Fig. 5A.2. The browser default is to set the organism to human and the default assembly set to the most recent build, but both of these can easily be changed

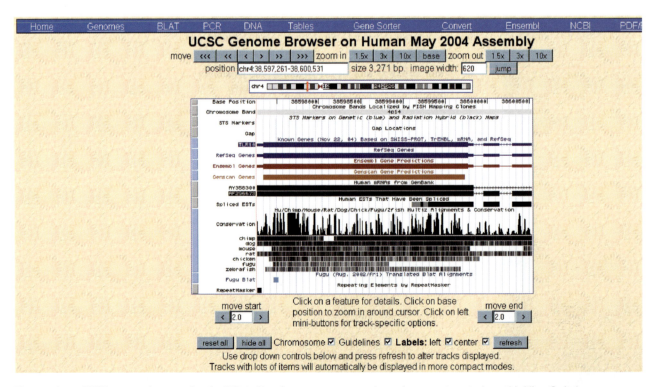

**Figure 5A.2**  *UCSC genome browser showing TLR10. Note browser move, zoom in, and zoom out controls on third line. Switches controlling annotation tracks are below the screen section shown here. Reproduced with permission from http://genome.ucsc.edu. See also Kent WJ, Sugnet CW, Furey TS et al. The human genome browser at UCSC.* Genome Res. *2002;* **12***: 996–1006.*

using 'drop down' lists. The browser is an extensible and flexible way to visualize genomic data. While examining any specific region, the user can interactively control the position and scale, and can specify genomic features or annotations to be included in or excluded from the view. There is a potentially bewildering list of annotations (termed 'tracks') or features to view including phylogenetic conservation scores, known genes, and SNPs. Users can add external annotation sources and even share their own specialized annotations. However, with a little guidance, the interface is remarkably flexible and easy to use. Fortunately, the quality of documentation is excellent with tutorials and other assistance readily available on-line. Some simple tasks using the UCSC browser and tools are described in the next section.

## Ensembl: www.ensembl.org

Ensembl is another specialized web-based genome and annotation browser for metazoan genomes, offering a consistent, internet-accessible interface, jointly maintained by the European Molecular Biology Laboratory and the Sanger Institute. As in the UCSC browser, the Ensembl

interface is extensive and complex, but again, a simple interface in the form of an exact match text search is immediately available from the top of the main Ensemble page at www.ensembl.org, allowing even inexperienced users to navigate directly to genes or regions. Figure 5A.3 shows part of the contig view for *TLR10*. As in the UCSC browser, the number of annotations available is enormous and users can easily add and share their own using the Distributed Annotation System (DAS – see http://biodas.org/). The main page offers links to tutorials and help is available for the deeper layers of complexity from the relevant pages.

## Summary

Presenting complex genomic annotation on a web browser screen is a technical challenge which Entrez, Ensembl, and GoldenPath each deal with superbly, using different styles and perspectives. While the underlying data and many of the annotations are the same, the facilities and interfaces are very different and each has particular strengths. Some researchers feel most comfortable learning to use just one of these resources for all tasks, but more experienced researchers are more likely to pick and choose, using each

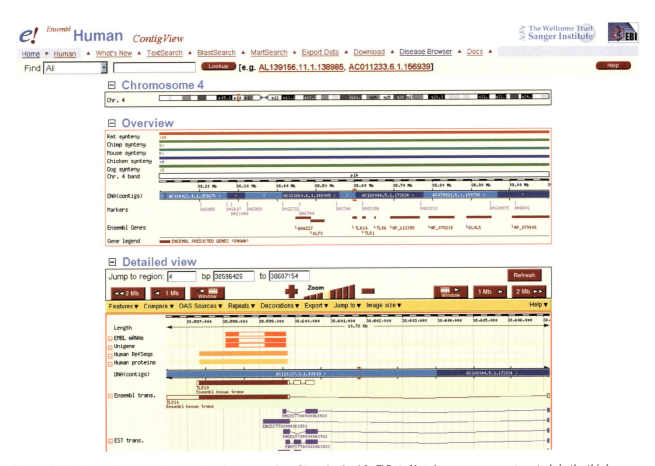

**Figure 5A.3**    *Ensembl genome browser showing top section of 'contig view' for* TLR10. *Note browser movement controls in the third ('Detailed view') section and 'Help' link upper right.*

resource for particular functions, depending on the specific task at hand. While it may be natural to ask which one is the 'best,' there are so many different potential tasks and so many individual differences in terms of taste and experience, that the answer is inevitably deeply personal and subjective. Wise researchers will experiment with them all to discover which ones work best in their own hands for specific aspects of their own research.

## BIOINFORMATIC RESOURCES FOR COMMON RESEARCH TASKS

### Finding and managing relevant literature

#### BACKGROUND

As in other types of health research, progress in respiratory genetics research usually begins from an understanding of what is already known. While textbooks such as this one provide an important source of comprehensive and summarized knowledge, recently published articles in the peer-reviewed literature are needed in order to understand the most recent developments and for specialized reviews. Arguably, the most comprehensive and 'user friendly' resource for gaining access to the biomedical peer reviewed literature is PubMed, maintained by the National Library of Medicine (NLM) and the National Institutes of Health (NIH) in the USA. PubMed is a freely available internet-accessible database of major sources of biomedical literature. Electronic citations from many of the major publishers are provided prior to, or immediately at, the time of publication, therefore, PubMed is kept up-to-date more or less automatically for the major journals – many new citations appear in PubMed at the same time as they appear electronically on the publisher's web site. As more publishers move to electronic publication, PubMed is becoming an increasingly convenient resource for quickly tracking down recent literature, because many citations for articles published in the past few years have hyperlinks to the publisher's web site for the specific article, if it is available electronically.

PubMed grew out of MEDLINE, the NLM's original bibliographic database, and currently contains more than 12 million citations from more than 4600 journals over a wide range of fields including medicine, veterinary medicine, and the healthcare system. The current PubMed service is conveniently integrated into the Entrez web gateway, and has evolved over many iterations to become a flexible and powerful window into the biomedical research literature.

Article abstracts are always freely accessible (and downloadable), but many publishers charge a fee to access the text of articles they publish – although an increasing number of publications is freely available such as those published on BioMedCentral (www.biomedcentral.com). Entrez search result pages (described in more detail below) contain a link to PubMedCentral results (just below the PubMed link), where full text of the citations are available free of charge. The free full-text access journals are a minority at present, but they offer the advantage of immediate on-line access to the entire research article.

#### GETTING THERE

Like all other Entrez resources, you can access PubMed from any internet-connected computer. Open a web browser window and type the main NCBI URL (www.ncbi.nlm. nih.gov) into the location bar (usually at the top of the browser screen). Clicking the 'Go' button (often to the right of the location bar) to request the web browser to open the page at that address.

The NCBI homepage may initially appear to offer a bewildering variety of links to rich resources, but it is actually very easy to use – particularly if you take advantage of the search options available from the search bar toward the top of the page shown in Fig. 5A.1. The default search engine is the most comprehensive and it is known as 'Entrez.' An Entrez search will return search results from (at the time of writing) 28 resources, categorized into three broad groups – literature, raw data, and information about data (termed 'metadata').

#### A TYPICAL TASK

As an illustration, a researcher might want to perform a literature review on asthma. One quick way to start is by searching Entrez, using the text term 'asthma' as the search term – every record in the NCBI databases which contains those six letters in that particular order will be matched. This is the simplest possible search and as we will see, the results are usually far too broad to be very useful. The search term is typed into the 'search bar' near the top of the Entrez home page to indicate that you are interested in all resources which precisely match 'asthma.' Leave 'Entrez' as the resource to be searched (it is possible to restrict the search to specific resources within Entrez using the 'drop down list' on the right hand side of the search bar, but that is usually not necessary as the next step will illustrate), and type 'asthma' as the search term (in the open area to the right of the word 'Entrez' in the search bar), then click on the button labeled 'Go' at the right hand side of the bar.

A summary of all of the Entrez resources which have 'asthma' in them will appear, allowing you to select the ones which are of particular interest – you may be shocked at how many resources there are and at how many resources have large number of 'hits' for asthma. Links to search results from the major Entrez databases, including PubMed (top of the left hand side column) which, at the time of writing had 81 124 entries matching 'asthma.' Follow the 'PubMed' link and your browser will show the first of many pages of articles which have the term 'asthma' in one of the fields indexed by PubMed. Reading without a break at an average of one abstract a minute, it would take a little more than 8 weeks to scan all these citations! Since the vast majority of them may not be of great interest, it is worth spending a little time learning how to refine a PubMed search so that the results are both sensitive and specific to your particular interests.

Fortunately, Entrez makes it very easy to narrow down the results returned by a generic text search. For example, when viewing the PubMed results for the asthma text word search, a researcher might prefer to limit the search to articles in English with abstracts. This is easily accomplished using the 'limits' link just below the search bar, which leads to a page containing options including language (select English) and a check box (click it to turn it 'on') for articles with abstracts. Select the 'Go' button again and the search will be repeated, but this time the results will be 'filtered' so only articles in English and with abstracts are included in the result. The number of articles drops dramatically – to less than half the size of the original unrestricted search result. Other useful limits on the 'limits' page include publication type (e.g., reviews or clinical trials only) and publication

date ranges, useful when seeking only the most recent articles to refresh a previously completed literature review.

Another useful strategy to make a search more specific is to add an additional text search term. The search interface allows Boolean logic using a simple convention. For example, to restrict the search to articles about asthma which also have the term 'SNP' in them, change the search term to read 'asthma AND snp' (note that the 'AND' should be in upper case to indicate that it is a Boolean logical connector for the two search terms). Select the 'Go' button again and you should see the number of articles drop even more dramatically – to about a thousandth of the original number, as illustrated in Fig. 5A.4. Efficient PubMed searching requires much more experience and many more techniques than this simple example illustrates. Many more advanced search techniques are clearly described in the tutorial link in the navigation bar on the left side of the PubMed page.

Many of the more advanced search methods rely on the use of specially formatted search terms. Although PubMed has a full text index which allows simple matching text searches, it also allows much more sophisticated and specific searches using what are called 'search term tags.' One

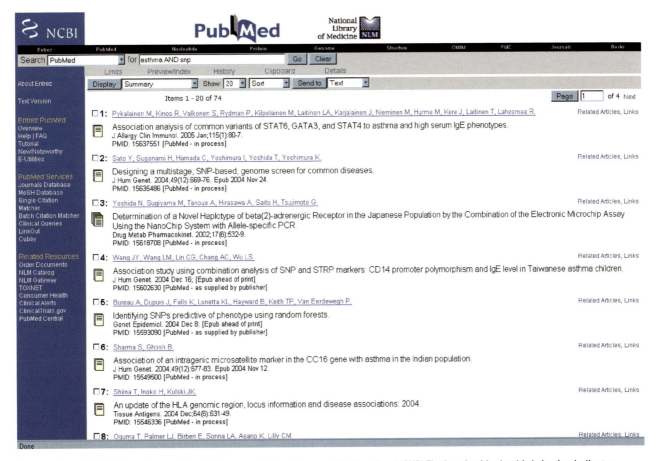

**Figure 5A.4** *PubMed search result for citations containing the words 'asthma' and 'SNP'. The icon beside the third citation indicates a link to free full text of the article.*

important group of these tags allow searches using terms from a specialized controlled vocabulary organized as an hierarchical tree of medical concepts – the medical subject headings (MeSH). Nearly all articles in PubMed are indexed by a human reader, who adds a set of MeSH terms to the article to categorize it. Once this has been done, the PubMed status field located next to the unique PubMed identifier for every article changes from 'PubMed – in process' to 'PubMed – indexed for MEDLINE.' As you use PubMed, you will soon discover that the most recent articles are nearly always 'in process' because the manual indexing process generally takes a month or two to complete. More details about MeSH are available from www.nlm.nih.gov/mesh/meshhome.html.

Entrez can help you to learn more about the MeSH headings relevant to your search. From the Entrez search page, perform the simple text search for the word 'asthma' as described above. The Entrez search result page is divided into three sections. The rightmost result in the lowest section has a tree icon and is entitled 'MeSH: detailed information about NLM's controlled vocabulary.' Clicking on that link will reveal a page with the MeSH terms which were matched by your text search term. The page shows hints about refining your search by selecting MeSH subheadings. For example, click on the 'Asthma' search term link and select the subheadings of interest by checking the relevant boxes with a mouse click, then click on the 'Send' button with the default option of 'Send to search box with AND.' A prewritten specialized PubMed query will appear in a text box (which you can change). Clicking the button labeled 'Search PubMed' will run the specialized MeSH term search.

PubMed citations can be viewed in many useful formats, for example, MeSH headings for any fully indexed article can be viewed on-line by changing the choice of display format (the default is 'Abstract') to 'Medline' while viewing an individual citation – to do this, click on the text box to the left of the 'Display' button while viewing an abstract and select the 'Medline' option. Click on the display button to reformat the abstract and look for terms which follow the abbreviation 'MH' (MeSH headings). A simple text search is often overwhelming in terms of the number of citations returned. Searching through the first few pages will often reveal some relevant abstracts – by viewing the MeSH headings for these, you may be able to quickly learn which MeSH headings are most relevant – using these headings as the search term (see the tutorial on using search tags) may provide a much more specific and sensitive search and save you valuable time.

One feature which is particularly helpful for literature reviews is that multiple citations from a PubMed search result can be manually selected and then manipulated as a group. Articles can be selected by clicking the box immediately to the left of the start of each citation as you scroll through the results of a search. Each selection is 'sticky' and stays in place until you start a new search, so you can work your way through multiple pages and your selections will all be remembered. (If necessary, selections from multiple searches can be saved in the 'clipboard' – see the PubMed tutorial for details.) The citations you have selected can then be emailed directly to your email inbox, from where they can be stored, organized, and manipulated with any text editor. When you have selected all the citations of interest, click the 'Send to' button toward the top of the page, and then select 'E-mail' from the drop-down list of options. A form will appear where you can type in your email address and select the format you would like to receive the citations – click the 'Mail' button and within a few minutes, an email will arrive containing the citations you selected in the specific format requested. Many commercial bibliography packages can be configured to automatically create citation entries from PubMed searches, making the task of preparing manuscripts for publication much easier and less prone to error. PubMed also provides a tool which can perform the reverse of this operation; the Batch Citation Matcher allows users to match a list of citations to PubMed entries by uploading fields including journal, volume, issue, page number, and year – the resulting matches can be expanded to include abstracts and even emailed back to the user for further processing.

## WHERE TO NEXT

All Entrez resources including PubMed provide built-in support and on-line user education services including tutorials, FAQs ('frequently asked questions'), and guides. These are all available through a web browser. For nearly all Entrez resource web pages including PubMed, the navigation bar on the left hand side of every page has links to an overview, a list of FAQ's and detailed tutorials. An hour spent working through the tutorials will help to save time by making more efficient use of the resource in future searches.

Like many other bioinformatic resources, PubMed is designed to be immediately useful to the first time visitor. However, it is a deep and complex resource which is highly configurable and flexible. Many advanced features and services are not immediately obvious. In fact, they are deliberately kept from immediate view in order to simplify the interface for first time visitors. New features are regularly added to Entrez resources, so even experienced users can occasionally learn new tricks by checking the on-line tutorials and guides. If you cannot find the answer you need from the support materials, help from a human is available by emailing your question to custserv@nlm.nih.gov.

The NCBI offers a program of on-site educational programs for institutions, including their well known 'field guide' sessions. Typically arranged as 1-day lecture and workshop sessions, these are delivered by very experienced teachers, targeted at busy researchers wanting to get the most out of the available resources. Further details may be found at www.ncbi.nlm.nih.gov/Class/FieldGuide/.

## Finding human disease-related information about a gene

### BACKGROUND

A central resource for genetic information about a specific human disease is the Online Mendelian Inheritance in Man (OMIM) database. This is the on-line version of Victor McKusick's book, *Mendelian Inheritance in Man*, which systematically describes human genes and human diseases with genetic associations. The on-line version is regularly updated, but unlike many other electronic resources, each individual entry is maintained by a select group of expert scientists. Through Entrez, OMIM has a flexible and simple text search interface. Like other Entrez resources, limits and special search tags can be used for more sophisticated searches. In many situations, a simple text search will provide a useful result leading to related terms to search.

### GETTING THERE

Since OMIM is integrated with Entrez, the easiest way to navigate to a gene of interest is to enter the gene HUGO symbol as an Entrez search term. The results page will include a record count and direct link to the gene entry in OMIM. For example, type 'TLR10' into the Entrez search bar and click the 'Go' button. The OMIM link is in the top panel of result links, on the right hand side of the screen showing the results for the text search for TLR10. Click the 'OMIM' link to see a series of links to all the OMIM pages which contain text exactly matching the search term TLR10. The first of these is a good place to start exploring.

### TYPICAL TASKS

When an OMIM page is displayed on a browser screen, other relevant OMIM pages are available as links when terms such as other genes or diseases, which are themselves elsewhere in OMIM, are encountered in the text. This internal linking within OMIM is a very powerful method for connecting all of the relevant information. Within the text on each page, all references are presented as a link which automatically scrolls the page down to the bibliography at the end. Within the bibliography for each page, every entry has a direct link (shown as the PubMed Id) to the relevant record in PubMed. Most OMIM record paragraphs end with a small image of a light bulb. Clicking this image will open a page containing the publications cited in the paragraph and other related material in a PubMed results page. This bibliography is carefully selected and maintained by experts in the field. While OMIM provides an excellent starting place, given the size of the field and the prodigious rate of publication, OMIM is often lacking the most recent published material. If you need the most up-to-date published material, an OMIM page can be quickly supplemented by exploring the results of an appropriate PubMed query with a period limit set so that only the most recent publications are returned (see previous section). The Edit History link on the left navigation bar of every OMIM page will show when the material was last updated.

### WHERE TO NEXT

As in all other Entrez resources, on-line help and tutorials are available for OMIM from the navigation bar on the left side of the browser screen. The main help document (click the 'OMIM Help' link in the second group of choices on the left side of the screen) contains a nicely graded introduction with simple examples, search strategies, and details on search options. The frequently asked questions are also a valuable source of both general and detailed information.

## Find human tissues in which a gene is expressed

In the positional cloning approach described elsewhere in this book, genomic regions of interest are identified using family-based linkage studies. A linked region may include many tens of millions of bases and this may potentially implicate hundreds of individual genes. Knowing that a particular gene is expressed in a tissue of interest (such as lung) may make that gene a more biologically plausible candidate for subsequent fine-mapping and genetic association studies.

### GETTING THERE

The UCSC GoldenPath genome browser provides annotation tracks for gene expression data. Like all UCSC browser annotation tracks, they can be switched on and off as needed.

### TYPICAL TASKS

While browsing any particular gene of interest with the UCSC browser, scroll down to the 'Expression and Regulation' group of annotation track options and change the 'GNF Atlas 2' selection to 'Full.' Refresh the browser display with the Refresh button and the screen will show a list of approximately 100 human tissues, partially visible in Fig. 5A.5. Expression levels are color coded with more intense red associated with higher levels of expression, and green associated with lower levels of expression. The list of tissues is fixed but sufficiently comprehensive for many purposes. Note that all tracks can be controlled in exactly the same manner – the UCSC browser uses tokens called 'cookies' to remember the configuration of tracks, so these are reinitialized the next time you return, making your personal selection 'sticky'.

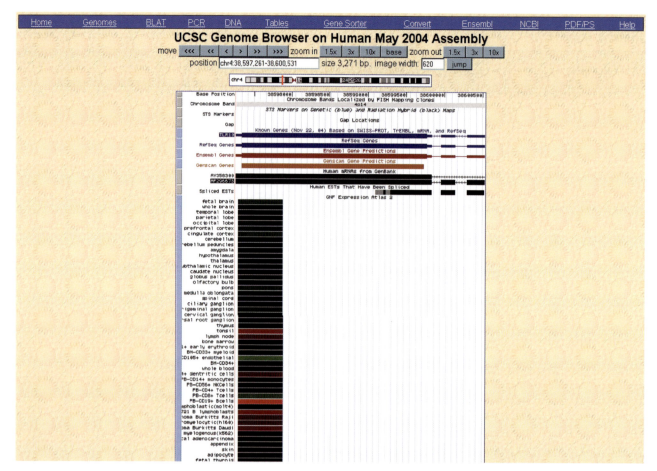

**Figure 5A.5** *USCS browser view of TLR10 with gene expression levels from the GNF Atlas track. Reproduced with permission from http://genome.ucsc.edu. See also Kent WJ, Sugnet CW, Furey TS et al. The human genome browser at UCSC. Genome Res. 2002; **12**: 996–1006.*

## WHERE TO NEXT

The GoldenPath gene expression track is well suited to many day-to-day purposes but may not always offer enough detail for more specialized tasks. There are many other resources which provide gene expression data including those accessible through the Ensembl and Entrez interfaces. They all have strengths and weaknesses depending on the purpose of the search.

For more detailed information, two specialized gene expression data repositories may be helpful. The first of these is called the Bodymap web site (http://bodymap.ims. u-tokyo.ac.jp). It is far less convenient to use than the UCSC browser, because the search interface is relatively primitive, detailed on-line help and tutorials are not available, and HUGO gene symbols are not supported in searches. Instead, a UniGene identifier or a GenBank accession number (these can be found using the gene search facility in SNPper as shown in Fig. 5A.6) must be used to identify the gene, and the search interface does not allow letter case changes, so 'HS.1074' will not be recognized if accidentally entered when searching for 'Hs.1074'. From the main Bodymap page, select the UniGene ID check box and enter

'Hs.1074' as the 'Input' field. This is the UniGene identifier for Surfactant, pulmonary-associated protein C (SFTPC). The UniGene ID must be entered precisely as shown for the search to work correctly. Click the submit button and a result page will appear. If the ID matches exactly to a UniGene in the Bodymap database a matching result will appear, otherwise there is no message, just an empty results list. The Bodymap GS identifier (GS02630) shown on the results screen is a link to a very useful summary of gene expression data for the gene, including evidence that this particular gene is expressed exclusively in lung tissue. Note that not all known UniGene genes are available, for example, TLR10 (UniGene Hs.120551) is not currently present in the Bodymap database.

The second specialized resource is the NCBI Gene Expression Omnibus (GEO) at www.ncbi.nlm.nih.gov/ entrez/query.fcgi?db=geo. It is easy to access and search through the Entrez search interface described above, and provides a great deal of detailed gene expression information. This, in turn, requires a substantial amount of user effort to organize into a simple summary of the type provided by the gene expression track for the UCSC browser.

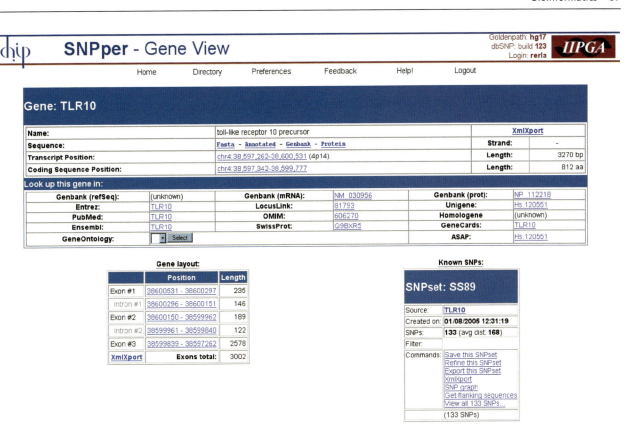

**Figure 5A.6** *SNPper 'Gene View' for* TLR10. *Note identifiers linking to external resources such as LocusLink, Genbank, and UniGene.*

However, GEO or the Bodymap may be the right tools for certain tasks requiring more deeply detailed gene expression results, whereas the integrated overview available from the UCSC browser is well suited for quickly checking expression data while viewing a gene of interest. As always, the wise researcher learns which tool is best suited to each task by experimenting.

## Finding conserved genomic regions

Phylogenetic conservation may offer clues about whether a SNP located in a particular part of a gene or a specific genomic region of an organism is functionally important. While there are no reliable rules, evidence of conservation over evolutionary time may offer clues about genomic features which have remained relatively unchanged over evolutionary time because they offer selective advantage. Research design methods taking advantage of evolutionary conservation are proving to be fruitful.[6]

### GETTING THERE

Although there are many, far more specialized tools available, as is often the case, the UCSC genome browser includes tracks which show various measures of conservation, and is very easy to use.

### TYPICAL TASKS

The default UCSC browser view of TLR10 includes a track labeled 'Conservation', visible in Fig. 5A.2. More detailed views can be added – while viewing a specific feature or region in the GoldenPath browser, scroll down to the 'Comparative Genomics' group of annotation track options. The options will vary with the assembly in use. At present, with the May 2004 assembly, the 'Conservation' and 'Most Conserved' tracks are a good place to start. Change these two options to 'Full.' Refresh the browser display with the Refresh button and the genome browser screen will show a global measure of evolutionary conservation in human, chimp, mouse, rat, dog, chicken, fugu, and zebrafish as a chart with higher levels of conservation shown as taller black filled regions. Below this will be pairwise comparisons between human and each individual species. Below these, the 'Most Conserved' track will display specific smaller conserved regions and a probability measure (log odds) derived from a phylogenetic hidden Markov model.[7] As with all GoldenPath tracks, detailed results and documentation are available by clicking on one of the label links or on the display itself.

# Find known SNPs in a gene

Many researchers are presented with the opportunity to design a study to test genetic variants in a candidate gene for association with disease. As described elsewhere in this book, candidate genes might come from family-based linkage studies or from expert knowledge of physiological pathways. Study design includes selecting an informative set of markers to measure and this can be most effectively performed by first identifying all known genetic variants in the gene or genomic region. Single nucleotide polymorphisms (SNPs) are generally used as genetic markers for association studies because they are abundant and relatively easy to measure using high throughput methods.[8] A PubMed search may locate some SNPs which have already been reported in the literature. However, only a small fraction of all known SNPs are likely to have been formally published in the peer reviewed literature covered by PubMed.

Fortunately, the NCBI maintains a database of SNPs called dbSNP, to which any research group performing SNP discovery can contribute. Like nearly all other NCBI databases, dbSNP is easily accessible through Entrez. dbSNP contains a wealth of information about each individual variant submitted, but the quantity and the reliability of this information varies, depending on the methods used to detect the variation, and ultimately, the quality of the work being carried out by the submitters. Not all SNPs reported to dbSNP will prove to be polymorphic in any given population sample. Some may be polymorphic only in the samples they were discovered in, and those samples may have come from populations where the SNP is far more common than the samples available to researchers elsewhere. Some dbSNP entries are discovered using sequence database mining and these in silico SNPs generally tend to be less reliable than those discovered by direct resequencing of multiple DNA samples.

The Boston Children's Hospital Informatics Program (CHIP) maintains a web-accessible bioinformatic resource called SNPper (http://snpper.chip.org) which integrates information from dbSNP with the annotated GoldenPath genome assembly from the UCSC.[9] While SNPper offers a detail page for every individual SNP in dbSNP which includes useful links and details, it also allows all of the SNPs in the region of a gene to be viewed together and managed as a set, which is particularly useful when designing association studies based on candidate genes.

SNPper also offers some very specific functions which are otherwise tedious and error-prone, such as extending a set of SNP flanks (the genomic sequence on each side or flank of a SNP) for primer design and identifying the gene relative coordinates for SNPs. SNPper allows sets of SNPs to be exported as machine-readable XML files which can be processed with appropriate software and incorporated into automated pipelines. When studying genes or SNPs (or SNPs in a gene), SNPper can serve as a convenient 'one-stop shop' because it offers hyperlinks directly into the relevant pages of many of the major relevant bioinformatic resources.

## GETTING THERE

SNPper may be accessed through a web browser on any internet connected computer by browsing to http://snpper. chip.org. SNPper allows users to register at no cost. Each registered user is permitted to choose their own private user name (assuming it is not already in use!) and associated password. Registered users maintain their own private configuration settings (including default SNP flank display length and email address for sending copies of SNP information), and a private space to store 'SNP sets.' Finally, the registered user database allows the maintainer of SNPper to obtain objective evidence of usefulness which can help ensure ongoing funding support. Although it is possible to use SNPper without registering (use the generic user id 'guest' with no password), if you find SNPper useful, you might consider registering not only so that you can store your own private SNP sets and configuration, but also to help provide evidence that the resource is worth maintaining. As a side benefit, providing a working email address with your registration allows SNPper to email your password if you forget it.

## TYPICAL TASKS

When planning a research project, or when reading the literature, it is often helpful to be able to quickly find core details including all known SNPs in a specific gene. For example, evidence that SNPs in *TLR10* were associated with asthma in a nested case control study, with supporting replication in a clinical trial sample, was recently published.[10] To obtain an overview of all public SNPs known in the gene *TLR10*, start at the SNPper home page (http://snpper.chip. org). Click on the SNPper link. A password dialog box will appear on your browser window. Either use your own private user name and password if you have one, or use 'guest' as the user name and leave the password field blank; then click on the 'OK' button of the password dialog box to log in.

From the main SNPper page, click on the 'Gene Finder' link. The Gene Finder page has four different ways to specify a gene (or genes) of interest. Click on the first field in the 'Find a gene' section, labeled 'Symbol.' Type the HUGO symbol for the gene of interest into the Symbol field ('TLR10' in this case) and click the Find button immediately to the right of the field. Figure 5A.6 shows the resulting page.

The SNPper *TLR10* gene view page is laid out as a table divided into three sections. Each section provides ready access to detailed information about the gene from major bioinformatic resources, as well as a variety of methods for exploring known SNPs in the region of the gene. For example, the top section of the page includes two links which show the position and length of the gene transcript (i.e., the region which is transcribed into messenger RNA) and the gene coding sequence (the region encoding amino acids which are found in the final TLR10 protein product after post-transcriptional processing is completed). Each of these links will open a window to the UCSC genome browser showing the selected region, together with an integrated view of a wide range of configurable genomic features, described in more detail below. The middle section of the SNPper gene page includes essential links to core NCBI and other bioinformatic databases containing information on TLR10 including GenBank (for reference genomic sequences), OMIM (for information about the role of this gene in human disease), and SwissProt (a protein database). The left side of the lower section of the page contains a section showing the layout of the gene in terms of exons and introns with their lengths and positions. Finally, the right hand side of the lower section contains a summary of all known *TLR10* SNPs together with links to an internal SNPper representation termed a 'SNP set'.

Clicking the link 'view all 113 snps' (that number will change with each new release of dbSNP!) closest to the end of the page on the right hand side, will reveal all of the SNPs in genomic order, laid out in a table with their dbSNP reference SNP (rs) number, their validation status, their position in the chromosome and within the gene itself, and a role designation such as 'coding sequence.' It is worth noting that SNPper may report that an SNP in the exon of one gene is also in the 3′ untranslated region (3′ UTR) of a nearby gene. This may seem confusing at first, but results from the fact that some genomic features are not easily defined precisely. For example, the boundaries for the genomic region containing a gene are not just defined by the extent of the coding region, since there may be nearby (but as yet undiscovered) regulatory elements and linkage disequilibrium may result in a distant SNP having an important effect on a disease. For these reasons, SNPper uses arbitrary limits to define some features and these limits may sometimes introduce ambiguity.

Clicking on any one of the SNP name links will take you to the SNPper detail page for that SNP which includes links to the NCBI dbSNP entry for the SNP, a link back to the SNPper TLR10 gene page and the SNP flanks which are needed for designing a genotyping assay to study the SNP. The flanks are the genomic sequence extending from each side of the SNP location. Assay design software varies in the number of flank bases required, but typically 50 or 100 base sequences are needed from each side ('flank') of the marker. The length of flank displayed on each side of the SNP can be configured to suit the needs of your own genotyping primer design software when you have your own registered user name for SNPper. These preferences can be viewed or changed by clicking the 'Preferences' link in the navigation bar toward the top of every SNPper page.

Once you have an SNP set available, SNPper offers two extremely useful features which can make the design of association studies much easier. The first is that in the same way a search result in PubMed can be 'limited' to review articles or articles with abstracts, in SNPper, a SNP set can

be 'filtered' so that it only contains SNPs matching certain criteria. The second is that like PubMed, any SNP set can be downloaded or sent to your own email inbox for further processing.

For example, it is well known that dbSNP entries which have been discovered by sequencing in more than one independent sample are far more likely to prove to be truly polymorphic when genotyped. In addition, you may want to select only SNPs which are in the coding region of the gene. From the SNPper TLR10 gene page, click on the command 'Refine this SNP set' in the box on the lower right. The page which then appears shows a variety of checkboxes in the second part of the table, including one labeled 'Validated SNPs' (these are SNPs which have been submitted by more than one submitter) and another labeled 'Coding sequence.' Check both of those boxes and then click the 'Apply filters' button. A listing of all validated coding SNPs will appear, where each SNP identifier is a link to the individual SNPper detail page for that SNP.

In order to design assays for an association study, you will need the flanks for each of these SNPs. Rather than laboriously viewing and cutting and pasting from each SNP detail page in turn, you can click the 'Export this SNP set' link from near the top of any SNP set page. The form which appears has a checkbox for each piece of information you would like included about each SNP. There are multiple output formats available including tab-delimited (which can be read by most spreadsheet programs), XML (which is a flexible computer readable format), or HTML which will give a page viewable in a web browser. You can view the results or you can provide an email address and have SNPper send the information in the format you have chosen to your own email inbox.

## Locate and identify an SNP from published flank sequence

Publications describing genetic associations with disease usually provide details such as the rs number of the SNPs involved, if these are known. Using SNPper, it is easy to find the SNP flanks by entering the rs number in the 'Find SNPs by name' box of the SNPper SNP finder page. However, in many cases, the researchers may not have provided an rs number. For example, the SNP may have been discovered by resequencing, and the discovery may not have been processed by dbSNP at the time of publication. In these cases, the SNP flanks are sometimes provided in the publication. Typically, published flank lengths are relatively short – 20 bases on each side of the SNP site for example. Unfortunately, 20 bases is usually not sufficient for genotype assay design, so a researcher wishing to design an assay might need to identify the genomic location of the SNP in order to obtain longer flanking sequences.

Many researchers are familiar with the NCBI BLAST program which is available at www.ncbi.nlm.nih.gov/BLAST

but the UCSC Blat program, which has been specifically optimized for locating short sequences (such as SNP flanks), is a more convenient tool for this particular task, particularly since the results are provided almost instantly and are integrated conveniently into the UCSC genome browser.

## GETTING THERE

Blat is available at http://genome.cse.ucsc.edu/cgi-bin/hgBlat which is a simple but flexible search page. Note that there are some important options along the top of the search page – the default genome is human, but chimp, dog, mouse, and many others are also available. The genome assembly is a crucial option, because the most recent genome assembly may not have SNP positions available until a few months after release – if the browser results page does not show an annotation section labeled 'Variation and repeats' with an SNPs option, try the search using the previous dated assembly.

## TYPICAL TASKS

Blat offers a deceptively simple interface but has some very useful and powerful options. Accepting the default set up will generally provide an appropriate search. Enter the published sequence into the text box and press the 'Submit' button. If possible, cut and paste the sequence (from a SNPper web page for example) to avoid introducing errors. Note that Blat works very well for sequence lengths around 40 to 50 bases – longer sequences can give more reliable matches, but in practice, there is generally very little marginal benefit beyond about 100 bases. If each flank is 50 or more bases, one flank is usually enough. For shorter flanks, you may get better results by submitting both flanks and inserting the major (common) SNP allele at the SNP position.

Note that Blat does not understand major/minor allele notation such as that used in SNPper flanks (e.g., [A/C]) – you must edit any SNP flanks containing both alleles, such as those you can cut and paste from SNPper, before submitting them to Blat. The search string must contain only the letters A, C, G, and T – letter case and spaces are ignored.

Blat will locate the sequence in the genome, so it is important to understand the position of the SNP in your search sequence and the location of the SNP in the matched location. If you submit only the 5′ flank (the sequence up to the '[' in a SNPper flank for example), your SNP location in the genome will be the base *after* the end of the region matched by Blat. If you submit the 3′ flank, the SNP is the base *before* the start of the region matched by your search sequence. Submitting both flanks, including the major allele in the center, will place the SNP locus where the major allele was, in the *center* of the

matched region. Note that Blat will also transparently check the reverse complement of your sequence and may find the best match that way.

The default Blat result display format is HTML – a web page with links for each match shown as 'Browse' which leads the UCSC genome browser centered on the region matched, and 'Details' which links to a Blat detailed report for the match. In order to find the SNP, use the UCSC genome browser link.

If there are no matches, check that you entered the correct flank – transcribing can lead to errors, so cut and paste from an electronic source if possible. If there is only one full length 100 percent matching 'hit,' the results are easy to interpret. However, if there are more than one matching regions, Blat provides some statistical measures (see the Blat help page for a detailed explanation) which can help to distinguish the closest match including the number of bases which match termed 'qsize' and the 'percent identity score', which represents the number of mismatches per thousand bases adjusted for insertions and deletions.

Generally, the region which has a qsize closest to the length of the entire sequence entered is a good first choice. If you entered both flanks, there may be a one base mismatch, depending on whether the SNP allele you included in your sequence was the major allele or not, but the entire sequence should otherwise match without error giving a qsize close to the length of your sequence. Often, small parts of the sequence you entered will have perfect matches in scattered parts of the genome, often on multiple chromosomes. These will have lower Blat qsize scores because they are only short fragments of the search sequence, although they may be perfect matches over those shorter lengths. In general, the longest match should be the entire flank length without any errors, suggesting that you found the correct place in the genome, so short matches can usually be safely ignored.

Click on the 'Browser' link for the best match as determined by qsize and identity scores – both of which should be as close to 100 percent as possible. The UCSC genome browser will appear with the search sequence showing as a black bar occupying the entire width of the display, labeled as 'Yourseq.' In order to see your sequence in a larger context, use one of the 'Zoom out' links near the top of the page – 1.5 or 3 times is usually sufficient. The UCSC browser offers a wide variety of annotations termed 'tracks.' These may be added to or removed from the browser display area by means of the long list of optional annotations below the display area.

Turn on the SNPs track by finding the annotation group labeled 'Variation and Repeats' which contains a SNPs track option. Use the drop down list to select 'Full' for the SNPs display. As described above, if there is no SNPs annotation track available on the USCS genome browser screen, you may need to repeat the Blat search after changing the Assembly option (drop down list at the upper part of the Blat search page) to the previous genome assembly. Refresh the browser display by clicking on the 'refresh' button on the right just above the chromosome color key. The browser window should now show an SNPs track. If there is a known SNP, it should be vertically below the place in the flank sequence where the variation was, either at the end if a single flank or in the center if both flanks were submitted.

Clicking on the SNP rs number shown on the left or on the small vertical bar in the browser window which corresponds to the SNP position will open a detail page with links to the detail record in dbSNP for that entry. Cut and paste the rs number and use SNPper's SNP finder for a detailed view of the SNP including flanks to confirm that you have found the one you were looking for.

Sometimes, publications list the PCR primers rather than the SNP flanks. It is much harder to unambiguously identify an SNP without flanks, because the primers will usually amplify a stretch of DNA rather than targeting a single base. Blat has a special search page for pairs of primers which will identify the region being amplified – the primer search link is toward the lower section of the main Blat page, labeled 'Electronic PCR.' While it may be possible to identify a single SNP within the range amplified by the primers, many SNPs may be found within the region, in which case unambiguous identification may not be possible.

## Determine sample size for a genetic association study: http://statgen.iop.kcl.ac.uk

As discussed in Chapter 3, the determination of an appropriate sample size is a crucial aspect of study design and planning. Recruiting more subjects than are needed gives rise to unnecessary costs, while studying too few subjects will provide inadequate statistical power and increase the chances of a false-negative finding. Statistical power for an association study is a measure of the probability of obtaining a statistically significant test result when there really is a true association between the outcome and the genetic variation under study. Typically, a researcher aims for at least 80 percent power, so if a negative study result is obtained, then there is a reasonable probability that there truly is no association. A study designed to give appropriate statistical power is useful even if it is negative. A negative underpowered study gives no useful information. For this reason, funding agencies are poorly disposed toward research proposals which do not provide a comprehensive assessment of statistical power. A well designed proposal will demonstrate that the study has a reasonable chance of finding true associations if they really exist.

There are a large number of general purpose epidemiological study design statistical power calculators and web sites, but the methods used in statistical genetics require assumptions about the genetic model, allele frequencies,

and disease penetrance, so specialized calculations are required.

### GETTING THERE

The web site at http://statgen.iop.kcl.ac.uk/gpc offers specialized calculators[11] for a wide variety of genetic study designs. Correct use of some of the specialized variance components calculators requires careful reading of the related publication,[12] but the calculator for case control genetic association designs is relatively straightforward.

### TYPICAL TASKS

For any given sample size, power tends to be higher when the minor allele is more frequent, so power calculations require estimates of the minor (risk) allele frequency expected in the general population. Of course, the minor allele cannot be more frequent than 0.5 (or it would be the major allele). Frequency data for some markers in some populations are available from public databases such as dbSNP through SNPper as described above, but in the majority of situations where the allele frequency is unknown, a series of power calculation should be performed using a plausible range of allele frequencies, as described below.

Estimates of population disease frequency (point prevalence) are needed for all calculations. For a common disease such as asthma, this might be 0.2 (i.e., assuming about 20 percent of the general population have asthma). Relative risks for the two genotypes containing the risk allele are also needed for the calculation. These, like the genetic model, are usually unknown when an experiment is being designed, so calculations should be performed over a range of plausible values. An additive genetic model is often assumed, where the risk for the minor allele homozygote (i.e., with genotype AA where A is the risk allele) is twice as high as the risk for the heterozygote (with only one copy of the risk allele). In a recessive genetic model, the heterozygote would have a relative risk of 1.0 (i.e., no additional risk) and only the minor allele homozygote relative risk would be elevated above 1.

Statistical power tends to increase with more cases, and to a lesser extent with higher ratios of control to case subject numbers, so the number of cases and the ratio of cases to controls are necessary elements for any power calculation. Power also varies with the probability chosen as the cutoff for rejecting the null hypothesis (usually defined as 'there is no association between the marker and disease risk'). Known as the type I error rate for the test, usually termed $\alpha$ in statistical text books, this is typically set at 0.05, although lower values may be more appropriate when many tests are to be performed.

When the number of subjects is fixed but the allele frequencies are not known in advance, it is useful to specify the lower limit of the range of minor allele frequencies with acceptable power. For example, when contemplating a case–control design, the number of cases and the control to case ratio may be already fixed if the genetic study is added on to an established clinical investigation.

From the page at http://statgen.iop.kcl.ac.uk/gpc, select the 'Case control for discrete traits' option. Enter the risk allele frequency (e.g., 0.1 for an SNP with a minor allele frequency of 10 percent), the estimated disease prevalence (e.g., 0.2 for asthma), then the estimated relative risk for the heterozygote and risk allele homozygote (e.g., 1.5 and 2.0, respectively). The next two fields are used to estimate power when the association is being tested using an SNP which is in linkage disequilibrium with the causal allele.[13,14] The marker allele refers to the allele being genotyped. The 'risk allele' refers to the (potentially unmeasured) causal SNP. For our purposes, setting D′ to 1.0 and the marker allele frequency to the same as the risk allele frequency, will ensure that the calculation is correct for the situation where the marker allele being studied is in fact the causal allele. Enter the number of cases and the control to case ratio (1.0 means there is 1:1 matching of cases to controls). The last two fields have reasonable default values for type I error rate and desired power, although these can be changed if necessary. Click the 'Process' button and a report will appear showing a variety of estimates. At the end of the page is a power table for a range of type I error rates and the number of cases required for attaining the specified desired power.

Values for a table showing differing allele frequencies, differing genetic models, and relative risks can be generated by systematically varying the risk allele frequency and the relative risks for the two risk genotypes over a range of plausible values, based on the biology and literature relevant to the specific research topic. Remember to change the marker allele frequency when you alter the risk allele frequency and leave the assumed D′ between them as 1.0.

## Visualizing SNP genotype data: www.pharmgat.net

As is often the case with complex biological data, important features can be discerned by visualizing experimental genotype data. For example, a graphical display of the pattern of pairwise linkage disequilibrium (LD) can help to understand the pattern of disease association statistical test results because SNPs which are in tight LD can be expected to have similar patterns of disease association.[13] A color-coded diagram showing individual subject genotype data can reveal important aspects of polymorphism frequency and can reveal missing data patterns, which can also help interpret disease association findings.

Tools for generating these images are highly specialized and are not as widely available as they might be, but methods for constructing two specific examples are described here – the visual genotype[15] and plots showing pairwise linkage disequilibrium values[16] between all markers, both of which can be quickly prepared along with many other simple but useful descriptive analyses from a single, freely available web tool.

### GETTING THERE

The PharmacoGenetics of Asthma Treatment (PharmGAT – www.pharmgat.net) project is part of the NIH-funded Pharmacogenetics Research Network (PGRN – www.pharmgkb.org/index.jsp) which makes data from sequencing and genotyping experiments freely available, together with many web accessible tools which can operate on the genotype data. Note that the visualization tools described here require individual subject genotypes – aggregate or summary data cannot be used to estimate pairwise LD or to prepare visual genotype diagrams. The data format required by the tools is very simple and is also the format in which subject level genotype data are made available from the PharmGAT site. In order to use experimental data from other sources, it must first be converted into the appropriate format, described below.

### TESTING THE TOOLS

A genotype data file may be obtained from the PharmGAT web site at www.pharmgat.net for testing the tools. From the main web site page, choose the 'Genes' link from the navigation bar near the top of the page. Click on the link for *ALOX15* to see the gene detail page and select the 'Prettybase' link from the top, left section of the 'Raw Data' group of options. The browser screen will show the contents of the file which contains 336 lines, each with four columns described in more detail below. To make a local copy of the raw data on your computer, click the 'Plain Text' link. The same lines will appear on the browser screen without any colored headers or other extraneous information, and can now be saved as a plain text file on the local computer hard disk. Use the browser 'Save as' option from the 'File' menu (usually the top line of the browser screen) to save a local copy of the prettybase file in a convenient local directory. Use the default name (ALOX15.prettybase.txt), and choose a directory which is easy to locate for the new file – it will be needed for the example exercises to follow.

The tools described below will be illustrated using the ALOX15 genotype data, but they will work with any experimental genotype data converted into the format illustrated by these data and described in more detail below. To view the contents of the file, open a copy downloaded from the web site in a text editor. If you use a word processing package to open the file, you may permanently damage it, because extraneous formatting information will be added unless you remember to save the file as plain text. It is much safer to use a non-wordprocessing text editor (such as Notepad). Notice that the file does not contain a 'header' line, so the first line is a line of data. Each line of data contains four fields, separated by a single 'tab' character. When preparing files containing your own data, a tab or any arbitrary number of spaces may be used to separate the fields on each line. The first column of each line contains a number which is the relative position of each marker – rs numbers or other identifiers containing non-numeric characters are not permitted. These relative positions may be negative or positive, as long as the number of bases between any two SNPs can be calculated as the difference between their relative offsets. All output tables and images are sorted by these numeric position values so SNPs will be seen in the order corresponding to these numbers. The second column contains an individual subject identifier. These can be a mixture of numbers and letters. The third and fourth columns must contain the two alleles of the individual subject's genotype at the specified relative position. Alleles can be provided as letter codes (e.g., A, C, G, or T) or as numbers. Letter codes are more convenient for preparing tables of allele and genotype distributions for publication.

It is often useful to ensure that each subject identifier starts with a letter designating race or subgroup if the data set contains multiple meaningful subgroups because the tools can provide separate reports based on these subject identifier prefixes. For example, it is usually not appropriate to combine subjects from different ethnic groups, or to combine parents and their offspring for estimating linkage disequilibrium. The default for these tools is to have European subject identifiers begin with the letter 'E' and African-American subject identifiers begin with the letter 'D'. Additional information is available from the on-line documentation for the tools linked from the main page.

## TYPICAL TASK 1: PREPARING A VISUAL GENOTYPE IMAGE

The visual genotype[15] is a simple but effective graphical representation of genotype data that facilitates assessment of the pattern of missing data and patterns of heterozygosity over the region. From the PharmGAT tools page, choose the link to the 'Prettybase reports' tool.

The first line on the form is for a gene name or other descriptive text which will appear on the report. Since all reports can be saved and printed, this is useful for remembering where the data came from. For the ALOX15 data, type 'ALOX15' as the gene name.

The second line has a 'Browse' button which is used to locate the data file on the local machine. Click that button to open a file browser window. Navigate to the folder where the ALOX15 example prettybase file was saved and click on that file to highlight it. Click the 'Open' button in the file browser window and the full path to that file will appear on the second line of the form. This is where the tool will take its genotype input.

The third line of the form is a drop down list containing a wide variety of report format options. To open the list, click on the small down-facing triangle to the left of the text

on the third form line. Choose the sixth option – 'Visual Genotype (ID order)'.

The fourth section of the form is the most complex. It contains information about how to interpret the first letter of each subject identifier. Leave it set to the default values for the ALOX15 prettybase file since the defaults are appropriate for that file.

The fifth section is a drop down list controlling the format in which the report will be delivered. Leave it as the default value ('HTML/Graphics') for this exercise. Other reports such as allele frequencies can be downloaded as spreadsheet-compatible files which are very handy for preparing material for publication.

The sixth section contains a filter for minor allele frequency (MAF). For this exercise, leave it set at the default value (0.0). Filtering out loci with MAF below 0.05 or even 0.1 can be helpful in many situations, for example, to see pairwise LD plots limited to the more common variants where LD is usually stronger (see below). The 'Download' check box is useful if you wish to save an image or spreadsheet-compatible report, for this exercise, leave it unchecked so that the image will appear in the browser window.

The final item on the form is the 'Submit' button. If necessary, the companion 'Reset' button can be used to clear the form back to default values in preparation for preparing reports for another gene. Click the 'Submit' button to view the report. Depending on the report type and the number of subjects and loci, the report may take some little time to prepare. When it is ready, the browser screen will automatically display it as shown in Fig. 5A.7.

The visual genotype shows each locus for each subject individually. Loci are columns and each subject is a single row. SNP loci offsets from the input file are shown at the top of each image in genomic order. Subjects are ordered by their ID number in the report formatted as described above. Missing data are shown as gray squares. Heterozygous loci are shown in red and the common and rare homozygous loci are blue and yellow, respectively. The samples may be ordered by a similarity measure rather than alphabetically, by choosing the 'Visual Genotype (Genotype order)' option on the form before submitting the job.

If you need to use an image for preparing a report or manuscript, check the 'Download' option and run the report. The image file will then be available to save on your local hard drive where it can be pasted into a word processed document.

## TYPICAL TASK 2: PREPARING A PAIRWISE LINKAGE DISEQUILIBRIUM IMAGE

Pairwise linkage disequilibrium (LD) is non-random association between the alleles of any two nearby SNPs.[13,17] It can be estimated in samples containing genotypes from multiple individuals but measures are biased and unreliable in small samples.[18] As described in Chapter 1, two commonly used measures of the strength of pairwise LD are

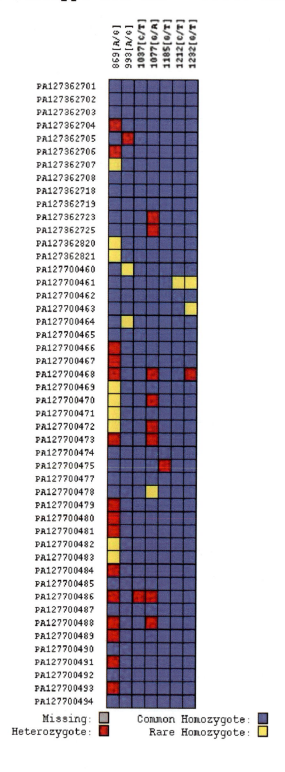

**Figure 5A.7**    *Visual genotype from the ALOX15 prettybase file downloaded from the PharmCAT website as described in the section entitled 'Visualizing SNP genotype data'.*

$D'$ (pronounced 'D prime') and $r^2$. These two quantities are related but have different properties and uses. Although both are scaled to a maximum value of 1.0, the $D'$ measure tends to be larger than the corresponding $r^2$, and $r^2$ can be interpreted as loss of effective sample size for indirect association studies.[14]

Pairwise LD provides a summary of association between markers in a region. If two SNPs have a high pairwise LD, then the genotype from one of them will be highly predictive of the genotype at the other. In practice, this means that only one of the two needs to be genotyped to gain information about disease association from both.[14] Disease association experiments can be designed with a small number of SNPs while still retaining good power to detect association over the region, using pairwise LD as a guide.[19,20] In practice, this is similar to well-known methods based on haplotype tagging SNPs,[21,22] but has the advantage of not requiring haplotype imputation which can be problematic over large regions.[23]

If there are N SNPs in a region, the matrix of pairwise LD values will contain $N^2$ cells, but the upper and lower triangular halves are symmetrical and contain the same values. In addition, there are no values along the diagonal because pairwise LD calculation requires two distinct SNPs. In total, there will be $(N^2 - N)/2$ distinct pairwise LD values for N SNPs. For large regions (e.g., more than 100 SNPs) this will require substantial calculation time since each value requires an iterative maximum likelihood procedure to determine the two locus haplotypes of individuals who have heterozygous genotypes at both SNP loci.[24] Note that there is no ambiguity for the haplotypes for all other individuals.

The prettybase reports tool from the PharmGAT web site (described above for visual genotypes) can also create an image showing pairwise LD values from a prettybase format input file. The steps are identical to those described above, but instead of choosing the Visual Genotype report, select one of the Pairwise LD reports – both $D'$ and $r^2$ calculations are available on the 'Report Type' drop-down list.

Options including downloading the image to a local hard disk, filtering out SNPs below a specified MAF, and grouping subjects according to the first letter of their ID number, are exactly the same for all of the reports from this particular tool. Choosing the 'Text' option for output format will provide the numerical LD values for each pair of SNPs as a text file if needed.

## Key learning points

- Bioinformatics may be defined as the rapidly evolving art and science of adding value to biological data in support of biological research.

- Many bioinformatic resources including vast and rapidly expanding repositories of genomic data are freely available via the internet.

- Many major genetic bioinformatic resources have been designed to be easy to use without requiring specific bioinformatic training or expertise.

- Integrative, web-based tools make these much easier to use.

- NCBI, UCSC, and Ensembl are three of the main integrative internet sites which make it easy to use an ordinary web browser to explore genomes, literature, and related data.

- SNPper automates many tasks when gathering information about SNPs for designing candidate gene disease association studies.

## REFERENCES

1 International Human Genome Sequencing Consortium. Finishing the euchromatic sequence of the human genome. *Nature* 2004; **431**: 931–45, doi: 10.1038/nature03001.

2 National Center for Biotechnology Information. GenBank statistics. In. NCBI web site documentation, http://www.ncbi.nlm.nih.gov/Genbank/genbankstats.html ed; 2004.

3 National Center for Biotechnology Information. GenBank Flat File Release 142.0. In: Distribution Release Notes. ftp://ftp.ncbi.nih.gov/genbank/gbrel.txt; 2004.

4 National Library of Medicine. PubMed: MEDLINE retrieval on the world wide web. In. Fact Sheet, http://www.nlm.nih.gov/pubs/factsheets/pubmed.html ed: National Institutes of Health; 2004.

5 National Center for Biotechnology Information. dbSNP. In: http://www.ncbi.nih.gov/SNP ed: Release 121; 2004.

6 Boffelli D, McAuliffe J, Ovcharenko D et al. Phylogenetic shadowing of primate sequences to find functional regions of the human genome. *Science* 2003; **299**: 1391–4.

7 Felsenstein J, Churchill G. A hidden Markov model approach to variation among sites in rate of evolution. *Mol Biol Evol* 1996; **13**: 93–104.

8 Botstein D, Risch N. Discovering genotypes underlying human phenotypes: past successes for mendelian disease, future approaches for complex disease. *Nat Genet* 2003; **33**(Suppl): 228–37.

9 Riva A, Kohane IS. SNPper: retrieval and analysis of human SNPs. *Bioinformatics* 2002; **18**: 1681–5.

10 Lazarus R, Raby BA, Lange C et al. Toll-like receptor 10 (TLR10) genetic variation is associated with asthma in two independent samples. *Am J Respir Crit Care Med* 2004; **170**: 594–600. doi: 10.1164/rccm.200404-491OC.

11 Purcell S, Sham PC. Genetic Power Calculator: design of linkage and association genetic mapping studies of complex traits. *Bioinformatics* 2003; **19**: 149–50.

12 Sham PC, Purcell S. Power of linkage versus association analysis of quantitative traits, by use of variance-components models, for sibship data. *Am J Hum Genet* 2000; **66**: 1616–30.

13  Ardlie KG, Kruglyak L, Seielstad M. Patterns of linkage
    disequilibrium in the human genome. *Nat Rev Genet* 2002; **3**:
    299–309.

14  Pritchard JK, Przeworski M. Linkage disequilibrium in humans:
    models and data. *Am J Hum Genet* 2001; **69**: 1–14.

15  Rieder MJ, Taylor SL, Clark AG, Nickerson DA. Sequence variation
    in the human angiotensin converting enzyme. *Nat Genet* 1999;
    **22**: 59–62.

16  Lazarus R, Vercelli D, Palmer LJ et al. Single nucleotide
    polymorphisms in innate immunity genes: abundant variation and
    potential role in complex human disease. *Immunol Rev* 2002;
    **190**: 9–25.

17  Devlin B, Risch N. A comparison of linkage disequilibrium
    measures for fine-scale mapping. *Genomics* 1995; **29**: 311–22.

18  Teare MD, Dunning AM, Durocher G et al. Sampling distribution
    of summary linkage disequilibrium measures. *Ann Hum Genet*
    2002; **66**: 223–33.

19  Byng MC, Whittaker JC, Cuthbert AP et al. SNP subset selection
    for genetic association studies. *Ann Hum Genet* 2003; **67**: 543–56.

20  Carlson CS, Eberle MA, Rieder MJ et al. Selecting a maximally
    informative set of SNPs for association analyses using linkage
    disequilibrium. *Am J Hum Genet* 2004; **74**: 106–20.

21  Johnson GCL, Esposito L, Barratt BJ et al. Haplotype tagging for
    the identification of common disease genes. *Nat Genet* 2001;
    **29**: 233–7.

22  Sebastiani P, Lazarus R, Weiss ST et al. Minimal haplotype
    tagging. *Proc Natl Acad Sci* 2003; **100**: 9900–5.

23  Schulze T, Zhang K, Chen Y et al. Defining haplotype blocks and
    tag single-nucleotide polymorphisms in the human genome.
    *Hum Mol Genet* 2004; **13**: 335–42.

24  Hill WG. Estimation of linkage disequilibrium in randomly mating
    populations. *Heredity* 1974; **33**: 229–39.

# Genomics and proteomics in lung disease: microarrays and bioinformatics issues

ISAAC S. KOHANE

## INTRODUCTION

Measurements of gene expression and protein levels have a long history in the investigation of pulmonary diseases, and applications of these insights have already had some clinical impact (e.g., in surfactant therapy for neonatal respiratory distress syndrome). Nonetheless, there is great excitement about current methods of protein and RNA measurement. The ability to measure, comprehensively and rapidly, the individual molecules making up a significant fraction of the entire transcriptome and proteome of a specified cell or tissue qualitatively changes the way that scientific questions can be posed, data are analyzed, and biological systems are modeled. Furthermore, the computational requirements of these massively parallel data, both in storage and in analysis, have required the development of new types of multidisciplinary teams well versed in the biological and computational sciences. This chapter section is intended to serve as a broad introduction to the application of genomics (and tangentially proteomics) to biomedical research and practice of pulmonary medicine.

## THE SINGULAR SUCCESS OF MICROARRAYS

Perhaps the most influential paper in functional genomics was published by Alizadeh et al. in 2000.[1] It should be noted that this experiment pertains to large B cell lymphoma, which is a malignancy and only occasionally a pulmonary disorder. As will be subsequently explained, cancer research was the first to benefit from functional genomics primarily because cancer is a disease in which the affected tissue is clearly identified, is often surgically removed, and in which transcriptional disorders are likely often very close to disease etiology. Subsequently, as genomic techniques have become more refined, cost-effective, and comprehensive, significant contributions have also been made in pulmonary medicine.[1a-1c]

In the study by Alizadeh and colleagues, gene expression profiles of the tumor tissue from a group of patients with large B cell lymphoma were studied. Specifically, the expression of over 10 000 genes was measured in each patient's sample. These data were then sorted in such a way (see discussion in the unsupervised clustering section below) that samples with similar expression profiles would be grouped together. See Fig. 5B.1(a), commonly called a 'dendrogram', where each leaf of the tree (dendrogram) represents a patient's sample. The visual shorthand used, which is a graphical representation of the data, is that the more similar two expression profiles are of two samples, the closer they are to each other on the tree. The investigators recognized that, based solely on these expression array results, there seemed to be two major groups in the data set with distinct expression profiles. When they reviewed the clinical data regarding these patients, it became apparent that there was an important and highly clinically relevant difference between the patients based on their expression profiles: their mortality. Shown in Fig. 5B.1(b) are the Kaplan–Meier survival curves corresponding to the two groups of patients identified by gene expression profile, with the number of years of survival on the x-axis and the probability of survival on the y-axis. Clearly, these two groups of patients have significantly different survival curves. This research made it abundantly clear that there were four new large clinical and research opportunities based on expression array data.

First, a new diagnostic classification was identified; previously, patients with B-cell lymphoma were treated as a monolithic group of patients, and clinically meaningful classification could not be performed. Second, new prognostic information was available to assist with clinical management. Previously, variations in outcome among B cell lymphoma patients could only be ascribed to individual variation of unknown origin. These microarray data led to the development of a biological, data-driven process by which patient outcome could be predicted. Thus, a patient with a gene

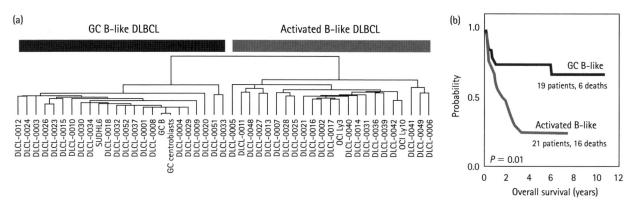

**Figure 5B.1** *Redefining large B-cell lymphoma by genomic profiling. On the left (a), a dendrogram has been constructed across the individual patient samples of B-cell lymphoma, using an unsupervised technique. The top branch essentially defines an even split between the category 'GC B-like DLBCL' and 'Activated B-like DLBCL,' but this distinction was never before made clinically. On the right (b), Kaplan–Meier survival curves of the patients providing samples are presented. Patients whose cancer matched the 'Activated B-like DLBCL' gene expression profile had significantly reduced survival.*

expression profile that resembled that of the high-risk group in (b) could be informed of a very different set of risks and expectations than a patient with an expression profile similar to the low risk group. Of course, this clinical application would require considerable validation prior to practicing this form of genomic prognostication. Nonetheless, the direction for future clinical application was clear. Third, a new therapeutic opportunity had been identified. Even without new therapeutic interventions, the change in prognostic information changes the therapeutic decision-making process. A patient that is in a cohort with a high mortality risk may warrant more aggressive application of available, potentially toxic chemotherapeutic agents. Additionally, the cellular profile of these patient groups (e.g., 'activated B cell') suggests a variety of pathways that can be explored to develop specific and novel therapies. Fourth, several new research opportunities had been identified. Determining the mechanistic differences, in the patient or the tumor, between the high and low risk groups was an obvious and important question. Although this remains unclear, the measurement of a significant fraction of the total number of human mRNA transcripts (the 'transcriptome') might provide important clues or hypotheses to test.

This was a remarkable set of results for a very modestly scaled clinical research effort, which included less than 100 patients. Subsequently, many clinical researchers have applied these techniques to their own areas of interest and expertise.

How did this come about? The recent astounding confluence of progress in robotics, fluorescence detection, photolithography, and the human genome project, have enabled the routine use of RNA expression microarray detection technologies in a variety of clinical and basic research applications. With commercially available tools, a single RNA expression detection microarray experiment can provide

systematic quantitative information on the expression of 60 000 unique RNAs. cDNA and oligonucleotide microarray technology can be used to determine, classify, and prognosticate disease states, and it can also be used to analyze complex systems, such as complex diseases influenced by multiple genes, gene × gene interactions, and gene × environment interactions.[2] RNA expression microarrays can also be used in time series to measure how a particular intervention[3,4] changes the expression of large numbers of genes in a reproducible pattern determined by inherent genetic regulatory networks. Whereas the former applications resemble the kinds of classification efforts that pulmonologists have previously applied to samples such as bronchoalveolar lavage fluid collections, the latter efforts are analogous to the dynamic and provocative testing of pulmonary function in response to environmental and pharmacological stimuli. However, by virtue of comprehensive rather than targeted measurements, these novel technologies do not fit well into the usual scientific method employed by pulmonologists.

As in genome-wide linkage or association studies, comprehensive measurement of RNA expression can reduce our dependence on a priori knowledge (with its attendant biases) and allow the biological processes to point us in potentially fruitful directions for research. Thus, much of bioinformatics and functional genomics is a *hypothesis-generating* effort, which has the potential to lead to a highly productive set of investigations using more conventional hypothesis-driven research. However, poorly controlled or performed measurements will not provide the high-yield hypotheses that have resulted from the more successful functional genomics experiments.

Gene expression microarrays are notable not because they can uniquely measure gene expression; quantitative or semi-quantitative measurement of gene expression has been available for decades. However, gene expression detection microarrays (and other genome-scale technologies) are uniquely capable of measuring tens of thousands of genes at a time; it is this *quantitative* change of the scale of gene measurement that has led to a *qualitative* change in our understanding of gene regulation.

Within this context, we will describe the features of a microarray that are suitable to large-scale genomic studies by the general scientific community. Other efforts that have also used the term 'microarray' are unlikely to be successful, at least in the near term. Optimally, a microarray should be low cost, such that hundreds of samples can be assayed within an individual laboratory with reasonable but not limitless funding. In addition, the cost of the equipment should be affordable by most investigational laboratories. The microarray should allow useful data to be generated with a routine set of procedures requiring no scientific judgment and using standard equipment. The process of data acquisition should be completely automated, or at least not require specialized intervention to generate useful data. The equipment required should easily fit into a standard laboratory bench format, and it should be usable by a clinical investigator without in-depth molecular biology knowledge. All items identified by the microarray technology (proteins or RNA species) should be automatically identified against standard reference nomenclatures (e.g., HUGO nomenclature). High throughput capacity is essential, with at least the capability to process hundreds of patient samples within days. Finally, there should be massively parallel measurements of the relevant analytes, such as members of transcriptome, members of the proteome, or members of the metabolome.

Expression microarray technology qualified fully for this microarray definition by 2001, although excellent science was carried out with microarrays previously. In contrast, proteomic technology has yet to achieve similar growth and applicability precisely because it does not meet these desirable criteria.

## PRAGMATICS OF GENE EXPRESSION MICROARRAYS

We will discuss the production, application, and data analysis of RNA detection microarrays, also referred to as DNA chips, biochips, or simply chips. There are several key components of these RNA detection microarrays:

1  *Probe*: The biochemical agent that is complementary to a specific sequence of RNA from a test sample.[5] Probes can be pieces of cDNA, synthesized oligonucleotides, or nucleotide fragments of a chromosome. The database of expressed sequence tags (ESTs) for serial analysis of gene expression (SAGE) can also be incorporated.

2  *Array*: The medium upon which the probes are placed. Current techniques to generate arrays include robotic spotting, electric guidance, photolithography, piezo-electricity, fiberoptics, and microbeads. This step also specifies the chemical constitution of the medium, such as glass slides, nylon meshes, silicon, nitrocellulose, or beads.

3  *Sample probe*: The RNA derived from test samples that is used in the assay. Total RNA may be used, or mRNA can be selected by binding its poly-adenine (poly-A) tail. Alternatively, mRNA may be copied into cDNA, typically using fluorescently labeled or biotinylated nucleotides. This tissue from which the RNA is derived requires careful consideration; the gene expression of a pathological end-stage of a lung disease such as chronic obstructive pulmonary disease (COPD) or idiopathic pulmonary fibrosis may differ considerably from earlier disease stages.

4  *Assay*: For microarrays in common use, the gene expression signal is measured by hybridization. For SAGE, gene expression is transduced into oligonucleotides via restriction enzymes and ligation.

5  *Readout*: The measurement of the expression signal and the representation of that signal comprise the readout of the array. Hybridization is typically measured using either fluorescent dyes or radioactive labels. For SAGE, the constructed oligonucleotides are assessed by sequencing.

For the microarrays in common use, one typically uses the five components listed above in the following manner. The process starts by taking a specific biological tissue of interest, extracting its mRNA (or total RNA), and making a fluorescence-tagged cDNA copy of this mRNA. This tagged cDNA copy, or *sample probe*, is then hybridized to a slide containing an array of single-strand cDNAs called *probes* which have been placed in specific locations on this grid. A *sample probe* will only hybridize with its complementary *probe*. A fluorescent detection signal is typically added to the sample probe either by: (1) fluorescent nucleotide bases are used when making the cDNA from the RNA, or (2) biotinylated nucleotides are first incorporated into the cDNA, followed by an application of fluorescence-labeled streptavidin which will bind to the biotin. The probe/sample probe hybridization process on a microarray typically occurs over several hours. All unhybridized sample probes are then washed off, and the microarray is lit under laser light and scanned using laser confocal microscopy; this generates the assay signal. A digital image scanner records the brightness level at each grid location on the microarray corresponding to particular RNA species, which creates the readout from the assay.

The brightness level detected by the digital image scanner is correlated with the absolute amount of mRNA in the original sample, and thus, the expression level of the gene encoding this mRNA.[6] Roughly, one microarray experiment is equivalent to many Northern blots that simultaneously assays a total RNA sample on a small common medium for many different unique mRNA species. However, the amount of total RNA required for one typical Northern blot is more than sufficient for one microarray experiment using current technologies. However, this analogy breaks down in that only a single hybridization condition (e.g., temperature, time) is used in hybridizing all of the mRNA assays in the microarray, and unless the probes are carefully chosen, this may not be the optimal condition for the assay of all RNA species.

Because microarray technologies allow the comprehensive measurement of the expression level of many genes simultaneously, typical applications include the comprehensive quantification of RNA expression profiles of a system under control versus test conditions. In addition, expression profiles of two systems under one or more conditions can be compared, such as different strains of organisms (e.g., wildtype versus knock-out mice). Microarrays can also be used to compare expression levels between neighboring cells within the same microscopic field, with appropriate amplification of the test sample mRNA.[7] As discussed in Chapter 4B, oligonucleotide microarrays have also been used for high throughput single nucleotide polymorphism (SNP) genotyping.

The performance of gene expression technology typically depends critically on the general validity of certain fundamental biological assumptions. The first key assumption is that there is a close correspondence between mRNA transcription and its associated protein translation. One would ideally measure the protein products of the gene, as in proteomics, or even better, the biologically functional activity of these products.[8] However, the field of proteomics is in its infancy, and there is no practical generic approach to assessing biological functionality. Fortunately, there is typically a close connection between the function of a gene product and its expression pattern. Of course, there are many exceptions to this assumption. For example, proteins that make up the lung extracellular matrix can considerably outlast the lifetime of their associated mRNA. Nevertheless, the initial successes in the application of gene expression microarrays in investigations of biological function suggest that this assumption frequently holds true.

The second key assumption of gene expression technology is that all mRNA transcripts have identical life spans. Again, there are well-known exceptions. For instance, it is known that the length of the 3′ poly-adenine (poly-A) tail of an mRNA species appears to be related to its stability.

The third key assumption in gene expression technology is that all cellular activities are entirely programmed by transcriptional events. There are many examples in which external stimuli cause biochemical changes within the cell *without* engaging the transcriptional machinery. There is also a much larger class of biological processes that do not primarily operate at the transcriptional level, such as muscular contraction, nerve excitation, and hormonal release. Eventually, all these events will cause some change in transcriptional activity, but such patterns of gene expression would probably not reveal the control processes that govern them.

There are currently two types of chip technologies in common usage: robotically spotted and photolithographic oligonucleotide microarrays.

## Robotically spotted microarrays

Robotically spotted microarrays are commonly used with cDNA probes on glass slides. This type of microarray, also known as a cDNA microarray, was first described in 1995.[6]

To make these arrays, a robotic spotter mechanically picks up a small volume of a solution containing a specific cDNA sequence and deposits this droplet at precise locations in a grid on a glass slide. The cDNA sequences that become these specific probes are typically amplified from vectors in bacterial clones using polymerase chain reaction. Each cDNA droplet should ideally have an equal number of cDNA molecules (see Fig. 5B.2). Although there are several commercially available versions, customized cDNA microarrays are often produced in individual laboratories, which poses challenges in the dual goals of background noise reduction and foreground RNA signal amplification. Designer-definable parameters exist to control spotting size, drying time, and the glass slide material used. Nonetheless, mastering this approach is quite challenging.

There are several important considerations in selecting robotically spotted microarrays. The first advantage is customizability. A large subsequence ($\approx$2000 base pairs long) complementary to the actual sequence that is to be probed is placed on the chip, and the designer has full control over the selection of probes to be used. The set up costs for this approach are approximately $20 000; detailed guidelines may be found at the Brown laboratory microarraying website (http://cmgm.stanford.edu/pbrown/mguide/index.html). Several companies sell robotic spotters-arrayer units. Glass slides for microarray construction are available from a variety of vendors. The notable disadvantage with greater customizability is that it may lead to greater potential for errors. For instance, poor quality control or nonuniformity in the construction of different probes, such as spot-basing size, will complicate the subsequent analysis and interpretation of the resulting data.

The second advantage of robotically spotted microarrays is that larger nucleotide fragments, including entire cDNAs, are placed on the chip, thus reducing the likelihood of nonspecific hybridization of labeled sample probes to the probe that was placed on the glass slide. Typically, a designer who wishes to have a particular gene probe on a chip will create a clone with 5′ and 3′ end of that particular gene of interest. These cDNA substrings of the original gene are approximately 100 to 200 base pairs in length. Although a long probing sequence ensures a unique representation of the original gene, it does not mean that hybridization conditions will be equally optimized for all cDNA subsequences.

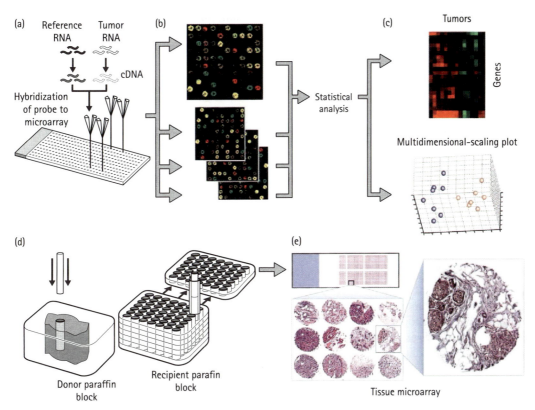

**Figure 5B.2**    *An overview of procedures for preparing and analyzing robotically spotted complementary DNA (cDNA) microarrays with breast-tumor tissue. (a) Reference RNA and tumor RNA are converted to cDNA by reverse transcription and labeled with different fluorescent dyes (green for the reference cells and red for the tumor cells), and hybridized to a cDNA microarray containing robotically placed cDNA clones on a glass slide. (b) The slides are analyzed with a confocal laser scanning microscope and color images are generated for each cDNA spot of hybridization with RNA from the tumor and reference cells. Genes with increased expression in the tumors appear red, whereas those with decreased expression in the tumors appear green. Genes with similar levels of expression in the two samples appear yellow. Genes of interest are selected on the basis of the differences in the level of expression by known tumor classes (e.g., BRCA1-mutation status). Statistical analysis determines whether the observed differences in the gene-expression profiles are greater than would be expected by chance. (c) The differences in gene expression patterns between tumor classes can be visualized in a color-coded plot, and the relations between tumors can be portrayed in a multidimensional-scaling plot. Tumors with similar gene-expression profiles cluster in the multidimensional-scaling plot. (d) Particular genes of interest can be studied in a histological context through the use of tissue microarrays, which include a large number of arrayed, paraffin-embedded tumor specimens. (e) Immunohistochemical analyses of many of these arrayed biopsy specimens can be performed in order to extend the cDNA microarray findings.[21]*

For example, probe/sample probe hybridization rate is known to vary depending upon the GC content of a transcript.

The third advantage of robotically spotted microarrays is that RNA from two different samples, usually a test and a control condition, can be hybridized onto a common cDNA microarray simultaneously. The two different RNA samples are typically labeled with different fluorescent dyes, such as Cy3 and Cy5. This two-dye system allows for the excitation of the microarray by laser light at two different frequencies; the hybridized RNA abundance can be scanned for both colors (corresponding to distinct samples) separately. Since the hybridization conditions, and thus the brightness, of each spot on the array are different, the absolute individual signals are not typically used. Instead, the *ratio* or *fold* difference in the brightness of the hybridized RNA

of one sample versus another is calculated; for example, the intensity of Cy3 versus Cy5 [(Cy3)/(Cy5)]. If the background intensity for each dye is measured and controlled for, the ratio becomes [(Cy3 measured-Cy3 background)/(Cy5 measured-Cy5 background)]. This provides a measurement of the relative abundance of the RNA, and thus the relative expression level, of one sample with respect to the other sample. However, it has been shown that not all cDNA sample probe sequences label symmetrically with Cy3 and Cy5[9] when paired dye-swapping experiments are performed (i.e., if the first hybridization is control (Cy3) versus test (Cy5), then switch dyes for the second hybridization).

Increasingly, rather than using cDNAs, robotic spotters are being used for oligonucleotide microarrays. These are arrays that use the two-dye methods described above but employ probe sequences, typically shorter than 80 bases, that hybridize with a specific portion of each gene. These have many of the benefits and disadvantages of the photolithographically constructed microarrays, described in the next section. They may be more cost-effective than photolithographically constructed microarrays, but they do require an experienced technical staff.

In summary, each robotically spotted microarray experiment has its own built-in control, and results are given in terms of fold change or difference from a control sample. However, the measurement of *absolute* quantities is quite challenging with this approach.

## Photolithographic microarrays

The second popular class of microarrays in use, photolithographic microarrays, has been most notably developed and marketed by Affymetrix. In current versions of these microarrays, more than one million oligonucleotides 25 base pairs in length, called *25-mers*, are selectively placed on a grid. These oligonucleotide chips, or oligochips, are constructed using a photolithographic masking technique similarly to the process that is used in microelectronics.[10] Currently, these microarrays are produced as a wafer containing between 40 and 400 microarrays; after this wafer is tested, it is broken into individual microarrays. Commercially produced oligochips exist that are disease- as well as species-specific, and custom microarrays can be produced rapidly.

The manufacturing technique for an Affymetrix oligochip is markedly different from robotically spotted arrays. Each wafer is built on an empty glass slide. Upon this slide, *25-mer* probes are created base-by-base using light-directed oligonucleotide synthesis. These oligonucleotides are constructed in parallel by selectively masking and unmasking specific coordinates of the array, and exposing the entire ensemble to ultraviolet light in between laying on the bases (A, T, G, or C) separately. Each applied photolithographic mask generates different areas of photodeprotection on the solid glass substrate. The combination of these masks with an intervening chemical coupling step allows the incorporation of additional nucleotides to existing strands only where desired.

The higher probe pair density of oligonucleotide microarrays, compared to robotically spotted arrays, allows more genes to be assayed on a single chip. A disadvantage is that current technology allows for only one experiment to be run on a single chip at a time. Thus, one does not obtain meaningful data from placing a control sample and test sample on an oligonucleotide microarray simultaneously. Instead, these two samples are measured on two separate oligochips. Thus, one typically has to apply a suitable normalization transformation across separate microarray data sets (i.e., *inter*-array) at the subsequent data analysis stage in order to make meaningful comparisons of reported expression changes in different samples. Oligochips are not as easily customizable at the user's end as robotically spotted microarrays, so if an oligochip is not available for a gene of interest, it cannot be easily interrogated with this approach.

Since each probe on the photolithographic microarray is limited to 25 base pairs in length, multiple probes are used to screen each gene. For each gene whose expression needs to be measured on an Affymetrix oligochip, a set of 16–20 25-mers are chosen that uniquely represent that particular gene, and that would hybridize under the same general conditions. The sample probe that is to be interrogated by cDNA probes on the Affymetrix microarray is referred to as the *target*. Every *perfect match* (PM) probe for a specific mRNA has a corresponding *mismatch* (MM) probe. A MM probe is constructed from the same nucleotide sequence as its PM probe partner, except that the middle (usually the 13th) base pair has been switched to result in a sequence mismatch.

The combination of a PM oligonucleotide probe and its associated MM oligonucleotide probe is called a *probe pair*. The MM probes serve two important functions. First, at low concentrations of the target (sample probe), the MM probes display greater sensitivity to changes in concentration. Second, MM probes are thought to bind to nonspecific sequences at the same rate as the PM probes, providing an internal control for *background* nonspecific hybridization. However, depending upon the total RNA sample, it is possible that the PM probe is already highly specific and the MM probes are simply binding to differently specific labeled subsequences in the sample. One has to be careful to distinguish between *nonspecific* hybridization and *differently specific* hybridization with regards to the use of MM probe data. These challenges have contributed to the expanding number of analytic programs that translate PM and MM values into expression levels (see Fig. 5B.3).

To synthesize an appropriate amount of target, sample probe is reverse transcribed from total RNA using an oligo-deoxythymidine (oligo-dT) primer containing a T7 polymerase site that allows 5′ to 3′ transcription. Amplification and labeling of the cDNA sample probe is achieved with an in vitro transcription reaction using biotinylated deoxynucleotide triphosphates (dNTPs), resulting in the linear amplification of the cDNA population. This linearity assumption becomes increasingly less valid with decreasing quantities of total RNA and increasing number of amplification cycles. The biotin-labeled cDNA probe is then hybridized to the oligonucleotide arrays, followed by binding to a streptavidin-conjugated fluorescent marker. Laser excitation of the hybridized sample, confocal microscopy, and image acquisition by an optical scanner, is performed. The data from these procedures are stored in an image file in which each oligonucleotide species is represented by a small rectangular area (approximately 50 $\mu^2$), called the *probe cell*. Each probe cell is composed of several image pixels, each of which occupies an area from 3 to 24 $\mu^2$. The image file is processed so that the intensity of the pixels in each probe cell recorded are stored in a .cel file, which reports a measure of

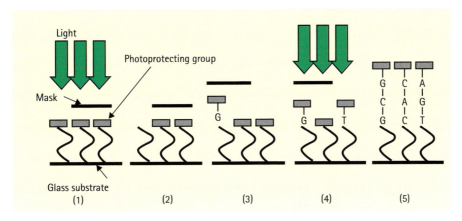

**Figure 5B.3** *High density oligonucleotide microarray synthesis using photolithography. Using selective masks, photo-labile protecting groups are light-activated for DNA synthesis (1, 2) and photoprotected DNA bases are coupled to the intended coordinates (3). This cycle is repeated (4) with the appropriate masks to allow for controlled parallel synthesis of oligonucleotide chains in all coordinates on the array (5).[21]*

hybridization per contiguous oligonucleotide surface on the microarray. The .cel files are processed to provide aggregate measures of expression for each *probe set*, the collection of probe pairs that are designed to measure a single mRNA species. These probe sets are referred to by an Affymetrix accession number that is in turn linked to a Genbank identifier, which typically is linked to a single gene.

There is a great deal of controversy regarding the best way to calculate the aggregate expression over a probe set from these .cel files.[11,12] Publicly available packages such as dCHIP or the algorithms developed by Affymetrix (the microarray array suite or MAS 5.0) are available options. Because MAS 5.0 is available with the Affymetrix data acquisition system and thus used most frequently, we will review it briefly here. In MAS 5.0, the measure of expression was designed to capture the difference in the hybridization of the perfect match probe cells versus the mismatch probe cells, to always return a non-negative value, and to be relatively insensitive to outlier values.[13] The MM probes are used as a measure of nonspecific hybridization signals and subtracted from the PM probe intensities; the resulting intensity values are then log transformed. The Tukey biweight[14] is then applied to the log-transformed intensities to provide a robust estimate of intensity, that is relatively insensitive to outlier values. MM probes that have higher intensities than the PM probes are replaced with several different estimates; all of them are less than that of the perfect match probes. In addition to this aggregate intensity measure for each probe set, MAS 5.0 also provides a 'detection' measure calculated from the contrast between PM and MM probe cells which is reported as *P* value (i.e., lower values are more significant and represent a more reliable measure). Furthermore, the *P* values are binned into three bins: the lowest *P* values are scored as *present*, the highest as *absent* and the ones in the middle as *marginal*. The boundaries between these bins can be adjusted by the user. In summary, for each probe set MAS

5.0 returns three types of measures: a measure of expression intensity, a *P* value for that measure, and a present/marginal/absent call. These measures are then used in multichip comparisons and calculations.

Before these are considered, however, the perspective and methods of proteomics are outlined.

## PROTEOMICS VERSUS GENOMICS

There is substantial enthusiasm about the emerging field of proteomics. The promise of proteomics is that we will be able to measure proteins in specific cells, tissues, and biological fluids in a similarly comprehensive and parallel fashion that RNA species are currently measured in microarray experiments. As noted above, one of the key assumptions in RNA expression microarray analysis is that the study of gene expression will provide insight into the basic regulatory rhythms of the cell. There are persuasive reasons why this assumption will not always hold. Most of the effector molecules in cellular metabolism are proteins. To the extent that the timing of protein synthesis and the half-life of proteins is not closely coupled to that of RNA expression, the assumption of the representativeness of RNA levels does not hold.

Nonetheless, in proteomics, there is a different but equally challenging set of assumptions. First, similar concentrations do not imply co-regulation. Given that proteins have markedly different half lives, even within a single cell (e.g., a structural protein in a pulmonary cartilage chondrocyte and a calcium receptor in the same cell) then the concentrations of protein molecules in a cell may only remotely reflect coordinated regulation. This problem is analogous to the wide range of stability/degradation rates of mRNA in RNA expression microarray analysis. Conversely, repeatedly different concentrations of two proteins may imply co-regulation or interactions. The two proteins could have quite variable concentrations and different mutual relationships over different stages of the life cycle. Yet, there is nothing about this to preclude important functional interactions between these proteins. Finally, unlike transcription of genes which occurs within the nucleus, protein activity has very distinct and heterogeneous functional significance in different cellular compartments, and therefore an essential part of understanding protein function and regulation from proteomic data will require detailed localization to cellular subcompartments.

These challenges will eventually be addressed by novel approaches to examine protein activity at different times and in different spatial locations. Nonetheless, at present, it is not possible to inexpensively and reliably obtain large numbers of parallel measurements of protein activity. When these challenges have been resolved, then data from proteomic arrays will be amenable to the same techniques of analysis as described in this chapter for RNA microarray data sets. At present, important proteomics data are being generated[15] but not without controversy.[16,17]

## WHY DOES FUNCTIONAL GENOMICS REQUIRE NEW ANALYTIC TECHNIQUES?

There has been a long history of the development of biostatistical techniques to analyze studies with large numbers of cases. The statistical issues in conventional epidemiological studies of disease risk factors superficially seem similar to many of those issues posed in gene expression analysis. Yet most of the bioinformatic/functional genomic analyses have been performed using techniques borrowed from the computational sciences and machine learning communities in particular rather than epidemiology. A high quality epidemiological study will involve tens of thousands of subjects as in the Nurses' Health Study[18] or the Framingham Heart Study,[19] and hundreds of variables are measured. In contrast, in a typical genomic study, there are only tens or, exceptionally, hundreds of cases, each with tens of thousands of measured variables. This fundamental difference in the amount of data per case has required different statistical approaches in genomics than epidemiology.

Initially, the low number of cases in genomics was related to the high cost of the microarrays (in 1999 on the order of several thousand dollars per microarray) but, increasingly, the scarcity of cases in a typical functional genomic study will relate to the scarcity of appropriate biological samples. As these experiments involve the measurement of gene expression, a particular tissue (e.g., brain, muscle, fat) has to be obtained under the right conditions for analysis.

Especially in human populations, suitable tissue samples are relatively rare. Yet even though there are only tens of cases, each case involves the measurements of tens of thousands of variables corresponding to the expression of tens of thousands of genes measurable with microarray technology. The result of the large number of variables compared to the number of cases is that we have highly underdetermined systems. Thus, there are many, many ways in which the variables being measured could be interrelated mechanistically, based on the relatively small number of observations. Due to this high dimensionality and the underdetermined nature of these systems, many of the assumptions that underlie conventional biostatistical techniques do not hold.

## THE INVESTIGATIONAL PIPELINE IN THE FUNCTIONAL GENOMIC ERA

Although functional genomic or proteomic experiments are usually not hypothesis driven, the more successful research efforts are question driven. The questions range from 'Is gene regulation of the stretch response altered in smooth muscle cells in asthma?' to 'What gene expression signatures best predict COPD in individuals with no smoking history?' to 'Which genes participate in glucocorticoid regulation in each of the specific cell types in the lung?' This crucial step is only the first one in a series of steps, often described as the functional genomics pipeline, and outlined in Fig. 5B.4.

The remainder of the pipeline is summarized in this section to frame the methodological challenges. For simplicity, only RNA analysis will be discussed, although similar issues are relevant for proteomics.

- *Selection of the right tissue.* Functional genomics experiments require selection of the functionally relevant tissue or cell type. In certain experiments, such as those using blood and solid cancers, the functionally relevant tissue is relatively obvious. In other analyses, the functionally relevant tissue may not be so easily ascertainable or available. For example, the clinical phenotype seen in asthma may involve the coordinated physiologic dysfunction of several organs and cell types, including cells of the immune system, endothelia, smooth muscle, or autonomic neural tissue. For some common diseases such as hypertension, it is not clear what the functionally relevant tissue is. A successful pipeline involves collaboration with a source of tissue, such as a surgical team, a laboratory with biologically relevant animals, or a laboratory with cell lines of interest.

- *Right conditions.* Even if the appropriate tissue is selected from the organism of interest, the conditions under which the tissue is obtained (e.g., number of hours post-mortem) can impact the outcome of the investigation. A stretch-sensitive tissue such as the lung will have a different metabolic and expression profile depending on the physiological state (e.g., mechanical ventilation, hypoxia, drug treatment) prior to the extraction of RNA. The time of day will influence the expression of genes in tissues that have endogenous

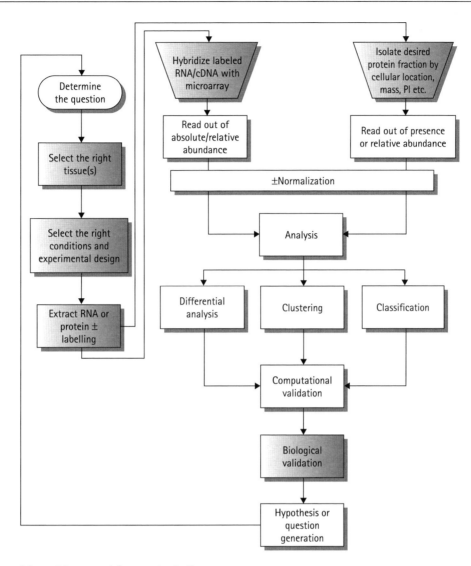

**Figure 5B.4** *Overall flow of the genomic/proteomic pipeline.*

circadian rhythms or that have processes entrained by physiological clocks. Awareness of these issues and cooperation from a surgeon, pathologist, or technician responsible for obtaining the tissue, is therefore an essential component to the success of the functional genomic pipeline. As expression array analysis involves the parallel measurement of thousands of analytes instead of the usual handful, many of these important physiological considerations have been omitted in most genomic studies. Other experimental design issues include whether the study is designed to determine the natural classes of samples, compare two or more conditions, or identify a predictor for a clinical state. Readers interested in more details on functional genomics or proteomics experimental design are referred to several recent books.[20,21]

- *Extract RNA.* Prepare RNA for hybridization to a robotically spotted or photolithographic microarray as previously described. Each of the steps in this 'wet

laboratory' component of a functional genomics pipeline is susceptible to operator error, which is a potential source of inaccurate measurements. The RNA extracted may be of poor quality, the hybridization conditions may vary (e.g., the room temperature), and the settings of the scanner that produces the digital image of the microarray may vary from one scan to another. Industrialization and standardization of this component has been the focus of the more successful and high-quality functional genomics efforts.

- *Read out of the raw data on abundance (absolute or relative) and/or presence of RNA.* Depending on the particular experimental set up, this step can be extremely arduous. Quality control of the data, or identification of which RNA corresponds to which measured value, are close to fully automated in commodity microarray systems.

- *Normalization.* Often before any further analysis is performed, the raw data from each experiment are adjusted so that the data are more comparable within a set of experiments. This highly controversial step is discussed below.

- *Differential expression.* This common analytical step is also often the most poorly performed. As described below, the large numbers of gene products measured have often led to overinterpretation of the very noisy data generated by these high throughput modalities.

- *Clustering and classification.* These 'dry laboratory' components of the functional genomics pipeline are often considered to be the bioinformatics components of genomics. However, bioinformatic issues are relevant throughout the entire pipeline.

- *Computational validation.* There are many reasons to perform bioinformatics analyses on functional genomics data sets, and many methods to perform such analyses. One unique problem with these types of data sets, alluded to above, is that they are 'short and wide,' meaning that many variables are measured on relatively few samples. This makes it all too easy for apparently significant findings to be obtained by chance. To avoid being misled, some computational validation is required immediately after the bioinformatics analysis so that computationally sound, but biologically improbable, hypotheses are screened out. The principal motivation for screening out improbable hypotheses is the time-intensive and expensive effort that follows a positive result. Each generated hypothesis that passes the computational validation step must be validated in a biological laboratory. Some laboratories may have the resources to pursue many hypotheses and tolerate the eventual refutation of large numbers of false-positive hypotheses. However, most biological laboratories are only able to validate a few. An ideal computational validation does not merely provide a 'yes' or 'no' answer as to potential validity of a hypothesis. Instead, it provides a continuum of validation, such as a receiver-operating characteristic curve, with which an investigative team can select the desired rates of sensitivity or specificity and true and false negatives and positives for generated hypotheses.

- *Biological validation.* Most biological questions will not be finally answered using microarrays. Instead, the most likely outcome from a successful functional genomics analysis is another interesting biological question to ask. As hypotheses are generated from bioinformatics analyses, biological validation is crucial to confirm these hypotheses. This verification may include, for instance, making sure that a particular set of genes is truly expressed at the proper time and place as hypothesized, using conventional biological techniques such as Northern blotting and in situ hybridization, to cell-line based over-expression and 'knockdown' experiments (see Chapter 6, Functional genomics) or whole animal models (see Chapter 7, Genomic physiology in animals).

In most settings, all of these steps, from asking the pertinent question to acquisition of source material, to microarray construction, to bioinformatics analysis to biological verification, cannot be performed by a single individual or laboratory. A successful functional genomics/proteomics pipeline brings together individuals and resources from many disciplines with varied backgrounds.

## Normalization

If you take a photograph of a person at two different times but at the same angle and distance, the two resulting pictures may well differ due to technical variables such as exposure time and lighting conditions. However, if you want to determine whether characteristics of that person have changed between the two pictures, then one reasonable approach would be to adjust the images using an image processing program to make the two pictures more alike and potentially more comparable. You might adjust the contrast, brightness, and color distribution of the two photographs to be more similar to one another, thus normalizing the two photographs which may enable detection of features that are different between the two pictures. This is essentially the process of normalizing the measurements performed in different experiments with expression microarray technology or quantitative proteomic measurements. Any normalization technique risks obscuring essential differences between the data sets that are compared, which could be biologically relevant. The goal of data normalization is to make the two data sets more comparable while preserving their essential differences. Different normalization methods will vary in their ability to achieve this goal with different data distributions. In addition, some methodologists contend that *any* normalization of the data will obscure the true biological differences and decrease the information that can be obtained from a study.

With these caveats in mind, the two most popular normalization methods are discussed below. The first method, linear regression, assumes that the change of intensity that will make two different microarrays more comparable is a linear effect, and the second method, lowess normalization, assumes that there are nonlinear effects that must be adjusted. In fact, there are dozens of alternative published normalization methods, each claiming improved relative performance.

## Linear regression

If duplicate experiments (referred to as B1 and B2) with the same sample probe were performed with the same type of expression microarray, the linear regression normalization process begins by selecting a reference data set. This reference data set is often chosen based on the experiment felt to have been the highest quality – let us assume that was experiment B1. Let $x_i$ and $y_i$ denote the reported expression intensity of gene $i$ in the duplicate experiments B1 and B2, respectively, with $I = 1, \ldots, N$, where $N$ is the total number of unique probes on the microarray. If microarray B2 has a systematic error in relation to the reference experiment B1, the expression level for every gene (referred to as $x_i$) in experiment B1 is remeasured in the B2 experiment as $y_i = a_1 x_i + a_0$. A global linear shift of this kind could arise, for instance, if chip B2 were scanned at a different uniform ambient brightness from chip B2. In this linear transformation, the slope $a_1$ is referred to as the *dilation* factor and the $y$-intercept $a_0$ is referred to as the *translation* factor. If chips B1 and B2 were ideal duplicates then the points ($x_i$, $y_i$) would be aligned on a line of slope one with a $y$-intercept at the origin (0,0), and without any scatter of the points.

After estimating the values for $a_1$ and $a_0$, the transformation $y' = (y_i - a_0)/(a_1)$ will correct this systematic difference in B2 with respect to B1 so that a plot of $x_i$ versus $y'_i$ is a line of slope one through the origin. In summary, this linear transformation for any number of chips, with regard to a reference experiment, is to calculate the slope and intercept using linear regression and then to use these values to adjust the slope and intercept of each of the nonreference experiments so that they have a slope of 1 and $y$-intercept at the origin with respect to the reference microarray.

## Lowess normalization

In a microarray expression experiment, if the logarithm of the ratio of Cy3 labeled RNA versus Cy5-labeled RNA is plotted against the logarithm of the product of the same measurements, then if the conditions and imaging on both the Cy3 and Cy5 measurements were identical, one would see a straight horizontal line. Instead, a curvilinear relationship is often observed, as shown in Fig. 5B.5a. A number of techniques have been proposed to normalize such nonlinear relationships by performing mathematical operations to straighten out the curve. Unlike linear regression, which makes the assumption that the 'curve' is a straight line, most of these methods minimize any assumptions regarding the shape of the curve. The most widely used of these nonlinear curve-fitting procedures is for the loess (aka lowess) curve.

The lowess curve fitting function draws a smooth curve through a scatter diagram that minimizes the variance of the residuals or prediction error (analogous to the minimization of residuals in linear regression). After replotting the points with respect to this lowess curve, as in Fig. 5B.5b, a straight line is observed.[22] This is the corresponding operation to subtracting the intercept and dividing by the slope for the linear regression method.

## DIFFERENTIAL EXPRESSION ANALYSIS

In routine, pregenomic pulmonary investigations, a question that is often asked is: 'How does the serum level of a cytokine change from one condition to another?' For example, what is the average serum IL-2 level in nonasthmatics versus asthmatic subjects? Similarly the comparison of the entire transcriptome or proteome across two conditions is the most frequently performed analysis in gene expression and proteomics. For example, questions often asked include:

- Which genes are differentially expressed between two tissues such as smooth muscle and respiratory epithelial cells?
- What is the gene expression in the same pulmonary muscle tissue exposed to two different doses of glucocorticoids?
- What is the difference in expression of the pulmonary tissue of mice with an allergen-induced decreased small airway diameter in IL-2 knockout versus 'wild-type' mice?

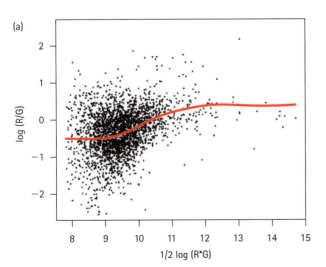
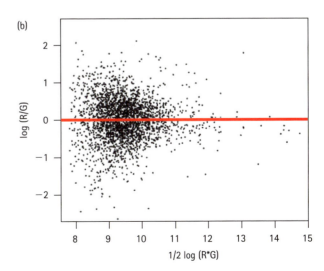

**Figure 5B.5** *(a) Typical microarray data before lowess normalization. R refers to the intensity of Cy3-labeled RNA and G refers to the intensity of Cy5-labeled RNA. The logarithm of the ratio of these intensities (y-axis) is plotted against the logarithm of the product of these intensities (x-axis). Substantial nonlinearity is seen. (b) Typical microarray data after lowess normalization. The plot now demonstrates a linear relationship between the logarithm of the ratio versus the logarithm of the product of Cy3 and Cy5 intensities.*

If only a single microarray is included for each of the two conditions of interest (i.e., two microarrays per question), the analysis is quite limited. The ratio of each gene's expression value in each condition can be calculated and sorted from highest to lowest. This use of microarrays, which continues to be applied, does not account for the measurement variation in gene expression techniques. To estimate the measurement error, multiple replicates for each condition must be obtained. Early in the development of microarray technology, the variance in the quality of the arrays was so extensive that the same extracted RNA for hybridization was used for multiple arrays; these 'technical replicates' were used to estimate variance due to the arrays. Currently, the quality of many of the commercial arrays is so high that technical replicates are not required; RNA from different samples are used for each microarray hybridization (i.e., biological replicates). Nonetheless, whether technical and/or biological replicates are used, the replicate measurements must be analyzed to obtain a more robust measure of differential expression (Fig. 5B.6).

Until recently, the most common approach for analyzing multiple replicate experiments was to pick an arbitrary threshold for the relative amount by which a gene's expression would have to change to have it be considered significant. For example, a two-fold increase or decrease in the expression of any gene across a set of conditions might be considered significant and reportable. As shown in Fig. 5B.6, at different expression levels these arbitrary thresholds would select different numbers of differentially expressed genes; thus, the true positive and false positive rates will vary with expression level. In response to the arbitrariness of this approach, a number of more rigorous measures for differential expression have been developed.[20,21,23] Here, we will focus on perhaps the most useful approach, the false discovery rate, although this is certainly debatable. It is important to keep in mind that microarray expression data are very noisy and false-positive and false-negative differential expression values cannot be avoided completely.

Applying a traditional statistical test of the difference of means in two groups, such as the Student's $t$-test, is problematic because the $P$ values obtained would have to be corrected for multiple hypothesis testing. Furthermore, a traditional correction for multiple hypothesis testing, such

as the Bonferroni correction, is unnecessarily stringent and would unnecessarily decrease the sensitivity of the differential analysis in order to achieve a desired specificity. To avoid overly conservative corrections for multiple testing, Hochberg and Benjamini[24] developed a procedure for controlling the false discovery rate. In the context of expression array analysis, the false discovery rate is the number of false positives that are found in the list of genes that appear to be differentially expressed in the microarray analysis. By controlling the false discovery rate, the probability of following up a false lead can be controlled by the investigator. The most popular automated method available for differential analysis of gene expression in microarrays that assesses the false discovery rate has been implemented in a program called SAM (significant analysis of microarrays).[25] In SAM, the difference between the group means is calculated as in a $t$-test but with a correction factor that improves the performance of this statistic for data sets with small numbers of microarrays. In addition, hundreds of permutations of the data set are performed, and the difference between the group means is recalculated across the two conditions for each permutation. This permutation procedure allows a direct estimate of the likelihood that the observed difference in gene expression intensity could be obtained by chance and thereby provides a built in correction for multiple hypotheses testing. Furthermore, ordering of the genes in the expression array by this score allows a list of genes to be generated with a predictable false discovery rate. This program is freely available to academic researchers at www.stat.stanford.edu/~tibs/SAM/. Recent work suggests that analysis of gene sets within pathways may provide biological insight even though individual gene expression differences are not statistically significant.[26]

Several differential analysis algorithms have been developed in addition to SAM, and it is likely that one or more of the new generation of differential analysis algorithms may provide superior performance. New algorithms such as Bayesian calculators, that take into account the distributional properties of microarray measurements, appear to be especially promising.

## CLUSTERING AND CLASSIFICATION

The central underlying assumption in all gene-clustering techniques for expression analysis is that genes that appear to be expressed in similar patterns are mechanistically related. Furthermore, although genes may distantly affect the function of other gene products, they fall into more tightly regulated groups. For instance, the genes that govern meiosis may be more tightly linked to each other than they are to the genes involved with another function, such as apoptosis. It is well known that groups of proteins can be organized into pathways such as glycolysis and the Krebs' cycle. Other functional clusters are those of structural

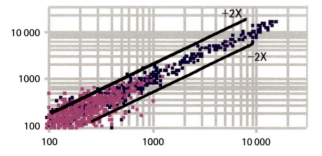

**Figure 5B.6**  *Using two-fold thresholds for determining differential expression in a microarray experiment.*

proteins which have to come together in a conserved and reproducible fashion in order to serve their purpose, such as the lung extracellular matrix. On this basis, if we can find genes whose expression patterns approximate one another, we can suggest that they are functionally clustered together.

There are several important caveats that are worth noting. First, it is unclear how commonly discrete functional groupings of genes exist within the cellular apparatus. Individual gene products may have many different roles under different circumstances. Second, the term 'functionally related' is vague. If the pattern of expression of one gene is similar to that of another, it could signify relationships ranging from 'two genes have gene products that physically interact,' to 'one gene encodes a transcriptional factor for the other gene,' to 'two genes have different functions but similar promoter sequences.' Of course at some level, *all* genes are functionally related in their role to keep the cell and organism alive, but below this level of abstraction, there are many alternate definitions of clustering. Therefore, we must be somewhat wary of the claim that similarity in expression corresponds to similarity in function. Nonetheless, it is a useful starting point for genomic analysis. The determination of what constitutes similar expression pattern also has multiple alternate definitions. For example, similarity could mean having similar patterns of change over time, similar absolute levels of expression at any given time, or perfectly opposite but well-choreographed patterns of expression. Which similarity measure is chosen for studying patterns of expression will influence the functional clusters that are observed.

## Supervised versus unsupervised learning

Because the data sets of expression array analysis are of high dimensionality with a relatively small number of cases, machine-learning techniques designed to explore high dimensional spaces (such as those of voice or face recognition) have been applied to genomic data sets.

Two broad categorizations of machine learning techniques are *supervised learning techniques* and *unsupervised learning techniques,* which are also commonly known as classification techniques and clustering techniques, respectively. The two techniques are easily distinguished by the presence of external labels for cases. For example, labeling lung tissue as obtained from a patient with asthma or COPD is required before applying a supervised learning technique to determine which combinations of variables predict those labels. In an unsupervised learning approach, such as finding those genes that are co-regulated across all of the lung tissue samples, the organization/clustering of the variables operates independently of any external labels. The types of variables, also known as *features* in machine learning jargon, that characterize each *case* in a data set can be quite varied. For example, measures of clinical outcome, gene expression, gene sequence, drug exposure, proteomic measurements, demographic characteristics, or any other discrete or continuous variable believed to be of relevance to the case, can be included.

Different types of questions are answered by the two types of machine learning. In supervised learning, the goal is typically to obtain a set of variables (e.g., expressed genes measured on a microarray) to categorize reliably that patient or tissue or animal as part of a class of interest (e.g., specific diagnostic group or prognostic implications). In unsupervised learning, the typical application is to find either a completely novel cluster of genes with putative common but previously unknown function, or to obtain a cluster of genes that appear to have similar patterns of expression to a gene already known to have an important well-defined function. Thus, in unsupervised learning, the goal is to learn about the mechanism by which the known gene works and to find other genes involved in that same mechanism in order to understand cellular physiology or, in the case of pharmacologically oriented research, other possible therapeutic targets.

However, the lists of genes that reliably divide the two states under study may have little to do with the actual pathophysiologic causes of the disease of interest and may not represent close relationships of those genes to functional consequences. The reasons for this disconnect include that it is quite possible that small amounts of change of some gene products, such as transcriptional activators, may cause large downstream changes in expression of many genes in different pathways. With only a subtle change, an important upstream gene may cause dramatic changes in the expression of genes in several pathways that are functionally only distantly related but are highly influenced by the same upstream gene. When applying a classification algorithm directly on the gene expression levels, the algorithm will naturally identify those genes that show the greatest change between the two or more states that are being classified. Thus, a study design geared towards the application of a supervised learning technique may generate a useful artifact for classification, diagnosis, or even prognosis, but it will not necessarily lead to valuable insights into the biology underlying the classes that are defined.

In more general situations, a case can include several thousand gene expression measurements but also several hundred phenotypic measurements such as $FEV_1$, second-hand smoke exposure, or the response to a smoking cessation regimen. A clustering algorithm can be used to find those features that are most tightly coupled in the observed data. However, when designing an experiment that includes various data types, it is worthwhile considering whether some kinds of features are more likely to cluster together, separately from the genomic data. After application of a clustering algorithm, the data set may reveal relationships between the nongenomic variables that are much more significant and stronger than any of those that involve genomic data. While that outcome may be interesting, it will not help to understand the contribution of genetic regulation to the observed phenomenon. As an example, if one looks at the effect of thousands of drugs on several cancer cell lines, then it would not be surprising if these drug effects were most tightly clustered around groups of pharmaceutical agents that were derived from one another through combinatorial chemistry. Similarly, phenotypic features that are highly interdependent, such as height and weight, will typically cluster together. The strength of these obvious clusters will often dominate those of heterogeneous clusters that contain both phenotypic measurements and gene expression measurements. This suggests that careful application of feature reduction to include only truly independent phenotypic measures for each case should be used. Systematic approaches to feature reduction have been reviewed.[27]

Because the wide range of techniques developed for both supervised and unsupervised learning fall considerably beyond the scope of this chapter, interested readers are referred to other excellent sources for information regarding principal component analysis,[28–32] nearest-neighbor clustering,[33] dendrogram algorithms,[31] divisive or partitional clustering,[34–38] network determination,[39–45] relevance networks,[46,47] Bayes classification and global relevance,[48–50] and multiple feature determination.[49,51–54]

## ANNOTATION

Whether the analysis involves clustering or classification, the key results are accession numbers and expression values. The accession numbers refer to either a cDNA clone or a set of oligonucleotides (in the case of the Affymetrix microarray platform). These cDNAs/oligonucleotides correspond to a stretch of expressed sequence, which usually identifies a specific gene. The manufacturer of the clone sets or microarrays will provide translation tables and software facilities to convert the accession numbers to gene names and Gene IDs (Gene IDs are the durable unique names for genes that are maintained by the National Center for Biotechnology Information at www.ncbi.nlm.nih.gov/entrez/query.fcgi?db=gene).

Even after identifying the gene names and identifier numbers, most researchers would then be unimpressed by the results. This is in marked contrast to a typical pulmonary investigation where most, if not all, of the analytes are well known and characterized. Because of the comprehensive nature of modern microarray technology, the entire transcriptome may be measured; consequently, most of the genes measured will be unfamiliar to the pulmonary investigator even though they clearly have some relevant activity in the experiment devised by that investigator. In 2001, or earlier, the most laborious part of the functional genomic experiment would begin – the determination of the biological significance of the up- or downregulation of each of the particular genes in the specified aforementioned list. This would typically require a search in PubMed (www.ncbi.nlm.nih.gov) to determine, from a review of the literature,

with which processes that gene was known to be involved. Based on this review, speculation would be made regarding the biological mechanism explaining why a particular gene co-clustered with other genes. Fortunately, the challenge of gene annotation became widely recognized, resulting in several efforts to generate compendia of gene annotations, some in the commercial sector and some in the public sector. Perhaps the single most successful such effort was called the 'gene ontology' (or more commonly simply GO).[55] The GO provides three kinds of annotations for genes, each organized in its own hierarchy. The first kind of annotation is a description of molecular function which describes the general biochemical activity of the entity such as whether it is a transcriptional factor, a transporter, or an enzyme. The second kind of annotation specifies the cellular component within which gene products are located. This provides a localization for a gene product's molecular function, such as the ribosome or mitochondrion. Localization can help to determine whether a purported function could occur through direct physical interaction between gene products or through an indirect mechanism. The final type of annotation in GO is the biological process implemented by the gene products. Biological process refers to a higher order process, such as protein translation or signal transduction. A view of a portion of this process hierarchy is shown in Fig. 5B.7.

A set of tools to browse this gene ontology is available at http://geneontology.org to allow the investigator to determine rapidly the processes, biochemical function, and locations of every annotated gene. Further, as a matter of convenience, these tools allow entire lists of genes to be submitted for annotation. Although this type of annotation can be quite useful, it is often quite simple to come up with a plausible but incorrect biological justification as to why this list of genes was found. One of the problems is that this annotation provides no insight regarding how likely this set of gene annotations would have arisen by chance. For example, because of their biological importance and complexity, cell cycle, protein synthesis, DNA synthesis, and other common cellular functions are highly represented as annotations in the gene ontology. Therefore, just based on random chance, any set of genes could include large numbers of genes annotated with the above functions. This realization led to an understanding that what investigators were really interested in determining was what characteristics of the genes obtained in a particular list are unlikely to be random events, and what biochemical function or cellular location characterize these genes? One way to address this problem is to determine whether a particular annotation is overrepresented in the experimental list compared to its frequency in the entire gene ontology. At http://geneontology.org there are several relevant tools such as DAVID available from the NIAID as well as Mappfinder from UCSF to assist with this process.

Although it is only the first decade of the research use of microarrays, these artifacts of the intersection of robotics,

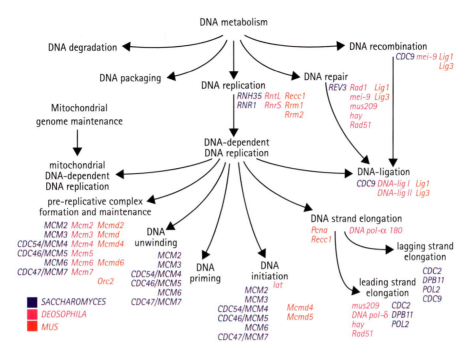

**Figure 5B.7** *Sample process hierarchy from GO.*

microelectronics, and molecular biology have enabled clinical researchers to avail themselves of insights into molecular physiology that include the measurement of the expression of the entire transcriptome. These insights provide a new level of breadth and precision of phenotyping that is much more closely related to the mechanisms of disease than many other phenotypes. Full exploitation of functional genomics data types, however, will require a level of quantitative and computational sophistication which will challenge our current means of biomedical training for years to come.

---

## Key learning points

- The differences in the measurements of expression in robotically spotted cDNA microarrays versus photolithographically constructed oligonucleotide microarrays.

- The distinction between supervised and unsupervised learning.

- Understand the Gene Ontology gene annotation system.

- Understand why a two- or three-fold threshold for differential gene expression is not useful. Understand the use of statistically robust differential measurement techniques.

- Understand the motivation for normalization of microarray measurements. Distinguish linear versus nonlinear methods.

## REFERENCES

●1 Alizadeh AA, Eisen MB, Davis RE et al. Distinct types of diffuse large B-cell lymphoma identified by gene expression profiling. *Nature* 2000; **403**: 503–11.

1a Chen JJ, Peck K, Hong TM et al. Global analysis of gene expression in invasion by a lung cancer model. *Cancer Res* 2001; **61**: 5223–30.

1b Powell CA, Xu G, Filmus J et al. Oligonucleotide microarray analysis of lung adenocarcinoma in smokers and nonsmokers identifies GPC3 as a potential lung tumor suppressor. *Chest* 2002; **121**(3 Suppl): 6S–7S.

1c Zimmermann N, King NE, Laporte J et al. Dissection of experimental asthma with DNA microarray analysis identifies arginase in asthma pathogenesis. *J Clin Invest* 2003; **111**: 1863–74.

●2 Butte AJ, Tamayo P, Slonim D et al. Discovering functional relationships between RNA expression and chemotherapeutic susceptibility using relevance networks. *Proc Natl Acad Sci USA* 2000; **97**: 12182–6.

●3 Spellman PT, Sherlock G, Zhang MQ et al. Comprehensive identification of cell cycle-regulated genes of the yeast Saccharomyces cerevisiae by microarray hybridization. *Mol Biol Cell* 1998; **9**: 3273–97.

●4 Iyer VR, Eisen MB, Ross DT et al. The transcriptional program in the response of human fibroblasts to serum. *Science* 1999; **283**: 83–7.

◆5 Anonymous. The chip challenge. *Nat Genet* 1999; **21**: 61–2.

6 Schena M, Shalon D, Davis RW, Brown PO. Quantitative monitoring of gene expression patterns with a complementary DNA microarray. *Science* 1995; **270**: 467–70.

7 Luo L, Salunga RC, Guo H et al. Gene expression profiles of laser-captured adjacent neuronal subtypes. *Nat Med* 1999; **5**: 117–22.

◆8　Brown PO, Botstein D. Exploring the new world of the genome with DNA microarrays. *Nat Genet* 1999; **21**(1 Suppl): 33–7.

9　Kerr M, Martin M, Churchill G. Analysis of variance for gene expression microarray data. *J Comput Biol* 2000; **7**: 819–37.

●10　Fodor SP, Read JL, Pirrung MC et al. Light-directed, spatially addressable parallel chemical synthesis. *Science* 1991; **251**: 767–73.

◆11　Rajagopalan D. A comparison of statistical methods for analysis of high density oligonucleotide array data. *Bioinformatics* 2003; **19**: 1469–76.

◆12　Lemon WJ, Liyanarachchi S, You M. A high performance test of differential gene expression for oligonucleotide arrays. *Genome Biol* 2003; **4**: R67.

13　Hubbell E, Liu WM, Mei R. Robust estimators for expression analysis. *Bioinformatics* 2002; **18**: 1585–92.

14　Hoaglin DC, Mosteller F, Tukey JW. *Understanding robust and exploratory data analysis.* New York: Wiley, 2000.

●15　Petricoin EF, Ardekani AM, Hitt BA et al. Use of proteomic patterns in serum to identify ovarian cancer. *Lancet* 2002; **359**: 572–7.

16　Diamandis EP. Analysis of serum proteomic patterns for early cancer diagnosis: drawing attention to potential problems. *J Natl Cancer Inst* 2004; **96**: 353–6.

17　Diamandis EP. OvaCheck: doubts voiced soon after publication. *Nature* 2004; **430**: 611.

18　Belanger C, Hennekens C, Rosner B, Speizer F. The Nurses' Health Study. *Am J Nurs* 1978; **78**: 1039–40.

19　Dawber T, Meadors G, Moore F. The Framingham Study: Epidemiological approaches to heart disease. *Am J Public Health* 1951; **41**: 279–86.

20　Speed TP. *Statistical analysis of gene expression microarray data.* Boca Raton, FL: Chapman & Hall/CRC, 2003.

21　Kohane IS, Kho AT, Butte AJ. *Microarrays for an integrative genomics.* Cambridge, MA: MIT Press, 2003.

22　Kauhanen H, Komi PV, Hakkinen K. Standardization and validation of the body weight adjustment regression equations in Olympic weightlifting. *J Strength Cond Res* 2002; **16**: 58–74.

23　Draeaghici S. *Data analysis tools for DNA microarrays.* Boca Raton: Chapman & Hall/CRC, 2003.

24　Hochberg Y, Benjamini Y. Controlling the false discovery rate: a practical and powerful approach to multiple testing. *J R Stat Soc V* 1995; **57**: 289–300.

●25　Tusher VG, Tibshirani R, Chu G. Significance analysis of microarrays applied to the ionizing radiation response. *Proc Natl Acad Sci USA* 2001; **98**: 5116–21.

●26　Mootha VK, Lindgren CM, Eriksson KF et al. PGC-1alpha-responsive genes involved in oxidative phosphorylation are coordinately downregulated in human diabetes. *Nat Genet* 2003; **34**: 267–73.

27　Weiss SM, Indurkhya N. *Predictive data mining: A practical guide.* San Francisco: Morgan Kaufmann, 1997.

28　Raychaudhuri S, Stuart JM, Altman RB. Principal components analysis to summarize microarray experiments: application to sporulation time series. *Pac Symp Biocomput* 2000: 455–66.

29　Alter O, Brown PO, Botstein D. Singular value decomposition for genome-wide expression data processing and modeling. *Proc Natl Acad Sci USA* 2000; **97**: 10101–6.

30　Hilsenbeck SG, Friedrichs WE, Schiff R et al. Statistical analysis of array expression data as applied to the problem of tamoxifen resistance. *J Natl Cancer Inst* 1999; **91**: 453–9.

31　Wen X, Fuhrman S, Michaels GS et al. Large-scale temporal gene expression mapping of central nervous system development. *Proc Natl Acad Sci USA* 1998; **95**: 334–9.

32　Fiehn O, Kopka J, Dormann P et al. Metabolite profiling for plant functional genomics. *Nat Biotechnol* 2000; **18**: 1157–61.

33　Ben-Dor A, Bruhn L, Friedman N et al. Tissue classification with gene expression profiles. *J Comput Biol* 2000; **7**: 559–83.

34　Kim JH, Ohno-Machado L, Kohane IS. Unsupervised learning from complex data: the Matrix Incision Tree Algorithm. In: *Pacific Symposium on Biocomputing,* Hawaii, 2001, pp. 30–41.

35　Alon U, Barkai N, Notterman DA et al. Broad patterns of gene expression revealed by clustering analysis of tumor and normal colon tissues probed by oligonucleotide arrays. *Proc Natl Acad Sci USA* 1999; **96**: 6745–50.

36　Getz G, Levine E, Domany E. Coupled two-way clustering analysis of gene microarray data. *Proc Natl Acad Sci USA* 2000; **97**: 12079–84.

37　Ben-Dor A, Shamir R, Yakhini Z. Clustering gene expression patterns. *J Comput Biol* 1999; **6**: 281–97.

38　Hastie T, Tibshirani R, Eisen MB et al. 'Gene shaving' as a method for identifying distinct sets of genes with similar expression patterns. *Genome Biol* 2000; **1**: RESEARCH0003.

39　Friedman N, Linial M, Nachman I, Pe'er D. Using Bayesian networks to analyze expression data. *J Comput Biol* 2000; **7**: 601–20.

40　Matsuno H, Doi A, Nagasaki M, Miyano S. Hybrid Petri net representation of gene regulatory network. *Pac Symp Biocomput* 2000: 341–52.

41　Liang S, Fuhrman S, Somogyi R. Reveal, a general reverse engineering algorithm for inference of genetic network architectures. *Pac Symp Biocomput* 1998: 18–29.

42　Wuensche A. Genomic regulation modeled as a network with basins of attraction. *Pac Symp Biocomput* 1998: 89–102.

43　Szallasi Z, Liang S. Modeling the normal and neoplastic cell cycle with 'realistic Boolean genetic networks': their application for understanding carcinogenesis and assessing therapeutic strategies. *Pac Symp Biocomput* 1998: 66–76.

44　Akutsu T, Miyano S, Kuhara S. Algorithms for identifying Boolean networks and related biological networks based on matrix multiplication and fingerprint function. *J Comput Biol* 2000; **7**: 331–43.

45　Akutsu T, Miyano S, Kuhara S. Inferring qualitative relations in genetic networks and metabolic pathways. *Bioinformatics* 2000; **16**: 727–34.

46　Butte A, Kohane I. Mutual information relevance networks: functional genomic clustering using pairwise entropy measurements. In: Altman R, Dunker K, Hunter L et al. (eds). *Pacific Symposium on Biocomputing, 2000.* Hawaii: World Scientific, 2000, 418–29.

47　Butte A, Kohane IS. Unsupervised knowledge discovery in medical databases using relevance networks. In: Lorenzi N (ed.). *Fall Symposium, American Medical Informatics Association, 1999.* Washington, DC: Hanley and Belfus, 1999, 711–15.

48　Ben-Dor A, Friedman N, Yakhini Z. Tissue classification with gene expression profiles. In: *RECOMB, 1999.* Tokyo, Japan: ACM; 1999, pp. 31–8.

49 Chow ML, Moler EJ, Mian IS. Identifying marker genes in transcription profiling data using a mixture of feature relevance experts. *Physiol Genomics* 2001; **5**: 99–111.

50 Moler EJ, Radisky DC, Mian IS. Integrating naive Bayes models and external knowledge to examine copper and iron homeostasis in *S. cerevisiae*. *Physiol Genomics* 2000; **4**: 127–35.

51 Dietterich TG. Approximate statistical tests for comparing supervised classification learning algorithms. *Neural Comput* 1998; **10**: 1895–923.

52 Furey TS, Cristianini N, Duffy N et al. Support vector machine classification and validation of cancer tissue samples using microarray expression data. *Bioinformatics* 2000; **16**: 906–14.

53 Brown MP, Grundy WN, Lin D et al. Knowledge-based analysis of microarray gene expression data by using support vector machines. *Proc Natl Acad Sci USA* 2000; **97**: 262–7.

54 Hastie T, Tibshirani R, Botstein D, Brown P. Supervised harvesting of expression trees. *Genome Biol* 2001; **2**: RESEARCH0003.

●55 Ashburner M, Ball CA, Blake JA et al. Gene ontology: tool for the unification of biology. The Gene Ontology Consortium. *Nat Genet* 2000; **25**: 25–9.

# 6

# Functional genomics

# Clinical functional genomics

DAVID J. HALSALL AND ELIZABETH A. DAVIDSON

## INTRODUCTION

The goal of clinical functional genomics is to use genetic variation to identify disease mechanisms and possible therapeutic targets. The tractable nature of nucleic acids analysis and the recent improvements in automated sequencing methodologies means it is usually easier to identify gene defects that associate with heritable diseases than the consequences of these changes. Having identified a sequence variation associated with a clinical phenotype, it is necessary to ascertain whether this change is responsible for the disease and, if so, how does the variant contribute to the disease mechanism.

The first point is usually addressed by segregation and association studies which can provide evidence, sometimes beyond reasonable doubt, that the sequence variation causes the clinical phenotype. These studies, however, rarely provide mechanistic insight. Such data are often much harder to obtain. RNA studies to detect transcribed genes can be limited by messenger RNA instability and the difficulty of obtaining tissue from human subjects, unlike genomic DNA that is readily available from peripheral blood lymphocytes. Purification of the gene product for functional and structural analysis can be greatly aided by activity assays, but usually requires the time-consuming and often frustrating search for a specific antibody. Ultimately describing a role of the gene or gene product in the integration of metabolism or the maintenance of cell structure will follow. This is now often achieved via transfection of cell lines or with transgenic animals. As all of these studies represent a considerable investment in time and resources so an attempt is usually made at the outset to predict ab initio whether a sequence variant is likely to contribute to disease. Typically two approaches are used, homology modeling which exploits phylogenetic databases to predict gene function and in silico modeling, which usually exploits prior data obtained from experimental structural and functional studies. Whilst modeling can never replace functional studies it can often provide a valuable insight into the most productive investigative strategy. Faced with a newly identified sequence variant three questions arise:

1 Is the sequence variation within a gene? The variation may be in an exon, intron, up or downstream untranslated region or a promotor
2 Does this gene have a known or predicted function?
3 Will the sequence variation affect gene function?

Gene prediction methods typically involve database searching or ab initio prediction based on the structure of known genes. Proof of gene prediction ultimately requires evidence of the gene transcript or product at the site of disease action. Homology modeling is a highly successful method for predicting gene function and it is likely that as many as 50–70 percent of the estimated 30 000 human protein-coding genes will be assigned a function in this manner. This method can also be used to predict whether function may be perturbed by mutation. In the case of gene deletions or premature termination of translation, predicting the potential effect of a mutation can be facile. However, ascertaining the effect of miss-sense mutations or sequence variations in putative gene regulation motifs can be much harder without experimental back-up. In addition to homology modeling, a further approach for protein coding genes is to attempt to predict the structure of the putative protein from primary sequence. It may be possible to predict how an amino acid change may perturb this. Naive conjecture based on amino acid size or charge changes in the absence of homology or structural data often leads to surprises when confirmatory studies are performed.

As methods for DNA analysis are applicable to the study of any heritable disease, there are considerable advantages to a systematic high throughput study of entire genomes rather than a piecemeal disease by disease approach. This is the cornerstone of the human genome project.[1] Functional genomics attempts the second phase of this project, that is to produce a systematic highly annotated and referenced

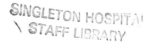

map of all human gene products and their functions. However, the vast array of gene functions and the variety of techniques needed to ascertain these functions makes a unified strategy less applicable. Expert manual sequence curation is recommended as the definitive method for gene annotation, and this will be required for a large number of genes if the functional genome map is to be of high quality. The current rate of progress with automated gene annotation and the excellent freely available clinical and mutation databases will mean the detection of sequence variation will soon be the first step in an investigation of heritable disease rather than a goal in itself. Invaluable resources include 'Entrez' (www.ncbi.nlm.nih.gov/Entrez) with links to OMIM and LocusLink, Swiss Prot (www.tw.expasy.org), and the Human Genome Mutation Database (http://archive.uwcm.ac.uk/uwcm/mg/hgmd0.html).

## CLASSICAL AND FUNCTIONAL GENOMIC APPROACHES

The investigative strategies used to study two common pulmonary diseases, $\alpha_1$-antitrypsin deficiency (OMIM No. 107400) and cystic fibrosis (OMIM No. 219700), are good examples of classical biochemistry and functional genomics (Fig. 6A.1). The gene encoding the cystic fibrosis transmembrane regulator was the first human disease-associated gene to be detected by positional cloning. This allowed identification of the protein product of the gene,

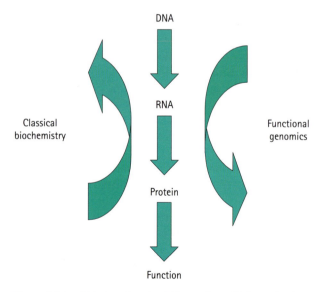

**Figure 6A.1**   *This describes the different flow of information in a classical and functional genomics approach. The classical approach uses a single biochemical functionality to identify a metabolic pathway and locate the genes responsible. Functional genomics attempts to use the sequence information provided by the Human Genome Project to describe the function of the entire proteome.*

an ideology that has revolutionized the study of human disease. Positional cloning is performed by co-segregation of genetic markers with disease in multiply affected pedigrees and crucially does not require an a priori hypothesis of gene function. The ability to clone and overexpress genes identified in this manner allows functional observations on vanishingly rare gene products. The now redundant term 'reverse genetics' was used to describe the direction of discovery from genetic material down, rather than from enzyme activity up.

A classical approach was used to identify the gene encoding $\alpha_1$-antitrypsin. As the protein is abundant and relatively straightforward to purify from human serum, the gene was identified using probes designed from protein sequencing experiments.[2] However, the correlation of $\alpha_1$-antitrypsin sequence variants with disease was noticed as early as 1963,[3] as the protein is present in sufficient quantity to be detected by nonspecific protein staining after agarose gel electrophoresis. Functional studies were still required to prove the hypothesis that lack of protease inhibitor in the lung was the cause of the emphysema associated with this condition.[4]

The successful use of homology modeling is also clearly demonstrated in the literature on cystic fibrosis, the paper that first describes cloning of the gene used homology modeling to correctly define one aspect of its functionality, that of an ATP binding motif.[5] The authors also correctly predict that the most common cystic fibrosis mutation (delF508) will disrupt this motif. However, it is also worth noting that concurrent functional studies had already defined the function of the cystic fibrosis gene product as a chloride channel (reviewed in Ref. 6). It is the power of this combined approach that has led to the rapid increase in understanding of the etiology and pathology of cystic fibrosis, culminating in the pioneering experiments for gene therapy in this condition.

The contrasting examples of $\alpha_1$-antitrypsin and cystic fibrosis are a testament to the success of the classical and positional cloning strategies. Both studies can be said to be problems solved by 'discovery genetics' in that they were diseases in search of causative genes. The next logical phase of the human genome project has been called 'discovery genomics,' as the discovery of each new human gene reveals a potential candidate for elucidation of as yet undetermined pathological processes.[7]

## SEQUENCE COMPARISON AND FUNCTIONAL PREDICTION

One of the most powerful tools currently available to molecular biologists is the comparison of a newly sequenced gene to other sequences, either nucleotide or protein, from a huge variety of organisms. Evaluation of a new gene sequence can include functional information, to which family the gene belongs, and even the evolutionary development of the gene. The power of this approach is based on the central premise of evolution; that is functional elements required for survival will be conserved.

Once a gene sequence has been determined, the first step is almost invariably to use a basic local alignment search tool (BLAST).[8] This enables the sequence similarity of the new gene sequence to those already available to be calculated. There are a number of different forms of BLAST available. The different tools can use a DNA sequence to search nucleotide databases (BLASTN), a DNA sequence translated in six frames to search protein databases (BLASTX), a protein sequence to search protein databases (BLASTP), and a protein sequence back-translated in six frames to search nucleotide databases (TBLASTX). PSI-BLAST and RPS-BLAST are additional tools for searching protein databases using iterative searches and protein domains, respectively.

A BLAST result is obtained by using an algorithm that performs a heuristic (self-refining) search of the available databases. In effect, the search time is reduced because rather than directly comparing the whole of the new sequence (query) to all the other sequences available, as is seen for global alignments, particular aspects of the query are chosen and used for searching. The BLAST algorithm identifies short adjacent segments or 'words' (the default setting for word size is three letters for proteins and eleven letters for nucleotides) within the query sequence. The database is then searched for sequences containing these words. Simplifying the description of the process enormously, the more closely the words from a query match in size, order, and number to a sequence from the database, the more likely the sequence is to be similar.

The BLAST algorithm can identify regions or motifs in the query sequence distant in the database sequences. For example, mRNA comparisons with genomic DNA would be far less sensitive if an alignment was attempted across the whole region of the gene. Likewise, proteins which contain specific motifs for binding or activity will not necessarily contain the same number or order of motifs found in different protein families or species.

After a query has been submitted to the database and the search results returned, the next step is to interpret them. Traditionally the BLAST report contains a header stating the size of the query, the type of sequence (protein or nucleotide) and the databases that were searched. This is followed by a list of which databases sequences have been identified by the search, two statistical estimates (bit score and expect E-value) of how good the alignments are, and finally the matched pairwise alignments of the query and the database sequences. The database sequences are listed with the sequence with the highest bit score first.

The statistical estimates can be used to provide an idea of how likely the alignment is to have arisen simply by chance or whether the two sequences may have a biological relationship. The bit score is generated by calculating the contributions of similar words (number and length) and any gaps that have had to be used. These are calculated using substitution matrices that generate a score based on the likelihood of aligning a given pair of residues. The higher the bit score, the better the alignment of the two sequences. It is important to check the alignments visually since a bit score can be attributed to a single region in the query sequence showing high identity to a particular motif, e.g., ATP-binding cassette transporter in cystic fibrosis *trans*-membrane regulator. The E-value takes into account the number of sequences searched and the length of sequence. A longer sequence is more likely to contain multiple distinct domains than a shorter one. An E-value of <0.001 indicates the likelihood of the alignment happening just by chance is less than 1 in 1000.

The functions of a particular gene product can be further investigated by studying conserved domains. The predicted protein sequence can be used to perform a search against multiple local alignments from three sources: SMART (simple modular architecture research tool),[9] Pfam (protein families database of alignments and hidden Markov models),[10] and COG (clusters of orthologous groups).[11] The local alignments are curated and compiled taking into account functional class, tertiary structures, and functionally important residues of protein families. This approach is inherently synergistic, as the more domain structures are discovered the better the database becomes for detecting function from new sequence.[12]

## GENE PREDICTION ALGORITHMS

The subset of genes that encode proteins have, to date, been the easiest to identify and assign function to, consequently these are almost exclusively the genes currently associated with disease. Although identifying which family a gene sequence belongs to is critical for predicting the function of a gene product, the use of BLAST searching is unlikely to reveal the effect a particular mutation will have, e.g., gene transcription rate and promoter regulation, splice sites, or alterations in product structure, even if the sequence of the whole gene is known. *Cis* regulatory elements necessary for coordinated protein expression can be far distant from the protein coding regions or buried in long intergenic regions or introns. Sequence variations in many of these elements have been shown to associate with disease processes. Consequently the ability to predict gene structure from sequence is vital to decipher the data obtained by genomic studies.[13]

Algorithms used to identify protein-coding genes can be classified into two groups, those that use the intrinsic features of genes (Fig. 6A.2) and those that use protein or mRNA sequences to bootstrap the gene structure.

Intrinsic gene features can be further divided into content terms which use sequence statistics such as G/C content or codon and hexamer usage that are typical to exonic regions

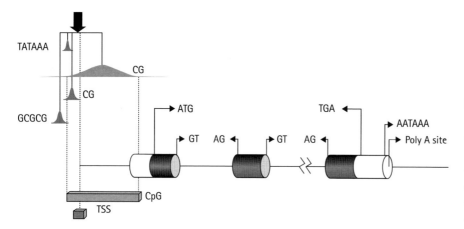

**Figure 6A.2**　*Diagram showing a full-length coding transcript. On the diagram is marked the CpG island, transcriptional start site (TSS), start (ATG), and stop (TGA) of translation, splice sites and polyadenylation signal (AATAAA), and site. (Taken from Ref. 27 with permission.)*

and signal terms which use motifs common to previously described genes. There are a number of public domain internet resources which enable the researcher to assess the probability that a DNA sequence of interest contains a particular gene feature (www.nslij-genetics.org/gene). A variety of approaches can be used, including a positional weight matrix (similar concept to the matrices used to calculate a BLAST score), analyzing the composition of 'words' contained within the DNA, and discriminant analysis which puts samples into two classes using statistical pattern recognition. The majority of these programs use data from known gene features sequences to train the algorithms to recognize particular features.

## Promoter sequences

Identification of gene promoter sequences is of paramount importance as it is this region of the genome that holds the key to the regulation of gene expression and ultimately the regulation of cell division and integration of metabolism. The transcriptional start site of a protein coding gene can be identified from the full length mRNA, although this can be technically difficult due to the fragility of RNA reverse transcription. Methodological improvements such as oligocapping make this easier.[14] The promoter region is upstream of the start site. Unfortunately these regions cannot be accurately identified by alignment procedures as they usually consist of multiple modular features separated by poorly conserved DNA sequences. Conserved features, such as CAAT or TATA boxes, exist but these are neither necessary nor sufficient for promoter identification. The major modules of the promoter are transcription factor binding sites. As there are around 2000 transcription factors and as each gene promoter has a unique combination of binding sites, there is tremendous potential for complex gene regulation. Similar to gene finding algorithms, promoter prediction algorithms rely on the identification of signals such as the TATA box, CpG islands or a transcription factor binding site with contextual information as triplet base-pair preferences around the transcription start site. The

most successful programs search for combinations of individual promoter elements. Once a putative promoter has been identified it becomes relatively straightforward to identify the *cis*-acting transcription factor binding elements, which are usually degenerate sequence motifs between 5 and 25 bp, although the relative frequency of these elements generates many false-positives.[15]

## Splice sites

The analysis of RNA sequence, as the intermediate between gene and protein, has been extremely useful in gene identification. The presence of an mRNA, however, cannot be used as proof as to the existence of a protein. A simple comparison between mRNA and its cognate DNA sequence can not only correctly identify a gene sequence, but also determine how the gene is spliced, which is the process by which introns are removed from RNA precursors. However, mRNA as a tool for gene analysis is confounded in two ways; first, many RNA molecules remain elusive due to temporal expression or expression at very low levels. Second, genes can be spliced in a variety of different ways. This may explain the C-value paradox, which refers to the difference in genome size between organisms of a similar complexity. As many as half of human genes are likely to have different splice variants, on average 2.5 per locus although over 30 000 splice variants have been predicted in some genes. As sequence variation in splice sites is likely to contribute to the maintenance of genetic diversity it also plays a role in the mechanism of human disease.[16]

The vast majority of splice sites contain conserved dinucleotides GT-AG that are likely to be essential for the precise removal of the intron. However, other exons use GC-AG pairs and a small number use other noncanonical splice sites. Taken together with the different contextual information of exonic DNA, algorithms can be determined to predict splice sites with reasonable accuracy. Sequence data from around the splice site may also contribute to the efficiency of splice site detection.[17] This situation has been further complicated by the presence of exonic splice site enhancers. These exonic sequences, which bind serine/arginine rich splicosome-associated proteins are essential for correct splicing. Silent mutations in these regions can leave the predicted protein sequence intact, and therefore be overlooked as potential causative mutations. However these 'silent' mutations can have catastrophic effects on gene translation and so represents a new mechanism for human genetic disease. Prediction algorithms for exonic splice enhancers are now available so these previously overlooked 'silent mutations' are being identified in human disease cohorts.[18]

## POLYA SIGNALS

Eukaryotic messages are polyadenylated usually 15–17 base-pairs downstream of the polyadenylation signal. The signal is most commonly AAUAAA, although at least 10 other signals can trigger message adenylation. The presence of alternate sites within genes contributes to differential message splicing. These forms are associated with differential tissue expression, possibly with tumorigenesis and viral infection mechanisms.[16,19] Whilst software packages are available to detect these motifs, the number of potential sites in the 3' untranslated region of some genes makes manual annotation based on experimental data the only reliable method.

## GLOBAL GENE PREDICTION

A combination of both intrinsic and protein or mRNA comparison methods have been used to annotate the draft human sequence (Ensembl www.ensembl.org[20] and Celera www.applera.com/celeradiagnostics[21]). Selection of an appropriate algorithm is a compromise between falsely detecting or missing genes or gene features. For example 'Ensembl' eliminates exons predicted ab initio that do not correspond to known vertebrate sequences. This increases specificity for gene detection to around 93 percent, so although some genes will be missing, most annotated genes (or at least parts of the gene) will be correctly assigned. Purely ab initio programs are more sensitive at the expense of a lower specificity. No program is entirely accurate and accuracy declines steeply with large genes.[22]

## Mutations which do not affect protein sequence

The classical definition of a gene is a heritable unit associated with a phenotype. A phenotypic change does not necessarily dictate a change in protein structure or concentration as the primary event. It has been estimated that 98 percent of RNA transcripts (98 percent) are not translated into proteins. The nature of these transcripts remains elusive as the motifs that are used to identify protein-coding genes are absent from these genes. Sequence variation within non-protein coding genes has been shown to associate with disease, the XIST gene (OMIN No. *314670) being the best described to date.

Mutations in this gene cause ineffective X chromosome inactivation and diseases associated with this, such as Snyder–Robinson mental retardation syndrome (OMIM No. *309583) and Prader–Willi syndrome (OMIM No. 176270).

Conversely, pseudogenes, which have many characteristic features of protein-coding genes but lack certain regulatory elements, are unlikely to have any direct function. The process of 'crossing over' with functional gene homologues causes gene duplications and rearrangements that may be advantageous for the maintenance of genetic diversity, but are better known as a significant cause of heritable human disease, such as Gaucher disease (OMIM No. *606463) and congenital adrenal hyperplasia (OMIM No. *201910).

## STRUCTURE PREDICTION ALGORITHMS

It is often quoted, particularly by structural biologists, that the human genome project will not be complete until we have a three-dimensional structure of every protein encoded by the human chromosomes. Originally, high-resolution structural determination was seen as the last part of the classical biochemical investigation, and was usually performed when detailed functional data on the protein were available. The field of structural genomics, in much the same as functional genomics, turns this approach on its head by attempting to use the inferred structure of a protein to predict its function. X-ray crystallographers have used homology modeling, exploiting data from a known structure to solve novel structures, to good effect for many years, despite concerns that this approach will bias the protein structure database to known rather than novel structural motifs. Taken a step further, a homologous protein structure can be used to predict the structure of a previously undescribed protein entirely from its primary sequence. It is hoped that the somewhat crude structures that these methods generate will be informative enough to predict function, without the high resolution data often required to establish a detailed molecular mechanism. Clearly the success of this approach will largely depend on technical advances in structure determination to provide an experimental database on which models can be built, the ultimate aim being to obtain structural data for all possible protein folds. There are several conceptual problems with this approach. First, the original premise that function can be determined from structure is by no means certain as in some situations even high-resolution structural data will not give insight into a protein's function. Second, proteins with the same function can have different folds. The converse, that individual proteins from homologous groups can have different functions, is also true. Despite these caveats, it has been suggested that two-thirds of proteins with the same fold will have the same function.

A good homology model relies on two facets. Clearly a homologue with a known high-resolution structure is an ideal starting point for structure prediction. Secondly, an extended family of gene homologues is essential, as accurate sequence alignment is usually the key to successful homology-based structure prediction. Whether the information gained from this process is more useful than the sequence alignment alone is debatable and attempts to refine the structure after homology modeling using molecular dynamics based packages is rarely successful.[23] If structural data from homologues are not available or homology is less than 30 percent, this approach is rarely successful. Two approaches can be used in this situation. The first assumes that all of the information pertaining to the tertiary structure is contained within the primary sequence and attempts to predict folding ab initio, starting from an unfolded protein with random conformation. The second approach called 'threading' is a compromise and uses information from the closest matching structures, which limits this method to predicting known structural elements. This method has been combined with an ab initio folding program to allow novel folds to be identified. Ab initio folding, despite the enormous number of conformers available to a nascent chain, has been successful to the extent that helical and $\alpha/\beta$ structures less than 100 residues can be 'folded' with reasonable accuracy.[24] The threading approach has also been successful in the correct identification of several families of previously uncharacterized bacterial enzymes, having considerably less false-positive scores than sequence-alone-based strategies.[25] However, it is clear that the ultimate goal of structural genomics has not been achieved, to the point where it has been said that the majority of folds will have been determined experimentally before proteins can be folded in silico.

Similar considerations, although less daunting, apply to predicting the functional consequence of an amino-acid change in a protein as to predicting a protein fold. An amino-acid change is most likely to be significant if the residue is highly conserved and has a molecular role assigned by previous structural or functional studies. A database of disease associated mutations described to date suggest that substitutions involving the amino acids cysteine and arginine are most likely to have a deleterious effect, with conservative changes such as leucine to methionine, leucine to isoleucine, alanine to serine, and phenylalanine to tyrosine more likely to be benign.[26] Even with access to high-resolution structural data, prediction of the effect of an amino acid substitution in a residue that does not have a defined molecular role or is poorly conserved within a gene family is unlikely to be much better than the simple rule of thumb described above.

## REFERENCES

1  Smith LM. Automated DNA sequencing and the analysis of the human genome. *Genome* 1989; **31**: 929–37.

2  Lai EC, Kao FT, Law ML, Woo SL. Assignment of the alpha 1-antitrypsin gene and a sequence-related gene to human chromosome 14 by molecular hybridization. *Am J Hum Genet* 1983; **35**: 385–92.

3  Laurell CB, Eriksson S. The electrophoretic alpha-1-globulin pattern of serum in alpha-1 antitrysin deficiency. *Scand J Clin Lab Invest* 1963; **15**: 132–40.

4  Weitz JI, Silverman EK, Thong B, Campbell EJ. Plasma levels of elastase-specific fibrinopeptides correlate with proteinase inhibitor phenotype. Evidence for increased elastase activity in subjects with homozygous and heterozygous deficiency of alpha 1-proteinase inhibitor. *J Clin Invest* 1992; **89**: 766–73.

5  Riordan JR, Rommens JM, Kerem B et al. Identification of the cystic fibrosis gene: cloning and characterization of complementary DNA. *Science* 1989; **245**: 1066–73.

6  Halley DJ, Bijman J, de Jonge HR et al. The cystic fibrosis defect approached from different angles – new perspectives on the gene, the chloride channel, diagnosis and therapy. *Eur J Pediatr* 1990; **149**: 670–7.

7  Roses AD. Pharmacogenetics and the practice of medicine. *Nature* 2000; **405**: 857–65.

8  Altschul SF, Gish W, Miller W et al. Basic local alignment search tool. *J Mol Biol* 1990; **215**: 403–10.

9  Letunic I, Goodstadt L, Dickens NJ et al. Recent improvements to the SMART domain-based sequence annotation resource. *Nucleic Acids Res* 2002; **30**: 242–4.

10  Bateman A, Birney E, Cerruti L et al. The Pfam protein families database. *Nucleic Acids Res* 2002; **30**: 276–80.

11  Tatusov RL, Natale DA, Garkavtsev IV et al. The COG database: new developments in phylogenetic classification of proteins from complete genomes. *Nucleic Acids Res* 2001; **29**: 22–8.

12  Thornton JW, DeSalle R. Gene family evolution and homology: genomics meets phylogenetics. *Annu Rev Genomics Hum Genet* 2000; **1**: 41–73.

13  Zhang MQ. Computational prediction of eukaryotic protein-coding genes. *Nat Rev Genet* 2002; **3**: 698–709.

14  Maruyama K, Sugano S. Oligo-capping: a simple method to replace the cap structure of eukaryotic mRNAs with oligoribonucleotides. *Gene* 1994; **138**: 171–4.

15  Qiu P. Recent advances in computational promoter analysis in understanding the transcriptional regulatory network. *Biochem Biophys Res Commun* 2003; **309**: 495–501.

16  Faustino NA, Cooper TA. Pre-mRNA splicing and human disease. *Genes Dev* 2003; **17**: 419–37.

17  Zhang L, Luo L. Splice site prediction with quadratic discriminant analysis using diversity measure. *Nucleic Acids Res* 2003; **31**: 6214–20.

18  Drabenstot SD, Kupfer DM, White JD et al. FELINES: a utility for extracting and examining EST-defined introns and exons. *Nucleic Acids Res* 2003; **31**: e141.

19  Scorilas A. Polyadenylate polymerase (PAP) and 3′ end pre-mRNA processing: function, assays, and association with disease. *Crit Rev Clin Lab Sci* 2002; **39**: 193–224.

20  Lander ES, Linton LM, Birren B et al. Initial sequencing and analysis of the human genome. *Nature* 2001; **409**: 860–921.

21  Venter JC, Adams MD, Myers EW et al. The sequence of the human genome. *Science* 2001; **291**: 1304–51.

22  Wang J, Li S, Zhang Y et al. Vertebrate gene predictions and the problem of large genes. *Nat Rev Genet* 2003; **4**: 741–9.

23  Schonbrun J, Wedemeyer WJ, Baker D. Protein structure prediction in 2002. *Curr Opin Struct Biol* 2002; **12**: 348–54.

24  Hardin C, Pogorelov TV, Luthey-Schulten Z. Ab initio protein structure prediction. *Curr Opin Struct Biol* 2002; **12**: 176–81.

25  Godzik A. Fold recognition methods. *Meth Biochem Anal* 2003; **44**: 525–46.

26  Goodstadt L, Ponting CP. Sequence variation and disease in the wake of the draft human genome. *Hum Mol Genet* 2001; **10**: 2209–14.

27  Ashurst JL, Collins JE. Gene annotation: prediction and testing. *Annu Rev Genom Hum Genet* 2003; **4**: 69–88.

# Expression and purification of recombinant proteins

DAMIAN C. CROWTHER

## INTRODUCTION

The understanding of protein structure and how it relates to function and disease has benefited greatly from the use of recombinant DNA technology to generate abundant quantities of proteins of interest. In the past, proteins were purified from biological samples, a process that was both laborious and often gave poor yields. By using micro-organisms, eukaryotic cell cultures, and even whole organisms, we can now purify large amounts of protein that are either rare or absent in nature.

This section will discuss the relative merits of various systems for recombinant protein expression and then describe each briefly. Finally, the techniques for protein purification will be discussed.

## THE RELATIVE MERITS OF THE VARIOUS PROTEIN EXPRESSION SYSTEMS

The most appropriate methods of expression and purification are determined by the experiments that one intends to perform on the protein of interest. For experiments requiring large quantities of the protein, for example $\alpha_1$-antitrypsin replacement therapy, then bacterial[1] or yeast expression may be most appropriate.[2] If the material is to be given to humans then stringent quality assurance is required and the absence of human-infecting viruses in *E. coli* and yeast makes them attractive. If the protein is to be used in an animal model, then expression in yeast has the advantage that yeasts do not produce endotoxin. *E. coli*-derived endotoxin contamination of test proteins can lead to problems interpreting data in animal and cell culture experiments.[3] The convenience and high yields from *E. coli* mean that protein crystallographers often try bacterial expression first; however, if the protein of interest has a complex structure, is prone to aggregation, needs pro-enzyme processing, or requires highly specific glycosylation or phosphorylation then one should consider expression

in a higher organism.[4,5] Yeast may be sufficient; however, insect or mammalian cell culture are likely to give better protein products.[6] Whole organism expression, such as secretion of recombinant protein into transgenic ovine milk, has been used where the combination of large quantities of product must be combined with the need for eukaryotic processing of the recombinant protein.[7,8]

At the opposite end of the scale from whole organism expression are the new commercial kits that allow protein expression in a cell-free system.[9] These kits conveniently produce small quantities of protein, sufficient to test for binding affinity or enzymic/inhibitor activity but the high cost prohibits scaling up even to the milligram range. Template DNA is usually plasmid-derived, however the generation of template DNA using PCR allows for flexible protein expression using sequence derived from genome databases and cDNA libraries.

Mutagenesis is a powerful and widely used tool for determining the relationship between protein structure and function, for example in the determination of a co-factor binding site.[10] Expression of mutant protein is most conveniently performed in *E. coli* unless eukaryotic glycosylation and/or folding are required, in which case yeast or eukaryotic expression may be required.[11] The most ambitious mutagenesis schemes aim to mimic evolution and ask how random mutations at one or more loci affect the function of a protein. In these protocols a large library of $>10^{10}$ uniquely mutated proteins are screened for a desired property, often binding affinity for another protein. Affinity chromatography is used to enrich the library in protein mutants that have an increased binding affinity. Bacteriophage-display and ribosome-display technologies have been developed to ensure that selection for the mutant protein also selects for the coding DNA. Thus expression of the protein of interest on the surface of bacteriophages[12] (phage-display systems) or more recently, using cell-free translation systems, on stalled ribosomes (ribosome-display) allows cloning and sequencing of the DNA that codes for high affinity mutants.[13]

## *Escherichia coli* expression systems

Plasmids used for expression in *E. coli* are almost all derived from the ColE1 replicon and are present in copy numbers of 15–200 per bacterium. The plasmid is passed on to daughter cells stochastically resulting in a rate of plasmid loss of $10^{-5}$–$10^{-6}$ per generation, a rate that increases if the expressed protein is toxic. Selection for the plasmid is provided by antibiotic resistance, often ampicillin. Transcription of the protein-coding sequence is directed classically by promoters derived from bacteriophage lambda, the *E. coli* lac operon or the *E. coli* trp operon. Recent plasmids combine the convenience and power of these systems in synthetic trc and tac promoters. Alternatively, the protein coding sequence may be put downstream of a T5 or T7 bacteriophage RNA polymerase-responsive promoter and expression is initiated by induction of RNA polymerase.[1]

Following expression, the bacteria must be disrupted to allow recovery of the protein. For analytical gels, boiling in SDS-PAGE loading buffer may be sufficient; however, for protein purification three main techniques are employed (Table 6B.1).

If expression levels are high then SDS-PAGE of the *E. coli* culture may show a protein band of the expected size; however, in most cases, expression is most conveniently detected and quantified using immunological techniques, including rocket immunoelectrophoresis,[14] Western blotting, and ELISA. It is important to determine the proportion of recombinant protein that is soluble by centrifuging the cell lysate at 14 000–16 000 g; insoluble protein being found in the pellet and soluble material in the supernatant. Insoluble protein found in inclusion bodies may be conveniently harvested by centrifugation, denatured using chaotropic agents such as urea or guanidinium HCl, and refolded to yield native protein.[15] Where solubility is essential, for example if the protein will not refold, then reducing the culture temperature following the addition of inducing agents or using a variable strength promoter, e.g., *araBAD*, may be appropriate.[16] Overexpression of chaperones may help solubility,[17] however, the number of candidates is large (e.g., GroES-GroEL, DnaK-DnaJ, peptidyl prolyl *cis/trans* isomerases) and the process is likely to be time consuming.

Knowledge of protein levels allows optimization of the expression protocol. Although this is an empirical process an initial protocol is described in Table 6B.2. The main variables that need optimizing are: (1) the density of the main culture when the inducing agents are added; (2) the duration of protein expression prior to harvesting; and (3) the temperature of the culture during expression.

Common problems encountered during protein expression include proteolysis, toxicity, and rare codon usage. Approaches to solving these problems are summarized in Table 6B.3.

## Yeast expression systems

The most common yeasts used for recombinant protein production are *Saccharomyces cerevisiae* (*S. cerevisiae*, baker's yeast) and *Pichia pastoris* (*P. pastoris*, a methylotrophic yeast). pYES, a commonly used vector in *S. cerevisiae*, is available with a promoter that is induced in the presence of galactose (Invitrogen). There are several vectors used with *P. pastoris* (for example, pHIL-D2, pPIC, and pMET), a convenient promoter for controlling protein expression is the alcohol oxidase that is activated in the presence of methanol. Selection markers in yeast plasmids usually allow the transformed yeast to grow in the absence of an otherwise essential substrate, examples include LEU2 (tolerant of leucine deficiency) or HIS4 (tolerant of histidine deficiency).[2]

Yeast cells are transformed by electroporation and incubated on selective agar at 30°C for a few days until colonies

**Table 6B.1** *Three main techniques for cell lysis prior to protein purification*

| Technique | Comments |
| --- | --- |
| Lysozyme followed by detergent or sonication | Lysozyme degrades the bacterial outer wall and the spheroplasts are subsequently lysed. DNase and RNase reduce viscosity |
| French Press or Manton-Gaulin homogenizer | Liquid sheer lyses bacterial cells |
| EDTA followed by hypotonic shock | Releases proteins from the periplasmic space without lysing the cells. Useful for secreted proteins |

**Table 6B.2** *Initial protocol for protein expression*

| Step | Conditions |
| --- | --- |
| Transformation | The plasmid is transformed into *E. coli* and incubated on selective agar overnight |
| Starter culture | A single colony from the transformation is inoculated into 50 mL of selective media in the absence of inducing agents. The culture is placed in a rotary shaker at 37°C |
| Main culture | 10 mL of the starter culture is inoculated into each litre of selective media. The culture is placed in a rotary shaker at 37°C. When the optical density at 600 nm reaches 0.6 then the inducing agents, e.g., IPTG for lac-based promoters, are added |
| Protein expression | The culture remains in the rotary shaker at 37°C for 6 h before harvesting of the bacteria |

are visible. Ten overnight cultures of separate clones are grown at 30°C with shaking in 5 mL cultures of selective media. One hundred microlitres of each culture is diluted into 50 mL of selective media containing the inducing agent. Samples are taken at intervals over the next 48 h to determine which clone expresses the most protein and what is the optimal duration of fermentation. Glycerol stocks of the best clone are stored at −80°C to provide material for subsequent fermentations. Protein can be detected by boiling a sample of the culture in SDS-PAGE loading buffer and subsequently Western blotting. Purification of proteins is most convenient when they are secreted into the medium because of the lower concentrations of contaminating yeast proteins and DNA. A yeast secretion signal

**Table 6B.3**   *Solutions to problems of proteolysis, toxicity, and rare codon usage*

| Problem | Solution |
| --- | --- |
| Proteolysis of recombinant protein by endogenous proteases such as *Lon* and *ClpYQ*. Particularly significant for protease inhibitors such as $\alpha_1$-antitrypsin | Cell lysis and purification performed at 4°C. Buffers should contain a broad-spectrum protease inhibitor cocktail including EDTA. Note that metal chelators must be absent when loading proteins onto metal-chelating chromatography media. Some bacterial strains such as BL21 are deficient in *Lon* and *OmpT* proteases |
| The protein is toxic to *E. coli* due to low level expression in the absence of inducing agents | Use a plasmid with a weaker promoter. Alternatively use a T7 promoter plasmid where the T7 polymerase is provided only when expression is required by infection with a bacteriophage, e.g., Novagen's pET with bacteriophage λCE6 |
| Use of codons that are rare in *E. coli* | Codons rarely used in *E. coli* have correspondingly low levels of tRNA. Bacterial strains that overexpress particular rare tRNAs are available (Novagen). Alternatively, the coding sequence can be mutated to a more common bacterial codon |

**Table 6B.4**   *Various techniques for lysing yeast cells intracellularly*

| Technique | Comments |
| --- | --- |
| French Press at high pressure (>12 000 psi) | Liquid sheer lyses yeast cells |
| Vortexing with glass beads | Glass beads sheer yeast cells |
| Zymolyase digestion followed by sonication | Spheroplasts ruptured by sonication. Only useful for small-scale protein production |

peptide from α-factor is commonly used at the N-terminus of the recombinant protein to promote secretion.[18] However, if the protein must be expressed intracellularly then there are various techniques for lysing yeast cells as described in Table 6B.4.

## Mammalian and insect cell culture expression systems

Mammalian and insect cells are able to perform all the complex post-translational modifications that may be required for successful expression of human proteins. In particular, eukaryotic cells are able to correctly glycosylate secreted proteins which may be essential for protein structure and function. There are many plasmids for expressing proteins in mammalian cells lines, but their common features are the presence of an antibiotic resistance gene (e.g., ampicillin) and origin of replication that permit cloning of the gene in *E. coli*. The plasmids usually contain a second antibiotic resistance gene (e.g., kanamycin) to permit selection in eukaryotic cells, as well as eukaryotic transcription promoters (e.g., CMV) and a polyadenylation signal.

Expression of proteins in cell lines such as Chinese hamster ovary (CHO) cells may be achieved using constitutively active plasmids, such as pcDNA3 (Invitrogen). Where the protein is toxic or the handling of the protein by cells is the focus of study then inducible plasmids may be useful, for example the pTet-on and pTet-off plasmids from Clontech allow expression to be turned on and off, respectively, in the presence of the antibiotic doxycycline. CHO cells have the added advantage that they can be grown in protein and peptide-free media which facilitates the process of purifying secreted recombinant proteins.

The expression of proteins in insect cells using *Baculovirus* vectors has become widely used because they offer the benefits of faithful eukaryotic post-translational processing with the promise of higher protein yields.[19] Commercial kits are available (Bac-to-Bac (Invitrogen) and BacPAK (Clontech)) that accelerate the process of protein expression. In summary, the gene of interest is cloned into a shuttle plasmid that is then incorporated into an engineered form of the *Autographa californica* nuclear polyhedrosis virus (AcNPV) (Fig. 6B.1). AcNPV is propagated in cell lines derived from the fall armyworm *Spodoptera frugiperda* or from the cabbage looper *Trichoplusia ni*. The cell lines grow well in culture and can be scaled up from flasks to large bioreactors. Proteins can be expressed within the cell; however, secretion into the culture medium facilitates purification.

## Cell–free protein expression systems

Cell-free translation systems using rabbit reticulocyte lysates have been available since their first description by

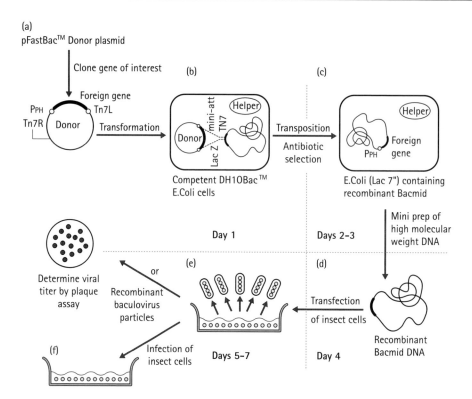

**Figure 6B.1**    *The gene of interest is cloned into the pFastBac plasmid (a) and transformed into DH10Bac E. coli cells that contain the Bacmid encoding the lacZ marker and expressing translocase from a helper plasmid (b). Tn7 transposon sites on pFastBac and the Bacmid mediate translocation of the gene of interest into the LacZ gene of the Bacmid resulting in generation of a white colony when the bacteria are grown on palates containing X-gal (c). Recombinant Bacmid DNA is prepared (d) and transfected into insect cells (e). Insect cells are used for protein production (f).*

Pelham and Jackson in 1976.[20] Commercially available kits now permit in vitro transcription of template DNA and subsequent translation of the mRNA.[9] These systems are suitable for applications where only a small amount of protein is required or where conventional expression using for example E. coli has yielded insoluble or inactive material. Several systems are available based on *E. coli* (Rapid Translation System, Roche Diagnostic), rabbit reticulocytes (TnT Coupled Reticulocyte Lysate System, Promega) and wheatgerm (TnT Coupled Wheatgerm Extract System, Promega). The problem of protein insolubility may be overcome by addition of detergents or chaperones to the reaction medium.[21] Template DNA is provided as a plasmid or as linear DNA, for example, a PCR product.

### Whole animal expression systems

Transgenic animals may be used as bioreactors for the industrial-scale production of proteins that require eukaryotic glycosylation, such as clotting factor VIII.[7] Other tissues that may be suitable for expressing proteins include egg white, blood, urine, and seminal plasma.[8] These approaches allow the production of recombinant protein in large amounts, essential when one considers replacement

therapy for patients with protein deficiencies, for example $\alpha_1$-antitrypsin deficiency.[22] Transgenic animals may also be used to express foreign proteins as a model for a human disease. Mouse models of Huntington's disease[23] and Alzheimer's disease[24] have been generated by overexpressing the pathogenic peptides or proteins in neurons. Recently, protein expression in *Drosophila melanogaster* has successfully modeled Huntington's[25] and Parkinson's disease.[26]

### PURIFICATION OF RECOMBINANT PROTEINS

Once the protein of interest has been expressed then we must purify the recombinant protein away from the endogenous host proteins. Purification may be facilitated if the (micro)organism can be induced to partition the recombinant protein away from other proteins. Most commonly, this is achieved by expressing high levels of recombinant protein in *E. coli* which results in insoluble inclusion bodies of almost pure protein which can then be purified and the protein denatured and refolded to yield native protein.[15] The secretion of a protein is another effective partitioning strategy requiring the addition of an N-terminal secretion signal peptide to the expressed

**Table 6B.5** *Commonly employed tags and partner proteins*

| Tag or partner protein | Chromatography media for immobilizing recombinant protein | References |
|---|---|---|
| 6x His | Nickel-chelating | 29 |
| FLAG tag | Monoclonal antibody chromatography media | 30 |
| GST (glutathione S-transferase) | Glutathione chromatography media | 31 |
| MBP (maltose binding protein) | Amylose resin | 32 |
| Thioredoxin | Phenylarsine oxide | 33 |

protein. Secretion of proteins from *E. coli* usually into the periplasm of the bacterium allows recovery of the recombinant protein with little contaminating bacterial protein using techniques such as osmotic shock.[27] Yeast can also be used to secrete proteins.[28] For some proteins, folding may be improved because of the similarity of the secretion pathway to the endoplasmic reticulum pathway of protein synthesis in the human. Indeed both bacteria and yeast have a limited system of chaperones to help with folding of secreted proteins; however, the yields from secreted protein expression in microorganisms are usually low. Secretion of proteins from eukaryotic cell culture, e.g., baculovirus expression in insect cells, or secretion of proteins into ovine milk are also effective methods of simplifying protein purification.

The main advances in recombinant protein purification, however, have related to tag or partner protein co-expression with the protein of interest. The most commonly employed tags and partner proteins are given in Table 6B.5. After affinity chromatography using one of these techniques, it is usually possible to purify the recombinant protein using ion exchange chromatography (e.g., Q-sepharose) followed, if required, by size exclusion chromatography (e.g., Sephacryl S200).

# REFERENCES

1 Bird PI, Pak SC, Worrall DM, Bottomley SP. Production of recombinant serpins in *Escherichia coli*. *Methods* 2004; **32**: 169–76.

2 Pemberton PA, Bird PI. Production of serpins using yeast expression systems. *Methods* 2004; **32**: 185–90.

3 Qahwash IM, Cassar CA, Radcliff RP, Smith GW. Bacterial lipopolysaccharide-induced coordinate downregulation of arginine vasopressin receptor V3 and corticotropin-releasing factor receptor 1 messenger ribonucleic acids in the anterior pituitary of endotoxemic steers. *Endocrine* 2002; **18**: 13–20.

4 Baneyx F. Recombinant protein expression in Escherichia coli. *Curr Opin Biotechnol* 1999; **10**: 411–21.

5 Swartz JR. Advances in *Escherichia coli* production of therapeutic proteins. *Curr Opin Biotechnol* 2001; **12**: 195–201.

6 Cooley J, Mathieu B, Remold-O'Donnell E, Mandle RJ. Production of recombinant human monocyte/neutrophil elastase inhibitor (rM/NEI). *Prot Expr Purif* 1998; **14**: 38–44.

7 Niemann H, Halter R, Carnwath JW et al. Expression of human blood clotting factor VIII in the mammary gland of transgenic sheep. *Transgenic Res* 1999; **8**: 237–47.

8 Houdebine LM. Transgenic animal bioreactors. *Transgenic Res* 2000; **9**: 305–20.

9 Luke CJ. Serpin production using rapid in vitro transcription/translation systems. *Methods* 2004; **32**: 191–8.

10 Belzar KJ, Zhou A, Carrell RW et al. Helix D elongation and allosteric activation of antithrombin. *J Biol Chem* 2002; **277**: 8551–8.

11 Tsiang M, Jain AK, Dunn KE et al. Functional mapping of the surface residues of human thrombin. *J Biol Chem* 1995; **270**: 16854–63.

12 Cloutier SM, Kundig C, Felber LM et al. Development of recombinant inhibitors specific to human kallikrein 2 using phage-display selected substrates. *Eur J Biochem* 2004; **271**: 607–13.

13 He M, Cooley N, Jackson A, Taussig MJ. Production of human single-chain antibodies by ribosome display. *Methods Mol Biol* 2004; **248**: 177–89.

14 Laurell C-B. Quantitative estimation of proteins by electrophoresis in agarose gel containing antibodies. *Anal Biochem* 1966; **15**: 45–52.

15 Belorgey D, Crowther DC, Mahadeva R, Lomas DA. Mutant neuroserpin (S49P) that causes familial encephalopathy with neuroserpin inclusion bodies is a poor proteinase inhibitor and readily forms polymers in vitro. *J Biol Chem* 2002; **277**: 17367–73.

16 Clark MA, Hammond FR, Papaioannou A et al. Regulation and expression of human Fabs under the control of the *Escherichia coli* arabinose promoter, PBAD. *Immunotechnology* 1997; **3**: 217–26.

17 Lee DH, Kim MD, Lee WH et al. Consortium of fold-catalyzing proteins increases soluble expression of cyclohexanone monooxygenase in recombinant *Escherichia coli*. *Appl Microbiol Biotechnol* 2004; **63**: 549–52.

18 Gurkan C, Symeonides SN, Ellar DJ. High-level production in *Pichia pastoris* of an anti-p185HER-2 single-chain antibody fragment using an alternative secretion expression vector. *Biotechnol Appl Biochem* 2004; **39** (Pt 1): 115–22.

19 Jayakumar A, Cataltepe S, Kang Y et al. Production of serpins using baculovirus expression systems. *Methods* 2004; **32**: 177–84.

20 Pelham HR, Jackson RJ. An efficient mRNA-dependent translation system from reticulocyte lysates. *Eur J Biochem* 1976; **67**: 247–56.

21 Rozema D, Gellman SH. Artificial chaperone-assisted refolding of denatured-reduced lysozyme; modulation of the competition between renaturation and aggregation. *Biochemistry* 1996; **35**: 15760–71.

22 Ward AC, Keogh BA. Intravenous alpha-1-antitrypsin replacement therapy; case report after one year of treatment. *Ir J Med Sci* 1997; **166**: 7–9.

23 Mangiarini L, Sathasivam K, Seller M et al. Exon 1 of the HD gene with an expanded CAG repeat is sufficient to cause a progressive neurological phenotype in transgenic mice. *Cell* 1996; **87**: 493–506.

24 Hsiao K, Chapman P, Nilsen S et al. Correlative memory deficits, Abeta elevation, and amyloid plaques in transgenic mice. *Science* 1996; **274**: 99–102.

25  Jackson GR, Salecker I, Dong X et al. Polyglutamine-expanded human huntingtin transgenes induce degeneration of Drosophila photoreceptor neurons. *Neuron* 1998; **21**: 633–42.

26  Feany MB, Bender WW. A Drosophila model of Parkinson's disease. *Nature* 2000; **404**: 394–8.

27  Shokri A, Sanden AM, Larsson G. Cell and process design for targeting of recombinant protein into the culture medium of *Escherichia coli*. *Appl Microbiol Biotechnol* 2003; **60**: 654–64.

28  Kjeldsen T. Yeast secretory expression of insulin precursors. *Appl Microbiol Biotechnol* 2000; **54**: 277–86.

29  Ljungquist C, Breitholtz A, Brink-Nilsson H et al. Immobilization and affinity purification of recombinant proteins using histidine peptide fusions. *Eur J Biochem* 1989; **186**: 563–9.

30  Prickett KS, Amberg DC, Hopp TP. A calcium-dependent antibody for identification and purification of recombinant proteins. *Biotechniques* 1989; **7**: 580–9.

31  Smith DB, Johnson KS. Single-step purification of polypeptides expressed in *Escherichia coli* as fusions with glutathione S-transferase. *Gene* 1988; **67**: 31–40.

32  Maina CV, Riggs PD, Grandea AG 3rd et al. An *Escherichia coli* vector to express and purify foreign proteins by fusion to and separation from maltose-binding protein. *Gene* 1988; **74**: 365–73.

33  LaVallie ER, DiBlasio EA, Kovacic S et al. A thioredoxin gene fusion expression system that circumvents inclusion body formation in the *E. coli* cytoplasm. *Biotechnology* (*NY*) 1993; **11**: 187–93.

# Functional characterization of a protein

DIDIER BELORGEY AND DAVID A. LOMAS

## INTRODUCTION

The advent of recombinant DNA technology allows a variety of in vitro techniques to be used to alter a specific sequence of DNA in order to study the effect of that alteration on a gene product or a regulatory element. In this chapter, we will focus our discussion on the utilization of those techniques and other biochemical and biophysical techniques to study the effect of a mutation on protein structure and function.

## SITE–DIRECTED MUTAGENESIS

There are numerous approaches to site-directed mutagenesis.[1–3] As we are interested in the effect of a mutation on protein structure and function, we will describe only the polymerase chain reaction (PCR)-based approaches to oligonucleotide-directed mutagenesis. A general introduction to PCR has been described in the previous chapters.

In oligonucleotide-directed mutagenesis, a nucleotide encoding the desired mutation(s) is annealed to one strand of DNA of interest and acts as a primer for initiation of DNA synthesis. The mutagenic oligonucleotide will then be incorporated in the newly synthesized strand. The oligonucleotides can be designed so that at least one base change will be introduced, but can also be designed to include more than one substitution, insertion, or deletion. Assuming the gene of interest had already been cloned to a plasmid (see Chapter 6B) the first step will be to denature the DNA to produce single-stranded regions. The synthetic oligonucleotide will anneal to the target strand and a DNA polymerase is used to synthesize a new complementary strand. There are numerous variations by which the PCR reaction is used to generate a mutation in DNA, but for the most part the approach to site-directed mutagenesis is based on the method of Higuchi et al. modified to produce multiple, overlapping PCR fragments with the mutation(s) in the overlap.[4–6] In the two-step polymerase reaction, two overlapping oligonucleotides containing the mutation(s) are produced and the DNA is amplified with one of the oligonucleotides and a second oligonucleotides that anneals to the DNA on the complementary strand (Fig. 6C.1). After amplification with DNA polymerase (preferably with a $3'->5'$ proofreading activity such as Vent or Pfu) the two PCR reactions are cleaned on an agarose gel and the two reactions are mixed together for a further round of PCR with only the $5'$ end and $3'$ end oligonucleotides containing the appropriate restriction enzyme sites. The gel-purified fragment is then cut with the two restrictions enzymes and cloned into the appropriate plasmid with the help of a DNA ligase such as T4 ligase.

There are now a number of commercially available kits to undertake site-directed mutagenesis. These kits have the advantage of being easy to use, as well as being optimized for particular conditions, such as when PCR of DNA fragments is challenging, as with large plasmid templates. In addition they often contain components to facilitate more efficient DNA replication and bacterial transformation.

## STABILITY OF PROTEINS

Mutations can affect the thermal and urea (or guanidine hydrochloride) stability of a protein. The thermal stability can be assessed by circular dichroism measurement and fluorescence spectroscopy (see Chapter 6D). The measurement of the enthalpy change ($\Delta H$) by microcalorimetry can also be a valuable tool to assess the reaction between two proteins or a protein and a ligand. Microcalorimetry can also help determine association constants even in the case of weak interactions.[7] This approach was, for example, used to investigate the binding of mucus proteinase inhibitor (MPI, also known as secretory leukoproteinase inhibitor (SLPI)) to heparin and the interaction of different serine protease inhibitors with proteinases, including the interaction of $\alpha_1$-proteinase inhibitor ($\alpha_1$-antitrypsin) with human neutrophil elastase (HNE).[7,8]

Stability can also be assessed by denaturation in the presence of urea or guanidine hydrochloride. Denaturation

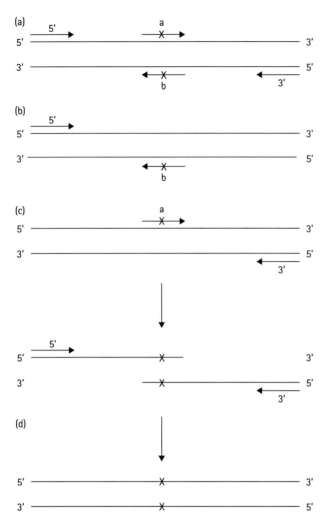

**Figure 6C.1**  *Site-directed mutagenesis: two step polymerase reaction. (a) 5' and a 3' end oligonucleotides and two complementary oligomers containing the mutation(x) are produced. (b) Two separate PCR reactions are performed with each of the complementary oligomers and the 5' and 3' end oligomers. (c) After cleaning on an agrose gel the two reactions are mixed together for a further round of PCR with only the 5' and 3' end oligomers containing the appropriate restriction enzyme sites. (d) The gel-purified fragment containing the desired mutation is then cloned into the appropriate plasmid.*

curves are an important tool to understand conformational changes that can occur with a single change in a protein sequence. When a protein unfolds, its physical properties change dramatically. This can be assessed using different techniques. The most common ones are circular dichroism, optical rotation, NMR, and fluorescence. For many proteins there is a measurable change in fluorescence emission between the native and the denatured state. This approach has been particularly useful in understanding the serine proteinase inhibitor (or serpin) superfamily of proteins, including ovalbumin[9] and serpins involved in respiratory disease, such as $\alpha_1$-antitrypsin and $\alpha_1$-antichymotrypsin.[10,11] In practice, fluorescence is the

technique of choice for convenience and due to the fact that relatively small amounts of protein (as low as 1 mg) can be used. Care must be taken as some batches of urea contain significant quantities of metallic impurities and cyanates and guanidine chloride may contain fluorescent impurities. Urea should be purified before use, as cyanates can chemically modify amino groups of proteins.[12] In practice, a typical denaturation curve is obtained by mixing the protein in a solution of urea ranging from 0 M to 8 M. It is important to obtain sufficient points (typically 10 to 20) in order to obtain an accurate measurement of denaturation, in particular around the transition point. It is also important to ensure that the reaction has reached equilibrium which can take from milliseconds to days.[13] The reaction will be temperature- and pH-dependent. Importantly, if the protein contains free sulfhydryl groups or disulfide bonds the pH dependence will need to be assessed thoroughly.[14] Once a denaturation curve has been obtained, the data can be analyzed to characterize the unfolding of a protein and determine if the process is a two-step mechanism or a more complex mechanism involving one or more intermediates. In the case of diseases associated with an incorrect folding of a protein, this can give an insight into the mechanism involved in the misfolding. This approach has been particularly useful in the investigation of genetic deficiency of $\alpha_1$-antitrypsin and $\alpha_1$-antichymotrypsin.[10,15] Denaturation curves can also be used to obtain an estimate of the conformational stability of a protein at 0 M of denaturant $\Delta G_D{}^{H_2O}$, allowing a comparison between two proteins or the same protein with amino acid variations due to mutation(s).[13,16]

## KINETIC ANALYSIS

When a mutation occurs in the gene coding for a protein known to be a protease or a protease inhibitor, a comparison of the kinetic properties of the protease or the inhibitor is a powerful way of assessing the effect of the mutation. If the substrate of the protease is known, then checking the ability of the mutant protein to cleave this substrate should be a first step. Many proteases cleave synthetic substrates allowing an assessment of their kinetic characteristics, such as the constants $K_m$ and $k_{cat}$ and their inhibition by proteinase inhibitors.[17,18] $K_m$ is an apparent dissociation constant related to the protease affinity for the substrate and $k_{cat}$ is a first order rate constant which represents the maximum number of molecules of substrate which can be converted into product per protease molecule per unit time (often known as the turnover number). The inhibitors involved in respiratory diseases are generally reversible tight-binding inhibitors (such as the mucus proteinase inhibitor) or irreversible tight-binding inhibitors, such as the serpins $\alpha_1$-antitrypsin and antichymotrypsin.[19–22] It is important to determine the detailed kinetic parameters describing a proteinase–inhibitor interaction such as the association rate constant $k_{ass}$ and equilibrium constant $K_i$. A percent of inhibition of an enzyme is an inadequate indicator of inhibitory function as it provides no information on the detailed interaction of enzyme with inhibitors.[23] Once the essential kinetics parameters are described, one can extrapolate the in vivo function of an inhibitor.[23,24]

The simplest reaction for a reversible inhibition is:

$$E + I \xrightleftharpoons[k_{diss}]{k_{ass}} EI$$

where $E$ is the enzyme, $I$ is the inhibitor, $EI$ is the enzyme–inhibitor complex, and $k_{ass}$ and $k_{diss}$ are the rate constants of complex formation and dissociation, respectively. In the case of an irreversible reaction only $k_{ass}$ is measurable. If the reaction is reversible one can determine $K_i$, the equilibrium dissociation constant of the enzyme–inhibitor complex. $K_i$ can be measured directly by incubating various amounts of inhibitor with a constant amount of enzyme,[24] but this is often not possible and in this case $K_i$ can be obtained by independently measuring $k_{ass}$ and $k_{diss}$ and applying the formula $K_i = k_{diss}/k_{ass}$. The association rate constant can be measured in a discontinuous assay by mixing equimolar concentrations of the enzyme and the inhibitor and measuring the activity of the enzyme at various times with an appropriate substrate (Fig. 6C.2a). It is also possible to measure the association rate constant in a pseudo-first order reaction when $[I]_0 \geqslant [E]_0$.[24,25] It is important to check that during the course of the experiment there is no dissociation of enzyme and inhibitor and only reactions with a half-time of at least 2 min can be measured for practical reasons. The amount of substrate required to stop the reaction needs to be $\geqslant 5 K_m$ which can be a problem when there is no substrate with a reasonable $K_m$ for the enzyme. Because of all of these factors, the value of $k_{ass}$ can sometimes only be a poor approximation of the real value.[23] The method of choice is therefore a continuous method which is called 'the progress curve method' (Fig. 6C.2b). In the progress curve method, the enzyme $E$ is added to a mixture of inhibitor $I$ and substrate $S$ and the release of product $P$ is continuously recorded.[26–29] In the case of a reversible competitive inhibition the simplest reaction will be:

$$E + S \xrightleftharpoons{K_m} ES \xrightarrow{k_{cat}} E + P$$
$$+$$
$$I$$
$$k_{diss} \Big\Updownarrow k_{ass}$$
$$EI$$

where $E$ is the enzyme, $I$ is the inhibitor, $S$ is the substrate, $EI$ is the enzyme–inhibitor complex, $ES$ is the enzyme–substrate

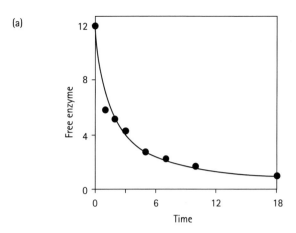

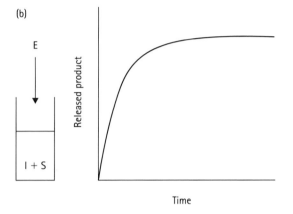

**Figure 6C.2**   *Measurement of an association rate constant. (a) Discontinuous assay. Equimolar concentration of the enzyme and the inhibitor are mixed together and the remaining activity is measured at various times. A plot of free enzyme versus time allows the calculation of an association rate constant by nonlinear regression analysis. (b) Progress curve assay. The enzyme and the appropriate substrate are mixed together and the enzyme is added to the mix. The release of cleaved substrate (released product) is then followed continuously over time and the association rate constant is calculated from this plot by nonlinear regression analysis.*

complex, $K_m$ and $k_{cat}$ represent the kinetic parameters of the enzyme for the substrate, and $k_{ass}$ and $k_{diss}$ are the rate constants of complex formation and dissociation, respectively. If $[I]_0 \geqslant [E]_0$, the initial concentration of inhibitor and enzyme, respectively, and if $[S]_0$, the initial concentration of substrate is not significantly depleted during the reaction, the biphasic release of product with time (progress curve) will allow the calculation of the constants $k_{ass}$ and $k_{diss}$.[23,26,27,29] The same method can be used to assess an irreversible inhibitor.[23,28] If the $k_{ass}$ is very high, as in the case of human neutrophil elastase inhibition by $\alpha_1$-antitrypsin ($k_{ass} = 1 \times 10^7 \, M^{-1} \, s^{-1}$), the use of a rapid kinetic apparatus (stopped flow) may be required. The measurement of $k_{diss}$ should in most cases be performed independently as the progress curve method does not allow an accurate measurement of this parameter. In this case the complex between the inhibitor and the enzyme should be prepared at high equimolar concentrations and diluted 100:1000-fold in an appropriate dissociating agent (for example, a high concentration of substrate).[23]

# LIGAND BINDING

Many proteins bind ligands in order to regulate gene expression, enzymatic activity, transport molecules, etc. Measurements of the binding affinity and binding stoichiometry between molecules and macromolecules provides essential information on the specificity and mechanism of action of these molecules. Binding of ligands is an important part of cell regulation and interactions of ligand and receptor are often associated with conformational changes. The interactions found between a protein and its ligand are generally the same as those found within proteins, i.e., hydrogen bounds, hydrophobic interactions, van der Waals' interactions, and electrostatic interaction. In the most simple case, the ligand will interact with the protein at only one site, but more than one site with a binding site per domain or two or more sites per domain are also fairly common. The binding affinity in the case of a single site will be measured by the association constant $K_a$ (also known as equilibrium constant $K_{eq}$ or affinity constant) for the binding of a ligand to a protein:

$$P + L \underset{}{\overset{K_a}{\rightleftharpoons}} PL$$

where $P$ is the protein, $L$ is the ligand, and $PL$ is the protein–ligand complex. The ratio of free protein to ligand-bound protein is directly proportional to the free ligand concentration and $K_a$ will be described by the following equation:

$$K_a = [PL]/[P][L]$$

and the greater the value of $K_a$ the greater the affinity. Usually the inverse of $K_a$, the dissociation constant $K_d$ will be considered. The most common way of determining the number of binding sites ($n$) and the value of $K_d$ is the construction of a Scatchard plot from experimental data (Fig. 6C.3).[30] Nowadays a nonlinear analysis of the data is the method of choice as it is less prone to errors caused by the linearization of data. Therefore, the Scatchard plot should be restricted to the presentation of the data for reasons of clarity. The concentration of $[PL]$ as a function of $[L]$ can also be obtained by equilibrium dialysis. In this case the protein in solution is placed inside a sealed bag composed of dialysis membrane and the bag placed in a buffer solution containing the ligand. The properties of the membrane allow free diffusion of the ligand across the membrane but not the protein. After the equilibrium is reached it is possible to measure the concentration of the ligand inside the bag

giving a measurement of $[PL] + [L]$ and the concentration of free ligand $[L]$ can be obtained from outside the bag. The ligand is often radiolabeled to allow measurement of its concentration. Another way of measuring $K_d$ is to monitor the change in the spectroscopic properties of the protein by exciting the tryptophan residues. In this case, increasing amounts of the ligand are added to the protein and the resulting change in tryptophan fluorescence is followed to equilibrium. This approach was used to determine the affinity of heparin for mucus proteinase inhibitor[31] or heparin to wildtype and mutant of antithrombin.[32,33] When the protein is a protease, it is also possible to use a synthetic substrate to obtain a stoichiometry and $K_d$ by measuring the difference of activity of the enzyme in the presence of an increasing amount of ligand.[34,35] Another way to obtain $K_d$ is to use the measure of $\Delta G$, as there is a direct relationship between the enthalpy of binding and $K_a$: $\Delta G = -RT\ln K_a$, where $K_a$ is the affinity constant, $\Delta G$ is the change in Gibbs free energy, $R$ is the gas constant, and $T$ is the temperature. This can be achieved by using microcalorimetry.[7] Over the past decade, a new technology based on surface plasmon resonance, utilizing Biacore® systems has been developed which allows the measurement of $K_d$ either by rate constant measurements or by measuring the steady-state level of binding as a function of sample concentration.[36] Surface plasmon resonance biosensors monitor interactions by measuring the mass concentration of a biomolecule close to a surface. In practice, one of the interacting partners is attached to a sensor chip covered by a thin layer of gold, itself covered with a matrix for covalent attachment of the ligand. The other partner is then passed over

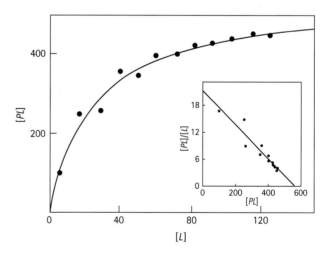

**Figure 6C.3** *Ligand binding and Scatchard plot. The amount of bound ligand (determined by radiolabeling, for example) was plotted against the amount of free ligand and a nonlinear regression analysis of the curve allowed the direct calculation of $K_d$, the dissociation constant and $B_{max}$, the maximum of bound ligand. The Scatchard plot (insert) is a good way to visualize saturation binding data. The Y intercept gives the value for $B_{max}/K_d$, the X intercept the value for $B_{max}$ and the slope the value for $-1/K_d$.*

the surface. The local concentration changes will produce a surface plasmon resonance response directly proportional to the mass of molecules that bind to the surface.[36–38]

It is not always the case that binding of one ligand to a protein has no effect on the subsequent binding of another ligand. In this case the binding is called allosteric and is observed when binding at one ligand-binding site affects the binding at another site on the protein, either by enhancing the binding or decreasing the binding of the second ligand. It can also be the case that the binding of one ligand to one site affects the binding of a second ligand (different from the first one) to the protein. This is called cooperativity and can be either positive (when the second ligand binding has higher affinity) or negative (when binding is at lower affinity). The degree of cooperativity can be assessed by plotting the data as a Hill plot and the determination of the Hill coefficient gives a quantitative measure of the degree of cooperativity.[39,40]

## GEL ELECTROPHORESIS OF PROTEINS

An easy way to assess the effect of a mutation on a protein conformation and/or some of its properties is to run polyacrylamide gels electrophoresis (PAGE) (Figure 6C.4). There are a number of techniques available and running one or more of these gels provides a great deal of useful information. The most common gels are one-dimensional sodium dodecyl sulfate PAGE (SDS-PAGE) and non-denaturing (native) PAGE.[41] Two dimension isoelectrofocusing (IEF) is also a good way to differentiate between

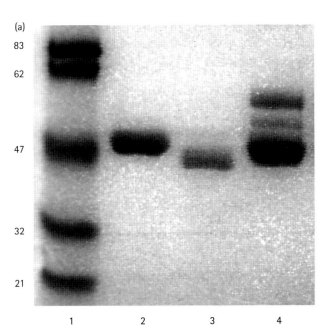

(a)

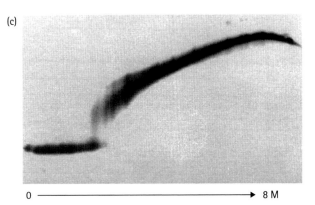

(b)

(c)

0 ————————————————————→ 8 M

**Figure 6C.4**  *Gel electrophoresis of proteins. (a) SDS-PAGE. Lane 1, Molecular mass markers; lane 2, 2 μg of α₁-antitrypsin; lane 3, 2 μg of reactive loop cleaved α₁-antitrypsin (which is lower in mass due to the loss of a small peptide); lane 4, α₁-antitrypsin-chymotrypsin complex (the lower band represents α₁-antitrypsin, the top band represents the complex, and the middle band a breakdown product of the complex).*

**Figure 6C.4**  *(continued) (b) Nondenaturing PAGE. Lane 1, 2 μg of α₁-antitrypsin; lane 2, polymers of α₁-antitrypsin (the ladder represents different size of polymers); lane 3, 2 μg of the Z mutant of α₁-antitrypsin (Glu342→Lys) which differs by only one amino acid; lane 4, polymers of Z α₁-antitrypsin. (c) Transverse urea gradient PAGE of α₁-antitrypsin. The left and right of the gel represent 0 and 8 M urea, respectively.*

different mutants of a protein and urea or transverse urea gradient (TUG) gels allow an assessment of conformational changes of some proteins.[42] The gels are usually stained by Coomassie Blue or silver to visualize the protein.

SDS-PAGE is usually carried out using a discontinuous buffer method according to the method of Laemmli.[43] In SDS-PAGE, the protein sample is mixed with SDS (usually 10 percent w/v) and boiled for 5 min leading to a denatured protein surrounded by negative charge. The protein will then run according to its charge on an acrylamide gel (6–20 percent w/v or a gradient) containing SDS. This method will not discriminate between two proteins that differ by only one or a few amino acids, but it is very useful in identifying SDS-stable complexes, as in the case of serpin–protease interactions such as $\alpha_1$-antitrypsin, antithrombin, or antichymotrypsin with their target proteases.

In the case of a nondenaturing gel, the protein is not denatured and the protein is separated on the gel on the basis of its charge and mass. Gels are usually run in basic or mildly acidic conditions, but the conditions need to be adjusted for basic proteins.[44] A difference of even one amino acid can be enough to separate two different proteins on a gel. This is the method of choice to separate polymers of proteins, thus investigating the effect of mutations on polymerization.

Transverse urea gradient gels are essentially run in the same conditions as non-denaturing gels, but consist of a polyacrylamide gel (usually around 7 percent w/v) with 0 to 8 M urea in a transverse linear gradient.[42] The shape of the stained protein and the eventual transition point will give a good indication of the protein(s) stability.

In addition to these techniques, there are methods combining immunodetection and agarose gels, such as crossed immunoelectrophoresis (CIE) or rocket electrophoresis. This last method had successfully been applied to identify mutant antithrombin with low heparin affinity.[45,46]

# ELECTRON MICROSCOPY

None of the techniques described above allow a direct view of the structure of a protein or the association of proteins. X-ray crystallography and electron microscopy are two techniques allowing such a structural view of the protein. X-ray crystallography is described in another chapter. The three-dimensional study of macromolecular assembly by transmission electron microscopy (TEM), in particular, has proven an important tool in understanding the process of protein aggregation and polymerization.[47,48] Electron microscopes use a beam of highly energetic electrons to examine objects on a very fine scale. In recent years, the use of electron microscopy had greatly improve our knowledge of conformational diseases, such as Alzheimer's disease,[49,50] Parkinson's disease,[50,51] diabetes type II,[52,53] and

of some complex multimeric enzyme inhibitors such as $\alpha_2$-macroglobulin.[54]

# REFERENCES

1  Botstein D, Shortle D. Strategies and applications of in vitro mutagenesis. *Science* 1985; **229**: 1193–201.

2.  Sambrook J, Fritsch EF, Maniatis T (eds). *Molecular cloning: a laboratory manual*, 2nd edn. Cold Spring Harbor: Cold Spring Harbor Laboratory Press, 1989.

3  Sambrook J, Russell DW (eds). *Molecular cloning: a laboratory manual*, 3rd edn. Cold Spring Harbor: Cold Spring Harbor Laboratory Press, 2001.

4  Higuchi R, Krummel B, Saiki RK. A general method of in vitro preparation and specific mutagenesis of DNA fragments: study of protein and DNA interactions. *Nucleic Acids Res* 1988; **16**: 7351–67.

5  Ho SN, Hunt HD, Horton RM et al. Site-directed mutagenesis by overlap extension using the polymerase chain reaction. *Gene* 1989; **77**: 51–59.

6  Horton RM, Hunt HD, Ho SN et al. Engineering hybrid genes without the use of restriction enzymes: gene splicing by overlap extension. *Gene* 1989; **77**: 61–68.

7  Cadène M, Morel-Desrosiers N, Morel JP, Bieth JG. Thermodynamic investigation of the heparin-mucus proteinase inhibitor binding. *J Am Chem Soc* 1995; **117**: 7882–6.

8  Boudier C, Bieth JG. The reaction of serpins with proteinases involves important enthalpy changes. *Biochemistry* 2001; **40**: 9962–7.

9  Onda M, Tatsumi E, Takahashi N, Hirose M. Refolding process of ovalbumin from urea-denatured state. Evidence for the involvement of nonproductive side chain interactions in an early intermediate. *J Biol Chem* 1997; **272**: 3973–9.

10  Pearce MC, Rubin H, Bottomley SP. Conformational change and intermediates in the unfolding of $\alpha_1$-antichymotrypsin. *J Biol Chem* 2000; **275**: 28513–8.

11  Tew DJ, Bottomley SP. Probing the equilibrium denaturation of the serpin $\alpha_1$-antitrypsin with single tryptophan mutants; evidence for structure in the urea unfolded state. *J Mol Biol* 2001; **313**: 1161–9.

12  Prakash V, Loucheux C, Scheufele S et al. Interactions of proteins with solvent components in 8 M urea. *Arch Biochem Biophys* 1981; **210**: 455–64.

13  Pace CN. Determination and analysis of urea and guanidine hydrochloride denaturation curves. *Methods Enzymol* 1986; **131**: 266–80.

14  Creighton TE. Experimental studies of protein folding and unfolding. *Prog Biophys Mol Biol* 1978; **33**: 231–97.

15  James EL, Whisstock JC, Gore MG, Bottomley SP. Probing the unfolding pathway of $\alpha_1$-antitrypsin. *J Biol Chem* 1999; **274**: 9482–8.

16  Pace CN. The stability of globular proteins. *Crit Rev Biochem* 1975; **3**: 1–43.

17  Fersht AR. Enzyme structure and mechanism. In: Fersht AR (ed.) *Enzyme structure and mechanism*. New York: Freeman WH, 1985: 155–94.

18  Michaelis L, Menten ML. Die kinetik der invertinwirkung. *Biochem Z* 1913; **49**: 333–69.

19  Boudier C, Bieth JG. Mucus proteinase inhibitor: a fast-acting inhibitor of leucocyte elastase. *Biochim Biophys Acta* 1989; **995**: 36–41.

20  Schiessler H, Hochstrasser K, Ohlsson K. Acid-stable inhibitors of granulocyte neutral proteases in human mucous secretions: biochemistry and possible biological function. In: Havemann K, Janoff A (eds). *Neutral proteases of human polymorphonuclear leukocytes.* Baltimore: Urban and Schwarzenberg, 1978: 185–207.

21  Schechter NM, Jordan LM, James AM et al. Reaction of human chymase with reactive site variants of $\alpha_1$-antichymotrypsin. Modulation of inhibitor *versus* substrate properties. *J Biol Chem* 1993; **268**: 23626–33.

22  Duranton J, Adam C, Bieth JG. Kinetic mechanism of the inhibition of cathepsin G by $\alpha_1$-antichymotrypsin and $\alpha_1$-proteinase inhibitor. *Biochemistry* 1998; **37**: 11239–45.

23  Bieth JG. Theoretical and practical aspects of proteinase inhibition kinetics. *Methods Enzymol* 1995; **248**: 59–84.

24  Bieth JG. In vivo significance of kinetic constants of protein proteinase inhibitors. *Biochem Med* 1984; **32**: 387–97.

25  Belorgey D, Dirrig S, Amouric M et al. Inhibition of human pancreatic proteinases by mucus proteinase inhibitor, eglin C and aprotinin. *Biochem J* 1996; **313**: 555–60.

26  Cha S. Tight-binding inhibitors I. Kinetic behavior. *Biochem Pharm* 1975; **24**: 2177–85.

27  Cha S. Tight-binding inhibitors I. Kinetic behavior (erratum). *Biochem Pharm* 1976; **25**: 1561.

28  Tian WX, Tsou C-L. Determination of the rate constant of enzyme modification by measuring the substrate reaction in the presence of the modifier. *Biochemistry* 1982; **21**: 1028–32.

29  Morrison JF, Walsh CT. The behavior and significance of slow-binding enzyme inhibitors. *Adv Enzymol Related Areas Mol Biol* 1988; **61**: 201–301.

30  Scatchard G. The attraction of proteins for small molecules and ions. *Ann NY Acad Sci* 1949; **51**: 660–72.

31  Faller B, Mély Y, Gérard D, Bieth JG. Heparin-induced conformational change and activation of mucus proteinase inhibitor. *Biochemistry* 1992; **31**: 8285–90.

32  Olson ST, Björk I, Shore JD. Kinetic characterization of heparin-catalyzed and uncatalyzed inhibition of blood coagulation proteinases by antithrombin. *Methods Enzymol* 1993; **222**: 525–59.

33  Belzar KJ, Zhou A, Carrell RW et al. Helix D elongation and allosteric activation of antithrombin. *J Biol Chem* 2002; **277**: 8551–8.

34  Szedlacsek SE, Ostafe V, Serban M, Vlad MO. A re-evaluation of the kinetic equations for hyperbolic tight binding inhibition. *Biochem J* 1988; **254**: 311–2.

35  Frommherz KJ, Faller B, Bieth JG. Heparin strongly decreases the rate of inhibition of neutrophil elastase by $\alpha_1$-proteinase inhibitor. *J Biol Chem* 1991; **266**: 15356–62.

36  Malmqvist M. BIACORE: an affinity biosensor system for characterization of biomolecular interactions. *Biochem Soc Trans* 1999; **27**: 335–40.

37  Myszka DG. Kinetic, equilibrium, and thermodynamic analysis of macromolecular interactions with BIACORE. *Methods Enzymol* 2000; **323**: 325–40.

38  Nagata K, Handa H. *Real-time analysis of biomolecular interactions: applications of BIACORE.* Tokyo: Springer-Verlag, 2000.

39  Morgan K, Scobie G, Marsters P, Kalsheker NA. Mutation in an $\alpha_1$-antitrypsin enhancer results in an interleukin-6 deficient acute-phase response due to loss of cooperativity between transcription factors. *Biochim Biophys Acta* 1997; **1362**: 67–76.

40  Kaslik G, Westler WM, Graf L, Markley JL. Properties of the His57-Asp102 dyad of rat trypsin D189S in the zymogen, activated enzyme, and $\alpha_1$-proteinase inhibitor complexed forms. *Arch Biochem Biophys* 1999; **362**: 254–64.

41  Hammes BD. One-dimensional polyacrylamide gel electrophoresis. In: Hammes BD, Rickwood D (eds). *Gel electrophoresis of proteins, a practical approach.* New York: Oxford University Press, 1990: 1–147.

42  Goldenberg DP. Analysis of protein conformation by gel electrophoresis. In: Creighton TE (ed.). *Protein structure: a practical approach.* Oxford: IRL Press, 1989: 225–50.

43  Laemmli UK. Cleavage of structural proteins during the assembly of the head of bacteriophage T4. *Nature* 1970; **227**: 680–5.

44  Reisfeld RA, Lewis VJ, Williams DE. Disk electrophoresis of basic proteins and peptides on polyacrylamide gels. *Nature* 1962; **195**: 281–3.

45  Sas G, Pepper DS, Cash JD. Investigations on antithrombin III in normal plasma and serum. *Br J Haematol* 1975; **30**: 265–72.

46  Corral J, Rivera J, Martinez C et al. Detection of conformational transformation of antithrombin in blood with crossed immunoelectrophoresis: new application for a classical method. *J Lab Clin Med* 2003; **142**: 298–305.

47  Frank J. *Three-dimensional electron microscopy of macro-molecular assemblies.* San Diego: Academic Press, 1996.

48  Williams DB, Carter CB. *Transmission electron microscopy: a textbook for materials science.* New York: Plenum Press, 1996.

49  Serpell LC, Smith JM. Direct visualisation of the beta-sheet structure of synthetic Alzheimer's amyloid. *J Mol Biol* 2000; **299**: 225–31.

50  Lashuel HA, Hartley D, Petre BM et al. Neurodegenerative disease: amyloid pores from pathogenic mutations. *Nature* 2002; **418**: 291.

51  Serpell LC, Berriman J, Jakes R et al. Fiber diffraction of synthetic $\alpha$-synuclein filaments shows amyloid-like cross-beta conformation. *Proc Natl Acad Sci USA* 2000; **97**: 4897–902.

52  Anguiano M, Nowak RJ, Lansbury PT Jr. Protofibrillar islet amyloid polypeptide permeabilizes synthetic vesicles by a pore-like mechanism that may be relevant to type II diabetes. *Biochemistry* 2002; **41**: 11338–43.

53  Makin OS, Serpell LC. Structural characterisation of islet amyloid polypeptide fibrils. *J Mol Biol* 2004; **335**: 1279–88.

54  Kolodziej SJ, Wagenknecht T, Strickland DK, Stoops JK. The three-dimensional structure of the human alpha 2-macroglobulin dimer reveals its structural organization in the tetrameric native and chymotrypsin $\alpha_2$-macroglobulin complexes. *J Biol Chem* 2002; **277**: 28031–7.

# Biophysical analysis of proteins and protein–protein interactions

TIMOTHY R. DAFFORN

## INTRODUCTION

Recent advances in molecular biology and its application to medicine have led to an ever improving understanding of the genetic lesions that underlie a large number of disease states. However, knowledge of the alteration in the genetic code that is linked to the illness tells us little about how the change affects underlying molecular mechanisms that leads to phenotype. To achieve this we must understand the functions and malfunctions of the protein coded by the mutant gene. In this section the details of some of the techniques commonly used to investigate protein form and function will be discussed with respect to a number of common respiratory syndromes.

Proteins are formed of one or more polypeptide chains that are folded into a single complex three-dimensional shape. The sequence of amino acids that make up the polypeptide chain provide the 'information' that allows the topology of the protein to be determined. Hence it becomes apparent that a mutation in the gene coding for the protein that leads to a change in the peptide sequence can result in an alteration in the shape and character of the resulting protein. In many cases, these changes produce little or no change in function of the protein. This is due to the redundancy in the make up of the protein structure and protein chaperones that exist in cells. These proteins aid the folding of polypeptides in cells and it has been shown that they act as a natural 'buffer' protecting against natural variance in protein sequence. However, in some cases mutations can lead to dramatic changes in the character of the protein. These changes can be broadly classified into two classes:

1  Mutation or deletion of a residue that directly alters protein function, e.g., mutations of residues in the active site of an enzyme
2  Mutation or deletion of a residue that directly effects the ability of the protein to be folded and transported to its cellular destination.

Examples of each of these classes can be readily observed in a number of common respiratory diseases. The Pittsburgh variant of $\alpha_1$-antitrypsin has an M358R mutation in the region of the protein that interacts with proteases and leads to the production of a protein that is able to inhibit thrombin,[1] factor XIa, kallikrein, and factor XIIf[2] in preference to elastase. This leads to episodic bleeding that is exacerbated by trauma as $\alpha_1$-antitrypsin is upregulated as part of the acute phase response.[1] Alternatively, the common mutation underlying cystic fibrosis (a deletion of residue 508) leads to a protein that aggregates in the endoplasmic reticulum, thus preventing its transport from the cell. The study of the effects of these mutations requires the use of techniques that allow us to compare the structure and stability of mutant and wildtype proteins. For the sake of clarity, these techniques can be divided into three sections: (1) those that can be used to study the structure of proteins; (2) those that examine its folding; and (3) those that provide information on protein–ligand interactions.

## ASSESSMENT OF PROTEIN STRUCTURE PETURBATION BY MUTATION

As has been discussed above, the direct result of an alteration in the genetic code of an organism is a change in the amino acid sequence of the protein coded by that gene. These alterations are often structurally silent (altering the three-dimensional structure of the protein in a way that does not effect its function), but in some cases they can alter the structure and dynamics of the protein substantially. In these cases, just how that sequence alteration alters the protein architecture needs to be studied. In this section, I detail a number of biophysical and biochemical techniques that allow the overall structure of the protein and its stability to be probed.

# Circular dichroism

Circular dichroism (CD) is an optical technique that measures the interaction of chiral components of a protein (the backbone peptide bond and chiral side chains) with circularly polarized light to provide information on what structures are present in a protein. The UV CD spectra of proteins are usually divided into the 'near' and 'far' regions. The near-UV region, also termed the aromatic region, is represented by wavelengths between 250 and 300 nm and provides information on the aromatic side chains (tyrosine, phenylalanine, and tryptophan) within proteins. The far-UV region consists of wavelengths less than 250 nm and is dominated by the peptide backbone (Fig. 6D.1). The structural information available from far-UV CD measurements provides direct quantitation of the secondary structures present in the protein (α-helix, β-sheet, and random coil) and as such has the potential to distinguish between different protein structural forms. The direct assignment of protein structure by CD although useful requires care due to a number of complicating factors that can cause problems in accurate measurement of CD spectra. CD is an absorbance-based optical technique and as such relies on the Beer–Lambert law for absorption of photons.

(a)

| Secondary structure | Near UV CD feature (nm) | |
|---|---|---|
| | Minima | Maxima |
| α-helix | 222 | 193 |
| | 208 | |
| β-sheet | 216 | 195 |
| Random coil | 198 | – |

(b) Ellipticity

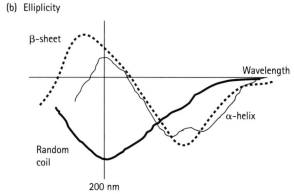

(c)

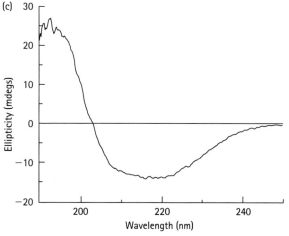

(d)

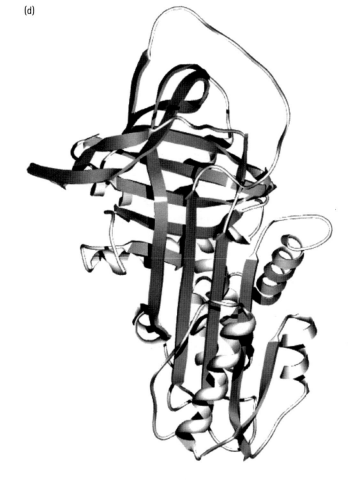

**Figure 6D.1**  *Determination of the secondary structure content of a protein using circular dichroism spectroscopy. (a) Each secondary structure element found within proteins has a particular circular dichroism spectrum with known features. (b) Examples of circular dichroism spectra of different protein secondary structure types. (c) CD spectrum of α₁-antitrypsin showing the effect of signals from each structure type combined. (d) The three-dimensional structure of α₁-antitrypsin confirms the presence of three β-sheets and nine α-helices.*

This means that the amplitude of the signal at any point in the spectra is directly related to protein concentration. Thus, in order to unequivocally assign a spectra of an unknown protein the concentration of that sample must be known to a high degree of accuracy (typically to within 2 percent). This sort of accuracy is greater than that required for the majority of other biochemical experiments and can be hard to obtain in most laboratories. If good quality data can be obtained, there are a range of different computer programs available for determining the percentage of different structural motifs from the CD spectrum of a protein. CD has also been successfully used for comparing the conformations of wildtype and mutant forms of a protein and, with good experimental technique, useful results can be obtained.

## ALTERATION OF THE PROTEIN FOLDING PATHWAY BY MUTATION

The effect of clinically relevant mutations on the stability of a protein can provide important information on both the mechanism and severity of a disease. Thus the accurate measurement of the stability of variants of a single protein becomes an important tool in molecular medicine. We will discuss the two most common methods of protein stability determination in this chapter, thermal denaturation monitored by CD and chemical denaturation monitored by intrinsic fluorescence. Other methods, such as differential scanning calorimetry, have also been employed and should certainly be considered during experimental design. In all cases, the result of such studies will be the discovery and characterization of one or more folding transitions for the protein of study. These transitions represent conditions over which a large reduction of protein structure occurs. For example, for $\alpha_1$-antitrypsin and $\alpha_1$-antichymotrypsin studies have shown two such transitions that represent the unfolding of two distinct parts of the protein.[3,4] Once the presence of these transitions has been characterized, the effect of mutations on these transitions can be analyzed. Such studies often show up mutants which have an extreme phenotype as those that have perturbed the unfolding and hence most likely the folding of the protein to the highest degree. Our own study of mutants of $\alpha_1$-antitrypsin that are implicated in deficiency showed that the stability of the mutation was directly linked to the ability of the protein to transform into the pathogenic polymeric conformation.[5]

## Thermal denaturation monitored by circular dichroism

The use of CD to directly measure the secondary structure content of a protein is not the only aspect of CD that can be useful in a laboratory. The CD signal of a protein indicates the secondary structures present and as a result acts as an excellent measure of the degree to which the protein is folded. This method has been employed in a number of systems directly related to respiratory disease, including work on the CFTR nucleotide binding domain,[6] the surfactant protein SP-A,[7,8] and $\alpha_1$-antityrpsin.[5] Thus by monitoring the CD signal of a protein a specific wavelengths (222 or 208 nm for $\alpha$-helix and 216 nm for $\beta$-sheet), while increasing the sample temperature, the thermal denaturation of the sample may be measured (Fig. 6D.2). It can be seen from Figure 6D.2 that as the temperature is increased, there is a loss of secondary structure.[5] In order to extract a numerical value for a denaturation of this kind a number of approaches can be taken. First and most simply, the temperature at which half the sample was unfolded can be measured.[7] Second, a second derivative plot of the data can be made to allow the inflexion point of the transition to be measured[5] and third, the data can be fitted to a version of the Van't Hoff equation to obtain the half point of denaturation analytically.[9]

### Chemical denaturation

One of the important driving forces in protein folding is the hydrophobic effect. This effect dictates that the hydrophobic residues of a protein sequence should ideally be buried, whereas the hydrophilic residues should be exposed. This is certainly the case that holds in the aqueous environment of the cell. However, alterations in the components of the solvent can greatly reduce this effect leading to unfolding protein. Such alterations are caused by chemicals (denaturants), such as urea and guanidinium hydrochloride. The properties of these solvents can be used to study the stability of the protein in a similar way to that demonstrated for temperature. If the structure of the protein is measured with respect to increasing concentrations of the denaturant, a

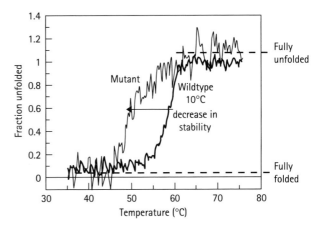

**Figure 6D.2** *An example of thermally induced unfolding of a protein as monitored by measuring its circular dichroism at 222 nm. The thick line represents the trace of a wildtype protein with a melting point of 59°C, the thin line is a mutant that is less stable by 10°C.*

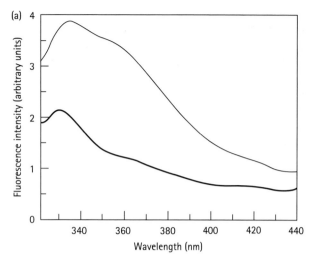

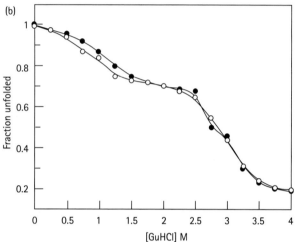

**Figure 6D.3**   *The effect of protein unfolding on intrinsic fluorescence. (a) Fluorescence emission spectra of a typical protein in the absence (thin line) and presence (thick line) of 4 M guanidinium HCl. The protein was excited with light at 290 nm ensuring that tyrosine, phenylalanine, and tryptophan residues produced fluorescence. The presence of 4 M guanidinium HCl produces a large reduction in the emitted fluorescence as the protein chain becomes more solvent exposed. (b) The unfolding of a typical protein by increasing concentration of guanidinium HCl monitored by intrinsic fluorescence (excited at 290 nm, emission detected at 340 nm). The trace shows two unfolding transitions centred on 1 and 3 M guanidinium HCl for the WT protein (filled circles). The trace for a mutant form (open circles) of the protein shows that the mutation alters the position of the first transition indicating that its presence has destabilized the structure of the protein.*

trace can be plotted that will provide information on the unfolding pathway of the protein. Such a study has been carried out on the Δ508 variant of the CFTR to investigate the effect of the mutation on the folding of the protein.[10] In this study, the structure of the protein was monitored using intrinsic fluorescence (Fig. 6D.3) (see later in the chapter); however, a range of techniques including CD

(although only urea should be used in this case as guanidinium hydrochloride absorbs light at this wavelength due to the presence of the chloride ion) can be used. In general, proteins tend to unfold between 0 and 6 M guanidinium hydrochloride or 0 and 8 M urea. An unfolding experiment is carried out by making a range of samples in which identical quantities of the protein have been dissolved in increasing concentrations of denaturant. It is important that these samples are then left to equilibrate for up to 12 h as the kinetics of unfolding can in some cases be very slow. It would be expected that the effect of the denaturant on the protein would manifest itself in a movement of the CD spectrum from a folded type trace towards that of random coil. Measurement of the same process using intrinsic fluorescence should show an overall change in both the intensity of the fluorescence and the wavelength of the maximum fluorescence signal. In general, the unfolding of the protein leads to the exposure of the residues that fluoresce to the solvent. This leads to a decrease (or quench of the fluorescence) with a resulting shift of the wavelength maximum for emission to higher wavelengths (red shift).

## ALTERATION IN PROTEIN–LIGAND INTERACTIONS BY MUTATION

Life is sustained by a complex array of interactions involving proteins: these interactions can be with small molecules, as is the case of many enzymes; nucleic acids, as with transcription factors; or other proteins, as with those involved in endocytosis. Mutations in these proteins that lead to a recognizable phenotype often alter these interactions leading to an inappropriate cellular response. It is thus important that anyone studying the effects of a genetic lesion in the clinical context should have the tools with which to dissect the protein–ligand interactions of both the wildtype and mutant forms of the protein. Discussed in this section are a range of biochemical and biophysical techniques that can be used for such an examination.

### Fluorescence

Protein–ligand interactions can be examined using a number of fluorescence-based techniques. These can be divided into two approaches: the use of fluorophores that are an intrinsic part of the protein itself and the use of artificially introduced fluorophores.

#### INTRINSIC FLUOROPHORES

Any protein that contains tryptophan, tyrosine, or phenylalanine residues has the ability to fluoresce when excited by ultraviolet light (Table 6D.1). This fluorescence contains no direct information on the secondary structure of a protein and so it cannot be used to definitively distinguish

**Table 6D.1** *The fluorescent amino acids found within proteins. The structures, excitation wavelength, and emission wavelengths of the free amino acids are shown*

| Side chain | R-group | Excitation wavelength (nm) | Emission wavelength (nm) |
|---|---|---|---|
| Phenylalanine | | 260 | 282 |
| Tyrosine | HO— | 275 | 304 |
| Tryptophan | | 295 | 353 |

between different protein types, unlike CD. However, the fluorescence of these residues is sensitive to alterations in the molecular environment that surrounds them. Thus these residues can report changes in the protein structure localized to the region around the residue. In some cases where the intrinsic fluorescence does not 'report' the binding of ligands the fluorescence of the ligand (e.g., NADH) or ligands that are modified to provide a fluorescence signal can be used. One such example is the extensive study of the nucleotide binding domain of CFTR where the fluorescent analogue of ATP, TNP-ATP has been used to measure nucleotide affinity.[6] Intrinsic fluorescence has an advantage over fluorescent ligands as they can provide information on both the strength and the position of the interaction (if the position of the fluorescent amino acids within the protein is known). For example, studies of the oligomerization of $\alpha_1$-antitrypsin have been carried out using the two tryptophans within its sequence to report the rate of formation of the polymers over time.[5]

## EXTRINSIC FLUOROPHORES

Extrinsic fluorophores have been developed with a number of properties that are not exhibited by the intrinsic fluorophores in protein. These chemicals include moieties that can be both covalently and noncovalently bound to proteins providing a plethora of options for investigations into protein–protein and protein–ligand interactions. Fluorophores that form covalent interactions with proteins do so via a limited number of well-understood chemistries to provide predictable labeling sites. For example, the iodoacetamide and maleimide conjugates of fluorophores form cysteine-specific linkages, whereas isothiocyanates and succinimidyl esters are specific for amines (e.g., the N terminus and lysine residues). The use of these sorts of chemicals combined with site-directed mutagenesis of the protein of interest allows the investigator to insert a fluorophore into any position of interest within the protein being studied. Such a study has used the red fluorophore rhodamine

derivatized with iodoacetamide to label cysteines in $\alpha_1$-antitrypsin. These cysteines had been engineered throughout the protein surface to monitor conformation changes upon oligomerization, as well as localize the monomer–monomer interaction site.[11–13] The use of extrinsic fluorophores in probing the interactions of proteins can also be extended further to provide quantitative structural information by application of a technique known as fluorescence resonance energy transfer (FRET) (Fig. 6D.4). This technique relies on the fact that if two fluorophores have complementary optical properties (the fluorescence emission spectra of one fluorophore overlaps the absorbance spectrum of a second) then when they are close in space (within angstroms) some of the energy from one fluorophore will be transferred to the second. The efficiency of this transfer can be related to the distance between the two moieties. Such a FRET experiment would involve taking two proteins which might interact with one another, and labeling them with different but complementary fluorophores. If a FRET signal is detected when the proteins are mixed then an interaction between the two proteins can be confirmed. Taking the theory of FRET further, if the efficiency of the FRET signal can be measured then a simple mathematical formula can be used to calculate the distance between the two fluorophores accurately. If this sort of information is combined with a three-dimensional structure of the two proteins, then FRET has the potential to provide information on the structure of the complex. Such a study has been carried out to examine the structure of the polymer of $\alpha_1$-antitrypsin formed as a result of the Z mutation underlying $\alpha_1$-antitrypsin deficiency.[11,13] In this study, a number of cysteines were engineered into various positions over the surface of the protein; these sites were then derivatized with fluorophores. Once the proteins had been labeled, each mutant was mixed with another and the FRET efficiency measured once they had been allowed to copolymerize. The data gained from a number of different copolymerizations were then used to triangulate the actual positions of the monomeric $\alpha_1$-antitrypsin units in the polymer.

Another common use of extrinsic fluorescence in protein chemistry involves the exploitation of the properties of a number of dyes that bind to specific chemical arrangements within proteins in a noncovalent manner. Two such dyes in common use are ANSA and Thioflavin T. ANSA is a hydrophobic dye that binds preferentially to exposed hydrophobic surfaces on proteins. In many cases these surfaces are part of binding sites, allowing the measurement of binding of a ligand by observing the perturbation of the bound ANSA induced by the presence of the ligand. Thioflavin T has been shown to specifically bind to β-sheet structures in proteins, in particular it has been used extensively to examine the formation of β-sheets during amyloidosis. Both dyes have been used in the study of the monomer–monomer association during serpin polymerization,[5] demonstrating a change in both hydrophobicity and β-sheet content as a result of polymerization.

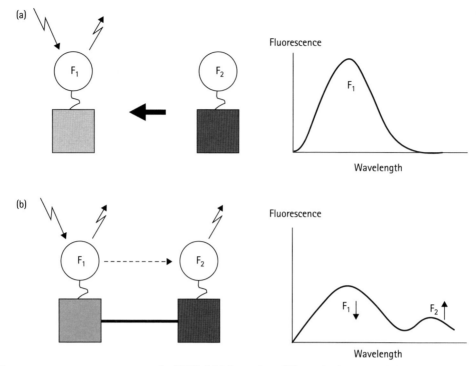

**Figure 6D.4**    *Fluorescence resonance energy transfer (FRET). (a) A fluorophore ($F_1$) attached to a protein is excited by an incident photon. The fluorophore reaches an excited electronic state that decays with the emission of a photon of lower energy (longer wavelength). An example of the fluorescence spectrum observed by the investigator is shown on the right. A second fluorophore ($F_2$) on a second protein distant from $F_1$ is unaffected by this process unless it binds to the protein carrying $F_1$ as in (b). In this case some of the energy from the excited state of $F_1$ is transferred nonradiatively to $F_2$ leading to a reduction in the observed fluorescence of $F_1$ and the appearance of fluorescence from $F_2$.*

**Table 6D.2**    *Summary of the physical characteristics and likely uses of a number of common extrinsic fluorophores*

| Name | Linkage | Emission wavelength (nm) | Emission wavelength (nm) | Usage |
|------|---------|--------------------------|--------------------------|-------|
| Tetramethylrhodamine-5-iodoacetamide dihydroiodide | Disulfide | 543 | 567 | FRET |
| 5-iodoacetamidofluorescein | Disulfide | 492 | 515 | FRET |
| Fluorescein-5-isothiocyanate | Amine | 494 | 519 | FRET |
| 1,5-IAEDANS | Disulfide | 336 | 490 | Sensitive to changes in local environment |
| 8-anilino-1-naphthalenesulfonic | Noncovalent to hydrophobic surfaces | 387 | ≈490 | Sensitive to acid (ANSA changes in hydrophobicity |
| Thioflavin T | Amyloids and β-sheet aggregates | 450 | ≈480 | Sensitive to changes in β-sheet content |

## CONCLUSION

Fully characterizing the effect of a mutation on a protein is not usually accomplished by the use of a single technique. Often the key to a truly comprehensive understanding of the perturbation is not the individual techniques used, but the careful choice of a combination of techniques that provides a 'collage' of data from which a solid hypothesis can be drawn (Table 6D.2). Flexibility and adaptability is thus the greatest strength of any researcher embarking on such a study.

## REFERENCES

1   Owen MC, Brennan SO, Lewis JH, Carrell RW. Mutations of antitrypsin to antithrombin: alpha 1-antitrypsin Pittsburgh (358 Met leads to Arg), a fatal bleeding disorder. *New Engl J Med* 1983; **309**: 694–8.

2   Scott CF, Carrell RW, Glaser CB et al. Alpha 1-antitrypsin-Pittsburgh. A potent inhibitor of human plasma factor XIa, kallikrein, and factor XIIf. *J Clin Invest* 1986; **77**: 631–4.

3   Pearce MC, Rubin H, Bottomley SP. Conformational change in intermediates in the unfolding of $\alpha_1$-antichymotrypsin. *J Biol Chem* 2000; **275**: 28513.

4   James EL, Whisstock JC, Gore MG, Bottomley SP. Probing the unfolding pathway of $\alpha_1$-antitrypsin. *J Biol Chem* 1999; **274**: 9482–8.

5   Dafforn TR, Mahadeva R, Elliott PR et al. A kinetic mechanism for the polymerization of $\alpha_1$-antitrypsin. *J Biol Chem* 1999; **274**: 9548–55.

6   Neville DCA, Rozanas CR, Tulk BM, Townsend RR, Verkman AS. Expression and characterisation of the NBD1-R domain region of CFTR: evidence for subunit–subunit interactions. *Biochemistry* 1998; **37**: 2401–9.

7   Garcia-Verdugo I, Sanchez-Barbero F, Bosch FU, Steinhilber W, Casals C. Effect of hydroxylation and N187-linked glycosylation on molecular and functional properties of recombinant human surfactant protein A. *Biochemistry* 2003; **42**: 9532–42.

8   Garcia-Verdugo I, Wang G, Floros J, Casals C. Structural analysis and lipid-binding properties of recombinant human surfactant protein A derived from one or both genes. *Biochemistry* 2002; **41**: 14041–53.

9   Lawrence DA, Olson ST, Palaniappan S, Ginsburg D. Engineering plasminogen activator inhibitor 1 mutants with increased functional stability. *Biochemistry* 1994; **33**: 3643–8.

10  Qu B-H, Thomas PJ. Alteration of the cystic fibrosis transmembrane conductance regulator folding pathway. *J Biol Chem* 1996; **271**: 7251–4.

11  Mahadeva R, Chang WSW, Dafforn TR et al. Heteropolymerization of S, I, and Z $\alpha_1$-antitrypsin and liver cirrhosis. *J Clin Invest* 1999; **103**: 999–1006.

12  Parfrey H, Mahadeva R, Ravenhill NA et al. Targeting a surface cavity of $\alpha_1$-antitrypsin to prevent conformational disease. *J Biol Chem* 2003; **278**: 33060–6.

13  Sivasothy P, Dafforn TR, Gettins PGW, Lomas DA. Pathogenic $\alpha_1$-antitrypsin polymers are formed by reactive loop-beta-sheet A linkage. *J Biol Chem* 2000; **275**: 33663–8.

# Crystallography, nuclear magnetic resonance, and modeling

ROGER B. DODD AND RANDY J. READ

## INTRODUCTION

The Human Genome Project has provided the biomedical research community with a wealth of information related to disease genetics. Increasingly, diseases are being associated with mutations within specific genes. To capitalize on this information will require the elucidation of the functions of the proteins encoded by these genes. The sequence of a protein determines the final conformation it will adopt, although the pathways through which protein folding occurs are only just beginning to be understood. In fact, the folding of proteins to their native conformations is so crucial that a set of proteins termed 'chaperones' functions to aid the folding process. The most powerful paradigm governing the study of protein function is that of the structure–function relationship – that protein function is determined by the precise three-dimensional shape of the folded polypeptide chain. Research into this relationship has given birth to a new field termed 'structural biology.'

Two techniques predominate when it comes to determining protein structures at the atomic level – X-ray crystallography and nuclear magnetic resonance (NMR). Structures determined by these methods are deposited in a publicly accessible database called the protein databank or pdb (www.rcsb.org/pdb). The number of structures being deposited is accelerating with almost 5000 structures deposited in 2003, compared to only 19 in 1980. The total number of structures stood at more than 31 000 in mid-2005, of which the majority (85 percent) were solved by crystallography and the remainder mostly by NMR. Often a protein structure will immediately suggest how a protein functions, especially when combined with prior biochemical data. In the case of the serine protease trypsin, the structure suggested an enzyme mechanism involving the conserved catalytic triad of residues (Fig. 6E.1). When a protein has unknown function, similarity of its structure to that of a previously characterized protein can imply function. The importance of classifying protein structures into related families has led to

(a)

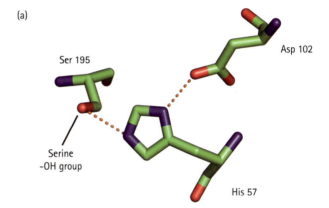

(b)

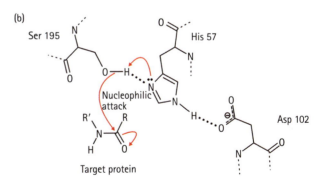

**Figure 6E.1** *(a) Spatial arrangement of the three residues of the trypsin catalytic triad and (b) the first step of the catalytic mechanism. Trypsin hydrolyzes peptide bonds in substrate proteins via a nucleophilic attack of the serine 195 hydroxyl group on the carbonyl carbon of the scissile bond. Histidine 57 is positioned by surrounding residues in an optimal orientation to accept a proton from the attacking –OH group, enhancing the nucleophilic nature of serine 195. Aspartate 102 is positioned such that it can form a very stable hydrogen bond that assists in delocalization of charge when histidine 57 becomes protonated. The enzyme can also stabilize the negative charge on the acylenzyme intermediate by interaction of the oxygen with the amide groups of serine 195 and glycine 193 (termed the oxyanion hole). (Carbon atoms, green; oxygen, red; nitrogen, blue)*

the development of databases, such as CATH and SCOP (www.biochem.ucl. ac.uk/bsm/cath/ and http://scop.mrc-lmb.cam.ac.uk/scop/ respectively). As the number of protein structures increases it becomes increasingly likely that a related protein structure will already have been solved.

When a structure exists for a protein associated with a disease-causing mutation, the mutation can be mapped onto the structure, which frequently explains at the molecular level how the mutation is deleterious to the correct functioning of the protein – for example, by reducing protein stability or disrupting an enzyme active site. A structure can also be used to direct the introduction of novel mutations at locations of interest, such as binding sites, using a process termed site-directed mutagenesis. The impact of these mutations on protein function can subsequently be dissected with biochemical assays specific to a protein's activity.

## Structure–based drug design

In addition to solving the structures of proteins in isolation, it is possible to determine the structures of protein–ligand complexes, whether with other macromolecules or with small molecules. Such structures open up a new avenue of drug development, where drugs are rationally designed to bind with high affinity to their targets. Prior to this approach, drug design relied principally on possession of large libraries of chemicals created through combinatorial chemistry and a high-throughput screening approach. Initially, structure-based drug design was applied to the optimization of previously identified candidate drug molecules in an iterative process where structure was used to direct alterations in drugs to enable tighter binding to target proteins. Advances in the rapidity of structure determination and in the development of computational tools mean that structure-based drug design is now one of the methods of choice for lead compound identification as well as for optimization. Computer docking programs are capable of conducting simulated binding experiments against large databases of small molecules and functional groups, in effect allowing virtual screening to be performed against a chemical library. The results from docking simulations can subsequently be used to build molecules with combinatorial chemistry that are likely to interact with a protein. The process of rational drug design can therefore narrow the search for drug compounds and avoid some of the expense associated with screening large libraries of chemicals.

The first drug produced using structure-based drug design was Relenza (zanamivir), which is used to treat influenza infection. Influenza virions possess two surface glycoproteins – hemagglutinin and neuraminidase. Hemagglutinin enables the entry of the virus to host cells through binding of terminal sialic acid residues from cell surface glycoproteins and glycolipids. The viral neuraminidase protein functions as an enzyme and catalyzes the cleavage of sialic acid residues from cell surface oligosaccharides, which allows the release of mature virus particles from a cell, enabling them to infect neighboring cells. In 1992, the structure of the neuraminidase catalytic head region in complex with sialic acid was determined.[1,2] This structure demonstrated that the sialic acid molecule was bound centrally within the neuraminidase molecule and all the sugar ring substituents are positioned equatorially (i.e., projecting outwards from the ring) and are recognized by a set of specific active site residues (Fig. 6E.2a). Analysis of the mode of binding and binding-site architecture led to the development of Relenza,[3,4] which is closely related in structural terms to sialic acid (Fig. 6E.2b) but binds with a significantly higher affinity and can block infectivity in vivo. The process of structure-based drug design has also been successful in the production of improved inhibitors of the HIV protease, vital in the treatment of AIDS.[5]

## X–RAY CRYSTALLOGRAPHY

In order to determine the shape of a protein at the atomic level, it is necessary to image features that are on the order of 1 Å ($10^{-10}$ M or 0.1 nm) apart – the approximate separation of two covalently bonded atoms. Usually, the shapes of small objects can be observed using a light microscope to magnify the image. However, the wavelength of visible light, which ranges from approximately 400 to 700 nm, is too long to resolve features on the scale of covalent bonds. Instead, electromagnetic radiation with a wavelength on the order of 1 Å is required: X-rays. When X-rays encounter matter they can become scattered due to interaction with the electrons surrounding atoms. This scattering – or diffraction – is much the same as occurs when visible light strikes an object, but in the case of visible light a lens can be used to refocus the diffracted light waves to form an image (Fig. 6E.3a). Unfortunately, it has not been possible to create an X-ray lens, so instead an image of the protein must be reconstructed mathematically from the information present in the diffracted X-rays (outlined in Fig. 6E.3b).

The X-rays for protein crystallography can be produced in two different ways. Each separate laboratory where crystallography is performed often has its own in-house X-ray generator, which produces X-rays through bombardment of a rotating copper target with high-energy electrons. One of the X-ray wavelengths created is termed CuKα (1.5418 Å wavelength) and is selected for use in protein crystallography. X-rays are also generated at national and international facilities termed 'synchrotrons,' where charged particles – typically electrons – are accelerated at speeds near to the speed of light. The particles are accelerated within a storage ring and emit very intense X-rays when they are forced to change direction by powerful magnets that steer the particle beam within the ring. The generation of highly intense synchrotron radiation has revolutionized protein crystallography, allowing smaller crystals to be used and often producing superior quality data. Synchrotron

(a)

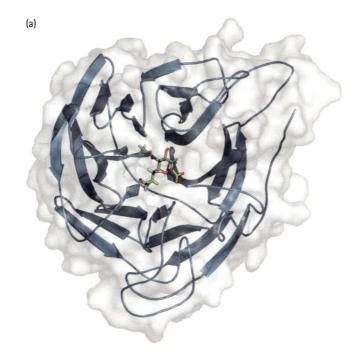

(b)

(c)

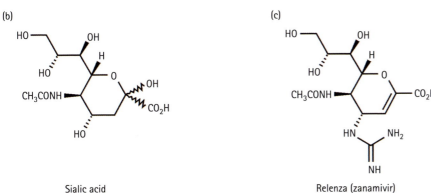

Sialic acid

Relenza (zanamivir)

**Figure 6E.2**   *(a) Structure of the complex between the influenza neuraminidase head region and the substrate molecule sialic acid. The sugar binds within the center of the approximately six-fold symmetric protein, with its groups arranged equatorially for interaction with protein side chains. This and all other structural figures were prepared using PyMOL[20] (http://pymol.sourceforge.net). (b) Molecular structure of sialic acid and Relenza. The structures of the two molecules are very similar, but certain ring substituents have been altered in the case of Relenza to increase binding affinity.*

(a)

(b)

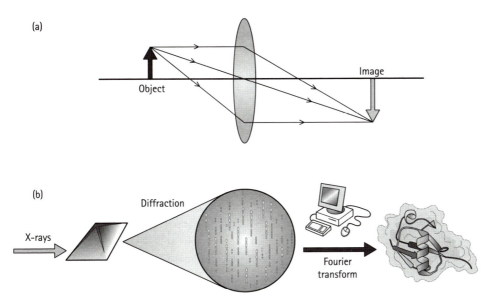

**Figure 6E.3**   *(a) Schematic of observation of an object by visible light. The light rays scattered by an object can be refocussed by a suitable lens, allowing them to be brought together again to form an image. (b) In the case of an X-ray diffraction experiment, no suitable X-ray focussing lens exists, such that the diffraction pattern itself must be collected. An image of the protein can be produced through the use of a Fourier transform applied to the diffraction data.*

technology is being constantly refined and improved to allow further advances in crystallography to be made.

X-ray diffraction of proteins cannot be studied one molecule at a time because the scattering of X-rays by a single molecule is very weak. The growth of a protein crystal results in a structure where large numbers of individual protein molecules (on the order of trillions) are arranged in the same orientation (Fig. 6E.4). The scattering from all the aligned proteins in a crystal adds up to a detectable level, such that the crystal in effect operates as an amplifier. The growth of protein crystals is probably the greatest bottleneck in the crystallographic process. In order to grow protein crystals, a very concentrated solution of highly purified protein is required. Crystallization is usually achieved through the method of vapor diffusion, where small volumes (typically 1 μL or less) of a protein solution and precipitant are mixed and equilibrated against a larger volume of the precipitant solution. Over time, the protein drop becomes supersaturated and the protein is forced from solution, in ideal circumstances forming a crystal. However, there are many variables that can affect crystallization, including whether the protein itself is folded and stable and environmental factors such as pH and temperature. Membrane proteins present a particular problem because they must be kept in solution using detergents and are often very challenging when it comes to crystallization. However, membrane proteins are frequently very important drug targets and structures of several important proteins have now been produced.

When the diffraction from a crystal is observed it is found to occur in a pattern of discrete spots determined by the geometry of the crystal lattice. These spots are observed at positions where X-ray waves scattered from the crystal meet in phase – i.e., where the peaks and troughs of the waves are aligned exactly with one another (which occurs when the path taken by the scattered waves differs by a multiple of the wavelength). At other positions, the path taken by the scattered X-rays is such that they are out of phase and cancel each other out, resulting in no spot in the diffraction pattern. The intensity of the spots is related to the distribution of the atoms within the crystal and hence to the structure of the protein. The diffraction pattern recorded from a crystal is related to the distribution of electrons within the crystallized protein via a mathematical operation known as the Fourier transform. The properties of the Fourier transform are such that it can in turn be applied computationally to the diffraction pattern to obtain a map of the electron density within the crystal. However, there is a problem in the calculation of this map – both the amplitude and the phase of the diffracted X-rays waves are

(a)

(b)

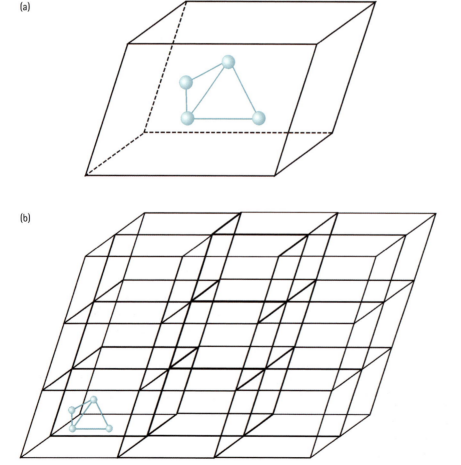

**Figure 6E.4** *(a) An object representing a protein is positioned within a unit cell. Many of these unit cells are repeated in three dimensions to produce a protein crystal (b) (molecule only shown for one unit cell for clarity). As all the unit cells contain the protein in the same orientation and are themselves arranged in a highly regular manner, all the protein molecules in the crystal are in the same orientation. The large number of orientated molecules enables a crystal to amplify the diffraction effect so that a measurable pattern results.*

required. Unfortunately, only the amplitude can be derived from the intensity of the diffraction spots (intensity is the square of the amplitude), resulting in what is termed the 'phase problem.'

The phase problem can be overcome through the application of one or more of three different methods to indirectly deduce the lost phase information:

- Isomorphous replacement: Crystals are produced that are very similar in shape to those being investigated, but with heavy atoms bound at a limited number of discrete sites. These heavy atoms have a high electron density and therefore perturb the diffraction pattern. This effect allows the positions of these few heavy atoms to be determined and initial estimates of phases to be derived.
- Multiple-wavelength anomalous dispersion (MAD): This technique is similar in some ways to isomorphous replacement, but only uses a single crystal that contains atoms termed 'anomalous scatterers.' These atoms interact differently with X-rays of differing wavelengths (which can be produced at synchrotrons) and hence their perturbation of the diffraction pattern can be altered, allowing their positions to be determined. The most popular way of performing MAD is with a sample where methionine has been replaced with seleno-methionine, because selenium has a strong anomalous signal at accessible X-ray wavelengths.
- Molecular replacement: This method relies on having a good starting model for the crystallized protein. Such a model can be obtained from a homologous protein (typically with >30 percent sequence identity) or from an example of the same protein in another crystal form. Such a model can be mathematically placed in the crystal to derive good starting estimates of the phase information.

Once phase information is obtained and an electron density map has been calculated, a model of atoms and bonds in the protein must be built (Fig. 6E.5). In the case of molecular replacement, the model for the homologous protein can be used as a starting point. In other cases a model must be built from scratch. In ideal cases with very good data, production of an initial model can be automated, but in most cases a model has to be built manually using a molecular graphics program. The first model produced generally has many errors in it and a final model is arrived at through an iterative process of model building and refinement. Refinement is an important process where the model is altered to agree better with the experimental diffraction data, while also restraining it to reasonable bond lengths and bond angles.

It is important to understand that a protein 'structure' is a model produced by human interpretation of the diffraction data and can contain errors. Therefore, it is important to validate the model to check for errors. Several methods are

(a)

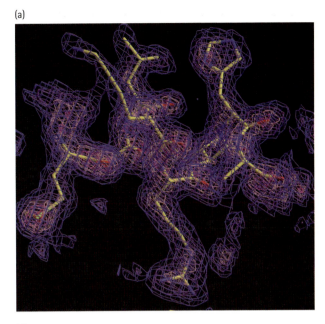

(b)

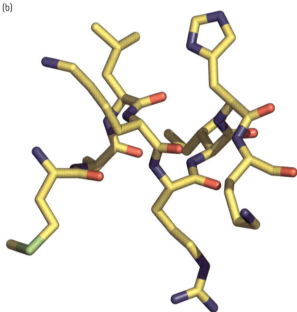

**Figure 6E.5**   *(a) Fitting of an atomic model to an electron density map (figure prepared with Xfit).[21] Here a section of an electron density map (blue, low density; pink, medium density; red, high density) is shown corresponding to an α-helix. The model of the protein in this region is shown within the density with carbon atoms colored yellow. This map is from a point near the end of refinement and the electron density corresponding to the side chains can be clearly observed. The sulfur atom of the methionine side chain (green atom, far left) has a particularly high electron density as it possesses approximately double the number of electrons to all the other atoms present. (b) A representation of the final model produced from fitting to this electron density map.*

available to do this, one of the most common being the Ramachandran plot showing the distribution of main chain torsion ($\phi$ and $\psi$) angles. Several caveats apply to the models produced by protein crystallography. First, hydrogen atoms have only a single electron and are therefore not usually seen in electron density maps. This limitation means that the side chains of certain residues may be modeled incorrectly. The packing of protein molecules into a crystal can introduce structural artefacts where the protein structure has become altered. However, protein crystals are usually highly hydrated, with a typical solvent content of 50 percent, meaning that the crystalline environment is often not vastly different from that in solution. Where examples exist of proteins being studied by both crystallography and NMR, the models produced are generally very similar suggesting that incorporation into a crystal has little effect on structure.

## Hemoglobinopathies

Since the earliest days of structural biology, one of the primary goals has been to understand the molecular pathology of inherited diseases. Within about 10 years of determining the structure of hemoglobin, Max Perutz and colleagues[6] could explain the structural basis of the phenotype of many abnormal hemoglobins. In some variant hemoglobins, oxygen affinity is altered because of changes in the environment of the binding site, while in others the cooperativity of oxygen binding is altered because of changes in the residues that mediate conformational change on oxygen binding.[6] Most strikingly, the pathology of sickle cell anemia (Glu6Val substitution in the $\beta$-chain) could be explained by the introduction of a 'sticky' hydrophobic patch on the surface, which can interact with another hydrophobic patch exposed in the deoxy state of hemoglobin to form polymers.[7]

In most cases, insights into molecular pathology can be gained from an examination of the structure(s) of the wild-type protein. Molecular graphics programs allow examination of the interactions of the amino acid residue before and, if desired, after substitution with the mutated residue. For proteins that undergo significant conformational change as part of their mechanism of action (such as hemoglobin), a proper understanding will require knowledge of the different structural states.

## $\alpha_1$-Antitrypsin

One well-studied example, relevant to respiratory genetics, is the serine protease inhibitor $\alpha_1$-antitrypsin. A number of mutations of $\alpha_1$-antitrypsin reduce its capacity to inhibit neutrophil elastase, through a reduction in either inherent activity, secretion, or stability; the consequent increase in levels of active neutrophil elastase can lead to emphysema. $\alpha_1$-Antitrypsin is a member of the serpin family of serine protease inhibitors, which share a remarkable inhibitory

mechanism. In their active form, serpins exist in a metastable state with an exposed reactive center loop that acts as bait for a target protease. On initial attack by a protease, the reactive center loop is broken, and the attacking protease is attached to the long end of the loop as an acylenzyme intermediate. The loop inserts as a strand in the central $\beta$-sheet, converting the serpin to a hyperstable state. As the loop inserts completely, the attacking serine residue of the protease is pulled out of the active site, inactivating the protease and blocking further catalysis. The steps along this pathway have been studied crystallographically. The first structure of $\alpha_1$-antitrypsin[8] showed the cleaved state where, strikingly, the residues on either side of the cleaved peptide bond end up about 70 Å apart. The structure of the active state[9] followed, showing the reactive center loop and the major $\beta$-sheet before insertion. Finally, the structure of an inhibited complex of $\alpha_1$-antitrypsin and trypsin[10] showed how the attacking protease is crushed against the body of the serpin.

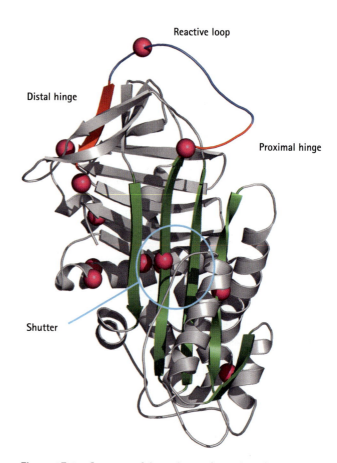

**Figure 6E.6** *Structure of the active conformation of $\alpha_1$-antitrypsin with disease causing mutations highlighted by magenta spheres. The reactive loop is colored blue and the two hinge regions that influence loop insertion kinetics in red. The central $\beta$-sheet into which the reactive loop inserts is colored green. The shutter region is circled in blue and maintains the sheet in its active conformation prior to loop insertion. Several mutations in this shutter region are pathogenic and result in the formation of antitrypsin polymers.*

The complicated mechanism of serpins makes them extremely sensitive to disruption through mutation (summarized in a review by Stein and Carrell[11]). For a serpin to inhibit a target protease, it must first bind as a substrate and undergo the first step in cleavage, the formation of the acylenzyme intermediate, but then the insertion of the reactive center loop must take place quickly, so that the protease active site is disrupted before the hydrolysis step can take place. Mutations that interfere with the kinetics of loop insertion, for instance, reduce the efficiency of inhibition when the serpin loses the race with the hydrolysis step of the protease. These mutations define so-called hinge domains.[11]

The delicate balance of the metastable active state is also easily disrupted. The central β-sheet is stabilized by the insertion of the reactive center loop, but it can also be stabilized by the addition of exogenous peptides or by the insertion of the reactive center loop from another molecule. This last mechanism leads to polymerization, a common feature of variants of $\alpha_1$-antitrypsin.[12] A cluster of mutations that lead to polymerization defines what has been termed the shutter domain,[11] which maintains the central β-sheet in its active conformation, but allows opening for strand insertion during inhibition. Mutants that readily undergo polymerization lead not only to emphysema, because of $\alpha_1$-antitrypsin deficiency, but also to liver disease, as the polymers accumulate in the cells synthesizing $\alpha_1$-antitrypsin.

Figure 6E.6 shows the structure of $\alpha_1$-antitrypsin in its active conformation, highlighting residues mutated in variant forms and indicating the hinge and shutter domains.

# NUCLEAR MAGNETIC RESONANCE SPECTROSCOPY

Nuclear magnetic resonance (NMR) is entirely different from crystallography in its route to structure determination and relies on a quantum property of nuclei termed 'spin'. The spin of a nucleus results in it behaving like a small magnet whose alignment is restricted to two possible orientations. NMR is performed by placing a protein solution in a strong magnetic field (typically on the order of 10–20 Tesla, compared with the Earth's field of 50 microTesla) and then perturbing the sample with a pulse of radiofrequency (RF) radiation. The RF pulse interacts with the nuclear spins and causes transitions between the two orientations creating a net magnetization in the sample. In many NMR experiments, the spins of the hydrogen nuclei (protons) are investigated. The measurement of the magnetization and its relaxation to equilibrium by induction in a coil surrounding the sample forms the basis for NMR. A high protein concentration – generally greater than 5 mg/mL – is required for NMR due to the very weak signal from each individual protein molecule. Each nucleus in a protein gives a unique frequency signal in an NMR

spectrum – termed its chemical shift – dependent on its local magnetic environment.

The process just described is termed 'one-dimensional NMR,' but is not directly applicable to protein structure solution because the number of signals is so great that they become overlapped and indistinguishable. In order to investigate protein structure the techniques of 2D, and in some cases even 3D and 4D NMR, must be applied. In certain cases these multidimensional methods must be applied to protein samples isotopically labeled with $^{15}N$ and $^{13}C$. These techniques rely on complex sequences of RF pulses to transfer the magnetization within a protein between nuclei connected either through bonds or through space. 2D spectra produced from these experiments consist of two frequency axes and the peaks in them demonstrate connectivities of two nuclei that have different chemical shifts. There are two basic types of 2D spectroscopy used in protein structure determination (Fig. 6E.7a):

- Correlated spectroscopy (COSY): This spectrum contains peaks that correspond to interaction between nuclei joined through up to three bonds. Variants on COSY, such as TOCSY, are able to detect coupling of nuclear spins throughout an entire amino acid side chain. Connections through peptide bonds are undetectable by COSY-related methods.
- Nuclear Overhauser effect spectroscopy (NOESY): Detects magnetization transfer between nuclei through space. The intensity of peaks on a NOESY spectrum is distant-dependent and connection through space cannot be detected at distances greater than 5 Å.

Determination of a structure using this information takes place in several stages. The first step in spectral analysis is to assign peaks within amino acid residues, which is done using COSY spectra. Different amino acids give characteristic sets of peaks in these spectra, although ambiguities can occur that are cleared up by the next stage of the process. This stage involves sequential assignment of the peaks along the protein backbone making use of the NOESY spectrum and the predetermined protein sequence. The strongest peaks in the NOESY spectrum are used, which correspond to the connections between the NH and αCH proton of a residue and the NH proton of the next residue in the sequence (Fig. 6E.7a). The majority of the strong peaks in the NOESY spectrum remaining after sequential assignment correspond to interactions between residues close to one another in the protein sequence. These peaks have characteristic patterns that are diagnostic of local secondary structure and provide important information for determination of protein structure.

Once these more local structural details have been identified, structural constraints on a more global level must be found. This is done using the remaining NOESY peaks. These arise due to nuclei in close proximity in space and

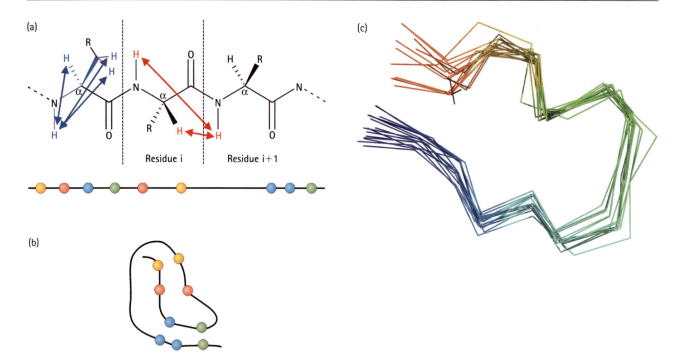

**Figure 6E.7**    *(a) Illustration of the types of information resulting from COSY and NOESY experiments. A section of polypeptide corresponding to three residues is shown. Through bond connections between protons within a single amino acid residue, as detected by COSY and related techniques, are shown for the leftmost residue in blue. Through space connectivities detected by a NOESY experiment are shown in red, identifying connections between sequential residues. Connectivities between the NH and αCH protons of residue i and the NH proton of residue I + 1 are indicated. (b) Schematic showing how NOESY-derived distance restraints can be used to derive a structural model. The horizontal line represents a polypeptide chain and similarly colored circles indicate protons NOESY has detected as being in close proximity. This information can be used to produce a model, such as the one shown, where all the distance constraints are satisfied. (c) In a real NMR experiment, a large number of distance constraints must be identified. These constraints are then used to calculate a family of structures (or conformers) that all agree with the data. A conformer family for the structure of glycoproteins G from respiratory syncytial virus is shown colored from blue at the N-terminus to red at the C-terminus. Panel (b) inspired by a figure in an NMR review by Gerhard Wider.[22]*

hence correspond to protons from residues far apart in sequence but near each other in three-dimensional space and tertiary structure. Definition of these contacts is clearly vital in determining the overall fold of the protein and the conformations of the side chains. Based on the size of the NOESY peak intensity, constraints can be placed on the distance between two specific protons (Fig. 6E.7b). Using all the constraints derived from the NOESY spectrum and constraints derived from the basic covalent geometry of proteins (such as bond lengths, bond angles, planarity of peptide bonds, and avoidance of steric clashes) a set of models is constructed computationally. Following construction of the initial models, they are refined further to minimize their energy in order to produce a family of models (referred to as conformers) that are consistent with all the data (Fig. 6E.7c).

Although NMR results in a family of models, if the data collected are sufficiently good the resulting structure can be of comparable quality to an X-ray model. Comparative studies of proteins with NMR and X-ray crystallography demonstrate that in most cases the techniques produce very similar structural models. The real limitation with

NMR spectroscopy is the ceiling on the size of protein that can be studied. Larger proteins give greater numbers of peaks in an NMR spectrum and these peaks are also wider than for smaller proteins, with the result that peaks begin to overlap and are impossible to resolve and assign correctly. Typically, NMR structure determination is limited to proteins of 30–40 kDa ($\approx$250–350 amino acids) and even in ideal circumstances with multidimensional NMR and isotopically labeled protein the absolute limit is on the order of 50 kDa. However, NMR can still be applied to individual domains from larger proteins. Despite this drawback, NMR has numerous advantages over X-ray crystallography related to its ability to detect information on dynamic processes. If $^{15}$N-labeled protein is available then NMR can be used to determine the motion of individual residues within a protein and identify regions with greater flexibility or the ability to change shape. NMR can also be used to detect binding of ligands or other proteins and to map the region of the protein involved in binding. NMR is one of the main techniques used for protein folding experiments where the pathways proteins follow to assume their final native shape are studied.

# FURTHER TECHNIQUES FOR PROBING PROTEIN STRUCTURE

## Neutron diffraction

This technique is conceptually similar to X-ray crystallography and requires the growth of a protein crystal. Neutrons are scattered by atomic nuclei, meaning that hydrogen atoms can be detected. The method has not been widely used and is limited by the requirement for a neutron reactor and large protein crystals.

## Electron microscopy

Electrons are also diffracted by matter, but unlike neutrons and X-rays they can be focussed by electromagnets, allowing the direct observation of an image. In most cases the resolution in electron microscopy (EM) is lower than X-ray crystallography, but it can be used successfully to produce low-resolution models of large protein assemblies that do not generally yield to crystallographic study. EM can be a particularly powerful technique when it is used to dock several X-ray models into a model of a larger multiprotein complex.

## Electron crystallography

Rather than directly forming an image in an electron microscope, it is possible to collect a diffraction pattern. The technique is not applicable to normal protein crystals because samples must be thin to allow electron penetration. However, some proteins – particularly membrane proteins – can form two-dimensional crystals which are amenable to the method. In ideal cases the data are of sufficient resolution to allow construction of an atomic model.

# MOLECULAR MODELING

## Comparative (homology–based) modeling

At present, molecular modeling techniques are not sufficiently powerful to predict the structure of a protein from its sequence alone, at least at the level of accuracy required to understand the consequences of a mutation. It is necessary to use the known structure of a reasonably close relative as a template, typically one sharing more than 30–40 percent identity in its amino acid sequence. In such cases, a comparative (homology-based) model can be constructed. To construct a model, possible templates are first identified by sequence comparison with proteins of known structure, the amino acid sequences are aligned, then a model is constructed by reproducing the backbone in conserved (core)

regions of the structure, replacing the side chains of nonidentical residues (using the conformations that are most commonly observed in other protein structures), and (optionally) constructing models of the less highly-conserved regions, such as surface loops with low sequence identity or regions with significant insertions or deletions.

Comparative modeling is a technique under active development in a number of groups. Progress in the field is evaluated in the CASP (critical assessment of structure prediction) exercises held every 2 years. The most recent exercise, CASP5, was held in 2002 and reported in 2003. There has been a steady but slow improvement in results over the years,[13] but even today comparative models are only accurate in regions where the template is conserved.[13,14] It can be very difficult to align the sequences correctly in regions where the level of homology is low, and local errors in sequence alignment account for much of the error in comparative models. There is still a great need for improvement of methods to predict the conformations of divergent regions, such as surface loops with insertions or deletions. The best comparative models are constructed with expert human intervention, but automated servers are catching up. In the CAFASP3 (critical assessment of fully automated structure prediction 3) exercise held in conjunction with CASP5, it was found that individual comparative modeling programs do not do as well as human predictors; however, meta-servers (which collate and analyze results from several prediction servers) can do as well as all but the very best human predictors.[15]

For the purpose of assessing the impact of a disease-associated mutation, the template structure must be conserved in sequence (and hence in structure and probably function) in the region surrounding the mutation, if a homology model is to be useful. Fortunately, it is often found that disease-associated mutations are indeed located in conserved regions of the protein. Wang and Moult[16] have looked into the question of whether it is possible to assign a structure-based mechanism by which single nucleotide polymorphisms (SNPs) cause inherited diseases. They examined missense mutations caused by SNPs in the coding region of proteins for which there was a known structure or the structure was known for a close homologue (better than 40 percent amino acid sequence identity). They found that in about 90 percent of cases, the amino acid substitution would be predicted to disrupt the structure or function of the protein. Most disease-associated mutations were predicted to affect protein stability, either by disrupting favorable interactions or by introducing strain. In other cases the mutated residues were associated with the active site (binding ligands or carrying out the chemistry) or involved in allosteric regulation. On the other hand, 70 percent of SNPs that are not definitely associated with disease were predicted to be neutral in their effects. Updated analyses for individual proteins are available at the SNPs 3D web server (www.snps3d.org). Similarly, Steward et al.[17] have shown that the effects of many disease-causing mutations can be rationalized from structure. They point out that, even when the structure is known, an examination of evolutionary sequence conservation within the family of related proteins provides valuable complementary information.

## Dynamic modeling

Some interesting mutations exert their effects by changing the dynamic properties of the protein. As discussed above, a number of mutations of hemoglobin and of $\alpha_1$-antitrypsin are believed to act by changing their dynamic behavior. Such mutations cannot be studied properly by examination of static pictures, and there is room for the application of new techniques such as molecular dynamics, in which the motion of the molecule is simulated over time. However, dynamics trajectories are extremely complicated; simpler pictures of motion and flexibility are therefore of great value. Such pictures can be obtained by methods that describe 'collective motions,'[18] i.e., large-scale motions of sets of atoms that, combined, describe most of the conformational freedom. Collective motions can be defined by analyzing molecular dynamics trajectories, to see which atomic motions are correlated (principal components analysis) or by determining from the energy function which atomic forces are correlated (normal mode analysis). One example of how this type of analysis can be used to understand the behavior of a point mutant comes from the study of a mutant (Met190Ala) of $\alpha$-lytic protease, in which the substrate specificity is broadened. A normal mode analysis suggests that this mutation changes the dynamic behavior of the active site pocket, so that movements opening the pocket are more easily allowed.[19]

## Fold recognition and secondary structure prediction

Even in the absence of an experimentally derived structure or detectable homology to a protein with a structure determined, predictions can be made about the nature of a protein's structure from its sequence alone. A method termed 'protein fold recognition' (or threading) attempts to predict structure when no homologues are identifiable. Several different methodologies are applied, but they all try to find folds that are compatible with a particular sequence. Variables used by fold recognition include the predicted secondary structure of the sequence and the preference for burying hydrophobic residues within the core of a protein. Examples of fold recognition web servers include 3D-PSSM (www.sbg.bio.ic.ac.uk/~3dpssm/) and UCLA-DOE Fold Server (http://fold.doe-mbi.ucla.edu/). In effect, fold recognition attempts to detect very remote homology using structural information. When no methods are available to successfully predict a protein's tertiary structure, it is possible to predict secondary structure. Secondary structure

prediction programs analyze multiple sequence alignments and predict whether a particular residue is most likely to adopt an $\alpha$-helical, $\beta$-sheet or random coil conformation (e.g., Jpred: www.compbio.dundee.ac.uk/~www-jpred/). Regions of a sequence that are expected to form transmembrane $\alpha$-helices can be predicted through analysis of the sequence for stretches of hydrophobic residues, as is performed by the TMHMM server (www.cbs.dtu.dk/services/TMHMM/). Many further tools for analyzing protein sequences and predicting protein structure are listed on the ExPASy proteomic tools page at www.expasy.org/tools/.

## STRUCTURAL GENOMICS

Due to the correlation between structure and function, structural genomics is a vital component of functional genomics. As discussed earlier, proteins can be organized into families of related structures. Structural genomics aims to determine the structures of one or more representative examples from each family, with the total number of representative models estimated to be approximately 10 000. The underlying principle of this approach is that these representative structures can subsequently be used in the computational modeling of other members of the same protein families, in turn allowing information about their functions to be inferred. Some sections of the structural genomics initiative are more focussed on determining all the protein structures from a particular pathogen or all structures pertaining to a disease. For example, the *Mycobacterium tuberculosis* Structural Genomic Consortium (www.doe-mbi.ucla.edu/TB/) aims to determine TB protein structures and from these learn about TB biology and develop methods of treating TB infection. The determination of such a large number of protein structures in an organized and timely manner has required the application of a high-throughput methodology, where as much of the process as possible is automated. Advances have been made in automating every stage of the process, including production and purification of proteins, protein crystallization, collection of data at synchrotrons, and the subsequent determination of protein structures from these data. Structural genomics consortia have already produced large numbers of protein structures, but the interpretation of these structures is going to require further, targeted structural and functional investigation.

## REFERENCES

1 Burmeister WP, Ruigrok RW, Cusack S. The 2.2 Å resolution crystal structure of influenza B neuraminidase and its complex with sialic acid. *Embo J* 1992; **11**: 49–56.

2 Varghese JN, McKimm-Breschkin JL, Caldwell JB, Kortt AA, Colman PM. The structure of the complex between influenza

virus neuraminidase and sialic acid, the viral receptor. *Proteins* 1992; **14**: 327–32.

3   Taylor NR, Cleasby A, Singh O et al. Dihydropyrancarboxamides related to zanamivir: a new series of inhibitors of influenza virus sialidases. 2. Crystallographic and molecular modeling study of complexes of 4-amino-4H-pyran-6-carboxamides and sialidase from influenza virus types A and B. *J Med Chem* 1998; **41**: 798–807.

4   Smith PW, Sollis SL, Howes PD et al. Dihydropyrancarboxamides related to zanamivir: a new series of inhibitors of influenza virus sialidases. 1. Discovery, synthesis, biological activity, and structure–activity relationships of 4-guanidino- and 4-amino-4H-pyran-6-carboxamides. *J Med Chem* 1998; **41**: 787–97.

5   Kempf DJ, Marsh KC, Denissen JF et al. ABT-538 is a potent inhibitor of human immunodeficiency virus protease and has high oral bioavailability in humans. *Proc Natl Acad Sci USA* 1995; **92**: 2484–8.

6   Perutz MF, Wilkinson AJ, Paoli M, Dodson GG. The stereochemical mechanism of the cooperative effects in hemoglobin revisited. *Annu Rev Biophys Biomol Struct* 1998; **27**: 1–34.

7   Finch JT, Perutz MF, Bertles JF, Dobler J. Structure of sickled erythrocytes and of sickle-cell hemoglobin fibers. *Proc Natl Acad Sci USA* 1973; **70**: 718–22.

8   Loebermann H, Tokuoka R, Deisenhofer J, Huber R. Human alpha 1-proteinase inhibitor. Crystal structure analysis of two crystal modifications, molecular model and preliminary analysis of the implications for function. *J Mol Biol* 1984; **177**: 531–57.

9   Elliott PR, Lomas DA, Carrell RW, Abrahams JP. Inhibitory conformation of the reactive loop of alpha 1-antitrypsin. *Nat Struct Biol* 1996; **3**: 676–81.

10  Huntington JA, Read RJ, Carrell RW. Structure of a serpin-protease complex shows inhibition by deformation. *Nature* 2000; **407**: 923–6.

11  Stein PE, Carrell RW. What do dysfunctional serpins tell us about molecular mobility and disease? *Nat Struct Biol* 1995; **2**: 96–113.

12  Lomas DA, Evans DL, Finch JT, Carrell RW. The mechanism of Z alpha 1-antitrypsin accumulation in the liver. *Nature* 1992; **357**: 605–7.

13  Venclovas C, Zemla A, Fidelis K, Moult J. Assessment of progress over the CASP experiments. *Proteins* 2003; **53** (Suppl. 6): 585–95.

14  Tramontano A, Morea V. Assessment of homology-based predictions in CASP5. *Proteins* 2003; **53** (Suppl. 6): 352–68.

15  Fischer D, Rychlewski L, Dunbrack RL Jr, Ortiz AR, Elofsson A. CAFASP3: the third critical assessment of fully automated structure prediction methods. *Proteins* 2003; **53** (Suppl. 6): 503–16.

16  Wang Z, Moult J. SNPs, protein structure, and disease. *Hum Mutat* 2001; **17**: 263–70.

17  Steward RE, MacArthur MW, Laskowski RA, Thornton JM. Molecular basis of inherited diseases: a structural perspective. *Trends Genet* 2003; **19**: 505–13.

18  Berendsen HJ, Hayward S. Collective protein dynamics in relation to function. *Curr Opin Struct Biol* 2000; **10**: 165–9.

19  Miller DW, Agard DA. Enzyme specificity under dynamic control: a normal mode analysis of alpha-lytic protease. *J Mol Biol* 1999; **286**: 267–78.

20  DeLano WL. *The PyMOL user's manual.* San Carlos, CA: DeLano Scientific, 2002.

21  McRee DE. XtalView/Xfit – A versatile program for manipulating atomic coordinates and electron density. *J Struct Biol* 1999; **125**: 156–65.

22  Wider G. Structure determination of biological macromolecules in solution using nuclear magnetic resonance spectroscopy. *Biotechniques* 2000; **29**: 1278–82, 1284–90, 1292.

# Functional analysis of mutant proteins in cells

PAUL D. UPTON AND NICHOLAS W. MORRELL

## INTRODUCTION

The preceding sections have dealt with the biochemical and biophysical characterization of a gene product thought to be involved in a particular disease process. These approaches may provide valuable insight into disease pathogenesis. However, frequently, the effect of a mutation in a gene can only be determined by study of the gene product in its cellular context. This may be because the gene is only expressed in certain organs or tissues. Alternatively, the nature of any defect in protein function may only be appreciated when the protein is expressed in cells. For example, mutations in the ligand binding domain of the bone morphogenetic protein type II receptor (BMPR-II), which underlie many cases of familial primary pulmonary hypertension,[1] would be predicted on the basis of modeling and biochemical studies to lead to reduced ligand binding at the cell surface. In fact, transfection studies in relevant cells have shown that trafficking of these mutants is held up within the endoplasmic reticulum and mutant receptors never attain the cell surface.[2]

## TECHNIQUES FOR EXPRESSING PROTEINS IN CELLS

Characterization of mutant protein function in a cellular context is usually tackled using transfection-based approaches in which the DNA encoding the protein of interest is introduced into a cell, where it will be transcribed and translated. Some cell types are more easily transfected than others. In general, immortalized cell lines are easier to transfect than primary cultured cells. Various strategies are available to encourage cells to take up plasmid DNA containing the construct of interest. For example, lipid-based transfection reagents rely on the ability of lipids to fuse with the cell membrane releasing their contents into the cell. Electroporation causes pores to open up in the cell membrane though which plasmid DNA then enters. Often it is a matter of trial and error to decide the best technique to use in a particular

cell type. Viruses offer another approach to attain high level transfection in cells and are particularly useful to increase the efficiency of protein expression in primary cultured cells. Adenoviral vectors are the most commonly used, but tend to transfect only dividing cells for a relatively short period of time (days) and can induce an inflammatory response in the transfected cell which may influence the results. The use of lentivirus offers advantages, since it is a retrovirus that leads to incorporation of the gene of interest into the cell's genome, leading to long-term expression (weeks). In addition, lentivirus produces less of an inflammatory response and can be used to transfect nondividing cells.[3]

Another novel method used to introduce proteins into cells difficult to transfect with other methods (e.g., neutrophils) is the use of cell-permeable peptides, for example HIV-TAT protein, linked to the protein of interest.[4]

Once the gene of interest is introduced into the cell it is vital to confirm that the protein is being expressed at the appropriate site, for example in the case of a receptor, at the cell surface. This is conveniently achieved by including a coding sequence for a small readily identified label or tag in the expression vector, which becomes attached to the translated protein. Commonly used tags are hemaglutinin (HA), c-myc, or histidine (HIS). Tags, and hence the protein of interest, can then be detected by immunohistochemistry using antibodies directed against the tag. This overcomes the problem of distinguishing between naturally occurring protein and the protein introduced in the transfected cells. In addition, by using different tags on different proteins, two or more proteins can be transfected and their location identified independently.

## MECHANISMS OF RECEPTOR SYNTHESIS AND TRAFFICKING

The mode of de novo synthesis of receptor molecules and their trafficking to the plasma membrane is achieved via an integrated process of translation and folding. As the receptor is synthesized by the membrane-bound ribosomes of the rough endoplasmic reticulum (ER), it partly translocates into the ER where it becomes embedded. All proteins that translocate to the ER possess a C-terminal signal peptide sequence, KDEL (Lys-Asp-Glu-Leu). The KDEL peptide is thought to bind a specific cytosolic signal recognition protein that mediates binding of the KDEL sequence to a specific KDEL receptor expressed only on the ER surface. The resulting complex drives translation and combines with an ER-bound protein translocator pore through which the receptor protein is embedded into the ER. Once synthesis is complete, the KDEL sequence is cleaved. During protein synthesis, structural proteins termed 'molecular chaperones' that are resident in the ER, control the folding of the receptor. Proteins demonstrated to have this role include the members of the prolyl disulfide isomerase (PDI) family[5,6] and ATP-dependent enzymes, such as BiP (GRP78, related to hsp70) and GroE proteins.[7,8] As a consequence of the dynamic folding required for large proteins, a proportion of nascent native protein will be misfolded. In addition, mutant proteins may also misfold. It is thought that chaperones bind the exposed amino acids of misfolded proteins to either (1) prevent aggregation; (2) direct the misfolded protein for export for proteosomal degradation; (3) enable the protein to fold properly; or (4) a combination of these roles.[9,10] However, it has been demonstrated that substoichiometric concentrations of PDIs or BiP may actually facilitate aggregation, an effect termed 'antichaperone activity.'[11,12] As well as controlling the dynamics of protein folding, the majority of PDIs possess a catalytic domain, which effects the oxidation of free sulfhydryl groups to form disulfide bonds and thus, cysteine bridges within or between proteins.[5] Either during and/or post-synthesis, most proteins synthesized in the rough ER are then glycosylated at specific serine/threonine residues with N-acetylglucosamine and also at the side chain -NH2 group of arginine residues (N-linked sugars) with a 14-sugar oligosaccharide.

Once the protein has been translated, folded, 'proofread', and glycosylated, some glycosyl residues are 'trimmed' from the oligosaccharide chains. The protein is then transferred via budding of ER vesicles containing protein and their transport to the Golgi apparatus. The Golgi apparatus is the site of further N-linked glycosylation, as well as the less prevalent O-linked glycosylation of the hydroxyl groups on the side chains of serine, threonine, or hydroxylysine. After stepwise processing in the Golgi network, the protein is transferred to the cell membrane by transport vesicles, which bud off the trans-Golgi network.

## RECEPTOR BINDING, INTERNALIZATION, AND CYCLING WITHIN CELLS

There is a vast array of different cell-surface receptors and modes of pharmacological and intracellular signal transduction these receptors may utilize. However, these can be summarized using a simple scheme that begins with the binding of a ligand (growth factor or peptide) to the binding site of the extracellular domain of the receptor. The receptor may already be associated with other cell-surface proteins that define its affinity for a particular ligand, examples of which are G-protein coupled receptors (GPCRs). It has recently been discovered that three receptor activity-modulating proteins (RAMPs) dictate the pharmacologies of a number of vasoactive peptide GPCRs.[13] Alternatively, ligand binding may stimulate association of the receptor with other homologous or heterologous receptors to form a signaling complex. For example, bone morphogenetic protein-4 (BMP4) binds to a type I receptor (BMPR-IA or BMP-RIB) leading to recruitment of a type II receptor (BMP-RII) to form the signaling complex. Generally, when the ligand binds, it causes a conformational change in the receptor and initiates the activity of the intracellular domain of the receptor or signaling complex to activate either stimulatory or inhibitory pathways within the cell. The majority of receptor–ligand complexes are cleared from the plasma membrane via endocytosis. This involves the accumulation of these complexes at pits on the cell surface which are associated with proteins, such as clathrin and caveolins. These bud off internally to form endocytotic vesicles which fuse into a larger body termed an 'early endosome.' The lumen of the early endosome contains the ligand and extracellular domain of the receptor and the intracellular domain of the receptor projects into the cytosol. From the endosome, the receptor will usually have two fates. The first involves loss of the ligand and subsequent recycling of the unoccupied receptor to the plasma membrane via transport vesicles which bud off the endosome. The second pathway involves the early endosome being converted to a late endosome and then a lysosome, and the receptors then being degraded. A third scenario also exists in polarized cells such as epithelial cells, where occupied receptors derived from the apical plasma membrane may be trafficked from the endosome to the basolateral plasma membrane in a process termed 'transcytosis.' This is thought to be a means of transporting ligands or soluble factors across epithelial barriers.

## ANALYSIS OF CELLULAR RECEPTOR LOCALIZATION AND TRAFFICKING

Disease-causing mutations can alter the trafficking or functionality of receptors through interfering with protein structure or altering the affinity of domains important for ligand binding, coupling to signal transduction, or association with other members of a receptor signaling complex. There are now over 45 mutations in the bone morphogenetic protein type II receptor (BMP-RII or BMPRZ) identified as disease-causing in primary pulmonary hypertension.[14] Using these as a model, we shall discuss how an array of molecular tools can be utilized to dissect the effects of different mutations on BMP-RII trafficking, binding, and signaling. In rare diseases such as primary pulmonary hypertension (PPH), studies of endogenous mutant receptors are limited by the availability of cells from patients. The construction of plasmids containing native or mutant receptors and their transfection into cultured cells provides an invaluable model for studying the effect of mutations. To enable visualization of the receptors, the constructs can be cloned into plasmids designed to attach fluorescent tags such as green fluorescent protein (GFP). These tags enable visualization of the tagged receptors in the cells by fluorescence confocal microscopy. In addition, receptors can also be tagged with other nonfluorescent markers, such as myc or hemagglutinin. Commercially available fluorescently labeled antibodies against these tags can be used to immunolabel myc-, FLAG- or HA-tagged receptors. Localization of tagged receptors can complement studies of GFP-labeled receptors, excluding the possibility that the relatively large GFP tag interferes with receptor trafficking or in cases where high levels of GFP expression may be cyotoxic. In the case of BMP-RII, this approach has highlighted the effects of different classes of mutations on receptor trafficking.[2] Native BMP-RII transfected into HeLa cells produces a GFP signal at the expected location of the plasma membrane. In contrast, introduction of disease-causing mutations, which substitute other amino acids for cysteine residues in the extracellular or transmembrane domains (C-E/T BMP-RII mutants) result in the fluorescent signal being retained intracellularly (Fig. 6F.1). Double immunostaining methods are very useful for elucidating the intracellular compartments 'trapping' the mutant receptors. In the case of BMP-RII, we have utilized red wavelength fluorescent antibodies against KDEL, which specifically label the endoplasmic reticulum. When cells transfected with GFP-tagged cysteine-mutant BMP-RII are stained for KDEL, the colocalization of mutant receptors and KDEL antibody produces a yellow wavelength fluorescent signal (Fig. 6F.1). A variety of markers for cell compartment identification are available, such as Lysotracker Red, which specifically labels lysosomes.

Radioligand binding is an invaluable tool for characterizing the pharmacology and density of receptors for a ligand at the cell surface. The ligand is labeled, usually with $^{125}$I, which is a high-energy gamma radiation emitter and thus enables even low density ligand binding sites to be characterized. Once a radioligand has been prepared and is known to bind in equilibrium, it can be used in different ways to gain information about the effects of mutations. The difference between binding of radioligand alone (total) and in the presence of a 100-fold molar excess of unlabeled ligand (nonspecific binding) is termed the specific binding. If mutations in receptors abolish ligand binding compared to mutant receptors, this implies either a failure of the mutants to traffick to the cell surface or a loss of affinity of the binding site. For example, HeLa cells demonstrate endogenous $^{125}$I-BMP4 ligand binding, and the amount of specific binding per cell is increased after transfection of wildtype BMP-RII or cytoplasmic tail mutants. In contrast, transfection of C-E/T BMP-RII mutants decreases specific binding, implying a possible 'dominant negative' effect on the native receptor complex. Cotransfection of GFP-tagged C-E/T mutants with HA-tagged native BMP-RII demonstrated that although the mutant receptor is retained in the cell, the native receptor was expressed at the cell surface. However, when the GFP-tagged C-E/T mutants are

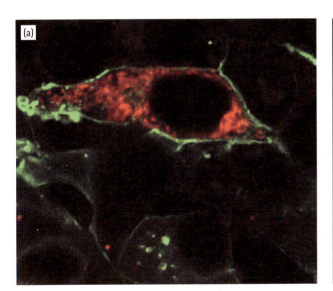
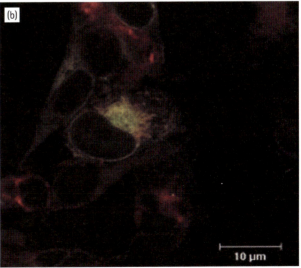

**Figure 6F.1**  *HeLa cells transfected with constructs encoding wildtype BMPR-II (a) and mutant (C118W) BMPR-II (b). The receptors have been tagged with green fluorescent protein (GFP) which appears green under the fluorescence microscope. The cells have then been counterstained with an anti-KDEL antibody which labels the endoplasmic reticulum (ER). The wildtype receptor is shown to be mainly present on the cell surface (a) with the ER stained red within the cytoplasm. The mutant receptor in (b) is held up within the ER and the colocalization of mutant receptor with ER appears as yellow staining.*

cotransfected with the HA-tagged native type I receptor (BMP-R1A), both receptors colocalize intracellularly. Adjacent cells transfected with BMP-R1A alone trafficked this receptor to the cell surface. Thus the dominant negative effect of mutant BMPR-II retained in the ER would appear to be due to coretention of the type I receptor.

Although total/nonspecific binding can be useful as a crude indicator of cell surface binding, two complementary radioligand binding methodologies can be applied to examine the pharmacology of receptors and the density of receptors at the surface of live cells, in cell membrane preparations, or using in vitro translated receptor protein. Competition binding studies involve incubation of cells/protein with a fixed low concentration of $^{125}$I-ligand in the presence of increasing concentrations of unlabeled ligand. The affinity of the binding site ($K_d$) can be estimated fairly accurately from the resulting single or multisite competition curve, and the relative affinities of related ligands ($IC_{50}$) can be determined. This method has the advantage that the amount of radioactivity required is relatively low, and the estimate of $IC_{50}$ usually reflects the true affinity of the receptor. The second method, saturation binding, requires greater quantities of $^{125}$I-ligand, but is considered to be a more accurate value for determination of the affinity of the receptor for the ligand. In addition, this method enables accurate calculation of the density of binding sites. This method involves the incubation of cells/protein with increasing concentrations of $^{125}$I-ligand in the presence/absence of at least 100-fold excess of unlabeled ligand. The nonspecific binding (NSB) values are subtracted from the total values and a hyperbolic curve should be produced. This curve can be used to calculate the density ($B_{max}$) and affinity ($K_d$) of the binding sites. The latter protocol is very useful for examining the affinity of radioligand binding of receptor protein produced by in vitro translation. By examining radioligand binding of native and C-E/T BMP-RII, we can demonstrate that the cysteine substitutions that result in failure of these mutants to traffick, have little effect on the affinity of these mutant receptors for BMP-RII. Therefore, if these mutants function properly, strategies to restore normal trafficking to the plasma membrane may restore normal cell function.

## ANALYZING LIGAND BINDING TO CELL SURFACE RECEPTORS

From the approaches discussed so far, we have examined whether mutant receptors are trafficked normally to the cell surface. For those retained in the cell, there is a possibility that they may be functional if they can be encouraged to the cell surface. For those that are expressed at the cell surface, if their affinity for radioligand binding is reduced or abolished, this may imply failure to bind or failure to form a signaling complex. However, intact binding does not preclude the latter. Two methods are useful for determining whether

the cell surface signaling complex formation is intact. For the first, BMP-RII mutants are a good example. Cells are cotransfected with myc-tagged native or mutant BMP-RII constructs and HA-tagged BMP-R1A. Protein extracts are prepared and these are either immunoprecipitated with anti-myc or anti-Ha antibodies. The immunoprecipitated proteins are then separated by SDS-PAGE and subjected to Western blotting. Probing blots of protein extracted for myc with an anti-HA primary antibody demonstrates whether BMP-R1A has coimmunoprecipitated with the myc-tagged BMP-RII receptors. Conversely, probing blots of protein extracted for HA with an anti-myc primary antibody demonstrates whether BMP-RII receptors have coimmunoprecipitated with the HA-tagged BMP-RIA. In the case of BMP-RII mutants, they all associate normally with the BMP-R1A receptor (Fig. 6F.2).

A second approach to examine this involves covalent crosslinking of the ligand to the cell-surface binding sites using reagents such as disuccinimidyl suberate (DSS). Excess ligand is then washed off and the total cell protein is separated by sodium dodecyl sulfate polyacrylamide gel electrophoresis (SDS-PAGE) and the gel dried and exposed to autoradiographic film. This protocol will produce a distinct pattern of bands corresponding to the components of the receptor complex that are in close proximity to the ligand when it binds. The relative pattern of bands in cells expressing mutant receptors will reflect whether the signaling complex is still intact. Furthermore, the protein can be immunoprecipitated with antibodies to receptors or expression tags to produce a more specific signal.

## EXAMINING RECEPTOR–MEDIATED INTRACELLULAR SIGNALING PATHWAYS

BMPRII and the other type II receptors of the TGFβ receptor superfamily contain a tyrosine kinase domain, which phosphorylates the type I receptor. The activity of this domain can be examined in vitro by incubating native or mutant BMP-RII receptors with HA-tagged BMP-RIA in the presence of $^{32}$P-ATP and immunoprecipitating the protein for HA, separating this on an SDS-PAGE, and then exposing the gel to autoradiographic film. Native BMP-RII, C-E/T BMP-RII mutants are able to phosphorylate BMP-RIA. In contrast, there is a failure of kinase domain BMP-RII mutants to phosphorylate BMP-RII and mutants involving the cytoplasmic tail also have reduced kinase activity.

Even if a mutant receptor is expressed at the cell surface, binds ligand normally, and forms an intact signaling complex, the intracellular signaling pathways coupled to receptor activation may be impaired or even enhanced. An example of the latter is increased as in the case of C and C mutants of the Ret proto-oncogene in MEN 2A. In the example of BMP-RII, both examples may occur concurrently for different pathways. A recent tool that has proven useful

| Lane | 1 | 2 | 3 | 4 | 5 | 6 | 7 | 8 | 9 |
|---|---|---|---|---|---|---|---|---|---|
| pcDNA3.0 | + | + | + | − | − | − | − | − | − |
| myc–BMPR-II | − | − | Wt | Wt | L1 | K1 | K2 | C1 | T1 |
| BMPR-IA-HA | − | + | − | + | + | + | + | + | + |

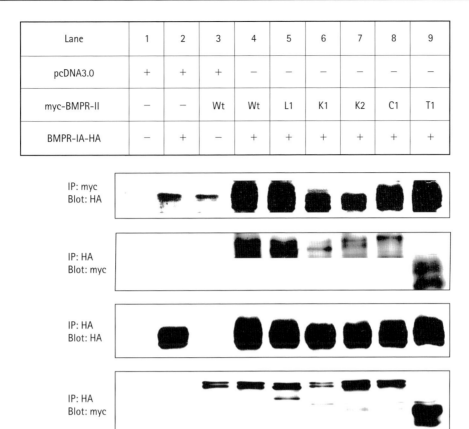

**Figure 6F.2** *Coimmunoprecipitation of myc-tagged wildtype or mutant BMPR-II with HA-tagged BMPR-IA from transfected HeLa cells. Top two panels, cell lysates were immunoprecipitated for one epitope tag followed by immunoblotting for the second epitope tag. Thus both wildtype and mutant BMPR-II are capable of forming complexes with BMPR-IA. Note that T1 is a short splice variant of BMPR-II and runs at a lower molecular weight on the gel. The bottom two panels confirm the presence of tagged BMPR-IA and BMPR-II protein by immunoprecipitation followed by immunoblotting with anti-HA and anti-myc antibodies, respectively. Wt, wildtype; L1, C118W; K1, C483R; K2, D485G; C1, N519K; T1, S532X.*

in the examination of the functional consequences of mutations in BMP-RII is the luciferase reporter gene assay. The BMP receptor complex is known to phosphorylate specific proteins, Smad2, Smad3, or Smad8. When phosphorylated, these associate with the co-Smad, Smad4 and the resulting complex translocates to the nucleus of the cell, where it can bind to specific consensus sequences in gene promoters (response elements) and modulate gene transcription. These response elements are inserted into a plasmid construct containing the gene for firefly luciferase and the construct is transfected into cells. Activation of the Smad pathway thus drives production of the luciferase enzyme in these cells and luciferase activity can then be assayed. When cells are cotransfected with native BMP-RII and the reporter construct, a luciferase response can be seen when cells are stimulated with BMP4, indicating intact signaling. BMP-RII mutants with mutations in the extracellular domain, transmembrane domain, or kinase domain all fail to drive the luciferase response when cotransfected with the reporter construct (Fig. 6F.3). In contrast, mutations in the cytoplasmic tail are still able to drive Smad signaling.[2] These

mutants are disease causing, but seem to possess normal characteristics.

Western blotting is still a key component of examining signal transduction pathways and this technique has helped in elucidating another possible effect of mutations in BMP-RII. There are now a vast number of commercially available antibodies directed against specific components of signal transduction pathways. In addition, many of these components are enzymes that are activated or inhibited by phosphorylation of specific amino acid residues in their structures, for which phosphospecific antibodies are also available. Alternatively, phosphorylation of signal transduction components can be examined by stimulating cells in the presence of $^{32}$P-ATP and immunoprecipitating for the component of interest. The gel is then blotted and the blot exposed to autoradiography film to assess the degree of phosphorylation. With respect to BMP-RII signaling, mitogen activated protein kinases (MAPKs), in particular p38 MAPK, have been implicated in signal transduction.

In summary, there is a vast array of technologies currently available which can be utilized for comprehensive studies

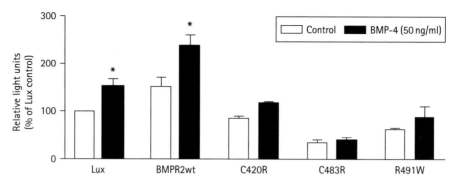

**Figure 6F.3**    *A normal mouse mammary gland epithelial cell line (NMuMG) was transfected with a reporter gene construct representing a Smad binding element fused to the luciferase gene. When BMP-4 is added to the control (Lux) cells, luciferase activity can be measured suggesting functional Smad signaling in these cells. In cells cotransfected with a wildtype BMPR-II receptor and the luciferase reporter, an enhanced luciferase signal can be seen. In contrast, cells cotransfected with mutant BMPR-II, in this case harboring mutations in the kinase domain of BMPR-II, there is a marked inhibition of BMP-4-stimulated luciferase activity. With some mutants (e.g., C483R) the baseline luciferase activity is reduced below the control, indicating a possible dominant-negative effect on Smad signaling.*

of the functional consequences of disease-causing mutations in receptors. The outcome of these investigations provides a basis for examining potential therapies. Our observation that BMP-RII mutation results in constitutive p38 MAPK activation suggests that this pathway may be a potential target for therapeutic intervention. Mutation of the cystic fibrosis conductance regulator (CFTR), a membrane chloride channel that causes cystic fibrosis, is the most studied genetic disease with respect to gene therapy. The most promising studies relating to therapeutic rescue of CFTR have employed relatively small compounds, such as sodium 4-phenylbutyrate (4PBA), that reduce the interaction of the mutant protein with endogenous chaperones that drive the receptor towards degradation.[15] Once at the cell surface, CFTR demonstrates intact functional responses[16] and some restoration of function has been shown in a pilot clinical trial of 4PBA.[17] From the perspective of BMP-RII, the C-E/T BMP-RII mutants are fully functional, but their trafficking is impaired. Therefore, a similar rescue strategy for these mutants may enable restoration of cellular responses to BMPs.

# REFERENCES

1  The International PPH Consortium. Heterozygous germ-line mutations in BMPR2, encoding a TGF-b receptor, cause familial primary pulmonary hypertension. *Nat Genet* 2000; **26**: 81–84.

2  Rudarakanchana N, Flanagan JA, Chen H et al. Functional analysis of bone morphogenetic protein type II receptor mutations underlying primary pulmonary hypertension. *Hum Mol Genet* 2002; **11**: 1517–25.

3  Lever AM. Lentiviral vectors: progress and potential. *Curr Opin Mol Ther* 2000; **2**: 488–96.

4  Joliot A, Prochiantz A. Transduction peptides: from technology to physiology. *Nature Cell Biol* 2004; **6**: 189–95.

5  Ferrari DM, Soling HD. The protein disulphide-isomerase family: unravelling a string of folds. *Biochem J* 1999; **339** (Pt 1): 1–10.

6  Gillece P, Luz JM, Lennarz WJ, de La Cruz FJ, Romisch K. Export of a cysteine-free misfolded secretory protein from the endoplasmic reticulum for degradation requires interaction with protein disulfide isomerase. *J Cell Biol* 1999; **147**: 1443–56.

7  Buchner J, Schmidt M, Fuchs M et al. GroE facilitates refolding of citrate synthase by suppressing aggregation. *Biochemistry* 1991; **30**: 1586–91.

8  Weissman JS, Kim PS. Efficient catalysis of disulphide bond rearrangements by protein disulphide isomerase. *Nature* 1993; **365**: 185–8.

9  Brodsky JL, Werner ED, Dubas ME et al. The requirement for molecular chaperones during endoplasmic reticulum-associated protein degradation demonstrates that protein export and import are mechanistically distinct. *J Biol Chem* 1999; **274**: 3453–60.

10  Fewell SW, Travers KJ, Weissman JS, Brodsky JL. The action of molecular chaperones in the early secretory pathway. *Annu Rev Genet* 2001; **35**: 149–91.

11  Giaid A, Polak JM, Gaitonde V et al. Distribution of endothelin-like immunoreactivity and mRNA in the developing and adult human lung. *Am J Respir Cell Mol Biol* 1991; **4**: 50–58.

12  Puig A, Gilbert HF. Anti-chaperone behavior of BiP during the protein disulphide isomerase-catalyzed refolding of reduced denatured lysozyme. *J Biol Chem* 1994; **269**: 25889–96.

13  Sexton PM, Albiston A, Morfis M, Tilakaratne N. Receptor activity modifying proteins. *Cell Signal* 2001; **13**: 73–83.

14  Machado RD, Pauciulo MW, Thomson JR et al. BMPR2 Haploinsufficiency as the inherited molecular mechanism for primary pulmonary hypertension. *Am J Hum Genet* 2001; **68**: 92–102.

15  Brodsky JL. Chaperoning the maturation of the cystic fibrosis transmembrane conductance regulator. *Am J Physiol Lung Cell Mol Physiol* 2001; **281**: L39–42.

16  Rubenstein RC, Zeitlin PL. A pilot clinical trial of oral sodium 4-phenylbutyrate (buphenyl) in deltaF508-homozygous cystic fibrosis patients: partial restoration of nasal epithelial CFTR function. *Am J Respir Crit Care Med* 1998; **157**: 484–90.

17  Rubenstein RC, Egan ME, Zeitlin PL. In vitro pharmacologic restoration of CFTR-mediated chloride transport with sodium 4-phenylbutyrate in cystic fibrosis epithelial cells containing delta F508-CFTR. *J Clin Invest* 1997; **100**: 2457–65.

## Key learning points

- It is important to characterize the functional consequences of mutations in order to understand their role in the pathogenesis of disease.

- Homology and in silico modeling can be used to make predictions of the effect of a mutation on the expression and function of a gene product.

- Wildtype protein and protein carrying a point mutation can be expressed using microorganisms, eukaryotic cell cultures, and even whole animals in order to purify large amounts of protein that can be characterized in vitro.

- The effect of a pathogenic mutation on the structure and function of a protein may be determined using biochemical and biophysical techniques.

- The precise effect of a mutation on the structure of a protein is best defined by crystallography or NMR spectroscopy.

- The effect of a mutation that disrupts trafficking and secretion of a protein needs to be assessed in cell models of disease.

# 7

# Genomic physiology in animals

STEVEN D. SHAPIRO AND DAWN L. DEMEO

## INTRODUCTION

### Importance of animal models to understand human (patho)biology

The human genome has now been sequenced; however, the functions of the proteins encoded by the vast majority of these genes remain a mystery. Use of animal models, particularly using transgenic and gene targeted mice, combined with genetics, functional genomics, and analytical tools such as imaging and physiology, provides a multidisciplinary approach loosely termed genomic physiology that allows one to determine protein function and dissect (patho)biological pathways in mammals in vivo.

Alternatively, one can think about genomic physiology as a means of using models to determine phenotype–genotype relationships. Following careful characterization of a phenotype, that being the structural and functional changes associated with the model, one can then determine the genes that contribute to that phenotype. This is most often done using genetic engineering (gain or loss of function models in mice). These techniques allow investigators to change single variables and perform controlled experiments in mammals and thus help determine both physiologic functions of proteins as well as dissect mechanisms of disease. One can also use classic genetics by defining the phenotype of interest, then determine phenotypic differences between genotypically distinct strains to determine the genetic basis for that phenotype.

## GENETIC ENGINEERING IN MICE

Transgenic and gene-targeted mice provide powerful techniques to determine protein function in vivo.[1–5] As mentioned above, gain of function models may be achieved by overexpression of proteins in transgenic mice, and loss of function models achieved by targeted mutagenesis or gene targeting with a null mutation, often referred to as 'knockout' mice. These gain of function and loss of function models can result in a spontaneous phenotype that suggests protein function. Alternatively, one can apply loss of function null mutant mice to specific disease models. Comparing wildtype and null mutant mice allows one to determine the contribution of the protein to the disease processes and tease out the biological pathway.

The main advantage of mice is that one can isolate and manipulate their embryonic stem cells and reintroduce them into blastocysts with retention of the capacity of the ES cell to contribute to the germline of offspring.[6] Other advantages of mice are that more is known about the mouse genome than any other animal and cDNA and antibody probes are abundant. They also offer the practical benefits of short breeding times, large litters, and relatively cheap housing. The main issue confounding the use of mice and other animals as a template for human disease is that we do not know how accurately they reflect human biology and pathology. Mouse and man clearly share many basic physiologic processes, but the details of how gas exchange is achieved will determine how closely findings in mice can be applied to man. Each animal model should be viewed as one component of the process for studying human disease and not viewed in isolation or extrapolated directly to humans.

### Generation of gene–targeted mice

#### TARGETING CONSTRUCTS

The general strategy is to first isolate isogenic genomic DNA and either insert or replace exonic DNA of the gene of interest with a selectable marker such as neomycin phosphotransferase gene driven by the phosphoglycerate kinase 1 promoter (PGK-neo).[7–14] This will cause a mutation preventing the generation of a functional protein and often results in loss of stable mRNA as well. Moreover, use of a positive selection marker will allow one to select clones that allowed integration of the construct into chromosomal DNA as described below. Thymidine kinase (TK) is often included at the 5′ and/or 3′ end as a negative selection marker to prevent nonhomologous recombination in the presence of gancyclovir. Thus, a typical construct consists of 5′ genomic DNA–PGK-neo–3′ genomic DNA–TK. One generally uses at least 6 kb of genomic DNA total for the 5′ and 3′ arms with at least 2 kb on the shorter arm.

## GENE TARGETING IN EMBRYONIC STEM CELLS

Targeting vectors are transfected into embryonic stem cells (ES cells) by electroporation.[15] ES cells are cultured in the presence of neomycin to select only colonies that incorporated the neomycin resistance gene by recombination. Gancyclovir, if used for negative selection, kills clones that have undergone nonhomologous recombination incorporating thymidine kinase. To identify clones that underwent appropriate homologous recombination, one can use polymerase chain reaction (PCR) or Southern strategies. Usually, one performs Southern hybridization, because it is difficult to perform PCR over the several kilobases that are required to assess incorporation of the mutation (PGK-neo) extending beyond the vector arms to unique sequence outside the construct. Once homologous recombination is confirmed, one often uses PCR for routine genotyping of mice. Electroporation targeting frequency is highly variable, but generally $\approx$1–25 percent of clones that grow in the presence of G418 have undergone correctly targeted homologous recombination.

## GENERATION OF GENE-TARGETED, NULL MUTANT MICE

Targeted ES clones (usually from 129/Sv mice which are agouti, i.e., yellow coat pigment) are injected into blastocysts that are most often derived from C57BL/6 females (black color) and inserted into receptive females (often Swiss–Webster). Highly chimeric male pups, that contain a significant amount of agouti ($\approx$30–80 percent), are raised and bred with C57BL/6 females. Pure agouti mice resulting from these matings demonstrate that the ES cell, which has an agouti coat pigment, has been incorporated into the germline; one-half of which should carry the mutant allele. These heterozygous mice are then bred to obtain homozygous 'knockouts,' that is, animals in which both alleles have been disrupted. One may also breed chimeras that show a tendency to 'go germline' to mice in the background of the ES cell to quickly obtain mice in a pure genetic background without laborious backcrossing.

## 'KNOCK-IN' AND CONDITIONAL/TISSUE SPECIFIC 'KNOCK-OUT' MICE

Newer techniques basically allow one to place any gene product under the gene regulatory control of another. To achieve this, one can put a cDNA in the translation start site of another. Thus, the new gene has all the regulatory sequences of the original gene (that is now disrupted). Cre-lox technology is used to remove PGK-neo to avoid transcriptional interference with the 'knocked-in' protein. This is done by placing LoxP sites around the PGK-neo sequence. Addition of Cre recombinase (either in ES cells or in mice expressing Cre) will excise LoxP and remove sequences within the two LoxP sites. Newer strategies to generate inducible and/or tissue specific 'knockouts' are possible using Cre-lox technology. This is most often achieved by placing LoxP sites within introns bracketing exonic sequence of the targeted gene, and, upon crossing these mice with those that express Cre recombinase in an inducible or tissue specific fashion, one achieves loss of function during the conditions where Cre expression has been engineered.

## Limitations of gene targeting

While the strengths of gene targeting are many, one must also recognize limitations of gene targeted mice including:[16] (1) Loss of a protein from the blastocyst stage onward might alter complex biological processes leading to what is commonly referred to as compensation; (2) due to redundancy, mutation of a gene may not unmask the true biological function of the protein it encodes; and (3) despite comments above, mice are not humans, and direct translation from mouse to human biology requires knowledge of similarities and differences between these species. One must also be aware of potential strain differences and the possibility of 'neighborhood knockout' effects, which refers to inhibition of expression of physically linked genes, related to retaining the phosphoglycerate kinase (PGK) promoter used to drive selectable markers.[4] The PGK promoter may act as a 'transcriptional sink' preventing activation of transcription of the targeted and linked genes. Removal of the PGK-neo by Cre technology eliminates this possibility.

## Generation of transgenic mice

### DNA CONSTRUCT

For protein overexpression, the gene of interest or cDNA is linked to either a strong nonspecific promoter or a cell-specific promoter for more precise targeting of gene expression.[17–22] If a cDNA is used, intronic sequence and a polyadenylation signal (often from growth hormone) is helpful to assure expression.[6,7] If the goal is to test promoter sequences required for gene regulation, promoter fragments are linked to reporter genes such as beta-galactosidase or green fluorescent protein (GFP).

## EGG MICROINJECTION

The double-stranded DNA construct is microinjected into the pronucleus of fertilized mammalian eggs to integrate the DNA into the genome and hence transfer the genetic material to offspring.[9] For this reason, DNA is introduced into the zygote as early as possible, i.e., at the pronuclear stage soon after fertilization. Females are often treated with hormones (PMS and hCG) to induce superovulation upon fertilization with a fertile male. Eggs are harvested and small amounts of DNA (1–2 picoliters at 200 ng/μL) is directly injected into eggs which are then reimplanted into pseudopregnant females (that have been mated with vasectomized males the day before). Fifteen to 20 eggs are implanted into each oviduct. Twenty days later, gestation is complete and offspring, termed founders (F0), are derived. Usually C3H and other strains are used to achieve best results, however, one can obtain mice in the C57BL/6 background, which is commonly used for many animal models.

## GENERATION OF LINES OF TRANSGENIC MICE

Litter sizes vary depending upon strains of mice used and mothering abilities. Generally, if the gene does not cause lethality, approximately 15 percent of offspring should carry the transgene DNA. Often, the DNA is inserted from one to hundreds of copies as concatemers in a single random site within the genome. If the transgene has been stably incorporated into the genome within the germ cells, then F0 mice will transmit the transgene to all future offspring. Because of the random nature of integration, several lines of transgenic mice should be bred to assure that the phenotype is integration site independent. While it is simpler to generate transgenic than gene targeted mice, it is often difficult to obtain reproducible tissue/cell-specific expression without unwanted integration-dependent effects.

## GENERATION OF INDUCIBLE AND CONDITIONAL TRANSGENIC MICE

Mice can be generated using cell-specific promoters such as Clara cell protein 10 (CC10) or surfactant protein C (SP-C), and inducible systems such as the tetracycline/doxycycline activating system.[23,24] Combining the two is frequently done, such that upon induction, the transgene is expressed in specific cells of the lung. To achieve this, one can simply co-inject the two constructs. The first construct determines cell specificity. To achieve expression in the small airways one can use the promoter of CC10, while the SP-C promoter directs expression in type II alveolar cells. The promoter is linked to the reverse tetracycline transactivator (rtTA) as well as a portion of the human growth hormone (hGH) known for reliable expression (CC10-rtTA(hGH)). The second construct utilizes a promoter driven by the tetracycline response element (active only in the presence of rtTA and tetracycline) that is linked to the gene of interest to be expressed (TetO (TRE)-gene of interest (SV40)). Since integration usually contains concatemers of DNA, both proteins should be expressed in founder mice.

Founder lines should have integration of both transgenes and inducible and/or tissue specific expression. For doxycycline inducible expression, mice are given doxycycline (200 mg/mL) daily in their drinking water and a brief time course of mRNA and protein expression is performed. Several founder lines with different lung-specific expression levels may be useful.

## Limitations of transgenic mice

One must be careful that random introduction of the gene of interest does not interfere with other gene functions, and thus, as discussed above, multiple founders are advised. For both techniques one must be cognizant of strain differences between mice and obtaining or breeding genetically engineered mice into a pure strain aids subsequent phenotype interpretation.

Distinction between transgenic overexpression and gene deletion deserves comment. If overexpression of a particular protein results in a phenotype characteristic of that in a disease process, then one may conclude that this protein is capable of causing a lesion similar to the actual disease state. If such a protein is expressed in the actual disease state, then it is likely that it contributes to the disease. A more direct approach is application of gene targeted null mutant mice to appropriate models of the disease. For example, exposure of mice to an etiologic agent such as an allergen results in a disease phenotype, here asthma. Thus, if application of mice that are identical except for the absence of an individual protein protects the mice from manifestations of allergic asthma, then one can directly infer that this protein participates in disease pathogenesis, at least in this model. This assumes that, in the absence of the particular protein in the null mutant, one has not interfered with normal lung development or function in such a way so as to preclude analysis in disease models.

## ANIMAL MODELS OF DISEASE

The ability to determine pathogenetic mechanisms of disease in mammals requires animal models that replicate the human disease. It is impossible to develop a model that perfectly mirrors human disease since mice and other animals differ from man. However, basic structure–function and response to injury are largely maintained between species. Thus, results from animal models often, but not always, predict mechanisms in humans.

With respect to specific diseases, the lung is unique in that most things that can go awry in the body can involve the lung. Thus, in addition to common primary lung diseases – such as asthma, chronic obstructive pulmonary disease

(COPD), lung cancer, pneumonia, pulmonary fibrosis, and acute lung injury – the lung is affected by manifestations of systemic diseases including cancer and infection, and collagen vascular diseases. Pulmonary edema may be cardiac in origin with increased hydrostatic pressure, or noncardiogenic due to increased vascular permeability. Severe noncardiogenic pulmonary edema, termed acute respiratory distress syndrome (ARDS), may be secondary to a variety of systemic or pulmonary insults; most commonly it is a manifestation of sepsis.

Many of these diseases can be modeled in animals. Most animal models are generated by applying relevant environmental insults resulting in a lung phenotype that replicates aspects of the human disease. Alternatively, as discussed above, genetic expression of a particular protein may also result in a disease phenotype, suggesting that this protein might be involved in the disease process. Models for specific lung diseases are discussed in each disease-related chapter. Below is a brief description of the most commonly used models – OVA-mediated allergic inflammation and bleomycin-induced lung injury/pulmonary fibrosis. This will be followed by a more comprehensive discussion of models for COPD, which will serve as an illustration of how one approaches models and interpretation.

Asthma, while often easy to diagnose, is difficult to model since we do not fully understand its etiology. Nevertheless, likely the most commonly used model in pulmonary research involves exposure of mice to allergens, most commonly ovalbumin (OVA), resulting in allergic inflammation and airway hyper-reactivity[25] (Fig. 7.1). This model is performed by first systemically sensitizing mice to an allergen which is then followed by repeated airway challenge (Fig. 7.1). In susceptible strains, this results in elevated IgE, eosinophilia, and a Th2-like response with increased levels of IL-4, IL-5, IL-13, eotaxin, and RANTES. Reversible airway obstruction is also an important feature of this model.

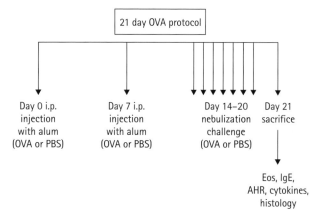

**Figure 7.1** *Murine model of allergic hyperresponsiveness. Standard ova protocol with ovalbumin sensitization at days 1 and 7 followed by airway challenge (days 14–20). This is followed by acute Th2 inflammation and airway hyperresponsiveness.*

Based on studies of gene targeted mice, more than 100 different genes have been identified that modulate experimental asthma. These genes are from multiple functional classes[26–28] including cytokines, chemokines, immunoglobulin superfamily, costimulatory molecules, adhesion receptors, enzymes, complement components, proteases, and innate immune receptors. In these studies, the deletion of each of these individual genes has been shown to decrease pulmonary inflammation, suggesting that a complex network of immune interactions in vivo mediates allergic inflammation. These observations are consistent with studies demonstrating that clinical asthma is a polygenic disease. While many of the pathways uncovered in this model likely contribute to human asthma, there have been striking differences noted between species. For example, using mouse models of asthma IL-5$-/-$ mice were protected both from acute allergic inflammation, airway hyperresponsiveness,[29] and chronic airway remodeling.[30] However, clinical trials utilizing IL-5 antagonists in both mild acute asthma[31] and chronic severe asthma[32] failed to provide a clinical benefit. Of note, the number of patients in the studies were few and there were other technical concerns as well – most notably, analysis of lung tissue following IL-5 antagonism caused less than a 50 percent depletion of tissue eosinophils.[33] Thus, the importance of IL-5 and eosinophils in asthma remains controversial, as does the utility of the murine models of asthma.[34]

Acute induction of inflammation and airway hyperresponsiveness is a useful model for investigating short-term, Th2-biased immune response within the lung. However, some of the pathologic changes that occur within the lung in chronic asthma including small airway remodeling (inflammation, goblet cell hyperplasia, and subepithelial fibrosis) do not occur in the acute model. While recurrent antigen challenge led to loss of allergic inflammation initially, it has become apparent that some strains have persistent inflammation with airway remodeling. One critical aspect of development of chronic inflammation following repeated OVA administration is the need for interrupted OVA challenge, as continuous challenge can lead to a diminished inflammatory response due to tolerance.[35] IL-13 generation seems to be required for induction of airway remodeling, perhaps through its effects on MMP expression.[36–38]

Pulmonary fibrosis is most often modeled using bleomycin as the instigating agent. Bleomycin produces lung epithelial cell death, followed by acute neutrophilic influx, subsequent chronic inflammation, and parenchymal fibrosis within 4 weeks in susceptible strains of mice.[39] In some ways, these changes mimic adult respiratory distress syndrome better than pulmonary fibrosis. However, the model does replicate some key pathologic features of human idiopathic pulmonary fibrosis (IPF), including fibroproliferation within the lung parenchyma, hence pathological mechanisms discerned in the mouse are worthy of consideration in humans. While bleomycin has been shown to be a cause of pulmonary fibrosis in humans as well, most often the clinical diagnosis of IPF is made late in the disease course only when symptoms intervene or following an incidental finding on a chest radiograph.[40] Hence, causative factors and early natural history are largely unknown, making this a difficult disease to model. This model has been used to generate novel concepts. For example, the model originally suggested the activated myofibroblast as the collagen producing cell causing pulmonary fibrosis.[41,42] However, recent use of this model combined with bone marrow replacement with tagged cells has shown that the majority of the collagen producing cells in the fibrotic lung are largely of bone marrow origin and may[43] or may not be myofibroblasts.[44]

With respect to COPD, animal models were fundamental in ushering in the elastase:antielastase hypothesis formulated over 40 years ago that remains a cornerstone of COPD pathogenesis. At that time, Gross instilled papain into experimental animals resulting in airspace enlargement that defines emphysema.[45] Subsequently, a variety of animal models have been used to further our understanding of COPD. Models include exposure of animals to molecular, chemical, and environmental agents that lead to airspace enlargement.[46] In particular, elastases,[47–52] cigarette smoke,[53,54] and more recently inducers of apoptosis, have been most informative.[55] Mouse genetic mutants have been extremely useful in exploring the pathogenesis of COPD.[16,56,57]

No single animal model recapitulates human COPD in its entirety, but several result in features associated with the disease (Fig. 7.2). An advantage of COPD as compared to many other diseases is that we know what causes it – cigarette smoke exposure. Many species of mammals have been exposed to cigarette smoke using a variety of smoking chambers. While the guinea pig is most susceptible, mice are often used because of the ability to manipulate gene expression. Mice are able to tolerate at least two cigarettes per day for a year with nontoxic carboxyhemoglobin levels, and minimal effects on body weight.[54] The mouse lung structure is not identical to humans. For example, mice have few submucosal glands, they have much less airway branching, and do no contain respiratory bronchioles – the initial site of centriacinar emphysema. However, upon exposure to cigarette smoke, mice do develop important changes similar to humans including inflammation with neutrophils, macrophages, and T cells followed by airspace enlargement

that is easily detectable in some strains at 6 months. With respect to the airway, mice lose cilia upon cigarette smoke exposure, and they develop goblet cell hypertophy.[57]

Instillation of elastases, particularly porcine pancreatic elastase (PPE),[47,48] has been a reliable means of quickly generating airspace enlargement. Not only has this established the importance of elastin in maintaining lung structure and function, but it has been most useful to test agents that have the capacity to restore lung structure such as retinoic acid.[58] It has been less helpful in determining the precise proteinases that lead to inflammation and lung destruction, however, as this model continues to be explored, it is apparent that following the initial elastolytic injury by PPE, inflammation (macrophage and neutrophil) with release of endogenous proteinases leads to further airspace enlargement over the ensuing weeks.[59] Thus, although mediators, cells, and proteinases might differ from authentic COPD, there do appear to be more similarities upstream of lung destruction, making this a more useful model than previously anticipated. Further study will determine how well it replicates COPD.

Intrapulmonary challenge with injurious proteins, chemicals, particulates, and other compounds into lungs of animals has been used to directly cause emphysema.[53,54] Administration of endotoxin results in neutrophilia and chronic administration leads to airspace enlargement. However, while a convenient model, the relevance of this type of inflammation and injury to COPD is questionable. Other environmental agents such as nitrogen dioxide and ozone cause mild lung injury. These and other factors might be modifying environmental factors, but certainly not the primary environmental factor leading to COPD. Administration of cadmium chloride,[60] a constituent of cigarette smoke, also results in primarily interstitial fibrosis with tethering open of airspaces simulating emphysema. While this mechanism differs from airspace enlargement secondary to matrix destruction that characterizes emphysema, we now appreciate that airway fibrosis is a significant factor in centrilobular emphysema seen in human smokers.

Recently, investigators have found that exposure to agents that initiate either endothelial cell death (via VEGFRII inhibition),[55] or epithelial cell death (via caspase 3 delivery),[61] lead to noninflammatory airspace enlargement. Clearly, to

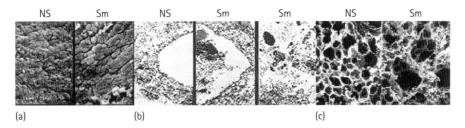

**Figure 7.2** *Changes in mouse lung following cigarette smoke exposure. (a) Scanning electron microscopy following 2 months of cigarette smoke shows decrease in ciliated epithelial cells in smoke exposed mice (Sm) as compared to non-smoke exposed mice (NS). (b) Transmission electron microscopy demonstrates obstruction in (some) small airways by inflammatory cells and debris with smoking (Sm) for 6 months as compared to NS. (c) Cigarette smoke exposure (6 months) results in airspace destruction and enlargement by SEM.*

lose an acinar unit, one must destroy both extracellular matrix (ECM) and the structural cells. Traditionally, we believed that inflammatory cell proteinases destroy ECM and cells unable to attach to the ECM float away and die. The apoptotic models suggest death of structural cells may be an initiating event, with subsequent release of matrix degrading proteinases. Whether this occurs in human COPD as a primary event is uncertain, but does raise interesting testable possibilities.

Manipulation of the mouse genome via natural genetic mutants, transgenic, and gene targeted mice, has resulted either in spontaneous airspace enlargement of developmental origin or emphysema acquired spontaneously over time (following either normal or abnormal development). Examples are too numerous to describe in detail but have been reviewed recently.[62] The important point is that overexpression or underexpression of a protein during development that leads to failed alveogenesis and enlarged airspaces is very informative regarding pathways required for normal lung development and hence repair in emphysema. However, this is very different from destruction and enlargement of normal mature alveoli that defines pulmonary emphysema. On the other hand, some gene targeted mice are not only normal but are resistant to COPD upon exposure to disease-inducing stimuli such as cigarette smoke, strongly implicating the deleted protein as playing a role in disease pathogenesis.

Emphysema acquired upon gene overexpression in adult mice (after development is complete) does lend insight into the disease process. Examples of this include transgenic inducible overexpression of IL-13[63] and IFN$\gamma$,[64] both of which surprisingly lead to inflammation and airspace enlargement. IFN$\gamma$ also has a marked element of structural cell apoptosis. Several knockouts including $\alpha_v\beta_6 -/-$[65] also develop acquired spontaneous emphysema over time. Further investigation has shown that $\alpha_v\beta_6 -/-$ mice fail to activate TGF$\beta$ which normally acts to inhibit macrophage elastase (MMP-12), suggesting a surprising role for TGF$\beta$ in maintenance of normal lung structure. The importance of MMP-12 in development of emphysema in mice had previously been demonstrated since upon exposure to cigarette smoke, MMP-12 $-/-$ mice failed to develop emphysema.[54] Whether MMP-12 is the sole enzyme in humans that causes emphysema is unlikely since, unlike mouse lung macrophages, human macrophages have more prominent expression of MMP-9 and other proteinases. These studies do confirm basic pathways of disease that can be attacked to develop therapy.

## PHENOTYPIC ANALYSIS OF MODELS

### Lung structure and biology

Careful phenotypic analysis of a model is critical both to determine its relevance to human pathobiology and to dissect

mechanisms of disease.[66] Phenotypic analysis usually begins by examination of gross lung morphology (and survey of other tissues), followed by microscopic analysis. Messenger RNA and protein expression can be studied on fixed tissue using in situ hybridization and immunohistochemistry (IHC), respectively. Alternatively, one can apply total lung tissue or isolated cells to other techniques, such as reverse transcription/real time polymerase chain reaction, to quantify mRNA levels. A variety of techniques can be used to measure protein content including Westen blots and ELISA.

Scanning and transmission electron microscopy are invaluable in providing extremely high resolution of lung structure and cellular detail. Newer noninvasive imaging techniques such as CT scans and PET scans are becoming applicable to small rodent models, further aiding in analysis of lung structure. Pulmonary function testing has been adapted to small animals allowing investigators to assess lung mechanics and volumes.

Lung morphometry is a term used to describe quantification of aspects of lung structure.[67-69] Computer-aided programs allow one to determine airspace dimensions such as the mean linear intercept, which is the average distance between alveoli, a measure of abnormal lung development and emphysema. Other common measurements include surface area, quantification of cell numbers, and vascular density.

One can more carefully assess the extracellular matrix by staining slides with Trichrome and Hart's to determine collagen and elastin content, respectively. Antibodies to individual matrix proteins allow one to identify spatial expression by IHC or quantify total protein from isolated tissue. Measurement of hydroxyproline and desmosine provide the most quantitative assessments of total lung collagen and elastin, respectively.

A variety of techniques are available to determine the cellular composition, state of activation, and health of individual cells. One is often interested in determining the effect of injury on lung cell damage and repair. A variety of techniques are available to assess apoptosis and cell proliferation. Specific cellular markers are available to determine the state of differentiation of structural cells of the lung. For example, smooth muscle actin staining is often used to identify these activated myofibroblast cells. However, as discussed above, the role of the myofibroblast in fibrosis has been questioned.

Inflammation is a hallmark of many pulmonary diseases. There are a variety of ways to assess inflammatory and immune cell types and their state of activation. One can obtain a general understanding of inflammation by hematoxylin and eosin (H&E) staining. Using fixed tissue, one can specifically stain for macrophages (mac-3, F4/80), and T cells (CD3 for total T cells – frozen sections needed for CD4, CD8 staining), and neutrophils (frozen tissue for Gr1), eosinophils (major basic protein and others), and mast cells (tryptase). Counting the number of cells per high power field gives information about total cells in a given location, for example a mid-sagittal section which is often used to reflect total lung burden. One can also perform bronchoalveolar lavage (BAL) which allows one to determine the total number of different inflammatory cells more precisely, with the caveat being that one is only counting those cells that are loose in the alveolar space. While this is often a reflection of total inflammation, it is best used in combination with examination of fixed tissue. For example, in asthma models one can observe decreases in BAL eosinophilia and conclude that the intervention inhibited eosinophils in the lung, only to find excessive eosinophil accumulations within obstructing the airways. The proper interpretation in that case is that the intervention prevented migration from tissue to airspace and actually may be detrimental not helpful. Ideally, one would like to assess total numbers of all inflammatory cells in the whole lung. One can perform tissue digestion followed by flow cytometry to achieve this goal. While potentially useful, it should be noted that the technique is cumbersome, expensive, and difficult to reproduce identical cell numbers from each isolation.

Newer techniques such as expression profiling can be applied to determine all mRNA species altered in a cell or organ in response to a stimulus.[70–75] Specific techniques are described elsewhere in this text, but in general, the strength of this methodology is to give a global view of molecular changes, allowing one to construct biochemical pathways of disease. Limitations include the fact that not all mRNAs are translated to proteins. Proteomic techniques are emerging, but at present total proteome analysis of complex tissue is beyond the capacity of the technology. Also, if one uses total lung tissue, results might be skewed merely by differing compositions of cell types between the two samples being compared. One can obtain individual cell types to study, but this can be complicated by lengthy isolation procedures altering mRNA levels, or small yield. Isolation of cells directly from tissue using laser capture microdissection is a powerful technique. Small yield (with laser capture, for instance) can be overcome by amplification of mRNA. Amplification leads to the potential problem of nonuniform amplification of different mRNAs. However, techniques are improving, making this an increasingly appealing approach.

## Lung function

Unrestrained whole body plethysmography (Buxco) is often used to indirectly measure airway resistance. The validity of this measurement to reflect airway resistance is controversial.[76] Mice are placed in individual chambers and increasing doses of nebulized methacholine (0–100 mg/mL) are introduced via an inlet. The whole-body plethysmograph measures changes in box pressure during expiration and inspiration, peak expiratory and inspiratory pressures, inspiratory and expiratory time, and a relaxation time, and generates a value called enhanced pause (Penh) which has been shown to be primarily related to ventilatory timing

and perhaps to airway resistance. The basis for this usage stems from studies that have shown changes in Penh to sometimes correlate with changes in pulmonary resistance in small experimental animals.[77–80] However, several others have shown that changes in Penh and respiratory resistance often do not correlate.[81–83] Penh measurements may be suitable as a preliminary technique, particularly when one is screening large numbers of mice or needs serial measurements. Validation using direct measurements of airway mechanics is recommended.

A direct dynamic measurement system consists of a computer-controlled volume displacement ventilator (Flexivent) that can be driven by a user-specified input signal. This technique has been applied to large[84,85] and small animals[86] including mice.[87] The signal developed to characterize murine lung impedance (i.e., the ratio of pressure to flow) is a sum of six sine waves that was designed to minimize harmonic distortion (i.e., nonlinear signal distortion) and nonlinearities (due to turbulence) associated with making measurements in the murine respiratory tract. Such a waveform is known as an optimal ventilation waveform (OVW). The OVW method provides information about the mechanical properties of the lung during conditions that mimic normal breathing, since the tidal volumes delivered, and transpulmonary pressures generated, are similar to those during normal spontaneous breathing.

Pressure, volume, and flow recordings are read into the computer from the ventilator system and using Fourier analysis one obtains an impedance function that provides information about lung resistance and elastance over the entire range of frequencies spanned by the input waveform (providing information about heterogeneity of airway narrowing/closure). Application of increasing doses of methacholine allows one to plot changes in airway resistance (Raw) as functions of the log of the methacholine dose administered. Results are expressed as the PC100%, the dose of methacholine that produces a 100 percent increase in Raw. The lower the PC100%, the greater the airway reactivity.[88] Quasistatic deflation pressure–volume data allow one to determine lung volumes and dynamic tissue elastic recoil, important measurements in emphysema.

# MOUSE GENETICS

## Investigation of quantitative trait loci

Success in mapping human disease complex traits has been, in part, due to the successful use of animal models of disease and mapping of quantitative trait loci. As reviewed below, in diseases such as asthma, replicated quantitative trait locus (QTL) associations in animal models have been demonstrated to be orthologous to regions identified through human linkage studies in some cases. It is through the intersection of QTL data in animals and human linkage studies that much progress will be achieved in understanding genetic bases of susceptibilities of humans to lung injury and disease. The publication of the mouse genome sequence (and the understanding of syntenic regions between mice and human genomes) has increased the utility of murine models for investigation of genetic contributions to complex human diseases, such as asthma or chronic obstructive pulmonary disease. Under laboratory conditions, investigation with murine models provides genetic homogeneity, environmental control, and controlled breeding. The investigation of complex traits in mice has been accelerated by the development of statistical methods and software, and bioinformatic approaches to QTL analysis using in silico gene mapping.[89]

## GENERAL ISSUES IN QTL MAPPING

Quantitative traits, whether they represent health or disease, are generally manifestations of the net effect of multiple genes with a small or moderate effect. QTL mapping is the laboratory-based approach to identify the location of the genes that may contribute to quantitative phenotypic manifestations. Successful mapping of a QTL requires that linkage is present between the QTL and genetically informative markers. Inbred mice including recombinant inbred strains, recombinant congenic strains, and consomic strains, all may be used in QTL analysis. Reviews of experimental designs can be helpful to select the best approach.[90,91] $F_1$ crosses between different strains of inbred mice are heterozygous at all loci that differ between the parental strains and share the same linkage phase; as such, all of the individuals in an inbred mouse strain are informative for linkage analysis. Environmental control limits confounding variables in these experiments, thus maximizing the effect of genetic influences on phenotypic expression.

In designing a QTL experiment, the greater the degree of discordance between phenotypes of different mouse strains, the greater the possibility of identifying QTLs of biologic importance. The power of a QTL analysis is influenced not only by the total number of mice phenotyped, but also the variance of the phenotype, the number of QTL influencing the phenotype of interest, as well as the variance related to each QTL.[92] Detection of QTLs of smaller effects generally requires larger cohorts of mice. Selective genotyping may be carried out on mice with the most extreme phenotypes. Pooling strategies for genotyping may be useful, but it may limit the power to reveal QTL of smaller effect.[93]

## GENERAL ISSUES IN STATISTICAL ANALYSIS

After phenotyping and genotyping are completed in classic QTL experiments, statistical software packages are used to identify, map, and determine the statistical significance of any QTL identified. Although an extensive review of each software program is beyond the scope of this chapter, several common publicly available programs for data analysis are listed in Table 7.1.[94] The statistical results from a QTL analysis suggest both the presence and approximate location of a gene influencing a trait of interest. The most common metric of the strength of linkage between the genetic markers tested and the QTL for the phenotype of interest is the LOD score. The LOD score is a likelihood based statistic for estimating the recombination fraction between an ungenotyped genetic susceptibility locus and tested genetic markers, and is further described in Chapter 1.

Stringent statistical criteria have been suggested for the interpretation of QTL results to minimize both type I (false positive) and type II (false negative) errors. A type I error may be the more critical of the two as finding statistical evidence for a QTL generally leads to further efforts at fine mapping a region of interest. The criteria proposed by Lander and Kruglyak for the mapping of complex traits and reporting of linkage results have been utilized in mouse QTL analysis as well as in human linkage studies, with LOD score criteria for suggestive (LOD >1.9) and significant (LOD >3.3) linkage of trait and genetic locus.[95] Although permutation tests may provide further confidence that a QTL is real and not a false positive finding, replication is the standard to strive for in complex trait genetics.

The width of the genomic region supporting linkage to a QTL depends upon the spacing of the genetic markers, the number of animals investigated, the existence of more than one gene under the QTL peak, and the distance between the genetic markers tested and the actual QTL. Once

**Table 7.1**   *Representative software available for QTL analysis*

| Name | URL |
| --- | --- |
| MAPMAKER/QTL | http://www.braod.mit.edu/genome-software |
| QTL Cartographer | http://statgen.ncsu.edu/qtlcart |
| Map Manager QT/QTX | http://www.mapmanager.org/ |
| MapQTL | http://www.kyazma.nl/ |
| PLABQTL | http://www.uni-hohenheim.de/~ipspwww/soft.html |
| MQTL | ftp://gnome.agrenv.mcgill.ca/dm/software/htm/ |
| Multimapper | http://www.rni.helsinki.fi/~mjs/ |
| Epistat | http://larklab.4biz.net/epistat.htm |

This table provides a sample of software suites available and is not an endorsement of any particular software package; website addresses current as of 11/2004 but may be subject to change.

significant linkage evidence for a QTL is identified, efforts to fine map the region are generally undertaken. The goal is to narrow the region of interest, followed by positional cloning or the selection of positional candidate genes.

## QTLS IN PULMONARY DISEASE

Multiple regions of chromosomal linkage for asthma have been described in human studies of the disease and its intermediate phenotypes,[96] with regions on 2q, 5q, 6p, 12q, and 13q being most frequently demonstrated to replicate in human asthma linkage studies. Identification of genes predisposing to asthma in humans has been slowed by issues of genetic heterogeneity, phenotypic heterogeneity, and confounding by environmental influences. Inbred mouse models of asthma have provided useful information to further hone in on the susceptibility loci suggested by human asthma linkage studies. Although the mouse does not spontaneously develop asthma, airway hyperresponsiveness can be induced by chemical and allergen challenge. Early work on mouse airway hyperresponsiveness focused on evaluation of airway pressure time index across nine inbred mouse strains; AJ and AKR/J mice demonstrated the most significant degree of hyper-responsiveness while C57BL6/J and CeH/HEJ strains demonstrated the least response to acetylcholine.[97–99] Subsequently, other approaches to identifying QTLs in asthma have been pursued using chemical airway challenge (methacholine, acetylcholine) or allergens.

Homology maps exist between mice and human genomes and syntenic regions of the human genome can be demonstrated for most QTLs described in murine models. For asthma QTLs, syntenic regions of mouse QTLs can be identified in humans (using bioinformatics tools such as that at www.ncbi.nlm.nih.gov/Homology), and these results can then be intersected with regions of human asthma linkage studies to prioritize genomic regions for fine mapping.

A summary of mouse QTLs for asthma phenotypes that intersect with human linkage studies is presented in Table 7.2. Further fine mapping in these regions is underway to identify asthma susceptibility genes.

QTL studies have been performed for modifiers of *Mycobacterium tuberculosis* infections[100,101] and cystic fibrosis.[102,103] Other groups have described QTLs for nickel-induced acute lung injury,[104,105] radiation fibrosis,[106,107] and lung tumor susceptibility loci.[108,109] QTL analysis has been used to assess strain susceptibility to ozone through in silico mapping as described below.

## IN SILICO QTL ANALYSIS

In silico methods for mapping quantitative trait loci are in their infancy but hold tremendous potential for speeding the discovery of human disease genes. Grupe and colleagues[89] utilized an in silico strategy that requires inputting phenotypic information from inbred mouse strains. This information is analyzed with the known genotypic single nucleotide polymorphism variation between inbred strains to predict chromosomal regions that may be involved in regulating the phenotype. This analysis involves a linkage prediction program which scans a murine single nucleotide polymorphism (SNP) database and, only on the basis of known inbred strain phenotypes and genotypes, predicts QTLs.[89] This tool is publicly available at http://mouse SNP.roche.com. From a rapid in silico analysis, syntenic chromosomal regions in humans can be considered for further investigation through fine mapping.

This in silico approach has been used to map QTLs for ozone-induced pulmonary injury in inbred mouse strains and will likely prove useful in further QTL studies for asthma, COPD, and other complex pulmonary diseases influenced by multiple genes. Analyses of strain differences between inbred strains of mice suggest that the response to

**Table 7.2**  *Genomic regions linked to asthma-related phenotypes in murine QTL and human linkage studies*

| Mouse QTL chromosome | Mouse strains | Mouse phenotype | LOD | Human population | Human phenotype | Human syntenic chromosome |
|---|---|---|---|---|---|---|
| 7 | (A/JxC3H/HeJ) F₁ by A/J | BHR(allergen)[114] | 1.9 | Hutterites[115] | BHR | 19q |
|  | (A/JxC3H/HeJ)F₁ by C3H/HeJ | BHR[116] | 3.8 | Chinese[117] | BHR |  |
| 10 | BALBc x BP2F₂ | BHR[118] | 3.8 | Dutch[119,120] | Total IgE | 12q |
|  |  |  |  | French[121] | Eosinophils |  |
|  |  |  |  | Japanese[122] | Asthma |  |
|  |  |  |  | Japanese[123] | Total IgE |  |
| 11 | BALBc x BP2F₂ | Eosinophils in airway[118] | 2.5 | Dutch[119,120] | IgE | 5q |
|  |  |  |  | Hutterites[115] | Asthma |  |
|  |  |  |  | Japanese[122] | Allergic asthma |  |
|  |  |  |  | Japanese[123] | IgE |  |
| 17 | BALBc x BP2F₂ | BHR[118] | 2.1 | Japanese[122] | Allergic asthma | 6p |
|  | (A/JxC3H/HeJ)F1 by C3H/HeJ | BHR[116] | 1.7 | Caucasions[124,125] | Asthma |  |
|  | C57BL/6JxA/JF1 by C56BL/6J | BHR[126] | 2.83 | Busselton[127] | Allergy phenotypes |  |
|  |  |  |  | German[128] | Allergy and asthma |  |

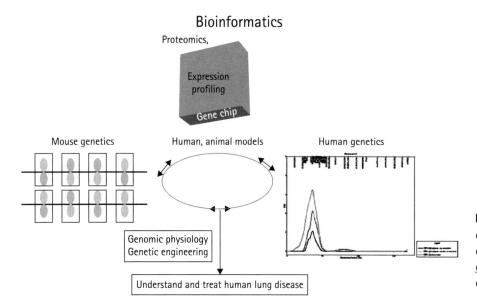

**Figure 7.3**   *Model of an integrated approach to the genetics of lung disease, which combines genetic and genomic approaches in animal models and humans.*

ozone may be genetically determined,[110] and experiments using classic techniques have identified potentially important QTLs on chromosomes 4, 11, and 17.[111,112] Using a standard model of lung injury induced by ozone, ozone-resistant (C3H/HeJ, A/J) and ozone-sensitive (C57BL/6J and 129/Svlm) strains of mice were observed. The phenotypic results for six total strains of mice were utilized for in silico mapping. This bioinformatic and computational approach suggested that chromosomes 1, 7, and 15 likely harbor loci for susceptibility to ozone.[113] As susceptibility to air pollution (for example, as measured by spirometry) is variable among humans and may be genetically determined,[129] candidate genes of ozone susceptibility identified in the mouse through traditional and in silico QTL experiments may provide an insight into the variable influences of air pollution in human populations.

In summary, the identification of genes that control complex traits in humans (QTLs) has been challenging due to locus heterogeneity, phenotypic heterogeneity, variable penetrance, and expressivity of traits, epistasis, pleiotropy, and limited statistical power. New strides in genetic and genomic resources should speed progress, and the development of congenic and consomic strains may speed the localization of QTLs to particular chromosomes and chromosomal regions. Comparative SNP maps between inbred strains will further speed progress, especially when combined with in silico and bioinformatics tools. Intersecting the results from QTL investigation in laboratory animals with human linkage for diseases such as asthma and COPD will provide important insights into the genetic susceptibility to common lung diseases.

## CONCLUSIONS

While hypotheses and mechanisms of lung function in health and disease can be addressed in the test tube and cell

culture, ultimately, these ideas need to be tested in mammals, to dissect the complex pathophysiology. Indeed, animal studies have been critical in shaping contemporary views regarding the pathogenesis of lung diseases for many years. The advent of genetic engineering, knowledge of genomic sequences in many mouse strains, and new techniques to interrogate the entire genome, combined with improved imaging of small animals, all have combined to provide unprecedented opportunity to determine the genetic and environmental influences and pathways leading to lung disease. Thus, animal models combined with genomic physiology provide a critical step in testing hypotheses and pathways determined from classical cell and molecular biology on the way toward translation to the treatment of human disease. A multidisciplinary approach, combining human genetics with genetics and genomic physiology in mice, integrated with proteomics and expression profiling, and supported by bioinformatics, provides a model for understanding and treating human disease (Fig. 7.3).

### Key learning points

- The fine art of phenotyping mouse lung structure and function is a critical component of any study utilizing murine models of disease.

- Structural and functional responses to lung stress and injury are generally maintained across species, but results from animal models may not necessarily recapitulate mechanisms of lung disease in humans.

- Genomic physiology is best used as part of a multidisciplinary approach to understand lung disease and lung biology. The integration of animal models of lung disease with insights from human genetics, proteomics, expression profiling, and bioinformatics provides a model for dissecting human lung disease pathways.

- Classical and in silico QTL analyses are complementary approaches for QTL investigation.

- The intersection of animal and human QTL analyses may speed advances in understanding the genetic basis of many human lung diseases.

# REFERENCES

1  Barinaga M. Knockout mice: Round two. *Science* 1994; **265**: 26–8.

2  Hogan B, Constantini F, Lacy E. *Manipulating the mouse embryo, a laboratory manual.* Cold Spring Harbor Laboratory, 1986.

3  Green E. (ed.) *Biology of the laboratory mouse 975.* Dover, UK: Dover Publications, 1975.

4  Whitten W, Champlin A. Pheromones, estrus, ovulation, and mating. In: Daniel J (ed.) *Methods in mammalian reproduction.* New York: Academic Press, 1978, 403–17.

5  Coussens L, Shapiro S, Soloway P, Werb Z. Models for gain-of-function and loss-of-function of MMPs: Transgenic and gene targeted mice. In: Clark IM (ed.) *Matrix metalloproteinase protocols.* Totawa, NJ: Humana Press, 149–79.

6  Paigen K. A miracle enough: the power of mice. *Nat Med* 1995; **1**: 215–20.

7  Jaenisch R, Mintz B. Simian virus 40 DNA sequences in DNA of healthy adult mice derived from preimplantation blastocysts injected with viral DNA. *Proc Natl Acad Sci USA* 1974; **71**: 1250–4.

8  Cappecchi M. High efficiency transformation by direct microinjection of DNA into cultured mammalian cells. *Cell* 1980; **22**: 479–488.

9  Brinster R, Chen H, Trumbauer M et al. Somatic expression of herpes thymidine kinase in mice following injection of a fusion gene into eggs. *Cell* 1981; **27**: 223–31.

10  Constantini F, Lacy E. Introduction of a rabbit globin gene into the mouse germline. *Nature* 1981; **294**: 92–4.

11  Bradley A. Modifying the mammalian genome by gene targeting. *Curr Opin Biotechnol* 1991; **2**: 823–9.

12  Thomas K, Deng C, Capecchi M. High-fidelity gene targeting in embryonic stem cells by using sequence replacement vectors. *Mol Cell Biol* 1992; **12**: 2919–23.

13  Hasty P, Rivera-Perez J, Bradley A. The length of homology required for gene targeting in embryonic stem cells. *Mol Cell Biol* 1991; **11**: 5586–91.

14  Hasty P, Rivera-Perez J, Chang C, Bradley A. Target frequency and integration pattern for insertion and replacement vectors in embryonic stem cells. *Mol Cell Biol* 1991; **11**: 4509–17.

15  Robertson EJ (ed.) *Teratocarcinomas and embryonic stem cells: A practical approach.* Oxford, UK: IRL Press, 1987.

16  Shapiro SD. Application of transgenic and gene-targeted mice to dissect mechanisms of lung disease. In: Stockley RA (ed.) *Molecular biology of the lung.* Switzerland: Birkhauser Press, 1998: 1–15.

17  Gordon J, Ruddle F. Integration and stable germline transmission of genes injected into mouse pronuclei. *Science* 1981; **214**: 1244–6.

18  Palmiter R, Brinster R, Hammer R et al. Dramatic growth of mice that develop from eggs microinjected with metallothione in growth hormone fusion gene. *Nature* 1982; **300**: 611–15.

19  Brinster R, Chen H, Messing A et al. Transgenic mice harboring SV40 T antigen genes develop characteristic brain tumors. *Cell* 1984; **37**: 359–65.

20  Swift G, Hammer R, MacDonald R, Brinster R. Tissue specific expression of the rat pancreatic elastase I gene in transgenic mice. *Cell* 1984; **38**: 639–46.

21  Hanahan D. Heritable formation of pancreatic beta cell tumors in transgenic mice expressing recombinant insulin/simian virus 40 oncogenes. *Nature* 1985; **315**: 115–22.

22  Chada K, Magrau J, Raphael K et al. Specific expression of a foreign globin gene in erythroid cells of transgenic mice. *Nature* 1984; **314**: 377–80.

23  Perl A, Tichelaar J, Whitsett J. Conditional gene expression in the respiratory epithelium of the mouse. *Transgenic Res* 2002; **11**: 21–9.

24  Whitsett J, Glasser S, Tichelaar J et al. Transgenic models for study of lung morphogenesis and repair: Parker B. Francis lecture. *Chest* 2001; **120**: 27S–30S.

25  Kung T, Jones H, Adams G et al. Characterization of a murine model of allergic pulmonary inflammation. *Int Arch Allergy Immunol* 1994; **105**: 83–90.

26  Gavett S, Chen X, Finkelman F, Willis-Karp M. Depletion of murine CD4+ T lymphocytes prevents antigen-induced airway hyperreactivity and pulmonary eosinophilia. *Am J Respir Cell Mol Biol* 1994; **10**: 587–93.

27  Brusselle G, Kips, J, Tavernier J et al. Attenuation of allergic airway inflammation in IL-4 deficient mice. *Clin Exp Allergy* 1994; **24**: 73–80.

28  Nakajima H, Sano H, Nishimura T et al. Role of VCAM-1/VLA-4/LFA-1 interactions in antigen-induced eosinophil and T-cell recruitment into the tissue. *J Exp Med* 1994; **179**: 1145–54.

29  Foster P, Hogan S, Ramsay A, Matthaei K, Young I. Interleukin-5 deficiency abolishes eosinophilia, airways hyperreactivity, and lung damage in a mouse asthma model. *J Exp Med*, 1996. **183**: 195–201.

30  Cho Y, Miller M, Baek K et al. Inhibition of airway remodeling in IL-5-deficient mice. *J Clin Invest* 2004; **113**: 551–60.

31  Leckie M, ten Brinke A, Khan J et al. Effects of an interleukin-5 blocking monoclonal antibody on eosinophils, airway hyper-responsiveness, and the late asthmatic response. *Lancet* 2000; **356**: 2144–8.

32  Kips J, O'Connor B, Langley S et al. Effect of SCH55700, a humanized anti-human interleukin-5 antibody, in severe persistent asthma: a pilot study. *Am J Respir Crit Care Med* 2003; **167**:1655–9.

33  Flood-Page P, Menzies-Gow A, Kay A, Robinson D. Eosinophil's role remains uncertain as anti-interleukin-5 only partially depletes numbers in asthmatic airway. *Am J Respir Crit Care Med* 2003; **167**: 199–204.

34  Williams T. The eosinophil enigma. *J Clin Invest* 2004; **113**: 507–9.

35  Lambrecht B, Salomon B, Klatzmann D, Pauwels R. Dendritic cells are required for the development of chronic eosinophilic airway inflammation in response to inhaled antigen in sensitized mice. *J Immunol* 1998; **160**: 4090–7.

36  Kumar R, Herbert C, Yang M et al. Role of interleukin-13 in eosinophil accumulation and airway remodelling in a mouse model of chronic asthma. *Clin Exp Allergy* 2002; **32**: 1104–11.

37  Lee C, Homer R, Zhu Z et al. Interleukin-13 induces tissue fibrosis by selectively stimulating and activating transforming growth factor beta(1). *J Exp Med* 2001; **194**: 809–21.

38  Corbel M, Caulet-Maugendre S, Germain N et al. Enhancement of gelatinase activity during development of subepithelial fibrosis in a murine model of asthma. *Clin Exp Allergy* 2003; **33**: 696–704.

39  Schrier D, Kunkel R, Phan S. The role of strain variation in murine bleomycin-induced pulmonary fibrosis. *Am Rev Respir Dis* 1983; **127**: 63–6.

40  Gross T, Hunninghake G. Idiopathic pulmonary fibrosis. *N Engl J Med* 2001; **345**: 517–25.

41  Kuhn C, McDonald J. The roles of the myofibroblast in idiopathic pulmonary fibrosis. Ultrastructural and immunohistochemical features of sites of active extracellular matrix synthesis. *Am J Pathol* 1991; **138**: 1257–65.

42  Zhang K, Rekhter M, Gordon D, Phan S. Myofibroblasts and their role in lung collagen gene expression during pulmonary fibrosis. A combined immunohistochemical and in situ hybridization study. *Am J Pathol* 1994; **145**: 114–25.

43  Epperly M, Guo H, Gretton J, Greenberger J. Bone marrow origin of myofibroblasts in irradiation pulmonary fibrosis. *Am J Respir Cell Mol Biol* 2003; **29**: 213–24.

44  Hashimoto N, Jin H, Liu TT et al. Bone marrow-derived progenitor cells in pulmonary fibrosis. *J Clin Invest* 2004; **113**: 243–52.

45  Gross P, Pfitzer E, Tolker E et al. Experimental emphysema: its production with papain in normal and silicotic rats. *Arch Environ Health* 1965; **11**: 50–8.

46  Snider GL, Lucey EC, Stone PJ. Animal models of emphysema. *Am Rev Respir Dis* 1986; **133**: 149–69.

47  Kuhn C, Yu S, Chraplyvy M et al. The induction of emphysema with elastase. Changes in connective tissue. *Lab Invest* 1976; **34**: 372–80.

48  Kuhn C, Starcher B. The effect of lathyrogens on the evolution of elastase-induced emphysema. *Am Rev Respir Dis* 1980; **122**: 453–60.

49  Janoff A, Sloan B, Weinbaum G et al. Experimental emphysema induced with purified human neutrophil elastase: tissue localization of the instilled protease. *Am Rev Respir Dis* 1977; **115**: 461–78.

50  Senior RM, Tegner H, Kuhn C et al. The induction of pulmonary emphysema induced with human leukocyte elastase. *Am Rev Respir Dis* 1977; **116**: 469–75.

51  Snider GL, Lucey EC, Christensen TG et al. Emphysema and bronchial secretory cell metaplasia induced in hamsters by human neutrophil products. *Am Rev Respir Dis* 1984; **129**: 155–60.

52  Kao RC, Wehner NG, Skubitz KM et al. Proteinase 3: A distinct human polymorphonuclear leukocyte proteinase that produces emphysema in hamsters. *J Clin Invest* 1988; **82**: 1963–73.

53  Wright JL, Churg A. Cigarette smoke causes physiologic and morphologic changes of emphysema in the guinea pig. *Am Rev Respir Dis* 1990; **142**: 1422–8.

54  Hautamaki RD, Kobayashi DK, Senior RM, Shapiro SD. Macrophage elastase is required for cigarette smoke-induced emphysema in mice. *Science* 1997; **277**: 2002–4.

55  Kasahara Y, Tuder RM, Taraseviciene-Stewart L et al. Inhibition of VEGF receptors causes lung cell apoptosis and emphysema. *J Clin Invest* 2000; **106**: 1311–19.

56  Shapiro SD. Mighty mice: transgenic technology 'knocks out' questions of matrix metalloproteinase function. *Matrix Biol* 1997; **15**: 527–33.

57  Shapiro SD. Animal models for COPD. *Chest* 2000; **117**: 223S–7S.

58  Massaro GD, Massaro D. Retinoic acid treatment abrogates elastase-induced pulmonary emphysema in rats. *Nature Med* 1997; **3**: 675–7.

59  Lucey E, Keane J, Kuang P et al. Severity of elastase-induced emphysema is decreased in tumor necrosis factor-alpha and interleukin-1beta receptor-deficient mice. *Lab Invest* 2002; **82**: 79–85.

60  Snider GL, Lucey EC, Faris B et al. Cadmium-chloride-induced air-space enlargement with interstitial pulmonary fibrosis is not associated with destruction of lung elastin. Implications for the pathogenesis of human emphysema. *Am Rev Respir Dis* 1988; **137**: 918–23.

61  Aoshiba K, Yokohori N, Nagai A. Alveolar wall apoptosis causes lung destruction and emphysematous changes. *Am J Respir Cell Mol Biol* 2003; **28**: 555–62.

62  Mahadeva R, Shapiro S. Chronic obstructive pulmonary disease: Experimental animal models. *Thorax* 2002; **57**: 908–14.

63  Zheng T, Zhu Z, Wang Z et al. Inducible targeting of IL-13 to the adult lung causes matrix metalloproteinase- and cathepsin-dependent emphysema. *J Clin Invest* 2000; **106**: 1081–93.

64  Wang Z, Zheng T, Zhu Z et al. Interferon gamma induction of pulmonary emphysema in the adult murine lung. *J Exp Med* 2000; **192**: 1587–600.

65  Morris D, Huang X, Kaminski N et al. Loss of integrin-mediated TGFb activation causes MMP-12 dependent pulmonary emphysema. *Nature* 2003; **422**: 169–73.

66  Rogers D, Donnelly L (eds) *Human airway inflammation: Sampling techniques and analytical protocols.* Totowa, NJ: Humana Press, 2001.

67  Weibel E. Morphometry of the human lung: the state of the art after two decades. *Bull Eur Physiopathol Respir* 1979; **15**: 999–1013.

68  Bolender R, Hyde D, Dehoff R. Lung morphometry: a new generation of tools and experiments for organ, tissue, cell, and molecular biology. *Am J Physiol* 1993; **265**: L521–8.

69  Dunnill MS. Evaluation of a simple method of sampling the lungs for quantitative histological analysis. *Thorax* 1964; **19**: 443–8.

70  Iyer V, Eisen M, Ross D et al. The transcriptional program in the response of human fibroblasts to serum. *Science* 1999; **283**: 83–7.

71  Golub T, Ionim D, Tamayo P et al. Molecular classification of cancer: class discovery and class prediction by gene expression monitoring. *Science* 1999; **286**: 531–7.

72  Sherloc G. Analysis of large-scale gene expression data. *Curr Opin Immunol* 2000; **12**: 201–5.

73  Hill A, Hunter C, Tsung B et al. Genomic analysis of gene expression in *C. elegans*. *Science* 2000; **290**: 809–12.

74  White K, Rifkin S, Hurban P, Hogness D. Microarray analysis of *Drosophila* development during metamorphosis. *Science* 1999; **286**: 2179–84.

75  Eisen M, Spellman P, Brown P, Botstein D. Cluster analysis and display of genome-wide expression patterns. *Proc Natl Acad Sci USA* 1998; **95**: 14863–8.

76 Mitzner W, Tankersley C, Lundblad L et al. Interpreting Penh in mice. *J Appl Physiol* 2003; **94**: 526–632.

77 Hamelmann E, Schwarze J, Takeda K et al. Noninvasive measurement of airway responsiveness in allergic mice using barometric plethysmography. *Am J Respir Crit Care Med* 1997; **156**: 766–75.

78 Mitzner W, Tankersley C. Noninvasive measurement of airway responsiveness in allergic mice using barometric plethysmography. *Am J Respir Crit Care Med* 1998; **158**: 340–1.

79 Chong B, Agrawal D, Romero F, Townley R. Measurement of bronchoconstriction using whole-body plethysmograph: comparison of freely moving versus restrained guinea pigs. *J Pharmacol Toxicol Methods* 1998; **39**: 163–8.

80 Bergren D. Chronic tobacco smoke exposure increases airway sensitivity to capsaicin in awake guinea pigs. *J Appl Physiol* 2001; **90**: 695–704.

81 Flandre T, Leroy P, Desmecht D. Effect of somatic growth, strain, and sex on double-chamber plethysmographic respiratory function values in healthy mice. *J Appl Physiol* 2003; **94**: 1129–36.

82 Petak F, Habre W, Donati Y et al. Hyperoxia-induced changes in mouse lung mechanics: forced oscillations vs. barometric plethysmography. *J Appl Physiol* 2001; **90**: 2221–30.

83 DeLorme M, Moss O. Pulmonary function assessment by whole-body plethysmography in restrained versus unrestrained mice. *J Pharmacol Toxicol Methods* 2002; **47**: 1–10.

84 Kaczka D, Ingenito E, Bella S. Partitioning airway and lung tissue resistances in humans: effects of bronchoconstriction. *J Appl Physiol* 1997; **82**: 1531–41.

85 Kaczka D, Ingenito E, Lutchen KA. A technique for determining inspiratory impedance during mechanical ventilation: implications for flow limited patients. *Ann Biomed Engin* 1999; **27**: 1–16.

86 Hantos Z, Adamicza A, Govaerts E. Mechanical impedances of lungs and chest wall in the cat. *J Appl Physiol* 1992; **73**: 427–33.

87 Tankersley C, Rabold R, Mitzner W. Differential lung mechanics are genetically determined in inbred murine strains. *J Appl Physiol* 1999; **86**: 1764–9.

88 American Thoracic Society Official Statement. Guidelines for methacholine and exercise challenge testing. *Am J Resp Crit Care Med* 2000; **161**: 309–29.

89 Grupe A, Germer S, Usuka J et al. In silico mapping of complex disease-related traits in mice. *Science* 2001; **292**: 1915–8.

90 Shalom A, Darvasi A. Experimental designs for QTL fine mapping in rodents. *Methods Mol Biol* 2002; **195**: 199–223.

91 Darvasi A. Experimental strategies for the genetic dissection of complex traits in animal models. *Nat Genet* 1998; **18**: 19–24.

92 Darvasi A, Soller M. A simple method to calculate resolving power and confidence interval of QTL map location. *Behav Genet* 1997; **27**: 125–32.

93 Darvasi A, Soller M. Selective DNA pooling for determination of linkage between a molecular marker and a quantitative trait locus. *Genetics* 1994; **138**: 1365–73.

94 Manly KF, Olson JM. Overview of QTL mapping software and introduction to map manager QT. *Mamm Genome* 1999; **10**: 327–34.

95 Lander E, Kruglyak L. Genetic dissection of complex traits: guidelines for interpreting and reporting linkage results. *Nat Genet* 1995; **11**: 241–7.

96 Hoffjan S, Ober C. Present status on the genetic studies of asthma. *Curr Opin Immunol* 2002; **14**: 709–17.

97 Levitt RC, Mitzner W. Expression of airway hyperreactivity to acetylcholine as a simple autosomal recessive trait in mice. *FASEB J* 1988; **2**: 2605–8.

98 Levitt RC, Mitzner W. Autosomal recessive inheritance of airway hyperreactivity to 5-hydroxytryptamine. *J Appl Physiol* 1989; **67**: 1125–32.

99 Levitt RC, Mitzner W, Kleeberger SR. A genetic approach to the study of lung physiology: understanding biological variability in airway responsiveness. *Am J Physiol* 1990; **258**(4 Pt 1): L157–64.

100 Mitsos LM, Cardon LR, Fortin A et al. Genetic control of susceptibility to infection with *Mycobacterium tuberculosis* in mice. *Genes Immun* 2000; **1**: 467–77.

101 Mitsos LM, Cardon LR, Ryan L et al. Susceptibility to tuberculosis: a locus on mouse chromosome 19 (Trl-4) regulates *Mycobacterium tuberculosis* replication in the lungs. *Proc Natl Acad Sci USA* 2003; **100**: 6610–5.

102 Haston CK, McKerlie C, Newbigging S et al. Detection of modifier loci influencing the lung phenotype of cystic fibrosis knockout mice. *Mamm Genome* 2002; **13**: 605–13.

103 Haston CK, Corey M, Tsui LC. Mapping of genetic factors influencing the weight of cystic fibrosis knockout mice. *Mamm Genome* 2002; **13**: 614–8.

104 Prows DR, McDowell SA, Aronow BJ, Leikauf GD. Genetic susceptibility to nickel-induced acute lung injury. *Chemosphere* 2003; **51**: 1139–48.

105 Prows DR, Leikauf GD. Quantitative trait analysis of nickel-induced acute lung injury in mice. *Am J Respir Cell Mol Biol* 2001; **24**: 740–6.

106 Haston CK, Travis EL. Murine susceptibility to radiation-induced pulmonary fibrosis is influenced by a genetic factor implicated in susceptibility to bleomycin-induced pulmonary fibrosis. *Cancer Res* 1997; **57**: 5286–91.

107 Haston CK, Zhou X, Gumbiner-Russo L et al. Universal and radiation-specific loci influence murine susceptibility to radiation-induced pulmonary fibrosis. *Cancer Res* 2002; **62**: 3782–8.

108 Wang D, Lemon WJ, You M. Linkage disequilibrium mapping of novel lung tumor susceptibility quantitative trait loci in mice. *Oncogene* 2002; **21**: 6858–65.

109 Devereux TR, Kaplan NL. Use of quantitative trait loci to map murine lung tumor susceptibility genes. *Exp Lung Res* 1998; **24**: 407–17.

110 Prows DR, Shertzer HG, Daly MJ et al. Genetic analysis of ozone-induced acute lung injury in sensitive and resistant strains of mice. *Nat Genet* 1997; **17**: 471–4.

111 Kleeberger SR, Levitt RC, Zhang LY et al. Linkage analysis of susceptibility to ozone-induced lung inflammation in inbred mice. *Nat Genet* 1997; **17**: 475–8.

112 Kleeberger SR, Reddy S, Zhang LY, Jedlicka AE. Genetic susceptibility to ozone-induced lung hyperpermeability: role of toll-like receptor 4. *Am J Respir Cell Mol Biol* 2000; **22**: 620–7.

113 Savov JD, Whitehead GS, Wang J et al. Ozone-induced acute pulmonary injury in inbred mouse strains. *Am J Respir Cell Mol Biol* 2004; **31**: 69–77.

114 Ewart SL, Kuperman D, Schadt E et al. Quantitative trait loci controlling allergen-induced airway hyperresponsiveness in inbred mice. *Am J Respir Cell Mol Biol* 2000; **23**: 537–45.

115  Ober C, Tsalenko A, Parry R, Cox NJ. A second-generation genomewide screen for asthma-susceptibility alleles in a founder population. *Am J Hum Genet* 2000; **67**: 1154–62.

116  De Sanctis GT, Singer JB, Jiao A et al. Quantitative trait locus mapping of airway responsiveness to chromosomes 6 and 7 in inbred mice. *Am J Physiol* 1999; **277**(6 Pt 1): L1118–23.

117  Xu X, Fang Z, Wang B et al. A genomewide search for quantitative-trait loci underlying asthma. *Am J Hum Genet* 2001; **69**: 1271–7.

118  Zhang Y, Lefort J, Kearsey V et al. A genome-wide screen for asthma-associated quantitative trait loci in a mouse model of allergic asthma. *Hum Mol Genet* 1999; **8**: 601–5.

119  Xu J, Postma DS, Howard TD et al. Major genes regulating total serum immunoglobulin E levels in families with asthma. *Am J Hum Genet* 2000; **67**: 1163–73.

120  Koppelman GH, Stine OC, Xu J et al. Genome-wide search for atopy susceptibility genes in Dutch families with asthma. *J Allergy Clin Immunol* 2002; **109**: 498–506.

121  Dizier MH, Besse-Schmittler C, Guilloud-Bataille M et al. Genome screen for asthma and related phenotypes in the French EGEA study. *Am J Respir Crit Care Med* 2000; **162**: 1812–8.

122  Yokouchi Y, Nukaga Y, Shibasaki M et al. Significant evidence for linkage of mite-sensitive childhood asthma to chromosome 5q31-q33 near the interleukin 12B locus by a genome-wide search in Japanese families. *Genomics* 2000; **66**: 152–60.

123  Yokouchi Y, Shibasaki M, Noguchi E et al. A genome-wide linkage analysis of orchard grass-sensitive childhood seasonal allergic rhinitis in Japanese families. *Genes Immun* 2002; **3**: 9–13.

124  Xu J, Meyers DA, Ober C et al. Genomewide screen and identification of gene–gene interactions for asthma-susceptibility loci in three US populations: collaborative study on the genetics of asthma. *Am J Hum Genet* 2001; **68**: 1437–46.

125  Mathias RA, Freidhoff LR, Blumenthal MN et al. Genome-wide linkage analyses of total serum IgE using variance components analysis in asthmatic families. *Genet Epidemiol* 2001; **20**: 340–55.

126  De Sanctis GT, Merchant M, Beier DR et al. Quantitative locus analysis of airway hyperresponsiveness in A/J and C57BL/6J mice. *Nat Genet* 1995; **11**: 150–4.

127  Daniels SE, Bhattacharrya S, James A et al. A genome-wide search for quantitative trait loci underlying asthma. *Nature* 1996; **383**: 247–50.

128  Wjst M, Fischer G, Immervoll T et al. A genome-wide search for linkage to asthma. German Asthma Genetics Group. *Genomics* 1999; **58**: 1–8.

129  Bergamaschi E, De Palma G, Mozzoni P et al. Polymorphism of quinone-metabolizing enzymes and susceptibility to ozone-induced acute effects. *Am J Respir Crit Care Med* 2001; **163**: 1426–31.

# 8

# Pharmacogenetics

## KELAN G. TANTISIRA AND JEFFREY M. DRAZEN

*What is one man's meat is another man's poison*

A. E. Garrod, 1902

## OVERVIEW OF PHARMACOGENETICS

### Introduction

The response to pharmacologic agents varies tremendously by individual. For instance, the plasma level of a given medication can vary more than 1000-fold between two individuals having the same weight when treated with the same drug dosage.[1] On average for a given drug, 30 percent of patients show beneficial effects, 30 percent fail to improve, 10 percent only experience side effects, and 30 percent are noncompliant (which may be related to either lack of efficacy or side effects).[2] Therefore, as many as 70 percent of all patients are unnecessarily exposed to the potential to develop adverse drug reactions (ADRs).[3–5] In 1994, over 2 million 'serious ADRs' and over 100 000 fatal ADRs were noted, ranking ADRs between the fourth and the sixth leading cause of death in the USA.[6] Overall, the cost of drug-related morbidity and mortality exceeded $177.4 billion in 2000,[7] a figure more than double the estimate from 1995.[8] As enormous as these figures are, some authorities feel that the burden due to lack of therapeutic response to drug therapy is much greater.[9]

Although many ADRs may be preventable, there are others that appear idiosyncratic; the ability to effectively prevent such ADRs, and to optimize therapeutic response to medications, may lie in the recognition of genetic factors influencing these outcomes. For example, of 2227 ADRs identified in a large teaching hospital, less than 50 percent had readily identified causes.[10] Genetic factors also likely contribute to treatment response; since the intra-individual response to a given therapeutic agent is highly repeatable.[11] In fact, genetic variability in drug absorption, drug metabolism, and drug action at the receptor level is well known. Overall, it is estimated that genetics can account for 20 to 95 percent of variability in drug disposition and effects.[12]

Pharmacogenetics is the study of variability in drug response due to heredity. That is, pharmacogenetics seeks to determine the role of genetic determinants in an individual's response to therapy. The related term, pharmacogenomics, refers to the development of novel drugs based upon the evolving knowledge of the genome. The two terms, however, are frequently used interchangeably. Ideally, pharmacogenetics will allow for 'individualized therapy' based upon an individual's genetic make-up that will maximize the potential for therapeutic benefit, while minimizing the risk of adverse effects. The potential for cost savings and for decreasing morbidity and mortality is immense.

This chapter provides a practical overview of the field of pharmacogenetics, beginning with a historical overview, proceeding through types of pharmacogenetic responses, and emphasizing approaches to pharmacogenetic study design and analysis. The chapter continues with a review of two classes of pharmacogenetic responses that have been well characterized in the respiratory literature and concludes with some thoughts on areas of respiratory pharmacogenetics of ongoing and future interest.

### Historical overview

The roots of pharmacogenetics may date back to as early as the sixth century BC, when Pythagoras is said to have recognized that eating fava beans caused some, but not all, individuals to become ill.[13–15] In the 1940s, the immunochemist William Boyd noted that the British, in contrast to Mediterranean populations, almost never developed hemolytic anemia on ingestion of fava beans, and suggested a genetic difference as the probable explanation.[14] It is now known that the hemolytic anemia associated with fava bean ingestion may also be caused by a variety of pharmacologic agents and is due to the X-linked glucose-6-phosphate dehydrogenase (G6PD) deficiency.[13,14] Other pioneers in the thought processes regarding inter-individual differences in drug response include Garrod's recognition of a subset of psychiatric patients who developed porphyria upon administration of sulphonal,[16,17] published in 1902, and Snyder's 1932 recognition that the 'phenolthiourea nontaster' phenotype was inherited as an autosomal recessive trait and varied by ethnicity.[15,18] In the 1950s, patients with an inherited deficiency of plasma cholinesterase were noted to have a prolonged paralytic response to suxamethonium.[19] In 1957, Motulsky suggested that interindividual differences in drug efficacy, as well as adverse drug reactions, were at least partially attributable to genetic differences.[20] Frederich Vogel, a German geneticist, first coined the term 'pharmacogenetics' in 1959.[21] Vessel and Page conducted a series of twin studies in the 1960s, noting that plasma half-lives of many drugs were very similar in monozygotic twins, but varied significantly among dizygotic twins, siblings, and the general population.[22–28] These studies reinforced the role of genetics in the inter-individual variation in drug responses.

In the late 1970s, two independent groups associated autosomal recessive deficiencies in drug metabolism with markedly increased side effects in certain volunteers taking the antihypertensive debrisoquine[29] and the antiarrhythmic sparteine.[30] In 1988, the metabolism of both of these drugs was subsequently shown to result from allelic variation at the cytochrome P450 2D6 (CYP2D6) locus.[31] This was the first example of applied genotyping in the field of pharmacogenetics. Since that time, advances in genetic technology and an increased understanding of the molecular basis of drug metabolism, transport, and receptor activity have led to the characterization of dozens of functional pharmacogenetic polymorphisms.

## Pharmacogenetics as a gene by environment interaction

The potential for efficacy and toxicity of a drug within a given individual can be modified by a variety of factors, including those endogenous to the host, environmental exposures, and genetics (Table 8.1). Genetic variation may account for between 20 and 95 percent of variability in drug disposition and effects.[1,12] Two functionally distinct classes of genetic response to a drug exposure may be made based upon the underlying biological variance.[17] In one class, the genetic variation is in itself not disease-causing or contributory and becomes relevant only in response to the

**Table 8.1**  *Factors affecting therapeutic levels and clinical response to medications*

| Environmental/ non-genetic host factors | Genetic |
| --- | --- |
| Host characteristics <br>• Age <br>• Sex <br>• Body mass <br>• Fat distribution | Related to therapeutic agent <br>• Drug absorption <br>• Drug metabolizing enzymes <br>• Drug transporters <br>• Drug receptors |
| Major organ function <br>• Liver <br>• Kidney <br>• Heart <br>• Lungs <br>• Gastrointestinal | Related to disease properties <br>• Susceptibility <br>• Disease modifying |
| Environmental exposures <br>• Cigarette smoking <br>• Alcohol consumption <br>• Other medications/remedies <br>• Environmental pollutants | Idiosyncratic |

exposure to the drug in question. That is, the genetic variant exerts its pharmacogenetic effect primarily through interaction with properties related to the drug, its metabolism, or its mechanism of action. In the other class, the genetic variation is directly related to disease causality or pathogenesis. In this case, the differential response to the drug is related to how well it is matched to the underlying pathophysiological mechanism underlying the disease.

The two functional classes of genetic response above have direct relevance to the study design and analysis of pharmacogenetic studies. Pharmacogenetics can be thought of as a classic example of gene by environment interactions. That is, in pharmacogenetics, one assesses the modification of the impact of an environmental exposure (the therapeutic agent) by genetic variation on disease outcome or severity. However, the origins and foundations of pharmacogenetics have been centered primarily around genetic differences determining drug metabolism, drug disposition, or drug-specific side effects.[12,32] In these instances, the therapeutic agent serves as both a necessary environmental exposure and the basis of the measured outcomes (i.e., one measures the level of a drug or one of its metabolites). These are examples of functional class 1 pharmacogenetic responses and comprise the vast majority of pharmacogenetic studies performed to date. For ease, we will refer to functional class 1 as the 'drug response' pharmacogenetic class throughout this chapter. Formal interaction analyses may be inappropriate in this context as the interaction of genetics with environmental exposure is assumed. However, complex secondary environmental effects such as those of smoking or other drugs may be appropriate. The inheritance pattern underlying these pharmacogenetic effects can often be defined as Mendelian, such as the X-linked inheritance underlying G6PD deficiency. In this chapter, the sections on warfarin pharmacogenetics, the pharmacogenetics of smoking cessation, and lung cancer pharmacogenetics will serve as extended discussions of this response class.

In functional class 2 pharmacogenetic responses, genetic factors may affect drug interactions with disease, disease course, or intermediate phenotypes associated with disease outcome or symptomatology. Improvement in disease status, therefore, may be attributable to either therapeutic effect or to the natural history of the underlying disease. We refer to this functional class as 'target response' pharmacogenetics. The inheritance patterns of these pharmacogenetic effects do not tend to be classically Mendelian. Instead, the target response tends to be determined by polygenic or gene–environment interactions. As pharmacogenetic analyses of complex diseases become more prevalent, an increasing number of pharmacogenetic associations will fall into this category. Since multiple treatment options exist for many of these complex diseases, including the administration of no regular medications, formal pharmacogenetic interaction analyses are appropriate and provide assurances that: (a) genotypes alter the effect of the therapy of interest, and (b) the genetic association noted is not just a marker for the natural history of the disease. In this chapter, the section on asthma pharmacogenetics will provide an extended discussion of this response class.

## Pharmacogenetic categories

In addition to the two functional response classes denoted above, pharmacogenetics has traditionally also been divided into four categories based upon the effects of genetic variability on the pharmacologic properties of a drug (Fig. 8.1). These categories include variation related to pharmacokinetics, pharmacodynamics, idiosyncratic reactions, and disease pathogenesis.[33] Pharmacokinetics studies the effect of the body upon an administered drug, including consideration of the absorption, distribution, tissue localization, biotransformation, and excretion of drugs.[34] The vast majority of pharmacogenetic investigations reported in the literature to date have been in this area. The major areas of pharmacokinetic investigations in the field of pharmacogenetics have been in the evaluation of genetic differences in drug metabolizing enzymes and drug transporters. There are two phases of xenobiotic metabolism controlled by an estimated several hundred drug metabolizing enzyme genes. In phase I, the compound is subjected to oxidation, reduction, and hydrolysis to other transformations of its structure. In phase II, conjugation of the compound with endogenous substances increases its solubility in water and thereby facilitates its elimination.[9] In addition to the cytochrome p450 (CYP) enzymes, examples of polymorphic phase I drug metabolizing enzymes relevant to the field of respiratory medicine include butyrylcholinesterase, which prolongs paralysis upon

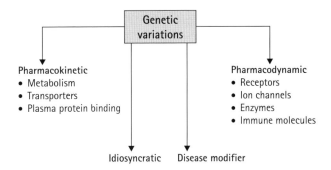

**Figure 8.1** *Pharmacogenetic categories. Traditionally, genetic differences have been classified to affect response to therapeutic agents in four distinct fashions. These include effects on pharmacokinetics (overall level of drug reaching the target), pharmacodynamics (interactions of the drug with its target), idiosyncratic reactions, and genetic variation related to disease pathogenesis.*

administration of succinylcholine,[19,35] and dihydropyrimidine dehydrogenase, which metabolizes the chemotherapeutic agent, 5-fluorouracil.[36,37] An example of polymorphic phase II drug metabolizing enzymes is the metabolism of azathioprine by thiopurine-*S*-methyltransferase.[38,39] Additional examples will be detailed in the section on drug response pharmacogenetics. Given the evolving knowledge of pharmacokinetic pharmacogenetics, preliminary dosing recommendations have been made based upon known genetic variations in drug metabolizing enzymes.[9,40,41]

Variance in drug transporters influencing drug absorption, distribution, and excretion make up the second major area of pharmacogenetic investigations in pharmacokinetics to date. Members of the adenosine triphosphate (ATP)-binding cassette family of membrane transporters are among the most extensively studied transporters in terms of disposition and effects.[12] A member of the ATP-binding cassette family, P-glycoprotein, is encoded by the human *ABCB1* gene. P-glycoprotein functions to enhance the energy-dependent cellular efflux of substrates, including bilirubin, several anticancer drugs, immunosuppressive agents, glucocorticoids, and other medications.[12,42–44]

Pharmacodynamics is the study of the biochemical and physiological consequences of the administration of a drug and its mechanism of action,[34] i.e., the effect of a drug at its therapeutic target. Genetic variation may lead to interindividual differences in the response to a drug despite the presence of appropriate concentrations of the drug at its intended target. In this category, the genetic variation is typically present at the site of the target or one of the downstream participants in the target's mechanistic pathway, thereby modulating the effects of the drug. One example of the pharmacodynamic category is the enhanced inhibition of platelets in subjects with the $Pl^{A2}$ polymorphism which encodes for a Leu → Pro substitution at position 33 of the GPIIIa subunit of the GPIIb-IIIa fibrinogen receptor (*ITGB3*) upon the administration of aspirin.[45,46]

No differences in platelet aggregation were noted with this genetic variant in the absence of aspirin. The field of asthma pharmacogenetics and several additional examples of drug–gene–target interactions will be reviewed below.

While studies of pharmacogenetic predictors of efficacy at therapeutic target sites are slated to eventually become the primary basis for 'individualized therapy,' to date there remain relatively few examples of replicable pharmacodynamic pharmacogenetic associations, compared with those related to pharmacokinetics.[47] At least two reasons exist for the prominence of pharmacokinetic studies. The first is that the biology of drug metabolism and drug transport is relatively straightforward. For instance, each compound typically has one principle enzyme responsible for its metabolism. However, the physiology of most drug target pathways is fairly complex, providing multiple pathways that may require investigation prior to the discovery of an interaction between the drug and genetic differences in part of the target pathway. The second is that differences in metabolism related to genetics can be as high as 10 000-fold, whereas differences in target binding related to genetics are generally less than 20-fold.[15,48–50] The resultant ability (power) to detect differences in metabolism within a population given a compound is clearly far greater than the ability to detect variance in drug targets.

The idiosyncratic category of pharmacogenetic response to drugs includes the individuals that experience an ADR to a therapeutic agent that could not be anticipated based upon the known drug target. Examples of the idiosyncratic category include some compounds that are metabolized by arylamine-*N*-acetyltransferase 2 (*NAT2*). Genetic differences in *NAT2* have been associated with predisposition to the development of peripheral neuropathy in certain individuals taking isoniazid[51–53] and hypersensitivity reactions to trimethoprim-sulfamethoxazole (including rash, granulocytopenia, and abnormal liver function tests).[52,54,55] Interestingly, the *NAT2* acetylator phenotype (based upon the metabolized level of drugs) may correlate poorly with *NAT2* genotype,[56–58] suggesting that factors other than drug level may explain these idiosyncratic reactions associated with genetic variation.

The final pharmacogenetic category is that of genetic factors influencing disease pathogenesis. This can be exemplified by variation of the angiotensin converting enzyme (*ACE*) gene and its effect on the progression of disease related to systemic hypertension. The *ACE* gene carries a 287 nucleotide insertion (I)/deletion (D) polymorphism in intron 16; the D allele has consistently been associated with higher *ACE* activity and higher angiotensin II levels.[9,59] The prognosis of patients with systolic dysfunction is significantly worse in heterozygous and homozygous carriers of the *ACE D* allele than in *I* allele homozygotes.[59] However, the *ACE D* allele also impacts therapeutic interactions on the converting enzyme itself. In a study comparing 12 homozygous *ACE DD* individuals with 11 homozygous for *ACE II*, enalapralat (an *ACE* inhibiting anti-hypertensive drug) had a significantly greater and longer lasting effect in subjects with the *ACE II* genotype than in those with the *ACE DD* genotype.[60] Overall, *ACE (I/D)* genotype and plasma angiotensin II levels were predictive of >50 percent of the variation in response to *ACE* inhibition.[60]

How do these categories of pharmacogenetic responses fit into our described classes above? In general, the pharmacokinetic and idiosyncratic categories fit into the drug response class, while pharmacodynamic and disease pathogenesis categories fit into the target response class.

## METHODOLOGIC APPROACHES TO PHARMACOGENETICS

The primary objective of studies in pharmacogenetics is to relate the response to the therapeutic agent of interest (drug phenotype) to genotype, at either the single nucleotide polymorphism (SNP) level, the level of a candidate gene (as with haplotype analyses), or at the level of the entire genome (as in genome-wide association tests). Of primary importance is the definition of accurate, repeatable phenotypes. Second, one needs to define the type of genetic relationship that a given variant has with the phenotype (pharmacogenetic study design). Finally, the relationship needs to be better defined, either through the demonstration of a functional change associated with the genetic change, through replication of the association results, or through demonstration of the impact that a variation has on the population of interest (explained phenotypic variance).

## Pharmacogenetic phenotypes

With the advances in knowledge of the human genome, the need for better documentation and determination of phenotypic responses has been noted, with a call for the development of a new field of 'phenomics'[61] as part of a proposed 'Human Phenome Project'.[62] The crux of the identified problem is that, while there has been enormous effort focused on the genotypic basis for phenotypic variation, little is known about how to integrate this effort with the environmental influences on phenotypes, or even how to accurately measure phenotypic features.[62] Accurate phenotypic definition is crucial in genetic studies in order to avoid diagnostic misclassification.[63–66] Two types of misclassification commonly occur in genetic studies: (1) nondifferential misclassification, in which the probability of error as to phenotype (in this case, a drug response or ADR) does not depend on exposure (genetic status), and (2) differential misclassification, in which it does. Nondifferential misclassification of phenotype reduces the observed genetic relative risk towards the null value, sometimes quite dramatically. An example of nondifferential misclassification is measurement error. For instance, let us assume that one were interested in studying the association

**Table 8.2** *Example of non-differential misclassification*

|  | Significant response | No significant response |
|---|---|---|
| *A. Actual* | | |
| SNP present | 40 | 40 |
| SNP absent | 120 | 200 |
| OR 1.67, 95% CI 1.00–2.81 (*P* = 0.04) | | |
| *B. Misclassification of 1 in 5 as responders* | | |
| SNP present | 48 | 32 |
| SNP absent | 160 | 160 |
| OR 1.50, 95% CI 0.89–2.54 (*P* = 0.11) | | |
| *C. Misclassification of 1 in 5 as nonresponders* | | |
| SNP present | 32 | 48 |
| SNP absent | 96 | 224 |
| OR 1.56, 95% CI 0.91–2.66 (*P* = 0.08) | | |

An association of an SNP with a 20 percent minor allele frequency with bronchodilator response is shown. If accurately measured, the SNP is significantly associated with the phenotype of interest. However, if, due to measurement error, one in five individuals is mistakenly classified as either 'Responder' or 'Nonresponder', there is a bias towards the null in the ability to detect a significant association, even if one actually exists.

of a candidate gene with bronchodilator response, with a significant response calculated as a 15 percent improvement from baseline. However, for each participant, the post-bronchodilator measurement is read as 5 percent higher than the actual value. In this case, an increased number of individuals both with and without the genetic variant of interest would be placed into the 'significant response' category. Therefore, there would be a decreased likelihood of detecting an association of the genetic variant with a significant bronchodilator response, if such an association actually existed (Table 8.2).

Differential misclassification can bias the observed relative risk in either direction, depending on the different values of sensitivity and specificity among cases and controls. An example of differential misclassification would be an attempt to compare CYP genotypes (see section on Drug response pharmacogenetics below) in lifelong smoker cases over the age of 50 to those of teenager smoking controls in relation to response to smoking cessation therapy. In this case, variant CYP genotypes may actually be a predictor of true nicotine addiction and therefore would be expected to be more prevalent in the lifelong smokers when compared to the teenagers. Therefore, the relative odds of response to smoking cessation therapy given a variant allele may appear to be falsely low in the lifelong smokers when compared to the controls. The problem of phenotypic misclassification is especially prominent in complex disease traits, including asthma,[67,68] and in studies of gene–environment interactions,[65,66] including pharmacogenetics.

All pharmacogenetic analyses are inherently longitudinal in nature. That is, for a given individual genotype, one measures the phenotypic characteristic of interest before and after the administration of a therapeutic agent. In the case where a property of the drug effect forms the basis of measurement after its administration, it is assumed that the baseline, prior to administration, is zero. In the case of the target response class, an intermediate phenotype or a measure of disease severity is obtained preceding and following the administration of the drug. The use of intermediate phenotypes, such as changes in a biochemical or physiological marker that are more proximal to the molecular basis of disease, has been advocated as a way to enhance phenotypic definitions.[61,62]

The field of pharmacogenetics began with the observations that there were clinically important inherited variations in drug metabolism.[32] These variations typically led to overly functional, poorly functional, nonfunctional, or absent proteins, leading to distinct phenotypes that were recognized prior to the understanding of the genetic basis for the phenotype.[69] While rates of metabolism of a drug can be quantified through direct assays of drug or drug metabolite concentrations with varying degrees of difficulty, most of the clinically relevant phenotypes have traditionally been considered as groups, since the functional genetic variants result in population distributions that tend to be bimodal or multimodal. For instance, patients with differential responses in the metabolism within the CYP system are frequently assigned designations such as 'poor', 'intermediate', 'extensive', and 'ultrarapid' metabolizers,[70] while those responding differently to N-acetylation of isoniazid are denoted 'slow' or 'fast' acetylators.[32] The basis of these designations has been to provide, through genetic testing, a safe, effective dosing regimen for drugs with narrow therapeutic indexes – drugs for which differences between toxic and therapeutic doses are relatively small.[32] For this type of variable drug response, inter-individual variation can usually be assessed after a single dose of the drug of interest. The categorical phenotypes of interest for the drug response class are thus usually easy to define.

In contrast, for our target response class, examples of drug receptor/effector gene polymorphisms that lead to a complete lack of protein have not been identified to date.[47] Functionally, the response to these variations tends to be spread across a unimodal distribution.[69] This indicates that either multiple genes each with multiple polymorphisms may influence the overall response, or that the phenotypic assessment itself is inherently noisy. In these cases the effect of a single polymorphism is small and the required sample sizes to detect significant pharmacogenetic associations are large. Moreover, the measurement of drug response or disease modifying phenotypes is often imprecise, highly variable over time, or may be inappropriate for modeling pharmacologic response.[47] Therefore, the identification of a valid drug response phenotype that is repeatable over time, and is able to be measured accurately and precisely, is

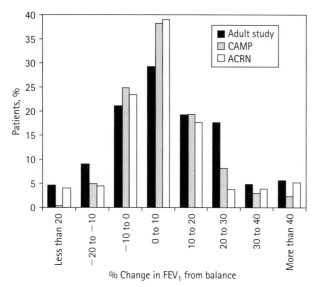

**Figure 8.2** *Response to inhaled corticosteroids in three populations. In each of the three populations shown, the quantitative response to inhaled corticosteroids is approximately normal, with a significant number of both very good responders and nonresponders. This suggests that factors other than the medications, including genetic factors contribute to the therapeutic response (from Tantisira et al.[268]) study groups are defined on page 207.*

especially important for target response pharmacogenetic studies.

How do we best define such a phenotype? To start, one needs to find a measure that best defines a differential response to the drug. This is best accomplished by way of an easily measured, quantitative trait. For instance, the response to inhaled corticosteroids in asthma can be assessed by the change in $FEV_1$ over time (Fig. 8.2). Once a reproducible measure of drug response is available, the next question is whether to further divide the population responses into discrete categories. The term 'extreme discordant phenotype' (EDP) has been applied to this categorization process.[71] To define an EDP, one simply takes the individuals at the highest and lowest ends of the response distribution, allowing them to represent 'sensitive outliers' (individuals that demonstrate a large response to the drug) and 'resistant outliers' (those that demonstrate little to no response to the drug).[15,71] The cutoffs for these outliers are based upon reasonable biological or physiological bounds, adequate to differentiate unequivocally between the response groups. In some cases, one would analyze the highest and lowest quartiles, whereas with others, only the highest and lowest 2.5 percent; usually the size of the treated population dictates what proportion of the population is studied.

The alternative to defining an EDP is to treat the response to the drug as a continuous phenotype, e.g., all blood pressure responses, and to perform quantitative trait analysis. This approach is appealing in that one utilizes all of the subject data available for any given analysis. The particular advantages of the EDP are that it does not depend

on the actual values of the quantitative trait, but only on the fact that patient pairs can exhibit extreme values.[71] EDP may be the analytic approach of greatest power given a proven functional mutation.[71] Overall, EDP analysis is best done given a functional mutation, with additional assumptions of complete penetrance, a dominant or recessive model, and limited epistatic (gene–gene or gene–environment) interactions. However, complex traits are often characterized by the degree of epistatic interactions[72] and causative polymorphisms in pharmacogenetic studies usually occur at low penetrance.[73] Continuous phenotypes may be analyzed in the context of epistatic interactions and incomplete penetrance, and they have greater power than case–control methodology if no genetic model is specified or if the model is incorrectly specified. Continuous phenotypic traits are also best utilized in the analysis of genetic studies under the assumption of an additive model, since that model assumes a response profile for heterozygous individuals intermediate between that of those homozygous for the variant allele and those homozygous for the wildtype allele. The choice of the qualitative (EDP) versus. quantitative phenotype is thus optimally dependent upon the expected differences in response based upon genotype status. Since this is not usually known prior to the start of a study, it is reasonable to define and analyze both qualitative and quantitative phenotypes based upon the same drug response distribution of interest.

In evaluating a phenotype based upon change in a quantitative trait over time, including the categorization of an EDP phenotype, it is of utmost importance to account for the baseline value in the definition of the phenotype or in the analytic phase. Subjects at the extremes of the response distribution at baseline may be there because they truly represent the extremes of the drug response trait distribution for a given study. Alternatively, others at the extremes may be there only because they happened, through random variation, to have an extreme value when they were first measured. Thus, on subsequent measurements, these subjects would be expected to have less extreme values, i.e., closer to the population mean. This phenomenon is known as 'regression to the mean'.[74,75] It is also possible that a patient's response may be due to a placebo effect of the active medication; there is no easy way to distinguish true responses and placebo responses.

Poor correlation of the trait of interest within an individual, also known as the intraclass correlation, determines an increased potential for regression to the mean to exist. The more extreme the initial observed value from the population mean, the larger the potential magnitude of the regression to the mean. In the examination of change in the drug response trait over time, as with pharmacogenetic phenotypes, change over time may be related to either a response to a drug or changes expected due to regression to the mean, with those at the extremes of the baseline distribution by chance, rather than by true therapeutic effect (or lack thereof), statistically most likely to demonstrate the

**Table 8.3** *Pharmacogenetic study designs*

| Study design type | Pros | Cons |
|---|---|---|
| Familial linkage | Allows localization of genetic loci of interest in an unbiased fashion | Requires phenotypic information about drug response on all individuals in the pedigree, even in those for whom the drug is not indicated |
| Familial association | Immune from population stratification<br>Requires DNA from individuals other than the drug-exposed proband<br>Can analyze haplotypic and interaction associations | Generally less powerful than case–control studies, requiring increases in sample size |
| Cross-sectional | Easiest of the study designs to implement | Subject to bias<br>Must limit to situations that entail a very well established response phenotype for a given drug |
| Cohort[a] | Amenable to both qualitative and quantitative analyses<br>Can readily analyze haplotypes and interactions<br>Generally one of the best study designs for optimal statistical power<br>Amenable to longitudinal designs and analyses | Possible population stratification |
| Case–control[a] | Similar to cohort studies | Similar to cohort studies |
| Case only | Allows for interrogation of response if all that is available are probands taking the medication | Possible population stratification<br><br>Difficult to ascertain interaction effects |
| Whole genome association | Like linkage studies, requires no a priori hypotheses | Uncertainty about how many SNPs are required<br>Cost<br>Can localize, but will still require follow-up candidate gene interrogation<br>Analytical methods still need to be standardized |

[a]Currently espoused as the most suitable study designs for pharmacogenetic analyses (see text).

largest change due to regression to the mean.[75] Accounting for baseline value in either the formative definition of a drug response phenotype or in the statistical analyses of the trait of interest over time, is therefore necessary to minimize the effects of regression to the mean. An example of accounting for baseline value in the definition of a phenotype would be defining the change in lung function over time as a percent of baseline, or using the baseline value as a covariate in a multivariate analysis.

## Pharmacogenetic study designs

Pharmacogenetic studies have the advantage that the phenotype is usually easy to measure as it is the outcome of a drug treatment. This allows patients to be proportioned categorically, i.e., into those who 'respond' and those who fail to do so, or quantitatively, i.e., by the magnitude of response. These outcomes can be used in linkage studies and population-based studies. (Readers interested in the specifics of these study designs are referred to Chapters 1 and 3 of this book.) The pros and cons of various study designs as they apply to pharmacogenetic analyses are outlined in Table 8.3 and in the text that follows.

Linkage studies in the context of pharmacogenetics would be applied to families where there is a clustering of a specific drug response. To date, there have been few linkage studies performed to assess drug response within families, and none in the respiratory pharmacogenetics literature. One example of a drug response linkage study is the study by Schuckit et al.[76] This group studied the low level of response to alcohol as a phenotype in 745 subjects participating in the Collaborative Study on the Genetics of Alcoholism. Using 336 markers across the genome, they identified four chromosomal regions with LOD scores $\geq 2.0$.[76] One practical pharmacogenetic linkage approach is in the determination of how phenotypic drug response may help to better define and map an underlying disease locus, such as the strong linkage evidence (LOD score of 3.46 on chromosome 15q14) noted for the diagnosis of bipolar disorder in patients who demonstrate good clinical response to lithium.[77] While some may view this approach as a way to optimize disease mapping, it may also represent a way to genetically localize drug treatment response. As an extension of this, methodologic considerations of the impact of gene–environment interactions in linkage analyses have been studied.[78,79] As a practical example, Colilla et al.[80] studied the impact of including environmental tobacco smoke (ETS) on a linkage study for the diagnosis of asthma. Three regions with nominal evidence for linkage when stratified on the basis of ETS exposure were identified; all demonstrated a significant increase from baseline LOD scores.[80] Pharmacogenetic investigations of asthma could proceed along similar lines, incorporating drug response in place of ETS.

In contrast to linkage studies, association studies typically test hypotheses about a specific gene or set of genes (e.g., a drug receptor pathway). Since we mentioned that linkage studies in pharmacogenetics are rare, the genes tested in these association studies are typically biological candidate genes, rather than positional candidate genes. These candidate genes can be selected based upon knowledge of the gene's biological action or by utilizing expression array data demonstrating up- or down-regulation of a gene in a phenotypically relevant fashion upon exposure to the drug of interest.[73,81] Family-based association studies, which would assess for differential transmission of a genetic variant of interest in relationship to drug response, are similarly rare in the pharmacogenetics literature. Although there are no overt reasons that studies involving trios (two parents and a child but where only the child needs to be phenotyped) or sib-pairs cannot be performed to ascertain drug response, from a practical point of view these studies may prove difficult to establish.[82]

Most epidemiologic studies of pharmacogenetic response have been population-based. All traditional and some nontraditional population-based epidemiological study designs can be used in pharmacogenetic studies, including cross-sectional, cohort, case–control, case only, and longitudinal studies. Population-based, genome-wide association studies are also now feasible. Cross-sectional studies are vulnerable to bias since the temporal relationship of exposure to outcome is not ascertained. In pharmacogenetics, this type of study is appropriate only if there is a well-established drug response phenotype, ascertained at one point in time while the subject is on the drug. In a cohort study, a population of exposed and unexposed individuals (on and off the pharmaceutical agent) is followed over time. The incidence of the drug response phenotype is ascertained in both groups, allowing for a calculation of relative risk. This approach is amenable to evaluation with both quantitative and qualitative outcomes, and, for the target response functional class of pharmacogenetic analyses, allows for calculation of a formal interaction term.

Case–control studies assess the proportion of individuals on and off a drug, given a drug response outcome of interest and a sample of controls without the outcome. Case–control studies have been espoused as the most suitable for pharmacogenetic studies for the following reasons:[2]

- Genetic markers are stable indicators of host susceptibility over time.
- Uncommon disease outcomes, including ADRs, can be readily assessed.
- The relative statistical power of the case–control study is good.
- This type of study also allows for the calculation of epistatic interactions, including those involving gene–gene and gene–environment.

Case-only studies focusing on gene–environment interactions are unique to genetic epidemiology.[83–87] In this study design, investigators use case subjects only (those with the drug response outcome of interest) to assess the magnitude of the exposure of interest and the genotype. If the genetic and environmental exposures are independent in the population and the risk of the drug response of interest is small (as for a rare ADR), the cross-product ratio (that is, the relative odds ratio for the response given a genotype of interest and a drug exposure of interest) of the case-only study is approximately equal to the odds ratio of the gene–environment interaction computed from case–control data.[86,88] While these studies are more powerful for the detection of gene by environment interactions than a case–control study of comparable size,[83,86] they cannot be used to ascertain the effects of the genotype or environmental exposure on the outcome of interest independent of the interaction.[87,89] Moreover, the assumption of independence of genetic and environmental exposures may lead to biased estimates if this assumption is violated.[90]

Although the advantage of utilizing longitudinal studies in genetic analyses has been recognized,[91] very little work has been carried out on evaluating the relationship of genetic architecture to longitudinal phenotypes in either respiratory genetics or in pharmacogenetics. For instance, to evaluate a drug metabolizing enzyme, one can measure serial drug levels at times following the administration of a medication. However, it is in the area of target response phenotypes that longitudinal trials may be of most benefit. In this instance, subjects are often enrolled in a clinical trial to ascertain response to an agent, often compared to placebo, over time. Multiple measurements of the outcome of interest are often obtained over the course of the trial. For instance, in an asthma clinical trial, peak flow measurements may be obtained daily and $FEV_1$ measurements every 4 weeks over the course of a 12-week clinical trial. By developing models that incorporate these repeated measures, one can best elicit the 'true responders' to therapy.[91] Moreover, longitudinal analysis is a more powerful approach to data analysis[92] and may help to alleviate concerns about sample sizes in genetic association studies.[93]

The prospects for whole genome association studies are just beginning to be realized.[94–98] In contrast to all of the other population-based study designs noted above, whole genome association studies do not require a priori hypotheses to select candidate genes. Instead, whole-genome linkage disequilibrium studies to map common disease genes employ a dense map of SNPs to detect association between a marker and disease. Proof-of-principle experiments have demonstrated that high density SNP maps in chromosomal regions of genetic linkage facilitate the identification of susceptibility disease genes.[96–98] The major question that remains unanswered is 'how many SNPs will it actually take to map a disease?' Various authors have estimated the number of SNPs required to be as few as 100 000[94] to as many as 500 000.[95] Still others feel that it is impossible to estimate the number of SNPs at this time, until measurement of allele frequency and linkage disequilibrium relationships for all SNPs in dbSNP is performed for any ethnic population utilized in the whole genome association study.[94]

## Common pharmacogenetic study problems

Pharmacogenetic studies are susceptible to all of the problems associated with other population-based (case–control) genetic study designs. The potential problems of chance (including the role of multiple comparisons), selection bias, confounders of the drug–genotype relationship, inappropriate control groups, population stratification, and genotyping error have all been adequately discussed in this text and elsewhere.[2,9,99–102] The need for accurate phenotyping and the role of diagnostic misclassification and regression to the mean in pharmacogenetic studies have been detailed above. However, the potential roles for inadequate sample size in pharmacogenetic studies cannot be emphasized enough.[103–105] Power and sample size calculations suggest that allele frequency and type of gene action can have a dramatic impact on trial sample sizes, in that under some conditions the required sample sizes are too large to be applicable in a costly clinical trial setting.[103] Many pharmacogenetic clinical trial studies are also 'spin-offs.' That is, studies are designed to be powered to detect genetic effects for the entire group, rather than for the treatment arm of interest. Finally, in keeping with the gene-by-environment interaction paradigm for pharmacogenetic studies, such studies focusing on interaction have generally been underpowered with inadequate sample sizes.[106,107] Indeed, it will likely be hard to detect a pharmacogenetic variant that occurs with a minor allele frequency of less than 0.15 without huge populations for study. Methods for calculation of adequate sample sizes for gene–environment interaction study design have been reviewed,[108] leading to the creation of a freely distributed software program, *Power*, by the National Cancer Institute to assist with the determination of sample sizes for pharmacogenetic investigation (http://dceg2.cancer.gov/POWER).

## Enhancing the pharmacogenetic association

Once an initial valid association has been established utilizing one of the study methods above and excluding the roles of chance, bias, and confounding, the relationship needs to be better defined, either through the demonstration of a functional change associated with the genetic change, through replication of the association results, or through demonstration of the impact that a variation has on the population of interest (explained phenotypic variance). The goal of the pursuit of an enhanced relationship is to determine the probability that the observed association is a causal one. In 1965, Sir Austin Bradford-Hill proposed a set of criteria to ascertain whether a relationship between a sickness and environmental factor is causal or just an association.[109] These criteria analyze the relationship's temporality, strength, dose-response, reversibility, consistency, biologic plausibility, specificity, and analogy. These criteria are applicable to pharmacogenetic associations, with a few caveats. In genetic studies, temporality is assumed, since an individual's genetic make-up is present at birth. Similarly, dose-response and reversibility may be noted only if an assumed additive model is correct.

The strength of the association is usually derived from the association study results, although haplotype analyses may be used to increase the strength, power, and proportion of the phenotypic variability in the drug response explained by genetics.[47,110,111] This proportion of the phenotypic variance is, by itself, a measure of the strength of a pharmacogenetic association. The stronger the genetic influence on the drug response, the more of that response is affected by genetic alterations. To analyze the population-based proportion of the variability of a given quantitative trait attributed to a genetic variant, several methods have been outlined.[112–115] Other methods estimating a proportion of variability in a trait for a given predictor[116] from non-genetics literature may also be applicable to pharmacogenetics. One intuitive method for estimating genetic proportion of explained phenotypic variance has been cited by Risch.[115] While this method assumes equality of variances for subjects with differing genotypes for the traits of interest, it is a reasonable method for relatively common SNPs in sample sizes appropriate for pharmacogenetic analyses. In brief, for a single locus $L$ with two variant alleles $A$ and $a$ with population frequencies $p$ and $q = 1 - p$ respectively, two important measures can be defined.[117] The first is termed displacement, denoted by $t$, which is the number of standard deviations difference between the mean values of the two homozygotes $AA$ and $aa$ (we assume, for simplicity, that the variance within genotype is the same for each genotype). There is an additional parameter, $d$, representing the mean value of heterozygotes $Aa$ relative to the two homozygotes. Thus, a value of $d = 1$ corresponds to equal means for genotypes $AA$ and $Aa$ ($A$ is dominant), whereas $d = 0$ corresponds to equal means for genotypes $Aa$ and $aa$ ($A$ is recessive). A value of $d = 0.5$ corresponds to the heterozygotes being exactly intermediate between the two homozygotes (as in an additive model). The second important measure of gene effect is the population variance attributable to segregation of the gene. This is given by $VG(L) = VA(L) + VD(L)$, where $VA(L) = 2pqt^2(p(1 - d) + qd)^2$ is the 'additive' genetic variance and $VD(L) = p^2q^2t^2(d - 0.5)^2$ is the 'dominance' genetic variance. The proportion of total variance attributable to locus $A$, which we denote $h_L^2$, is then given by $VG(L)/(1 + VG(L))$, assuming the variance within genotype to be 1.0. It is important to note that $h_L^2$ is a function of both displacement $t$ and the allele frequency $p$.

As an example, let us assume that we are studying a hypothetical SNP with alleles [A/T] and a minor allele frequency (T) of 0.30 that is felt relevant to the 6-month asthmatic response to inhaled corticosteroids. At the end of the 6 months, the mean improvement in $FEV_1$ for those homozygous AA is $5 \pm 10$ percent and for TT $15 \pm 10$ percent. The AT individuals demonstrate a 10 percent improvement. Thus, for the above calculations, $p = 0.7$, $q = 0.3$, $t = 1$, and $d = 0.5$. Completing the equations, $VA(L) = 0.105$, $VD(L) = 0$ (we assume a fully additive model), and $VG(L) = 0.105$. The calculated proportion explained phenotypic variance, $h_L^2$ is 0.095. That is, this one SNP would explain 9.5 percent of the overall variability in the response to inhaled corticosteroids in asthma. The calculation of the percent explained phenotypic variance can underscore the relative importance of any given polymorphism, or group of polymorphisms, and will be vitally important in the designation of diagnostic tests (e.g., a panel of SNPs) in pharmacogenetics.

In genetics, Bradford-Hill's 'consistency' criteria essentially refers to replication of the association. A major criticism of genetic association studies, including pharmacogenetic studies, has been the failure to provide demonstrable replication of findings.[118–120] Failure to replicate findings in genetic association studies has been attributed to variations in study design, including differing study populations and definitions of phenotypes.[119,120] Conversely, the replication of associations in populations with differing clinical characteristics supports both the validity and generalizability of the reported associations.

The final, and perhaps most important, causal criteria in genetic association studies is biologic plausibility. We mentioned previously that pharmacogenetic candidate genes are usually biologic candidates, specifically related to properties of the drug, its action, or its effect on a portion of the disease pathway. However, in genetics, biologic plausibility normally extends to functionality. That is, does the polymorphism associated with the drug response phenotype encode for a change in the gene's predicted protein, mRNA stability, splice site, transcriptional activity, or interactions with other genes? If not, is the SNP in LD with another functional SNP within the gene or a nearby gene? To address these questions, resequencing of the candidate genes initially associated with the drug response followed by a functional evaluation of the SNPs discovered has been recommended.[15,28,71]

Despite the above, in pharmacogenetics, the need to identify the functional variant can be debated. We mentioned above the benefits of haplotype analyses and the prospects for whole genome association studies. Both of these utilize linkage disequilibrium, rather than functional association, as the basis of their analyses. In haplotypes, limited diversity across a candidate gene or region allows for the generation of haplotype-tag SNPs. These haplotype-tag SNPs represent the sum of LD across the gene and may be analyzed for association with the drug response phenotype.[47,121,122] Whole genome association studies are based on linkage disequilibrium mapping across the genome.[94,95] SNP 'fingerprints' based on the SNP mapping characteristics are anticipated to be used to identify patients at greater risk of an ADR, or those patients with a greater chance of demonstrating a positive treatment response to a medicine.[97] Despite the advantages and promises of these association study techniques, basing associations consistently on LD patterns alone will still require extensive, ethnic-specific mapping efforts.[94] This variability in LD patterns between ethnic groups is well recognized and may extend to ethnic subgroups[123–126] and will need to be adequately addressed prior to the assignment of a 'predictive panel' to any individual. Until then, we recommend that any pharmacogenetic association with a candidate gene undergoes investigation to fulfil criteria for biologic plausibility.

## Summary

The ability to successfully conduct studies relating genetic variation to drug treatment response is contingent upon the understanding and application of appropriate phenotypic definitions, study designs, and genetic methodology. A list of common methodologic problems associated with pharmacogenetic studies is shown in Table 8.4. Careful attention to these methodologic issues will maximize one's ability to successfully address pharmacogenetic and other studies involving gene by environment interactions. Active investigation of epistatic interactions and polygenic effects, based upon relative amounts of phenotypic variation explained, will be required in order to facilitate the development of a true diagnostic test.

## DRUG RESPONSE PHARMACOGENETICS

In this section, we will highlight the features of the drug response class of pharmacogenetics, focusing on drug metabolism by the CYP system. We shall first review the CYPs as the largest class of drug metabolizing enzymes. Subsequently, we shall focus on drug metabolism of the anti-coagulant drug, warfarin, followed by a discussion of the pharmacogenetics of smoking cessation, and conclude

**Table 8.4**   *Common methodological problems in pharmacogenetic studies[a]*

| Problem | Potential solution |
|---------|-------------------|
| Phenotypic misclassification | Carefully define a readily measured phenotype |
| | Use a central laboratory or standardized measurement techniques |
| | Verify with repeat measurements for quality control |
| Regression to the mean | Account for baseline measurement in the analytic phase |
| | Evaluate potential for regression to the mean by use of the intraclass correlation |
| Small sample size | Power the study design based upon the assumption of an interaction term, rather than upon a simple genetic effect |
| | Optimize power through the use of quantitative phenotypes, where appropriate and possible |
| | If a functional locus is not known, consider increased power by utilizing haplotypic analyses |
| Replication not demonstrated | Consider any reported finding, even those involving functional SNPs, as preliminary until replication studies are performed |
| | Replication in several different populations enhances generalizability |
| Function not demonstrated | Select only biologically relevant candidate genes |
| | Once association is identified, full resequencing of gene is carried out, followed by molecular studies |
| | Acknowledge that an association may represent linkage disequilibrium with another nearby gene |

[a]Note: The potential problems associated with all genetic case–control studies, such as population stratification, genetic heterogeneity, confounding, and multiple comparisons are also equally relevant to pharmacogenetic studies. The items presented may be especially problematic in pharmacogenetic studies.

with an overview and example of the pharmacogenetics of lung cancer therapeutics.

## CYP metabolism

The CYPs are members of a superfamily of oxidative enzymes, sometimes also referred to as microsomal oxidative enzymes. This family forms the major system for oxidative metabolism of therapeutic substances.[41] Sequencing of the human genome revealed 58 different human CYP genes.[1] Of these, the majority of the CYP genes encoding for enzymes active in xenobiotic metabolism are polymorphic. Due to the importance of these genes, a website that is continuously updated for CYP polymorphisms has been created (www.imm.ki.se/CYP-alleles).[1] The frequency of each of these polymorphisms varies by ethnic background. The clinically most important polymorphisms variations in hepatic CYPs are seen in the *CYP2C9*, *CYP2D6*, and *CYP3A4* genes. These genes encode for approximately 60–70 percent of all phase I dependent metabolism of available medications. A visual example of how variation in the CYP genes might affect therapeutic efficacy and potential for side effects is shown in Fig. 8.3.

## Warfarin pharmacogenetics

The incidence of acute pulmonary embolism in the USA is approximately 200 000 cases per year.[127] Warfarin is the most commonly used oral anticoagulant in North America and Asia.[128] It is a vitamin K antagonist that is used for the long-term treatment of patients with venous thromboembolic disease, including pulmonary embolism. In these patients, warfarin is usually started within 24 hours after diagnosis, with a target international normalized ratio (INR) of 2.0–3.0. The INR is a ratio of the time required for a patient's blood to coagulate relative to a standardized coagulation time. Values higher than 3.0 are associated with increased bleeding risk, but no greater efficacy.[129] Patient to patient variability in warfarin requirements and responsiveness is common, necessitating regular monitoring of the INR. It is clear that many drugs, including antibiotics, can interact with warfarin, altering INR levels.[128] Patients with idiopathic thromboembolic disease are treated for 3–6 months, and those with underlying malignancies or with recurrent thromboembolism may be treated indefinitely. The major complication of warfarin therapy remains risk of bleeding. Overall, the bleeding rate is 7.6–16.5 per hundred patient-years, while major or life-threatening bleeds occur at a rate of 1.3–2.7 per hundred patient-years.[130–132]

Warfarin is a racemic mixture of R- and S-enantiomers. The S-enantiomer of warfarin is approximately three times as potent as the R-enantiomer and is metabolized by *CYP2C9*, with subsequent renal elimination of the inactive hydroxyl-metabolites.[133–135] The warfarin dose required to achieve a target INR may vary by as much as 120-fold between individuals.[136,137] Given the recognized variability in this gene, and the decreased in vitro activity of the gene associated with its major polymorphic variants, studies have been undertaken to assess the relevance of *CYP2C9* polymorphisms to response to warfarin, as manifested by the INR and by risk of bleeding complications.

*CYP2C9* is the principal *CYP2C* in the human liver and catalyzes oxidative metabolism of many common drugs, including warfarin, phenytoin, losartan, non-steroidal anti-inflammatory agents (e.g., ibuprofen), and oral hypoglycemic agents (e.g., glyburide).[9,40,138,139] The genomic cluster of human *CYP2C* genes spans about 500 kb on

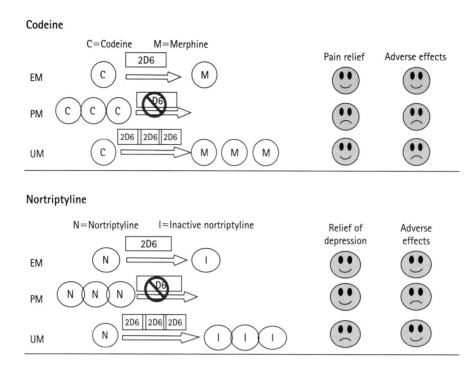

**Figure 8.3** *Effect of variation in CYP2D6 metabolism with clinical response to two therapeutic agents. Based upon genetic make-up and the resultant ability to metabolize therapeutic agents, individuals can be classified as extensive (normal) metabolizers (EM), poor metabolizers (PM), or ultrarapid metabolizers (UM). Since codeine is metabolized into an active agent (morphine), poor metabolizers may require increased dosing for a given therapeutic effect, while ultrarapid metabolizers may build up excessive levels of morphine, leading to adverse sequelae. In the lower panel, nortriptyline is the active therapeutic agent and is metabolized to an inactive form. In this case, poor metabolism leads to adequate therapy but an increased incidence of side effects, while extensive metabolizers may require increased dosing for therapeutic effect. (From PharmGKB, http://www.pharmgkb.org/resources/education/cyp2d6.jsp)*

chromosome 10q24.[140] The *CYP2C9* gene product is approximately a 55.6-kDa protein of 490 amino acids.[9] A common characteristic of the drugs catalyzed by *CYP2C9* is the distance of approximately 8 Å between the anionic group and the oxidized carbon moiety.[141,142] Many of these agents have a narrow therapeutic window and are frequently associated with side effects. To date, 11 functional polymorphisms have been identified (http://www.imm.ki.se/CYPalleles/cyp2c9.htm). The best characterized of the variant alleles are the *CYP2C9*2* allele (allele frequency of about 10 percent in Caucasians), a [C/T] at cDNA position 416 which encodes for a replacement of arginine by cysteine at amino acid residue 144 and *CYP2C9*3* (allele frequency of about 7 percent in Caucasians), an [A/C] at cDNA position 1061 which encodes for a replacement of isoleucine by leucine at residue 359. In vitro studies of both of these alleles demonstrate impaired enzymatic activity resulting in significantly reduced intrinsic clearance rates compared to the wildtype allele. The *CYP2C9*2* protein product expressed in vitro demonstrates about 12 percent of the wild-type protein activity,[133] whereas the *CYP2C9*3* protein product demonstrates only about 5 percent of the wildtype protein activity in vitro.[143,144]

Furuya et al.[145] noted an association between *CYP2C9* genotype and dose requirement of warfarin. They demonstrated, in 94 Caucasians, that subjects heterozygous for the *CYP2C9*2* allele (*CYP2C9*2/CYP2C9*1*) required a 20 percent reduction in warfarin dose (3.8 versus 4.7 mg/day) to achieve a therapeutic INR in the range of 2.0–4.0. Moreover, 90 percent of subjects requiring the lowest dosage to achieve this INR were heterozygous *CYP2C9*2/ CYP2C9*1*. No evaluation of the *CYP2C9*3* allele was performed.

In a second study[146] of Caucasians with a targeted INR of 2.0–3.0 on warfarin, 81 percent of the 31 subjects in the low dosage extreme (≤1.5 mg/day) had at least one *CYP2C9*2* or *CYP2C9*3* allele compared to only 40 percent of 100 individuals in a community-based control group not on warfarin. The calculated odds ratio for at least one of these *CYP2C9* variants was 6.21 (95 percent CI: 2.48–15.6). Moreover, compared to 52 randomly selected anticoagulation clinic controls, the patients in the low dosage group were significantly more likely to have an initial INR peak outside the therapeutic upper limits (>4.0) (OR 5.97, 95 percent CI: 2.26–15.82) and to have major bleeding complications during induction of therapy (rate ratio 3.68, 95 percent CI: 1.43–9.50). Margaglione et al.[147] confirmed these findings in 180 Caucasians on warfarin therapy, noting significantly decreased dosing requirements for those individuals with at least one

CYP2C9*2 or CYP2C9*3 allele. These patients also demonstrated a significantly higher risk of bleeding complications (OR: 2.57, 95 percent CI: 1.16–5.73).

Taube et al.[148] evaluated a much larger cohort of patients to verify the above findings and to evaluate risk of bleeding over the long term. These patients had a median duration of treatment of 2.4 years and were genotyped for the CYP2C9*1, CYP2C9*2, and CYP2C9*3 alleles. In evaluating the 561 patients meeting a target INR of 2.5, the presence of any variant allele was significantly related to genotype (P = 0.001). The mean maintenance doses of warfarin in patients with a variant allele averaged 61–86 percent of those patients homozygous for the wildtype CYP2C9*1 allele. The odds ratio for the CYP2C9*2 allele in patients with maintenance dose requirements ≤1.5 mg/day was 5.42 (95 percent CI: 1.68–17.4). While the mean dose of those heterozygous for the CYP2C9*3 allele was less than that of those heterozygous for the CYP2C9*2 and for the wildtype, (mean dose of 3.97, 4.31, and 5.01 mg/day, respectively), these individuals were not more likely to be in the low dose group (OR1.49, 95 percent CI: 0.17–13.0). There was no association of genotype with risk of high INRs (>8.0) in this study of patients on stable doses of anticoagulant. It has been suggested that the reason for the differences in bleeding risk across these studies might be related to variability in the pharmacodynamic response to warfarin, which may be under different genetic influences.[135] One alternative explanation is that the study designs are sufficiently different and that there may be a risk for bleeding associated with genotype during the induction phase, but not the maintenance phase of anticoagulant therapy.

While the above studies have all been performed in Caucasians, the pharmacogenetics of warfarin therapy has also been studied in two small studies of Japanese subjects.[149,150] The CYP2C9*2 allele has not been detected in Asians and the CYP2C9*3 allele has a much lower minor allele frequency in the Japanese (approximately 2 percent).[135] Nonetheless, these studies demonstrated an in vitro reduction of 63–66 percent and 90 percent in the clearance of the S-enantiomer of warfarin associated with the presence of a CYP2C9*3 allele compared to those homozygous for the wildtype CYP2C9*1 allele.[149,150] The median warfarin dosing requirement was reduced by 40 percent (1.75 mg/day versus 3 mg/day) with the presence of the heterozygous CYP2C9*1/CYP2C9*3 genotype and by 90 percent (to 0.4 mg/day) in the single individual homozygous for the CYP2C9*3 allele.[135]

## The pharmacogenetics of smoking cessation

Cigarette smoking is the single most preventable cause of disease and death in the USA.[151,152] It is well established that smoking cessation has substantial immediate and long-term health benefits, regardless of the age or relative health of the individual.[153] As discussed in Chapter 10, there is evolving evidence that smoking behavior and response to pharmacologic therapy designed to assist with smoking cessation may be influenced by genetics. Nicotine as a drug is known to exert its addictive effects through activation of the mesolimbic dopaminergic pathway.[154–156] Since nicotine is metabolized to cotinine by CYP2D6, it was hypothesized a decade ago that nicotine dependence might be modified by variation in this enzyme.[157] Additionally, CYP2D6 also catalyzes the conversion of tyramine to dopamine;[158] increased levels of dopamine available for the dopaminergic receptors would then be associated with decreased nicotine binding, forming another mechanism by which variation in CYP2D6 might influence smoking behavior. As with many drug metabolizing enzymes, studies focusing on CYP2D6 have combined genetic variations into groups, focusing on the variant ability to metabolize compared to the wild type. Homozygotes for the CYP2D6*5, CYP2D6*4, and CYP2D6*3 alleles are associated with poor metabolism,[159] whereas those for CYP2D6*2 and CYP2D6*1 are associated with ultrarapid metabolism.[160] Overall, studies generally support the hypothesis that level of metabolism correlates with addiction to cigarettes, with rapid metabolizers more likely to become nicotine dependent than slow metabolizers.[161–164] For instance, Saarikoski et al.[163] examined 976 individuals (302 never smokers, 383 variable smokers, and 292 heavy smokers). The odds ratio for the presence of an ultrarapid CYP2D6 metabolism phenotype in heavy smokers versus never smokers was 4.2 (95 percent CI: 1.8–9.8).

Recently, there has also been interest in how drug metabolism genetics might affect pharmacologic efforts at smoking cessation. The most common pharmacologic interventions for smoking cessation are alternative forms of nicotine replacement, including gums, inhalational sprays, lozenges, and transdermal patches.[165] It is reasonable to hypothesize, then, that CYP2D6 metabolism could have a direct association with the ability to respond to nicotine replacement therapy, with ultra-rapid metabolizers having the greatest therapeutic need and, therefore, the least likelihood of responding to this form of treatment. Unfortunately, this hypothesis has not yet been tested.

Bupropion is an antidepressant that inhibits reuptake of dopamine, noradrenaline, and serotonin in the central nervous system, is a noncompetitive nicotine receptor antagonist, and at high concentrations inhibits the firing of noradrenergic neurons in the locus caeruleus.[166] It is not clear which of these effects accounts for the antismoking activity of the drug, but inhibition of the reductions in levels of dopamine and noradrenaline levels in the central nervous system that occur in nicotine withdrawal is likely to be important. In double-blind, placebo-controlled trials of bupropion versus placebo, the 1-year rates of smoking abstinence were significantly greater for individuals who took bupropion than for placebo.[167,168] However, the majority of individuals for all therapies relapsed. Bupropion is metabolized by CYP2B6.[169,170] A CYP2B6 polymorphism (1459C > T) and its association with success of bupropion therapy for smoking cessation, has been evaluated. This SNP has been associated with decreased *CYP2B6* protein expression.[171] Lerman et al.[172] examined the 1459C > T variant in a trial of 197 subjects taking bupropion along with 229 placebo controls. Overall, the minor allele (lower activity variant) was associated with less abstinence at the end of therapy than the wild type variant (OR 1.56, 95 percent CI: 1.01–2.41 for relapse). At the end of 6 months, the men, but not women, harboring the variant allele had a significantly higher relapse rate in those taking bupropion.

## Cancer pharmacogenetics

No discussion of drug response pharmacogenetics in general, and drug metabolizing enzymes in specific, would be complete without mentioning the pharmacogenetics of cancer therapeutics. Administration of 'standard' doses of chemotherapy to patients with inherited deficiencies in enzymes responsible for their metabolism and disposition can result in marked toxicity, which at times can be lethal. Conversely, patients who have increased enzymatic activity may be at risk for underdosing resulting in treatment failure. Traditionally, anticancer drug doses for a given individual are determined by the use of body surface area measurements and weight-based dosing.[173] However, dosing in this manner may not reliably account for the variability in clearance of most chemotherapeutic drugs.[174]

A number of excellent reviews of the pharmacogenetics of cancer therapeutics have recently been published.[175–182] With regards to respiratory genetics, an extensive review of pharmacogenetics of lung cancer was recently published,[183] as well as several reviews focusing on the application of genomic technologies to the therapy of lung cancer.[184,185] To fully elucidate all of the described genetic variants affecting the disposition of agents utilized in lung cancer chemotherapy is beyond the scope of this chapter. However, an illustrative example follows.

Irinotecan is a topoisomerase I inhibitor that has been demonstrated to have activity against a variety of malignancies[186–188] including both non-small cell[189–191] and small cell[192–196] carcinoma of the lung. Irinotecan is a prodrug that is metabolized to the active 7-ethyl-10-hydroxycamptothecin (SN-38).[197] SN-38 is primarily eliminated via glucuronidation to the inactive SN-38 glucuronide[198] (SN-38G). Reduction in the glucuronidation of SN-38 is associated with an increase in the two severe toxicities associated with irinotecan, diarrhea and neutropenia.[197,199,200]

Uridine diphosphate glucuronosyltransferases are microsomal enzymes that catalyze glucuronidation of a wide number of substrates.[201] SN-38 glucuronidation is catalyzed by the polymorphic uridine diphosphate glucuronosyltransferase 1A1 (*UGT1A1*). *UGT1A1* has over 30 known genetic variants. Activity of the enzyme appears to be inversely related to the number of dinucleotide (TA) repeats in the promoter region; compared to the wildtype (TA)$_6$ the homozygous (TA)$_7$ (*UGT1A1\*28*) leads to a 70 percent reduction in *UGT1A1* gene expression.[202–204] In a retrospective study of 118 patients taking irinotecan,[205] 26 patients were noted to have severe toxicity, defined as severe neutropenia and/or diarrhea. The frequency of any *UGT1A1\*28* variant was 3.5 times higher in patients with severe toxicity compared to those without (odds ratio, 7.23; 95 percent confidence interval, 2.52–22.3, $P < 0.001$). These investigators also noted that all three individuals heterozygous for the *UGT1A1\*27* variant demonstrated toxicity.

In a prospective study of irinotecan toxicity, *UGT1A1\*28* carriers demonstrated lower SN-38G/SN-38 AUC ratios compared to *UGT1A1\*1* subjects. Since SN-38 AUC was inversely related to absolute neutrophil count nadir ($r = -0.81$, $P < 0.001$), severe neutropenia was reported in a greater number of *UGT1A1\*28* subjects compared to *UGT1A1\*1* ($P = 0.04$).[200] Subsequent enrolment of 60 patients confirmed that, of the 28 patients homozygous for the *UGT1A1\*1* allele, none experienced grade 4 neutropenia, whereas three of the six patients homozygous for the variant *UGT1A1\*28* did ($P < 0.001$).[197,206] Thus, genetic variation leading to decreased metabolism of the active form of irinotecan has been consistently associated with increased toxicity due to the drug. Whether dosing guidelines should be altered in relationship to *UGT1A1\*28* status or other genetic variation has yet to be determined.

## TARGET RESPONSE PHARMACOGENETICS

In this section, we focus on the features of the target response class of pharmacogenetics, concentrating on examples drawn from three therapeutic pathways in the management of asthma.

### The pharmacogenetics of asthma

Asthma is a genetically complex syndrome affecting over 155 million individuals in the developed world.[207] In evaluating asthma therapy response, measures of lung function, as manifested by the forced expiratory volume in the first second (FEV$_1$), and of airway responsiveness, as measured by the provocative concentration of methacholine causing a 20 percent decrement in FEV$_1$ (PC$_{20}$) are commonly used. However, there is large inter-individual variation in the FEV$_1$ and PC$_{20}$ responses to asthma treatment[208,209] (Fig. 8.2). Since the intra-individual response to inhaled corticosteroid treatment in patients with asthma is highly repeatable[11] and since both FEV$_1$ and PC$_{20}$ are heritable traits,[210,211] a genetic basis for the heterogeneity of this therapeutic response is plausible.

Given that the variation in the response to therapy may largely be due to genetic causes, the field of asthma is well suited to pharmacogenetic investigations. Prior investigations in the field of asthma pharmacogenetics have focused on $\beta_2$-agonists, leukotriene inhibitors, and corticosteroid pathways. Altogether, the data summarized below provide evolving evidence that response to asthma therapy is highly variable between individuals with asthma, and genetic differences can help to predict the response to treatment in asthma.

## THE $\beta_2$-ADRENERGIC RECEPTOR PATHWAY

Beta-adrenergic receptor agonists are the most commonly used class of medication in the treatment of asthma worldwide.[212] From a pharmacogenetics perspective, inter-individual variability in the response to these agents has been recognized for over 60 years. For instance, the 1942 edition of Osler's *Principles and Practice of Medicine* noted, on the treatment of asthma, 'Hypodermics of epinephrine, Mv to xv (0.3 to 1 cc) of a 1:1000 solution or of atropine, gr. 1/100 (0.6 mgm.), may give prompt relief, but individual cases vary greatly'.[213]

In the $\beta_2$-agonist pathway, two nonsynonymous SNPs encoding for amino acid changes from arginine to glycine at position 16 (Arg16 $\rightarrow$ Gly) and from glutamic acid to glutamine at position 27 (Glu27 $\rightarrow$ Gln) of the $\beta_2$-adrenergic receptor gene (*ADRB2*) have been well characterized.[214] These SNPs are common, with reported allele frequencies between 40–50 percent in large cohort studies. The pharmacogenetic effects of the $\beta_2$AR 16 and 27 loci have been examined in six trials. The six studies differ substantially from one another with respect to study design, chemical nature of agonist assessed, and outcome measurement employed.[212] Not surprisingly, there is marked inconsistency in results between trials. Two studies assessed responsiveness with respect to the $\beta_2$-agonist's ability to attenuate methacholine-induced constrictor responses ($\beta_2$-agonist bronchoprotection). The two studies, both of small sample size, produced conflicting results: one showed a correlation between genotype and degree of bronchoconstriction attenuation,[215] while the second did not.[216] A third trial examining the long-term use of fenoterol showed no difference in bronchodilator response (change in FEV$_1$ from baseline) between genotype groups.[217]

In contrast to the previous studies, three larger studies have demonstrated important effects of these variants. In a longitudinal birth cohort of 269 children from Tucson, Arizona, Martinez et al.[218] examined the change in FEV$_1$ at 30 min following albuterol administration (180 $\mu$g). 39.7 percent of subjects were asthmatic and only 11.5 percent were regular $\beta_2$-agonist users. A linear relationship between Arg16 allele number and prevalence of response to $\beta_2$-agonist was noted. After adjustment for asthma and wheeze, subjects who were Arg16 homozygotes were 5.3 times more likely to show a bronchodilator response than Gly16 homozygotes (CI: 1.6–17.7). Heterozygotes showed intermediate response. Of note, the Arg16 allele was in strong LD with the Gln27 allele. Similar findings were demonstrated

by Lima et al. who assessed response in FEV$_1$ to an oral albuterol challenge. Bronchodilator responses were higher (18 percent versus 4.9 percent, $P < 0.03$) and more rapid among Arg16 homozygotes as compared to Gly16 homozygotes and heterozygotes.[219] In a study of molecular haplotypes of the $\beta_2$-adrenergic receptor gene, acute bronchodilator response to inhaled albuterol was approximately twice as high in individuals homozygous for the most common haplotype when compared to those homozygous for the second most common haplotype ($P = 0.046$).[110] Importantly, haplotypic analysis was more powerful in detecting associations in this population compared to single SNP analyses.[110] However, the haplotype containing the Arg16 allele actually exhibited lower albuterol responsiveness compared to those that did not. From these data, along with in vitro work, it appears that genetic variation at the $\beta_2$AR locus does influence beta-agonist response, but the precise relationship between genotype, haplotype and acute $\beta$-agonist response remains poorly understood.

A more consistent finding that appears to have important clinical implications is the relationship between $\beta_2$AR genotype and the development of residual bronchoconstriction following the acute bronchodilation caused by a $\beta$-agonist. The Asthma Clinical Research Network (ACRN) was established to address the safety of regular beta-agonist use in the treatment of asthma. In this multicentered trial, 255 asthmatics of mild severity were randomized to either regular (180 $\mu$g qid) or as-needed albuterol use and were assessed over a 16-week period for evidence of physiological deterioration (as measured by fall in AM peak expiratory flow rate (PEFR)). No difference in PEFR variation was observed between treatment groups.[220] However, a subset of subjects in the regular albuterol group was noted to have a significant decline in pulmonary function over the course of the trial. Arg16 homozygotes significantly decreased their peak expiratory flow rates with regular utilization of albuterol therapy, compared to both Arg16 homozygotes receiving prn (as needed) albuterol and Gly16 homozygotes in either treatment group.[221,222] The difference in evening peak flow rates between these groups was $31.6 \pm 10.2$ l/min comparing Arg16 homozygous regular users versus. Gly16 homozygous regular users ($P = 0.002$) and $31.1 \pm 13.0$ l/min versus the Arg16 homozygous prn group ($P = 0.02$).[221] Similar differences in morning peak flow rates were noted (Fig. 8.4). This may be the result of basal downregulation of Gly16 homozygotes.[223] Several studies have demonstrated that falls in PEFR similar to that observed in the ACRN are associated with adverse outcome.[224,225] Further support for a correlation between Arg16 and increased in vivo $\beta_2$AR desensitization was recently provided in a study examining the vascular response to intravenous $\beta_2$-agonist exposure. In this study of 26 healthy subjects, Arg16 homozygotes demonstrated almost complete physiological desensitization within 90 min of constant infusion of isoproterenol, as compared to individuals with

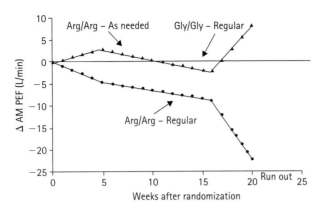

**Figure 8.4**  *Response to chronic beta-agonist therapy in asthma, stratified by ADRB2 genotype. Regular use of albuterol results in decrements in peak flow rates in asthmatics, when compared to as-needed therapy, but only in those homozygous for arginine at position 16 of the $\beta_2$-adrenergic receptor protein (from Israel et al.[221]).*

homozygous Gly16 receptors, who showed only 50 percent desensitization as late as 120 min ($P = 0.006$).[226] Overall, the weight of the evidence suggests that the Arg16 allele is an important determinant of in vivo $\beta_2$AR desensitization.

To specifically address the impact of genotype on the rate of adverse outcome with regular $\beta_2$-agonist use, Taylor performed a post-hoc analysis of a clinical trial comparing the efficacy of short- and long-acting beta-agonists in the management of asthma.[227] Using a three-way crossover design, 157 patients with mild to moderately severe asthma were randomized to receive either salbutamol 400 μg qid, salmeterol 50 μg bid or placebo for 24 weeks each. Among Arg16 homozygotes, the rate of major asthma exacerbation was significantly higher with regular salbutamol use (1.9 major events per year) as compared to placebo (0.8 exacerbations per year) ($P = 0.005$). This association was not observed in other genotype groups. Moreover, during regular salbutamol use, the total exacerbation rate (major and minor) was higher among Arg16 homozygotes (3.57) compared to Gly16 homozygotes (1.19) and heterozygotes (0.72) ($P = 0.033$ and $P = 0.003$, respectively). Genotype also had a significant impact on response to long-acting beta-agonist use. The total number of exacerbations with salmeterol was reduced among Gly16 homozygotes (0.34 versus 1.49 for placebo, $P < 0.003$) and heterozygous subjects (0.49 versus 1.41, $P < 0.04$), but not in the Arg16 group (0.64 versus 1.91, $P = 0.16$). Need for corticosteroids was also significantly greater among Arg16 individuals ($P = 0.02$).

Recently, additional data further corroborates the association of the Arg16Gly polymorphism in its relationship to lung function. In the first prospective, genotype-stratified study of the effect of polymorphisms of the *ADRB2* gene on treatment related changes in lung function, Israel et al.[228] matched asthmatic individuals homozygous Arg/Arg ($n = 37$) at position 16 to those Gly/Gly ($n = 41$), by level of FEV$_1$. The investigators of this trial (named BARGE for the β-Agonist Response by Genotype) then randomized all of the individuals in a double-blind, cross-over study of regularly scheduled albuterol therapy (four times daily) versus placebo over two 16-week periods with an intervening 8 week wash-out period. The major findings somewhat parallel those that they had previously reported for clinical trials genotyped retrospectively. Those Arg/Arg had lower morning peak flow rates during regularly scheduled treatment versus placebo ($-10$ L/min, $P = 0.02$), while those Gly/Gly had higher rates during those times (14 L/min, $P = 0.02$). The Arg/Arg minus Gly/Gly difference was very significant for morning peak flow ($-24$ L/min, $P = 0.0003$) and also reported to be significantly different while on treatment in regards to evening peak flow, FEV$_1$, morning symptom score, and need for rescue medication.

The accompanying editorial to this manuscript pointed out three interesting data issues whose significance remains to be determined.[229] First, the improvement in the morning peak flow with regularly scheduled albuterol in the Gly/Gly group continued during the washout period. Interestingly, there was an improvement in peak flow during the washout for those homozygous for Gly/Gly at position 16 in a previous study as well.[221] Next, it was noted that no deterioration of the Arg/Arg individuals in BARGE occurred while on regularly scheduled albuterol.[229] Instead, increases on placebo occurred after the run-in or wash-out periods. This is distinct from previously reported findings.[221] Finally, the editorial noted that the Arg/Arg group experienced a large increase in peak flow during the initial run-in period, despite averaging only one puff of β-agonist daily prior to the run-in.[229] Clearly, these findings need to be replicated. The possibility that such a common variant may portend to basal deterioration in the peak flow rates of asthmatics given even minimal exposure to β-agonist medications, may suggest huge implications. However, limitations not mentioned in the editorial including the relatively small sample size, the use of multi-ethnic populations without being able to investigate epistatic or haplotypic interactions, and the actual very small percent of the phenotypic variance (in this case morning peak flow interindividual variability) explained would argue against making too large generalizations from this data at this early time.

In summary, studies on the $\beta_2$AR gene provide compelling evidence that the gene is associated with bronchodilator response. Additionally, individuals homozygous for Arg16 demonstrate significant $\beta_2$AR downregulation and these individuals (approximately 15 percent of the population) are at risk of asthma deterioration with regular use of $\beta_2$-agonists. This response does not appear to be predictable from currently available clinical or physiological parameters, and suggests that $\beta_2$AR genotyping may have an important role in future clinical practice. Further work, including better characterization of the other genes involved in the β-agonist pathway and their association with clinical outcomes, is underway.

## THE LEUKOTRIENE ANTAGONIST PATHWAY

Leukotrienes are a family of eicosatetraenoic acids with profound effects on airway biology.[230,231] The cysteinyl-leukotrienes ($LTC_4$, $LTD_4$, $LTE_4$) are among the most potent bronchoconstrictors ever identified,[232] and their effects are mediated by binding to the $Cys-LT_1$ receptor.[233] $LTB_4$ is not a bronchoconstrictor but a chemotactic agent that attracts neutrophils, eosinophils, and monocytes.[234] Asthmatics have increased levels of $LTB_4$ and cysteinyl-leukotrienes in their airways[235] and anti-leukotriene therapy has been associated with improvement in various types of asthma.[236] Currently, two classes of anti-leukotriene drugs have been approved for asthma treatment, the leukotriene $Cys-LT_1$ receptor antagonists (e.g., pranlukast, zafirlukast, and montelukast) and the 5-lipoxygenase (5-LO) inhibitor (zileuton). Despite the overall improvement versus placebo with anti-leukotriene drugs, the inter-individual response is highly variable;[209] genetic factors may be responsible for some of this heterogeneity.[11]

Expression of 5-LO protein is regulated at a number of levels.[237] At the transcriptional level, binding of different transcription factors to specific consensus binding sites in the 5-LO gene (ALOX5) promoter region has been shown to be important for expression in vitro. Two transcription factors, Sp1 and early growth response factor-1 (Egr-1), bind to the promoter in a series of tandem consensus sites located in a G + C-rich core promoter region between −179 to −56 bp relative to the transcriptional start site.[238] The Sp1 binding sites share the same DNA sequence as the Egr-1 binding sites, and Egr-1 can displace Sp1 from this promoter region and increase transcription above basal levels by recruiting the transcriptional coactivator CREB-binding protein (CBP).[239] A family of ALOX5 polymorphisms has been identified in this region that consists of a deletion of one or two Egr-1-GGGCGG- consensus binding sites or the addition of one of these sites.[240] Approximately 78 percent of subjects have the wildtype allele at this microsatellite locus. Lack of the wildtype allele has been associated with decrements in $FEV_1$ upon receipt of leukotriene antagonists in two different studies.[105,241,242] In a clinical drug trial of the zileuton-like 5-lipoxygenase inhibitor, ABT-761, asthmatics with at least one wildtype allele had an average improvement in their $FEV_1$ of 19 percent, while patients with any two of the mutant alleles had an average decrement in their $FEV_1$ of 1 percent (Fig. 8.5).[242] Data demonstrating replication of these findings in a study of asthmatics on zafirlukast has been published in abstract form.[241] A second leukotriene pathway pharmacogenetic locus has been described. A transversion SNP (A to C) at position −444

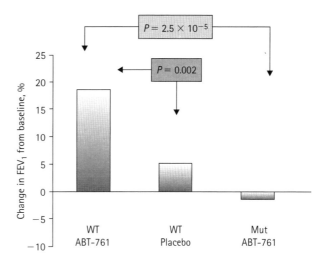

**Figure 8.5** *Response to leukotriene antagonist therapy in asthma, stratified by presence or absence of 5-LO promoter wildtype tandem repeat. Those individuals with any copies of the wildtype (five repeats) exhibit significant response to therapy with leukotriene antagonists, while those with two variant forms of the promoter do not respond to this class of therapy. (from Drazen et al.)[242]*

in the $LTC_4$ synthase gene (LTC4S) promoter results in the creation of an activator protein binding site that may be associated with enhanced production of cysteinyl-leukotrienes.[243] In a small case–control study, the presence of any C allele ($n = 13$) at this polymorphic site was associated with an increased $FEV_1$ response to zafirlukast therapy compared to those asthmatic individuals homozygous for the A allele ($n = 10$).[243] Of interest, Sanak et al.[244] have shown that this polymorphism may be associated with the diagnosis of aspirin-induced asthma; this may represent the first example of the idiosyncratic category of pharmacogenetic response to asthma therapy.

## THE CORTICOSTEROID PATHWAY

Inhaled corticosteroids are effective and commonly used drugs for the chronic treatment of asthma but may be associated with serious adverse effects.[245–251] While many of the major benefits are achieved within the first 2 weeks of therapy, some patients require more than a year of treatment before the therapeutic response plateaus.[252] There is large inter-individual variation in the treatment response to each of the major classes of asthma medications,[209,253] including corticosteroids. Twenty-two percent of individuals in one study of asthmatics taking inhaled beclomethasone had decrements in their forced expiratory volume at 1 second ($FEV_1$)[209] after 12 weeks of therapy, while in a second study 38 percent of patients randomized to either budesonide or fluticasone demonstrated $FEV_1$ improvements of under 5 percent over the course of 24 weeks.[253] As noted previously, since the intra-individual response to inhaled corticosteroid treatment in patients with asthma is highly repeatable,[11] it is reasonable to postulate a genetic difference for the response to inhaled corticosteroids in asthma.

Glucocorticoid resistance, defined in asthma as the failure to improve baseline morning pre-bronchodilator $FEV_1$ values by more than 15 percent after 7–14 days of 20 mg oral prednisone twice daily,[254] is prevalent in approximately 25 percent of patients with difficult to control asthma.[255] One study evaluating the role of interleukin-4 (*IL-4*) in glucocorticoid resistant asthma performed genotyping of the *IL4* C-589T SNP in case–control fashion, comparing 24 patients with glucocorticoid-resistant asthma to 682 glucocorticoid sensitive asthmatics.[256] The *IL4* C-589T SNP is associated with increased *IL4* gene transcription.[257] Overexpression of the T allele was significantly associated with glucocorticoid resistant asthma ($P = 0.009$).

A number of family and twin studies have demonstrated consistent evidence that endogenous levels of glucocorticoids, usually measured as plasma cortisol levels at certain times of the day, are heritable.[258–264] In turn, decrements in endogenous plasma cortisol levels at night[265–267] and during periods of stress[268] have been associated with nocturnal and stress-related asthma, respectively. Furthermore, cortisol levels in nocturnal asthma may be partially resistant to the effects of corticotropin.[265] In adults, subjects with morning cortisol levels one standard deviation below normal have been associated with longitudinal decrements in $FEV_1$ comparable to the effects of smoking, when compared to individuals with morning cortisol levels one standard deviation above normal.[269] Overall, these studies suggest a potential role for genetic factors regulating endogenous cortisol production in the pathogenesis and long-term treatment response of asthma.

In a study of 14 candidate genes selected for their biologic relevance to the entire corticosteroid pathway, including synthesis, binding, and metabolism, we found a significant association between 8-week response to inhaled steroids and SNPs from the corticotropin releasing hormone receptor 1 (*CRHR1*) gene in adult asthmatics.[270] *CRHR1* was also significantly associated with 8-week response to inhaled steroids in a clinical trial of children with asthma. Moreover, one particular SNP and one specific haplotype (utilizing haplotype-tag SNPs[122]) in the *CRHR1* gene that predicted good response to inhaled steroids in both populations was noted. The SNP, rs242941 (minor allele frequency approximately 30 percent) was associated with positive treatment response in both the adult study and the pediatric study, CAMP ($P = 0.025$ and $0.006$, respectively). In the adult study, the mean percent change in $FEV_1$ for those homozygous for the minor allele was $13.28 \pm 3.11$, compared to $5.49 \pm 1.40$ for those homozygous for the wildtype allele. Similarly, in CAMP, the percent change was $17.80 \pm 6.77$ versus $7.57 \pm 1.50$ for the variant and wildtype homozygotes, respectively. In CAMP, evaluation of the placebo arm revealed no association of rs242941 or any of

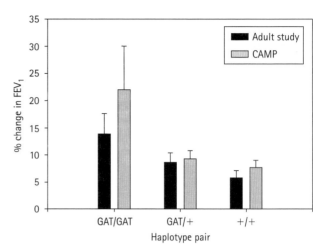

**Figure 8.6**   *Eight-week response to inhaled corticosteroids, stratified by* CRHR1 *GAT haplotype status in the adult study and CAMP. Utilizing the htSNPs rs1876828, rs242939, and rs242941, the mean* $FEV_1$ *improvement in an adult and a pediatric population was 2–3 times as great for those imputed with the GAT/GAT homozygous haplotype compared to those homozygous for two non-GAT haplotypes. Improvement in those heterozygous for the GAT haplotype was intermediate between the two groups, suggesting an additive effect. Mean values* $\pm$ *SEM are shown (from Tantisira et al.[270]).*

the other genotyped SNPs with change in lung function. Moreover, while inhaled corticosteroid usage was associated with improved $FEV_1$ at 8 weeks ($P < 0.001$), variation in rs242941 significantly enhanced the improvement in lung function associated with this form of therapy (interaction $P = 0.02$).

The haplotype of interest had similar, but larger, improvements on inhaled steroids. On average, those imputed to have the haplotype of interest had two to three times the short-term response to inhaled steroids compared to those without the haplotype (Fig. 8.6). The overall explained phenotypic variance was small ($<5$ percent in both populations), however, suggesting that multiple other factors (including additional genes) are responsible for the variability in the response to inhaled corticosteroids. Since *CRHR1* is the primary receptor for corticotropin releasing factor in the brain, and thereby modulates adrenocorticotropic hormone (*ACTH*) and endogenous cortisol levels, these results confirm the role of genetics in the asthma outcomes related to endogenous steroid levels.

## CONCLUSION

Variation in the response to drugs has a significant heritable component. Although the time required to decipher the genetics of drug response is likely to be many years, we are making progress toward the goal of individualized medicine.

## Key learning points

- Pharmacogenetics is the study of variability in drug response due to heredity.

- There are two major functional classes of pharmacogenetic studies.
  1 Drug response – evaluates properties of the therapeutic agent (such as levels) as the outcome that varies by genetics. Often Mendelian.
  2 Target response – evaluates differences in disease expression or intermediate phenotypes as the outcome that varies by genetics. Likely to be polygenic or depend upon epistatic interactions.

- There are four principle categories of pharmacogenetic variation.
  1 Pharmacokinetic
  2 Pharmacodynamic
  3 Idiosyncratic
  4 Disease modifying

- Careful attention to the development of pharmacogenetic phenotypes must precede any analysis.

- Population-based case–control and cohort studies remain the most suitable study designs for pharmacogenetic analyses.

- Misclassification, regression to the mean, small sample size, failure to replicate, and failure to localize a functional variant are common methodologic problems in pharmacogenetic studies.

- Although examples are readily available for both types of functional classes in respiratory pharmacogenetics, the field is still young. Individualized medicine remains a viable, but future goal.

## REFERENCES

◆1 Ingelman-Sundberg M. Pharmacogenetics: an opportunity for a safer and more efficient pharmacotherapy. *J Intern Med* 2001; **250**: 186–200.

2 Maitland-van der Zee AH, de Boer A, Leufkens HG. The interface between pharmacoepidemiology and pharmacogenetics. *Eur J Pharmacol* 2000; **410**: 121–30.

3 Vesell ES. Therapeutic lessons from pharmacogenetics. *Ann Intern Med* 1997; **126**: 653–5.

◆4 Evans WE, Relling MV. Pharmacogenomics: translating functional genomics into rational therapeutics. *Science* 1999; **286**: 487–91.

5 Mancinelli L, Cronin M, Sadee W. Pharmacogenomics: the promise of personalized medicine. *AAPS PharmSci* 2000; **2**: E4.

6 Lazarou J, Pomeranz BH, Corey PN. Incidence of adverse drug reactions in hospitalized patients: a meta-analysis of prospective studies. *JAMA* 1998; **279**: 1200–5.

7 Ernst FR, Grizzle AJ. Drug-related morbidity and mortality: updating the cost-of-illness model. *J Am Pharm Assoc (Wash)* 2001; **41**: 192–9.

8 Johnson JA, Bootman JL. Drug-related morbidity and mortality. A cost-of-illness model. *Arch Intern Med* 1995; **155**: 1949–56.

9 Meisel C, Gerloff T, Kirchheiner J et al. Implications of pharmacogenetics for individualizing drug treatment and for study design. *J Mol Med* 2003; **81**: 154–67.

10 Classen DC, Pestotnik SL, Evans RS et al. Adverse drug events in hospitalized patients. Excess length of stay, extra costs, and attributable mortality. *J Am Med Assoc* 1997; **277**: 301–6.

11 Drazen JM, Silverman EK, Lee TH. Heterogeneity of therapeutic responses in asthma. *Br Med Bull* 2000; **56**: 1054–70.

◆12 Evans WE, McLeod HL. Pharmacogenomics-drug disposition, drug targets, and side effects. *N Engl J Med* 2003; **348**: 538–49.

13 Luzatto L, Mehta A. Glucose-6-phosphate dehydrogenase deficiency. In: Scriver CR, Beaudet AL, Sly WS, Valle D (eds). *The metabolic and molecular basis of inherited disease.* New York: McGraw-Hill, 1995: 5024.

14 Davidson RG. Pharmacogenetics: pharmacogenomics. In: *PDQ medical genetics.* Oxford: Elsevier, 2002: 232.

15 Nebert DW. Pharmacogenetics and pharmacogenomics: why is this relevant to the clinical geneticist? *Clin Genet* 1999; **56**: 247–58.

●16 Garrod AE. The incidence of alkaptonuria: a study in chemical individuality. *Lancet* 1902; 160: 1616–20.

17 Lindpainter K. Pharmacogenetics and the future of medical practice. *J Mol Med* 2003; **81**: 141–53.

●18 Snyder LH. Studies in human inheritance. IX. The inheritance of taste deficiency in man. *Ohio J Sci* 1932; **32**: 436–68.

●19 Kalow W. Familial incidence of low pseudocholinesterase level. *Lancet* 1956; **271**: 576.

●20 Motulsky AG. Drug reactions, enzymes and biochemical genetics. *J Am Med Assoc* 1957; **165**: 835–7.

●21 Vogel F. Moderne Probleme der Humangenetik. *Ergeb Inn Med Kinderheilkd* 1959; **12**: 52–125.

22 Vesell ES, Page JG. Genetic control of drug levels in man: phenylbutazone. *Science* 1968; **159**: 1479–80.

23 Vesell ES, Page JG. Genetic control of drug levels in man: antipyrine. *Science* 1968; **161**: 72–3.

24 Vesell ES, Page JG. Genetic control of dicumarol levels in man. *J Clin Invest* 1968; **47**: 2657–63.

25 Vesell ES, Page JG. Genetic control of the phenobarbital-induced shortening of plasma antipyrine half-lives in man. *J Clin Invest* 1969; **48**: 2202–9.

26 Vesell ES, Page JG, Passananti GT. Genetic and environmental factors affecting ethanol metabolism in man. *Clin Pharmacol Ther* 1971; **12**: 192–201.

27 Vesell ES, Passananti GT, Greene FE, Page JG. Genetic control of drug levels and of the induction of drug-metabolizing enzymes in man: individual variability in the extent of allopurinol and nortriptyline inhibition of drug metabolism. *Ann NY Acad Sci* 1971; **179**: 752–73.

28 Rusnak JM, Kisabeth RM, Herbert DP, McNeil DM. Pharmacogenomics: a clinician's primer on emerging technologies for improved patient care. *Mayo Clin Proc* 2001; **76**: 299–309.

29 Mahgoub A, Idle JR, Dring LG et al. Polymorphic hydroxylation of debrisoquine in man. *Lancet* 1977; **2**: 584–6.

30   Eichelbaum M, Spannbrucker N, Steincke B, Dengler HJ. Defective N-oxidation of sparteine in man: a new pharmacogenetic defect. *Eur J Clin Pharmacol* 1979; **16**: 183–7.

●31   Gonzalez FJ, Skoda RC, Kimura S et al. Characterization of the common genetic defect in humans deficient in debrisoquine metabolism. *Nature* 1988; **331**: 442–6.

◆32   Weinshilboum R. Inheritance and drug response. *N Engl J Med* 2003; **348**: 529–37.

33   Silverman ES, Hjoberg J, Palmer LJ et al. Application of pharmacogenetics to the therapeutics of asthma. In: Eissa NT, Huston D (eds). *Therapeutic targets of airway inflammation*. New York: Marcel Dekker, 2003: 1000.

34   Steimer W, Potter JM. Pharmacogenetic screening and therapeutic drugs. *Clin Chim Acta* 2002; **315**: 137–55.

35   Barta C, Sasvari-Szekely M, Devai A et al. Analysis of mutations in the plasma cholinesterase gene of patients with a history of prolonged neuromuscular block during anesthesia. *Mol Genet Metab* 2001; **74**: 484–8.

36   Harris BE, Carpenter JT, Diasio RB. Severe 5-fluorouracil toxicity secondary to dihydropyrimidine dehydrogenase deficiency. A potentially more common pharmacogenetic syndrome. *Cancer* 1991; **68**: 499–501.

37   Wei X, McLeod HL, McMurrough J et al. Molecular basis of the human dihydropyrimidine dehydrogenase deficiency and 5-fluorouracil toxicity. *J Clin Invest* 1996; **98**: 610–5.

38   Yates CR, Krynetski EY, Loennechen T et al. Molecular diagnosis of thiopurine S-methyltransferase deficiency: genetic basis for azathioprine and mercaptopurine intolerance. *Ann Intern Med* 1997; **126**: 608–14.

39   Evans WE, Hon YY, Bomgaars L et al. Preponderance of thiopurine S-methyltransferase deficiency and heterozygosity among patients intolerant to mercaptopurine or azathioprine. *J Clin Oncol* 2001; **19**: 2293–301.

40   Brockmoller J, Kirchheiner J, Meisel C, Roots I. Pharmacogenetic diagnostics of cytochrome P450 polymorphisms in clinical drug development and in drug treatment. *Pharmacogenomics* 2000; **1**: 125–51.

41   Kirchheiner J, Brosen K, Dahl ML et al. CYP2D6 and CYP2C19 genotype-based dose recommendations for antidepressants: a first step towards subpopulation-specific dosages. *Acta Psychiatr Scand* 2001; **104**: 173–92.

42   Brinkmann U, Roots I, Eichelbaum M. Pharmacogenetics of the human drug-transporter gene MDR1: impact of polymorphisms on pharmacotherapy. *Drug Discov Today* 2001; **6**: 835–9.

43   Choo EF, Leake B, Wandel C et al. Pharmacological inhibition of P-glycoprotein transport enhances the distribution of HIV-1 protease inhibitors into brain and testes. *Drug Metab Dispos* 2000; **28**:655–60.

44   Borst P, Evers R, Kool M, Wijnholds J. A family of drug transporters: the multidrug resistance-associated proteins. *J Natl Cancer Inst* 2000; **92**: 1295–302.

45   Michelson AD, Furman MI, Goldschmidt-Clermont P et al. Platelet GP IIIa PI(A) polymorphisms display different sensitivities to agonists. *Circulation* 2000; **101**: 1013–8.

46   Cooke GE, Bray PF, Hamlington JD et al. PIA2 polymorphism and efficacy of aspirin. *Lancet* 1998; **351**: 1253.

47   Johnson JA, Lima JJ. Drug receptor/effector polymorphisms and pharmacogenetics: current status and challenges. *Pharmacogenetics* 2003; **13**: 525–34.

48   Meyer UA. Pharmacogenetics: the slow, the rapid, and the ultrarapid. *Proc Natl Acad Sci USA* 1994; **91**: 1983–4.

49   Nebert DW, McKinnon RA, Puga A. Human drug-metabolizing enzyme polymorphisms: effects on risk of toxicity and cancer. *DNA Cell Biol* 1996; **15**: 273–80.

50   Nebert DW, Ingelman-Sundberg M, Daly AK. Genetic epidemiology of environmental toxicity and cancer susceptibility: human allelic polymorphisms in drug-metabolizing enzyme genes, their functional importance, and nomenclature issues. *Drug Metab Rev* 1999; **31**: 467–87.

●51   Hughes HB, Biehl JP, Jones AP, Schmidt LH. Metabolism of isoniazid in man as related to the occurrence of peripheral neuritis. *Am Rev Tuberc* 1954; **70**: 266–73.

52   Spielberg SP. N-acetyltransferases: pharmacogenetics and clinical consequences of polymorphic drug metabolism. *J Pharmacokinet Biopharm* 1996; **24**: 509–19.

●53   Evans DAP, Manley KA, McKusick VA. Genetic control of isoniazid metabolism in man. *Br Med J* 1960; **2**.

54   Zielinska E, Niewiarowski W, Bodalski J et al. Genotyping of the arylamine N-acetyltransferase polymorphism in the prediction of idiosyncratic reactions to trimethoprim-sulfamethoxazole in infants. *Pharm World Sci* 1998; **20**: 123–30.

55   Zielinska E, Niewiarowski W, Bodalski J. The arylamine N-acetyltransferase (NAT2) polymorphism and the risk of adverse reactions to co-trimoxazole in children. *Eur J Clin Pharmacol* 1998; **54**: 779–85.

56   O'Neil WM, Drobitch RK, MacArthur RD et al. Acetylator phenotype and genotype in patients infected with HIV: discordance between methods for phenotype determination and genotype. *Pharmacogenetics* 2000; **10**: 171–82.

57   O'Neil WM, MacArthur RD, Farrough MJ et al. Acetylator phenotype and genotype in HIV-infected patients with and without sulfonamide hypersensitivity. *J Clin Pharmacol* 2002; **42**: 613–9.

58   Zielinska E, Bodalski J, Niewiarowski W et al. Comparison of acetylation phenotype with genotype coding for N-acetyltransferase (NAT2) in children. *Pediatr Res* 1999; **45**: 403–8.

59   McNamara DM, Holubkov R, Janosko K et al. Pharmacogenetic interactions between beta-blocker therapy and the angiotensin-converting enzyme deletion polymorphism in patients with congestive heart failure. *Circulation* 2001; **103**: 1644–8.

60   Ueda S, Meredith PA, Morton JJ et al. ACE (I/D) genotype as a predictor of the magnitude and duration of the response to an ACE inhibitor drug (enalaprilat) in humans. *Circulation* 1998; **98**: 2148–53.

◆61   Schork NJ. Genetics of complex disease: approaches, problems, and solutions. *Am J Respir Crit Care Med* 1997; **156**: S103–9.

62   Freimer N, Sabatti C. The human phenome project. *Nat Genet* 2003; **34**: 15–21.

63   Tsuang MT, Lyons MJ, Faraone SV. Problems of diagnoses in family studies. *J Psychiatr Res* 1987; **21**: 391–9.

64   Szatmari P, Jones MB. Effects of misclassification on estimates of relative risk in family history studies. *Genet Epidemiol* 1999; **16**: 368–81.

65   Garcia-Closas M, Rothman N, Lubin J. Misclassification in case–control studies of gene–environment interactions: assessment of bias and sample size. *Cancer Epidemiol Biomarkers Prev* 1999; **8**: 1043–50.

66  Rothman N, Garcia-Closas M, Stewart WT, Lubin J. The impact of misclassification in case-control studies of gene-environment interactions. *IARC Sci Publ* 1999; **148**: 89-96.

67  Clough JB. Phenotype stability in asthma and atopy in childhood. *Clin Exp Allergy* 1998; **28** Suppl 1: 22-5; discussion 32-6.

68  Panhuysen CI, Bleecker ER, Koeter GH et al. Characterization of obstructive airway disease in family members of probands with asthma. An algorithm for the diagnosis of asthma. *Am J Respir Crit Care Med* 1998; **157**: 1734-42.

69  Evans WE, Johnson JA. Pharmacogenomics: the inherited basis for interindividual differences in drug response. *Annu Rev Genomics Hum Genet* 2001; **2**: 9-39.

70  Rogers JF, Nafziger AN, Bertino JS Jr. Pharmacogenetics affects dosing, efficacy, and toxicity of cytochrome P450-metabolized drugs. *Am J Med* 2002; **113**: 746-50.

71  Nebert DW. Extreme discordant phenotype methodology: an intuitive approach to clinical pharmacogenetics. *Eur J Pharmacol* 2000; **410**: 107-20.

72  Yi N, Xu S, Allison DB. Bayesian model choice and search strategies for mapping interacting quantitative trait Loci. *Genetics* 2003; **165**: 867-83.

73  Lash LH, Hines RN, Gonzalez FJ et al. Genetics and susceptibility to toxic chemicals: do you (or should you) know your genetic profile? *J Pharmacol Exp Ther* 2003; **305**: 403-9.

74  Morton V, Torgerson DJ. Effect of regression to the mean on decision making in health care. *Br Med J* 2003; **326**: 1083-4.

75  Zhang X, Tomblin JB. Explaining and controlling regression to the mean in longitudinal research designs. *J Speech Lang Hear Res* 2003; **46**: 1340-51.

76  Schuckit MA, Edenberg HJ, Kalmijn J et al. A genome-wide search for genes that relate to a low level of response to alcohol. *Alcohol Clin Exp Res* 2001; **25**: 323-9.

77  Turecki G, Grof P, Grof E et al. Mapping susceptibility genes for bipolar disorder: a pharmacogenetic approach based on excellent response to lithium. *Mol Psychiatry* 2001; **6**: 570-8.

78  Mosley J, Conti DV, Elston RC, Witte JS. Impact of preadjusting a quantitative phenotype prior to sib-pair linkage analysis when gene x environment interaction exists. *Genet Epidemiol* 2001; **21** Suppl 1: S837-42.

79  Gauderman WJ, Morrison JL, Siegmund KD. Should we consider gene x environment interaction in the hunt for quantitative trait loci? *Genet Epidemiol* 2001; **21** Suppl 1: S831-6.

80  Colilla S, Nicolae D, Pluzhnikov A et al. Evidence for gene-environment interactions in a linkage study of asthma and smoking exposure. *J Allergy Clin Immunol* 2003; **111**: 840-6.

81  Oestreicher JL, Walters IB, Kikuchi T et al. Molecular classification of psoriasis disease-associated genes through pharmacogenomic expression profiling. *Pharmacogenomics J* 2001; **1**: 272-87.

82  Kleyn PW, Vesell ES. Genetic variation as a guide to drug development. *Science* 1998; **281**: 1820-1.

83  Yang Q, Khoury MJ, Flanders WD. Sample size requirements in case-only designs to detect gene-environment interaction. *Am J Epidemiol* 1997; **146**: 713-20.

84  Khoury MJ, Flanders WD. Nontraditional epidemiologic approaches in the analysis of gene-environment interaction: case-control studies with no controls! *Am J Epidemiol* 1996; **144**: 207-13.

85  Piegorsch WW, Weinberg CR, Taylor JA. Non-hierarchical logistic models and case-only designs for assessing susceptibility in population-based case-control studies. *Stat Med* 1994; **13**: 153-62.

86  Liu X, Fallin MD, Kao WH. Genetic dissection methods: designs used for tests of gene-environment interaction. *Curr Opin Genet Dev* 2004; **14**: 241-5.

87  Deng Y, Newman B, Dunne MP et al. Case-only study of interactions between genetic polymorphisms of GSTM1, P1, T1 and Z1 and smoking in Parkinson's disease. *Neurosci Lett* 2004; **366**: 326-31.

88  Schmidt S, Schaid DJ. Potential misinterpretation of the case-only study to assess gene-environment interaction. *Am J Epidemiol* 1999; **150**: 878-85.

89  Hamajima N, Yuasa H, Matsuo K, Kurobe Y. Detection of gene-environment interaction by case-only studies. *Jpn J Clin Oncol* 1999; **29**: 490-3.

90  Albert PS, Ratnasinghe D, Tangrea J, Wacholder S. Limitations of the case-only design for identifying gene-environment interactions. *Am J Epidemiol* 2001; **154**: 687-93.

91  Le Souef P. Use of cohorts with extensive longitudinal data in investigating the molecular genetics of asthma. *Clin Exp Allergy* 1998; **28** Suppl 1: 46-50; discussion 65-6.

92  Burton P, Gurrin L, Sly P. Extending the simple linear regression model to account for correlated responses: an introduction to generalized estimating equations and multi-level mixed modelling. *Stat Med* 1998; **17**: 1261-91.

93  Schmitz S, Cherny SS, Fulker DW. Increase in power through multivariate analyses. *Behav Genet* 1998; **28**: 357-63.

94  Carlson CS, Eberle MA, Rieder MJ et al. Additional SNPs and linkage-disequilibrium analyses are necessary for whole-genome association studies in humans. *Nat Genet* 2003; **33**: 518-21.

95  Kruglyak L. Prospects for whole-genome linkage disequilibrium mapping of common disease genes. *Nat Genet* 1999; **22**: 139-44.

96  Schmith VD, Campbell DA, Sehgal S et al. Pharmacogenetics and disease genetics of complex diseases. *Cell Mol Life Sci* 2003; **60**: 1636-46.

97  Roses AD. Pharmacogenetics. *Hum Mol Genet* 2001; **10**: 2261-7.

98  Roses AD. Pharmacogenetics place in modern medical science and practice. *Life Sci* 2002; **70**: 1471-80.

99  Silverman EK, Palmer LJ. Case-control association studies for the genetics of complex respiratory diseases. *Am J Respir Cell Mol Biol* 2000; **22**: 645-8.

◆100  Weiss ST, Silverman EK, Palmer LJ. Case-control association studies in pharmacogenetics. *Pharmacogenomics J* 2001; **1**: 157-8.

101  Pritchard JK, Rosenberg NA. Use of unlinked genetic markers to detect population stratification in association studies. *Am J Hum Genet* 1999; **65**: 220-8.

102  Pritchard JK, Stephens M, Rosenberg NA, Donnelly P. Association mapping in structured populations. *Am J Hum Genet* 2000; **67**: 170-81.

103  Cardon LR, Idury RM, Harris TJ et al. Testing drug response in the presence of genetic information: sampling issues for clinical trials. *Pharmacogenetics* 2000; **10**: 503-10.

104  Elston RC, Idury RM, Cardon LR, Lichter JB. The study of candidate genes in drug trials: sample size considerations. *Stat Med* 1999; **18**: 741-51.

105  Palmer LJ, Silverman ES, Weiss ST, Drazen JM. Pharmacogenetics of asthma. *Am J Respir Crit Care Med* 2002; **165**: 861–6.

106  Foppa I, Spiegelman D. Power and sample size calculations for case–control studies of gene–environment interactions with a polytomous exposure variable. *Am J Epidemiol* 1997; **146**: 596–604.

107  Weiss ST. Gene by environment interaction and asthma. *Clin Exp Allergy* 1999; **29** Suppl 2: 96–9.

108  Garcia-Closas M, Lubin JH. Power and sample size calculations in case–control studies of gene–environment interactions: comments on different approaches. *Am J Epidemiol* 1999; **149**: 689–92.

109  Bradford-Hill AB. The environment and disease: association and causation. *Proc R Soc Med* 1965; **58**: 295–300.

●110  Drysdale CM, McGraw DW, Stack CB et al. Complex promoter and coding region beta 2-adrenergic receptor haplotypes alter receptor expression and predict in vivo responsiveness. *Proc Natl Acad Sci USA* 2000; **97**: 10483–8.

111  Johnson JA, Zineh I, Puckett BJ et al. Beta 1-adrenergic receptor polymorphisms and antihypertensive response to metoprolol. *Clin Pharmacol Ther* 2003; **74**: 44–52.

112  Boerwinkle E, Chakraborty R, Sing CF. The use of measured genotype information in the analysis of quantitative phenotypes in man. I. Models and analytical methods. *Ann Hum Genet* 1986; **50**(Pt 2): 181–94.

113  Templeton AR, Boerwinkle E, Sing CF. A cladistic analysis of phenotypic associations with haplotypes inferred from restriction endonuclease mapping. I. Basic theory and an analysis of alcohol dehydrogenase activity in Drosophila. *Genetics* 1987; **117**: 343–51.

114  Kamboh MI, Evans RW, Aston CE. Genetic effect of apolipoprotein(a) and apolipoprotein E polymorphisms on plasma quantitative risk factors for coronary heart disease in American black women. *Atherosclerosis* 1995; **117**: 73–81.

◆115  Risch NJ. Searching for genetic determinants in the new millennium. *Nature* 2000; **405**: 847–56.

116  Olejnik S, Algina J. Generalized eta and omega squared statistics: measures of effect size for some common research designs. *Psychol Methods* 2003; **8**: 434–47.

117  Kempthorne O. *An introduction to genetic statistics.* Ames: Iowa University Press, 1969.

118  Cardon LR, Bell JI. Association study designs for complex diseases. *Nat Rev Genet* 2001; **2**: 91–9.

119  Hirschhorn JN, Altshuler D. Once and again-issues surrounding replication in genetic association studies. *J Clin Endocrinol Metab* 2002; **87**: 4438–41.

120  Tabor HK, Risch NJ, Myers RM. Opinion: Candidate-gene approaches for studying complex genetic traits: practical considerations. *Nat Rev Genet* 2002; **3**: 391–7.

121  Sebastiani P, Lazarus R, Weiss ST et al. Minimal haplotype tagging. *Proc Natl Acad Sci USA* 2003; **100**: 9900–5.

●122  Johnson GC, Esposito L, Barratt BJ et al. Haplotype tagging for the identification of common disease genes. *Nat Genet* 2001; **29**: 233–7.

123  Wilson JF, Weale ME, Smith AC et al. Population genetic structure of variable drug response. *Nat Genet* 2001; **29**: 265–9.

124  Evans DA, McLeod HL, Pritchard S et al. Interethnic variability in human drug responses. *Drug Metab Dispos* 2001; **29**: 606–10.

125  Lonjou C, Zhang W, Collins A et al. Linkage disequilibrium in human populations. *Proc Natl Acad Sci USA* 2003; **100**: 6069–74.

126  Tian W, Boggs DA, Uko G et al. MICA, HLA-B haplotypic variation in five population groups of sub-Saharan African ancestry. *Genes Immun* 2003; **4**: 500–5.

127  Sobieszczyk P, Fishbein MC, Goldhaber SZ. Acute pulmonary embolism: don't ignore the platelet. *Circulation* 2002; **106**: 1748–9.

128  Ginsberg JS. Management of venous thromboembolism. *N Engl J Med* 1996; **335**: 1816–28.

129  Hull R, Hirsh J, Jay R et al. Different intensities of oral anticoagulant therapy in the treatment of proximal-vein thrombosis. *N Engl J Med* 1982; **307**: 1676–81.

130  van der Meer FJ, Rosendaal FR, Vandenbroucke JP, Briet E. Bleeding complications in oral anticoagulant therapy. An analysis of risk factors. *Arch Intern Med* 1993; **153**: 1557–62.

131  Cannegieter SC, Rosendaal FR, Wintzen AR et al. Optimal oral anticoagulant therapy in patients with mechanical heart valves. *N Engl J Med* 1995; **333**: 11–7.

132  Palareti G, Leali N, Coccheri S et al. Bleeding complications of oral anticoagulant treatment: an inception-cohort, prospective collaborative study (ISCOAT). Italian Study on Complications of Oral Anticoagulant Therapy. *Lancet* 1996; **348**: 423–8.

133  Rettie AE, Wienkers LC, Gonzalez FJ et al. Impaired (S)-warfarin metabolism catalysed by the R144C allelic variant of CYP2C9. *Pharmacogenetics* 1994; **4**: 39–42.

134  Linder MW. Genetic mechanisms for hypersensitivity and resistance to the anticoagulant warfarin. *Clin Chim Acta* 2001; **308**: 9–15.

135  Takahashi H, Echizen H. Pharmacogenetics of warfarin elimination and its clinical implications. *Clin Pharmacokinet* 2001; **40**: 587–603.

136  Hallak HO, Wedlund PJ, Modi MW et al. High clearance of (S)-warfarin in a warfarin-resistant subject. *Br J Clin Pharmacol* 1993; **35**: 327–30.

137  James AH, Britt RP, Raskino CL, Thompson SG. Factors affecting the maintenance dose of warfarin. *J Clin Pathol* 1992; **45**: 704–6.

138  Miners JO, Birkett DJ. Cytochrome P450 2C9: an enzyme of major importance in human drug metabolism. *Br J Clin Pharmacol* 1998; **45**: 525–38.

139  Goldstein JA, de Morais SM. Biochemistry and molecular biology of the human CYP2C subfamily. *Pharmacogenetics* 1994; **4**: 285–99.

140  Gray IC, Nobile C, Muresu R et al. A 2.4-megabase physical map spanning the CYP2C gene cluster on chromosome 10q24. *Genomics* 1995; **28**: 328–32.

141  Mancy A, Broto P, Dijols S et al. The substrate binding site of human liver cytochrome P450 2C9: an approach using designed tienilic acid derivatives and molecular modeling. *Biochemistry* 1995; **34**: 10365–75.

142  Jones BC, Hawksworth G, Horne VA et al. Putative active site template model for cytochrome P4502C9 (tolbutamide hydroxylase). *Drug Metab Dispos* 1996; **24**: 260–6.

143  Haining RL, Hunter AP, Veronese ME et al. Allelic variants of human cytochrome P450 2C9: baculovirus-mediated expression, purification, structural characterization, substrate stereoselectivity, and prochiral selectivity of the wild-type and I359L mutant forms. *Arch Biochem Biophys* 1996; **333**: 447–58.

144 Sullivan-Klose TH, Ghanayem BI, Bell DA et al. The role of the CYP2C9-Leu359 allelic variant in the tolbutamide polymorphism. *Pharmacogenetics* 1996; **6**: 341–9.

●145 Furuya H, Fernandez-Salguero P, Gregory W et al. Genetic polymorphism of CYP2C9 and its effect on warfarin maintenance dose requirement in patients undergoing anticoagulation therapy. *Pharmacogenetics* 1995; **5**: 389–92.

146 Aithal GP, Day CP, Kesteven PJ, Daly AK. Association of polymorphisms in the cytochrome P450 CYP2C9 with warfarin dose requirement and risk of bleeding complications. *Lancet* 1999; **353**: 717–9.

147 Margaglione M, Colaizzo D, D'Andrea G et al. Genetic modulation of oral anticoagulation with warfarin. *Thromb Haemost* 2000; **84**: 775–8.

148 Taube J, Halsall D, Baglin T. Influence of cytochrome P-450 CYP2C9 polymorphisms on warfarin sensitivity and risk of over-anticoagulation in patients on long-term treatment. *Blood* 2000; **96**: 1816–9.

149 Takahashi H, Kashima T, Nomoto S et al. Comparisons between in vitro and in vivo metabolism of (S)-warfarin: catalytic activities of cDNA-expressed CYP2C9, its Leu359 variant and their mixture versus unbound clearance in patients with the corresponding CYP2C9 genotypes. *Pharmacogenetics* 1998; **8**: 365–73.

150 Takahashi H, Kashima T, Nomizo Y et al. Metabolism of warfarin enantiomers in Japanese patients with heart disease having different CYP2C9 and CYP2C19 genotypes. *Clin Pharmacol Ther* 1998; **63**: 519–28.

151 US Department of Health and Human Services. Healthy People 2010: Understanding and improving health, 2nd edn. Washington, DC: US Government Printing Office, 2000.

152 Mokdad AH, Marks JS, Stroup DF, Gerberding JL. Actual causes of death in the United States, 2000. *J Am Med Assoc* 2004; **291**: 1238–45.

153 Edwards R. The problem of tobacco smoking. *Br Med J* 2004; **328**: 217–9.

154 Corrigall WA. Understanding brain mechanisms in nicotine reinforcement. *Br J Addict* 1991; **86**: 507–10.

155 Stolerman IP, Shoaib M. The neurobiology of tobacco addiction. *Trends Pharmacol Sci* 1991; **12**: 467–73.

156 Dani JA, Heinemann S. Molecular and cellular aspects of nicotine abuse. *Neuron* 1996; **16**: 905–8.

●157 Cholerton S, Arpanahi A, McCracken N et al. Poor metabolisers of nicotine and CYP2D6 polymorphism. *Lancet* 1994; **343**: 62–3.

158 Hiroi T, Imaoka S, Funae Y. Dopamine formation from tyramine by CYP2D6. *Biochem Biophys Res Commun* 1998; **249**: 838–43.

159 Daly AK, Brockmoller J, Broly F et al. Nomenclature for human CYP2D6 alleles. *Pharmacogenetics* 1996; **6**: 193–201.

160 Johansson I, Lundqvist E, Bertilsson L et al. Inherited amplification of an active gene in the cytochrome P450 CYP2D locus as a cause of ultrarapid metabolism of debrisoquine. *Proc Natl Acad Sci USA* 1993; **90**: 11825–9.

161 Cholerton S, Boustead C, Taber H et al. CYP2D6 genotypes in cigarette smokers and non-tobacco users. *Pharmacogenetics* 1996; **6**: 261–3.

162 Boustead C, Taber H, Idle JR, Cholerton S. CYP2D6 genotype and smoking behaviour in cigarette smokers. *Pharmacogenetics* 1997; **7**: 411–4.

163 Saarikoski ST, Sata F, Husgafvel-Pursiainen K et al. CYP2D6 ultrarapid metabolizer genotype as a potential modifier of smoking behaviour. *Pharmacogenetics* 2000; **10**: 5–10.

164 Walton R, Johnstone E, Munafo M et al. Genetic clues to the molecular basis of tobacco addiction and progress towards personalized therapy. *Trends Mol Med* 2001; **7**: 70–6.

165 Molyneux A. Nicotine replacement therapy. *Br Med J* 2004; **328**: 454–6.

166 Roddy E. Bupropion and other non-nicotine pharmacotherapies. *Br Med J* 2004; **328**: 509–11.

167 Jorenby DE, Leischow SJ, Nides MA et al. A controlled trial of sustained-release bupropion, a nicotine patch, or both for smoking cessation. *N Engl J Med* 1999; **340**: 685–91.

168 Hurt RD, Sachs DP, Glover ED et al. A comparison of sustained-release bupropion and placebo for smoking cessation. *N Engl J Med* 1997; **337**: 1195–202.

169 Court MH, Duan SX, Hesse LM et al. Cytochrome P-450 2B6 is responsible for interindividual variability of propofol hydroxylation by human liver microsomes. *Anesthesiology* 2001; **94**: 110–9.

170 Faucette SR, Hawke RL, Lecluyse EL et al. Validation of bupropion hydroxylation as a selective marker of human cytochrome P450 2B6 catalytic activity. *Drug Metab Dispos* 2000; **28**: 1222–30.

171 Lang T, Klein K, Fischer J et al. Extensive genetic polymorphism in the human CYP2B6 gene with impact on expression and function in human liver. *Pharmacogenetics* 2001; **11**: 399–415.

172 Lerman C, Shields PG, Wileyto EP et al. Pharmacogenetic investigation of smoking cessation treatment. *Pharmacogenetics* 2002; **12**: 627–34.

173 Gurney H. Dose calculation of anticancer drugs: a review of the current practice and introduction of an alternative. *J Clin Oncol* 1996; **14**: 2590–611.

174 Baker SD, Verweij J, Rowinsky EK et al. Role of body surface area in dosing of investigational anticancer agents in adults, 1991–2001. *J Natl Cancer Inst* 2002; **94**: 1883–8.

175 Goetz MP, Ames MM, Weinshilboum RM. Primer on medical genomics. Part XII: Pharmacogenomics – general principles with cancer as a model. *Mayo Clin Proc* 2004; **79**: 376–84.

◆176 Ulrich CM, Robien K, McLeod HL. Cancer pharmacogenetics: polymorphisms, pathways and beyond. *Nat Rev Cancer* 2003; **3**: 912–20.

177 McLeod HL, Yu J. Cancer pharmacogenomics: SNPs, chips, and the individual patient. *Cancer Invest* 2003; **21**: 630–40.

178 Veal GJ, Coulthard SA, Boddy AV. Chemotherapy individualization. *Invest New Drugs* 2003; **21**: 149–56.

179 Watters JW, McLeod HL. Cancer pharmacogenomics: current and future applications. *Biochim Biophys Acta* 2003; **1603**: 99–111.

180 Nagasubramanian R, Innocenti F, Ratain MJ. Pharmacogenetics in cancer treatment. *Annu Rev Med* 2003; **54**: 437–52.

181 Daly AK, Hall AG. Pharmacogenetics of cytotoxic drugs. *Exp Rev Anticancer Ther* 2001; **1**: 301–8.

182 Relling MV, Dervieux T. Pharmacogenetics and cancer therapy. *Nat Rev Cancer* 2001; **1**: 99–108.

183 Danesi R, de Braud F, Fogli S et al. Pharmacogenetics of anticancer drug sensitivity in non-small cell lung cancer. *Pharmacol Rev* 2003; **55**: 57–103.

184 Franklin WA, Carbone DP. Molecular staging and pharmacogenomics. Clinical implications: from lab to patients and back. *Lung Cancer* 2003; **41** Suppl 1: S147–54.

185   Sarries C, Haura EB, Roig B et al. Pharmacogenomic strategies for developing customized chemotherapy in non-small cell lung cancer. *Pharmacogenomics* 2002; **3**: 763–80.

186   Reardon DA, Friedman HS, Powell JB Jr et al. Irinotecan: promising activity in the treatment of malignant glioma. *Oncology (Huntingt)* 2003; **17**: 9–14.

187   Fuchs CS, Moore MR, Harker G et al. Phase III comparison of two irinotecan dosing regimens in second-line therapy of metastatic colorectal cancer. *J Clin Oncol* 2003; **21**: 807–14.

188   Pizzolato JF, Saltz LB. Irinotecan (Campto) in the treatment of pancreatic cancer. *Exp Rev Anticancer Ther* 2003; **3**: 587–93.

189   Negoro S, Masuda N, Takada Y et al. Randomised phase III trial of irinotecan combined with cisplatin for advanced non-small-cell lung cancer. *Br J Cancer* 2003; **88**: 335–41.

190   Choy H, Kim JS, Pyo H, MacRae R. Topoisomerase I inhibitors in the combined modality therapy of lung cancer. *Clin Lung Cancer* 2001; **2** Suppl 2: S34–40.

191   Rocha Lima CM, Rizvi NA, Zhang C et al. Randomized phase II trial of gemcitabine plus irinotecan or docetaxel in stage IIIB or stage IV NSCLC. *Ann Oncol* 2004; **15**: 410–8.

192   Noda K, Nishiwaki Y, Kawahara M et al. Irinotecan plus cisplatin compared with etoposide plus cisplatin for extensive small-cell lung cancer. *N Engl J Med* 2002; **346**: 85–91.

193   Ichiki M, Gohara R, Rikimaru T et al. Combination chemotherapy with irinotecan and ifosfamide as second-line treatment of refractory or sensitive relapsed small cell lung cancer: a phase II study. *Chemotherapy* 2003; **49**: 200–5.

194   Saijo N. Progress in treatment of small-cell lung cancer: role of CPT-11. *Br J Cancer* 2003; **89**: 2178–83.

195   Fisher MD, D'Orazio A. Irinotecan and cisplatin versus etoposide and cisplatin in small-cell lung cancer: *JCOG* 9511. *Clin Lung Cancer* 2000; 2: 23–4.

196   Ando M, Kobayashi K, Yoshimura A et al. Weekly administration of irinotecan (CPT-11) plus cisplatin for refractory or relapsed small cell lung cancer. *Lung Cancer* 2004; **44**: 121–7.

197   Desai AA, Innocenti F, Ratain MJ. Pharmacogenomics: road to anticancer therapeutics nirvana? *Oncogene* 2003; **22**: 6621–8.

198   Iyer L, King CD, Whitington PF et al. Genetic predisposition to the metabolism of irinotecan (CPT-11). Role of uridine diphosphate glucuronosyltransferase isoform 1A1 in the glucuronidation of its active metabolite (SN-38) in human liver microsomes. *J Clin Invest* 1998; **101**: 847–54.

199   Gupta E, Lestingi TM, Mick R et al. Metabolic fate of irinotecan in humans: correlation of glucuronidation with diarrhea. *Cancer Res* 1994; **54**: 3723–5.

200   Iyer L, Das S, Janisch L et al. UGT1A1*28 polymorphism as a determinant of irinotecan disposition and toxicity. *Pharmacogenomics J* 2002; **2**: 43–7.

201   Burchell B, Brierley CH, Rance D. Specificity of human UDP-glucuronosyltransferases and xenobiotic glucuronidation. *Life Sci* 1995; **57**: 1819–31.

●202   Bosma PJ, Chowdhury JR, Bakker C et al. The genetic basis of the reduced expression of bilirubin UDP-glucuronosyl-transferase 1 in Gilbert's syndrome. *N Engl J Med* 1995; **333**: 1171–5.

203   Monaghan G, Ryan M, Seddon R et al. Genetic variation in bilirubin UPD-glucuronosyltransferase gene promoter and Gilbert's syndrome. *Lancet* 1996; **347**: 578–81.

204   Beutler E, Gelbart T, Demina A. Racial variability in the UDP-glucuronosyltransferase 1 (UGT1A1) promoter: a balanced polymorphism for regulation of bilirubin metabolism? *Proc Natl Acad Sci USA* 1998; **95**: 8170–4.

●205   Ando Y, Saka H, Ando M et al. Polymorphisms of UDP-glucuronosyltransferase gene and irinotecan toxicity: a pharmacogenetic analysis. *Cancer Res* 2000; **60**: 6921–6.

206   Innocenti F, Ratain MJ. Irinotecan treatment in cancer patients with UGT1A1 polymorphisms. *Oncology (Huntingt)* 2003; **17**: 52–5.

207   Palmer LJ, Cookson WO. Genomic approaches to understanding asthma. *Genome Res* 2000; **10**: 1280–7.

208   Lemanske RF Jr, Allen DB. Choosing a long-term controller medication in childhood asthma. The proverbial two-edged sword. *Am J Respir Crit Care Med* 1997; **156**: 685–7.

209   Malmstrom K, Rodriguez-Gomez G, Guerra J et al. Oral montelukast, inhaled beclomethasone, and placebo for chronic asthma. A randomized, controlled trial. Montelukast/Beclomethasone Study Group. *Ann Intern Med* 1999; **130**: 487–95.

210   Wilk JB, Djousse L, Arnett DK et al. Evidence for major genes influencing pulmonary function in the NHLBI family heart study. *Genet Epidemiol* 2000; **19**: 81–94.

211   Palmer LJ, Burton PR, James AL et al. Familial aggregation and heritability of asthma-associated quantitative traits in a population-based sample of nuclear families. *Eur J Hum Genet* 2000; **8**: 853–60.

◆212   Raby BA, Weiss ST. Beta2-adrenergic receptor genetics. *Curr Pin Mol Ther* 2001; **3**: 554–66.

213   Osler W. *Principles and practice of medicine*, 14th edn. New York: D. Appleton-Century Company, 1942.

●214   Reihsaus E, Innis M, MacIntyre N, Liggett SB. Mutations in the gene encoding for the beta 2-adrenergic receptor in normal and asthmatic subjects. *Am J Respir Cell Mol Biol* 1993; **8**: 334–9.

215   Ohe M, Munakata M, Hizawa N et al. Beta 2 adrenergic receptor gene restriction fragment length polymorphism and bronchial asthma. *Thorax* 1995; **50**: 353–9.

216   Aziz I, McFarlane LC, Lipworth BJ. Comparative trough effects of formoterol and salmeterol on lymphocyte beta2-adrenoceptor – regulation and bronchodilatation. *Eur J Clin Pharmacol* 1999; **55**: 431–6.

217   Hancox RJ, Sears MR, Taylor DR. Polymorphism of the beta2-adrenoceptor and the response to long-term beta2-agonist therapy in asthma. *Eur Respir J* 1998; **11**: 589–93.

218   Martinez FD, Graves PE, Baldini M et al. Association between genetic polymorphisms of the beta2-adrenoceptor and response to albuterol in children with and without a history of wheezing. *J Clin Invest* 1997; **100**: 3184–8.

219   Lima JJ, Thomason DB, Mohamed MH et al. Impact of genetic polymorphisms of the beta 2-adrenergic receptor on albuterol bronchodilator pharmacodynamics. *Clin Pharmacol Ther* 1999; **65**: 519–25.

●220   Drazen JM, Israel E, Boushey HA et al. Comparison of regularly scheduled with as-needed use of albuterol in mild asthma. Asthma Clinical Research Network. *N Engl J Med* 1996; **335**: 841–7.

●221   Israel E, Drazen JM, Liggett SB et al. The effect of polymorphisms of the beta(2)-adrenergic receptor on the response to regular use of albuterol in asthma. *Am J Respir Crit Care Med* 2000; **162**: 75–80.

222   Israel E, Drazen JM, Liggett SB et al. Effect of polymorphism of the beta(2)-adrenergic receptor on response to regular use

of albuterol in asthma. *Int Arch Allergy Immunol* 2001; **124**: 183–6.

223  Liggett SB. Pharmacogenetics of beta-1- and beta-2-adrenergic receptors. *Pharmacology* 2000; **61**: 167–73.

224  Haahtela T, Jarvinen M, Kava T et al. Comparison of a beta 2-agonist, terbutaline, with an inhaled corticosteroid, budesonide, in newly detected asthma. *N Engl J Med* 1991; **325**: 388–392.

225  Chervinsky P, van As A, Bronsky EA et al. Fluticasone propionate aerosol for the treatment of adults with mild to moderate asthma. The Fluticasone Propionate Asthma Study Group. *J Allergy Clin Immunol* 1994; **94**: 676–83.

●226  Dishy V, Sofowora GG, Xie HG et al. The effect of common polymorphisms of the beta2-adrenergic receptor on agonist-mediated vascular desensitization. *N Engl J Med* 2001; **345**: 1030–5.

227  Taylor DR, Drazen JM, Herbison GP et al. Asthma exacerbations during long term beta agonist use: influence of beta(2) adrenoceptor polymorphism. *Thorax* 2000; **55**: 762–7.

228  Israel E, Chinchilli VM, Ford JG et al. Use of regularly scheduled albuterol treatment in asthma: genotype-stratified, randomised, placebo-controlled cross-over trial. *Lancet* 2004; **364**: 1505–12.

229  Tattersfield AE, Hall IP. Are beta2-adrenoceptor polymorphisms important in asthma – an unravelling story. *Lancet* 2004; **364**: 1464–6.

●230  Samuelsson B. Leukotrienes: mediators of immediate hypersensitivity reactions and inflammation. *Science* 1983; 220: 568–75.

231  Samuelsson B, Dahlen SE, Lindgren JA et al. Leukotrienes and lipoxins: structures, biosynthesis, and biological effects. *Science* 1987; **237**: 1171–6.

232  Drazen JM. Cysteinyl leukotrienes. In: Barnes PJ, Rodger IW, Thomson NC (eds). *Asthma: Basic mechanisms and clinical management.* San Diego: Academic Press, 1998: 281–95.

233  Figueroa DJ, Breyer RM, Defoe SK et al. Expression of the cysteinyl leukotriene 1 receptor in normal human lung and peripheral blood leukocytes. *Am J Respir Crit Care Med* 2001; **163**: 226–33.

234  Lewis RA, Austen KF, Soberman RJ. Leukotrienes and other products of the 5-lipoxygenase pathway. Biochemistry and relation to pathobiology in human diseases. *N Engl J Med* 1990; **323**: 645–55.

235  Holgate ST, Bradding P, Sampson AP. Leukotriene antagonists and synthesis inhibitors: new directions in asthma therapy. *J Allergy Clin Immunol* 1996; **98**: 1–13.

●236  Drazen JM, Israel E, O'Byrne PM. Treatment of asthma with drugs modifying the leukotriene pathway. *N Engl J Med* 1999; **340**: 197–206.

237  Silverman ES, Drazen JM. The biology of 5-lipoxygenase: function, structure, and regulatory mechanisms. *Proc Assoc Am Phys* 1999; **111**: 525–36.

238  Silverman ES, Du J, De Sanctis GT et al. Egr-1 and Sp1 interact functionally with the 5-lipoxygenase promoter and its naturally occurring mutants. *Am J Respir Cell Mol Biol* 1998; **19**: 316–23.

239  Silverman ES, Du J, Williams AJ et al. cAMP-response-element-binding-protein-binding protein (CBP) and p300 are transcriptional co-activators of early growth response factor-1 (Egr-1). *Biochem J* 1998; **336** (Pt 1): 183–9.

●240  In KH, Asano K, Beier D et al. Naturally occurring mutations in the human 5-lipoxygenase gene promoter that modify transcription factor binding and reporter gene transcription. *J Clin Invest* 1997; **99**: 1130–7.

241  Anderson W, Kalberg C, Edwards L et al. Effects of polymorphisms in the promoter region of 5-lipoxygenase and LTC4 synthase on the clinical response to zafirlukast and fluticasone. *Eur Resir J* 2000; **16** (Suppl B): 183s.

●242  Drazen JM, Yandava CN, Dube L et al. Pharmacogenetic association between ALOX5 promoter genotype and the response to anti-asthma treatment. *Nat Genet* 1999; **22**: 168–70.

243  Sampson AP, Siddiqui S, Buchanan D et al. Variant LTC(4) synthase allele modifies cysteinyl leukotriene synthesis in eosinophils and predicts clinical response to zafirlukast. *Thorax* 2000; **55** (Suppl 2): S28–31.

244  Sanak M, Pierzchalska M, Bazan-Socha S, Szczeklik A. Enhanced expression of the leukotriene C(4) synthase due to overactive transcription of an allelic variant associated with aspirin intolerant asthma. *Am J Respir Cell Mol Biol* 2000; **23**: 290–6.

✱245  NHLBI. Highlights of the Expert Panel Report 2. *Guidelines for the diagnosis and management of asthma.* Bethesda: NIH Publications, 1997: 50.

246  Von Mutius E. Presentation of new GINA guidelines for paediatrics. The global initiative on asthma. *Clin Exp Allergy* 2000; **30** (Suppl 1): 6–10.

247  Rossi N, Dalfino T, Verrotti A et al. Third International Pediatric Consensus statement on the management of childhood asthma. International Pediatric Asthma Consensus Group. *Allergy Asthma Proc* 2001; **22**: 297–302.

248  Guidelines on the management of asthma. Statement by the British Thoracic Society, the British Paediatric Association, the Research Unit of the Royal College of Physicians of London, the King's Fund Centre, the National Asthma Campaign, the Royal College of General Practitioners, the General Practitioners in Asthma Group, the British Association of Accident and Emergency Medicine, and the British Paediatric Respiratory Group [erratum appears in *Thorax* 1994; **49**: 386; *Thorax* 1994; **49**: 96.]. *Thorax* 1993; **48**: S1–24.

✱249  Bousquet J. Global initiative for asthma (GINA) and its objectives. *Clin Exp Allergy* 2000; **30** (Suppl 1): 2–5.

250  Chung KF, O'Byrne P. Pharmacological agents used to treat asthma. In: Chung KF, Fabbri LM (eds). *Asthma.* Sheffield: European Respiratory Society Journals Ltd, 2003: 458.

251  Barnes PJ. Corticosteroids. In: Sampson AP, Church MK (eds) *Anti-inflammatory drugs in asthma.* Basal: Birkhauser Berlag, 1999: 33–85.

252  Barnes PJ, Grunstein MM, Leff AR, Woolcock AJ. *Asthma.* Philadelphia: Lippincott-Raven, 1997.

253  Szefler SJ, Martin RJ, King TS et al. Significant variability in response to inhaled corticosteroids for persistent asthma. *J Allergy Clin Immunol* 2002; **109**: 410–8.

254  Sher ER, Leung DY, Surs W et al. Steroid-resistant asthma. Cellular mechanisms contributing to inadequate response to glucocorticoid therapy. *J Clin Invest* 1994; **93**: 33–9.

255  Chan MT, Leung DY, Szefler SJ, Spahn JD. Difficult-to-control asthma: clinical characteristics of steroid-insensitive asthma. *J Allergy Clin Immunol* 1998; **101**: 594–601.

256  Rosenwasser L, Klemm JD, Klemm DJ et al. Association of asthmatic steroid insensitivity with an IL-4 gene promoter

polymorphism [abstract 771]. *J Allergy Clin Immunol* 2001; **107**: S235.

257 Leung DY, Bloom JW. Update on glucocorticoid action and resistance. *J Allergy Clin Immunol* 2003; **111**: 3–22; quiz 23.

258 Levene RZ, Schwartz B, Workman PL. Heritability of plasma cortisol. *Arch Ophthalmol* 1972; **87**: 389–91.

259 Meikle AW, Stringham JD, Woodward MG, Bishop DT. Heritability of variation of plasma cortisol levels. *Metabolism* 1988; **37**: 514–7.

260 Kirschbaum C, Wust S, Faig HG, Hellhammer DH. Heritability of cortisol responses to human corticotropin-releasing hormone, ergometry, and psychological stress in humans. *J Clin Endocrinol Metab* 1992; **75**: 1526–30.

261 Inglis GC, Ingram MC, Holloway CD et al. Familial pattern of corticosteroids and their metabolism in adult human subjects – the Scottish Adult Twin Study. *J Clin Endocrinol Metab* 1999; **84**: 4132–7.

262 Wust S, Federenko I, Hellhammer DH, Kirschbaum C. Genetic factors, perceived chronic stress, and the free cortisol response to awakening. *Psychoneuroendocrinology* 2000; **25**: 707–20.

263 Ober C, Abney M, McPeek MS. The genetic dissection of complex traits in a founder population. *Am J Hum Genet* 2001; **69**: 1068–79.

264 Bartels M, Van den Berg M, Sluyter F et al. Heritability of cortisol levels: review and simultaneous analysis of twin studies. *Psychoneuroendocrinology* 2003; **28**: 121–37.

265 Sutherland ER, Ellison MC, Kraft M, Martin RJ. Altered pituitary–adrenal interaction in nocturnal asthma. *J Allergy Clin Immunol* 2003; **112**: 52–7.

266 Landstra AM, Boezen HM, Postma DS, van Aalderen WM. Effect of intravenous hydrocortisone on nocturnal airflow limitation in childhood asthma. *Eur Respir J* 2003; **21**: 627–32.

267 Landstra AM, Postma DS, Boezen HM, van Aalderen WM. Role of serum cortisol levels in children with asthma. *Am J Respir Crit Care Med* 2002; **165**: 708–12.

268 Laube BL, Curbow BA, Costello RW, Fitzgerald ST. A pilot study examining the relationship between stress and serum cortisol concentrations in women with asthma. *Respir Med* 2002; **96**: 823–8.

269 Sparrow D, O'Connor GT, Rosner B et al. A longitudinal study of plasma cortisol concentration and pulmonary function decline in men. The Normative Aging Study. *Am Rev Respir Dis* 1993; **147**: 1345–8.

●270 Tantisira KG, Lake S, Silverman ES et al. Corticosteroid pharmacogenetics: Association of sequence variants in CRHR1 with improved lung function in asthmatics treated with inhaled corticosteroids. *Hum Mol Genet* 2004; **13**: 1353–9.

# PART 2

# Obstructive lung diseases

# 9

# Asthma genetics

JUAN C. CELEDON, BENJAMIN A. RABY, AND SCOTT T. WEISS

## DEFINITION OF ASTHMA

Asthma is a clinical syndrome of unknown etiology characterized by reversible episodes of airflow obstruction, airway hyper-responsiveness, and a chronic inflammatory process of the airways in which mast cells, eosinophils, T-lymphocytes, epithelial cells, and airway smooth muscle cells play a prominent role.[1] Figure 9.1 shows important pathobiologic features of asthma. CD4 lymphocytes produce IL-3, IL-4, IL-5, IL-13, and GM-CSF and thereby promote

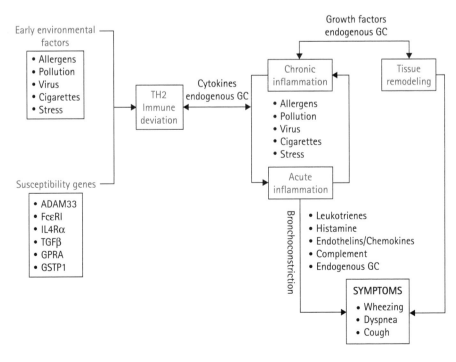

**Figure 9.1** *Asthma pathobiology. Schematic diagram relating genes and environmental exposures to inflammation and lung structural remodeling (courtesy of Eric S. Silverman).*

the synthesis of IgE, an important allergic effector molecule. Chemokines, such as eotaxin, RANTES, and IL-8 produced by epithelial and inflammatory cells, serve to amplify and perpetuate the inflammatory events. Several bronchoactive mediators, such as histamine, leukotrienes, and neuropeptides are released into the airways and precipitate an asthma attack by causing airway smooth muscle constriction, mucus secretion, and edema. Over time, there is smooth muscle growth and the deposition of subepithelial connective tissue, a process referred to as airway remodeling. Understanding the basic pathobiology of asthma is important, because it is clear that many genes may be involved. Clinically, asthmatics have difficulty exhaling air because of an increase in airway resistance that is a consequence of smooth muscle contraction, inflammation, and remodeling. In clinical practice, the degree of resistance and physiological impairment is quantitated most commonly by the forced vital capacity in 1 second ($FEV_1$) (See Chapter 2).[2]

During an asthma attack, patients experience shortness of breath, cough, and/or wheezing. Between attacks, patients may be asymptomatic, or they may have chronic symptoms of breathlessness with mild-to-moderate exertion or episodes of nocturnal awakening due to airway narrowing at night. Most importantly for genetic studies, there is no single defining feature of the disease that is a global standard for diagnosis.

## EPIDEMIOLOGY AND NATURAL HISTORY OF ASTHMA

Asthma is a complex disease affecting over 300 million individuals in the developed world. Ninety percent of all asthma cases, including asthma in adults, have their origins in childhood.[3] The strongest links are with prematurity and low birth weight; roughly 40 percent of children born at term have wheezing symptoms in the first year of life. This decreases to 20 percent at age 3 and remains at 20 percent through age 6, after which time wheezing gradually decreases to a prevalence of approximately 10 percent throughout pre-puberty childhood.[3] Factors associated with an asthma diagnosis in early childhood are the presence of atopic dermatitis, allergic rhinitis, and parental history of asthma or allergy. Eighty percent of all childhood asthma is associated with allergy, although allergy is neither necessary nor sufficient to cause the disease. Gender is an important predictor of asthma occurrence with asthma in early childhood being more common in males, whereas asthma post-puberty and persistence of the disease into adult life are more common in females. The relationship of childhood asthma to adult asthma is uncertain, although it is clear that a large percentage of children outgrow their symptoms in adulthood; however, they do not lose the intermediate phenotypes of airway responsiveness or allergy, and they are susceptible to a recrudescence of the disease in adult life as

a result of cigarette smoking, severe viral respiratory illness, or occupational exposure. Increased airway responsiveness is an important predictor of accelerated decline in lung function in adult life and the development of chronic obstructive pulmonary disease (COPD). Whether childhood asthma is, in fact, a predictor of COPD remains unproven. The central features of asthma epidemiology have been the marked recent increases in asthma prevalence and hospitalization rates in western developed countries. In the USA, between 1980–1994, the self reported prevalence of asthma increased from 30.7 to 53.8/1000 persons, an increase of 75 percent.[4] This increase was accompanied by a similar increase in healthcare utilization and mortality over the same period. An estimated $12.6 billion was spent on the diagnosis and management of asthma in the USA in 1998, of which 58 percent were direct medical expenses.[5] Medication costs are the largest component of direct medical expenditures. Asthma is the most common cause of hospitalization in children in the USA, the most common cause for days lost from school, and the most common cause of emergency room visits.[4]

## IDENTIFIED SYNDROMES WITH ASTHMA–RELATED FEATURES

### Hyperimmunoglobulin E syndrome

#### CLINICAL MANIFESTATIONS

Hyperimmunoglobulin E Syndrome (HIES, Job's syndrome, MIM No. 147060 and MIM No. 243700) is a rare genetic syndrome. In 1966, Davis and colleagues[6] described the first cases of HIES in two unrelated girls with recurrent cutaneous staphylococcal abscesses, reminiscent of the curse placed on the biblical character Job: '{Satan} smote Job with sore boils from the sole of his foot unto his crown' (Job 2:7). To date, more than 200 cases of HIES have been reported.[7–12] The most prominent features of this syndrome are the result of immunologic abnormalities, including moderate-to-severe eczema, recurrent cutaneous and pulmonary infections, elevated total serum immunoglobulin E (IgE) levels, and eosinophilia.[7,13,14] Necrotizing pulmonary infection, typically caused by *Staphlococcus aureus*, complicates the majority of cases and often leads to formation of pneumatoceles. Additional clinical manifestations that underscore the severity of impairment of the immune system in HIES include chronic mucocutaneous candidiasis, *Pneumocystis carinii* pneumonia, and deep tissue-invasive fungal infections. Although total serum IgE levels greater than 2000 IU/ml are present in nearly all patients with HIES, lower IgE levels have been observed, particularly among adults.[7] Hypereosinophilia is common, although not universal. There does not appear to be a strong correlation between clinical severity of disease, total serum IgE levels, and peripheral blood eosinophilia.[7] Importantly, asthma does not appear to be a prominent manifestation of this syndrome. Patients with HIES also display characteristic skeletal, dental, and facial abnormalities that are useful in identifying unknowingly affected individuals.

## FUNCTIONAL DEFECTS

Although the primary defect in HIES remains unidentified, several important immune-related functional abnormalities have been observed. Defective granulocyte chemotaxis is a common feature of HIES.[15,16] In one report, three patients with HIES-like features demonstrated impaired neutrophil chemotactic responsiveness to 'bacterial chemotactic factors' isolated from E. coli culture, but preserved mobility, phagocytosis, and bactericidal activity.[17] Witemeyer and Van Epps[18] observed similar abnormal neutrophil chemotaxis in two subjects with HIES, but not among their family members. Because of the variability in the expression of this phenotype, defective neutrophil chemotaxis is not considered a reliable marker of the HIES. There is evidence that this defect may be due to the production of an inhibitor, as sera from affected individuals can inhibit neutrophil chemotaxis from normal controls.[19] This may be due to circulating immune-complexes,[16,20] and anti-IgE IgG antibodies directed against the Fc portion of IgE have been observed in subjects with HIES.[21] Abnormalities in T cell function, including selective deficiency of suppressor (CD8[+]) T cells and enhanced in vitro production of total serum IgE, have also been observed in patients with HIES.[22] Others have noted impaired T cell response to cytokines, suggesting an underlying defect in T cell signaling.[23–26]

## GENETICS

A significant genetic etiology of HIES is supported by a number of studies showing familial aggregation of this disease.[12,15,16] Although most cases of HIES appear to be sporadic, detailed examination of relatives of affected individuals often reveals evidence of subclinical disease in these individuals, including elevated serum immunoglobulin E levels, dental abnormalities, or distinct facies.

Current evidence suggests that chromosome 4q21 contains a susceptibility gene(s) for HIES. A supernumerary marker chromosome resulting from a 15 to 20 cM interstitial deletion in chromosome 4q21 was observed in a patient with HIES, autism, and mental retardation.[27] On the basis of this finding, Grimbacher et al.[28] performed a directed analysis of linkage between markers on chromosome 4 and HIES in 19 families with multiple affected members. This analysis revealed significant evidence of linkage between chromosome 4q and HIES (LOD = 3.61), with the strongest signal for linkage located within 8 cM of the proximal boundary of the previously described interstitial deletion. To date, the precise nature of the locus (or loci) on chromosome 4q21 remains unidentified. Reports of association between a common atopy-associated Q576R variant in the IL4 receptor and HIES have not been confirmed in follow-up studies.[29,30]

# Hypereosinophilic syndrome

## CLINICAL MANIFESTATIONS

The most common causes of elevated peripheral blood eosinophilia are secondary responses to parasitic infection or allergen exposure. Although less common, there is a long list of primary (non-reactive) eosinophilias relating to myeloid or lymphoproliferative disorders that includes myeloid leukemias, T-cell associated disorders, and myelodysplasias. The hypereosinophilic syndrome (HES – OMIM No. 607685) is characterized by a sustained peripheral blood eosinophilia (greater than $1500 \times 10^6$ cells per liter for at least 6 months) with secondary tissue infiltration and organ damage that is not due to exposure to parasites or allergens.[31] White blood cell counts range between 20 000 and 30 000/mm$^3$, with 30–70 percent eosinophils. Typical sites of organ infiltration include the heart, lungs, skin, and nervous system. Bone marrow and peripheral blood eosinophils display a mature morphology without increased representation of myeloid precursors, thus distinguishing this condition from eosinophilic leukemia. Although most patients present in adulthood, pediatric cases have been reported.[32,33] A male predominance is observed, with a 9:1 male:female ratio.

While HES cases are typically sporadic, several families have been described with heritable peripheral eosinophilia with or without secondary tissue infiltration (see Familial eosinophilia, page 222). This familial form of hypereosinophilia portends a more benign clinical course than sporadic HES. Linkage analyses of families with this more benign disorder have identified genomic regions that are distinct from those implicated in the more severe disease HES, suggesting that familial eosinophilia and HES are two distinct disorders.[34] Early reports of HES suggested nearly universal mortality related to cardiac or pulmonary compromise,[31] yet a more recent survey reported a 42 percent survival rate at 15 years.[35] Therapies aimed at reducing tissue infiltration including corticosteroids and immunosuppressants typically delay disease progression. Subsets of HES patients demonstrate clinical and molecular remissions in response to the tyrosine kinase inhibitor imatinib mesylate (Gleevec), anti-IL5 antibodies, and platelet-derived growth factor receptor inhibitors, implicating their target molecules in HES pathobiology.[36–38]

## GENETICS

The wide variability in the clinical, pathologic, cytogenetic, and molecular features of HES suggests important genetic heterogeneity. Although eosinophil clonality has been observed in many cases of HES, a ubiquitous clonal karyotype has not been observed in most of these cases.[39,40]

Most patients with HES have normal karyotypes. However, karyotype abnormalities such as trisomy 8, and translocations involving chromosome 4q, have been reported, with most trisomy 8 positive cases demonstrating leukemic features.[36,41–46] Genes mapping to chromosome 4q12 include

KIT and the platelet-derived growth factor receptor alpha subunit (PDGFRA), two molecular targets of imatinib mesylate, first described as a tyrosine kinase inhibitor approved for the treatment of BRC-ABL-positive chronic myelogenous leukemia.[47,48] On the basis of variation in clinical responsiveness to imatinib in patients with HES, Cools and colleagues[36] surveyed the genomic structure of its known targets, including PDGFRA and PDGFRB, in 10 imatinib responders. Evidence of chromosomal rearrangement involving the PDGFRA locus on chromosome 4q12 was observed in one of 10 patients surveyed. Resequencing of 5′ RACE products encoding the PDGFRA kinase domain revealed that this chromosomal rearrangement resulted in a fusion of the PDGFRA locus to the Fip1-like 1 (FIP1L1) locus, leading to an in-frame fusion of the first 233 amino acids of FIP1L1 to the terminal 523 amino acids of PDGFRA, within the PDGFRA kinase domain (exon 12). The fusion product was identified in four of the remaining nine patients, and also in four of six additional HES patients. Transfection of a murine hematopoietic cell line Ba/F3 with FIP1L1-PDGFRA resulted in interleukin-3-independent cell growth, with constitutive tyrosine-phosphorylation. Mutation analysis confirmed that a segment of FIP1L1 was responsible for kinase activation; sequence analysis of the PDGFRA kinase domain in one FIP1L1-PDGFRA patient who relapsed during imatinib treatment revealed the presence of a non-synonymous mutation (T674I) in the ATP-binding region of PDGFRA. A similar mutation in the BCR-ABL fusion protein confers resistance to imatinib in CML, suggesting that the FIP1L1-PDGFRA T674I mutation was responsible for the treatment failure in this patient. Dose-response studies confirmed that concentrations of imatinib required to inhibit T674I-FIP1L1-PDGFRA transfected Ba/F3 cell lines were substantially greater than for cell lines transfected with wildtype FIP1L1-PDGFRA. These findings provide compelling evidence that FIP1L1-PDGFRA is a molecular target among imatinib-responsive patients presenting with primary hypereosinophilia. However, because not all imatinib responders are FIP1L1-PDGFRA positive, it is likely that HES cases can also result from aberrations at other loci.

An important byproduct of the identification of FIP1L1-PDGFRA is the recognition that the current clinical classification of primary eosinophilia is not appropriate.[49] FIP1L1-PDGFRA genotype–phenotype correlation studies suggest that FIP1L1-PDGFRA-positive HES represents a distinct clinicopathologic entity. A subset of HES characterized by bone marrow mast cell infiltration, elevated serum tryptase levels, and myelodysplastic features (including splenomegaly and elevated B12 levels with anemia and/or thrombocytopenia) has been described, and termed myelodysplastic HES.[50] FIP1L1-PDGFRA was detected in these patients and clinical response to imatinib was observed, with complete clinical remission in all treated patients.[51] In a survey of 89 patients with primary eosinophilia, FIP1L1-PDGFRA was identified in 10 of 19 patients with myelodysplastic HES (also referred as systemic mast cell disease – SMCD).[52] FIP1L1-PDGFRA was also detected in one patient with clonal eosinophilia. Notably, these 11 FIP1L1-PDGFRA positive patients all demonstrated clinical response with imatinib therapy. Of 57 patients with HES in whom SMCD was excluded, none carried the FIP1L1-PDGFRA mutation, and all had a normal karyotype. Only four of 10 FIP1L1-PDGFRA-negative imatinib-treated patients demonstrated clinical response, and all required higher doses to achieve partial response. It is likely that additional molecular defects will be identified to enable further classification of these FIP1L1-PDGFRA-negative cases.

## Familial eosinophilia

Large extended pedigrees and small nuclear families with multiple members affected with peripheral blood eosinophilia (eosinophil levels >500 cells/mm³) have been reported.[53–56] Of these families, the most extensively characterized is a multigenerational pedigree from the USA ascertained through a male proband with asymptomatic eosinophilia, who later succumbed to progressive cardiac failure due to endomyocardial fibrosis with eosinophilic infiltration.[57] In this family, five of 19 affected members (here defined as $>1500 \times 10^6$ eosinophils/L) demonstrated cardiac involvement (echocardiographic evidence of valvular abnormalities with or without conduction abnormalities). Two of these five also had evidence of mononeuritis multiplex.[57] A follow-up study of 15 affected individuals from this kindred reported that a second affected family member died of complications relating to myocardial fibrosis. Of interest, obstructive pulmonary disease (defined as either a history of asthma or spirometric evidence of airflow obstruction) was observed in a disproportionate number of unaffected family members (7/16 compared to 1/15 affected individuals). There were no differences in smoking history or atopic status to explain this paradox, and it remains unclear whether this inverse association of airways disease with familial eosinophilia is unique to this pedigree.[34]

Eosinophil morphology is typically normal in subjects with familial eosinophilia. Whereas eosinophil activation is common in non-familial HES, circulating eosinophils are not activated in familial eosinophilia. Serum levels of eosinophil-derived granular proteins are elevated in familial eosinophilia, but to a lesser degree than in non-familial HES.

### GENETICS

Karyotype analysis performed on eight of 19 affected members of the large USA familial eosinophilia pedigree. Two individuals (both with cardiac involvement) carried a pericentric inversion of chromosome 10 (inv(10)(p11.2q21.2)). In their report, the investigators noted that other cytogenetic abnormalities on chromosome 10 have been observed in cases of hypereosinophilia, although most commonly in patients with eosinophilia associated with myeloproliferative disorders.[57] Linkage analysis performed in this kindred (see subsequent discussion) did not identify evidence for a familial eosinophilia locus on chromosome 10, suggesting the pericentric inversion is not related to familial eosinophilia.[58] To localize genomic regions containing a gene(s) influencing familial eosinophilia, Rioux and colleagues performed a non-parametric genome-wide linkage analysis for familial eosinophilia in the large USA pedigree described above and identified a single linkage peak on chromosome 5q (LOD = 2.12). Subsequent typing of additional markers and parametric linkage analysis specifying a dominant mode of inheritance with near-complete penetrance (0.9 for heterozygotes, 1.0 for homozygotes) found significant evidence of linkage to hypereosinophilia ($>1500 \times 10^6$ eosinophils/L) for an 18 cM genomic region on chromosome 5q between markers D5S462 and D5S1480 (LOD = 3.28).[58] This genomic region, which includes the cytokine cluster on chromosome 5q31–33, has been linked to asthma and asthma-related phenotypes in several genome scans.[59–61] In addition, chromosome 5q is frequently involved in chromosomal translocations in hematologic malignancies with eosinophilic predominance.[58] Among the many transcripts mapped to this region are IL3, GM-CSF, and IL5, all of which are implicated in eosinophil signaling. However, resequencing of the aforementioned candidate genes on chromosome 5q in affected family members failed to identify disease-causing mutations. To date, no susceptibility genes for familial eosinophilia have been identified.

## Systemic mastocytosis

### CLINICAL FEATURES

Pathologic infiltration of mast cells in various organs is observed in mast cell disorders of varying involvement and severity, including relatively benign cutaneous disease manifested by urticaria pigmentosa and systemic disease.[62] The latter group of disorders can be broadly categorized into systemic mastocytoses and mast cell leukemias based on mast cell morphology and clinical course. Whereas cutaneous mastocytosis often presents in childhood and remits or resolves in early life, systemic mastocytosis is primarily a progressive disease of adulthood. Symptoms relate to direct infiltration of involved tissues and to effects of mast-cell degranulation, including flushing, gastrointestinal symptoms, and hypotension. The most common organs affected include the bone marrow, lymphopoietic tissues, and the gastrointestinal tract. In the bone marrow, mast cells form structured aggregates with or without accompanying lymphocytes.[63,64] Eosinophilic infiltration and peripheral eosinophilia are often observed, making differentiation from HES difficult at times. Elevated serum tryptase levels ($>20$ ng/ml) are observed in most subjects with systemic mastocytosis, including patients with the mast cell-associated myelodysplastic form of HES.[50,65] Additional findings present in a variable percentage of cases include atypical mast cell morphology or altered cell surface marker profiles, including CD2, CD25, and CD35.[66]

### GENETICS

Studies of familial aggregation in nuclear families and twins suggest that there is a significant genetic contribution to the etiology of both cutaneous and systemic mast cell disease.[67–71] Pedigrees with transmission patterns consistent with dominant and recessive inheritance with incomplete penetrance have been described. In several affected pedigree members, identical immunophenotype profiles have been observed.[72,73]

Mast cell clonality is a common feature in most forms of systemic mast cell disease, including those with more benign clinical presentations. A diverse spectrum of karyotypic abnormalities has been described, particularly among more aggressive and malignant forms of the disease.[46,74–76] A unique feature common to most cases is a point mutation in the cKIT protooncogene (KIT), an A → T substitution at nucleotide 2468, that results in substitution of aspartate 816 for valine. The cKIT gene encodes a type III transmembrane tyrosine kinase receptor that is the principal receptor for stem cell factor (aka mast-cell growth factor, KITLG). cKIT has been implicated in many hematologic malignancies, including mast cell leukemia[77] and murine models of both cKIT and KITLG mutation demonstrate impaired mast-cell production.[78] Furitsu and colleagues first described the Asp816Val mutation in a human mast cell leukemia cell line HMC-1, which exhibited constitutive phosphorylation of cKIT. This mutation has subsequently been observed in cases of both primary and malignancy-associated systemic mastocytosis.[79–81] Of note, point mutations at codon 816 that result in alternate amino acid substitutions (Asp816Tyr and Asp816Phe) have also been reported,[80] as have mutations at other codons in the cKIT gene (Phe522Cys, Asp820Gly, and Glu839Lys).[80,82,83] Several studies have demonstrated the presence of the Asp816Val mutation in cKIT in most cases of systemic mastocytosis in adults, particularly those exhibiting an indolent course.[80,84,85] Although children with systemic mastocytosis can carry the Val816Asp mutation in cKIT, pediatric cases of systemic mastocytosis can have normal cKIT, carry the Tyr816 or Phe816 variants, or have an inactivating mutation (Glu839Lys).[80] Lack of cKIT involvement has been documented in familial cases of systemic mastocytosis,[86] although germline mutations have recently been described.[87] Although imatinib may be useful in treating cases of systemic mastocytosis bearing wildtype cKIT, cKIT mutations appear to induce resistance to treatment with imatinib.[88]

## Netherton syndrome

Netherton syndrome (OMIM 256500) is a severe autosomal recessive disorder characterized by abnormal 'bamboo' hair (trichorrhexis invaginata), congenital ichthyosiform erythroderma (redness, blistering, and scaling hypertrophy of the skin), and atopic diathesis.[89,90] Dermatologic manifestations of Netherton syndrome are typified by a generalized scaly erythroderma that is refractory to topical corticosteroid therapy and that often leads to dehydration and superinfection of the skin, thus contributing to the high infant mortality observed in this condition. The atopic manifestations of Netherton syndrome are severe and include atopic dermatitis, allergic rhinitis, asthma, and elevated total serum IgE levels. Phenotypic expression of Netherton syndrome was initially thought to be restricted to females, but more recent reports confirm that the disease is fully penetrant in males as well, confirming autosomal inheritance.[91,92]

The gene causing Netherton syndrome has been identified as SPINK5, a serine protease inhibitor localizing to chromosome 5q32. Highly significant evidence for linkage (maximum multipoint LOD score 10.11) between a 3.5-cM genetic interval telomeric to the cytokine gene cluster and Netherton syndrome was observed in 20 families of affected individuals.[93] Mutation discovery efforts focusing on the coding regions of SPINK5 identified 11 mutations in 13 families of subjects with Netherton syndrome.[94] Of these 11 mutations, nine alter the SPINK5 reading frame and two were found in multiple families, including several known to be related. All affected subjects were either homozygous for mutations in SPINK5 or were compound heterozygotes, while unaffected family members were either heterozygous or homozygous for the wildtype alleles of SPINK5. Mutation screening of SPINK5 as a candidate gene for Netherton was motivated by its tissue distribution in thymus and mucosal epithelium, its role as a serine-protease,[95] and the observation that SPINK5 mRNA levels were markedly reduced in patient-derived extracts from cultured epidermal keratinocytes.[94] Since the original report, four additional common nonsynonymous coding polymorphisms have been identified in patients with Netherton syndrome or atopic dermatitis. Walley and colleagues[96] found evidence of association of maternally derived alleles in two of these polymorphisms with common atopic dermatitis, IgE levels and asthma, suggesting that more common variation in SPINK5 affects less severe atopic disease. Replication of these associations has been reported.[97–99]

## Churg–Strauss syndrome

In 1951, Churg and Strauss described a series of patients with severe asthma and rhinitis who subsequently developed hypereosinophilia, pneumonia, and eosinophilic arteritis and granulomas in multiple organs;[100] the presence of asthma and allergies in all of these patients distinguished this disorder from other vasculitides. Vasculitic involvement in Churg–Strauss syndrome (CSS) is most commonly observed in the heart, lungs, sinuses, skin, gastrointestinal tract, kidneys, and both the central and peripheral nervous systems. Although several sets of criteria have been used to define this condition, all include a diagnosis of asthma,

peripheral blood eosinophilia, and clinical or pathological evidence of systemic eosinophilic vasculitis.[101–103] Asthma is a defining feature of Churg–Strauss syndrome; however, as many as 2 percent of patients may develop airway symptoms after the onset of systemic vasculitis.[104] Symptom onset is typically in adulthood and often occurs in individuals who have no family history of atopy. Although rare in the general population (incidence ranging from 2–4 cases per million patient-years), asthmatic populations are at much greater risk, with reported incidence rates of 60 cases per million patient-years.[105,106] Although there has been a recent increase in case reports of Churg–Strauss syndrome in association with leukotriene modifier treatment,[105,107] it is unclear whether introduction of these agents caused the disease or simply unmasked the vasculitic manifestations upon concomitant steroid withdrawal.[108,109]

Very little is known about the pathogenesis of CSS, but several lines of evidence suggest that aberrant eosinophil regulation plays a central underlying role. Churg–Strauss syndrome is associated with circulating anti-neutrophil cytoplasmic antibodies (predominantly the perinuclear, p-ANCA antibodies); markedly increased levels of circulating soluble IL-2 receptor, eosinophil cationic protein, and thrombomodulin;[110] and increased production of IL-10, IL-4, IL-13, and interferon-gamma.[111,112] Evidence of defective eosinophil and lymphocyte apoptosis has been provided by Muschen and colleagues,[113] who demonstrated enhanced expression of a soluble splice variant of CD95 in eight CSS patients. Soluble CD95 is known to rescue eosinophils from apoptosis, and has been implicated in other vasculitic and lymphoproliperative disease states. Patients with CSS can have severe asthma, requiring high doses of oral corticosteroids for adequate symptom control. The vasculitis associated with CSS is also responsive to corticosteroid therapy, with documented clinical remission obtained in over 90 percent of subjects treated.[104] Approximately 25 percent of treated subjects may relapse, often due to corticosteroid tapering, with a rising eosinophil count heralding the relapse.[104]

Although familial clustering of CSS has not been commonly reported, one report of a father with typical CSS whose son developed Wegener's granulomatosis suggests that a hereditary basis for a subset of vasculitis may exist.[114] To date, no studies have examined the genetics of CSS and there is no conclusive evidence that CSS has genetic antecedents. Since asthma and eosinophic vasculitis are prominent features of the syndrome, should genetics prove a cause of the syndrome, it may have relevance to asthma genetics generally.

## Asthma as a complex disease

### ENVIRONMENTAL FACTORS

The strongest predictors of asthma development are maternal history of asthma, prematurity, and environmental tobacco smoke. A substantial body of data supports each of these three risk factors as clear-cut predictors of the disease very early in life.[115–117] Subepithelial fibrosis, which is characteristic of asthma as a disease, can be directly traced to in utero cigarette smoke exposure of the fetus. This lesion is present at birth and airway remodeling may be a phenomenon of in utero fetal programming in response to this environmental exposure.[118] A list of potential environmental influences on asthma development and progression is provided in Table 9.1. Some environmental exposures noted to be important predictors of asthma risk are of such importance that they appear to overwhelm other factors – an example might be cigarette smoking. In addition, some of these factors may be risk factors for the development of the allergy phenotype but may be protective against asthma and vice versa. For example, there is no evidence that environmental tobacco smoke exposure influences the development of allergy in children. One of the mechanisms by which environmental exposures exert their influence on the disease is through their impact on the ontogeny of the immune system, specifically, the development of a Th2 phenotype in the asthma. The dose, route of administration, and timing of exposure may all be important in determining whether certain antigens tolerize and lead to normal immune system development or result in immune system deviation with the development of a pathologic response.

There are three known key prevalent environmental exposures involved in disease persistence and severity in early childhood: (1) allergen exposure, (2) viral respiratory illness, and (3) environmental tobacco smoke exposure or personal smoking. These factors may have a detrimental

**Table 9.1** *Potential environmental factors in asthma*

| Factors |
| --- |
| Diet/bottle feeding |
| Tobacco smoke (active and passive) |
| Respiratory infection |
| Day care |
| Endotoxin exposure |
| Allergen exposure |
| Stress |
| Farming |
| Pets (cats, dogs) |
| Parasites |

effect on the persistence of the disease or its recrudescence after a period of quiescence.[119]

## Familial aggregation and twin studies

### EVIDENCE FOR A HERITABLE COMPONENT OF ASTHMA AND LUNG FUNCTION PHENOTYPES

#### Bronchial asthma

Data from a significant number of studies indicate familial aggregation of asthma.[120–125] As discussed in Chapter 1, a method frequently used to establish the existence of familial aggregation of a trait is to calculate the recurrence risk to relatives of a particular type, such as siblings or all first-degree relatives. Sibbald et al.[124] found the prevalence of asthma to be 13 percent among first-degree relatives of 77 asthmatic children and 4 percent among first-degree relatives of 87 control children, resulting in a relative risk (often referred to as $\lambda$) in first-degree relatives of 3.3. Familial aggregation, however, could result from genetic factors or a shared environment. The twin study design is useful to separate the relative contributions of genetic and environmental factors. In a large study of 3800 Australian twins, the concordance rate for self-reported asthma was 30 percent in monozygotic (MZ) twins, whereas it was 12 percent in dizygotic (DZ) twins,[126] suggesting a significant genetic component for asthma.

Heritability, the proportion of phenotypic variance that can be attributed to genetic factors, can also be estimated from twin studies. Estimates of the heritability of asthma in several twin studies conducted around the world have ranged from 36 to 79 percent,[126–130] with the highest values coming from studies that had a more comprehensive phenotypic assessment of asthma.[131] Twin studies of asthma are summarized in Table 9.2.

### AIRWAY RESPONSIVENESS

Konig and Godfried[132] conducted an early study of airway responsiveness with eight MZ and seven DZ twins using a standard exercise challenge. Six of the MZ pairs had similar levels of airway responsiveness, but only one of the DZ pairs had similar responses to this nonpharmacologic challenge. Although this study had a small sample size, its results suggest the existence of a heritable component to

**Table 9.2** *Summary table of twin studies of asthma*

| Author | Year | Country | Phenotype | MZ | MZ Correlation | DZ | DZ Correlation | H | Comments |
| --- | --- | --- | --- | --- | --- | --- | --- | --- | --- |
| Edfors–Lubs | 1971 | Sweden | Asthma | 2434 | 0.65 | 4302 | 0.25 | – | Pop-based |
| Niemienen | 1991 | Finland | Asthma | 4307 | 0.43 | 9581 | 0.25 | 0.36 | Pop-based adults |
| Duffy | 1990 | Australia | Asthma | 1799 | 0.65 | 2009 | 0.25 | 0.60–0.75 | Pop-based |
| Harris | 1997 | Norway | Asthma | 939 | 0.75 | 1620 | 0.21 | 0.75 | Pop-based aged 18–25 |
| Laitinen | 1998 | Finland | Asthma | 535 | 0.76 | 1178 | 0.45 | 0.79 | Prenatal/twins |
| Lichtenstein | 1997 | Sweden | Asthma | 421 | 0.64–0.79 | 856 | 0.25–0.27 | 0.62–0.76 | Pop-based aged 7–9 |
| Skadhauger | 1999 | Denmark | Asthma | 3690 | 0.65–0.81 | 7998 | 0.05–0.47 | 0.73 | Pop-based aged 12–41 |

MZ = Number of monozygotic twin pairs; DZ = Number of dizygotic twin pairs; H = heritability. Table adapted from Los H, Koppleman GH, Postma DS. The importance of genetic influence in asthma. *Eur Resp J* 1999; **14**: 1210–27.

**Table 9.3** *Summary table of twin studies of asthma intermediate phenotypes*

| Author | Year | Country | Phenotype | MZ | MZ Correlation | DZ | DZ Correlation | H | Comments |
|--------|------|---------|-----------|-----|----------------|-----|----------------|-----|----------|
| Hopp | 1984 | USA | IgE | 56 | 82 | 43 | 0.32 | 0.61 | |
| Hanson | 1991 | USA | IgE | 34 | 0.42 | 27 | 0.26 | | Together |
| Hanson | 1991 | USA | IgE | 49 | 0.64 | 21 | 0.49 | | Apart |
| Hanson | 1991 | Finland | IgE | 76 | 0.56 | 82 | 0.37 | | Together |
| Duffy | 1998 | Australia | IgE | – | – | – | – | | CoTwin control study |
| Duffy | 1998 | Australia | ST | – | – | – | – | | CoTwin control study |
| Hanson | 1991 | USA | ST | – | – | – | – | | Together/apart |
| Hanson | 1991 | USA | Specific IgE | – | – | – | – | | Together/apart |
| Hopp | 1984 | USA | AHR | 61 | 0.67 | 44 | 0.34 | 0.66 | |

Table adapted from Los H, Koppleman GH, Postma DS. The importance of genetic influence in asthma. *Eur Resp J* 1999; **14**: 1210–27. See Table 9.2 for abbreviations.

airway responsiveness. Hopp et al.[128] conducted a study where methacholine challenge tests were used to measure airway responsiveness in 107 twin pairs (61 MZ and 46 DZ). The intrapair correlation coefficient for the area under the dose-response curve for methacholine was 0.67 for MZ twin pairs, but only 0.34 for DZ twin pairs, and the heritability of airway responsiveness was estimated to be 66 percent. However, no adjustments were made for differences in lung size among subjects or cigarette smoking. Twin studies of airway responsiveness and IgE are summarized in Table 9.3.

### FORCED EXPIRATORY VOLUME IN ONE SECOND (FEV₁)

The measurement of $FEV_1$ from a forced vital capacity maneuver is depicted in Fig. 2.1 of Chapter 2. The role of genetic factors in normal pulmonary function is discussed in detail in Chapter 10. In brief, several studies have reported familial aggregation of $FEV_1$ as a measure of lung function.[133,134] In a study of 15 pairs of MZ twins raised apart, Hankins and co-workers[135] found that intrapair differences in $FEV_1$ were small and virtually identical in concordant smoking and nonsmoking pairs. The high heritability of $FEV_1$ was confirmed in a study of 127 MZ and 141 DZ white male twin pairs from the NHLBI twin study.[136] A study from the Channing Laboratory assessed both genetic and non-genetic influences on 1635 members of 414 families of adult twins from the Greater Boston Twin Registry.[137] After adjusting for age, sex, height, and smoking status, intrapair correlation coefficients were 0.71 for MZ twins and 0.16 for DZ twins. Furthermore, intrapair correlation coefficients for $FEV_1$ among pairs of relatives with the same fraction of shared ancestry (e.g., dizygotic twins, parent–offspring, MZ twin–niece/nephew) were similar despite differences in the degree of shared environment between these groups. Taken together, these findings suggest that genetic factors have a strong influence on $FEV_1$ levels.

### BRONCHODILATOR RESPONSIVENESS

Our group has recently found evidence for familial aggregation of bronchodilator responsiveness in a rural Chinese population.[138]

In summary, these data indicate a significant heritable component of asthma and asthma-related lung function phenotypes.

## GENOME–WIDE LINKAGE ANALYSIS FOR ASTHMA AND ASTHMA–RELATED PHENOTYPES

Eleven groups have reported results of genome-wide linkage analysis for asthma-related phenotypes.[139–149] Several of these groups have published second-generation surveys with larger numbers of subjects and markers.[150–156] An additional genome-wide linkage study for asthma reported only partial results.[157]

Daniels and colleagues[158] performed a genome-wide linkage analysis for quantitative (total serum IgE, skin test index, peripheral blood eosinophil count, and airway responsiveness to methacholine) and qualitative (atopy) phenotypes related to asthma in 172 sib-pairs in 80 families selected from a population-based study in Busselton (Western Australia). These investigators found suggestive evidence of linkage[159] ($P < 0.0005$) to total serum IgE (chromosomes 11q and 16q), skin test index (chromosome 11q), peripheral blood eosinophil count (chromosome 6p), airway responsiveness (chromosomes 4q and 7p), and atopy (chromosomes 6p and 13q).

The Collaborative Study on the Genetics of Asthma (CSGA) performed genome-wide linkage analyses for asthma and asthma-related phenotypes in families of siblings with asthma in each of three ethnic groups (European-Americans, African-Americans, and Hispanics) in the USA.[160–163] In that study, there was suggestive evidence of linkage to asthma in 129 European-American families (chromosome 6p, LOD = 1.9), 107 African-American families (chromosome 11q, LOD = 2.0), and 30 Hispanic families (chromosome 1p, LOD = 2.9).[161] There was only modest evidence of linkage ($P < 0.01$) to either total serum IgE or skin test reactivity to at least one allergen in each of the three ethnic groups included in the CSGA. After adjusting the analysis for gender, age, and a skin test index, the evidence of linkage between chromosome 18q and total serum IgE increased only among European-Americans (adjusted LOD = 2.75).[162]

Wjst and colleagues[143] conducted a genome-wide linkage analysis for asthma and asthma-related phenotypes in 415 members of 97 families of siblings with asthma in Germany and Sweden. In these families, there was modest evidence of linkage ($P < 0.01$) to asthma (on chromosomes 6p and 9q), total serum IgE (on chromosomes 1p, 2p, 2q, 6p, 9q, 15q, and Xq), increased airway responsiveness (on chromosome 2p and 9p), and peripheral blood eosinophil count (on chromosomes 1p, 6p, 6q, 11q, and Xq).

Among 424 members of nuclear families of atopic individuals in Denmark, a genome-wide linkage analysis showed suggestive evidence of linkage to asthma (on chromosomes 1p (LOD = 2.02), 5q (LOD = 2.20), and 6p (LOD = 2.66)); total serum IgE (on chromosomes 3q (LOD = 2.41), 5q (LOD = 2.12), and 6p (LOD = 2.61)); and sensitization to at least one allergen (on chromosome 6p (LOD = 2.27)).[148] In addition, there was modest evidence of linkage ($P < 0.01$) to asthma (on chromosomes 12q and Xp), total serum IgE (on chromosome 4q), and sensitization to at least one allergen (on chromosomes 3q, 4q, 5q, 22q, and Xp).

Dizier and colleagues[145] conducted a genome-wide linkage analysis for asthma and asthma-related phenotypes in 279 individuals in 107 families of siblings with asthma in France. These investigators found modest evidence of linkage ($P < 0.01$) to asthma (on chromosome 7q), total serum IgE (on chromosome 11p), peripheral blood eosinophil count (on chromosome 12q), and skin test reactivity to at least one allergen (on chromosome 17q).

Among 1174 members of 200 families of individuals with asthma in the Netherlands, a genome-wide analysis found significant evidence of linkage to total serum IgE (on chromosome 7q (LOD = 3.36)) and suggestive evidence of linkage to total serum IgE (on chromosomes 2q (LOD = 1.96), 3q (LOD = 2.11), 5q (LOD = 2.73), 12q (LOD = 2.46), and 13q (LOD = 2.28)) and peripheral blood eosinophil count (on chromosomes 15q (LOD = 2.19) and 17q (LOD = 1.97)). In addition, there was modest evidence of linkage ($P < 0.01$) to total serum IgE (on chromosome 6p), peripheral blood eosinophil count (on chromosome 2q), sensitization to house dust mite (on chromosomes 3q, 8p, and 11q), and sensitization to at least one allergen (chromosome 17q).[155] Of note, a genome-wide linkage analysis for airway responsiveness conducted in a subset of the families included in the study by Koppelman et al. was reported only in abstract form.[140] There was 'strong' evidence of linkage to airway hyper-responsiveness on chromosomes 5q (LOD not reported) and suggestive evidence of linkage to airway hyper-responsiveness on chromosome 3 (LOD = 2.8).

There have been two genome-wide linkage scans for asthma-related phenotypes in Asian populations. Yokouchi and colleagues[144] conducted a genome-wide linkage analysis for asthma-related phenotypes among 197 members of 47 Japanese families of siblings who had asthma and who were sensitized to house dust mite. There was significant evidence of linkage to mite-sensitive asthma on chromosome 5q (LOD = 4.73) and suggestive evidence of linkage to mite-sensitive asthma on chromosomes 4q (LOD = 2.74), 6p (LOD = 2.13), 12q (LOD = 1.92), and 13q (LOD = 2.41). Among 2551 Chinese subjects in 533 families of siblings with asthma, genome-wide linkage analysis showed significant evidence of linkage to airway responsiveness on chromosome 2p ($P = 0.00002$) and suggestive evidence of linkage to FVC (on chromosome 16p, $P = 0.0006$) and skin test reactivity to cockroach (on chromosome 4q, $P = 0.0003$).[147] In addition, there was some evidence of linkage ($P < 0.01$) to $FEV_1$ (on chromosomes 2p, 10p, and 22q), FVC (on chromosome 1q), airway responsiveness (on chromosome 19q), and total serum IgE (on chromosome 1q).

A potentially helpful strategy to identify genomic regions influencing asthma is to focus on genetically isolated populations, because in these populations the number of genes influencing a complex trait may be relatively small.[164] The Hutterite population of South Dakota (USA) is a religious isolate of European ancestry. Among 693 members of a large Hutterite family pedigree with high prevalence of asthma and atopy, there was suggestive evidence of linkage to asthma (chromosomes 1p and 8p), skin test reactivity to mold (chromosome 11p), and airway responsiveness (chromosome 19q).[165] In addition, there was modest evidence of linkage ($P < 0.01$) to skin test reactivity to house dust mite (chromosome 2q), skin test reactivity to mold (chromosomes 3q and 16q), skin test reactivity to at least one allergen (chromosome 8q), and airway responsiveness (chromosome 5p). Among 1107 members of 175 families of individuals with asthma in Iceland, Hakonarson and colleagues[149] found suggestive evidence of linkage to asthma on chromosomes 14q (LOD = 2.6) and 10 (LOD ≈ 2.1). In that study, the evidence for linkage to asthma on chromosome 14q increased markedly after genotyping additional markers (LOD = 4.0). Laitinen and colleagues[146] conducted a genome-wide linkage analysis for asthma in 443 members of 86 families of individuals with asthma in Finland. There was suggestive evidence of linkage to asthma on chromosomes 4q (LOD = 2.5) and 7p (LOD = 2.0). A repeat analysis after genotyping additional markers on chromosomes 4q and 7p showed increased evidence of linkage to asthma on chromosome 7p (LOD = 2.8) and significant evidence of linkage to total serum IgE on chromosome 7p (LOD = 3.9). The findings with regard to asthma were then replicated in an analysis of linkage between markers on chromosome 7p and asthma among families in a population isolate from Canada (LOD = 2.7). In a second population isolated from North Karelia (Finland), there was suggestive evidence of linkage between chromosome 7p and elevated total serum IgE level (LOD = 1.9).

Although van Eerdewegh and colleagues[157] conducted a genome-wide linkage analysis for asthma-related phenotypes on 460 sibling pairs affected with asthma in the

USA and the UK, they only reported their results for chromosome 20. There was suggestive evidence of linkage to asthma (defined as physician-diagnosed asthma and current medication use) on chromosome 20p (LOD = 2.94). Although using a more stringent definition of asthma (physician-diagnosed asthma and increased airway responsiveness) reduced the effective sample size to 218 affected sibling pairs, these investigators found significant evidence of linkage to asthma on chromosome 20p (LOD = 3.93).

Table 9.4 summarizes the results of fully reported genome-wide linkage analyses of asthma and/or asthma-related phenotypes by showing chromosomal regions linked to asthma and asthma phenotypes at the $\alpha < 0.01$ level. These studies varied widely with respect to the number of families and individuals assessed, methods used for ascertainment of probands, methods used for assessing asthma and asthma-related phenotypes, ethnicity of subjects, and definition of asthma and asthma-related phenotypes.

**Table 9.4** *Published genome-wide linkage analyses of asthma and asthma-related phenotypes[a]*

| Study group, year | Population | No. of families | No. of subjects | Linkage to asthma | Linkage to asthma phenotypes[b] |
|---|---|---|---|---|---|
| Oxford, 1996 | Western Australia | 80 | 203 | Not assessed | Western Australian population: AHR = 4q, 7p; eosinophil count = 6p; atopy (composite score) = 6p, 13q; skin test index = 11q; total serum IgE = 7p, 11q, 16q; British population: atopy = 13q |
| | | 77 | 215 | | |
| CSGA 2001, 2001, 2004 | US (white, Hispanic, African-American) | 266 | 885 | Whites: 6p; Hispanics: 1p; African-Americans: 11q | Total serum IgE: Whites = 4p; African-Americans = 2q, 4q; Skin test reactivity to ≥1 allergen: Whites = 3q, 14p; Hispanics = 1p, 20p, 21q; African Americans = 17p |
| Hutterites 2000 | Isolate originally from Tyrolean Alps | 1 large pedigree | 693 | 1p, 8p | AHR: 5p, 19q; skin test reactivity to ≥1 allergen: 8q; skin test reactivity to house dust mite: 2q; skin test reactivity to mold: 3q, 11p, 16q |
| German Asthma Genetics Group 1999 | Families from Germany/Sweden | 97 | 415 | 2p, 6p, 9q | AHR: 2p, 9p; total serum IgE: 1p, 2p, 2q, 6p, 9q, 15q, Xq; eosinophil count: 1p, 6p, 6q, 11q, Xq |
| Netherlands 1999, 2002 | Families from the Netherlands | 200 | 1,174 | Not assessed | AHR[c]: 3, 5q; total serum IgE: 2q, 3q, 5q, 6p, 7q, 12q, 13q; skin test to reactivity to ≥1 allergen: 17q; sensitization to house dust mite: 3q, 8p, 11q; eosinophils: 2q, 15q, 17q |
| Japanese 2000 | Dust-mite sensitized asthmatics | 47 | 196 | 4q, 5q, 6p, 12q, 13q | Not assessed |
| French EGEA Study 2000 | Siblings and parents born in France | 107 | 279 sibs | 17q | Eosinophil count: 12q; total serum IgE: 11p; skin test reactivity to ≥1 allergen: 17q |
| Finnish 2001 | Population isolate from Finland | 86 | 443 | 4q, 7p | Total serum IgE: 7p |
| China 2001 | Cohort from Anqing, China | 533 | 2,551 | Not assessed | AHR: 2p, 19q; total serum IgE: 1q; FEV$_1$ = 2p, 10p, and 22q; FVC = 1q, 16p; skin test reactivity to cockroach = 4q |
| Danish 2002 | Danish families selected for atopy | 100 | 424 | 1p, 5q, 6p, 12q, Xp | Total serum IgE: 3q, 4q, 5q, 6p; Increased serum IgE to ≥1 allergen: 3q, 4q, 5q, 6p, 22q, Xp |
| Iceland 2002 | Population isolate from Iceland | 175 | 1,107 | 10, 14q | Not assessed |

[a]Loci included are those linked to asthma and asthma-related phenotypes at $\alpha < 0.01$.
[b]AHR = airway hyperresponsiveness.
[c]Complete linkage results for all chromosomes not published. AHR results based on 140 families.

Few of the findings of these studies met rigorous criteria for significant linkage in genome-wide analysis of complex traits.[159] In particular, two genome scans in individuals of European descent reported significant evidence of linkage to asthma on chromosomes 14q[149] and 20p,[157] and one genome scan in Japanese individuals reported significant evidence of linkage to mite-sensitive asthma on chromosome 5q.[144] In addition, two genome scans in individuals of European descent found significant evidence of linkage to total serum IgE on chromosomes 7p[146] and 7q,[155] and a genome scan in Chinese individuals showed significant evidence of linkage to increased airway responsiveness to methacholine on chromosome 2p.[151] It should be noted, however, that more than 20 chromosomal regions across the genome have shown some evidence for linkage to asthma phenotypes. Of these chromosomal regions, several have been associated with asthma (1p, 4q, 5q, 6p, 11q, 12q), increased airway responsiveness (2p and 19q), total serum IgE (2q, 3q, 4q, 5q, 6p, 7p), sensitization to ≥1 allergen (1p, 3q, 4q, 6p, 17q), and peripheral blood eosinophil count (6p) in at least two genome scans at the $\alpha < 0.01$ level.

The results of multiple genome-wide linkage analyses for asthma and asthma-related phenotypes suggest that multiple genomic regions contain genes that influence asthma phenotypes. In addition, potential explanations for the discrepant results of these analyses include differences in sample size and statistical power, genetic heterogeneity, gene-by-gene interactions, differences in exposure to environmental factors relevant to asthma and asthma-related phenotypes, and differences in phenotypic assessment of asthma and asthma-related phenotypes.

# CANDIDATE GENES FOR ASTHMA AND ASTHMA-RELATED PHENOTYPES

A large number of studies of genetic association for asthma phenotypes have been conducted, often yielding inconsistent results. Potential reasons for the conflicting findings of studies of genetic association in asthma include small sample sizes, failure to correct for multiple comparisons, genetic and environmental heterogeneity, and (for case–control studies) population stratification.[166] Although there are statistical methods to detect and correct for population stratification in case–control studies, few of the case–control studies of genetic association in asthma have accounted for possible population stratification. In spite of these problems, association studies have helped identify potential asthma susceptibility genes. To date, there have been reports of association between variants in over 70 genes and asthma phenotypes. Candidate genes for association studies of asthma phenotypes have been selected on the basis of the results of genome-wide linkage analyses ('positional') and/ or the biological plausibility that they influence asthma phenotypes ('functional').

# POTENTIAL ASTHMA–SUSCEPTIBILITY LOCI IDENTIFIED BY POSITIONAL CLONING

Four potential asthma susceptibility genes (ADAM33, PHF11, DPP10, and GPRA (also known as GPR154)) have been identified using a positional cloning approach.[157,167–169] In all cases, significant linkage between a chromosomal region and asthma phenotypes was found in a genome-wide linkage analysis, and fine-mapping studies of linkage and association were then performed in the linked genomic region. Following the fine-mapping studies, associations between variants in a specific gene and asthma phenotypes were identified in at least two populations.

## ADAM33

In 2002, van Eerdewegh and coworkers[157] reported the identification of the ADAM33 gene (ADAM33) as a susceptibility gene for asthma and airway hyperresponsiveness on chromosome 20p13. In a genome scan on 460 Caucasian families, these investigators found evidence of linkage between chromosome 20p13 and both physician-diagnosed asthma (LOD = 2.94) and a stringent definition of asthma that included airways hyper-responsiveness (LOD = 3.93). The 1-LOD-support interval for the genomic region linked to asthma spanned 2.5 megabases (Mb) and included more than 40 genes. As an initial screen of candidate genes in this region, 135 single nucleotide polymorphisms (SNPs) in 23 genes were genotyped in a case–control association study composed of the probands of families showing evidence for linkage to asthma and 'hypernormal' controls. Although variants in several candidate genes were associated with asthma, a relatively large number of SNPs in a specific gene (ADAM33) were associated with asthma. The association between SNPs in ADAM33 and asthma was then confirmed using family-based association methods in the pedigrees included in the genome-wide linkage analysis.

Although ADAM33 is expressed in multiple tissues, it is highly expressed in bronchial smooth muscle and lung fibroblasts, two cells critical in the processes of airway responsiveness and airway remodeling. ADAM33 belongs to a large family of molecules (disintegrin-containing zinc-dependent metalloproteinases) implicated in diverse biological processes, including cell fusion, myofibroblast proliferation, proteolysis, and cell-signaling.[157] The murine homolog of ADAM33 maps to mouse chromosome 2, a region linked to native airways responsiveness in C57BL/6J × A/J crossbreeds.[170] Taken together with the results of association studies in humans, these findings support a role for ADAM33 in the pathogenesis of asthma and airway responsiveness.

Although there is evidence to support that ADAM33 is an asthma susceptibility gene, there is also substantial evidence to refute a major role of ADAM33 in asthma pathogenesis. First, linkage between chromosome 20p and asthma has not been observed in most genome scans for asthma and asthma-related phenotypes (see above), raising concerns about the generalizability of the original findings. Second, most of the polymorphisms in *ADAM33* that were associated with asthma in the original report do not reside within coding regions but are located in introns. Although it is conceivable that these intronic variants alter gene expression or splicing profile, there is no data to support this hypothesis. Third, several groups have attempted to replicate the association between variants in ADAM33 and asthma, obtaining mixed results. Howard and colleagues[171] reported evidence of association between variants in *ADAM33* and asthma in four distinct cohorts: a US Caucasian cohort, a Dutch Caucasian cohort, an African-American cohort, and a Hispanic cohort. Although several SNPs in ADAM33 were associated with asthma-related phenotypes in each of the four cohorts, none of the SNPs included in the study was associated with asthma-related phenotypes in all of the cohorts. In addition, there was no consistency of the associations in populations included in the study by Howard et al. and those reported by van Eerdewegh and colleagues. Among 583 Hispanic (Mexican-American and Puerto Rican) nuclear families of subjects with asthma, Lind and colleagues[172] found no significant association between six SNPs in *ADAM33* and asthma or asthma-related phenotypes. In a third replication study, Raby and colleagues[173] examined the association between 17 polymorphisms in ADAM33 and asthma and asthma-related phenotypes in 587 nuclear families of asthmatic children. Among European-Americans and African-Americans, there was no association between any of the 17 SNPs in *ADAM33* and asthma. Among Hispanics, two markers in strong linkage disequilibrium (LD) (T1 and T+1) demonstrated very weak evidence of association with asthma, total serum IgE levels, and peripheral blood eosinophilia. The lack of replication of linkage between chromosome 20p and asthma, the lack of data to support a functional role of the SNPs in *ADAM33* that have been associated with asthma, and the inconsistent results of association studies raise concerns about a significant role of ADAM33 in the pathogenesis of asthma. Further work needs to be performed, both in terms of replication of genetic association as well as attempts to determine gene function, before any firm conclusions can be made regarding the importance of *ADAM33* in the pathobiology of asthma.

## DPP10

Chromosome 2q has been linked to asthma in several human populations (see above), and the homologous region in mouse includes a quantitative trait locus (QTL) for airway responsiveness.[170] Among 244 Caucasian families in whom associations between variants in the interleukin 1 gene (*IL1*) cluster and asthma had been previously identified, Allen and colleagues[169] reported an association between asthma

and a microsatellite marker (D2S308, allele 3) located on chromosome 2q14 (800 kb distal to the IL1 gene cluster). Marker D2S308 localizes to one of four distinct LD blocks across chromosome 2q14-q32. Asthma was most strongly associated with SNPs localizing to this block (Block B), including marker WTC122, which is adjacent to D2S308. SNPs in an adjacent but distinct LD block (Block A) were associated with total serum IgE levels, and multivariate analysis suggested that each associated allele on chromosome 2q14-q32 contributed independently to variation in total serum IgE levels. Although the observed associations between alleles and haplotypes on chromosome 2q14-q32 were replicated in a second cohort of German schoolchildren, the risk-conferring haplotypes differed from those found in the original population. In a third cohort tested, the WTC122-D2S308 haplotype was associated with asthma severity, but not with asthma per se. The authors then concluded that the interaction between loci on chromosome 2q14-q32 and asthma-related phenotypes is complex, and that genes within chromosome 2q14-q32 may interact with other unidentified susceptibility alleles.

By screening a panel of cDNA libraries for all potential exons within this region, a novel gene was identified that spans across more than 1.4 Mb of genomic DNA, including the LD block that contained the variants associated with asthma. The protein coded by this gene (*DPP10*) shares features with members of the S9B family of DPP serine proteases such as DPP4, which has been implicated in chemokine processing as part of the innate immune system.[174] *DPP10* displays a complex pattern of transcript splicing, with eight alternate first exons; four of these exons are within the LD block that was strongly associated with asthma. Although no coding variants were identified in *DPP10*, the SNP WTC122 alters the sequence of a known promoter element (CdxA) adjacent to one of the alternative exons of DPP10. Allen and colleagues presented some functional evaluation of this polymorphism, demonstrating that the CdxA promoter sequence differentially binds nuclear protein extract depending on which allele is present. It is unclear, however, if WTC122 alters DPP10 expression.

## PHF11

PHF11 (PDH finger protein 11) is located on chromosome 13q14,[168] a region linked to asthma[144] and total serum IgE levels.[156] Cookson and colleagues found evidence of linkage between chromosome 13q14 and atopy and atopy-related phenotypes among Australian families selected to be informative for atopy. In these families, a strong association between a short-tandem repeat marker in the linked region and total serum IgE levels suggested that an atopy-susceptibility locus was in close proximity.[168] Further characterization of the structure of LD surrounding this marker demonstrated clustering of SNPs into four islands (or blocks). Evidence for association with total serum IgE level was observed with variants in two adjacent blocks of LD, centering on one gene – PHF11. Although a haplotype that included the two markers in PHF11 that were most strongly associated with total serum IgE levels in the Australian families was associated with either total serum IgE level or atopic dermatitis in three additional populations, evidence of single-SNP association was not reported for the replication populations. Although there were associations between variants in PHF11 and asthma and asthma severity, they were less impressive than the observed associations between variants in PHF11 and atopy-related phenotypes.

PHF11 encodes the NY-REN-34 protein and may play a role in transcriptional regulation.[175] The gene is expressed in most tissues, including the lung and B-lymphocytes. Although the evidence from association studies and the gene expression in B-lymphocytes supports a potential role of PHF11 in regulation of total serum IgE levels, two genes that are both adjacent to PHF11 and within the same LD blocks (SETDB2 and RCBTB1) may also be important in IgE regulation. In particular, SETDB2 has an expression profile in cells of the immune system that is similar to PHF11.[168]

## GPR154

Chromosome 7p has been linked to total serum IgE levels,[146,158] asthma,[146] and airway responsiveness.[158] To localize the asthma susceptibility gene on chromosome 7p, Laitinen and colleagues performed hierarchical genotyping in families in a genetically isolated population in Finland (the Kainuu). Sequential rounds of genotyping across a 20 cM region on chromosome 7p identified a 46-kb segment that demonstrated differential haplotype distributions between individuals with asthma and family-matched controls. Genotyping of additional variants discovered upon resequencing of an asthmatic homozygous for the segregating haplotype resulted in extension of the conserved haplotype over 133 kb. Association between this extended haplotype and asthma was then demonstrated in two genetically isolated populations from French Canada and Finland (the North Karelians). Within the 77 kb region most conserved across the three populations of interest, seven common haplotypes (frequency ≥2 percent) were observed; three of these haplotypes conferred increased risks for asthma and elevated total serum high IgE levels. Haplotypes H4 and H5 were associated with high total serum IgE levels in the Kainuu (relative risk 1.4, 95 percent CI 1.1–1.9) and haplotype H2 was associated with asthma in French Canadians (RR 2.5, 95 percent CI 2.0–3.1). Interestingly, phylogenetic analysis suggested that these three haplotypes were closely related and clustered at a distance from the other four non-risk haplotypes, suggesting that the susceptibility variants initially arose on a common founder haplotype.

Two previously uncharacterized genes map within the boundaries of the asthma risk haplotypes, and were named a G-protein coupled receptor for asthma susceptibility (GPRA, HUGO name GPR154) and asthma-associated alternatively spliced gene 1 (AAA1). GPR154 shares homology with other members of the g-protein family of receptors and is expressed in bronchial smooth muscle and epithelium. The locus spans 10 exons, of which exons 3 through 5 reside within the haplotype associated with asthma. Among the many variants in GPR154 identified across this haplotype, only one (Asn107Ile) is coding. GPR154 displays differential splicing, with only one of the two terminal exons included in mature protein, resulting in protein isoforms of 371 (isoform A) or 377 (isoform B) amino acids in size. Immunohistochemical analysis of bronchial biopsies revealed that isoform A of GPR154 was expressed in bronchial smooth muscle of asthmatic subjects and that isoform B of GPR154 was expressed in bronchial smooth muscle of non-asthmatic subjects; similar patterns were observed in bronchial epithelium. Taken together with the studies of association and gene expression in humans, the finding that GPR154 is upregulated in the murine airway following ovalbumin challenge in sensitized mice provides convincing evidence that GPR154 contributes to asthma susceptibility. Although haplotype-specific differences in the pattern of splicing of AAA1 have been demonstrated, there is substantially less evidence supporting AAA1 in asthma pathobiology and there is little evidence that the gene encodes mature protein.

## Summary

Four potential asthma-susceptibility genes have been identified by positional cloning. The biochemical mechanisms linking three of these genes (PHF11, DPP10, and ADAM33) to asthma phenotypes are poorly understood, and replication studies of the association between ADAM33 and asthma phenotypes have yielded conflicting results. Functional studies supporting the association between GPR154 and asthma suggest that this gene is the most likely to influence asthma pathogenesis. To date, there has been no replication of the associations between GPR154, PHF11, and DPP10 and asthma phenotypes by groups independent from those publishing the original reports.

## SELECTED CANDIDATE GENES FOR ASTHMA AND ASTHMA-RELATED PHENOTYPES

Of the reported associations between candidate genes and asthma and/or asthma-related phenotypes, 40 associations were replicated in at least two populations.[157,167–169,176] Ten candidate genes (IL4, IL4RA, IL10, IL13, ADRB2, CD14, TNF, LTA, HLA-DRB1, and FCERIB) have been associated with asthma and/or asthma-related phenotypes in at least five populations. We discuss the findings for these 10 genes below. Particular attention is given to two genes (ADRB2 and FCERIB) that have been extensively studied, as they illustrate some of the challenges found in interpreting the findings from association studies of asthma.

## IL4 and IL4RA

Through activation of its receptor, interleukin 4 induces polarization of naive T cells towards Th2 cells and stimulates production of total serum IgE by Th2 cells.[177] The genes for interleukin 4 (IL4) and IL4 receptor α chain (IL4RA) are in genomic regions linked to asthma phenotypes (5q31 for IL4 and 16p12 for IL4RA).

A potentially functional SNP (−589 C/T) in the promoter of the gene coding for IL-4 (IL4) has been associated with asthma[178–183] and/or asthma-related phenotypes[178,180,182,184–187] in most[178–187] but not all studies.[165,184,188–190] Basehore et al. recently resequenced most of IL4 in 16 white subjects and identified 19 SNPs;[183] 11 of these 19 SNPs were then genotyped in subjects with (n = 233) and without (n = 245) asthma. Of the 11 SNPs in IL4, nine were associated with total serum IgE and five were associated with asthma. All of the three common haplotypes in IL4 were associated with total serum IgE.

Two potentially functional SNPs (Ser478Pro and Ile50Val) in coding regions of IL4RA have been associated with asthma[181,188,191–193] and/or asthma-related phenotypes[191,192,194] in some studies,[181,188,191–194] but not in others.[184,195–197] A functional haplotype in IL4RA (one SNP in the promoter and two in coding regions, including Ile50Val) was recently associated with asthma and asthma severity among Finnish individuals with (n = 170) and without (n = 350) asthma.[198]

## IL10

Production of the cytokine IL-10 by T-regulatory cells (Tregs) downregulates Th1 and Th2 immune responses.[199] Thus, IL-10 may influence the pathogenesis of allergic diseases such as atopic asthma. Potentially functional SNPs (−627C/A) and/or haplotypes of the promoter of the gene for IL-10 (IL10) have been associated with asthma[200,201] and/or asthma phenotypes[200,202–205] in most,[200–205] but not all,[189,206] studies.

## IL13

Experiments in rodents and humans support a critical role of IL-13 in asthma pathogenesis.[207–209] Potentially functional SNPs in the promoter and coding regions of the gene for IL-13 (IL13) have been associated with asthma[210–213] and/or asthma-related phenotypes[211,212,214–223] in most,[210–223] but not all,[165,189,224] studies. Of interest, findings from studies of genetic association,[191] and recent experiments in rodents,[209] support an interaction between functional variants in IL13

and IL4RA in the pathogenesis of asthma and airway responsiveness.

## ADRB2

The β2-adrenergic receptor (β2AR) gene (ADRB2) is the most extensively studied gene in asthma genetics and pharmacogenetics. The gene maps to chromosome 5q31-33, a genomic region linked to asthma,[144,148] increased airway responsiveness,[140] and total serum IgE.[148] Airway smooth muscle cells and lymphocytes isolated from asthmatics demonstrate reduced response and enhanced downregulation of β2-ARs, supporting the notion of partial beta-adrenergic blockade as a potential cause of asthma.[225] β2AR-agonists are the mainstay of asthma therapy and it is possible that β2AR sequence variation explains inter-individual clinical differences in response to these medications.

ADRB2 has only one exon and encodes a 413 amino acid protein that bears similar structural resemblance to other members of the G protein-coupled receptor superfamily.[226] This protein consists of an extracellular amino-terminus, seven transmembrane domains, three intracellular and three extracellular loops, and an intracellular carboxy-terminus. The transmembrane domains are essential for normal ligand binding and subsequent signal transduction,[227,228] and the amino-terminus plays an important role in receptor trafficking through post-translational glycosylation.[229] Signal transduction is mediated through Gs coupled adenylyl cyclase activation. Sixteen polymorphisms have been identified in both the coding and 5′ upstream regions of ADRB2. Four variants result in amino-acid variation: Arg16Gly and Gln27Glu in the extracellular amino-terminus, and Val34Met and Thr164Ile in the transmembrane domains.[230] An additional coding variant of arginine for cysteine is found in the beta upstream regulator (BUP),[231] a protein situated immediately 5′ to the β2AR that inhibits normal receptor translation,[232] and SNPs located further upstream (positions −1023, −654, −468, −367) may affect β2AR transcription rates.[233]

The four common coding variants of ADRB2 may have functional consequences. Although Ile164 reduces receptor ligand-binding affinity and adenylyl-cyclase activity compared to Thr164-bearing receptors,[234–236] this variant has not been evaluated in most association studies of asthma due to its relatively low allele frequency (2.5–3.0 percent). The loci situated in the amino-terminus likely impact down-regulation of the β2AR. Green[237] observed marked differences in the degree of agonist-mediated down-regulation using constructs representing the four possible isoforms at the 16 and 27 positions, with Gly16-Gln27 and Gly16-Glu27 Chinese hamster fibroblast cell lines demonstrating enhanced receptor downregulation. Similar results were obtained in studies of human airway smooth muscle cells, with Gly16-bearing receptors demonstrating enhanced in vitro desensitization.[238] An altered degradation profile of receptors with amino-terminus variation is consistent with deletion studies that demonstrated the amino-terminus' importance in receptor trafficking.[228,229] In contrast to these findings, other studies of human airway smooth muscle have found that the Glu27 allele, not Gly16, was associated with enhanced acute and long-term β₂AR desensitization to beta-agonists. The Cys19Arg BUP variant also impacts β₂AR function by enhancing cell surface β₂AR density.[231,239]

There is strong LD across *ADRB2*, with a limited set of haplotypes observed in numerous ethnic populations.[233] In this context, the diverse functional effects of these common variants may have very different effects in combination. Drysdale and colleagues[233] demonstrated that common 13-allele haplotypes showed significant differences in their in vivo response to albuterol. These haplotypes varied from one another at eight of 13 loci, including four situated upstream from BUP. mRNA expression levels of *ADRB2* differed by more than two-fold between common haplotypes. The Cys19 BUP variant, associated with increased regulation, was on the haplotype associated with lower expression, suggesting that other upstream variants confer the differences in transcription, and argue that the β₂AR variants may interact with each other as a meta-haplotype.

There have been more than 20 studies of association between SNPs and/or haplotypes in *ADRB2* and asthma and/or asthma-related phenotypes.[176] There is conflicting evidence to support an association between *ADRB2* and asthma per se, as some studies have found a positive association between variants in *ADRB2* and asthma,[200,240,241] and others have not.[165,189,242–247] Of the studies that found an association between variants in *ADRB2* and asthma, two were population-based and did not adequately account for potential population stratification,[240,241] and one family-based study found a weak association.[200] On the other hand, most of the studies that showed no association between *ADRB2* and asthma could not exclude weak to moderate genetic effects due to relatively small sample sizes.[165,189,245–247] In a relatively large study of 650 nuclear families of children with well-characterized asthma, there was no association between *ADRB2* and asthma.[242] Thus, the cumulative evidence does not support the hypothesis that *ADRB2* is a major susceptibility gene for asthma. However, a minor role of *ADRB2* in the pathogenesis of asthma cannot be excluded on the basis of the available literature.

There is evidence to support and refute the hypothesis that variants in *ADRB2* act as disease modifiers in asthma and/or influence asthma-related phenotypes. In the initial report describing polymorphisms in *ADRB2*, it was noted that of the patients requiring continuous oral steroids, 75 percent were homozygous at Gly16 (compared to 53 percent in the asthma group as a whole).[230] Others have found evidence of association of the Gly16 allele with nocturnal asthma.[248] Although these results and others[230,248–252] suggest that the *ADRB2* locus may be an important modifier of asthma severity, there is evidence to refute this theory.[248,253]

Several studies have found an association between variants in *ADRB2* and airways responsiveness, with most showing increased airways responsiveness either in subjects homozygous for Gln27 or among individuals bearing the Gly16-Gln27 haplotype.[254–256] Other studies provide contradictory evidence to this effect.[243,244] Polymorphisms and/or haplotypes in *ADRB2* have been associated with total serum IgE,[257] response to inhaled beta2-agonists,[242,251,258–261] and FEV₁.[242,243] Other studies have shown no association between variants in *ADRB2* and total serum IgE,[262] atopy,[165] and response to inhaled beta2-agonists.[263] Among nuclear families of children with asthma, there was evidence that variants in or near *ADRB2* influence lung function and bronchodilator responsiveness, but that different regions of *ADRB2* influence these phenotypes.[242] In particular, variants in the 5′ end of *ADRB2* were associated with spirometric measures of lung function and a variant in the 3′ end of the gene was associated with bronchodilator responsiveness. Although Silverman et al. found an association between homozygosity for Arg16 and lung function, it was in the opposite direction of that shown by Summerhill and colleagues. Overall, the findings of Silverman and colleagues suggest that yet-unidentified polymorphisms in or near *ADRB2* may ultimately explain the observed associations between SNPs and/or haplotypes in *ADRB2* and lung function and bronchodilator responsiveness.

In summary, *ADRB2* is not likely to be a major susceptibility gene for asthma. The observed associations between variants in *ADRB2* and asthma-related phenotypes (e.g., total serum IgE, airway responsiveness, asthma severity) may be due to the influence of *ADRB2* on other asthma-related phenotypes (e.g., bronchodilator responsiveness, lung function), to the interaction between *ADRB2* with other asthma-susceptibility genes, and/or to LD with adjacent genes. Although variants in *ADRB2* may influence lung function and response to beta2-agonists, the functional mutations responsible for the observed associations have yet to be confidently identified.

## CD14

The monocyte differentiation antigen CD14 (*CD14*) gene is on chromosome 5q31-33, a region repeatedly linked to asthma-related phenotypes. CD14 is a receptor for bacterial cell wall components that may influence immune responses.[264] A functional SNP in the promoter of CD14 has been associated with total serum IgE[265–268] and/or atopy,[165,200,266,269,270] in most,[165,200,265–270] but not all,[189,271,272] studies.

## TNF, LTA, and HLA–DRB1

The tumor necrosis factor alpha (*TNF*), lymphotoxin alpha (*LTA*), and human leukocyte antigen DRB1 (*HLA-DRB1*) genes are on chromosome 6p21, a genomic region linked to asthma-related phenotypes. A functional variant in the promoter of *TNF* has been associated with asthma[273–279] and/or asthma-related phenotypes[273,279–281] in some,[273–281] but not all,[282–287] studies. Variants in *LTA* have been associated with asthma,[273,274,277,288,289] and/or asthma-related phenotypes[273,282,284,288] in some,[273,274,277,282,284,288,289] but not all, studies.[202,271,280,281,283,286,287,290] Potentially functional SNPs and/or haplotypes in *HLA-DRB1* have been associated with sensitization to specific allergens[271,289,291–304] atopy,[305–307] asthma,[289,306–308] and total serum IgE,[271,289,297,299,308] in some, studies, but not in others.[309–311]

## HIGH–AFFINITY IGE RECEPTOR

Human chromosome 11q13 has received considerable attention as an asthma and atopy locus.[312–314] In 1989, Cookson and colleagues reported strong evidence for linkage (LOD score = 5.58) on chromosome 11q13 (marker D11S97) with atopy in seven extended pedigrees using parametric linkage analysis.[315] Atopy was defined as either a positive skin test to a series of common allergens, an elevated specific IgE to at least one tested antigen, or an elevated total serum IgE. The bulk of the linkage was driven by one of the seven pedigrees, where recombination between the marker and disease phenotype was observed in only two of 23 informative meioses (LOD = 3.14). Linkage to this marker with atopy was later observed in 32 additional informative nuclear families (LOD = 3.80), suggesting that the original findings were more broadly generalizable.[316] Combining the extended pedigree and nuclear family data resulted in a LOD score greater than 8.0, suggesting that a gene within 0.2 cM of D11S97 was the major genetic determinant of atopy. Despite the strength of these initial reports, attempts to replicate linkage have been mixed. Evidence for linkage of this region with asthma and atopy phenotypes have been observed in several genome-wide surveys.[317,318] Additional regional linkage studies have supported evidence for linkage to chromosome 11q13 with atopy phenotypes, asthma and airway responsiveness,[312,319–322] while others have not.[323–327]

Among the many genes that localize to chromosome 11q13, the most obvious positional candidate in this region is the beta-chain of the high-affinity IgE receptor (FCER1B, otherwise known as membrane-spanning 4 domains, subfamily A, member 2; MS4A2). The type I, or allergic, hypersensitivity reaction is a hallmark of atopic diseases. The reaction is initiated by the interaction of allergen-bound immunoglobulin E with its high-affinity IgE receptor, with subsequent activation of macrophages and degranulation of basophils through a series of diverse cellular processes.[328] The high-affinity IgE receptor (FcεRI) is constitutively expressed on basophils and mast cells as a tetrameric structure, composed of an alpha chain, a beta chain, and two gamma chains. Although the beta-chain does not appear to be critical either for initiating or propagating the allergic response, it provides an important amplifier function, whereby the expression of the beta-subunit results in an increase in FcεRI cell surface expression.[329,330] It is thought that the FcεRIβ subunit stabilizes and facilitates intracellular processing of immature FcεRIα chains to the cell surface.[331]

In light of the importance of FCER1B in allergic response signaling, and the linkage evidence described, mutation discovery efforts across this locus have been performed, with identified coding variants demonstrating association with atopy and asthma phenotypes. Three coding variants have been described: Ile181Leu, Val183Leu, and Glu237Gly. Leu183 and Gly237 result from single base-pair substitutions. Ile181Leu results from two nucleotide substitutions of codon 181 (TTA → GTT). All three variants were initially described in the British atopic families linked to chromosome 11q13.[319,332] The Leu183 variant was observed only once among 175 individuals, but Leu181 and Gly237 were observed at frequencies of 8 and 5.4 percent, respectively. These latter two variants were significantly associated with atopy and asthma phenotypes. Additional reports of association of Gly237 with atopic asthma and with elevated serum IgE in the Japanese population have been reported,[333,334] suggesting that genetic variation in FCER1B is responsible for the observed linkages on chromosome 11q13. However, these variants are not present in all populations, including several asthmatic or atopic cohorts,[335–338] and additional association studies have failed to demonstrate association with these coding variants and atopy or asthma.[339] Moreover, there is little evidence that these variants have any pertinent functional impact on receptor signaling. Specifically, neither Leu181 nor Gly237 appear to affect the amplification functions of the beta-subunit,[340] or the downstream activation of mast cells following IgE stimulation.[341] Overall, it appears that these coding variants are not responsible for the atopy linkage to chromosome 11q13.

Given the inconsistencies noted in the associations with coding variants, it is probable that, if genetic variation related to FCER1B is responsible for the observed linkage, the susceptibility variants in this region are noncoding and regulatory. Noncoding variants have been associated with atopy and asthma, including two *RsaI* restriction sites located in intron 2 and exon 7. Using variance-component modeling, the exon 7 *RsaI* variant was associated with total serum IgE levels in a population of endemically parasitized Australian aborigines, explaining percent of the total residual variation in serum total IgE and exhibiting a significant ($P < 0.0001$) additive relationship with total serum IgE levels.[342] In a second study of Australian Caucasians, both the intron 2 and exon 7 *RsaI* variants were associated with total serum IgE levels and the combined RAST index.[338] Associations of exon 7 *RsaI* with specific IgE responses to pollen and dust mite, but not atopy or asthma, were observed in a population of Swedish farmers.[343] These variants were evaluated because of the availability of known restriction sites. It is likely that these variants have no functional importance, given their location deep within intronic sequence, and that they are in linkage disequilibrium with causative alleles. In an attempt to identify putative susceptibility alleles across the FCR locus, Traherne and colleagues[344] performed an extensive variation discovery search across 18 kb (including 3.7 kb of flanking sequence) in 12 unrelated Caucasians. Thirty-eight variants were identified, including 237Gly, RsaI-int2, and RsaI-ex7. Leu181 and Leu183 were not observed. Thirty-one of these polymorphisms were genotyped in two panels of atopic families, including the British nuclear families with which the initial linkages to FCER1B were described. LD plots across the locus suggested that LD of the genomic region upstream from the transcript was discrete from that surrounding the transcript. In these two panels of families, four clusters of SNPs demonstrated significant associations with measures of atopy, including skin test indices and RAST index. The strongest associations were observed in SNPs that localized to the LD blocks within the gene, not upstream. The most significant associations were with SNPs in intron 3, where four SNPs demonstrated evidence of association ($P = 0.04$–$0.005$). Sequence analysis for promoter elements identified two clusters of interferon regulatory factor 2 (IRF-2) sites that are altered by several significantly associated SNPs, suggesting that these variants may alter FCR expression. Importantly, stepwise regression analysis and haplotype analysis suggested that the associations observed at the most significant loci were largely independent from each other. If true, this allelic heterogeneity would explain the difficulties in replicating association findings when evaluating only a handful of coding variants.

Heterogeneity of results of linkage and association studies for complex trait susceptibility loci is not uncommon, and can result through a variety of mechanisms, including true genetic or phenotypic differences across populations and issues relating to study design (i.e., ascertainment scheme, sample size, population substructure). Epigenetic effects, including allelic imprinting, can also introduce important heterogeneity across studies, and may contribute to observed inconsistencies in linkage and association results. Because there is evidence that maternal history of allergic disease (compared to paternal history) has more influence over subsequent allergic phenotypes in offspring,[345–347] this latter possibility of genetic imprinting of genes related to atopy has received considerable attention, particularly with regard to chromosome 11q13. Using statistical models that consider allelic parent-of-origin effects, several groups have demonstrated strengthened evidence of either linkage or association with FCER1B when considering maternally derived alleles.[312,319,344,348–350] In certain instances, maternally derived effects were detected without evidence of primary association. Although an intriguing possible mechanism, there is no molecular evidence that chromosome 11q13 demonstrates imprinting, and the observed associations may simply reflect post-hoc analysis and type I error inflation.

## Summary

There is contradictory evidence to support an association between each of the 10 genes discussed above (IL4, IL4RA, IL10, IL13, ADRB2, CD14, TNFA, LTA, HLA-DRB1, and FCERIB) and asthma and/or asthma-related phenotypes, suggesting that none of these genes is a major susceptibility gene for asthma. However, the relatively high number of positive association studies, and the fact that potentially functional SNPs in eight of these genes (IL4, IL4RA, IL10, IL13, ADRB2, CD14, TNFA, and HLA-DRB1) are associated with asthma and/or asthma-related phenotypes, suggests that these genes are either true susceptibility genes for asthma-related phenotypes with minor to moderate effect, or that they are in LD with genes that influence asthma-related phenotypes.

## OTHER CANDIDATE GENES

Experimental evidence in rodents[351] and data from genome-wide linkage scans in humans support a potential role of the prostanoid D receptor in asthma pathogenesis. Oguma et al.[352] conducted a recent study of association between functional variants in the promoter of the prostanoid D receptor gene (PTGDR) and asthma and total serum IgE. Among whites with ($n = 518$) and without ($n = 175$) asthma, genotypes containing the C allele of the T-549C SNP and the T allele of the C-441T allele were associated with asthma. Among African-Americans with ($n = 80$) and without ($n = 45$) asthma, genotypes containing the C allele of the T-549C SNP were weakly associated with asthma ($P = 0.04$). Haplotypes of PTGDR with low transcriptional efficiency were inversely associated with asthma in whites and in African-Americans. These findings have not yet been replicated by other investigators.

## MOUSE MODELS IN ASTHMA GENETICS

As discussed in Chapter 7, animal models have been instrumental in elucidating the cellular and molecular mechanisms of asthma and allergic disease. Among the many species that have been used to develop such models, none has been used as widely, particularly for genetic studies, as has the mouse. Although the mouse does not develop asthma-like features spontaneously, several inbred strains develop histologic and physiologic changes following allergen sensitization and subsequent allergen challenge that are reminiscent of asthma in humans, including eosinophilic and lymphocytic infiltration of the airways and perivascular spaces, and secretion of inflammatory cytokines.[353,354] This acute inflammatory response is followed by increased airway resistance and airway hyperresponsiveness.

Although the mouse does not spontaneously develop asthma, sensitization to allergens and airway challenge results in a typical asthmatic inflammatory response that includes increases in IL-4, IL-5, and IL-13 levels with a decrease in IL-10. The inflammatory response is also typical of human asthma with a transient neutrophilic infiltration followed by sustained eosinophilic and lymphocytic inflammatory response, goblet cell metaplasia, and mucous hyperproduction. Increases in airway responsiveness and airway resistance are also described.[355] Thus, the acute allergic asthmatic response in the mouse is very similar to the responses observed in humans. Chronic challenge protocols induce airway remodeling with sub-basement membrane fibrosis and smooth muscle hyperplasia.[356] Although murine eosinophils do not release granules to the usual stimuli that cause human eosinophils to do so,[357] the model does appear to mimic human asthma both acutely and chronically. This has led to the use of the mouse for genetic purposes. The asthma phenotype that has been most widely studied in the mouse is airway responsiveness. As discussed in more detail below, initial studies by Levitt and Mintzer[358] reported significant strain variation in airway responsiveness to acetylcholine and serotonin assessed by the airway pressure time index (APTI) across nine standard inbred strains of mice. The A/J and AKR/J strains showed the greatest degree of airway responsiveness to acetylcholine while the C57 BL6/J and C3H/HEJ strains were the least responsive. This work formed the basis for various QTL analyses relating to airway responsiveness in the mouse. Of importance, virtually every region identified in the mouse for both baseline and allergen-induced airway responsiveness corresponds to a linked region for asthma and airway responsiveness in humans.

Work in this area has been plagued by lack of consistency in determining the airway responsiveness phenotype in the mouse. When airway resistance was examined by DeSanctis and coworkers,[359] mouse chromosomal regions 2, 15, and 17 were identified; however, using a different strain of mouse and a different technique of phenotyping, Ewart and coworkers[360] identified a QTL on mouse chromosome 6. When De Sanctis and coworkers[361] repeated their work, utilizing a similar technique to that of Ewart and focused on pulmonary resistance, they confirmed the chromosome 6 linkage and identified two more regions on chromosome 7 and 17 (the locus on chromosome 17 was the same as that identified by them previously). Although these data suggest that the choice of phenotyping protocols and the mouse strains crossed impact which linkages are identified, there is evidence that several of these identified QTLs have human correlates. For example, chromosome 17 (identified as an airway responsiveness QTL in three separate backcross experiments) is syntenic with human chromosome 6p21, which has been repeatedly identified in human genome linkage studies as being linked with airway responsiveness in asthmatic cohorts. In addition, the QTL on mouse chromosome 2 identified by De Sanctis is syntenic with human

chromosome 20p13. In both species, this genomic region includes ADAM33.

In summary, the mouse QTL data show surprising homology to the human linkage data and when different investigators utilize similar phenotyping approaches, similar loci have been identified.

## MURINE STRAIN DIFFERENCES IN ASTHMA-RELATED PHENOTYPES

Mice demonstrate significant between-strain variability in several asthma-related phenotypes, including both native and allergen-induced airway responsiveness,[361,362] and patterns of airway inflammation[363] and airway remodeling.[364] Of these, airway responsiveness has been most extensively studied, with significant differences in native airway responsiveness demonstrated in response to several nonspecific bronchoconstrictors, including acetylcholine,[365–367] methacholine,[368] serotonin,[358,366,368] and atracurium.[369] Although different measures of constrictor response were used across studies, and some differences in strain rank-order of constrictor response are noted depending on the constrictor agent used, fairly consistent patterns in constrictor response are observed, with strains broadly categorized into high-responders and low-responders (see Table 9.5). Across studies, the A strain consistently demonstrates the greatest constrictor response, while C57BL6, SJL, and C3H/He strains consistently demonstrated minimal responsiveness to all agents. Other strains evaluated show less consistent patterns of responsiveness: DBA/2 is highly responsive to serotonin and atracurium but less so to acetylcholine, while AKR demonstrated high responsiveness to acetylcholine and atricurium but low responsiveness to serotonin. Strain differences in airway responsiveness are highly correlated with airway smooth-muscle shortening velocity, with A/J-derived smooth muscle demonstrating faster contraction than that derived from either C3H/HeJ or C57BL/6J strain (BALB/C-derived airway smooth muscle has an intermediate rate of shortening).[370]

In a series of crossbreeding experiments, Levitt and Mitzner[365] proposed that airway responsiveness to intravenous infusions of acetylcholine and serotonin segregate as autosomal recessive traits. Progeny of hyper-responsive A/J and hypo-responsive C3H/HeJ crossbreeding all expressed the hypo-responsive trait, as did C3H/HeJ × (C3H/HeJ × A/J) backcross progeny. However, airway hyper-responsiveness was observed in one quarter of F2 intercross progeny ((A/J × C3H/HeJ) × (C3H/HeJ × A/J)), suggestive of recessive segregation. Similar patterns were observed in responsiveness to serotonin among offspring of DBA/2J (hyper-responsive) and C57BL/6J (hypo-responsive) crossbreeding: F1 progeny and C57BL/6J backcross progeny were uniformly hypo-responsive, 58 percent of DBA/2J backcross progeny, and 31 percent of the F2 intercross progeny

**Table 9.5**  *Strain-differences in native airway responsiveness*

| Airway responsiveness | Acetylcholine | Serotonin | Atricurium | Methacholine |
|---|---|---|---|---|
| High | A/J<br>AKR/J | A/J<br>DBA/2J<br>WB/ReJ | DBA/2NCr<br>AKR/NCr<br>A/J | A/J<br>DBA/2 |
| Medium | DBA/2J | WBB6F1-W/Wv | | WBB6F1-W/Wv |
| Low | WB/ReJ<br>BALB/cJ<br>CBA/J<br>C57BL/6J<br>SJL/J<br>C3H/HeJ | AKR/J<br>BALB/cJ<br>CBA/J<br>C57BL/6J<br>SJL/J<br>C3H/HeJ | CBA/JCr<br>C3H/HeJ<br>C57BL/6NCr<br>BALB/CanNCr<br>SJL/JCr<br>SWR/J | C3H/HeN<br>C57BL/6 |

Acetylcholine data abstracted from Levitt[366] and Ewart.[372] Serotonin data abstracted from Levitt[366] and Konno.[368] Atricurium data abstracted from Levitt.[369] Methacholine data abstracted from Konno.[368]

were hyper-responsive, consistent with an autosomal recessive mode of inheritance. Cosegregation analysis suggested that the loci conferring responsiveness to acetylcholine and serotonin are inherited separately, as a substantial proportion of A/J × C3H/HeJ F2 progeny were discordant with respect to their responsiveness to both agents.[358] Subsequent segregation studies have demonstrated different results suggesting more complex patterns of inheritance. A second report of A/J and C3H/HeJ crosses by Levitt[360] suggested that the segregation pattern observed in F1 and F2 progeny was more consistent with a major airway responsiveness locus plus polygenic inheritance. A third study of A/J and C3H/HeJ crosses supports a polygenic model.[371] Studies assessing the segregation of methacholine responsiveness in A/J × C57BL/6J crosses also suggest polygenic inheritance. Using a different measure of hyper-responsiveness (the effective dose of methacholine causing a doubling in pulmonary resistance – $ED_{200}R_L$), De Sanctis and colleagues[359] demonstrated that both A/J × C57BL/6J and C57BL/6J × A/J F1 crosses exhibited a distribution of methacholine responsiveness similar to the A/J (responsive) strain, suggesting an autosomal dominant mode of inheritance. Moreover, F2 intercross progeny had a unimodal, almost normal distribution of methacholine responsiveness, suggesting a polygenic mode of inheritance.

Complementing studies of native, or non-inflammatory, airways responsiveness are those studies that have focused on airway responsiveness following allergen sensitization and rechallenge. These protocols are more labor intensive and subject to greater between-study variability due to differences in the sensitization protocols and readouts of inflammatory response. As a consequence, discrepant results regarding strain-related profiles of both airway responsiveness and the accompanying inflammatory response have been reported.[363,364,372,373] Surveys in multiple strains have demonstrated significant between-strain variability in the development of allergen-induced airway responsiveness.[363,372,373] Ewart and coworkers found that the distribution of airway responsiveness 72 h following inhalational ovalbumin challenge in five strains mirrored the native distribution, with the native hyper-responsive A/J and AKR/J strains demonstrating the greatest increases ($\approx$2.5-fold) in airway responsiveness, and C57BL/6J and C3H/HeJ demonstrating no increase from their minimal baseline airway responsiveness. Airway responsiveness in the BALB/cJ strain (whose native responsiveness is variable across studies) significantly increased following allergen challenge, but to a lesser degree than in the A/J and AKR/J strains. Similar results have been observed in other studies although some differences were noted, probably relating to methods of sensitization and routes of allergen challenge.[363,373]

These studies also provided important information regarding the patterns of distribution of allergic response across strains, demonstrating that allergen-induced changes in airway inflammation, cytokine expression, and OVA-specific serum IgE levels are strain dependent, and likely under genetic influence. Moreover, they suggest that allergen-induced airway responsiveness, and the accompanying systemic and local (pulmonary) allergic responses, are controlled by distinct genetic mechanisms, as the patterns of strain distribution for these immune/inflammatory phenotypes were very different from those for airway responsiveness. For example, Ewart showed that only A/J and C57BL/6J strains demonstrated concordant responses across phenotypes. A/J mice demonstrated the greatest increase in both bronchoalveolar lavage (BAL) eosinophilia and IgE levels, concomitant with the dramatic rise in airway responsiveness, reminiscent of allergy-induced asthma exacerbation. However, C57BL/6J mice showed no evidence of allergic response, with only a minimal (nonsignificant) rise in BAL eosinophils and no increase in either airway responsiveness or OVA-specific IgE levels. The other three strains studied revealed more discordant patterns of allergic response: AKH/J mice displayed the greatest increase in airway responsiveness but had no increase in either BAL eosinophils or IgE; C3H/HeJ mice had a significant influx of BAL eosinophils but lacked an accompanying increase in airway responsiveness; BALB/cJ mice had a modest rise in BAL eosinophila but no concomitant increase in IgE.[372] The observed differences in pulmonary eosinophilia may relate to differences in the localization of eosinophils within the lung, as C57BL/6J strains mount a diffuse pulmonary eosinophilia that, conspicuously, does not involve the airways, while the response seen in BALB/cJ strains has a prominent peribronchial component.[374] This dissociation of airway inflammation and airway responsiveness has been observed in several laboratories, reinforcing the notion of differential genetic control of these phenotypes.[363,375] Evidence that allergen-induced airway responsiveness may relate to altered neural control of the airways independent from direct inflammatory changes, may provide an explanation for this phenomenon in some strains.[376]

## AIRWAY HYPER-RESPONSIVENESS QTL MAPPING

There are six published reports of QTL mapping using murine models of airway responsiveness (see Table 9.6). Four examined the native airway responsiveness phenotype,[359,360,371,377] while two employed models of allergen-induced airway responsiveness.[372,378] Consistent with the majority of available segregation analysis data, multiple QTLs were identified which contribute to the variance of both native and allergen-induced airway responsiveness, supporting polygenic inheritance. Several loci demonstrate linkage in two or more studies, including loci on mouse chromosome 6, chromosome 7, and chromosome 17. The locus on chromosome 6, syntenic to portions of human chromosomes 2p11-13 and 3p24-26, was demonstrated in two studies of native airway responsiveness in crosses of C3H/HeJ and A/J. Although differing in breeding strategies and phenotypic assessment, both demonstrated a 'genome-wide' level of linkage statistical significance, suggesting that a major native airway responsiveness locus resides in this region. Similar evidence of replication was noted for a locus on chromosome 7 in models of both native and allergy-induced airway responsiveness, although genome-wide evidence of linkage was observed in only one study. The chromosome 7 QTL is syntenic with human chromosome 19q13, a region linked to asthma in several populations.[379,380] The third replicated locus, residing on mouse chromosome 17 and harboring the major histocompatibility locus, showed suggestive evidence for linkage (LOD 1.7–2.8) with both native and allergic phenotypes in three studies using crossbred strains with diverse genetic backgrounds. The human MHC locus on chromosome 6p21 has been linked to asthma in multiple cohorts,[59,61,379,381] and associations of asthma with polymorphisms across this region have been demonstrated.[382–384] In addition to these replicated QTLs, four others have demonstrated highly significant evidence for linkage with airway responsiveness, including loci on mouse chromosomes 2, 10, 11, and 15. The loci on mouse chromosomes

10 and 15 are syntenic with human chromosome 12q12-24, a region that has been linked with asthma and related phenotypes in many populations (see Table 9.4 of this chapter and Ref. 385). Although this region is quite broad ($\approx$40 Mb), two interesting candidate genes mapping to this region are interferon gamma (IFNG) and the vitamin D receptor (VDR), both of which are strongly implicated in Th1/Th2 differentiation and the development of allergy.[386–390] While genetic data supporting a relationship between asthma and IFNG polymorphisms are sparse,[391,392] genetic associations between VDR polymorphisms and asthma and atopy phenotypes have been observed in three populations.[393,394] The airway responsiveness locus on chromosome 2 is homologous with the region of human chromosome 20p that harbors ADAM33; as noted above, ADAM33 has been implicated as an asthma and airway responsiveness locus. However, evidence of interstrain sequence variation in the murine Adam33 homolog correlating with interstrain variability in airway responsiveness has not been demonstrated.

Like linkage analysis in human populations, QTL mapping by crossbreeding has been helpful in identifying broad chromosomal regions that influence phenotype, but is limited in its ability to more precisely narrow these regions due to the large number of recombinants that would be required, and the complications introduced by genetic heterogeneity and genetic epistasis often seen in polygenic traits. To overcome these limitations, alternative approaches have been used including the use of congenic or YAC transgenic mice strains, and expression profile analysis. QTL mapping in congenic mouse strains is advantageous in the study of polygenic traits because progeny genotype differs only at the one congenic locus, thereby eliminating the complications of genetic heterogeneity and genetic epistasis that blur single-locus genotype–phenotype correlations in crossbreeding studies using two unrelated strains. Using this strategy, McIntyre screened congenic BALB/c mice strains bearing individual DBA/2 chromosomal segments, and identified one strain with a DBA/2-inherited segment of chromosome 11 homologous to human chromosome 5q23-35 (the strain was termed HBA), linked with asthma in multiple studies (see Genome-wide linkage analysis for asthma and asthma-related phenotypes, page 226). Whereas BALB/c mice demonstrated a Th2-like immune response and allergen-induced airway responsiveness, HBA strains, differing from BALB/c only at this one locus, did not manifest these features, as in DBA/2 strains.[395] BALB/c × HBA progeny manifest BALB/c-like Th2 profiles, suggesting that the chromosomal region regulating the T-cell and airway responsiveness (named Tapr) segregates in a recessive fashion. HBA backcross experiments employing more than 1000 progeny narrowed the location of Tapr to a 0.3–0.5 cM segment near Kim1 (a homolog of rat kidney injury molecule 1). Despite being linked to the Tapr response (IL4 and IL13 levels), this gene maps to a region of human chromosome 5q at a distance from the region containing the cytokine gene cluster (IL4, IL5, and IL13). Subsequent characterization of this

**Table 9.6**  *Summary of mouse QTL data for airway responsiveness*

| Author/year | Strains crossed | Phenotype | Mouse region | LOD score | Human synteny | Human candidate genes |
|---|---|---|---|---|---|---|
| Levitt 1995[377] | C57BL6/J × DBA/2J | Baseline AR (atracurium) | 13 | 2.43 | 5q13-q33 | SPINK5 ADRB2 |
| De Sanctis 1995[359] | C57BL/6J × A/J | Baseline AR (methacholine) | 2 | 3.00 | 20p13 | ADAM33 |
| | | | 15 | 3.70 | 22q13 | PPARA FBLN1 |
| | | | | | 12q12-13 | VDR AQP |
| | | | 17 | 2.83 | 6p21 | MHC TNFA |
| | | | | | 16p13 | MCPT |
| Ewart 1996[360] | C3H/HeJ × A/J | Baseline AR (acetylcholine) | 6 | N/A | 2p11-13 3p24-26 10q11 12p11-13 | IL1RN IL5RA GATA3 CD4 TNFRSF1A |
| De Sanctis 1999[371] | A/J × C3H/HeJ | Baseline AR (methacholine) | 6 | 3.30 | 2p11-13 3p24-26 | Same as Ewart 1996 |
| | | | 7 | 3.80 | 19q13 | IL11 CEBPA |
| | | | 17 | 1.70 | 6p21, 16p13 | same as DeSanctis 1995 |
| Zhang 1999[378] | BP2 × BALB/c | Allergen-induced AR (methacholine) | 9 | 2.50 | 11q22-23 | IL10R |
| | | | 10 | 3.80 | 12q21 | IFNG |
| | | | 11 | 3.65 | 17p11-13 | NOS2A CCL11 |
| | | | 17 | 2.10 | 6p21 | same as De Sanctis 1995 |
| Ewart 2000[372] | C3H/HeJ × A/J | Allergen-induced AR (acetylcholine) | 2 | 4.20 | 2q12-14 9q22-34 10p11-13 | IL1RN PTGES2 GATA3 |
| | | | 2 | 3.70 | 2q14-24 9q33-34 | – C5, PTGS1 |
| | | | 7 | 1.90 | 19q13 | IL11 |

ADRB2: Beta-2-Adrenergic Receptor; AQP: Aquaporin gene cluster (AQP2, AQP5, AQP6); C5: Complement Component 5; CCL11: Chemokine CCMotif, Ligand 11 (Eotaxin); CD4: CD4 antigen; CEBPA: CCAAT/enhancer binding protein alpha; FBLN1: Fibulin 1; GATA3: GATA-Binding Protein 3; IL1RN: Interleukin 1 Receptor Inhibitor; IL5RA: Interleukin 5 Receptor Alpha; IL11: Interleukin 11; IFNG: Interferon gamma; IRAK4: Interleukin 1 Receptor Associated Kinase; MCPT cluster: Mast Cell Protease gene cluster (MCPT6, MCPT7); MHC: Major histocompatibility Complex; NOS2A: Nitric Oxide Synthase 2; PPARA: peroxisome proliferator activated receptor alpha; PTGES2: Prostaglandin E Synthase 2; PTGS1: Prostaglandin-Endoperoxide Synthase 1; SPINK5: Serine Protease Inhibitor, Kazal-Type 5; TNFA: Tumor Necrosis Factor Alpha; TNFRSF1A: Tumor Necrosis Factor Receptor Superfamily 1A; VDR: Vitamin D Receptor.

locus revealed Kim1 as the rat ortholog of the mouse hepatitis A virus cellular receptor 1 (Havcr1, otherwise known as Tim1). A significant polymorphism in Tim1 (a 15 amino acid deletion), and a second variant in the adjacent Tim3 gene, segregated with the Tapr phenotype in backcross progeny, and were also present in C57BL/6J Th2-unresponsive strains. Ecologic data suggest that infection with hepatitis A may protect individuals from developing atopy.[396] In a follow up study, McIntyre et al.[397] evaluated whether variation in human HAVCR1 was associated with atopy, and whether these effects were modified by HAV– antibody seropositivity.

No associations were found between atopic status and a six amino-acid HAVCR1 variant. Stratification by HAV-seropositivity demonstrated that seropositive individuals carrying the insertion variant had a 74 percent reduced odds of atopy compared to those not carrying the variant. While suggesting a complex gene-by-environment interaction, these findings require corroboration.

Using an alternative approach, Symula and colleagues[398] screened the adjacent cytokine cluster on chromosome 5q for additional loci contributing to serum IgE levels and bronchoconstriction using humanized YAC transgenic mice. A panel of transgenic mice were constructed using three YACs from the 5q31 cytokine cluster. Bronchoconstrictor response was not altered in the three strains, but two of the three strains demonstrated reduced IgE production following allergen challenge. These two YACs shared a common region with five genes, including IL4 and IL13. While human IL4 and IL13 mRNA was expressed at high levels in these strains, murine IL4 and IL13 expression was reduced, suggesting that the human transcripts interfered with murine gene expression and that these genes regulate IgE production. Targeted pulmonary overexpression of IL13 in transgenic mouse models results in an eosinophilic response reminiscent of human asthma,[399] and polymorphisms in both IL4 and IL13 have been associated with serum IgE levels and other atopic features in asthmatic populations.[183,217,400]

Karp and colleagues[401] used expression profiling analysis to identify complement factor 5 (C5) as a positional candidate in the chromosome 2 airway responsiveness locus. Expression profiles of whole lung explants from post-ovalbumin challenged $(A/J \times C3H/HeJ) \times A/J$ backcross progeny were compared, resulting in the identification of 21 genes that were differentially expressed between eight extreme high and low acetylcholine responsive progeny. Of these 21 genes, C5 on chromosome 2 was the only differentially expressed gene that localized to a known airway responsiveness QTL. High negative correlation $(r^2 = -0.66)$ between degree of airway responsiveness and C5 mRNA expression was observed in backcross progeny and the inbred parental strains. A 2-bp deletion in a 5' C5 exon that results in deficient C5 mRNA and protein production and that is present in A/J but not C3H/HeJ strains, was significantly correlated with airway responsiveness in 172 backcross progeny. These data provided further support that C5 genetic variation is responsible for the QTL linkage to this region, but in itself are not conclusive, as any variant from this region present in only one of the two parental strains would probably show similar results because segregation patterns would be identical over non-recombinant regions. Observations that the C5-del is present in multiple acetylcholine-responsive strains (A/J and AKR/J) and absent in low-responders (C57BL/6J, BALB/cJ, and C3H/HeJ) suggest that the variation is a determinant of interstrain airway responsiveness. Differences in C5 expression have been observed in BAL specimens following segmental airway allergen challenge,[402] and human C5 maps to chromosome 9q34, a region linked to asthma in German and Hutterite asthma populations.[380,381] Associations with common C5 polymorphisms and asthma have been described in two cohorts, further supporting this molecule's role in asthma pathogenesis.[200,403]

## FUTURE DIRECTIONS FOR RESEARCH

More asthma genes have been identified both by positional cloning (four) and by replicated genetic association (at least 10) than have been identified for most complex traits. What is unclear at the present is how variation in these genes functionally relates to the pathobiology of asthma, and the relative importance of the identified genes in terms of attributable risk. It is anticipated that the rate of gene identification will accelerate over the next several years as the cost of genotyping drops. Asthma is also one of the disease areas where there is a substantial opportunity to integrate mouse genetics, human genetics, and mouse functional genomics into an integrated program to assess novel genes and their potential importance for disease risk. Finally, another area that will develop rapidly over the next several years will be the use of genetic markers for prediction of disease risk which will potentially prove useful for asthma where wheezing in early life is common and clinical prediction of future disease risk is poor.

## Key learning points

- Asthma is a very common complex disease with its origins in childhood.

- The disorder is characterized by reversible airflow obstruction and airway inflammation.

- There are a small number of monogenic disorders with clinical features that overlap with asthma and atopy. Asthma may share common molecular origins with these syndromes.

- There are many environmental exposures that contribute to the development of asthma. Of these, the most important and consistent is environmental tobacco smoke.

- Familial aggregation, twin studies, and risk to relatives all demonstrate that there is substantial heritability for asthma and its intermediate phenotypes.

- Four potential asthma-susceptibility genes have been identified by positional cloning, and there are 40 asthma candidate genes that have been replicated two or more times.

- Although mouse models of both acute and chronic allergen exposure are not perfect models of human asthma, use of inbred mouse strains for QTL mapping has been helpful in identifying loci that contribute to innate and allergen-induced airway responsiveness.

## REFERENCES

1  Elias JA, Lee CG, Zheng T et al. New insights into the pathogenesis of asthma. *J Clin Invest* 2003; 111: 291–7.
2  Standardization of Spirometry, 1994 Update. American Thoracic Society. *Am J Respir Crit Care Med* 1995; **152**: 1107–36.

3 Yunginger JW, Reed CE, O'Connell EJ et al. A community-based study of the epidemiology of asthma. Incidence rates, 1964–1983. *Am Rev Respir Dis* 1992; **146**: 888–94.

4 Mannino DM, Homa DM, Akinbami LJ et al. Surveillance for asthma – United States, 1980–1999. *MMWR Surveill Summ* 2002; **51**: 1–13.

5 Weiss KB, Sullivan SD. The health economics of asthma and rhinitis. I. Assessing the economic impact. *J Allergy Clin Immunol* 2001; **107**: 3–8.

6 Davis EC, Mecham RP. Selective degradation of accumulated secretory proteins in the endoplasmic reticulum. A possible clearance pathway for abnormal tropoelastin. *J Biol Chem* 1996; **271**: 3787–94.

7 Grimbacher B, Holland SM, Gallin JI et al. Hyper-IgE syndrome with recurrent infections – an autosomal dominant multisystem disorder. *N Engl J Med* 1999; **340**: 692–702.

8 Daumling S, Buriot D, Trung PH et al. The Buckley syndrome: recurring, severe staphylococcal infections, eczema and hyperimmunoglobulinemia E (author's translation). *Infection* 1980; **8** (Suppl 3): 248–54.

9 Donabedian H, Gallin JI. The hyperimmunoglobulin E recurrent-infection (Job's) syndrome. A review of the NIH experience and the literature. *Medicine (Balt)* 1983; **62**: 195–208.

10 Belohradsky BH, Daumling S, Kiess W, Griscelli C. The hyper-IgE-syndrome (Buckley- or Job-syndrome). *Ergeb Inn Med Kinderheilkd* 1987; **55**: 1–39.

11 Gahr M, Muller W, Allgeier B, Speer CP. A boy with recurrent infections, impaired PMN-chemotaxis, increased IgE concentrations and cranial synostosis – a variant of the hyper-IgE syndrome? *Helv Paediatr Acta* 1987; **42**: 185–90.

12 Buckley RH, Becker WG. Abnormalities in the regulation of human IgE synthesis. *Immunol Rev* 1978; **41**: 288–314.

13 Leung DY, Frankel R, Wood N, Geha RS. Potentiation of human immunoglobulin E synthesis by plasma immunoglobulin E binding factors from patients with the hyperimmunoglobulin E syndrome. *J Clin Invest* 1986; **77**: 952–7.

14 Geha RS, Leung DY. Regulation of the human allergic response. *Int Arch Allergy Appl Immunol* 1987; **82**: 389–91.

15 Van Scoy RE, Hill HR, Ritts RE, Quie PG. Familial neutrophil chemotaxis defect, recurrent bacterial infections, mucocutaneous candidiasis, and hyperimmunoglobulinemia E. *Ann Intern Med* 1975; **82**: 766–71.

16 Robinson MF, McGregor R, Collins R, Cheung K. Combined neutrophil and T-cell deficiency: initial report of a kindred with features of the hyper-IgE syndrome and chronic granulomatous disease. *Am J Med* 1982; **73**: 63–70.

17 Hill HR, Quie PG. Raised serum-IgE levels and defective neutrophil chemotaxis in three children with eczema and recurrent bacterial infections. *Lancet* 1974; **1**: 183–7.

18 Witemeyer S, Van Epps DE. A familial defect in cellular chemotaxis associated with redheadedness and recurrent infection. *J Pediatr* 1976; **89**: 33–7.

19 Donabedian H, Gallin JI. Mononuclear cells from patients with the hyperimmunoglobulin E-recurrent infection syndrome produce an inhibitor of leukocyte chemotaxis. *J Clin Invest* 1982; **69**: 1155–63.

20 Ito S, Shinomiya K, Mikawa H. Suppressive effect of IgE soluble immune complex on neutrophil chemotaxis. *Clin Exp Immunol* 1983; **51**: 407–12.

21 Quinti I, Brozek C, Wood N et al. Circulating IgG autoantibodies to IgE in atopic syndromes. *J Allergy Clin Immunol* 1986; **77**: 586–94.

22 Geha RS, Reinherz E, Leung D et al. Deficiency of suppressor T cells in the hyperimmunoglobulin E syndrome. *J Clin Invest* 1981; **68**: 783–91.

23 King CL, Gallin JI, Malech HL et al. Regulation of immunoglobulin production in hyperimmunoglobulin E recurrent-infection syndrome by interferon gamma. *Proc Natl Acad Sci USA* 1989; **86**: 10085–9.

24 Paganelli R, Scala E, Capobianchi MR et al. Selective deficiency of interferon-gamma production in the hyper-IgE syndrome. Relationship to in vitro IgE synthesis. *Clin Exp Immunol* 1991; **84**: 28–33.

25 Rousset F, Robert J, Andary M et al. Shifts in interleukin-4 and interferon-gamma production by T cells of patients with elevated serum IgE levels and the modulatory effects of these lymphokines on spontaneous IgE synthesis. *J Allergy Clin Immunol* 1991; **87**: 58–69.

26 Claasen JJ, Levine AD, Schiff SE, Buckley RH. Mononuclear cells from patients with the hyper-IgE syndrome produce little IgE when they are stimulated with recombinant human interleukin-4. *J Allergy Clin Immunol* 1991; **88**: 713–21.

27 Grimbacher B, Dutra AS, Holland SM et al. Analphoid marker chromosome in a patient with hyper-IgE syndrome, autism, and mild mental retardation. *Genet Med* 1999; **1**: 213–8.

28 Grimbacher B, Schaffer AA, Holland SM et al. Genetic linkage of hyper-IgE syndrome to chromosome 4. *Am J Hum Genet* 1999; **65**: 735–44.

29 Hershey GK, Friedrich MF, Esswein LA et al. The association of atopy with a gain-of-function mutation in the alpha subunit of the interleukin-4 receptor. *N Engl J Med* 1997; **337**: 1720–5.

30 Grimbacher B, Holland SM, Puck JM. The interleukin-4 receptor variant Q576R in hyper-IgE syndrome. *N Engl J Med* 1998; **338**: 1073–4.

31 Chusid MJ, Dale DC, West BC, Wolff SM. The hypereosinophilic syndrome: analysis of fourteen cases with review of the literature. *Medicine (Balt)* 1975; **54**: 1–27.

32 Kao CC, Ou LS, Lin SJ, Huang JL. Childhood idiopathic hypereosinophilic syndrome: report of a case. *Asian Pac J Allergy Immunol* 2002; **20**: 121–6.

33 Marshall GM, White L. Effective therapy for a severe case of the idiopathic hypereosinophilic syndrome. *Am J Pediatr Hematol Oncol* 1989; **11**: 178–83.

34 Klion AD, Law MA, Riemenschneider W et al. Familial eosinophilia: a benign disorder? *Blood* 2004; **103**: 4050–5.

35 Lefebvre C, Bletry O, Degoulet P et al. Prognostic factors of hypereosinophilic syndrome. Study of 40 cases. *Ann Med Interne (Paris)* 1989; **140**: 253–7.

36 Cools J, DeAngelo DJ, Gotlib J et al. A tyrosine kinase created by fusion of the PDGFRA and FIP1L1 genes as a therapeutic target of imatinib in idiopathic hypereosinophilic syndrome. *N Engl J Med* 2003; **348**: 1201–14.

37 Klion AD, Law MA, Noel P et al. Safety and efficacy of the monoclonal anti-interleukin-5 antibody SCH55700 in the treatment of patients with hypereosinophilic syndrome. *Blood* 2004; **103**: 2939–41.

38 Stone RM, Gilliland DG, Klion AD. Platelet-derived growth factor receptor inhibition to treat idiopathic hypereosinophilic syndrome. *Semin Oncol* 2004; **31**: 12–7.

39 Luppi M, Marasca R, Morselli M et al. Clonal nature of hypereosinophilic syndrome. *Blood* 1994; **84**: 349–50.

40 Chang HW, Leong KH, Koh DR, Lee SH. Clonality of isolated eosinophils in the hypereosinophilic syndrome. *Blood* 1999; **93**: 1651–7.

41 Weinfeld A, Westin J, Swolin B. Ph1-negative eosinophilic leukaemia with trisomy 8. Case report and review of cytogenetic studies. *Scand J Haematol* 1977; **18**: 413–20.

42 Guitard AM, Horschowski N, Mozziconacci MJ et al. Hypereosinophilic syndrome in childhood: trisomy 8 and transformation to mixed acute leukaemia. *Nouv Rev Fr Hematol* 1994; **35**: 555–9.

43 Quiquandon I, Claisse JF, Capiod JC et al. alpha-Interferon and hypereosinophilic syndrome with trisomy 8: karyotypic remission. *Blood* 1995; **85**: 2284–5.

44 Myint H, Chacko J, Mould S et al. Karyotypic evolution in a granulocytic sarcoma developing in a myeloproliferative disorder with a novel (3;4) translocation. *Br J Haematol* 1995; **90**: 462–4.

45 Duell T, Mittermuller J, Schmetzer HM et al. Chronic myeloid leukemia associated hypereosinophilic syndrome with a clonal t(4;7)(q11;q32). *Cancer Genet Cytogenet* 1997; **94**: 91–4.

46 Jost E, Michaux L, Vanden Abeele M et al. Complex karyotype and absence of mutation in the c-kit receptor in aggressive mastocytosis presenting with pelvic osteolysis, eosinophilia and brain damage. *Ann Hematol* 2001; **80**: 302–7.

47 Carroll M, Ohno-Jones S, Tamura S et al. CGP 57148, a tyrosine kinase inhibitor, inhibits the growth of cells expressing BCR-ABL, TEL-ABL, and TEL-PDGFR fusion proteins. *Blood* 1997; **90**: 4947–52.

48 Buchdunger E, Cioffi CL, Law N et al. Abl protein-tyrosine kinase inhibitor STI571 inhibits in vitro signal transduction mediated by c-kit and platelet-derived growth factor receptors. *J Pharmacol Exp Ther* 2000; **295**: 139–45.

49 Gotlib J, Cools J, Malone JM 3rd et al. The FIP1L1-PDGFRalpha fusion tyrosine kinase in hypereosinophilic syndrome and chronic eosinophilic leukemia: implications for diagnosis, classification, and management. *Blood* 2004; **103**: 2879–91.

50 Klion AD, Noel P, Akin C et al. Elevated serum tryptase levels identify a subset of patients with a myeloproliferative variant of idiopathic hypereosinophilic syndrome associated with tissue fibrosis, poor prognosis, and imatinib responsiveness. *Blood* 2003; **101**: 4660–6.

51 Klion AD, Robyn J, Akin C et al. Molecular remission and reversal of myelofibrosis in response to imatinib mesylate treatment in patients with the myeloproliferative variant of hypereosinophilic syndrome. *Blood* 2004; **103**: 473–8.

52 Pardanani A, Brockman SR, Paternoster SF et al. FIP1L1-PDGFRA fusion: Prevalence and clinicopathologic correlates in 89 consecutive patients with moderate to severe eosinophilia. *Blood* 2004; **104**: 3038–45.

53 Naiman JL, Oski FA, Allen FH Jr, Diamond LK. Hereditary eosinophilia: Report of a family and review of the literature. *Am J Hum Genet* 1964; **16**: 195–203.

54 Zeni G, Nardi F, Frezza M. In tema di ipereosinofilia constituzionale familiare idiopatica. *Acta Med Patav* 1964; **24**: 589–602.

55 Zuelzer WW, Apt L. Disseminated visceral lesions associated with extreme eosinophilia: pathological and clinical observations on syndrome of young children. *Am J Dis Child* 1949; **78**: 153–81.

56 Sparrevohn S. Disseminated eosinophilic collagenosis and familial eosinophilia. *Acta Paediatr Scand* 1967; **56**: 307–12.

57 Lin AY, Nutman TB, Kaslow D et al. Familial eosinophilia: clinical and laboratory results on a US kindred. *Am J Med Genet* 1998; **76**: 229–37.

58 Rioux JD, Stone VA, Daly MJ et al. Familial eosinophilia maps to the cytokine gene cluster on human chromosomal region 5q31-q33. *Am J Hum Genet* 1998; **63**: 1086–94.

59 Haagerup A, Bjerke T, Schiotz PO et al. Asthma and atopy – a total genome scan for susceptibility genes. *Allergy* 2002; **57**: 680–6.

60 Koppelman GH, Stine OC, Xu J et al. Genome-wide search for atopy susceptibility genes in Dutch families with asthma. *J Allergy Clin Immunol* 2002; **109**: 498–506.

61 Yokouchi Y, Nukaga Y, Shibasaki M et al. Significant evidence for linkage of mite-sensitive childhood asthma to chromosome 5q31-q33 near the interleukin 12 B locus by a genome-wide search in Japanese families. *Genomics* 2000; **66**: 152–60.

62 Akin C, Metcalfe DD. Systemic mastocytosis. *Annu Rev Med* 2004; **55**: 419–32.

63 Parker RI. Hematologic aspects of mastocytosis: I: Bone marrow pathology in adult and pediatric systemic mast cell disease. *J Invest Dermatol* 1991; **96**: 47S–51S.

64 Akin C, Jaffe ES, Raffeld M et al. An immunohistochemical study of the bone marrow lesions of systemic mastocytosis: expression of stem cell factor by lesional mast cells. *Am J Clin Pathol* 2002; **118**: 242–7.

65 Schwartz LB, Sakai K, Bradford TR et al. The alpha form of human tryptase is the predominant type present in blood at baseline in normal subjects and is elevated in those with systemic mastocytosis. *J Clin Invest* 1995; **96**: 2702–10.

66 Escribano L, Orfao A, Diaz-Agustin B et al. Indolent systemic mast cell disease in adults: immunophenotypic characterization of bone marrow mast cells and its diagnostic implications. *Blood* 1998; **91**: 2731–6.

67 Burgoon CF Jr, Graham JH, McCaffree DL. Mast cell disease. A cutaneous variant with multisystem involvement. *Arch Dermatol* 1968; **98**: 590–605.

68 Selmanowitz VJ, Orentreich N. Mastocytosis. A clinical genetic evaluation. *J Hered* 1970; **61**: 91–4.

69 Shaw JM. Genetic aspects of urticaria pigmentosa. *Arch Dermatol* 1968; **97**: 137–8.

70 Boyano T, Carrascosa T, Val J et al. Urticaria pigmentosa in monozygotic twins. *Arch Dermatol* 1990; **126**: 1375–6.

71 Clark DP, Buescher L, Havey A. Familial urticaria pigmentosa. *Arch Intern Med* 1990; **150**: 1742–4.

72 Anstey A, Lowe DG, Kirby JD, Horton MA. Familial mastocytosis: a clinical, immunophenotypic, light and electron microscopic study. *Br J Dermatol* 1991; **125**: 583–7.

73 James MP, Eady RA. Familial urticaria pigmentosa with giant mast cell granules. A clinical, light, and electron microscopic study. *Arch Dermatol* 1981; **117**: 713–8.

74 Sundstrom M, Vliagoftis H, Karlberg P et al. Functional and phenotypic studies of two variants of a human mast cell line with a distinct set of mutations in the c-kit proto-oncogene. *Immunology* 2003; **108**: 89–97.

75 Beghini A, Ripamonti CB, Castorina P et al. Trisomy 4 leading to duplication of a mutated KIT allele in acute myeloid leukemia with mast cell involvement. *Cancer Genet Cytogenet* 2000; **119**: 26–31.

76 Lishner M, Confino-Cohen R, Mekori YA et al. Trisomies 9 and 8 detected by fluorescence in situ hybridization in patients with systemic mastocytosis. *J Allergy Clin Immunol* 1996; **98**: 199–204.

77 Sillaber C, Strobl H, Bevec D et al. IL-4 regulates c-kit proto-oncogene product expression in human mast and myeloid progenitor cells. *J Immunol* 1991; **147**: 4224–8.

78 Galli SJ, Kitamura Y. Genetically mast-cell-deficient W/Wv and Sl/Sld mice. Their value for the analysis of the roles of mast cells in biologic responses in vivo. *Am J Pathol* 1987; **127**: 191–8.

79 Nagata H, Worobec AS, Oh CK et al. Identification of a point mutation in the catalytic domain of the protooncogene c-kit in

peripheral blood mononuclear cells of patients who have mastocytosis with an associated hematologic disorder. *Proc Natl Acad Sci USA* 1995; **92**: 10560–4.

80 Longley BJ Jr, Metcalfe DD, Tharp M et al. Activating and dominant inactivating c-KIT catalytic domain mutations in distinct clinical forms of human mastocytosis. *Proc Natl Acad Sci USA* 1999; **96**: 1609–14.

81 Akin C, Kirshenbaum AS, Semere T et al. Analysis of the surface expression of c-kit and occurrence of the c-kit Asp816Val activating mutation in T cells, B cells, and myelomonocytic cells in patients with mastocytosis. *Exp Hematol* 2000; **28**: 140–7.

82 Akin C, Fumo G, Yavuz AS et al. A novel form of mastocytosis associated with a transmembrane c-kit mutation and response to imatinib. *Blood* 2004; **103**: 3222–5.

83 Pignon JM, Giraudier S, Duquesnoy P et al. A new c-kit mutation in a case of aggressive mast cell disease. *Br J Haematol* 1997; **96**: 374–6.

84 Worobec AS, Semere T, Nagata H, Metcalfe DD. Clinical correlates of the presence of the Asp816Val c-kit mutation in the peripheral blood mononuclear cells of patients with mastocytosis. *Cancer* 1998; **83**: 2120–9.

85 Fritsche-Polanz R, Jordan JH, Feix A et al. Mutation analysis of C-KIT in patients with myelodysplastic syndromes without mastocytosis and cases of systemic mastocytosis. *Br J Haematol* 2001; **113**: 357–64.

86 Rosbotham JL, Malik NM, Syrris P et al. Lack of c-kit mutation in familial urticaria pigmentosa. *Br J Dermatol* 1999; **140**: 849–52.

87 Tang X, Boxer M, Drummond A et al. A germline mutation in KIT in familial diffuse cutaneous mastocytosis. *J Med Genet* 2004; **41**: e88.

88 Akin C, Brockow K, D'Ambrosio C et al. Effects of tyrosine kinase inhibitor STI571 on human mast cells bearing wild-type or mutated c-kit. *Exp Hematol* 2003; **31**: 686–92.

89 Netherton EW. A unique case of trichorrhexis nodosa; bamboo hairs. *AMA Arch Derm* 1958; **78**: 483–7.

90 Altman J, Stroud J. Netherton's syndrome and ichthyosis linearis circumflexa. *Arch Dermatol* 1969; **100**: 550–8.

91 Julius CE, Keeran M. Netherton's syndrome in a male. *Arch Dermatol* 1971; **104**: 422–4.

92 Smith DL, Smith JG, Wong SW, deShazo RD. Netherton's syndrome: a syndrome of elevated IgE and characteristic skin and hair findings. *J Allergy Clin Immunol* 1995; **95**: 116–23.

93 Chavanas S, Garner C, Bodemer C et al. Localization of the Netherton syndrome gene to chromosome 5q32, by linkage analysis and homozygosity mapping. *Am J Hum Genet* 2000; **66**: 914–21.

94 Chavanas S, Bodemer C, Rochat A et al. Mutations in SPINK5, encoding a serine protease inhibitor, cause Netherton syndrome. *Nat Genet* 2000; **25**: 141–2.

95 Magert HJ, Standker L, Kreutzmann P et al. LEKTI, a novel 15-domain type of human serine proteinase inhibitor. *J Biol Chem* 1999; **274**: 21499–502.

96 Walley AJ, Chavanas S, Moffatt MF et al. Gene polymorphism in Netherton and common atopic disease. *Nat Genet* 2001; **29**: 175–8.

97 Kato A, Fukai K, Oiso N et al. Association of SPINK5 gene polymorphisms with atopic dermatitis in the Japanese population. *Br J Dermatol* 2003; **148**: 665–9.

98 Nishio Y, Noguchi E, Shibasaki M et al. Association between polymorphisms in the SPINK5 gene and atopic dermatitis in the Japanese. *Genes Immun* 2003; **4**: 515–7.

99 Kabesch M, Carr D, Weiland SK, von Mutius E. Association between polymorphisms in serine protease inhibitor, kazal type 5 and asthma phenotypes in a large German population sample. *Clin Exp Allergy* 2004; **34**: 340–5.

100 Churg J, Strauss L. Allergic granulomatosis, allergic angiitis, and periarteritis nodosa. *Am J Pathol* 1951; **27**: 277–301.

101 Finan MC, Winkelmann RK. The cutaneous extravascular necrotizing granuloma (Churg–Strauss granuloma) and systemic disease: a review of 27 cases. *Medicine (Balt)* 1983; **62**: 142–58.

102 Masi AT, Hunder GG, Lie JT et al. The American College of Rheumatology 1990 criteria for the classification of Churg–Strauss syndrome (allergic granulomatosis and angiitis). *Arthritis Rheum* 1990; **33**: 1094–100.

103 Jennette JC, Falk RJ, Andrassy K et al. Nomenclature of systemic vasculitides. Proposal of an international consensus conference. *Arthritis Rheum* 1994; **37**: 187–92.

104 Guillevin L, Cohen P, Gayraud M et al. Churg–Strauss syndrome. Clinical study and long-term follow-up of 96 patients. *Medicine (Balt)* 1999; **78**: 26–37.

105 Wechsler ME, Finn D, Gunawardena D et al. Churg–Strauss syndrome in patients receiving montelukast as treatment for asthma. *Chest* 2000; **117**: 708–13.

106 Martin RM, Wilton LV, Mann RD. Prevalence of Churg–Strauss syndrome, vasculitis, eosinophilia and associated conditions: retrospective analysis of 58 prescription-event monitoring cohort studies. *Pharmacoepidemiol Drug Saf* 1999; **8**: 179–89.

107 Wechsler ME, Garpestad E, Flier SR et al. Pulmonary infiltrates, eosinophilia, and cardiomyopathy following corticosteroid withdrawal in patients with asthma receiving zafirlukast. *J Am Med Assoc* 1998; **279**: 455–7.

108 Le Gall C, Pham S, Vignes S et al. Inhaled corticosteroids and Churg–Strauss syndrome: a report of five cases. *Eur Respir J* 2000; **15**: 978–81.

109 Churg A, Brallas M, Cronin SR, Churg J. Formes frustes of Churg–Strauss syndrome. *Chest* 1995; **108**: 320–3.

110 Schmitt WH, Csernok E, Kobayashi S et al. Churg–Strauss syndrome: serum markers of lymphocyte activation and endothelial damage. *Arthritis Rheum* 1998; **41**: 445–52.

111 Schonermarck U, Csernok E, Trabandt A et al. Circulating cytokines and soluble CD23, CD26 and CD30 in ANCA-associated vasculitides. *Clin Exp Rheumatol* 2000; **18**: 457–63.

112 Kiene M, Csernok E, Muller A et al. Elevated interleukin-4 and interleukin-13 production by T cell lines from patients with Churg–Strauss syndrome. *Arthritis Rheum* 2001; **44**: 469–73.

113 Muschen M, Warskulat U, Perniok A et al. Involvement of soluble CD95 in Churg–Strauss syndrome. *Am J Pathol* 1999; **155**: 915–25.

114 Manganelli P, Giacosa R, Fietta P et al. Familial vasculitides: Churg–Strauss syndrome and Wegener's granulomatosis in two first-degree relatives. *J Rheumatol* 2003; **30**: 618–21.

115 Steffensen FH, Sorensen HT, Gillman MW et al. Low birth weight and preterm delivery as risk factors for asthma and atopic dermatitis in young adult males. *Epidemiology* 2000; **11**: 185–8.

116 Litonjua AA, Carey VJ, Burge HA et al. Parental history and the risk for childhood asthma. Does mother confer more risk than father? *Am J Respir Crit Care Med* 1998; **158**: 176–81.

117 Li YF, Gilliland FD, Berhane K et al. Effects of in utero and environmental tobacco smoke exposure on lung function in boys and girls with and without asthma. *Am J Respir Crit Care Med* 2000; **162**: 2097–104.

118  Dejmek J, Solansky I, Podrazilova K, Sram RJ. The exposure of nonsmoking and smoking mothers to environmental tobacco smoke during different gestational phases and fetal growth. *Environ Health Perspect* 2002; **110**: 601–6.

119  Gilliland FD, Berhane K, Li YF et al. Effects of early onset asthma and in utero exposure to maternal smoking on childhood lung function. *Am J Respir Crit Care Med* 2003; **167**: 917–24.

120  Dold S, Wjst M, von Mutius E, Reitmeir P, Stiepel E. Genetic risk for asthma, allergic rhinitis, and atopic dermatitis. *Arch Dis Child* 1992; **67**: 1018–22.

121  Longo G, Strinati R, Poli F, Fumi F. Genetic factors in nonspecific bronchial hyperreactivity. An epidemiologic study. *Am J Dis Child* 1987; **141**: 331–4.

122  Greally M, Jagoe WS, Greally J. The genetics of asthma. *Ir Med J* 1982; **75**: 403–5.

123  Van Arsdel PP Jr, Motulsky AG. Frequency and hereditability of asthma and allergic rhinitis in college students. *Acta Genet Stat Med* 1959; **9**: 101–14.

124  Sibbald B, Horn ME, Brain EA, Gregg I. Genetic factors in childhood asthma. *Thorax* 1980; **35**: 671–4.

125  Jenkins MA, Hopper JL, Giles GG. Regressive logistic modeling of familial aggregation for asthma in 7394 population-based nuclear families. *Genet Epidemiol* 1997; **14**: 317–32.

126  Duffy DL, Martin NG, Battistutta D et al. Genetics of asthma and hay fever in Australian twins. *Am Rev Respir Dis* 1990; **142**: 1351–8.

127  Nieminen MM, Kaprio J, Koskenvuo M. A population-based study of bronchial asthma in adult twin pairs. *Chest* 1991; **100**: 70–5.

128  Hopp RJ, Bewtra AK, Watt GD et al. Genetic analysis of allergic disease in twins. *J Allergy Clin Immunol* 1984; **73**: 265–70.

129  Lubs ML. Emperic risks for genetic counseling in families with allergy. *J Pediatr* 1972; **80**: 26–31.

130  Edfors-Lubs ML. Allergy in 7000 twin pairs. *Acta Allergol* 1971; **26**: 249–85.

131  Sandford A, Weir T, Pare P. The genetics of asthma. *Am J Respir Crit Care Med* 1996; **153**: 1749–65.

132  Konig P, Godfrey S. Exercise-induced bronchial lability and atopic status of families of infants with wheezy bronchitis. *Arch Dis Child* 1973; **48**: 942–6.

133  Lewitter FI, Tager IB, McGue M et al. Genetic and environmental determinants of level of pulmonary function. *Am J Epidemiol* 1984; **120**: 518–30.

134  Tager IB, Rosner B, Tishler PV et al. Household aggregation of pulmonary function and chronic bronchitis. *Am Rev Respir Dis* 1976; **114**: 485–92.

135  Hankins D, Drage C, Zamel N, Kronenberg R. Pulmonary function in identical twins raised apart. *Am Rev Respir Dis* 1982; **125**: 119–21.

136  Hubert HB, Fabsitz RR, Feinleib M, Gwinn C. Genetic and environmental influences on pulmonary function in adult twins. *Am Rev Respir Dis* 1982; **125**: 409–15.

137  Redline S, Tishler PV, Rosner B et al. Genotypic and phenotypic similarities in pulmonary function among family members of adult monozygotic and dizygotic twins. *Am J Epidemiol* 1989; **129**: 827–36.

138  Niu T, Rogus JJ, Chen C et al. Familial aggregation of bronchodilator response: a community-based study. *Am J Respir Crit Care Med* 2000; **162**: 1833–7.

139  Daniels SE, Bhattacharrya S, James A et al. A genome-wide search for quantitative trait loci underlying asthma. *Nature* 1996; **383**: 247–50.

140  Bleecker ER, Postma DS, Howard TD et al. Genome screen for susceptibility loci in a genetically homogeneous Dutch population. *Am J Respir Crit Care Med* 1999; **159**: A645 (Abstract).

141  A genome-wide search for asthma susceptibility loci in ethnically diverse populations. The Collaborative Study on the Genetics of Asthma (CSGA). *Nat Genet* 1997; **15**: 389–92.

142  Ober C, Cox NJ, Abney M et al. Genome-wide search for asthma susceptibility loci in a founder population. The Collaborative Study on the Genetics of Asthma. *Hum Mol Genet* 1998; **7**: 1393–8.

143  Wjst M, Fischer G, Immervoll T et al. A genome-wide search for linkage to asthma. German Asthma Genetics Group. *Genomics* 1999; **58**: 1–8.

144  Yokouchi Y, Nukaga Y, Shibasaki M et al. Significant evidence for linkage of mite-sensitive childhood asthma to chromosome 5q31-q33 near the interleukin 12 B locus by a genome-wide search in Japanese families. *Genomics* 2000; **66**: 152–60.

145  Dizier MH, Besse-Schmittler C, Guilloud-Bataille M et al. Genome screen for asthma and related phenotypes in the French EGEA study. *Am J Respir Crit Care Med* 2000; **162**: 1812–8.

146  Laitinen T, Daly MJ, Rioux JD et al. A susceptibility locus for asthma-related traits on chromosome 7 revealed by genome-wide scan in a founder population. *Nat Genet* 2001; **28**: 87–91.

147  Xu X, Fang Z, Wang B et al. A genomewide search for quantitative-trait loci underlying asthma. *Am J Hum Genet* 2001; **69**: 1271–7.

148  Haagerup A, Bjerke T, Schiotz PO et al. Asthma and atopy – a total genome scan for susceptibility genes. *Allergy* 2002; **57**: 680–6.

149  Hakonarson H, Bjornsdottir US, Halapi E et al. A major susceptibility gene for asthma maps to chromosome 14q24. *Am J Hum Genet* 2002; **71**: 483–91.

150  Huang SK, Mathias RA, Ehrlich E et al. Evidence for asthma susceptibility genes on chromosome 11 in an African-American population. *Hum Genet* 2003; **113**: 71–5.

151  Xu J, Meyers DA, Ober C et al. Genomewide screen and identification of gene–gene interactions for asthma-susceptibility loci in three US populations: collaborative study on the genetics of asthma. *Am J Hum Genet* 2001; **68**: 1437–46.

152  Mathias RA, Freidhoff LR, Blumenthal MN et al. Genome-wide linkage analyses of total serum IgE using variance components analysis in asthmatic families. *Genet Epidemiol* 2001; **20**: 340–55.

153  Blumenthal MN, Langefeld CD, Beaty TH et al. A genome-wide search for allergic response (atopy) genes in three ethnic groups: Collaborative Study on the Genetics of Asthma. *Hum Genet* 2004; **114**: 157–64.

154  Ober C, Tsalenko A, Willadsen S et al. Genome-wide screen for atopy susceptibility alleles in the Hutterites. *Clin Exp Allergy* 1999; **29**: 11–5.

155  Koppelman GH, Stine OC, Xu J et al. Genome-wide search for atopy susceptibility genes in Dutch families with asthma. *J Allergy Clin Immunol* 2002; **109**: 498–506.

156  Xu J, Postma DS, Howard TD et al. Major genes regulating total serum immunoglobulin E levels in families with asthma. *Am J Hum Genet* 2000; **67**: 1163–73.

157  Van Eerdewegh P, Little RD, Dupuis J et al. Association of the ADAM33 gene with asthma and bronchial hyperresponsiveness. *Nature* 2002; **418**: 426–30.

158  Daniels SE, Bhattacharrya S, James A et al. A genome-wide search for quantitative trait loci underlying asthma. *Nature* 1996; **383**: 247–50.

159 Lander E, Kruglyak L. Genetic dissection of complex traits: guidelines for interpreting and reporting linkage results. *Nat Genet* 1995; **11**: 241–7.

160 Collaborative Study on the Genetics of Asthma. A genome-wide search for asthma susceptibility loci in ethnically diverse populations. *Nat Genet* 1997; **15**: 389–392.

161 Xu J, Meyers DA, Ober C et al. Genomewide screen and identification of gene-gene interactions for asthma-susceptibility loci in three US populations: collaborative study on the genetics of asthma. *Am J Hum Genet* 2001; **68**: 1437–46.

162 Mathias RA, Freidhoff LR, Blumenthal MN et al. Genome-wide linkage analyses of total serum IgE using variance components analysis in asthmatic families. *Genet Epidemiol* 2001; **20**: 340–55.

163 Blumenthal MN, Ober C, Beaty TH et al. Genome scan for loci linked to mite sensitivity: the Collaborative Study on the Genetics of Asthma (CSGA). *Genes Immun* 2004; **5**: 226–31.

164 Lander ES, Schork N. Genetic dissection of complex traits. *Science* 1994; **265**: 2037–48.

165 Ober C, Tsalenko A, Parry R, Cox NJ. A second-generation genomewide screen for asthma-susceptibility alleles in a founder population. *Am J Hum Genet* 2000; **67**: 1154–62.

166 Silverman EK, Palmer LJ. Case-control association studies for the genetics of complex respiratory diseases. *Am J Respir Cell Mol Biol* 2000; **22**: 645–8.

167 Laitinen T, Polvi A, Rydman P et al. Characterization of a common susceptibility locus for asthma-related traits. *Science* 2004; **304**: 300–4.

168 Zhang Y, Leaves NI, Anderson GG et al. Positional cloning of a quantitative trait locus on chromosome 13q14 that influences immunoglobulin E levels and asthma. *Nat Genet* 2003; **34**: 181–6.

169 Allen M, Heinzmann A, Noguchi E et al. Positional cloning of a novel gene influencing asthma from chromosome 2q14. *Nat Genet* 2003; **35**: 258–63.

170 DeSanctis GT, Merchant M, Beier DR et al. Quantitative locus analysis of airway hyperresponsiveness in A/J and C57BL/6J mice. *Nat Genet* 1995; **11**: 150–154.

171 Howard TD, Postma DS, Jongepier H et al. Association of a disintegrin and metalloprotease 33 (ADAM33) gene with asthma in ethnically diverse populations. *J Allergy Clin Immunol* 2003; **112**: 717–22.

172 Lind DL, Choudhry S, Ung N et al. ADAM33 is not associated with asthma in Puerto Rican or Mexican populations. *Am J Respir Crit Care Med* 2003; **168**: 1312–6.

173 Raby BA, Silverman EK, Kwiatkowski DJ et al. ADAM33 polymorphisms and phenotype associations in childhood asthma. *J Allergy Clin Immunol* 2004; **113**: 1071–8.

174 Qi SY, Riviere PJ, Trojnar J et al. Cloning and characterization of dipetidyl peptidase 10, a new member of an emerging subgroup of serine proteases. *Biochem J* 2003; **373**: 179–189.

175 Scanlan MJ, Gordan JD, Williamson B et al. Antigens recognized by autologous antibody in patients with renal-cell carcinoma. *Int J Cancer* 1999; **83**: 456–64.

176 Hoffjan S, Nicolae D, Ober C. Association studies for asthma and atopic diseases: a comprehensive review of the literature. *Respir Res* 2003; **4**: 14.

177 Wahl SM, Vazquez N, Chen W. Regulatory T cells and transcription factors: gatekeepers in allergic inflammation. *Curr Opin Immunol* 2004; **16**: 768–74.

178 Rosenwasser LJ, Klemm DJ, Dresback JK et al. Promoter polymorphisms in the chromosome 5 gene cluster in asthma and atopy. *Clin Exp Aller* 1995; **25**(Suppl 2): 74–8; discussion 95–6.

179 Noguchi E, Shibasaki M, Arinami T et al. Association of asthma and the interleukin-4 promoter gene in Japanese. *Clin Exp Allergy* 1998; **28**: 449–53.

180 Zhu S, Chan-Yeung M, Becker AB et al. Polymorphisms of the IL-4, TNF-alpha, and Fcepsilon RIbeta genes and the risk of allergic disorders in at-risk infants. *Am J Respir Crit Care Med* 2000; **161**: 1655–9.

181 Beghe B, Barton S, Rorke S et al. Polymorphisms in the interleukin-4 and interleukin-4 receptor alpha chain genes confer susceptibility to asthma and atopy in a Caucasian population. *Clin Exp Allergy* 2003; **33**: 1111–7.

182 Kabesch M, Tzotcheva I, Carr D et al. A complete screening of the IL4 gene: novel polymorphisms and their association with asthma and IgE in childhood. *J Allergy Clin Immunol* 2003; **112**: 893–8.

183 Basehore MJ, Howard TD, Lange LA et al. A comprehensive evaluation of IL4 variants in ethnically diverse populations: association of total serum IgE levels and asthma in white subjects. *J Allergy Clin Immunol* 2004; **114**: 80–7.

184 Tanaka K, Sugiura H, Uehara M et al. Lack of association between atopic eczema and the genetic variants of interleukin-4 and the interleukin-4 receptor alpha chain gene: heterogeneity of genetic backgrounds on immunoglobulin E production in atopic eczema patients. *Clin Exp Allergy* 2001; **31**: 1522–7.

185 Sandford AJ, Chagani T, Zhu S et al. Polymorphisms in the IL4, IL4RA, and FCERIB genes and asthma severity. *J Allergy Clin Immunol* 2000; **106**: 135–40.

186 Burchard EG, Silverman EK, Rosenwasser LJ et al. Association between a sequence variant in the IL-4 gene promoter and FEV(1) in asthma. *Am J Respir Crit Care Med* 1999; **160**: 919–22.

187 Novak N, Kruse S, Kraft S et al. Dichotomic nature of atopic dermatitis reflected by combined analysis of monocyte immunophenotyping and single nucleotide polymorphisms of the interleukin-4/interleukin-13 receptor gene: the dichotomy of extrinsic and intrinsic atopic dermatitis. *J Invest Dermatol* 2002; **119**: 870–5.

188 Takabayashi A, Ihara K, Sasaki Y et al. Childhood atopic asthma: positive association with a polymorphism of IL-4 receptor alpha gene but not with that of IL-4 promoter or Fc epsilon receptor I beta gene. *Exp Clin Immunogenet* 2000; **17**: 63–70.

189 Hakonarson H, Bjornsdottir US, Ostermann E et al. Allelic frequencies and patterns of single-nucleotide polymorphisms in candidate genes for asthma and atopy in Iceland. *Am J Respir Crit Care Med* 2001; **164**: 2036–44.

190 Elliott K, Fitzpatrick E, Hill D et al. The -590C/T and -34C/T interleukin-4 promoter polymorphisms are not associated with atopic eczema in childhood. *J Allergy Clin Immunol* 2001; **108**: 285–7.

191 Howard TD, Koppelman GH, Zheng SL et al. Gene–gene interaction in asthma: IL4RA and IL13 in a Dutch population with asthma. *Am J Hum Genet* 2002; **70**: 230–6.

192 Mitsuyasu H, Izuhara K, Mao XQ et al. Ile50Val variant of IL4R alpha upregulates IgE synthesis and associates with atopic asthma. *Nat Genet* 1998; **19**: 119–20.

193 Izuhara K, Yanagihara Y, Hamasaki N et al. Atopy and the human IL-4 receptor alpha chain. *J Allergy Clin Immunol* 2000; **106**: S65–71.

194  Kruse S, Japha T, Tedner M et al. The polymorphisms S503P and Q576R in the interleukin-4 receptor alpha gene are associated with atopy and influence the signal transduction. *Immunology* 1999; **96**: 365–71.

195  Noguchi E, Shibasaki M, Arinami T et al. No association between atopy/asthma and the ILe50Val polymorphism of IL-4 receptor. *Am J Respir Crit Care Med* 1999; **160**: 342–5.

196  Migliaccio C, Patuzzo C, Malerba G et al. No linkage or association of five polymorphisms in the interleukin-4 receptor alpha gene with atopic asthma in Italian families. *Eur J Immunogenet* 2003; **30**: 349–53.

197  Tan EC, Lee BW, Chew FT et al. IL-4Ralpha gene Ile50Val polymorphism. *Allergy* 1999; **54**: 1005–7.

198  Hytonen AM, Lowhagen O, Arvidsson M et al. Haplotypes of the interleukin-4 receptor alpha chain gene associate with susceptibility to and severity of atopic asthma. *Clin Exp Allergy* 2004; **34**: 1570–5.

199  Fehervari Z, Sakaguchi S. CD4+ Tregs and immune control. *J Clin Invest* 2004; **114**: 1209–17.

200  Bourgain C, Hoffjan S, Nicolae R et al. Novel case–control test in a founder population identifies P-selectin as an atopy-susceptibility locus. *Am J Hum Genet* 2003; **73**: 612–26.

201  Hang LW, Hsia TC, Chen WC et al. Interleukin-10 gene -627 allele variants, not interleukin-I beta gene and receptor antagonist gene polymorphisms, are associated with atopic bronchial asthma. *J Clin Lab Anal* 2003; **17**: 168–73.

202  Immervoll T, Loesgen S, Dutsch G et al. Fine mapping and single nucleotide polymorphism association results of candidate genes for asthma and related phenotypes. *Hum Mutat* 2001; **18**: 327–36.

203  Hobbs K, Negri J, Klinnert M et al. Interleukin-10 and transforming growth factor-beta promoter polymorphisms in allergies and asthma. *Am J Respir Crit Care Med* 1998; **158**: 1958–62.

204  Karjalainen J, Hulkkonen J, Nieminen MM et al. Interleukin-10 gene promoter region polymorphism is associated with eosinophil count and circulating immunoglobulin E in adult asthma. *Clin Exp Allergy* 2003; **33**: 78–83.

205  Lyon H, Lange C, Lake S et al. IL10 gene polymorphisms are associated with asthma phenotypes in children. *Genet Epidemiol* 2004; **26**: 155–65.

206  Unoki M, Furuta S, Onouchi Y et al. Association studies of 33 single nucleotide polymorphisms (SNPs) in 29 candidate genes for bronchial asthma: positive association a T924C polymorphism in the thromboxane A2 receptor gene. *Hum Genet* 2000; **106**: 440–6.

207  Grunig G, Warnock M, Wakil AE et al. Requirement for IL-13 independently of IL-4 in experimental asthma. *Science* 1998; **282**: 2261–3.

208  de Vries JE. The role of IL-13 and its receptor in allergy and inflammatory responses. *J Allergy Clin Immun* 1998; **102**: 165–9.

209  Chen W, Ericksen MB, Levin LS, Khurana Hershey GK. Functional effect of the R110Q IL13 genetic variant alone and in combination with IL4RA genetic variants. *J Allergy Clin Immunol* 2004; **114**: 553–60.

210  van der Pouw Kraan TC, van Veen A, Boeije LC et al. An IL-13 promotor polymorphism associated with increased risk of allergic asthma. *Genes Immun* 1999; **1**: 61–5.

211  Howard TD, Whittaker PA, Zaiman AL et al. Identification and association of polymorphisms in the interleukin-13 gene with asthma and atopy in a Dutch population. *Am J Respir Cell Mol Biol* 2001; **25**: 377–84.

212  Heinzmann A, Jerkic SP, Ganter K et al. Association study of the IL13 variant Arg110Gln in atopic diseases and juvenile idiopathic arthritis. *J Allergy Clin Immunol* 2003; **112**: 735–9.

213  Heinzmann A, Mao XQ, Akaiwa M et al. Genetic variants of IL-13 signalling and human asthma and atopy. *Hum Mol Genet* 2000; **9**: 549–59.

214  Liu X, Nickel R, Beyer K et al. An IL13 coding region variant is associated with a high total serum IgE level and atopic dermatitis in the German multicenter atopy study (MAS-90). *J Allergy Clin Immunol* 2000; **106**: 167–70.

215  Leung TF, Tang NL, Chan IH et al. A polymorphism in the coding region of interleukin-13 gene is associated with atopy but not asthma in Chinese children. *Clin Exp Allergy* 2001; **31**: 1515–21.

216  Tsunemi Y, Saeki H, Nakamura K et al. Interleukin-13 gene polymorphism G4257A is associated with atopic dermatitis in Japanese patients. *J Dermatol Sci* 2002; **30**: 100–7.

217  DeMeo DL, Lange C, Silverman EK et al. Univariate and multivariate family-based association analysis of the IL-13 ARG130GLN polymorphism in the Childhood Asthma Management Program. *Genet Epidemiol* 2002; **23**: 335–48.

218  Liu X, Beaty TH, Deindl P et al. Associations between specific serum IgE response and 6 variants within the genes IL4, IL13, and IL4RA in German children: the German Multicenter Atopy Study. *J Allergy Clin Immunol* 2004; **113**: 489–95.

219  Liu X, Beaty TH, Deindl P et al. Associations between total serum IgE levels and the 6 potentially functional variants within the genes IL4, IL13, and IL4RA in German children: the German Multicenter Atopy Study. *J Allergy Clin Immunol* 2003; **112**: 382–8.

220  Hummelshoj T, Bodtger U, Datta P et al. Association between an interleukin-13 promoter polymorphism and atopy. *Eur J Immunogenet* 2003; **30**: 355–9.

221  Wang M, Xing ZM, Lu C et al. A common IL-13 Arg130Gln single nucleotide polymorphism among Chinese atopy patients with allergic rhinitis. *Hum Genet* 2003; **113**: 387–90.

222  Graves PE, Kabesch M, Halonen M et al. A cluster of seven tightly linked polymorphisms in the IL-13 gene is associated with total serum IgE levels in three populations of white children. *J Allergy Clin Immunol* 2000; **105**: 506–13.

223  He JQ, Chan-Yeung M, Becker AB et al. Genetic variants of the IL13 and IL4 genes and atopic diseases in at-risk children. *Genes Immun* 2003; **4**: 385–9.

224  Celedón JC, Soto-Quiros ME, Palmer LJ et al. Lack of association between a polymorphism in the IL-13 gene and total serum IgE among nuclear families in Costa Rica. *Clin Exp Allergy* 2002; **32**: 387–90.

225  Szentivayni A. The β-adrenergic theory of the atopic abnormality in bronchial asthma. *J Allergy* 1968; **42**: 203–232.

226  Kobilka BK, Dixon RA, Frielle T et al. cDNA for the human beta 2-adrenergic receptor: a protein with multiple membrane-spanning domains and encoded by a gene whose chromosomal location is shared with that of the receptor for platelet-derived growth factor. *Proc Natl Acad Sci USA* 1987; **84**: 46–50.

227  Strader CD, Candelore MR, Hill WS et al. A single amino acid substitution in the beta-adrenergic receptor promotes partial agonist activity from antagonists. *J Biol Chem* 1989; **264**: 16470–7.

228 Dixon RA, Sigal IS, Candelore MR et al. Structural features required for ligand binding to the beta-adrenergic receptor. *EMBO J* 1987; **6**: 3269–75.

229 Rands E, Candelore MR, Cheung AH et al. Mutational analysis of beta-adrenergic receptor glycosylation. *J Biol Chem* 1990; **265**: 10759–64.

230 Reihsaus E, Innis M, MacIntyre N, Liggett SB. Mutations in the gene encoding for the beta 2-adrenergic receptor in normal and asthmatic subjects. *Am J Respir Cell Mol Biol* 1993; **8**: 334–9.

231 McGraw DW, Forbes SL, Kramer LA, Liggett SB. Polymorphisms of the 5′ leader cistron of the human beta2-adrenergic receptor regulate receptor expression. *J Clin Invest* 1998; **102**: 1927–32.

232 Parola AL, Kobilka BK. The peptide product of a 5′ leader cistron in the beta 2 adrenergic receptor mRNA inhibits receptor synthesis. *J Biol Chem* 1994; **269**: 4497–505.

233 Drysdale C, McGraw D, Stack C et al. Complex promoter and coding region beta 2-adrenergic receptor haplotypes alter receptor expression and predict in vivo responsiveness. *Proc Natl Acad Sci USA* 2000; **97**: 10483–8.

234 Green SA, Cole G, Jacinto M et al. A polymorphism of the human beta 2-adrenergic receptor within the fourth transmembrane domain alters ligand binding and functional properties of the receptor. *J Biol Chem* 1993; **268**: 23116–21.

235 Green SA, Rathz DA, Schuster AJ, Liggett SB. The Ile164 beta(2)-adrenoceptor polymorphism alters salmeterol exosite binding and conventional agonist coupling to G(s). *Eur J Pharmacol* 2001; **421**: 141–7.

236 Turki J, Lorenz JN, Green SA et al. Myocardial signaling defects and impaired cardiac function of a human beta 2-adrenergic receptor polymorphism expressed in transgenic mice. *Proc Natl Acad Sci USA* 1996; **93**: 10483–8.

237 Green SA, Turki J, Innis M, Liggett SB. Amino-terminal polymorphisms of the human beta 2-adrenergic receptor impart distinct agonist-promoted regulatory properties. *Biochemistry* 1994; **33**: 9414–9.

238 Green SA, Turki J, Bejarano P et al. Influence of beta 2-adrenergic receptor genotypes on signal transduction in human airway smooth muscle cells. *Am J Respir Cell Mol Biol* 1995; **13**: 25–33.

239 Moore PE, Laporte JD, Abraham JH et al. Polymorphism of the beta(2)-adrenergic receptor gene and desensitization in human airway smooth muscle. *Am J Respir Crit Care Med* 2000; **162**: 2117–24.

240 Hopes E, McDougall C, Christie G et al. Association of glutamine 27 polymorphism of beta 2 adrenoceptor with reported childhood asthma: population based study. *Br Med J* 1998; **316**: 664.

241 Santillan AA, Camargo CA Jr, Ramirez-Rivera A et al. Association between beta2-adrenoceptor polymorphisms and asthma diagnosis among Mexican adults. *J Allergy Clin Immunol* 2003; **112**: 1095–100.

242 Silverman EK, Kwiatkowski DJ, Sylvia JS et al. Family-based association analysis of beta2-adrenergic receptor polymorphisms in the childhood asthma management program. *J Allergy Clin Immunol* 2003; **112**: 870–6.

243 Summerhill E, Leavitt SA, Gidley H et al. Beta(2)-adrenergic receptor Arg16/Arg16 genotype is associated with reduced lung function, but not with asthma, in the Hutterites. *Am J Respir Crit Care Med* 2000; **162**: 599–602.

244 Dewar JC, Wheatley AP, Venn A et al. Beta2-adrenoceptor polymorphisms are in linkage disequilibrium, but are not associated with asthma in an adult population. *Clin Exp Allergy* 1998; **28**: 442–8.

245 Wang Z, Chen C, Niu T et al. Association of asthma with beta(2)-adrenergic receptor gene polymorphism and cigarette smoking. *Am J Respir Crit Care Med* 2001; **163**: 1404–9.

246 Martinez FD, Graves PE, Baldini M et al. Association between genetic polymorphisms of the beta2-adrenoceptor and response to albuterol in children with and without a history of wheezing. *J Clin Invest* 1997; **100**: 3184–8.

247 Ramsay CE, Hayden CM, Tiller KJ et al. Polymorphisms in the beta2-adrenoreceptor gene are associated with decreased airway responsiveness. *Clin Exp Allergy* 1999; **29**: 1195–203.

248 Turki J, Pak J, Green SA et al. Genetic polymorphisms of the beta 2-adrenergic receptor in nocturnal and nonnocturnal asthma. Evidence that Gly16 correlates with the nocturnal phenotype. *J Clin Invest* 1995; **95**: 1635–41.

249 Holloway JW, Dunbar PR, Riley GA et al. Association of beta2-adrenergic receptor polymorphisms with severe asthma. *Clin Exp Allergy* 2000; **30**: 1097–103.

250 Binaei S, Christensen M, Murphy C et al. Beta2-adrenergic receptor polymorphisms in children with status asthmaticus. *Chest* 2003; **123**: 375S.

251 Kotani Y, Nishimura Y, Maeda H, Yokoyama M. Beta2-adrenergic receptor polymorphisms affect airway responsiveness to salbutamol in asthmatics. *J Asthma* 1999; **36**: 583–90.

252 Kim SH, Oh SY, Oh HB et al. Association of beta2-adrenoreceptor polymorphisms with nocturnal cough among atopic subjects but not with atopy and nonspecific bronchial hyperresponsiveness. *J Allergy Clin Immunol* 2002; **109**: 630–5.

253 Weir TD, Mallek N, Sandford AJ et al. Beta2-adrenergic receptor haplotypes in mild, moderate and fatal/near fatal asthma. *Am J Respir Crit Care Med* 1998; **158**: 787–91.

254 Hall IP, Wheatley A, Wilding P, Liggett SB. Association of Glu 27 beta 2-adrenoceptor polymorphism with lower airway reactivity in asthmatic subjects. *Lancet* 1995; **345**: 1213–4.

255 D'Amato M, Vitiani LR, Petrelli G et al. Association of persistent bronchial hyperresponsiveness with beta2-adrenoceptor (ADRB2) haplotypes. A population study. *Am J Respir Crit Care Med* 1998; **158**: 1968–73.

256 Ulbrecht M, Hergeth MT, Wjst M et al. Association of beta(2)-adrenoreceptor variants with bronchial hyperresponsiveness. *Am J Respir Crit Care Med* 2000; **161**: 469–74.

257 Dewar JC, Wilkinson J, Wheatley A et al. The glutamine 27 B2-adrenoceptor polymorphism is associated with elevated IgE levels in asthmatic families. *J Aller Clin Immun* 1997; **100**: 261–5.

258 Tan S, Hall IP, Dewar J et al. Association between B2-adrenoceptor polymorphism and susceptibility to bronchodilator desensitisation in moderately severe stable asthmatics. *Lancet* 1997; **350**: 995–9.

259 Martinez FD, Graves PE, Baldini M et al. Association between genetic polymorphisms of the B2-adrenoceptor and response to albuterol in children with and without a history of wheezing. *J Clin Invest* 1997; **100**: 3184–8.

260 Drysdale CM, McGraw DW, Stack CB et al. Complex promoter and coding region beta 2-adrenergic receptor haplotypes alter receptor expression and predict in vivo responsiveness. *Proc Natl Acad Sci USA* 2000; **97**: 10483–8.

261 Israel E, Drazen JM, Liggett SB et al. The effect of polymorphisms of the beta(2)-adrenergic receptor on the response to regular use of albuterol in asthma. *Am J Respir Crit Care Med* 2000; **162**: 75–80.

262 Deichmann KA, Schmidt A, Heinzmann A et al. Association studies on beta2-adrenoceptor polymorphisms and enhanced

IgE responsiveness in an atopic population. *Clin Exp Allergy* 1999; **29**: 794–9.

263  Lipworth BJ, Hall IP, Aziz I et al. Beta2-adrenoceptor polymorphism and bronchoprotective sensitivity with regular short- and long-acting beta2-agonist therapy. *Clin Sci (Lond)* 1999; **96**: 253–9.

264  Guerra S, Lohman IC, Halonen M et al. Reduced interferon gamma production and soluble CD14 levels in early life predict recurrent wheezing by 1 year of age. *Am J Respir Crit Care Med* 2004; **169**: 70–6.

265  Baldini M, Lohman IC, Halonen M et al. A polymorphism* in the 5′ flanking region of the CD14 gene is associated with circulating soluble CD14 levels and with total serum immunoglobulin E. *Am J Respir Cell Mol Biol* 1999; **20**: 976–83.

266  Koppelman GH, Reijmerink NE, Colin Stine O et al. Association of a promoter polymorphism of the CD14 gene and atopy. *Am J Respir Crit Care Med* 2001; **163**: 965–9.

267  Leung TF, Tang NL, Sung YM et al. The C-159T polymorphism in the CD14 promoter is associated with serum total IgE concentration in atopic Chinese children. *Pediatr Allergy Immunol* 2003; **14**: 255–60.

268  Gao PS, Mao XQ, Kawai M et al. Lack of association between ACE gene polymorphisms and atopy and asthma in British and Japanese populations. *Clin Genet* 1998; **54**: 245–7.

269  O'Donnell AR, Toelle BG, Marks GB et al. Age-specific relationship between CD14 and atopy in a cohort assessed from age 8 to 25 years. *Am J Respir Crit Care Med* 2004; **169**: 615–22.

270  Buckova D, Holla LI, Schuller M et al. Two CD14 promoter polymorphisms and atopic phenotypes in Czech patients with IgE-mediated allergy. *Allergy* 2003; **58**: 1023–6.

271  Cardaba B, Moffatt MF, Fernandez E et al. Allergy to dermatophagoides in a group of Spanish gypsies: genetic restrictions. *Int Arch Allergy Immunol* 2001; **125**: 297–306.

272  Sengler C, Haider A, Sommerfeld C et al. Evaluation of the CD14 C-159 T polymorphism in the German Multicenter Allergy Study cohort. *Clin Exp Allergy* 2003; **33**: 166–9.

273  Moffatt MF, Cookson WO. Tumour necrosis factor haplotypes and asthma. *Hum Mol Genet* 1997; **6**: 551–4.

274  Albuquerque RV, Hayden CM, Palmer LJ et al. Association of polymorphisms within the tumour necrosis factor (TNF) genes and childhood asthma. *Clin Exp Allergy* 1998; **28**: 578–84.

275  Chagani T, Pare PD, Zhu S et al. Prevalence of tumor necrosis factor-alpha and angiotensin converting enzyme polymorphisms in mild/moderate and fatal/near-fatal asthma. *Am J Respir Crit Care Med* 1999; **160**: 278–82.

276  Winchester EC, Millwood IY, Rand L et al. Association of the TNF-alpha-308 (G7A) polymorphism with self-reported history of childhood asthma. *Hum Genet* 2000; **107**: 591–6.

277  Witte JS, Palmer LJ, O'Connor RD et al. Relation between tumour necrosis factor polymorphism TNFalpha-308 and risk of asthma. *Eur J Hum Genet* 2002; **10**: 82–5.

278  Wang TN, Chen WY, Wang TH et al. Gene–gene synergistic effect on atopic asthma: tumour necrosis factor-alpha-308 and lymphotoxin-alpha-NcoI in Taiwan's children. *Clin Exp Allergy* 2004; **34**: 184–8.

279  Shin HD, Park BL, Kim LH et al. Association of tumor necrosis factor polymorphisms with asthma and serum total IgE. *Hum Mol Genet* 2004; **13**: 397–403.

280  Li Kam Wa TC, Mansur AH, Britton J et al. Association between -308 tumour necrosis factor promoter polymorphism and bronchial hyperreactivity in asthma. *Clin Exp Allergy* 1999; **29**: 1204–8.

281  Castro J, Telleria JJ, Linares P, Blanco-Quiros A. Increased TNFA*2, but not TNFB*1, allele frequency in Spanish atopic patients. *J Investig Allergol Clin Immunol* 2000; **10**: 149–54.

282  Trabetti E, Patuzzo C, Malerba G et al. Association of a lymphotoxin alpha gene polymorphism and atopy in Italian families. *J Med Genet* 1999; **36**: 323–5.

283  Tan EC, Lee BW, Tay AW et al. Asthma and TNF variants in Chinese and Malays. *Allergy* 1999; **54**: 402–3.

284  Malerba G, Trabetti E, Patuzzo C et al. Candidate genes and a genome-wide search in Italian families with atopic asthmatic children. *Clin Exp Allergy* 1999; **29**(Suppl 4): 27–30.

285  Louis R, Leyder E, Malaise M et al. Lack of association between adult asthma and the tumour necrosis factor alpha-308 polymorphism gene. *Eur Respir J* 2000; **16**: 604–8.

286  El Bahlawan L, Christensen M, Binaei S et al. Lack of association between the tumor necrosis factor-alpha regulatory region genetic polymorphisms associated with elevated tumor necrosis factor-alpha levels and children with asthma. *Chest* 2003; **123**: 374S–5S.

287  Buckova D, Holla LI, Vasku A et al. Lack of association between atopic asthma and the tumor necrosis factor alpha-308 gene polymorphism in a Czech population. *J Invest Allerg Clin Immunol* 2002; **12**: 192–7.

288  Moffatt MF, James A, Ryan G et al. Extended tumour necrosis factor/HLA-DR haplotypes and asthma in an Australian population sample. *Thorax* 1999; **54**: 757–61.

289  Lin YC, Lu CC, Su HJ et al. The association between tumor necrosis factor, HLA-DR alleles, and IgE-mediated asthma in Taiwanese adolescents. *Allergy* 2002; **57**: 831–4.

290  Izakovicova Holla L, Vasku A, Izakovic V, Znojil V. The interaction of the polymorphisms in transporter of antigen peptides (TAP) and lymphotoxin alpha (LT-alpha) genes and atopic diseases in the Czech population. *Clin Exp Allergy* 2001; **31**: 1418–23.

291  Ansari AA, Freidhoff LR, Meyers DA et al. Human immune responsiveness to Lolium perenne pollen allergen Lol p III (rye III) is associated with HLA-DR3 and DR5. *Hum Immunol* 1989; **25**: 59–71.

292  Fischer GF, Pickl WF, Fae I et al. Association between IgE response against Bet v I, the major allergen of birch pollen, and HLA-DRB alleles. *Hum Immunol* 1992; **33**: 259–65.

293  D'Amato M, Scotto d'Abusco A, Maggi E et al. Association of responsiveness to the major pollen allergen of *Parietaria officinalis* with HLA-DRB1* alleles: a multicenter study. *Hum Immun* 1996; **46**: 100–6.

294  Stephan V, Kuehr J, Seibt A et al. Genetic linkage of HLA-class II locus to mite-specific IgE immune responsiveness. *Clin Exp Allergy* 1999; **29**: 1049–54.

295  Donfack J, Tsalenko A, Hoki DM et al. HLA-DRB1*01 alleles are associated with sensitization to cockroach allergens. *J Aller Clin Immun* 2000; **105**: 960–6.

296  Hu C, Hsu PN, Lin RH et al. HLA DPB1*0201 allele is negatively associated with immunoglobulin E responsiveness specific for house dust mite allergens in Taiwan. *Clin Exp Allergy* 2000; **30**: 538–45.

297  Moffatt MF, Schou C, Faux JA et al. Association between quantitative traits underlying asthma and the HLA-DRB1 locus in a family-based population sample. *Eur J Hum Genet* 2001; **9**: 341–6.

298  Kim YK, Oh HB, Oh SY et al. HLA-DRB1*07 may have a susceptibility and DRB1*04 a protective effect upon the development of a sensitization to house dust mite

*Dermatophagoides pteronyssinus. Clin Exp Allergy* 2001; **31**: 110–5.

299 Moffatt MF, Faux JA, Lester S et al. Atopy, respiratory function and HLA-DR in Aboriginal Australians. *Hum Mol Genet* 2003; **12**: 625–30.

300 Marsh DG, Hsu SH, Roebber M et al. HLA-Dw2: a genetic marker for human immune response to short ragweed pollen allergen Ra5. I. Response resulting primarily from natural antigenic exposure. *J Exp Med* 1982; **155**: 1439–51.

301 Marsh DG, Freidhoff LR, Ehrlich-Kautzky E et al. Immune responsiveness to *Ambrosia artemisiifolia* (short ragweed) pollen allergen Amb a VI (Ra6) is associated with HLA-DR5 in allergic humans. *Immunogenetics* 1987; **26**: 230–6.

302 Freidhoff LR, Ehrlich-Kautzky E, Meyers DA et al. Association of HLA-DR3 with human immune response to Lol p I and Lol p II allergens in allergic subjects. *Tissue Antigens* 1988; **31**: 211–9.

303 Cardaba B, Vilches C, Martin E et al. DR7 and DQ2 are positively associated with immunoglobulin-E response to the main antigen of olive pollen (Ole e I) in allergic patients. *Hum Immunol* 1993; **38**: 293–9.

304 Kalpaklioglu AF, Turan M. Possible association between cockroach allergy and HLA class II antigens. *Ann Allergy Asthma Immunol* 2002; **89**: 155–8.

305 Aron Y, Desmazes-Dufeu N, Matran R et al. Evidence of a strong positive association between atopy and the HLA class II alleles DR4 and DR7. *Clin Exp Allergy* 1996; **26**: 821–826.

306 Di Somma C, Charron D, Deichmann K et al. Atopic asthma and TNF-308 alleles: linkage disequilibrium and association analyses. *Hum Immunol* 2003; **64**: 359–65.

307 Howell WM, Standring P, Warner JA, Warner JO. HLA class II genotype, HLA-DR B cell surface expression and allergen specific IgE production in atopic and non-atopic members of asthmatic family pedigrees. *Clin Exp Allergy* 1999; **29** (Suppl 4): 35–8.

308 Woszczek G, Kowalski ML, Borowiec M. Association of asthma and total IgE levels with human leucocyte antigen-DR in patients with grass allergy. *Eur Respir J* 2002; **20**: 79–85.

309 Holloway JW, Doull I, Begishvili B et al. Lack of evidence of a significant association between HLA-DR, DQ and DP genotypes and atopy in families with HDM allergy. *Clin Exp Allergy* 1996; **26**: 1142–9.

310 Dekker JW, Nizankowska E, Schmitz-Schumann M et al. Aspirin-induced asthma and HLA-DRB1 and HLA-DPB1 genotypes. *Clin Exp Allergy* 1997; **27**: 574–7.

311 Young RP, Dekker JW, Wordsworth BP et al. HLA-DR and HLA-DP genotypes and immunoglobulin E responses to common major allergens. *Clin Exp Allergy* 1994; **24**: 431–9.

312 Sandford AJ, Shirakawa T, Moffatt MF et al. Localisation of atopy and beta subunit of high-affinity IgE receptor (Fc epsilon RI) on chromosome 11q. *Lancet* 1993; **341**: 332–4.

313 Szepetowski P, Gaudray P. FCER1B, a candidate gene for atopy, is located in 11q13 between CD20 and TCN1. *Genomics* 1994; **19**: 399–400.

314 Kuster H, Zhang L, Brini AT et al. The gene and cDNA for the human high affinity immunoglobulin E receptor beta chain and expression of the complete human receptor. *J Biol Chem* 1992; **267**: 12782–7.

315 Cookson WO, Sharp PA, Faux JA, Hopkin JM. Linkage between immunoglobulin E responses underlying asthma and rhinitis and chromosome 11q. *Lancet* 1989; **1**: 1292–5.

316 Young RP, Sharp PA, Lynch JR et al. Confirmation of genetic linkage between atopic IgE responses and chromosome 11q13. *J Med Genet* 1992; **29**: 236–8.

317 The Collaborative Study on the Genetics of Asthma. A genome-wide search for asthma susceptibility loci in ethnically diverse populations. The Collaborative Study on the Genetics of Asthma (CSGA). *Nat Genet* 1997; **15**: 389–92.

318 Daniels S, Bhattacharrya S, James A et al. A genome-wide search for quantitative trait loci underlying asthma. *Nature* 1996; **383**: 247–50.

319 Shirakawa T, Li A, Dubowitz M et al. Association between atopy and variants of the beta subunit of the high-affinity immunoglobulin E receptor. *Nat Genet* 1994; **7**: 125–9.

320 Folster-Holst R, Moises HW, Yang L et al. Linkage between atopy and the IgE high-affinity receptor gene at 11q13 in atopic dermatitis families. *Hum Genet* 1998; **102**: 236–9.

321 van Herwerden L, Harrap SB, Wong ZY et al. Linkage of high-affinity IgE receptor gene with bronchial hyperreactivity, even in absence of atopy. *Lancet* 1995; **346**: 1262–5.

322 Trabetti E, Cusin V, Malerba G et al. Association of the FcepsilonRIbeta gene with bronchial hyper-responsiveness in an Italian population. *J Med Genet* 1998; **35**: 680–1.

323 Hizawa N, Yamaguchi E, Ohe M et al. Lack of linkage between atopy and locus 11q13. *Clin Exp Allergy* 1992; **22**: 1065–9.

324 Rich SS, Roitman-Johnson B, Greenberg B et al. Genetic analysis of atopy in three large kindreds: no evidence of linkage to D11S97. *Clin Exp Allergy* 1992; **22**: 1070–6.

325 Amelung PJ, Panhuysen CI, Postma DS et al. Atopy and bronchial hyperresponsiveness: exclusion of linkage to markers on chromosomes 11q and 6p. *Clin Exp Allergy* 1992; **22**: 1077–84.

326 Lympany P, Welsh KI, Cochrane GM et al. Genetic analysis of the linkage between chromosome 11q and atopy. *Clin Exp Allergy* 1992; **22**: 1085–92.

327 Simon Thomas N, Wilkinson J, Lonjou C et al. Linkage analysis of markers on chromosome 11q13 with asthma and atopy in a United Kingdom population. *Am J Respir Crit Care Med* 2000; **162**: 1268–72.

328 Ishizaka K, Ishizaka T. Physicochemical properties of reaginic antibody. 1. Association of reaginic activity with an immunoglobulin other than gammaA- or gammaG-globulin. *J Allergy* 1966; **37**: 169–85.

329 Lin S, Cicala C, Scharenberg AM, Kinet JP. The Fc(epsilon)RIbeta subunit functions as an amplifier of Fc(epsilon)RIgamma-mediated cell activation signals. *Cell* 1996; **85**: 985–95.

330 Donnadieu E, Jouvin MH, Kinet JP. A second amplifier function for the allergy-associated Fc(epsilon)RI-beta subunit. *Immunity* 2000; **12**: 515–23.

331 Saini SS, Richardson JJ, Wofsy C et al. Expression and modulation of FcepsilonRIalpha and FcepsilonRIbeta in human blood basophils. *J Allergy Clin Immunol* 2001; **107**: 832–41.

332 Hill MR, Cookson WO. A new variant of the beta subunit of the high-affinity receptor for immunoglobulin E (Fc epsilon RI-beta E237G): associations with measures of atopy and bronchial hyper-responsiveness. *Hum Mol Genet* 1996; **5**: 959–62.

333 Shirakawa T, Mao XQ, Sasaki S et al. Association between Fc epsilon RI beta and atopic disorder in a Japanese population. *Lancet* 1996; **347**: 394–5.

334 Nagata H, Mutoh H, Kumahara K et al. Association between nasal allergy and a coding variant of the Fc epsilon RI beta gene Glu237Gly in a Japanese population. *Hum Genet* 2001; **109**: 262–6.

335  Dickson PW, Wong ZY, Harrap SB et al. Mutational analysis of the high affinity immunoglobulin E receptor beta subunit gene in asthma. *Thorax* 1999; **54**: 409–12.

336  Hizawa N, Yamaguchi E, Furuya K et al. Association between high serum total IgE levels and D11S97 on chromosome 11q13 in Japanese subjects. *J Med Genet* 1995; **32**: 363–9.

337  Rohrbach M, Kraemer R, Liechti-Gallati S. Screening of the Fc epsilon RI-beta-gene in a Swiss population of asthmatic children: no association with E237G and identification of new sequence variations. *Dis Markers* 1998; **14**: 177–86.

338  Palmer LJ, Rye PJ, Gibson NA et al. Association of FcepsilonR1-beta polymorphisms with asthma and associated traits in Australian asthmatic families. *Clin Exp Allergy* 1999; **29**: 1555–62.

339  Green SL, Gaillard MC, Song E et al. Polymorphisms of the beta chain of the high-affinity immunoglobulin E receptor (Fcepsilon RI-beta) in South African black and white asthmatic and nonasthmatic individuals. *Am J Respir Crit Care Med* 1998; **158**: 1487–92.

340  Donnadieu E, Cookson WO, Jouvin MH, Kinet JP. Allergy-associated polymorphisms of the Fc epsilon RI beta subunit do not impact its two amplification functions. *J Immunol* 2000; **165**: 3917–22.

341  Furumoto Y, Hiraoka S, Kawamoto K et al. Polymorphisms in FcepsilonRI beta chain do not affect IgE-mediated mast cell activation. *Biochem Biophys Res Commun* 2000; **273**: 765–71.

342  Palmer LJ, Pare PD, Faux JA et al. Fc epsilon R1-beta polymorphism and total serum IgE levels in endemically parasitized Australian aborigines. *Am J Hum Genet* 1997; **61**: 182–8.

343  van Hage-Hamsten M, Johansson E, Kronqvist M et al. Associations of Fc epsilon R1-beta polymorphisms with immunoglobin E antibody responses to common inhalant allergens in a rural population. *Clin Exp Allergy* 2002; **32**: 838–42.

344  Traherne JA, Hill MR, Hysi P et al. LD mapping of maternally and non-maternally derived alleles and atopy in FcepsilonRI-beta. *Hum Mol Genet* 2003; **12**: 2577–85.

345  Moffatt MF, Cookson WO. The genetics of asthma. Maternal effects in atopic disease. *Clin Exp Allergy* 1998; **28**(Suppl 1): 56–61; discussion 65–6.

346  Kuehr J, Karmaus W, Forster J et al. Sensitization to four common inhalant allergens within 302 nuclear families. *Clin Exp Allergy* 1993; **23**: 600–5.

347  Bray GW. The heredity factor in hypersensitiveness, anaphylaxis and allergy. *J Allergy* 1931; **2**: 203–4.

348  Collee JM, ten Kate LP, de Vries HG et al. Allele sharing on chromosome 11q13 in sibs with asthma and atopy. *Lancet* 1993; **342**: 936.

349  Deichmann KA, Starke B, Schlenther S et al. Linkage and association studies of atopy and the chromosome 11q13 region. *J Med Genet* 1999; **36**: 379–82.

350  Cox HE, Moffatt MF, Faux JA et al. Association of atopic dermatitis to the beta subunit of the high affinity immunoglobulin E receptor. *Br J Dermatol* 1998; **138**: 182–7.

351  Matsuoka T, Hirata M, Tanaka H et al. Prostaglandin D2 as a mediator of allergic asthma. *Science* 2000; **287**: 2013–7.

352  Oguma T, Palmer LJ, Birben E et al. Role of prostanoid DP receptor variants in susceptibility to asthma. *N Engl J Med* 2004; **351**: 1752–63.

353  Tomkinson A, Cieslewicz G, Duez C et al. Temporal association between airway hyperresponsiveness and airway eosinophilia in ovalbumin-sensitized mice. *Am J Respir Crit Care Med* 2001; **163**: 721–30.

354  Takeda K, Hamelmann E, Joetham A et al. Development of eosinophilic airway inflammation and airway hyperresponsiveness in mast cell-deficient mice. *J Exp Med* 1997; **186**: 449–54.

355  Wills-Karp M. Murine models of asthma in understanding immune dysregulation in human asthma. *Immunopharmacology* 2000; **48**: 263–8.

356  Henderson WR Jr, Tang LO, Chu SJ et al. A role for cysteinyl leukotrienes in airway remodeling in a mouse asthma model. *Am J Respir Crit Care Med* 2002; **165**: 108–16.

357  Erjefalt JS, Greiff L, Andersson M et al. Degranulation patterns of eosinophil granulocytes as determinants of eosinophil driven disease. *Thorax* 2001; **56**: 341–4.

358  Levitt RC, Mitzner W. Autosomal recessive inheritance of airway hyperreactivity to 5-hydroxytryptamine. *J Appl Physiol* 1989; **67**: 1125–32.

359  De Sanctis GT, Merchant M, Beier DR et al. Quantitative locus analysis of airway hyperresponsiveness in A/J and C57BL/6J mice. *Nat Genet* 1995; **11**: 150–4.

360  Ewart SL, Mitzner W, DiSilvestre DA et al. Airway hyperresponsiveness to acetylcholine: segregation analysis and evidence for linkage to murine chromosome 6. *Am J Respir Cell Mol Biol* 1996; **14**: 487–95.

361  De Sanctis GT, Drazen JM. Genetics of native airway responsiveness in mice. *Am J Respir Crit Care Med* 1997; **156**: S82–8.

362  Wills-Karp M, Ewart SL. The genetics of allergen-induced airway hyperresponsiveness in mice. *Am J Respir Crit Care Med* 1997; **156**: S89–96.

363  Whitehead GS, Walker JK, Berman KG et al. Allergen-induced airway disease is mouse strain dependent. *Am J Physiol Lung Cell Mol Physiol* 2003; **285**: L32–42.

364  Shinagawa K, Kojima M. Mouse model of airway remodeling: strain differences. *Am J Respir Crit Care Med* 2003; **168**: 959–67.

365  Levitt RC, Mitzner W. Expression of airway hyperreactivity to acetylcholine as a simple autosomal recessive trait in mice. *FASEB J* 1988; **2**: 2605–8.

366  Levitt RC, Mitzner W, Kleeberger SR. A genetic approach to the study of lung physiology: understanding biological variability in airway responsiveness. *Am J Physiol* 1990; **258**: L157–64.

367  Longphre M, Kleeberger SR. Susceptibility to platelet-activating factor-induced airway hyperreactivity and hyperpermeability: interstrain variation and genetic control. *Am J Respir Cell Mol Biol* 1995; **13**: 586–94.

368  Konno S, Adachi M, Matsuura T et al. Bronchial reactivity to methacholine and serotonin in six inbred mouse strains. *Arerugi* 1993; **42**: 42–7.

369  Levitt RC, Ewart SL. Genetic susceptibility to atracurium-induced bronchoconstriction. *Am J Respir Crit Care Med* 1995; **151**: 1537–42.

370  Duguet A, Biyah K, Minshall E et al. Bronchial responsiveness among inbred mouse strains. Role of airway smooth-muscle shortening velocity. *Am J Respir Crit Care Med* 2000; **161**: 839–48.

371  De Sanctis GT, Singer JB, Jiao A et al. Quantitative trait locus mapping of airway responsiveness to chromosomes 6 and 7 in inbred mice. *Am J Physiol* 1999; **277**: L1118–23.

372  Ewart SL, Kuperman D, Schadt E et al. Quantitative trait loci controlling allergen-induced airway hyperresponsiveness in inbred mice. *Am J Respir Cell Mol Biol* 2000; **23**: 537–545.

373 Brewer JP, Kisselgof AB, Martin TR. Genetic variability in pulmonary physiological, cellular, and antibody responses to antigen in mice. *Am J Respir Crit Care Med* 1999; **160**: 1150–6.

374 Takeda K, Haczku A, Lee JJ et al. Strain dependence of airway hyperresponsiveness reflects differences in eosinophil localization in the lung. *Am J Physiol Lung Cell Mol Physiol* 2001; **281**: L394–402.

375 Wilder JA, Collie DD, Wilson BS et al. Dissociation of airway hyperresponsiveness from immunoglobulin E and airway eosinophilia in a murine model of allergic asthma. *Am J Respir Cell Mol Biol* 1999; **20**: 1326–34.

376 Larsen GL, Renz H, Loader JE et al. Airway response to electrical field stimulation in sensitized inbred mice. Passive transfer of increased responsiveness with peribronchial lymph nodes. *J Clin Invest* 1992; **89**: 747–52.

377 Levitt RC, Eleff SM, Zhang LY et al. Linkage homology for bronchial hyperresponsiveness between DNA markers on human chromosome 5q31-q33 and mouse chromosome 13. *Clin Exp Allergy* 1995; **25**(Suppl 2): 61–3.

378 Zhang Y, Lefort J, Kearsey V et al. A genome-wide screen for asthma-associated quantitative trait loci in a mouse model of allergic asthma. *Hum Mol Genet* 1999; **8**: 601–5.

379 The Collaborative Study on the Genetics of Asthma (CSGA). A genome-wide search for asthma susceptibility loci in ethnically diverse populations. *Nat Genet* 1997; **15**: 389–92.

380 Ober C, Cox NJ, Abney M et al. Genome-wide search for asthma susceptibility loci in a founder population. The Collaborative Study on the Genetics of Asthma. *Hum Mol Genet* 1998; **7**: 1393–8.

381 Wjst M, Fischer G, Immervoll T et al. A genome-wide search for linkage to asthma. German Asthma Genetics Group. *Genomics* 1999; **58**: 1–8.

382 Leaves NI, Bhattacharyya S, Wiltshire S, Cookson WO. A detailed genetic map of the chromosome 7 bronchial hyper-responsiveness locus. *Eur J Hum Genet* 2002; **10**: 177–82.

383 Noguchi E, Yokouchi Y, Shibasaki M et al. Association between TNFA polymorphism and the development of asthma in the Japanese population. *Am J Respir Crit Care Med* 2002; **166**: 43–6.

384 Herbon N, Werner M, Braig C et al. High-resolution SNP scan of chromosome 6p21 in pooled samples from patients with complex diseases. *Genomics* 2003; **81**: 510–8.

385 Raby BA, Silverman EK, Lazarus R et al. Chromosome 12q harbors multiple genetic loci related to asthma and asthma-related phenotypes. *Hum Mol Genet* 2003; **12**: 1973–9.

386 Szabo SJ, Sullivan BM, Peng SL, Glimcher LH. Molecular mechanisms regulating Th1 immune responses. *Ann Rev Immunol* 2003; **21**: 713–758.

387 D'Ambrosio D, Cippitelli M, Cocciolo MG et al. Inhibition of IL-12 production by 1,25-dihydroxyvitamin D3. Involvement of NF-kappaB downregulation in transcriptional repression of the p40 gene. *J Clin Invest* 1998; **101**: 252–62.

388 Lemire JM, Archer DC, Beck L, Spiegelberg HL. Immunosuppressive actions of 1,25-dihydroxyvitamin D3: preferential inhibition of Th1 functions. *J Nutr* 1995; **125**: 1704S–8S.

389 O'Kelly J, Hisatake J, Hisatake Y et al. Normal myelopoiesis but abnormal T lymphocyte responses in vitamin D receptor knockout mice. *J Clin Invest* 2002; **109**: 1091–9.

390 Matheu V, Back O, Mondoc E, Issazadeh-Navikas S. Dual effects of vitamin D-induced alteration of TH1/TH2 cytokine expression: enhancing IgE production and decreasing airway eosinophilia in murine allergic airway disease. *J Allergy Clin Immunol* 2003; **112**: 585–92.

391 Nakao F, Ihara K, Kusuhara K et al. Association of IFN-gamma and IFN regulatory factor 1 polymorphisms with childhood atopic asthma. *J Allergy Clin Immunol* 2001; **107**: 499–504.

392 Ober C, Tsalenko A, Parry R, Cox NJ. A second-generation genomewide screen for asthma-susceptibility alleles in a founder population. *Am J Hum Genet* 2000; **67**: 1154–62.

393 Poon AH, Laprise C, Lemire M et al. Association of vitamin D receptor genetic variants with susceptibility to asthma and atopy. *Am J Respir Crit Care Med* 2004; **170**: 967–73.

394 Raby BA, Lazarus R, Silverman EK et al. Association of vitamin D receptor gene polymorphisms with childhood and adult asthma. *Am J Respir Crit Care Med* 2004; **170**: 1057–65.

395 McIntire JJ, Umetsu SE, Akbari O et al. Identification of Tapr (an airway hyperreactivity regulatory locus) and the linked Tim gene family. *Nat Immunol* 2001; **2**: 1109–16.

396 Matricardi PM, Rosmini F, Panetta V et al. Hay fever and asthma in relation to markers of infection in the United States. *J Allergy Clin Immunol* 2002; **110**: 381–7.

397 McIntire JJ, Umetsu SE, Macaubas C et al. Immunology: hepatitis A virus link to atopic disease. *Nature* 2003; **425**: 576.

398 Symula DJ, Frazer KA, Ueda Y et al. Functional screening of an asthma QTL in YAC transgenic mice. *Nat Genet* 1999; **23**: 241–4.

399 Zhu Z, Homer RJ, Wang Z et al. Pulmonary expression of interleukin-13 causes inflammation, mucus hypersecretion, subepithelial fibrosis, physiologic abnormalities, and eotaxin production. *J Clin Invest* 1999; **103**: 779–88.

400 Kauppi P, Lindblad-Toh K, Sevon P et al. A second-generation association study of the 5q31 cytokine gene cluster and the interleukin-4 receptor in asthma. *Genomics* 2001; **77**: 35–42.

401 Karp CL, Grupe A, Schadt E et al. Identification of complement factor 5 as a susceptibility locus for experimental allergic asthma. *Nat Immunol* 2000; **1**: 221–6.

402 Krug N, Tschernig T, Erpenbeck VJ et al. Complement factors C3a and C5a are increased in bronchoalveolar lavage fluid after segmental allergen provocation in subjects with asthma. *Am J Respir Crit Care Med* 2001; **164**: 1841–3.

403 Hasegawa K, Tamari M, Shao C et al. Variations in the C3, C3a receptor, and C5 genes affect susceptibility to bronchial asthma. *Hum Genet* 2004; **115**: 295–301.

The following references are duplicated: 141/160/317/319, 61/144, 139/158/318, 151/161, 60/155, 142/380, and 165/392.

# 10

# Chronic obstructive pulmonary disease

CRAIG P. HERSH, DAWN L. DEMEO, AND EDWIN K. SILVERMAN

## INTRODUCTION

The global initiative for chronic obstructive lung disease (GOLD) defines chronic obstructive pulmonary disease (COPD) as 'a disease state characterized by airflow limitation that is not fully reversible. The airflow limitation is usually both progressive and associated with an abnormal inflammatory response of the lungs to noxious particles or gases'.[1] The GOLD criteria rely on post-bronchodilator spirometric measures to define and stage the disease, and they include the concepts of host response and environmental exposures in the definition of disease itself, highlighting the fact that COPD is a complex disease.

Using these concepts as a framework, this chapter will start with a discussion of the genetic analysis of normal variation in pulmonary function, pointing out the steps necessary in the analysis of any complex trait in humans. The next section will introduce COPD as a disease entity, highlighting clinical definitions, relevant COPD-related phenotypes, and the effects of smoking and other exposures as they relate to genetic analysis. Alpha 1-antitrypsin deficiency, the most important known genetic cause of COPD, will be discussed in detail, and other rare genetic disorders with emphysema or related changes as part of their phenotypes will be mentioned. The genetic analysis of COPD as a complex disorder will be covered, reviewing familial aggregation, linkage, and association studies in humans. Lessons from animal models as well as implications of genetic research on disease management will be included. The final section of the chapter will cover genetic influences on nicotine addiction, because cigarette smoking is the most important environmental exposure for the development of COPD.

## PULMONARY FUNCTION IN THE GENERAL POPULATION

### Background

Measurements of pulmonary function, usually determined by spirometry, are integral to the diagnosis of COPD and are the most common intermediate phenotypes used in genetic studies of this disease. Commonly recorded values from the forced expiratory maneuver include the forced expiratory volume in 1 second ($FEV_1$), the forced vital capacity (FVC), the ratio of $FEV_1$ to FVC, the peak expiratory flow rate (PEFR), and the maximum mid-expiratory flow rate (MMEF or $FEF_{25-75}$). These values are often expressed as a percent of a predicted value derived from race-specific regression equations controlling for age, sex, and height.[2,3] The diffusing capacity for carbon monoxide (DLCO), also known as the gas transfer factor, has also been used in genetic studies, despite being technically more challenging to measure than spirometry. The various pulmonary function tests used in respiratory genetic studies are reviewed in Chapter 2.

The measurements yielded via spirometry demonstrate a broad range of quantitative variation in the general population, as well as in subjects with respiratory illnesses. Like other quantitative traits, such as height or blood pressure, genetic and environmental factors may affect their values in normal individuals. As noted in Chapter 1, the first step in identifying a genetic determinant of a complex trait is to demonstrate a genetic effect on the trait, using family-based study designs, including twin studies. Once evidence of significant familial correlation is shown, the proportion of phenotypic variation that is due to genetic effects, the heritability, can be estimated. Segregation analysis can be used to determine whether the pattern of phenotype distribution in families is consistent with a major gene effect and, if so, to assess the mode of inheritance. Linkage studies can then be performed to find chromosomal regions where genetic determinants of pulmonary function may be located. Finally, association studies can be carried out to test the relationship between a specific allele to variation in pulmonary function. The genetic epidemiology of lung function has been recently reviewed.[4]

## Familial aggregation

The demonstration of significant positive familial correlations is not necessarily proof of a genetic influence on the phenotype; familial similarity may result from shared genes, shared environmental exposures, or both. Twin studies can help to distinguish the genetic and environmental effects. If pulmonary function measures are more similar within pairs of monozygotic twins, who share all of their genes, than within pairs of dizygotic twins, who would be expected to share the same childhood environment but only half of their genes, then a genetic influence is likely. A large study of adult male twin pairs showed that the correlation in $FEV_1$ among monozygotic twins was twice that of dizygotic twins; this finding persisted even with adjustment for cigarette smoking.[5] With adjustment for smoking, the heritability of FVC was not significantly greater than zero.

In another large study of twin pairs of both sexes, Redline et al.[6] reported that the intrapair correlations in monozygotic twins for multiple spirometric measures were approximately twice the values in dizygotic twins. Other studies have found the intrapair differences in pulmonary function values to be smaller in monozygotic than in dizygotic twins.[7,8] However, one twin study found no evidence of a heritable effect on lung function.[9]

Webster and colleagues[10] examined maximal expiratory flow at 60 percent of total lung capacity in 45 pairs of monozygotic twins. They found that the intrapair differences were small in twin pairs concordant for cigarette smoking (both smokers or both nonsmokers), but larger in pairs discordant for smoking. This suggests that genetic effects may be involved in the susceptibility to smoking-related airflow obstruction. In a study of 15 pairs of monozygotic twins raised apart, intrapair differences in three pulmonary function measures were small in pairs with the same smoking status, but large in discordant pairs.[11] Because the twins were separated since infancy, the differences in susceptibility to cigarette smoke are likely genetic, and not determined by other shared environmental factors. In a large study of male twins, Tishler and coworkers[12] found a greater correlation in $FEV_1$ among monozygotic twins than among dizygotic twins. The highest correlations were found among twin pairs with similar smoking histories, though discordance in pack-years smoked had little effect on the correlation. This suggests the presence of a gene–environment interaction.

In studies of familial correlation in relatives who are not twins, the contributions of genetic and environmental influences are more difficult to determine. Simple correlations between lung function measures in a parent and a child or in two siblings will reflect both genetic and environmental effects. Various statistical methods have been used to address this issue. Higgins and Keller[13] found the correlation in $FEV_1$ to be greater in sibs of the same sex – who might be expected to share a similar environment – than in parent–child pairs. This study and others have shown the correlations to be greater between parent–child pairs than between spouses.[14,15] The spousal correlation has been used to indicate the contribution of the shared family environment, though assortative mating may also be a factor.

Multiple authors have used regression models to study familial aggregation of pulmonary function. In a cohort in East Boston, Tager and colleagues[14] found that the father's $FEV_1$ (percent predicted) was the strongest predictor of a child's, especially a daughter's, $FEV_1$ (percent predicted) in a model that controlled for father's and child's smoking habits. Just as linear regression is commonly used to calculate predicted values for pulmonary function parameters, regression models can be used to adjust for smoking status and other relevant environmental cofactors. The residual values yielded from these regressions can then be correlated between relatives; this method is also used in segregation analysis, discussed below. Redline and colleagues[16] used residual values in a study of monozygotic and dizygotic twins, as well as their family members. The strength of the correlation decreased as the degree of relatedness decreased. In a study of over 1000 French families, Kauffmann et al.[17] found significant correlations for residual values of $FEV_1$, FVC, and $FEF_{25-75}$. Environmental cofactors and body habitus could not explain the familial correlations. Other studies have found the correlations in spirometric measures to be attenuated[18] or to disappear[19] after adjustment for familial correlations in body habitus.

Most of the subjects in these studies have been Caucasian, but two studies have demonstrated familial correlation in pulmonary function in families of other races. Cotch et al.[20] used a novel regression method to estimate adjusted correlation coefficients for $FEV_1$ in Caucasian and African-American sibships. They concluded that familial aggregation of lung function might be stronger in whites than in African-Americans. Using data from a large genetic epidemiology study in China, Xu and coworkers[21] demonstrated significant correlation of $FEV_1$ and FVC in families ascertained through an asthma index case as well as in randomly sampled families. Generalized estimating equations were used to show that the father's, mother's, and first sibling's pulmonary function were each independently predictive of other siblings' values, even after adjustment for smoking and other cofactors.

Although regression methods can be used to adjust for various environmental effects on an individual's lung function, they require all potentially important environmental factors to be included in the model and accurately measured.

If an important variable is not included, then the estimate of familial correlation can reflect the effects of that shared exposure, as well as shared genes. An additional limitation is that many analyses do not assume the presence of a gene–environment interaction. Other statistical methods have been employed to address these issues and to estimate the heritability of pulmonary function.

## Heritability

Heritability may be overestimated by twin studies, since the environment is likely more similar for monozygotic than dizygotic twins. A unique solution to this problem was employed in a Swedish study of 230 twin pairs, of which 37 monozygotic and 72 dizygotic pairs had been reared apart.[22] Heritability estimates of 67 and 48 percent were found for $FEV_1$ and FVC, respectively.

Large studies of twins reared apart are exceedingly rare, so most investigators have relied on nontwin family studies. Path analysis is a common technique for estimating the heritability of a complex trait in families. In path analysis, the phenotype is modeled as a function of genetic factors and shared and nonshared environmental factors; the regression models have been extended to account for unmeasured or unknown environmental variables. Using the East Boston cohort, Lewitter and colleagues[23] estimated the heritability of $FEV_1$ and $FEF_{25-75}$ to be 41–47 percent. Other path analyses in Caucasian populations have confirmed that between 20–40 percent of the variance in $FEV_1$ is genetic.[24,25] A study of Hispanics in New Mexico also found similar results.[26]

In contrast to path analysis, variance component analysis models the variability about the mean of phenotypes of interest, as opposed to modeling the variables themselves;[27] nonetheless, these statistical methods are quite similar. Using control families from a genetic epidemiology study of obstructive lung disease performed at Johns Hopkins, Astemborski et al.[28] studied residual values for $FEV_1$ and $FEV_1/FVC$ ratio following adjustment for several variables including smoking. Heritability was estimated as 28 percent for residual $FEV_1$ and 24 percent for residual $FEV_1/FVC$. Corresponding heritability estimates of 9 and 25 percent for $FEV_1$ and $FEV_1/FVC$, respectively, were found in an analysis of families in the same study who were ascertained through a proband with COPD.[29] In an analysis of nuclear families participating in the Busselton (Australia) Health Study, the heritability of $FEV_1$ and FVC were both estimated to be close to 40 percent, after adjusting for age, sex, height, and smoking.[30]

The technique of segregation analysis seeks to determine the presence of a genetic effect on a phenotype, and whether that effect is best explained by a major gene or by polygenic inheritance. A series of hierarchical models is tested to find the model that best fits the data. Most of the published studies have failed to find evidence of a major gene influencing $FEV_1$;[31–35] the best fitting models have been consistent with polygenic inheritance and/or shared environmental effects.

In one of these studies, the authors performed separate analyses, with and without adjustment for cigarette smoking.[35] The similarity in results of the two analyses suggests that the familial correlations in current smoking status and pack-years do not account for the familial correlations in $FEV_1$. In contrast, Wilk and colleagues[36] found evidence for a major gene effect on $FEV_1$ in a segregation analysis of participants in the National Heart, Lung, and Blood Institute (NHLBI) Family Heart Study. Residual familial correlation was also consistent with additional polygenic and/or shared environmental effects. In that study, no support for a major gene effect on FVC was found. Other authors did report evidence of a major gene influencing FVC.[37]

Using data from longitudinal studies, several authors have used the rate of decline in $FEV_1$ as an outcome in respiratory genetics studies.[38,39] Kurzius-Spencer et al.[40] have shown that the slope of $FEV_1$ decline is significantly correlated in smoking-concordant sibling pairs, but not in discordant pairs. In a variance component analysis of families participating in the Framingham Heart Study, heritabilities of decline in $FEV_1$ and FVC were estimated to be 5 and 18 percent, respectively.[41] These values were greater in smoking-concordant subjects. The increased familial aggregation in smoking-concordant subjects in both of these studies suggests the effect of gene–environment interaction.

In a population-based study of families in Humboldt, Saskatchewan, Chen and colleagues[42] demonstrated familial aggregation of the maximal expiratory flow rate at 50 percent of vital capacity ($Vmax_{50}$) and $Vmax_{50}/VC$, a measure of airway-parenchymal dysanapsis. The heritability of $Vmax_{50}/VC$ was estimated to be 40 percent. Segregation analysis showed evidence for a major locus influencing dysanapsis.

## Linkage analysis

In genome-wide linkage analysis, a panel of genetic markers at approximately regular intervals across the genome is genotyped in families in order to determine which chromosomal locations co-segregate with the trait of interest. More details on the theory and applications of linkage analysis can be found in Chapter 1. To date, several groups have performed linkage analyses for lung function phenotypes in families from the general population.

Joost et al.[43] studied 1578 members of 330 families in the Framingham Heart Study; 345 were members of the original Framingham cohort, and 1233 were members of the offspring cohort. They estimated the following heritabilities: $FEV_1$ 35 percent, FVC 49 percent, and $FEV_1/FVC$ 26 percent. Based on a 10-cM genome-wide scan of short tandem repeat (STR) markers, multipoint variance component linkage analysis found the strongest evidence for linkage to $FEV_1$ on chromosome 6q (LOD = 2.4); the highest LOD score for $FEV_1/FVC$ co-localized to this region (LOD = 1.4). The next highest LOD score for $FEV_1$ (LOD = 1.6) was found on chromosome 4. The strongest linkage evidence for FVC was found on chromosome 21p (LOD = 2.6).

Subsequently, the same group genotyped three additional microsatellite markers on chromosome 6q.[44] Including these additional markers in a variance component linkage analysis in a subset of the families, the maximum multipoint LOD score for $FEV_1$ was 5.0 at 184.5 cM. LOD scores for both FVC and $FEV_1$/FVC ratio were also found to be greater than 1.0 in this region. Using the family-based association test (FBAT), they found evidence of association for $FEV_1$ and FVC with marker D6S281 at 190 cM.

This group also performed linkage analysis for pulmonary function in 391 pedigrees with 2178 individuals in the National Heart, Lung, and Blood Institute Family Heart Study (FHS).[45] FHS families were ascertained through individuals participating in three existing epidemiological studies, one of which was the Framingham Heart Study, though there were only 12 families with members included in both genome scans. Using variance component linkage analysis, regions with LOD scores above 2.5 were found on chromosomes 4 and 18; additional markers were genotyped in these regions. With the additional markers, the $FEV_1$/FVC ratio had a multipoint LOD score of 3.5 for linkage to chromosome 4 at 28 cM. The highest multipoint LOD scores for $FEV_1$ (2.4 at 31 cM) and FVC (2.9 at 79 cM) were found on chromosome 18.

Malhotra and colleagues performed a linkage analysis using 264 members of 26 families in Utah, which had been collected as part of the Centre d'Etude du Polymorphisme Humain (CEPH) genetic mapping project.[46,47] By using genotype data from the CEPH database (STR and restriction fragment length polymorphisms) as well as genotyping an additional set of 245 STR markers, Malhotra used over 1300 markers at an average spacing of 2.5 cM across the genome. The highest heritability estimate, 67 percent, was found for $FEV_1$/FVC ratio, and segregation analysis was consistent with a major gene effect, though the mode of inheritance could not be determined. Multipoint parametric linkage analysis for $FEV_1$/FVC ratio yielded parametric LOD scores of 2.36 on chromosome 2 (dominant model) and 2.23 on chromosome 5 (recessive). No LOD scores for $FEV_1$ or FVC exceeded 1.5.

Ober and colleagues have studied many complex traits in the Hutterites in South Dakota, an isolated population with a limited number of founders.[48] In a sample of 654 subjects, variance component analysis yielded an estimated heritability for $FEV_1$ (percent predicted) of 35 percent and $FEV_1$/FVC ratio of 41 percent. Because of the inbreeding present in the pedigrees, they were able to perform a genome-wide linkage and association study with a relatively sparse set of STR markers. $FEV_1$ was most strongly associated with a microsatellite marker on chromosome 11 at 43 cM ($P = 0.0017$), and $FEV_1$/FVC with a marker on chromosome 5 at 160 cM ($P = 0.0038$). Neither of these results reached genome-wide significance.

Perhaps the most striking features of these linkage analyses are that the chromosomal regions identified are found on multiple different autosomes. These results are not unique to studies of lung function; poor replication across multiple linkage analyses is common in studies of other complex diseases, as well.[49] Limited sample sizes, genetic and phenotypic heterogeneity, and incomplete penetrance are all possible explanations for this lack of replication.

To date, no genes within these loci or otherwise have been found to be associated with lung function in healthy individuals, and it still remains unclear whether genetic loci that affect lung function in healthy individuals will translate into effects on COPD susceptibility. Lung function phenotypes in adults may reflect the effects of genes acting at three distinct phases of the life cycle: genes involved in fetal lung development, genes important in childhood lung growth, and genes responsible for lung function decline in adulthood, including genes that only exert their effects in the presence of environmental cofactors, primarily cigarette smoke. All three aspects may be important in the development of chronic airflow obstruction later in life. Future research may focus on regions that show evidence of linkage to pulmonary function measures in both healthy and diseased populations. Genes that have been found to be potentially associated with COPD may be studied as determinants of lung function in healthy individuals, though the large sample sizes necessitated by the narrower range of spirometric values in normal subjects may make such studies more challenging.

# CHRONIC OBSTRUCTIVE PULMONARY DISEASE

## Epidemiology and definitions

In the USA, in 2000, approximately 10 million adults reported a physician-diagnosis of COPD;[50] however, the third National Health and Nutrition Examination Survey estimated that 24 million adults have abnormal pulmonary function consistent with COPD, suggesting substantial underdiagnosis.[50] In 2000, COPD was the fourth leading cause of death in the USA, and mortality due to COPD has been increasing over the past two decades.[51] Direct and indirect costs of COPD in the USA were estimated at nearly $24 billion in 1993.[52]

The definition of COPD from the Global Initiative for Chronic Obstructive Lung Disease (GOLD) was presented in the introduction to this chapter. The GOLD criteria highlight the importance of airflow obstruction in the diagnosis of COPD and the relevance of inflammation and environmental exposures to its development.[1] In the GOLD schema, airflow obstruction is measured using spirometry, with an $FEV_1$/FVC ratio less than 0.7 defining airflow obstruction. Post-bronchodilator pulmonary function measures are used in the GOLD criteria, to highlight that the airflow obstruction is not fully reversible. COPD severity is staged by $FEV_1$ (Table 10.1).[1,53] Individuals with symptoms of cough and

**Table 10.1**  *GOLD staging of COPD severity*[1,53]

| GOLD stage | Definition[a] |
|---|---|
| 0, At risk | Normal spirometry<br>Chronic symptoms (cough, sputum) |
| I, Mild | $FEV_1/FVC < 0.7$<br>$FEV_1 \geqslant 80\%$ predicted |
| II, Moderate | $FEV_1/FVC < 0.7$<br>$50\% \leqslant FEV_1 < 80\%$ predicted |
| III, Severe | $FEV_1/FVC < 0.7$<br>$30\% \leqslant FEV_1 < 50\%$ predicted |
| IV, Very severe | $FEV_1/FVC < 0.7$<br>$FEV_1 < 30\%$ predicted |

[a] Uses post-bronchodilator spirometry

sputum production but with normal spirometry are classified as stage 0, signifying a group potentially at risk for the development of COPD. However, whether GOLD stage 0 individuals really are at increased risk of developing COPD remains controversial.[54]

The GOLD definition of COPD also emphasizes the importance of environmental exposures. In developed nations, the most important risk factor for airflow obstruction is cigarette smoking. A dose–response relationship between cigarette smoking and pulmonary function has been convincingly demonstrated, yet significant variability in the individual response to cigarette smoking exists. In a study by Burrows et al.,[55] pack-years of smoking was shown to account for only about 15 percent of the variability in $FEV_1$. This suggests the importance of additional factors in the development of COPD. Occupational exposures, indoor and outdoor air pollution, and respiratory infections are other potential contributing environmental exposures.[1,56] Airway hyperresponsiveness, reduced maximal lung growth, and accelerated decline of pulmonary function – all of which may have genetic influences – are important host factors in the development of airflow obstruction.[1,57,58]

COPD is a heterogeneous disorder and previous definitions have stressed the contributions of emphysema, chronic bronchitis, and small airway disease.[59–61] Although combining these disorders under a single diagnosis may be useful for the clinical identification and management of COPD patients, it may complicate the genetic analysis of COPD. The phenotypes of emphysema, chronic bronchitis, and small airway disease share some similar pathophysiology and likely share some similar genetic determinants; however, there may also be divergent underlying pathways in their development. Combining these phenotypes may reduce the power to uncover specific genetic mechanisms.

## COPD-related phenotypes

The heterogeneity inherent in COPD might be reduced through the use of more detailed phenotypic measurements

for the genetic dissection of COPD. The discussions above and in Chapter 2 highlight the importance of quantitative measurements of pulmonary function in the genetic analysis of COPD and other respiratory diseases. Spirometric measurements have been commonly used, although the $FEV_1$ and $FEV_1/FVC$ cannot distinguish the relative effects of emphysema and airway disease on airflow obstruction. Spirometry performed after the administration of an inhaled bronchodilator may distinguish airflow obstruction that is not completely reversible, the hallmark of COPD.[1]

Other measurements must be used in order to assess the presence and degree of emphysema, chronic bronchitis, and small airway disease. Chronic bronchitis has traditionally been clinically defined by the presence of chronic cough and sputum production for at least 3 months in each of 2 consecutive years, in the absence of other diseases causing a chronic cough.[62] This definition does not require the presence of airflow obstruction, though it is often present in patients with chronic bronchitis.[63]

In contrast to the clinical diagnosis of chronic bronchitis, emphysema has classically been an anatomic diagnosis, characterized by abnormal permanent enlargement of distal airspaces, with associated destruction of alveolar walls.[59] The requirement for lung tissue to classify emphysema has limited the usefulness of this anatomic definition in epidemiological and genetic studies. Noninvasive methods, such as measurement of the DLCO, have been used as a correlate for the extent of emphysema. The measurement of DLCO is technically more challenging than spirometry, leading to substantial variability on repeated testing of the same individual.[64] The technical difficulties, coupled with a reduced sensitivity and specificity for the diagnosis of emphysema, have limited the usefulness of DLCO in genetic investigation.[65] Low sensitivity and specificity, along with high interobserver variation, have similarly limited the use of chest radiography in the diagnosis of emphysema.[66]

Computed tomography (CT) of the chest, specifically the use of thin-slice or high-resolution CT (HRCT) imaging, performs substantially better in the diagnosis of emphysema. Its use has been reviewed in Chapter 2.[66–68] HRCT allows for the qualitative assessment of presence, distribution, and severity of emphysema; such an approach has been used in the evaluation of patients for lung volume reduction surgery.[69,70] Different approaches to the quantitative assessment of emphysema on HRCT have been developed and continue to be refined. Serial CT scan assessments can be used to quantify loss of lung tissue over time, as was done in a randomized trial of alpha 1-antitrypsin augmentation therapy.[71]

Several impediments to the widespread use of HRCT in respiratory genetics must still be addressed, including standardization of imaging protocols across different sites and different models of CT scanners and determination of the most useful set of qualitative and quantitative phenotypes. The relatively high cost of CT imaging, compared to spirometry, for example, is another hurdle to be overcome. Measurement of airway dimensions has proven to be more challenging than assessment of emphysema.[66] The 1–2 mm small airways, the site of critical airflow obstruction in COPD, are smaller than the limits of resolution of the current generation of CT scanners. Further research will be necessary in order to determine how best to visualize and quantify the small airway disease of COPD.

Magnetic resonance imaging (MRI) with hyperpolarized [3]He gas is a novel technique to assess pulmonary ventilation.[72] Visualization of regional ventilation defects may serve as a means to assess small airway disease in COPD.[73] Measurements of [3]He diffusion may allow for identification of early emphysematous changes.[72] The future applications of MRI with hyperpolarized [3]He to the study of respiratory genetics remain to be seen.

Recent work has also addressed the noninvasive assessment of inflammation in COPD. Biomarkers in exhaled breath and in exhaled breath condensate, such as nitric oxide and cytokines, can be measured in order to assess airway inflammation.[74,75] Other exhaled biomarkers, such as carbon monoxide, hydrogen peroxide, and isoprostanes, can be used to measure oxidative stress.[76] The relevance of exhaled biomarkers to respiratory genetics is discussed in Chapter 2. Positron emission tomography may also play a role in the in vivo assessment of neutrophil and macrophage activity in the inflamed COPD airway.[77]

Progression of disease in COPD has traditionally been measured as the decline in FEV$_1$ over time. The classic study by Fletcher et al.[78] demonstrated the rate to be approximately 50 ml/year in smokers, compared to 25 ml/year in nonsmokers. The Six Cities study found the rate of decline in smokers to be 53 ml/year in men and 38 ml/year in women, which were larger than the rates in never-smokers (38 ml/year in men, 29 ml/year in women).[79] Demonstrating significant differences in rate of decline of FEV$_1$, due to different genotypes for example, may require a large study with extended follow-up time. Therefore, investigators have searched for other markers of disease progression.

The hypothesis that elastin breakdown is central to the development and progression of emphysema has led to assays of elastin breakdown products. Desmosine and isodesmosine are amino acids found only in elastin, and the presence of these amino acids in serum or urine is a specific marker of elastin degradation.[80] Stone and colleagues assayed urinary desmosine and isodesmosine in 21 COPD patients, 13 current smokers without airflow obstruction, and 22 never-smokers.[81] They found that the presence of COPD as well as current smoking were both associated with higher levels of elastin breakdown products in the urine. The same group demonstrated an association between urinary desmosine and rapid decline in lung function among 18 male current smokers.[82] Urinary desmosine has also shown to be elevated during acute exacerbations of COPD, implying an increase in lung elastin breakdown.[83] However, elastin breakdown products may also be derived from elastic fiber destruction in blood vessels and cartilage, so measurement of serum or urine desmosine is not specific for emphysema.[84] Measurement of desmosine in sputum is a potential solution,[84] though only preliminary human studies have been performed so far.[85] The ability to visualize directly the progression of emphysema using changes in lung density may make CT scanning a more attractive source of intermediate phenotypes in studies of COPD progression.

## Smoking

One unique feature of COPD as a complex disease is that the major environmental risk factor, tobacco smoking, is known and readily quantifiable. Smoking is often defined as categories, such as current, former, and never smokers, or as total smoking exposure, usually measured in pack-years (average number of packs per day multiplied by the number of years smoked). Although the risk for the development of airflow obstruction increases with increased smoking intensity, many individuals with significant smoking histories do not develop significant airflow obstruction. Active and passive smoking, along with other inhalation exposures such as indoor and outdoor air pollution, lead to cumulative injury in the lung, although the effects of each may vary depending on the intensity, type, and timing of the exposure, as well as individual host factors.

Discussion of all the effects of tobacco smoking is beyond the scope of this chapter; an extensive review of the health effects of smoking has been published.[86] Depending upon when an individual begins to smoke, airway obstruction can be a consequence of reduced lung growth, lower levels of maximally attained lung function, and early or accelerated lung function decline in adulthood. In adolescent smokers, both slowed growth of lung function and mild airway obstruction may contribute to abnormal lung function in adulthood.[87,88] Although the average slowing in lung growth observed is only 1–2 percent in adolescent smokers, large variability between individuals suggests that different susceptibilities (potentially genetic) to the effects of tobacco smoke are relevant during these early years of exposure.

## Other environmental exposures

The role of other environmental exposures – including second-hand (or environmental) tobacco smoke, air pollution, and occupational exposures – is more difficult to quantify. Maternal smoking during pregnancy has been associated with lower lung function in infancy.[89–91] The effect of this exposure is a result of both the intensity and timing of maternal smoking; genetic variants that influence maternal metabolism of tobacco smoke and programming of innate immune responses may be important.

Other exposures, such as air pollution, may act independently to influence the risk of COPD or may augment the effect of cigarette smoke. Similar to studies that have demonstrated differences between mouse strains for susceptibility to tobacco smoke,[92] differences between mouse strains for effects of ozone have also been demonstrated, supporting the fact that genetic susceptibility is also important in responses to other environmental exposures.[93] Among women, particulate air pollution produced by indoor cooking with biomass fuels has been associated with the development of COPD. This is particularly relevant in countries where this exposure is common and cigarette smoking is not.[94–99]

Genetic variation may affect susceptibility to occupational exposures, including dusts and fumes.[100–102] For example, cadmium exposure has been associated with emphysema in exposed workers.[103,104] Cadmium exposure has also been associated with the development of emphysema in rats.[105] Although ingested through vegetable matter, cigarette smoke is a major source of cadmium exposure due to accumulation in the tobacco leaf. In humans, higher blood and urine cadmium levels have been observed in smokers, although the precise role of cadmium in COPD development through tobacco exposure has been debated.[106–108] Urinary cadmium levels have been observed to predict lower lung function in current and former cigarette smokers.[109] Genetic factors likely regulate cadmium concentrations in blood and urine, with one study suggesting at least 10 percent of the variability in cadmium concentrations is due to genetic effects.[110] Variation in cadmium levels may have important implications for oxidative stress in the lung caused by tobacco smoke. The development of COPD in smokers may be influenced by polymorphisms in genes that modify susceptibility to oxidative stress and cadmium metabolism. Cadmium has been demonstrated to induce heme oxygenase,[111,112] and heme oxygenase-1 has been associated with emphysema in Japanese smokers.[113] More research is needed to clarify the genetic, environmental, and gene–environment interactions between cadmium from cigarette smoke and the development of COPD.

Viral exposures may also contribute to COPD susceptibility. Individuals with HIV are at risk for a variety of infectious and noninfectious complications, including emphysema.[114] CD4 and CD8 cells in the lung are decreased in HIV-positive smokers, and the CD4/CD8 ratio is reduced.[115] The development of emphysematous changes on CT is not universal, and the factors that determine who may develop destructive pulmonary parenchymal changes may be due to viral load and CD4/CD8 ratio, as well as underlying genetic susceptibility. HIV also infects alveolar macrophages,[116] so alterations in macrophage scavenger functions may also predispose individuals to emphysema. Although HIV may be directly pathogenic, more research is needed to understand the variable expression of HIV-related pulmonary emphysema; the alteration in CD4/CD8 ratios in HIV-positive individuals may provide insight into the innate and acquired immune responses associated with COPD in HIV-negative smokers.

## ALPHA 1–ANTITRYPSIN DEFICIENCY

### Pathophysiology

Severe alpha 1-antitrypsin deficiency is a proven genetic risk factor for COPD. Alpha 1-antitrypsin (AAT) is a 54 kDa glycoprotein encoded by SERPINA1 on chromosome 14q32. SERPINA1 is part of a serine proteinase inhibitor gene cluster, which includes corticosteroid binding globulin (SERPINA6), protein C inhibitor (SERPINA5), and alpha 1-antichymotrypsin (SERPINA3). SERPINA1 is 12.2 kb long; there are over 100 known genetic variants, with some variants leading to dysfunction and/or deficiency of the AAT protein. Most of the genetic variants do not change the serum protein level or function, but may lead to alterations in the overall molecular charge and isoelectric point, allowing for their characterization. AAT is an inhibitor of many serine proteinases, but its main target is human neutrophil elastase (ELA2). The active site of AAT, a methionine$^{358}$-serine$^{359}$ amino acid sequence, defines the specificity of AAT for neutrophil elastase. When neutrophil elastase binds to this active site it is irreversibly inactivated, and the AAT-neutrophil elastase complex is then cleared from the circulation.

The mode of inheritance of the common disease manifestations (COPD and liver disease) in AAT deficiency is autosomal recessive; the mode of inheritance of the serum AAT levels and serum protease inhibitor (PI) phenotypes is autosomal codominant. AAT variants were initially named on the basis of protein migration velocity using starch-gel electrophoresis, and the protein type observed is referred to as the PI phenotype. Subsequently, isoelectric focusing of serum in polyacrylamide gels has become the standard method to determine PI phenotype (Table 10.2). The use of the term 'phenotype' is technically correct, since the protein pattern that is visualized on the electrophoresis gel represents the observable expression of a genetic trait. The initially discovered AAT variants were named based on electrophoretic migration: M (medium), F (fast), S (slow), or Z (very slow).[117] The presence of null alleles is not detected on serum protein electrophoresis, and individuals with a Z pattern on PI phenotyping are referred to as PI Z to include both PI ZZ and PI Znull variants.

The most common AAT alleles are the M alleles (subtypes M1–M4), with 95 percent frequency in individuals of northern European descent. The M alleles are associated with normal serum AAT protein levels. The S and Z variants also occur in most Caucasian populations, with average allele frequencies of 2 and 1 percent, respectively. The peak prevalence of the PI*Z allele has been observed in Scandinavia, Denmark, the Netherlands, UK, and the northern part of France.[118–124] The worldwide distributions of the different variants have been reviewed elsewhere.[125]

**Table 10.2**  *Alpha 1-antitrypsin phenotype and genotype correlations. Modified from DeMeo and Silverman[534]*

| Alleles inherited | Phenotype (isoelectric focusing) | Serum level (nephelometry) | Molecular genotype (allele specific hybridization) |
|---|---|---|---|
| MM | M | Normal | non-S, non-Z/non-S, non-Z |
| ZZ | Z[a] | Very low | ZZ |
| Znull | Z[a] | Very low | Z/non-S, non-Z |
| MZ | MZ | Intermediate | Z/non-S, non-Z |
| Mnull | M | Intermediate | non-S, non-Z/non-S, non-Z |
| SZ | SZ[b] | Low | SZ |
| MS | MS | Low normal | S/non-S, non-Z |

[a]Appears as PI MZ phenotype on AAT augmentation therapy.
[b]Appears as PI MSZ phenotype on AAT augmentation therapy, although multiple bands make accurate phenotyping difficult.

AAT variants may be classified as normal, deficient, null, or dysfunctional. Normal variants have AAT plasma levels greater than 20 μmol/L or 150 mg/dL; clinical laboratories may use either scale. Deficiency alleles result in lower AAT levels (PI MZ 17–33 μmol/L, PI SS 15–33 μmol/L, PI SZ 8–16 μmol/L, PI ZZ 2.5–7 μmol/L);[126] null variants are associated with no detectable circulating levels of AAT. AAT plasma levels greater than 11 μmol/L (corresponding to approximately 50 mg/dL) are generally considered to be protective against the proteolytic stress of neutrophil elastase.[127]

Homozygotes for the Z allele account for the vast majority of cases of severe AAT deficiency and have protein levels approximately 15 percent of normal. Although gene transcription occurs normally, the point mutation in the Z allele leads to a glutamic acid to lysine amino acid change at position 342. This alteration causes a modest reduction of the protein association binding constant with neutrophil elastase.[128] Increased mobility in the active site leads to polymerization of the protein in the liver, which leads both to low serum protein levels and to an increased risk for cirrhosis.[129]

Null variants can be the result of multiple molecular mechanisms, including deletion of coding exons, premature stop codons, and splicing abnormalities,[130] and result in no detectable AAT in the blood. Some of the null mutations may also result in intracellular accumulation of protein in hepatocytes. For example, QO$_{hongkong}$ results from a 2-bp deletion resulting in both a truncated protein and intracellular accumulation.[131] Other null variants resulting in no detectable protein include QO$_{isola\ di\ procida}$, which is associated with a 17-kb deletion of most of the coding region, and QO$_{granite\ falls}$, in which a 1-bp deletion leads to a frameshift mutation and no detectable mRNA.[132,133] In addition to the null variants, several low expressing alleles have been associated with the development of lung and liver disease. Low expressing alleles generally have electrophoretic features similar to M or S alleles, but have very low serum protein levels. M$_{malton}$ and S$_{iiyama}$ result in intracellular accumulation of protein, whereas M$_{heerlen}$ and M$_{procida}$ are associated with protein degradation.[133–138]

Severe AAT deficiency, found in PI ZZ, PI Znull, and PI null-null individuals, leads to the highest risk of developing COPD, especially in the setting of cigarette smoking. The Z variant of the SERPINA1 gene leads to consistently low serum protein levels, but the development and severity of lung and liver disease varies markedly between individuals. The decline in lung function in both smokers and non-smokers is variable, suggesting the presence of genetic modifiers and gene–environment interactions in the development of COPD in AAT-deficient individuals. Investigation of genetic modifiers in AAT deficiency is currently underway, with the hope of providing insight into the variability of COPD both related and unrelated to AAT deficiency.

PI null homozygotes are rare but have been suggested to have the highest risk for early-onset emphysema.[139,140] The PI phenotype (from electrophoresis) does not distinguish between PI ZZ and PI Znull individuals; in addition, individuals receiving AAT augmentation appear as PI MZ. Molecular genotyping can assist in determining S and Z alleles, but molecular probes for null alleles are not in widespread use. PI MZ and PI Z null individuals will appear to have the same molecular genotype (Table 10.2). In this setting, a very low AAT level would suggest the presence of a null allele, but isoelectric focusing can assist in discriminating between these genotypes.

The initial evaluation of suspected AAT-deficient individuals may begin with an assessment of serum protein levels followed by isoelectric focusing by an experienced laboratory. Martin and colleagues[141] studied 114 pedigrees and observed that the PI locus was the major determinant of AAT serum levels. In families ascertained through a PI Z individual, Silverman and colleagues[142] noted that 72–92 percent of the variation in serum protein level was due to PI type. Although AAT is an acute phase reactant, the PI genotype is clearly the most important genetic determinant of measurable AAT levels in serum.

AAT deficiency can result from abnormalities in gene expression or translation as well as faulty intracellular protein processing. AAT protein may accumulate in the liver or may undergo degradation once released into the serum. The Z form of AAT polymerizes in the endoplasmic reticulum of hepatocytes, and low measured serum levels result from subsequent intracellular accumulation in the liver.[143]

Polymers of Z type AAT have also been detected in bronchoalveolar lavage fluid, suggesting that altered pulmonary defense to neutrophil elastase may be a result of local polymerization as well.[144,145]

Although AAT deficiency is generally regarded to be the defect in PI Z individuals, their AAT protein is dysfunctional as well. Z type AAT, when complexed with neutrophil elastase, is less stable than M type AAT-elastase complexes; elastase can be released from the Z complexes, propagating elastolytic injury. Z type AAT also has a rate of inhibition of neutrophil elastase that is twice as long as M type protein. These observations suggest that Z type protein can be both deficient and dysfunctional.[128,146] Acquired dysfunction and deficiency in the AAT protein in response to oxidative inactivation is also a possible contributor to lung function decline,[147] and variations between individuals for these acquired deficiency states may contribute to the variable susceptibility to cigarette smoke. Some dysfunctional proteins completely lack AAT inhibitory capacity and acquire functions of other serine protease inhibitors. For example, the PI Pittsburgh mutation results in a protein with antithrombin activity.[148] This dysfunctional variant has electrophoretic and antigenic features of AAT, resulting from a single base pair change, causing a methionine to arginine substitution at position 358.[149] The protein lacks all anti-elastase capacity but is a potent inhibitor of plasma kallikrein and activated factor XII,[150] and can lead to a bleeding diathesis.

## Screening and detection of AAT deficiency

Recent guidelines have been published grading the evidence for screening and detection of this genetic cause of COPD.[126] Testing for AAT deficiency may be used for diagnosis, assessment of susceptibility to disease (predispositional testing), carrier status evaluation, and population screening. Clinical presentations that should lead to a high suspicion for AAT deficiency are listed in Table 10.3. The main manifestations of AAT deficiency are pulmonary and hepatic disease. Individuals may be diagnosed with AAT deficiency after the development of disease symptoms or through family screening after the diagnosis of an index case. Among respiratory disorders, the highest grade of support for diagnostic testing is in symptomatic and asymptomatic adults with irreversible airflow obstruction. This includes all adults with COPD, as well as adult asthmatics with chronic airflow obstruction. Predispositional testing has been supported for siblings of individuals diagnosed with AAT deficiency. Presently, there is not adequate evidence to support widespread screening of neonates, adolescents, or adults, but a suggestion to consider screening has been proposed in countries where the prevalence of AAT deficiency exceeds 1/1500, where smoking is prevalent, and where genetic counseling services could be provided.[126]

Identifying an individual with AAT deficiency may result in genetic discrimination or in the psychological burden of

**Table 10.3** *Clinical presentations that may be consistent with AAT deficiency*

| Clinical presentations |
| --- |
| *Emphysema* |
| Early onset (onset age ≤ 45) |
| Without a history of smoking |
| Basilar predominance |
| Family history |
| *Other lung disease* |
| Bronchiectasis of unclear etiology |
| *Liver disease* |
| Cirrhosis of unclear etiology |
| Family history |
| *Other* |
| Necrotizing panniculitis |
| Anti-proteinase 3-positive vasculitis (C-ANCA) |

having a genetic disease. The decision to perform genetic testing should be based upon the clinical scenario and potential benefits of knowing the AAT phenotype. Genetic counseling may assist in decision-making regarding AAT testing. Prenatal screening for the PI ZZ genotype is possible, but it is not routinely recommended.

Evaluation of symptoms or family screening after the diagnosis of an affected relative may lead an individual to be diagnosed with AAT deficiency. Symptomatic individuals generally present with dyspnea, cough, phlegm, and/or wheeze.[151] Reports on the natural history of COPD and lung function decline in PI Z individuals may be biased by the ascertainment of study participants with lung disease; many individuals included in studies of AAT deficiency already had COPD. Silverman and colleagues[152] studied 52 PI Z individuals and noted that 20 out of 30 nonindex individuals (not ascertained on the basis of COPD) had $FEV_1$ values greater than 65 percent predicted. PI Z index cases identified with AAT because of a prior diagnosis of COPD all had low $FEV_1$ values. The variable natural history in the nonindex individuals suggests the presence of disease modifying factors.

Genetic modifiers in AAT deficiency may act through gene–smoking interactions. AAT-deficient individuals who smoke generally develop COPD earlier than nonsmoking deficient individuals.[153–155] The importance of modifying factors is illustrated by the observations that some current (and former) PI Z cigarette smokers maintain normal lung function[152] and that among some nonsmoking PI Z individuals, variability has been observed in pulmonary function and in respiratory symptoms.[156,157] In addition to lung function decline, severe AAT deficiency is associated with the development of early-onset emphysema, out of proportion to the amount of cigarette smoking. Although classically the distribution of emphysema has been described as lower lobe predominant, chest CT scanning has revealed other patterns of distribution of emphysema as well.

## Familial aggregation

Familial aggregation of lung function has been observed in individuals with AAT deficiency. Silverman and colleagues[158] investigated quantitative spirometric phenotypes in 82 PI MZ first-degree relatives of PI Z individuals with and without airflow obstruction. A trend for lower $FEV_1$ was observed in the PI MZ relatives of PI Z individuals with $FEV_1 \leq 65$ percent of predicted when compared with the $FEV_1$ of PI MZ relatives of PI Z individuals with $FEV_1 > 65$ percent of predicted (93 versus 101 percent predicted). $FEV_1$ measures were lower in parents of PI Z individuals in the lower lung function category compared to parents of PI Z individuals with higher lung function (75 versus 95 percent predicted).[158] In addition, segregation analysis on 44 nuclear families with AAT-deficient individuals suggested the presence of additional genetic factors that contribute to the phenotypic manifestations of disease.[159]

Positional cloning is one way to identify relevant modifier genes in a monogenic disorder like AAT deficiency. Linkage studies in AAT deficiency have not yet been reported, but research is underway to identify regions of the genome that may harbor modifier genes. Candidate genes can also be selected on the basis of the known pathophysiology of disease. This approach has not been widely used in AAT deficiency. Six polymorphisms in nitric oxide synthase 3 (NOS3) have been investigated in a case–control study of 55 PI Z individuals with severely reduced $FEV_1$ values and 122 PI Z subjects with less severe airflow obstruction.[160] Two coding region polymorphisms demonstrated association with severe airflow obstruction. These polymorphisms had no functional impact on the protein, which suggests that functional variants may be in nearby genomic regions.

## Heterozygote risk

Heterozygotes with only one M allele often have AAT levels less than PI MM individuals. PI MZ individuals have levels approximately 60 percent normal, PI MS individuals have levels about 80 percent of normal, and PI SZ individuals have levels about 35 percent of normal. Recent reports estimate that there are at least 116 million carriers of deficiency alleles (PI MZ, PI MS) worldwide and 3.4 million carriers of combined deficiency alleles (e.g., PI SZ),[161] so the controversy regarding heterozygote risk may have broad public health implications.

A number of different methodologies have been used to assess the risk of COPD in PI MZ heterozygotes, and the results have been inconsistent. Case–control studies have tended to find a moderate increase in risk.[162–169] In the largest case–control study, Lieberman used isoelectric focusing to determine PI types in 965 patients with severe COPD in California.[167] Eight percent of the cases were PI MZ heterozygotes, significantly more than the 2.9 percent of Caucasian junior high school students used as controls.

Population-based study designs have been used as well. PI phenotyping was conducted in a large community sample in Norway,[170] revealing that the diagnosis of COPD was no more common in PI MZ heterozygotes than in normal PI MM individuals. In a population sample in San Francisco, COPD prevalence was higher in heterozygotes,[171] although the difference was only noticed in smokers. Other investigators have measured lung function and PI types in a community sample. Two large studies of 500 subjects in Rochester, NY and of 2944 subjects in Tucson, AZ have shown no difference in lung function between PI MZ heterozygotes and PI MM individuals.[172,173]

Several recent longitudinal studies have tested whether the rate of lung function decline varies among PI phenotypes. In a population-based cohort of over 9000 adults in the Copenhagen City Heart Study, Dahl and coworkers[174] found a slightly increased rate of decline in $FEV_1$ in PI MZ heterozygotes compared to PI MM individuals (25 mL/year versus 21 mL/year, $P = 0.048$). The difference was more pronounced in nonsmokers. Sandford and colleagues[38] examined PI MZ heterozygotes in the Lung Health Study (LHS) population. The LHS recruited 5887 smokers, aged 35–60 years, with mild airflow obstruction on spirometry; they were followed over 5 years to examine the effects of smoking cessation intervention and ipratropium bromide on decline in lung function.[175] From this cohort, Sandford et al. identified 283 individuals with rapid decline in lung function ($\Delta FEV_1 = -154 \pm 3$ mL/year) and 308 individuals with no decline ($\Delta FEV_1 = +15 \pm 2$ mL/year); these two groups were used as cases and controls, respectively. Using this approach, they found more PI MZ heterozygotes among the rapid decliners than the nondecliners; the association was stronger in the subjects with a family history of COPD.

Silva and coworkers[39] analyzed the relationship between PI phenotype and decline in lung function in a community sample in Tucson. The study included over 2000 randomly sampled white individuals who were followed for an average of 15 years; more than half of the participants were current or former smokers. They found no differences in the rate of decline in $FEV_1$ between the PI phenotypes. In addition, PI MZ heterozygotes were not found to be more common among individuals with a rapid rate of $FEV_1$ decline compared to those with a slow decline, categories similar to those used in the Lung Health Study.

Hersh and colleagues[176] performed a meta-analysis of studies that addressed COPD risk in PI MZ heterozygotes. In 16 studies that defined COPD as a categorical outcome, there was a significantly elevated risk of COPD in PI MZ individuals compared to PI MM individuals (OR = 2.31; 95 percent CI 1.60, 3.35). The finding of an increased odds ratio was especially pronounced in case–control studies. However, there was no difference in mean $FEV_1$ between PI MM and PI MZ individuals in seven studies that reported $FEV_1$ as a continuous measure. These apparently discrepant findings are consistent with a small increase in risk of COPD in all PI MZ heterozygotes or a larger risk in a subset. The risk may be confined to smokers or to heterozygotes who also harbor other genetic polymorphisms.

## Other AAT variants

One of the initial case series concluded that the risk of COPD among PI SZ compound heterozygotes was similar to PI Z subjects.[177] Other uncontrolled studies have suggested that the increased risk in PI SZ individuals is confined to smokers only.[178–181] Some of the case–control and cross-sectional studies have demonstrated an increased risk of COPD[163,170] or rapid decline in $FEV_1$[174] among PI SZ individuals, but the results have not been universal.[167] All of these studies have been limited by small sample sizes, given the relative rarity of the PI SZ genotype. Most authors have not considered the PI MS genotype to be a risk factor for COPD.[38,164,169,173,174,182] However, several studies have suggested otherwise,[165,170,183] possibly warranting further investigation.

A polymorphism 3' to the SERPINA1 gene that leads to the loss of a *Taq*I restriction site has been described. Kalsheker et al.[184] found this polymorphism in 18 percent of 49 patients with emphysema, compared to 5 percent of 101 controls. Another study by this group, as well as a study by Poller et al. have replicated this association.[168,185] However, two other studies have not found the *Taq*I polymorphism to be associated with COPD,[186,187] and the polymorphism did not lead to more rapid decline in lung function in either the Lung Health Study[38] or the Copenhagen City Heart Study.[174]

The mechanism behind a possible effect of the 3' *Taq*I polymorphism on the development of COPD is still unclear, as the variant does not appear to affect serum AAT levels.[184] Morgan and colleagues sequenced the region; the polymorphism is a G to A transition that occurs in a regulatory sequence, possibly affecting an enhancer binding site.[188] In vitro, the 3' mutation leads to a decrease in interleukin-6 induced acute phase AAT expression.[189] However, Sandford and colleagues did not find an association between the 3' polymorphism and a reduced rise in AAT levels as part of the acute phase response to cardiac surgery.[190] They concluded that any increased susceptibility to COPD in carriers of the 3' *Taq*I mutation is not likely the result of a reduced AAT acute phase response. The observed associations between this polymorphism and COPD risk may be due to linkage disequilibrium with other variants in the AAT gene (not the Z or S mutations) or in a neighboring gene, such as alpha 1-antichymotrypsin (SERPINA3).

## Treatment

The treatment of COPD in AAT-deficient individuals is similar to that for COPD not associated with AAT deficiency, except for the consideration of intravenous augmentation therapy in severely AAT-deficient individuals (PI Z, PI null-null). AAT augmentation therapy is a partially purified plasma product that is given as an intravenous infusion, although aerosolized AAT is in development. There are currently three intravenous formulations that have been approved by the US Food and Drug Administration. These medications were approved on the basis of biochemical efficacy (demonstration of an increase in serum levels and bronchoalveolar lavage elastase inhibitory capacity); randomized trials showing reduction in lung function decline have not been reported.

Two observational studies suggested that augmentation therapy reduced the rate of $FEV_1$ decline in AAT-deficient individuals with moderate airflow obstruction.[191,192] In the National Heart Lung and Blood Institute (NHLBI) registry of patients with severe AAT deficiency, 1129 individuals with severe AAT deficiency were followed prospectively for 3.5–5 years, with spirometry every 6–12 months.[191] The overall mortality rate was 19 percent at the end of 5 years; subjects receiving augmentation therapy had a lower mortality rate than those not on therapy (RR 0.64, $P = 0.02$). In an overall analysis of the 927 participants who had at least two $FEV_1$ measurements, there was no difference in $FEV_1$ decline observed between subjects who were and were not receiving augmentation therapy. In a subgroup analysis of individuals with moderate COPD ($FEV_1$ 35–49 percent predicted), $FEV_1$ decline was 27 mL/year slower in those receiving augmentation therapy ($P = 0.03$).[126] Another observational study compared $FEV_1$ decline in 198 German AAT-deficient patients who received weekly AAT augmentation therapy and 97 Danish patients who did not.[192] Similar to the NHLBI study, individuals were included in the $FEV_1$ analysis if they had repeated spirometric measures at least 1 year apart. The investigators observed a slower decline in $FEV_1$ in individuals treated ($\Delta FEV_1 = 53$ mL/year) versus those not treated ($\Delta FEV_1 = 75$ mL/year). Stratification of the analysis by $FEV_1$ revealed that the major effect was in those with moderate COPD ($FEV_1$ 31–65 percent predicted); mortality was not an outcome measure in this study.[192]

One small randomized controlled trial showed a trend for reduction in the progression of chest CT scan assessment of emphysema.[71] This trial included 58 individuals who either received monthly AAT infusion or placebo. Although potentially underpowered to demonstrate a difference in $FEV_1$ decline for the randomized groups, a trend for significance ($P = 0.07$) was observed for attenuation in loss of lung density as measured by high resolution CT scanning of the chest.

Although it remains unclear if augmentation therapy slows the rate of $FEV_1$ decline in all AAT-deficient individuals, observational data do suggest a benefit of treating individuals with airflow obstruction and emphysema. The data from the two observational trials above favor augmentation in those individuals with moderate airflow obstruction. Although biweekly and monthly infusion regimens have been used, the FDA-approved regimen is a weekly infusion of 60 mg/kg. Augmentation therapy has generally been well tolerated with minimal side-effects; as with all blood products, there is a theoretical risk of anaphylaxis in IgA-deficient individuals. Although the processing of these medications appears to destroy HIV and hepatitis viruses, hepatitis B vaccination is recommended, and the possible transmission of undiscovered bloodborne pathogens remains a concern. A review of augmentation therapy has been published.[193]

## AAT animal models

Efforts at engineering a true knockout mouse that recapitulates human AAT deficiency have been challenging. However, lower AAT levels have been measured in C57BL/6J mice and the pallid, tight skin, and beige mice, three naturally occurring mutants on the C57BL/6J background (see Animal models, below).[194] Further understanding of AAT deficiency will likely result from the successful development of the AAT knockout mouse.

## OTHER RARE DISEASES

AAT deficiency is clearly the most common and the most widely studied single gene disorder causing COPD, but it is not the only genetic condition with emphysema or emphysema-like changes as part of its phenotype. These other genetic disorders are rare and account for only a small minority of the disease burden due to COPD. In many of the diseases, emphysema is only a minor contributor to disease morbidity and mortality. Yet these single gene disorders can be helpful in the search for genetic mechanisms involved in COPD. It has been much easier to discern the genes responsible for many of these Mendelian diseases. These genes may have important roles in lung development or in protection from alveolar destruction, as evidenced by emphysema-like phenotypes in diseased individuals. The information gained through study of these rare diseases may contribute to our understanding of COPD genetics and pathogenesis in the vast majority of COPD patients who do not have these monogenic conditions. For example, there may be a risk of COPD in carriers of one copy of a recessive mutation, as has been debated in PI MZ heterozygotes. Other variants in these genes – not necessarily the mutations implicated in the rare disorders – may increase susceptibility to COPD in the general population.

The rare genetic diseases associated with emphysema can be divided into three categories. First are the single gene disorders in which the causative gene has been identified. For the most part, the causal genes encode extracellular matrix proteins; examples include cutis laxa, Ehlers–Danlos syndrome, and Marfan syndrome. The second category contains Down syndrome, a major genetic syndrome with emphysema-like changes as one of its many manifestations. Last are the inherited conditions whose genetic mechanisms, if they exist, remain unknown. These conditions include

familial spontaneous pneumothorax, congenital lobar emphysema, and hypocomplementemic urticarial vasculitis.

## Cutis laxa

Cutis laxa is a heterogeneous clinical syndrome characterized by loose, sagging skin, giving the appearance of premature aging.[195] Histologic examination of skin biopsies reveals fragmented elastic fibers.[195] Autosomal dominant (OMIM (Online Mendelian Inheritance in Man) No. 123700),[196] autosomal recessive type I (No. 219100) and type II (No. 219200), and X-linked (No. 304150) genetic forms of cutis laxa, as well as an acquired form, have all been described.[197] Pulmonary emphysema is a frequently reported manifestation of type I autosomal recessive cutis laxa.[198–201] Cases have presented with emphysema in infancy, with a rapid progression to respiratory failure and death in early childhood.[202]

Two groups independently reported animal models that provided insight into the molecular mechanisms of autosomal recessive cutis laxa.[203, 204] Yanagisawa et al.[203] and Nakamura et al.[204] both described fibulin-5 knock-out mice that displayed a phenotype similar to the human phenotype of loose skin, vascular abnormalities, and pulmonary emphysema. Both groups showed that the fibulin-5-deficient mice had disorganized elastic fibers, pointing to the importance of the fibulin-5 protein for the organization and cross-linking of elastic fibers. In a study of a large Turkish family with four members with autosomal recessive cutis laxa type I, Loeys and colleagues[205] found a homozygous missense mutation (T998C, Ser227Pro) in fibulin-5 (FBLN5) in affected individuals; the mutation was not found in 100 control subjects. Skin histology showed disorganized elastic fibers. These findings, as well as the high conservation of the Serine 227 residue across species and across human fibulins, led the authors to conclude that the T998C mutation was causative in type I autosomal recessive cutis laxa.

In contrast to the autosomal recessive form, respiratory involvement is rare in autosomal dominant cutis laxa. However, Corbett and colleagues[206] described a 51-year-old mother and her 23-year-old daughter, both with early-onset emphysema; the mother required lung transplantation. Both were cigarette smokers and carried the alpha 1-antitrypsin PI MZ genotype. Three different frameshift mutations in elastin (ELN) have been described in three unrelated individuals with autosomal dominant cutis laxa.[207,208] The mutations consist of single base pair deletions in exons 30 and 32 in the coding region of the gene. Markova et al.[209] described a patient with autosomal dominant cutis laxa due to a heterozygous duplication within FBLN5, demonstrating genetic heterogeneity in this disorder. This patient had mild cutaneous and cardiovascular involvement, consistent with the less severe phenotype usually seen in the autosomal dominant type.

Emphysema has also been reported in Menkes disease (OMIM No. 309400), which is usually characterized by growth retardation, neurologic disorders, and kinky hair.[210] Menkes disease is an X-linked disorder of copper metabolism, due to mutations in ATP7A, the gene encoding the alpha subunit of the copper-transporting ATPase, the same gene implicated in X-linked cutis laxa. Abnormalities in collagen metabolism have been found in patients with Menkes disease.[211]

## Ehlers–Danlos syndrome

The Ehlers–Danlos syndromes (EDS) are a group of connective tissue disorders, which include hypermobile joints and extensible, fragile skin. At least 11 separate disorders have been described, classified into six major types.[212] Type IV (OMIM No. 130050), the arterial type, carries significant morbidity and mortality due to the spontaneous rupture of the bowel, the large arteries, or the gravid uterus.[213] Skin is thin, with visible veins and marked bruising. Joint extensibility is often normal. Type IV EDS displays autosomal dominant inheritance and is caused by heterozygosity for one of multiple mutations in COL3A1, the gene encoding type III procollagen.[213] Dowton and colleagues[214] reported a 20-year-old man with EDS type IV who was found to have bilateral cystic lung changes on a chest CT scan which was obtained when he presented with hemoptysis and a right hemopneumothorax. A review of the literature demonstrated six additional EDS type IV patients with cystic or bullous lung disease, and five others presenting with pneumothorax.

## Marfan syndrome and related disorders

Marfan syndrome (OMIM No. 154700) is a heritable connective tissue disorder with variable clinical features including tall stature, long limbs, pectus and spinal deformities, joint laxity, aortic dilation and dissection, ectopia lentis, and dural ectasia.[215] Spontaneous pneumothorax occurs in about 5 percent of Marfan patients; rupture of an apical bleb is the usual mechanism.[215] In a review of 100 Marfan cases from Brompton Hospital, Wood and colleagues[216] documented pneumothorax in 11 patients and emphysematous bullae in five. Emphysematous changes and bullae have been reported by other authors, as early as in infancy.[217–219]

Marfan syndrome displays autosomal dominant inheritance and is caused by mutations in fibrillin-1 (FBN1), an extracellular matrix protein that is a major component of microfibrils.[220] Over 200 mutations have been described, with the majority found in only a single individual or family; up to one-third of cases may be due to spontaneous mutations.[215] Experiments with knock-out mice have shown that fibrillin-1 is predominantly involved in tissue homeostasis and not matrix assembly.[221] The fibrillin-1-deficient mice have abnormal postnatal lung development, leading to airspace enlargement, before the animals die from aortic dissection by postnatal day 10.[222] Dysfunction of transforming

growth factor-β signaling is an important mechanism in disease pathogenesis in these animals.[222]

Homocystinuria (OMIM No. 236200), due to homozygous mutations in cystathione beta-synthase (CBS), shares several clinical features with Marfan syndrome, including ectopia lentis and skeletal abnormalities. Collagen cross-linking has been shown to be disturbed in patients with homocystinuria.[223] Case reports have described spontaneous pneumothorax in individuals with homocystinuria.[224,225]

## Birt–Hogg–Dube syndrome

Birt–Hogg–Dube (BHD) syndrome (OMIM No. 135150) is a rare condition characterized by benign tumors of the hair follicle and by renal cancer. Spontaneous pneumothorax is a common complication.[226–228] Zbar and colleagues[228] described a series of 98 BHD patients and 112 of their unaffected family members. On high-resolution chest CT scan, 83 percent of affected individuals had cystic lung changes. Ten percent of unaffected family members also had lung cysts. Positional cloning has identified mutations in a novel protein, folliculin (FLCN), on chromosome 17p11.2, as the cause of BHD syndrome.[229] The folliculin DNA sequence is highly conserved across species, but its function is unknown.[229]

## Sialuria

Sialuria describes a group of disorders, characterized by the accumulation of free sialic acid. Salla disease (OMIM No. 604369) and infantile sialic acid storage disorder (No. 269920) are autosomal recessive neurodegenerative diseases that present in adulthood and infancy, respectively. Both are due to mutations in the SLC17A5 gene, on chromosome 6q14–15, which encodes a sodium/phosphate cotransporter.[230] Salla disease is also known as Finnish-type sialuria, since most cases are from northeastern Finland. The rapid development of severe emphysema has been reported in a nonsmoking man with Salla disease.[231] The French type of sialuria (OMIM No. 269921) is due to mutations in the gene encoding uridinediphosphate-N-acetylglucosamine 2-epimerase (GNE), the rate-limiting enzyme in sialic acid biosynthesis.[232] French-type sialuria is extremely rare; only six cases have been reported. Pulmonary function testing on a 10-year-old male patient was reported to demonstrate minimal small airway obstruction that was unresponsive to bronchodilators.[233]

## Niemann–Pick disease, type C

Niemann–Pick disease, type C encompasses two genetic subtypes of a phospholipid storage disorder. Niemann–Pick, type C2 (OMIM No. 60725) is a rare autosomal recessive disease, due to mutations in NPC2.[234] Neurodegenerative symptoms are the most frequent manifestation, but pulmonary disease due to massive infiltration of the lung with storage macrophages has been recognized. Elleder and colleagues[235] described a case with emphysema presenting in infancy. Histology revealed storage histiocytes infiltrating the bronchioles as well as the alveoli, leading to emphysema and small airway disease.

## Down syndrome

Down syndrome (OMIM No. 190685) is caused by trisomy 21; the major manifestations include dysmorphic features, mental retardation, congenital heart disease, gastrointestinal abnormalities, and an increased incidence of leukemia. Lungs cysts or blebs have been reported in children with Down syndrome, almost exclusively in patients with congenital heart disease.[236–240] Abnormal lung development leads to a diminished number of alveoli and a reduced alveolar surface area.[241] It is hypothesized that this reduction in alveoli combined with abnormal connective tissue leads to alveolar distention.[240] The cystic lung disease may increase the severity of cardiac disease and adversely affect the postoperative course in patients with Down syndrome.[236,240]

## Familial spontaneous pneumothorax

A spontaneous pneumothorax that occurs in an individual without clinically apparent lung disease is classified as a primary spontaneous pneumothorax.[242] However, a large majority of these patients are found to have subpleural bullous changes at surgery or on chest CT examination.[242] Familial clustering of primary spontaneous pneumothorax has been well described. Various modes of inheritance, including autosomal dominant, autosomal recessive, and X-linked recessive, have been proposed for familial spontaneous pneumothorax (OMIM No. 173600).[243–246] Examining a series of 15 families and reviewing 14 additional families from the literature, Abolnik and colleagues[244] proposed two possible inheritance models. The pedigrees were consistent with either autosomal dominant inheritance with incomplete penetrance, or a combination of X-linked recessive and autosomal dominant with incomplete penetrance. The penetrance is postulated to be lower in females, in order to explain the observed excess of males with this condition.

Spontaneous pneumothorax may occur in several of the diseases described above, including Ehlers–Danlos syndrome and Marfan syndrome. Several additional genetic associations have been proposed, though the data have not been conclusive. In a single pedigree of 23 members, Sharpe et al.[247] found that five out of six affected individuals carried the human leukocyte antigen (HLA) haplotype A2B40; four individuals with that haplotype were not affected, although two were children under 10 years old. Five out of the six affected cases were also found to have PI type M1M2, compared to three unaffected relatives. In a Japanese family, Yamada and coworkers[248] detected the HLA A2B61 haplotype

(which the authors suggest is equivalent to A2B40) in three of four affecteds who were tested, but in only one of four unaffected relatives; an association with the A2B70 haplotype was also suggested. Sugiyama et al.[249] reported two brothers with Marfan-like skeletal abnormalities, who presented with spontaneous pneumothorax. Both were found to have HLA type A2B15Cw3/A11Bw55. Studies in a three-generation Danish family and in two Taiwanese families failed to show an association with alpha 1-antitrypsin deficiency or HLA haplotypes.[250,251] Cardy and colleagues[252] studied haplotypes in fibrillin-1 (FBN1, the cause of Marfan syndrome) in two pedigrees with autosomal dominant spontaneous pneumothorax; genetic variants in FBN1 did not segregate with disease. A recent report identified folliculin (FLCH) mutations in two families with familial spontaneous pneumothorax.[252a]

## Congenital lobar emphysema

Congenital lobar emphysema (OMIM No. 13070) is a congenital malformation characterized by massive hyperinflation of one or more lobes of the lung, with the majority of cases presenting in the first month of life.[253] The most common abnormality is a deficiency of bronchial cartilage, leading to overinflation of the affected lobe.[253] However, true panlobular emphysema has been reported.[254] The molecular defect (or defects) has not been defined. Though most commonly a sporadic disorder, affected siblings have been described.[255,256] A mother and daughter both with congenital emphysema of the right middle lobe have been reported.[257]

## Hypocomplementemic urticarial vasculitis

Hypocomplementemic urticarial vasculitis (HUV) is a rare syndrome, with clinical manifestations similar to systemic lupus erythematosus, including small vessel vasculitis, arthritis, nephritis, and hypocomplementemia.[258] COPD is a frequent manifestation, especially in smokers.[258,259] Emphysema has been documented on pathology and chest CT scans.[258,260] HUV is due to IgG autoantibodies to the collagen-like region of complement C1q; in a series of 12 patients, cross-reactivity with type IV collagen was not found.[258] A case report of HUV in identical twin sisters suggests a genetic influence,[261] yet a specific genetic mechanism has not been identified. No association with HLA type was seen in 11 tested patients.[258]

# COPD AS A COMPLEX DISEASE

Alpha 1-antitrypsin deficiency and the other rare diseases above are instructive in the study of COPD genetics, yet they account for only a small fraction of COPD cases worldwide. Multiple environmental factors, including cigarette smoking, and genetic factors are likely to influence susceptibility

**Table 10.4**   *How genes may influence the susceptibility to develop COPD*

| The influence of genes |
| --- |
| *Development*<br>Influence on the development of the lungs: size of airways, and alveoli |
| *Clearance mechanisms and cilia function*<br>Response to particulate exposures/depositions |
| *Biotransformation pathways*<br>Relevant for the metabolism of toxic exposures (fumes, chemicals, tobacco smoke) |
| *Defense against biochemical stress*<br>Balance of oxidant–antioxidant stress and protease–antiprotease stress |
| *Response to inflammatory stress*<br>Profiles of cytokines and growth factors |
| *Immunological responses*<br>CD4 versus CD8 predominance |

to COPD. Earlier in this chapter, the approach to genetic analysis of lung function in the general population was reviewed, and the strategies used in the search for genetic influences on the development of COPD will follow the same progression. Genes may influence COPD susceptibility through a variety of mechanisms (Table 10.4), and uncovering the effects of specific genes may allow for a deeper understanding of pathways involved in COPD pathophysiology.

## Familial aggregation

A hereditary predisposition to emphysema had been observed in the early nineteenth century,[262] and the topic was revisited in the mid-twentieth century, in several reports that examined members of kindreds with multiple affected members.[263–266] In contrast to the numerous twin studies of lung function measurements, there have been far fewer twin studies of COPD. A large Swedish twin study demonstrated familial susceptibility to 'smoker's cough'.[267,268] There is only a single case report of bullous emphysema in monozygotic twins.[269]

Familial aggregation of chronic bronchitis has been described. In a large population study, Higgins and Keller[13] found that chronic bronchitis was more common among children of parents with chronic bronchitis than in children of parents without respiratory disease. Several studies have used a modification of the case–control design, comparing first-degree relatives of individuals with disease and of individuals without disease. Using this method, Speizer et al.[270] and Tager and colleagues[14,271] demonstrated familial aggregation of chronic bronchitis, using data from an East Boston cohort and from the US National Health Interview Survey. In a matched pair study, Kueppers and colleagues[166] found a higher frequency of COPD in siblings, but not parents, of COPD index cases compared to the siblings

and parents of controls. Larson et al.[272] suggested that the increased prevalence of COPD in first-degree relatives may be due to an excess of disease in female relatives.

In a large study of the genetic epidemiology of COPD conducted at Johns Hopkins, Cohen and coworkers[273–275] demonstrated a familial risk for COPD, not explained by smoking, alpha 1-antitrypsin phenotype, or socioeconomic status. In an additional analysis of this study population, male and female first-degree relatives of COPD cases were shown to have more than double the risk of airflow obstruction than relatives of controls.[276] The risk of chronic bronchitis was two-fold increased in female first-degree relatives, but was over four-fold increased in male relatives. In this cohort, a significant interaction was seen between smoking and family history, with a relative risk of 8.8 for airflow obstruction in heavy smokers (>30 pack-years) with a family history of chronic bronchitis.[277] A study in Sweden using a mailed questionnaire confirmed family history as a risk for self-reported chronic bronchitis and emphysema.[278] The interaction between smoking status (current or exsmokers) and family history was not significant.

In the Boston Early-Onset COPD Study, Silverman and colleagues[279] collected data on families ascertained through a proband with severe, early-onset COPD, based on the hypothesis that severe, early-onset disease is more likely to have genetic influences than later onset disease. Probands had physician-diagnosed COPD with an $FEV_1$ less than 40 percent of predicted, were younger than 53 years old, and did not have severe alpha 1-antitrypsin deficiency. More than 70 percent of the early-onset COPD probands were women, suggesting that gender may influence susceptibility at least in this unique subset of COPD patients. Compared to community controls, first-degree relatives of early-onset COPD probands had significantly increased risks of reduced $FEV_1$ and chronic bronchitis. This was especially prominent in current or exsmoking first-degree relatives, with odds ratios of 4.5 (95 percent CI, 1.8–11.5) for $FEV_1 < 80$ percent predicted and 3.6 (95 percent CI, 1.1–11.5) for chronic bronchitis.[279] Greater bronchodilator responsiveness was also found in current and exsmoking first-degree relatives of COPD probands, compared to current and exsmoking controls.[280] Further analysis has shown that the risk for reduced $FEV_1$ is greater in female first-degree relatives (current and exsmokers) than in male first-degree relatives.[281] First-degree relatives of early-onset COPD probands were also found to have lower values for $FEF_{25–75}$ and $FEF_{25–75}/FVC$.[282] Though this effect was stronger in smokers, it was also present in nonsmokers, suggesting that these measures may be markers of a genetic predisposition to airflow obstruction.

In a study conducted in the UK, McCloskey et al.[283] examined siblings of probands with airflow obstruction and a low gas transfer factor. The probands had severe COPD, defined by age-specific $FEV_1$ thresholds. They found an increased risk of COPD in current or exsmoking siblings of probands compared to matched controls. Nonsmoking siblings had normal spirometry. The probands recruited by McCloskey and colleagues did not show the female predominance that was seen in the Boston Early-Onset COPD Study.[281]

## Heritability

Two studies have calculated heritability of pulmonary function parameters in families ascertained through a proband with COPD. As discussed in the section Pulmonary function in the general population, Beatty et al.[29] used variance component analysis to derive estimates of 9 and 25 percent for the heritability of $FEV_1$ and $FEV_1/FVC$ ratio, respectively.[29] FVC was not significantly heritable.

In the Boston Early-Onset COPD Study, Silverman et al.[284] found significant heritability of $FEV_1$, FVC, and $FEV_1/FVC$ ratio; additive genetic effects explained greater than 30 percent of the variation in each of these measures in early-onset COPD families. Significant heritability has also been demonstrated for $FEF_{25-75}$ ($h^2 = 38$ percent) and $FEF_{25-75}/FVC$ ($h^2 = 45$ percent).[282]

## Linkage analysis

To date, the only published linkage analyses for qualitative and quantitative COPD-related phenotypes have been performed in the Boston Early-Onset COPD Study families.[284,285] Analyzing qualitative COPD-related traits, modest evidence for linkage was found on chromosomes 12 and 19 for moderate-to-severe airflow obstruction (defined as $FEV_1 < 60$ percent predicted with $FEV_1/FVC < 90$ percent predicted), on chromosomes 8 and 19 for mild-to-severe airflow obstruction ($FEV_1 < 80$ percent predicted with $FEV_1/FVC < 90$ percent predicted), and on chromosomes 19 and 22 for chronic bronchitis; restricting the analysis to smokers only increased the strength of the linkage evidence to several genomic regions.

A variance component analysis of quantitative prebronchodilator spirometric measures found more impressive evidence for linkage.[284] Significant evidence for linkage to $FEV_1/FVC$ was found on chromosome 2q (multipoint LOD score = 4.12 at 222 cM); suggestive evidence for linkage to $FEV_1/FVC$ on chromosomes 1 and 17 and to FVC on chromosome 1 was also demonstrated.[286] Additional

markers were genotyped on chromosome 12p, providing suggestive evidence for linkage of $FEV_1$ to this region (LOD = 2.43 at 37 cM).

Postbronchodilator lung function and bronchodilator responsiveness phenotypes were also studied.[287] Significant evidence of linkage for postbronchodilator $FEV_1$ was found on chromosome 8p, with a multipoint LOD score of 3.30 (at 2 cM), which represented a doubling of the LOD score for prebronchodilator $FEV_1$. Significant linkage for postbronchodilator $FEV_1/FVC$ was found on chromosome 2q (LOD score = 4.42 at 222 cM). Regions on chromosomes 3 and 4 showed modest evidence for linkage to measures of bronchodilator responsiveness.

Although lung function measurements in families ascertained through a proband affected with COPD and in families from the general population may not necessarily reflect the same phenotype, there are some common regions identified in these two types of linkage studies (Table 10.5). A region on chromosome 2q has LOD scores greater than two for $FEV_1/FVC$ ratio in the Utah CEPH families and the Boston Early-Onset COPD Study families.[47,284] This and the other regions of overlap may be more likely to harbor genes conferring risk for COPD and related phenotypes. A linkage study for COPD has been performed in the Icelandic families collected by deCODE Genetics, but results have only been published in abstract form.[288] If chromosomal regions identified in this population overlap with the previously identified regions, especially those in the Boston Early-Onset COPD Study families, then this would provide additional support for the presence of COPD-susceptibility genes in these loci.

The variable susceptibility to develop smoking-related lung disease suggests the importance of gene–environment interactions. In the Boston Early-Onset COPD Study, genomewide linkage analysis of $FEV_1$, $FEV_1/FVC$, $FEF_{25-75}$ and $FEF_{25-75}/FVC$ was performed excluding, including, and stratifying by cigarette smoking.[289] Models that demonstrated the highest LOD scores upon stratification by smoking were considered suggestive of a gene–smoking interaction. Focusing on chromosomes that had increased LOD scores in stratified models, chromosomes 2, 12, 16, 20, and 22 were identified as potentially harboring loci that may influence COPD-related traits through gene–environment interactions. This approach has also demonstrated increased evidence for linkage to chromosome 19q for COPD

**Table 10.5**  *Overlapping chromosomal regions in more than one linkage analysis of quantitative measures of pulmonary function.*

| Chromosome | Phenotype | Max LOD score | Location (cM) | Study |
|---|---|---|---|---|
| 1 | $FEV_1/FVC$ | 1.92 | 120 | Silverman[284] |
|   |   | 1.79 | 123 | Wilk[45] |
| 2 | $FEV_1/FVC$ | 4.12 | 222 | Silverman[284] |
|   |   | 2.36 | 216–251[a] | Malhotra[47] |
| 19 | $FEV_1/FVC$ | 1.47 | 61 | Silverman[284] |
|   |   | 1.3 | 78 | Joost[43] |

[a]1-lod support interval

phenotypes.[290] Stratification by tobacco smoking in linkage studies may lead to less heterogeneity of the phenotype of interest and more power to detect COPD susceptibility loci, but replication of these linkage studies is needed.

## COPD association studies

Similar to other complex diseases, the majority of association studies in COPD genetics have used the case–control design. Candidate genes have been identified based on prior knowledge of disease biology (Table 10.4), and polymorphisms in those genes have tested for association with COPD or related phenotypes. Association studies have largely focused on the genes in the following pathways: protease–antiprotease, oxidant–antioxidant and xenobiotic metabolism, atopy and asthma-related genes, inflammatory cytokines, innate immune system, as well as other candidate genes (Table 10.6).

**Table 10.6** *Candidate genes that have been associated with COPD or related phenotypes, with selected references*

**Candidate genes**

*Proteases and antiproteases*
Alpha 1-antitrypsin
    heterozygotes (PI MZ, PI MS, PI SZ)[163,167,170,174]
        3' Taq I polymorphism[184]
Alpha 1-antichymotrypsin[294]
Matrix metalloproteinases-1, 9, 12[309,310]
Tissue inhibitor of metalloproteinase-2[311]

*Antioxidants*
Heme oxygenase-1[113]

*Xenobiotic metabolism*
Microsomal epoxide hydrolase-1[38,320]
Glutathione S-transferases (M1, P1, T1)[317,331,335]
Cytochrome P450 (CYP1A1, CYP2A6)[338,339]

*Inflammatory mediators*
Tumor necrosis factor alpha[345,346]
Interleukin-1 and Interleukin-1 receptor antagonist[355]
Interleukin-11[535]

*Immune response*
Surfactant proteins A, B, D[358]
Human beta defensin-1[363]
Human leukocyte antigen (HLA)[368]
Vitamin D binding protein (Group specific complement)[370,371]

*Asthma-related*
Beta-2 adrenergic receptor[381]
Interleukin-13[385]
Interleukin-10[536]

*Others*
Cystic fibrosis transmembrane conductance regulator[388]
ABO, Lewis blood groups[274,403]
ABH secretor status[406]
Transforming growth factor beta-1[290,413]
Vascular endothelial growth factor[537]
Calcium activated chloride channel-1[538]

See text for additional references

## Proteases and antiproteases

### ALPHA 1-ANTICHYMOTRYPSIN

Alpha 1-antichymotrypsin, encoded by SERPINA3, is another member of the serine protease inhibitor family. It is located on 14q32.1, approximately 220 kb away from the alpha 1-antitrypsin gene (SERPINA1).[291] In 1986, Eriksson et al.[292] described a series of Swedish families with autosomal dominant alpha 1-antichymotrypsin (AACT) deficiency. Probands were ascertained from a liver biopsy series and from general population screening. The condition was rare, with a frequency of 0.7 percent in the screened population. Three of the eight AACT-deficient individuals over age 25 had abnormal spirometry, but there was no consistent obstructive pattern; liver dysfunction was a more common manifestation. Protein levels were reduced in deficient individuals, but electrophoretic properties were similar in normal and deficient individuals. Lindmark and colleagues[293] screened 1872 middle-aged Swedish women, identifying 12 women (0.64 percent) with hereditary AACT deficiency. There was no difference in respiratory symptoms or spirometry between these 12 women and 24 matched controls, but the mean post-bronchodilator residual volume (RV) and RV/TLC ratio were higher in the AACT-deficient subjects, possibly indicating subclinical airway obstruction.

Poller and colleagues[294] identified a sequence variant in a patient with AACT deficiency and chronic lung disease. The proline229alanine mutation, which they later termed Bonn-1, was found in four of 100 COPD cases, but none of 100 healthy controls. The carriers had reduced AACT levels, but normal isoelectric focusing of the protein. The Bonn-1 allele was not found in a screen of 102 Russian COPD patients.[295] Poller et al.[296] also identified a variant associated with an abnormal AACT protein. This leucine55 proline mutation, termed Bochum-1, was observed in three of the 100 COPD cases, but none of the 100 controls. The more common threonine-15alanine signal peptide polymorphism was found in similar frequency in cases and controls. In a North American study, Sandford and colleagues[297] did not find the Pro229Ala variant to be associated with COPD; no subjects had the Leu55Pro allele. Neither the Bonn-1 nor the Bochum-1 variants were seen among 232 Italian individuals, and the frequency of the signal peptide polymorphism was similar in COPD cases and controls.[187] A study in Tokyo found more Thr-15Ala homozygotes among 53 male COPD patients than 65 male current smokers with normal pulmonary function tests (odds ratio = 2.7).[298] The two previously described rare variants were not observed.

### ALPHA 2-MACROGLOBULIN

Alpha 2-macroglobulin (A2M) is a plasma inhibitor of a wide range of proteases and could be protective in the lung. A2M is a large tetrameric protein and may not be transported from the blood to the alveolar space in large amounts; however, synthesis by alveolar macrophages has been demonstrated.[299] A family with autosomal dominant A2M deficiency has been described, but there were no clinical effects.[300] Poller et al. described a 42-year-old man with A2M levels 50 percent of normal who had severe COPD;[301] he also had selective IgG subclass deficiencies. Restriction mapping was consistent with a major gene deletion in this subject, but no differences were found between 39 other COPD cases and 40 controls. The same group sequenced portions of the A2M gene in 30 COPD patients and 30 healthy controls.[302] A common nonsynonymous variant was seen in equal frequencies in both groups. Another variant (Cys972Tyr) was detected in one COPD case and no controls. The serum A2M level was normal in this patient; however, the polymorphism was predicted to affect protein function.

## MATRIX METALLOPROTEINASES

Members of the matrix metalloproteinase (MMP) family are involved in the degradation of connective tissue proteins. Several avenues of investigation have pointed to the importance of MMPs and the tissue inhibitors of metalloproteinases (TIMPs) in the pathogenesis of emphysema, including genetically engineered mouse models.[303–306] Alveolar macrophages from emphysema patients have been found to have increased expression of gelatinase B (MMP9) and interstitial collagenase (MMP1) compared to smokers without emphysema.[307]

An SNP in the MMP9 promoter (C-1562T) has been shown to increase gene expression due to loss of a transcription repressor binding site.[308] In a study of Japanese smokers, 45 with emphysema on CT and 65 without, the MMP9 promoter polymorphism was significantly associated with the diagnosis of emphysema;[309] the odds ratio was 2.7 for carriers of the variant allele. The MMP9 C–1562T polymorphism and an STR in the MMP9 promoter were not more frequent among individuals with a rapid decline in $FEV_1$ in the Lung Health Study population compared to those without a decline in lung function.[310] The MMP1 promoter G-1607GG insertion-deletion was associated with a fast rate of decline ($P = 0.02$). A haplotype consisting of the MMP1 promoter indel and a nonsynonymous SNP in MMP12 (Asn357Ser) showed a stronger association ($P = 0.0007$); an additional polymorphism in MMP12 was not predictive of rapid decline.

Two variants were studied in tissue inhibitor of metalloproteinases-2 (TIMP2) in 88 Japanese COPD patients and 40 smoking controls.[311] The allele frequency of a silent variant in exon 3 was significantly higher in COPD cases ($P < 0.0001$). A variant in the promoter region showed a borderline association ($P = 0.049$).

## Oxidants, antioxidants, and xenobiotic metabolizing enzymes

### HEME OXYGENASE-1

High concentrations of reactive oxygen species (ROS) are found in cigarette smoke; activated neutrophils and macrophages contribute additional free radicals to the smoker's lung.[312] ROS may exert a detrimental effect in the lung through direct epithelial injury, oxidation (and inactivation) of antiproteases, activation of proteases, sequestration of neutrophils, and upregulation of inflammatory genes.[312–314]

Heme oxygenase catalyzes the rate-limiting step in heme degradation. The final products of this pathway – bilirubin, carbon monoxide, and ferritin – all serve as antioxidants.[315] The inducible form of the enzyme, heme oxygenase-1 (HMOX1), has been the subject of the most intensive study. In patients undergoing surgical resections for lung cancer, alveolar macrophages with HMOX1 immunoreactivity were increased in smokers with COPD compared to nonsmokers; no differences were seen between COPD patients and smokers without airflow obstruction.[316]

Yamada et al.[113] genotyped a dinucleotide $(GT)_n$ repeat in the HMOX1 promoter region in 101 Japanese smokers with emphysema and 100 smoker controls. They observed a greater number of long repeats in the emphysema cases (OR = 2.4). In vitro studies revealed that increased size of the $(GT)_n$ repeat might reduce HMOX1 inducibility by ROS, suggesting a functional mechanism for this polymorphism. The promoter repeat was also genotyped in 299 individuals with rapid decline in $FEV_1$ and 322 nondecliners from the Lung Health Study.[317] There was no association between the number of HMOX1 $(GT)_n$ repeats and rate of decline in lung function in this Caucasian population.

### MICROSOMAL EPOXIDE HYDROLASE

Microsomal epoxide hydrolase (EPHX1) is involved in the first-pass metabolism of highly reactive epoxide intermediates, such as those found in cigarette smoke. Polymorphisms in exon 3 (Tyr113His) and exon 4 (His139Arg) have been suggested to decrease (slow allele) or increase (fast allele) enzyme activity, respectively.[318] Haplotypes carrying the exon 3 variant with the wildtype exon 4 allele or the exon 3 wildtype with the exon 4 variant are named slow or fast haplotypes, respectively. Individuals with slow EPHX1 activity may be at increased risk of cigarette smoke induced damage, and those with fast activity may be at a decreased risk, although the latter may also lead to higher production of certain toxic compounds.[319]

Smith and Harrison[320] genotyped the slow and fast polymorphisms in 68 patients with COPD from a respiratory clinic, 94 patients with emphysema confirmed in lung tissue specimens obtained at resection for lung cancer, and 203 blood donor controls. Homozygous slow individuals had increased risks for COPD (OR = 3.5) or emphysema (OR = 5.6). There were more carriers of the fast allele among COPD cases as well. Sandford et al.[38] found a higher frequency of individuals with the homozygous slow haplotype ($His^{113}$–$His^{139}$) among the rapid decliners compared to the nondecliners in the Lung Health Study (OR = 2.4). The effect was stronger in those with a family history of

COPD. The fast haplotype was not associated with rate of lung function decline.

Multiple studies of EPHX1 and COPD risk have been reported in Asian populations, with a predominance of negative results, compared to the two studies above, which were conducted in Europe and North America. In a study of 180 former workers in a Japanese poison gas factory, Yoshikawa and coworkers[321] found no difference in either slow or fast allele EPHX1 frequencies between individuals with and without COPD. However, the slow allele was more frequent in patients with severe COPD ($FEV_1 < 60$ percent predicted) compared to those with mild disease. Two other Japanese studies,[322,323] a Korean study,[324] and a Taiwanese study[325] found no association between either EPHX1 variant and COPD risk. Xiao and colleagues[326] found a higher proportion of slow EPHX1 heterozygotes in COPD patients than controls in a Chinese population (OR = 3.0). Allele frequencies were not different in a smaller study of Chinese COPD patients and smoking controls.[327]

## GLUTATHIONE S-TRANSFERASES (M1, P1, T1)

Enzymes in the glutathione S-transferase (GST) superfamily are important in the detoxification of hydrophobic and electrophilic compounds, including polycyclic aromatic hydrocarbons found in cigarette smoke. Homozygous deletion of the GST M1 gene can be found in 50 percent of individuals in some populations.[328] Several studies have reported an association between the homozygous GST M1 deletion and other smoking-related diseases, including lung and bladder cancer.[329,330] In 168 UK patients undergoing surgery for lung cancer, the frequency of the GST M1 homozygous deletion was significantly higher in those with pathological evidence of emphysema compared to blood donor controls (OR = 1.36); there was no difference in frequency of the homozygous deletion in those with lung cancer only, compared to controls.[331] In a French sample, the GST M1 homozygous deletion genotype was significantly more common among individuals with chronic bronchitis and either severe ($n = 87$) or moderate ($n = 102$) obstructive disease than among 172 controls with a heavy smoking history but no airflow obstruction or chronic bronchitis.[332] A study of 184 COPD cases and 212 controls from Taiwan also confirmed the association.[325]

No associations were seen between homozygous deletions of either GST M1 or GST T1 and the diagnosis of COPD in Korean[324] and Japanese populations.[323] When analyzed individually, deletions of GST M1 or T1 and a polymorphism in GST P1 were not associated with the rate of lung function decline in the Lung Health Study subjects.[317] When a combination of three GST variants was present, there was a borderline association ($P = 0.03$); the authors note that this may represent a type 1 error due to the multiple comparisons performed.

Of the GST gene family, GST P1 has been found to have the highest expression in the lung, localized to the alveoli, alveolar macrophages, and respiratory bronchioles.[333] An exon 5 polymorphism (Ile105Val) in GST P1 has been shown to confer increased activity towards certain substrates.[334] In a study of Japanese men, homozygosity for the wildtype GST P1 allele was found more frequently in COPD patients than in smoking controls (OR = 3.5).[335] This result has not been replicated in multiple studies in Asian populations.[323,325,326,336,337] In the Lung Health Study, the GST P1 polymorphism was associated with the rate of decline in lung function only in those individuals with a family history of COPD.[317]

Other genes involved in xenobiotic metabolism have been tested for association with COPD. Single studies have reported associations with variants in the cytochrome P-450 enzymes CYP1A1[338] and CYP2A6,[339] but not with a variant in the NADPH/NADH oxidase p22-phox subunit (CYBA).[340]

## Immune response and inflammatory mediators

### TUMOR NECROSIS FACTOR ALPHA

Tumor necrosis factor (TNF) alpha is a proinflammatory cytokine which is found in high concentrations in the sputum of COPD patients,[341] with even higher levels found during acute exacerbations.[342] A guanine to adenine polymorphism at position −308 in the promoter region (alleles referred to as TNF*1 and 2) has been described, with increased gene expression in vitro resulting from the variant TNF*2 allele.[343] TNF is located on chromosome 6p, adjacent to lymphotoxin-$\alpha$ (LTA), within the major histocompatibility complex class III region.[344]

Multiple authors have examined the association between TNF and COPD, with conflicting results. Huang and colleagues found a higher frequency of the TNF*2 allele in 42 Taiwanese men – both smokers and nonsmokers – with chronic bronchitis compared to matched controls (OR = 11.1) and compared to a second control group that included a population sample of 99 schoolchildren.[345] In a Japanese population, Sakao and coworkers[346] genotyped the TNF-308 polymorphism in 106 individuals with smoking-related airflow obstruction, 110 smokers/exsmokers with normal pulmonary function, and 129 blood donors; subjects with chronic bronchitis were excluded. The TNF*2 allele frequency was significantly higher in the cases than in either control group. The same authors found a trend towards association between the TNF*2 allele and low attenuation areas on high resolution computed tomography (HRCT) scans of COPD patients.[347]

Other studies in Caucasian[348–352] and Japanese[353] populations have failed to observe an association between the TNF-308 promoter polymorphism and COPD. The polymorphism was not associated with lung function decline in the Lung Health Study.[38] However, one group did find that COPD patients homozygous for the TNF*2 allele had less reversible airflow obstruction and greater mortality over 2 years of follow-up.[349] No associations have been found between a polymorphism in the lymphotoxin-$\alpha$ gene (LTA) and COPD or lung function decline.[38,350,351]

Interleukin-1$\beta$ (IL1B) is another proinflammatory cytokine, with some similar effects to TNF. IL1B has been postulated to be involved in COPD pathogenesis.[354] Joos et al.[355] genotyped polymorphisms in IL1B and in the IL-1 receptor antagonist (IL1RN) in the rapid and nondecliners in the Lung Health Study. Individually, neither variant was associated with rapid decline in lung function, but the haplotype distributions were significantly different between the two groups. These two polymorphisms were not found to be associated with COPD in a Japanese study.[353]

## Innate and adaptive immunity

### SURFACTANT PROTEINS

In addition to their roles in regulating surfactant structure and function, the surfactant proteins, specifically surfactant proteins A (SFTPA) and D (SFTPD), play an important role in innate immune defense in the lung.[356] Surprisingly, a surfactant protein D knockout mouse developed not just lung inflammation, but progressive emphysema with advancing age.[357] This was associated with increased MMP2 and MMP9 activity.

Surfactant protein variants have been tested for association with human COPD. Guo and coworkers[358] genotyped markers in the genes for surfactant proteins A1, A2, B, and D in 97 Mexican COPD patients and in 82 smoker and 99 nonsmoker controls. SNPs in SFTPA1 and SFTPB and an STR linked to SFTPB were all associated with COPD in a logistic regression model.

Mannose binding lectin (MBL2) is another member of the collectin family, structurally related to SFTPA and D, though found primarily in serum.[356] Variants in MBL2 may modify the severity of lung disease in cystic fibrosis (see Chapter 11).[359,360] No association was found between a functional variant in MBL2 and susceptibility to COPD, though it may be associated with increased risk of hospital admission for COPD exacerbations.[361]

### HUMAN BETA-DEFENSIN 1

Members of the $\beta$-defensin family are antimicrobial peptides, widely expressed on mucosal surfaces.[362] Human $\beta$-defensin 1 (DEFB1) is constitutively expressed in the airway. A nonsynonymous coding variant (Val38Ile) was significantly more frequent among 60 Japanese COPD patients than 213 blood donor controls;[363] five other variants in DEFB1 were not associated with COPD.

### IMMUNOGLOBULINS

Individuals with selective IgA deficiency are predisposed to recurrent sinopulmonary infections.[364] A large kindred has been described with concurrent IgA deficiency and early onset COPD.[365] Since IgA deficiency is one of the most common antibody deficiencies, this correlation does not necessarily imply a causal association. Another study found reduced lung function measures in individuals with IgA deficiency who also had concurrent IgG subclass deficiencies compared to those with normal IgG levels.[366] Total IgG levels were lower in COPD patients taking steroids compared to patients not taking steroids; total and IgG subclasses (IgG1, IgG2) were lower in those not taking steroids compared to healthy controls.[367] In a study by Kauffmann and coauthors,[368] immunoglobulin levels did not differ between a group of never-smokers with low $FEV_1$ values and a group of heavy smokers with preserved $FEV_1$.

### HUMAN LEUKOCYTE ANTIGEN LOCUS

Kauffmann et al.[368] also investigated HLA class I genes in the study mentioned above. Frequency of the HLA-B7 type was significantly increased in the never-smokers with low $FEV_1$ compared to the heavy smokers with high $FEV_1$ (OR = 3.8); HLA-Bw16 frequency was decreased in those with low $FEV_1$ (OR = 0.2). Increased frequencies of HLA-A1 and HLA-B17 were seen in 57 Greek patients with chronic bronchitis (only 17 with $FEV_1$ < 80 percent predicted) compared to 250 healthy smokers.[369]

### VITAMIN D BINDING PROTEIN

Vitamin D binding protein, also known as group-specific complement (GC), has three major serum isotypes (1F, 1S, 2), resulting from two separate point mutations in exon 11. It has been considered as a candidate gene for COPD, based on its role in C5a-mediated neutrophil chemotaxis. Early studies analyzed GC protein phenotypes using electrophoresis. In 114 matched pairs of COPD patients and controls, Kueppers et al.[166] found that homozygosity for GC-2 allele was protective against COPD (P = 0.049). Horne and colleagues[370] observed that even a single GC-2 allele was protective, and that homozygous GC-1F individuals were at increased risk of COPD (OR = 7.1). Kauffmann et al.[368] did not find a difference in GC allele frequencies between never-smokers with low $FEV_1$ and heavy smokers with normal $FEV_1$.[368]

More recent reports have determined genotypes at the GC locus in COPD and control populations. By comparing patients referred for lung cancer surgery who did and did not have evidence of airflow obstruction, Schellenberg et al.[371] found GC-2 homozygosity to be protective against COPD. In an in vitro analysis, they found no difference in neutrophil chemotaxis among the different serum isotypes, suggesting that the protective effect of the GC-2 variant relies on a different mechanism. Two analyses in the Lung Health Study population reported that GC isotypes were not associated with either baseline lung function[372] or rate of decline in lung function.[38] Two Japanese studies have found an increased risk of COPD in GC-1F homozygotes compared to healthy controls[373] or to smokers without airflow obstruction.[374] In both studies, the risk due to this genotype was doubled, but neither found an effect of the GC-2 allele. In the latter study by Ito and colleagues, the GC-1F allele was also predictive of a greater decline in $FEV_1$ and more emphysematous change on high resolution CT scan. In a study in Iceland, vitamin D binding protein variants were not associated with the diagnosis of COPD, but the GC-1F allele was overrepresented and the GC-2 allele underrepresented in 48 patients with chronic mucous hypersecretion.[375]

## Genes related to asthma and atopy

### BETA-2 ADRENERGIC RECEPTOR

The Dutch hypothesis proposes a common origin for asthma and COPD; the host factors of airways hyperresponsiveness and atopy are thought to predispose an individual to chronic respiratory symptoms and airflow obstruction.[57] Evidence supporting the Dutch hypothesis has been reviewed elsewhere.[376–378] Genetic variation, particularly in genes central to asthma-related traits, may help to clarify the connection between these diseases. The β2 adrenergic receptor (ADRB2) has two well-described coding variants (Arg16Gly, Gln27Glu) that have been extensively studied in asthma genetics.[379]

In a family study in the Hutterites, a founder population in South Dakota, Summerhill and colleagues[380] genotyped two ADRB2 polymorphisms. Neither was associated with asthma or airway hyperresponsiveness, but individuals homozygous for the Arg16 allele were found to have lower values for $FEV_1$ and FVC (both as a percent of predicted). This result was found only in those over age 12, suggesting that the gene may influence lung growth during adolescence or lung function decline with aging.

Comparing 65 Chinese COPD patients to 41 controls, Ho and coworkers[381] found the homozygous Arg16 genotype to be protective against COPD. The Gln27 variant was associated with COPD severity in this study. In the Lung Health Study population, neither the Arg16Gly nor the Gln27Glu polymorphisms were associated with bronchial hyperresponsiveness, bronchodilator response, or rate of lung function decline.[382]

### INTERLEUKIN-13

Two polymorphisms in interleukin-13 (IL13) have been associated with asthma in prior studies.[383] In the Lung Health Study population, these two polymorphisms (Arg130Gln, C-1112T) were not associated with rate of lung function decline.[384] However, the IL13 promoter polymorphism C-1055T (referred to as C-1112T in the previous reference) was found more frequently in COPD patients compared to smoking controls ($P = 0.01$) and to healthy individuals ($P = 0.002$) in a Dutch study.[385] Polymorphisms in another

asthma candidate gene, the high-affinity immunoglobulin E receptor, β-subunit (MS4A2), were not found to be associated with adult-onset airflow obstruction in another study.[386]

## Other genes

### CYSTIC FIBROSIS TRANSMEMBRANE CONDUCTANCE REGULATOR

Cystic fibrosis (CF) is one of the most common serious autosomal recessive diseases in Caucasians, with an incidence of one in 2000 to one in 4000 live births.[387] Even before the discovery of the cystic fibrosis transmembrane conductance regulator (CFTR) as the gene for CF, investigators had examined the risk of obstructive lung disease and chronic bronchitis in obligate heterozygotes, the parents of children with CF. One of the earliest publications demonstrated a high rate of abnormal pulmonary function among parents,[388] yet others failed to find differences in symptoms or pulmonary function when comparing parents of CF children to control parents.[389–391] Use of the case parent/control parent study design persisted until the cloning of CFTR allowed for more specific investigations, with one of the later studies showing increased symptoms of wheezing in CF heterozygous parents.[392]

Worldwide, the most common CF causing mutation is the deletion of phenylalanine at codon 508 (ΔF508),[387] and this mutation has been the most widely studied for COPD risk in heterozygotes. Most researchers have focused on the phenotype of chronic bronchitis, with some finding a higher than expected frequency of ΔF508 heterozygotes among chronic bronchitis patients[393,394] and others failing to replicate these results.[395] These studies were limited by the lack of a control group. Gervais and colleagues[396] showed a slight increase in frequency of ΔF508 in patients with chronic bronchitis who also had elevated values for sweat chloride. No information on smoking histories was provided, so it is not clear whether these patients have a usual form of COPD or a variant form of CF (e.g., one ΔF508 mutation and one other mutation). Dahl and coworkers identified ΔF508 heterozygotes in the Copenhagen City Heart Study cohort, finding an increased prevalence of asthma[397] as well as lower cross-sectional lung function measurements.[398] However, decline in lung function over time was not greater in carriers, so the connection between the ΔF508 mutation in CFTR and susceptibility to COPD remains unclear. One small study from Greece showed associations between COPD and two non-CF causing variants.[399]

### BLOOD GROUP ANTIGENS

The ABO blood group system is one of the first described genetic markers in humans, and largely because of the well-defined methodology for determining ABO status, it has been studied for association with many complex diseases. In one of the earliest studies, Cohen et al.[274] found blood group A to be a risk factor for COPD. The same investigators also showed that lung function decline over 5 years was greater in blood group A individuals, especially among women.[400] A Polish study showed a trend towards reduced decline in $FEV_1$ in those with blood group A.[401] Other authors have failed to confirm an association between ABO blood group and risk of airflow obstruction or chronic bronchitis.[166,368,402–404]

A plausible biologic link between COPD and antigens on red blood cells (RBC) is not readily apparent. However, the ABH antigens (the H antigen is expressed on blood group O cells) are expressed not just on RBCs, but also secreted into bodily fluids, including saliva and respiratory tract secretions. Approximately 80 percent of Caucasians are ABH secretors.[405] The trait is autosomal dominant, determined by the secretor gene (fucosyltransferase 2; FUT2) on chromosome 19q. In a cohort of over 1000 adults, Cohen and colleagues[406] found that nonsecretors had lower mean values for $FEV_1/FVC$ than secretors. A large occupational cohort in London showed a similar effect on peak expiratory flow rates;[407] the difference was larger among current smokers. Kauffmann and coworkers[368] found more nonsecretors of blood type O among never-smokers with low lung function than among heavy smokers with normal lung function. A cross-sectional study of 228 French coal miners confirmed lower values of $FEV_1$, as well as increased rates of asthma and wheezing, in nonsecretors of blood group O.[408] As is the case with ABO blood group, multiple studies have failed to show an association with ABH secretor status and lung function or COPD.[402–404,409] Other blood group antigens – including Lewis, Rhesus, and MNS – have been associated with COPD or related phenotypes in single studies.[403,404,410]

### TRANSFORMING GROWTH FACTOR BETA-1

Transforming growth factor beta-1 (TGFB1) belongs to a family of cytokine growth factors that are widely expressed in various organ systems.[411] Members of the TGF-β family have been implicated in the pathogenesis of a variety of interstitial, environmental, and obstructive lung diseases.[412] In a study from New Zealand, a coding polymorphism (Leu10Pro) in TGFB1 was significantly less common in 165 COPD patients than in 76 smokers with normal lung function (OR = 0.45, 95 percent CI 0.40, 0.88).[413] TGFB1 is located on chromosome 19q, a region linked to COPD-related traits in the Boston Early-Onset COPD Study.[290] In these families, a SNP in the promoter and two SNPs 3′ to the TGFB1 gene were significantly associated with $FEV_1$. The association with the promoter SNP was confirmed in an analysis comparing COPD cases from the National Emphysema Treatment Trial (NETT) with community controls. An additional promoter SNP and the Leu10Pro coding polymorphism were also significant in the case–control analysis.

## Interpretation of association studies

One theme that is evident in the discussion of candidate gene studies in COPD is that the initial published study often reports a positive association, but subsequent studies are often unable to replicate these associations. This lack of consistency is not unique to the study of COPD; it is a well-described occurrence throughout complex disease genetics.[414,415] As reviewed in Chapter 1, there are many possible explanations. One problem is phenotypic heterogeneity, with the variety of case definitions used in studies of COPD, an inherently heterogeneous disorder. Throughout the COPD genetics literature, different studies have included or excluded cases with various phenotypes, such as chronic bronchitis or bronchodilator responsiveness. If a gene were important in one particular phenotype, such as chronic bronchitis, then this association might be easily missed. Partly due to changes in consensus guidelines over time, different studies have used various parameters (e.g., $FEV_1/FVC < 0.7$ in GOLD) for defining airflow obstruction in COPD, which could also contribute to the inconsistent results. The typical case–control design forces authors to dichotomize a disease status (affected/unaffected), which usually is less powerful than using the full range of values of a quantitative trait, such as $FEV_1$. Many of the reported case–control association studies are limited by small sample sizes. Publication bias, genetic heterogeneity, and population stratification are additional potential contributors to inconsistent replication.

## Animal models

The application of animal models to the study of respiratory genetics has been detailed in Chapter 7. This section will highlight the animal models used to understand the genetic mechanisms of COPD; a topic that has also been reviewed elsewhere.[416,417] The history of animal models for COPD began in the 1960s when Gross and colleagues[418] discovered that intratracheal administration of papain, a plant-derived protease, produced emphysema in rats. Since those initial experiments, numerous proteases and other compounds have been shown to produce emphysema or related phenotypes when delivered to the lungs of experimental animals.[417] These experiments added support to the importance of protease–antiprotease balance in the pathogenesis of emphysema. The protease models are relatively straightforward and have been useful in the study of downstream events, such as tissue response to injury, and have served as a system to test novel therapies for emphysema. However, their applicability to the genetic mechanisms of human COPD has been limited.

Animal models of cigarette smoke induced COPD may have more direct relevance to the study of human disease. Wright and Churg[419] described the first such model in the guinea pig; they showed that exposure to 10 cigarettes per day resulted in progressive emphysema and pulmonary function changes similar to human COPD. More recently, investigators have preferred a murine model for cigarette smoke induced COPD for multiple reasons, including the large body of knowledge regarding mouse biology and the ability to perform genetic manipulations in the mouse.[416]

There are several naturally occurring mouse strains that develop emphysema or airspace enlargement. These models can be seen as analogous to the monogenic human diseases discussed in this chapter. For example, tight skin mice have a mutation in fibrillin-1, a structural protein important in the formation of elastic fibers.[420] Tight-skin mice have AAT levels of about half those of other strains, and have higher levels of neutrophil elastase.[194,421] Tight-skin mice have emphysematous lung lesions that may be observed between 2 and 4 weeks of age. The altered fibrillin protein may be associated with increased proteolytic stress and poor elastic fiber integrity, which together with low AAT levels contribute to emphysema in these mice (and may be a reasonable modifier gene to consider for investigation in human AAT disease). Mutations in human fibrillin-1 cause Marfan syndrome, yet emphysema is an uncommon manifestation of this disorder.

The pallid mutation occurs on a C57 background due to an alteration in the pallidin gene (*Pldn*) on chromosome 2.[422] The pallid phenotype includes a prolonged bleeding time, as well as AAT levels about 60 percent of other C57 mice;[423] the AAT deficiency results from a nonsense mutation at codon 69 of the gene. The overall result of this mutation is an inability to secrete AAT,[423] similar to human AAT deficiency. Pallid mice spontaneously develop emphysematous changes at 8–12 months of life, likely due to deficient AAT activity, increased elastase activity, and decreased lung elastin.[423]

Beige mice have a defect in the formation of lysosomes; their lungs show abnormal airspace enlargement starting in early life.[424] Beige mice may have abnormal levels of serine proteases, including a mild reduction in AAT. The development of emphysema may result from excessive recruitment and activation of neutrophils in the lungs. The beige gene has been identified as the lysosomal trafficking regulator.[425] Defects in the human homologue (CHS1) cause Chediak–Higashi syndrome (OMIM No. 214500), yet emphysema has not been reported in this disorder.

A genetic basis of susceptibility to tobacco smoke is also supported by experiments in multiple strains of mice, in which the development of emphysematous changes in response to cigarette smoke is strain dependent, likely due to differences in inflammatory and cytokine responses to exposure.[92] Further investigation of the genetic and phenotypic differences between susceptible and nonsusceptible strains should provide insight into some of the underlying genetic differences in humans.

Though the naturally occurring genetic variation can yield information regarding the pathways involved in human emphysema, the power of mouse genetics comes from the ability to develop genetically engineered animals. These models make possible the in vivo study of the effects of abnormal protein levels – overexpressed in transgenic mice or absent in 'knock-out' mice – or abnormal protein structure, in the case of targeted mutations. Models have been described that demonstrate abnormal fetal alveolar development. These animals are important to the understanding of human emphysema and have been reviewed in detail elsewhere.[417] Table 10.7 lists genetically engineered mice that either develop air space enlargement after birth or are protected from the development of emphysema when challenged. The insights gained from study of these animals may be more directly relevant to the pathophysiology of human COPD.

Mice with targeted ablation (knock-out) of the surfactant protein D, tissue inhibitor of metalloproteases-3, and the integrin β6 genes all spontaneously develop progressive

**Table 10.7** *Genetically engineered mouse models of emphysema. Adapted from Mahadeva and Shapiro[417]*

| Gene | Comments | Reference |
|---|---|---|
| *Gene knockouts causing emphysema-like changes* | | |
| Tissue inhibitor of metalloproteinases-3 −/− | Reduced amounts of collagen in alveolar insterstitium<br>Increased matrix metalloprotease (MMP) activity | 426 |
| Surfactant protein D −/− | Activated alveolar macrophages<br>Increased MMP activity, oxidant production | 357 |
| Integrin β6 −/− | Increased MMP12 expression<br>Abolished by transgenic TGF-β1 expression or MMP12 knockout | 427 |
| *Gene knockouts protecting against emphysema* | | |
| Macrophage elastase (MMP-12) −/− | Emphysema absent after long-term cigarette smoke exposure | 305 |
| Interleukin 1β type 1 receptor and TNFα type 1 and 2 receptors | Less severe porcine pancreatic elastase-induced emphysema<br>No protection in individual gene knock-out mice | 539 |
| *Transgene overexpression causing emphysema* | | |
| Interleukin-13 | Inducible overexpression in the adult lung<br>MMP- and cathepsin- dependent mechanism | 428 |
| Interferon-γ | Inducible overexpression in the adult lung<br>Increased MMP-9, -12 and cathepsins<br>Decreased secretory leukocyte protease inhibitor | 429 |
| Human interstitial collagenase (MMP-1) | Increased collagen degradation by collagenase(?) | 306 |

emphysema with age.[357,426,427] These animals show increased matrix metalloprotease (MMP) expression or activity. Conversely, mice lacking MMP-12 are protected from development of emphysema in response to chronic cigarette smoke exposure.[305] Evidence from these animal studies points to the importance of proteases, especially MMPs, in the pathogenesis of emphysema.

Evidence from transgenic mice also highlights the role of protease–antiprotease balance in the development of emphysema. Transgenic mice overexpressing the cytokine interleukin-13 (IL13) in the adult lung developed emphysema, mucus metaplasia, and inflammation, a phenotype similar to human COPD.[428] Matrix metalloproteinase- and cathepsin-dependent pathways are important in this model. The same group has also produced transgenic mice that inducibly overexpress interferon-$\gamma$ (IFN-$\gamma$) in the adult lung.[429] These mice also develop emphysema via a MMP- and cathepsin-dependent mechanism. These two cytokines, IL-13 and interferon-$\gamma$, are more widely discussed in the context of Th1 and Th2 balance in the pathogenesis of asthma and other immune diseases, yet they may also play a role in COPD.

The results from genetically engineered mice are crucial to the discovery and definition of pathways that may be important in the development of human emphysema and COPD. When the animal and human evidence is in agreement, this lends great support to the hypothesized importance of a particular gene or pathway. However, the gene alterations in mice leading to emphysema may not necessarily be the same as those responsible for the individual variation in susceptibility to COPD in humans. The large effect of knocking out a gene may not necessarily be comparable to the presumably smaller effects of single nucleotide polymorphisms as they relate to individual disease susceptibility. The use of animal models that provide more focused study of specific genetic variants is discussed in Chapter 7. The lack of concordance between the results of animal experiments and human association studies highlights the necessity of continued research along these complementary avenues.

## Disease management

The cornerstones of management of stable COPD include smoking cessation, symptomatic treatment with bronchodilators, pulmonary rehabilitation, and supplemental oxygen if needed.[1] The use of inhaled corticosteroids is controversial; inhaled steroids do not alter disease course, but may reduce the number of exacerbations.[430] Relatively little progress has been made in the medical treatment of COPD since the landmark Nocturnal Oxygen Therapy Trial (NOTT) and the Medical Research Council study both demonstrated the benefits of supplemental oxygen therapy for hypoxemic patients.[431,432] Tiotropium, a long-acting inhaled anticholinergic bronchodilator, was approved by the US Food and Drug Administration early in 2004; this medication is chemically related to ipratropium, which has been available since the mid-1980s.

One of the goals of study in the field of COPD genetics is to lead to improvements in therapy for COPD patients. Both human and animal genetic studies may elucidate important pathways in COPD pathogenesis, pathways that could be the targets of pharmacological intervention. One possibility includes the replacement of deficient proteins, similar to alpha 1-antitrypsin augmentation therapy. Alternatively, an inhibitor of a destructive protein, such as a metalloprotease, may be administered. New drug developments for COPD are ongoing.[433] Another potential application of human genetics to COPD therapy is in pharmacogenetics. The study of inherited variability in response to treatment is well underway in the field of asthma,[434] but its application in COPD has lagged behind. Although drugs such as bronchodilators and inhaled corticosteroids have not been shown to slow the decline in $FEV_1$ in COPD patients,[175,430] individual responses to these drugs may vary on the basis of genetic factors.

Two surgical approaches to the treatment of COPD have received recent attention. COPD is the most frequent indication for lung transplantation worldwide,[435] although it still remains unclear whether transplantation confers a survival benefit in patients with end-stage COPD.[436,437] On the other hand, the National Emphysema Treatment Trial (NETT) has demonstrated a survival benefit for lung volume reduction surgery (LVRS) in certain subgroups of emphysema patients, those with upper-lobe emphysema and low exercise capacity.[70] The procedure may prove to be cost-effective in reducing disability in other subgroups as well.[438] Studies are ongoing to determine whether these clinically-relevant phenotypes, such as upper-lobe predominant emphysema, have specific genetic determinants. Techniques of pharmacogenetics, though usually used to study genetic variation in response to drugs, may also be applied to determine if genetic differences underlie the highly variable individual response to LVRS.

## Future directions

Gene expression profiling using microarray technology is a promising tool in the identification of genetic risk factors for COPD.[439] This technique has already been used to demonstrate upregulation of antioxidant-related genes in airway epithelial cells of smokers collected via bronchoscopy.[440] Genomic approaches to COPD will require appropriate tissue samples, such as emphysematous lung excised during cancer resections or LVRS. However, this tool has great potential to uncover novel susceptibility genes and pathways involved in COPD pathogenesis.

Great advances have been made in reducing the cost and increasing the availability of various technologies for genetics and genomics, but advances in phenotyping have been much slower to develop. As discussed, most human

COPD genetic studies have relied on spirometry to define COPD and related phenotypes. However, COPD is an inherently heterogeneous disorder, and distinctions between parenchymal and large and small airway disease may be blurred using spirometry. Though there are likely to be common genetic mechanisms for all forms of COPD, especially those due to cigarette smoking, there are also likely to be different genetic mechanisms underlying the different subtypes. Failing to make distinctions between the various disorders encompassed under the diagnosis of COPD may reduce the power to find these genetic associations. High resolution CT scanning is a technology that has the potential to differentiate COPD-related subtypes and should serve an increasingly prominent role in COPD genetic investigations.

Serum or urine biomarkers may also be used for phenotype distinctions in future studies of COPD genetics.[74] Conversely, genetic studies may uncover genes whose products could be analyzed as biomarkers of COPD susceptibility or progression. This would be a welcome addition, since one of the major hindrances to investigations of novel therapies for COPD is the paucity of intermediate phenotypes that can be used to follow disease progression. In contrast to cardiovascular drug trials that can use measures such as blood pressure or serum lipid levels as surrogate markers, studies of COPD therapeutics have typically used decline in $FEV_1$ or mortality as endpoints. To find changes in these outcomes requires a large, long-term, and thus very expensive, trial. The use of other biomarkers of disease may allow for a proliferation of COPD clinical trials.

Included in the goals of genetic investigation of any complex disease are the improvement in care of patients with that disease and the prevention of the disease in susceptible individuals. Genes may influence the susceptibility to develop COPD through a variety of mechanisms (Table 10.4) and advances in COPD genetics may lead to the discovery of genetic or protein markers that may aid in diagnosis or help to determine prognosis, and better disease understanding will likely lead to novel therapies for COPD.

# GENETICS OF NICOTINE DEPENDENCE

## Introduction

Tobacco smoking is a leading cause of mortality in the USA and worldwide. In spite of the well-known adverse effects of smoking, in the year 2000, 46.5 million Americans were current smokers;[441] approximately 70 percent reported a desire to quit smoking. Nicotine is the addictive substance in tobacco and tobacco (nicotine) addiction (OMIM No. 188890) is classified as a disease. Because the major risk factor for chronic obstructive pulmonary disease is tobacco smoke, aspects of tobacco addiction are relevant to understanding genes that may influence the development of COPD. Environmental factors (peer pressures, stress,

influences of advertising) and secular trends are important to smoking initiation, addiction, and dependence. However, not all smokers experience nicotine addiction to the same extent, and individuals are able to desist from smoking at different rates. Variable genetic susceptibility to nicotine addiction may account for why some adolescent smokers become lifetime smokers despite repeated efforts to quit. As a modifiable risk factor for many diseases, understanding the biology that underlies nicotine dependence is essential.

Cigarette smoking is the main activity associated with nicotine addiction. Physiologically, smoking is associated with decreased irritability and increased attention and psychomotor functioning,[442] and it has been observed that individuals smoke to maintain specific nicotine levels.[443] Systemic levels of nicotine are determined by intake and metabolism. When the exposure is stopped or limited, a physical and psychological withdrawal syndrome is experienced, the severity of which varies by individual. Nicotine acts on nicotinic receptors on the surface of dopaminergic neurons in the mesolimbic or 'reward' pathways in the brain, increasing extracellular dopamine. Genetic variations leading to alterations in hepatic enzymes for nicotine metabolism, neuronal receptors, and neurotransmitter metabolizing enzymes could influence nicotine addiction. Studies of candidate genes and drug therapies to treat nicotine addiction have focused on these pathways.

Nicotine addiction and smoking-related behaviors are complex traits. Smoking initiation, smoking persistence, and smoking intensity, as well as the ability to quit and maintain long-term abstinence, probably have different combinations of genetic and environmental influences. Gene–gene and gene–environment interactions are likely to further modify smoking-related phenotypes. As with any complex trait, the challenge of identifying susceptibility genes is contingent upon precise and reproducible phenotypes. Intermediate phenotypes of nicotine addiction have included smoking initiation (captured incompletely by ever smoking variables and age at initiation of smoking), nicotine dependence (defined by number of daily cigarettes smoked), and total exposure to cigarettes (usually measured as pack-years); all of these characteristics have been demonstrated to be associated with nicotine dependence.[444–447] Efforts at codifying definitions have included the Fagerstrom Nicotine Dependence Scale and the DSM-IIIR nicotine dependence criteria.[444] Phenotypic heterogeneity may explain some of the lack of replication in linkage and association studies of nicotine addiction.

## Familial aggregation

Several key behaviors related to smoking have been demonstrated to aggregate within families, and it is likely that this clustering is due to both genetic and environmental factors.[448–452] Familial aggregation of smoking was first noted by Fisher who observed that concordance for smoking behavior was higher in monozygotic versus dizygotic male[453] and female[454] twins. Subsequently, many groups have proceeded to estimate heritability using the twin study approach. Sullivan and colleagues reviewed data from 17 500 twin pairs from 14 studies and calculated weighted heritability estimates of 0.56 for smoking initiation and 0.67 for nicotine dependence.[455] In a study of twins reared apart, it has been estimated that genetic factors explained 60 percent of the variance of smoking behavior.[456]

A comprehensive review of estimates of heritability across twin studies is available.[457] A meta-analysis analyzing the heritability of smoking-related behaviors has been published, suggesting the importance of considering sex-specific heritability estimates for smoking initiation and persistence.[458] For smoking initiation, heritability estimates (mean ± standard error of the mean) were 0.37 ± 0.04 for men and 0.55 ± 0.04 for women; for smoking persistence, heritability estimates of 0.59 ± 0.02 in men and 0.46 ± 0.12 in women were observed. The different heritabilities in the two sexes suggest that genetic and environmental effects on smoking-related traits may contribute differently in men and women.[458]

The data from twin studies support the fact that genetic factors contribute to smoking, but there are several important caveats. First, heritability estimates from twin studies may be inflated due to the potentially increased environmental sharing between monozygotic twins. Second, phenotypic heterogeneity between studies may account for the wide range of reported heritabilities. Last, most studies do not consider the general heritability of addictive tendencies and the potential confounding of heritability estimates for nicotine by genetic contributions from other aspects of addictive behavior (such as cross-addiction with alcohol), which may falsely elevate heritability estimates for nicotine alone.

## Linkage analysis

Linkage studies are valuable for localizing chromosomal regions that may harbor susceptibility genes for nicotine use and addiction. Straub and colleagues[459] conducted a genome scan in 343 individuals from 130 families in Christchurch, New Zealand. In this general population sample, defining nicotine dependence by the Fagerstrom tolerance questionnaire (FTQ), loci on chromosomes 2, 4, 10, 16, 17, and 18 were identified as potential regions of interest, though none of the regions reached genome-wide significance. The maximum LOD score of 2.63 was observed for nicotine dependence on chromosome 2 (at 149 cM). In an independent sample of 264 individuals from 91 families, attempts to replicate these findings failed, with a maximum LOD of 1.60 on chromosome 17 (at 66 cM). The replication sample likely had limited power to detect linkage due to the small sample size.[459]

Several other linkage studies have used data from the Collaborative Study on the Genetics of Alcoholism (COGA) provided as part of the Genetic Analysis Workshop 11 (GAW11).[460,461] Bergen and colleagues performed linkage analysis on sibling pairs for the phenotypes of 'ever smoking' (defined as a lifetime history of smoking daily for at least 1 month and smoking more than 100 cigarettes in a lifetime) and pack-years of cigarettes smoked.[461] For the qualitative phenotype 'ever smoking,' evidence for linkage was observed on chromosomes 6, 9, and 14; evidence for linkage with pack-years was found on chromosomes 3, 5, 17, and 18. Smoking history (defined as the average number of packs of cigarettes smoked per day for 1 year) was also assessed for linkage using 973 individuals across 105 families.[460] The maximum LOD was 3.2 on 5q, with minimal evidence for linkage on 4q, 15q, and 17p.

To investigate whether some of the linkage signal detected for nicotine-related phenotypes may reflect crossover loci for addiction with other substances such as alcohol,[462] an extension of genome scan linkage analyses was performed for smoking and smoking with alcohol dependence in families from the COGA study. A phenotype of 'habitual smoking' was defined as smoking one or more packs of cigarettes a day for 6 or more months. Individuals were ascertained through families with alcohol-dependent members, with an initial analysis in 67 families with 154 sibling pairs, followed by a replication analysis in 79 families with 173 sibling pairs. Loci on chromosomes 5, 9, 11, and 21 had LOD scores greater than 1, with the highest LOD score of 2.2 on chromosome 9 at 103 cM. When analyzed together with the alcoholism phenotypes, chromosomes 1, 2, 11, and 15 demonstrated modest linkage evidence, with the highest LOD score of 3.30 on chromosome 2 at 87 cM, suggesting that this chromosome 2 region may represent a susceptibility locus for combined nicotine and alcohol dependence.

Li and colleagues[463] studied smoking rates in 2583 participants in 313 extended pedigrees from the Framingham Heart Study (FHS) families, as part of GAW13. Significant linkage of smoking rate to chromosome 11 was found, with suggestive linkage on 9, 14, and 17. When the same FHS data were analyzed for 1389 sibling pairs from the 313 pedigrees, there was suggestive linkage of smoking rate to chromosomes 4, 7, and 17. Modest results for a variety of chromosomal regions between the different studies may be a result of phenotypic heterogeneity, epistasis, environmental factors, or the influence of comorbid addictions. Research designed to address these important issues is needed to identify quantitative trait loci for nicotine addiction.

## Candidate gene association studies

Multiple candidate genes for nicotine use and addiction have been investigated.[442,464,465] Genetic factors that contribute to drug metabolism and drug action are likely to influence addiction to drugs of abuse such as nicotine.[466] A major overview of pathways of addiction is beyond the scope of this chapter.[467] Addictive substances such as nicotine lead to positive reinforcement for further use, in part, through increasing dopamine release from the mesocorticolimbic systems of the brain,[468] although the effects of nicotine use are probably more complex.[469] Most of the candidate genes investigated in tobacco addiction have been genes coding for enzymes involved in the metabolism of nicotine or in dopaminergic neural transmission. However, there is evidence that serotonin pathways may be important for persistence of smoking behaviors, as nicotine exposure is associated with increases in brain serotonin and nicotine withdrawal is associated with reduced serotonin.[470,471]

## Nicotine metabolism

Nicotine metabolism rates vary substantially between individuals, suggesting that alterations in nicotine metabolism may be associated with addictive smoking behavior. The hepatic metabolism of nicotine may be increased or decreased by variants of genes encoding cytochrome P450 (CYP) enzymes. In turn, these enzymes may influence nicotine levels and dose–response characteristics of the effects of nicotine.

### CYTOCHROME P450

Cytochrome P450 2A6 (CYP2A6), located on 19q13.2, is the main enzyme involved in nicotine and cotinine metabolism and elimination.[472] It has been hypothesized that polymorphisms resulting in slower nicotine metabolism are associated with a reduced tendency to smoke due to less pleasurable and more adverse experiences with higher nicotine levels. Lower frequencies of slow metabolizing alleles have been observed among tobacco-dependent versus control individuals.[473] Individuals with slow metabolizing alleles smoked fewer cigarettes on a daily basis and were more likely to quit.[474] There is some preliminary data to suggest that inhibition of CYP2A6 alone or with oral nicotine might result in decreased smoking,[475,476] so this metabolic pathway may have some relevance to the pharmacogenetic approaches to treating tobacco dependence. Other groups who have studied CYP2A6 modulation of tobacco intake have been unable to replicate these findings. This has led to the suggestion that nicotine metabolism does not influence smoking behavior,[477,478] and that reduced metabolizing variants of CYP2A6 are not associated with less cigarette consumption among smokers.[479] A recent meta-analysis of 11 studies of CYP2A6 variants did not reveal an association with smoking status or cigarette consumption, but the phenotypes selected for analysis (ever versus never-smoking) may be too broad to allow for the detection of small genetic effects.[478]

Cytochrome P450 2D6 (CYP2D6), located on chromosome 22q13.2, is another enzyme in the cytochrome P450-mediated metabolism of nicotine to cotinine. Genetic variants and gene duplications affect the rate of debrisoquine metabolism. Individuals homozygous for the defective alleles

(CYP2D6*3, CYP2D6*4, or CYP2D6*5) are classified as poor metabolizers.[480] If one or two copies of the functional gene are present (CYP2D6*1 or CYP2D6*2), they are classified as extensive metabolizers, and if more than two copies of the functional gene are present, individuals are categorized as ultrarapid metabolizers.[481] Cholerton and colleagues[482] did not demonstrate a difference in CYP2D6 genotype frequencies between smokers and nonsmokers; however, they did observe that once an individual is already a smoker, CYP2D6 is associated with smoking behavior.[483] In a later study of CYP2D6 and smoking behavior, the odds of being an ultrarapid metabolizer were four-fold increased for heavy smokers compared to nonsmokers, and a trend test revealed an increased use of tobacco in genotypes associated with increased metabolism. The data suggest that variants in metabolic pathways of nicotine metabolism may be important in tobacco addiction, but replication of positive associations is needed.

## Neurotransmitter pathways

Nicotine stimulates the release of dopamine in the brain, and dopamine receptors might be involved in reinforcing behavior through reward pathways in the nucleus accumbens.[484] Variation in genes that code for enzymes involved in dopamine synthesis and metabolism and in genes that code for dopamine receptors and transporters might influence tobacco use and addiction. Further investigation of polymorphisms in this pathway may lead to insight into differential dopamine metabolism, with implications for the treatment of nicotine dependence.

### DOPAMINE RECEPTORS

There are five known dopamine receptor genes, with most research focusing on the dopamine D2 receptor (DRD2) gene, located on chromosome 11q23.2. A decreased number of DRD2 receptors in the brain has been associated with a TaqI restriction fragment polymorphism in the 3′ flanking region of the DRD2 gene.[485] This site has two allelic variants (DRD2*A1 and DRD2*A2); the A1 variant leads to decreased dopamine receptor binding and receptor density in the brain.[486,487] The DRD2*A1 allele has been associated with novelty-seeking behavior and categorized as a 'reward' gene; this has been suggested as a potential pharmacogenetic target.[488] Noble and colleagues[489] reported an elevated odds ratio of being a past (OR = 1.7) or current (OR = 2.2) smoker versus a never-smoker in individuals with the DRD2*A1 allele. Comings and colleagues[490] found a higher prevalence of the DRD2*A1 allele among individuals with higher total daily smoking and among those least successful in quitting; they demonstrated an inverse association between this polymorphism and age of onset of smoking. An association between the DRD2*A1 allele and smoking was demonstrated in individuals with low P300 evoked brain potentials, suggesting that some of the central nervous system effects of nicotine may be due to this genetic variant or a variant in linkage disequilibrium with DRD2*A1.[491,492]

Association of smoking phenotypes with DRD2 variants has not been consistently replicated.[493,494] Likely reasons include population stratification and the small sample sizes in the case–control studies performed to date. Phenotypic heterogeneity, as addressed below, is another important consideration. There have been other small studies of genetic variants in other dopamine receptors demonstrating association with smoking, but these have not been replicated.[495–497]

## DOPAMINE TRANSPORTER

The dopamine transporter is responsible for the reuptake and regulation of dopamine at the synaptic cleft, and this transporter protein is encoded by the solute carrier family 6, member 3 (SLC6A3) gene, located on chromosome 5p15.3. Variable tandem repeats in the 3′ untranslated region have been described, with a nine-repeat allele (SLC6A3-9) associated with dopamine excess.[498] The nine-repeat variant has been associated with a decreased risk of being a smoker; those smokers with the variant were less likely to start smoking before age 16 and had longer periods of sustained smoking cessation, suggesting that the gene may influence smoking initiation and tobacco dependence characteristics.[499] Although another group subsequently replicated the association of the SLC6A3-9 variant with successful smoking cessation, the association with age of smoking initiation was not replicated in a case–control study of former, current, and nonsmokers.[500] One study has observed an association of this variant with onset of smoking,[501] yet other groups have failed to replicate the associations with smoking initiation or cessation.[502,503]

## DOPAMINE SYNTHESIS AND METABOLISM

The synthesis and metabolism of dopamine is mediated through a variety of enzymes including tyrosine hydroxylase (TH, located on chromosome 11p15.5), catechol-O-methyl transferase (COMT, located on 22q11.2), and the monoamine oxidases (MAOA and MAOB, located on Xp11.23). The role of these genes in neurotransmission in relation to smoking has been summarized.[442] Replicated associations in these pathways could potentially lead to useful pharmacogenetic targets.

Tyrosine hyroxylase catalyzes the rate-limiting step in dopamine biosynthesis, and an association between a tetranucleotide repeat in the first intron of the TH gene has been associated with metabolism of dopamine in the brain.[504] Studies of this variant in association with smoking behavior have been pursued in Caucasian and African-American smokers and nonsmokers. No significant difference in allele frequencies was observed between smokers and nonsmokers in the overall cohort or when stratified by race, but there was a suggestion of an association with

lower smoking rate among smokers with the tetranucleotide repeat, suggesting that it might be protective against tobacco dependence.[505] Recently, another group investigated tobacco dependence among a small group of adolescents and concluded that there was a protective effect of this tetranucleotide repeat.[506] Studies investigating variants in MAOB,[507,508] MAOA,[509] and dopamine beta-hydroxylase[509] have demonstrated significant associations, but replication of these small studies is required. To date, the evidence for association of variants in these genes and smoking characteristics has been inconsistent.

## SEROTONERGIC PATHWAYS

The serotonin pathway has been suggested to be important in nicotine addiction and nicotine withdrawal symptoms.[510] Tryptophan hydrolase (TPH1) is the rate-limiting enzyme in the synthesis of serotonin. Two particular polymorphisms of the TPH1 gene have been identified in intron 7 (A218C and A779C).[511] In a population-based study of 780 individuals, Sullivan and colleagues[512] demonstrated an association of these polymorphisms with smoking initiation, but not with age of onset of smoking initiation, or progression to nicotine dependence. In an investigation of 249 smokers and 202 nonsmokers, no association was found with the intron 7 A779C TPH1 alleles and smoking status. However, those individuals with the AA genotype started smoking 1.5 years earlier than those with alternate genotypes.[513]

Other groups have investigated the serotonin transporter gene (SLC6A4, located on chromosome 17q11.1-12), because the transporter protein is important in regulating the duration and magnitude of serotonergic signals in the brain. A 44-bp insertion in the promoter region of the SLC6A4 leads to short/deletion (S) and long/insertion (L) alleles. The S variant has been associated with decreased transcription and decreased serotonergic expression and uptake.[514] Although one study found no association with cigarette smoking in Caucasians and African Americans,[515] another group has demonstrated an association of the L variant with smoking in Japanese men;[516] the L allele frequency was higher in smokers (37 percent) than nonsmokers (24 percent). An association has been described for the serotonin receptor 2A gene (5HT2A, chromosome 13q14-21) T102C polymorphism with maintenance but not initiation of smoking.[517]

Many of the candidate gene associations for tobacco dependence have failed to replicate, and many of the significant studies have examined only a single SNP in a candidate gene. Recently, SNPs in the nicotine acetylcholine receptor alpha4 subunit gene (CHRNA4) have been associated with protection against nicotine addiction in a family-based study of 901 individuals from 22 nuclear families.[518] This association study was extended to include a family-based haplotype analysis, demonstrating that the common GCTATA haplotype of the CHRNA4 gene was protective against nicotine addiction. Replication of associations and extension to include haplotype analyses are important next steps in identifying candidate genes for nicotine addiction.

## Pharmacogenetics

The neurotransmitter pathways of nicotine addiction have direct relevance to pharmacogenetic approaches to smoking cessation.[519] Identification of susceptibility genes may allow for targeted prevention and treatment of nicotine dependence and withdrawal. The major barrier to quitting smoking is nicotine addiction. Only about 20 percent of individuals respond to smoking cessation treatments with long-term abstinence,[520] suggesting that variability in the intensity of nicotine addiction may correlate with treatment efficacy. Pharmacotherapy and behavioral counseling are both effective approaches to managing nicotine addiction and smoking cessation.[520] Nicotine replacement products (gum, patch, lozenge, inhaler, or nasal spray) provide an alternative source of nicotine to the addicted individual allowing some smokers to quit successfully. Resulting from the understanding of the nicotine metabolism pathways, small studies of inhibitors of CYP2A6 enzyme have been demonstrated to reduce smoking intensity.[476] In the future, individuals in trials of nicotine replacement may be stratified by genetic variants that may predict response to nicotine replacement or enzyme inhibition.

Bupropion is an antidepressant that is an FDA-approved therapy for smoking cessation. Bupropion binds to the dopamine transporter protein and inhibits the reuptake of dopamine at the neuronal synaptic cleft. Based on this mechanism, potential candidate genes for smoking behaviors are the genes in the dopamine pathway that may influence the action of bupropion (SLC6A3, DRD2, DRD4, TH, COMT, MAOA, and MAOB).[521] The dopamine-enhancing aspects of bupropion decrease nicotine cravings, and the noradrenergic effects mitigate withdrawal symptoms.[521,522] Bupropion is metabolized by the cytochrome P450 2B6 enzyme (CYP2B6),[523] and polymorphisms in CYP2B6 have been associated with increased withdrawal symptoms and recidivism.[524] One group has observed a significant epistatic effect between DRD2 and SLC6A3 with abstinence time and time to relapse at the end of a drug trial (bupropion versus placebo) in both treatment groups; genotypic variants may predict smoking relapse regardless of treatment.[525]

Opioid receptors are novel targets for study in nicotine addiction. In a trial of 320 smokers, Lerman and colleagues[526] investigated the mu-opioid receptor (OPRM1) Asn40Asp variant and the efficacy of different forms of nicotine replacement therapy (transdermal versus nasal spray). They observed that smokers with an Asp40 variant ($n = 82$) were more likely to be abstinent from smoking at the end of the treatment trial, compared to individuals homozygous for the Asn40 variant ($n = 238$). This effect was most prominent in the subgroup of participants who received transdermal nicotine, which provided a constant level of nicotine.

## Future directions

Progress in understanding the genetic aspects of tobacco addiction must involve a multidisciplinary approach. For example, Sullivan and colleagues have integrated genome scan linkage analysis with data from microarray and candidate gene studies to identify potential pathways that might be involved in nicotine dependence.[527–529] So far, the mitogen-activated protein kinase system (MAPK), nuclear factor kappa B complex (NFKB), neuropeptide Y (NPY) signaling, the vesicular monoamine transporter (SLC18A2), a nicotinic receptor subunit (CHRNA2), and the mu-opioid receptor (OPRM1) have been identified for further study based on this integrated approach.[530]

As in other complex diseases, better phenotypes are necessary for linkage and association studies of nicotine addiction. Although there is likely correlation between the smoking-related traits, varying phenotype definitions limit comparability across studies. Differences in nicotine exposures (variability in cigarette nicotine content as well as nicotine metabolism) may be important confounders in these studies. The coexistence of smoking with other addictive behaviors may also confound linkage and association results. Imaging the brain may provide reproducible phenotypes for the study of nicotine addiction. Functional magnetic resonance imaging and positron emission tomography may assist in identifying relevant candidate genes and pathways involved in addiction.[531,532]

The ultimate goal of nicotine addiction research is to provide targeted interventions to individuals based upon their genetic susceptibilities. This approach requires knowledge of drug activities and dose–response characteristics (pharmacokinetics), as well as individual genetic differences that determine drug efficacy (pharmacogenetics). Smokers may be classified by their genetic predisposition to addiction and their genetic susceptibility to treatment drugs. For example, individuals with polymorphisms in dopamine pathways may smoke due to the pleasurable sensation mediated through reward pathways. Others may smoke and maintain addiction due to avoidance of withdrawal symptoms potentially mediated through noradrenergic pathways. Smokers in different categories may require treatments tailored to these unique features of addiction.[464]

Progress in identifying genetic loci that determine nicotine addiction will require multidisciplinary studies using reproducible phenotypes. Longitudinal family-based investigations are critical to dissect genetic and environmental aspects of tobacco initiation and dependence.[533] Integrated approaches to the study of nicotine addiction include studying genetic, behavioral, and pharmacological aspects of nicotine addiction along with the social, cultural, and psychological influences on cigarette smoking, as well as the complex interactions between all of these features.[533] Over the life span, the genetic and environmental influences on tobacco use are likely to vary.[449] The goal is to identify individual genetic risk profiles for prevention and treatment of nicotine addiction through the study of gene effects and gene–gene and gene–environment interactions.

## Key learning points

- Cigarette smoking is the major environmental risk factor for COPD; however, COPD is a complex disease with additional environmental and genetic factors influencing susceptibility.

- Alpha 1-antitrypsin (AAT) deficiency is a Mendelian disorder and the primary known genetic cause of emphysema. However, the severity of lung disease in AAT-deficient individuals is likely modified by other genetic and environmental factors.

- Familial aggregation of pulmonary function measures in both healthy individuals and COPD patients has been demonstrated. Linkage analysis has identified genomic regions that influence these traits.

- Many genes have been found to be associated with COPD, though many of these findings have not been replicated in subsequent studies. Better phenotypes that capture relevant features of COPD subtypes will be necessary in future research.

- Novel methods using animal models and gene expression analysis may be useful to uncover COPD susceptibility genes.

- Progress has been made in elucidating the genetic basis of tobacco addiction, a relevant disorder to respiratory medicine. These studies may also provide useful insight for the study of COPD genetics.

## ACKNOWLEDGEMENTS

Supported by US National Institutes of Health grants HL71393, HL075478, HL68926, T32 HL07427, and K08 HL072918, and by an American Lung Association Career Investigator Award.

## REFERENCES

✳1  Pauwels RA, Buist AS, Calverley PM et al. Global strategy for the diagnosis, management, and prevention of chronic obstructive pulmonary disease. NHLBI/WHO Global Initiative for Chronic Obstructive Lung Disease (GOLD) Workshop summary. *Am J Respir Crit Care Med* 2001; **163**: 1256–76.

●2  Crapo RO, Morris AH, Gardner RM. Reference spirometric values using techniques and equipment that meet ATS recommendations. *Am Rev Respir Dis* 1981; **123**: 659–64.

3  Hankinson JL, Odencrantz JR, Fedan KB. Spirometric reference values from a sample of the general US population. *Am J Respir Crit Care Med* 1999; **159**: 179–87.

◆4  Chen Y. Genetics and pulmonary medicine. 10: Genetic epidemiology of pulmonary function. *Thorax* 1999; **54**: 818–24.

5  Hubert HB, Fabsitz RR, Feinleib M, Gwinn C. Genetic and environmental influences on pulmonary function in adult twins. *Am Rev Respir Dis* 1982; **125**: 409–15.

6  Redline S, Tishler PV, Lewitter FI et al. Assessment of genetic and nongenetic influences on pulmonary function. A twin study. *Am Rev Respir Dis* 1987; **135**: 217–22.

7  Man SF, Zamel N. Genetic influence on normal variability of maximum expiratory flow-volume curves. *J Appl Physiol* 1976; **41**: 874–7.

8  Kawakami Y, Shida A, Yamamoto H, Yoshikawa T. Pattern of genetic influence on pulmonary function. *Chest* 1985; **87**: 507–11.

9  Ghio AJ, Crapo RO, Elliott CG et al. Heritability estimates of pulmonary function. *Chest* 1989; **96**: 743–6.

10  Webster PM, Lorimer EG, Man SF et al. Pulmonary function in identical twins: comparison of nonsmokers and smokers. *Am Rev Respir Dis* 1979; **119**: 223–8.

11  Hankins D, Drage C, Zamel N, Kronenberg R. Pulmonary function in identical twins raised apart. *Am Rev Respir Dis* 1982; **125**: 119–21.

12  Tishler PV, Carey VJ, Reed T, Fabsitz RR. The role of genotype in determining the effects of cigarette smoking on pulmonary function. *Genet Epidemiol* 2002; **22**: 272–82.

13  Higgins M, Keller J. Familial occurrence of chronic respiratory disease and familial resemblance in ventilatory capacity. *J Chronic Dis* 1975; **28**: 239–51.

14  Tager IB, Rosner B, Tishler PV et al. Household aggregation of pulmonary function and chronic bronchitis. *Am Rev Respir Dis* 1976; **114**: 485–92.

15  Perusse L, Leblanc C, Tremblay A et al. Familial aggregation in physical fitness, coronary heart disease risk factors, and pulmonary function measurements. *Prev Med* 1987; **16**: 607–15.

16  Redline S, Tishler PV, Rosner B et al. Genotypic and phenotypic similarities in pulmonary function among family members of adult monozygotic and dizygotic twins. *Am J Epidemiol* 1989; **129**: 827–36.

17  Kauffmann F, Tager IB, Munoz A, Speizer FE. Familial factors related to lung function in children aged 6–10 years. Results from the PAARC epidemiologic study. *Am J Epidemiol* 1989; **129**: 1289–99.

18  Schilling RS, Letai AD, Hui SL et al. Lung function, respiratory disease, and smoking in families. *Am J Epidemiol* 1977; **106**: 274–83.

19  Lebowitz MD, Knudson RJ, Burrows B. Family aggregation of pulmonary function measurements. *Am Rev Respir Dis* 1984; **129**: 8–11.

20  Cotch MF, Beaty TH, Munoz A, Cohen BH. Estimating familial aggregation while adjusting for covariates. Application to pulmonary function data from black and white sibships. *Ann Epidemiol* 1992; **2**: 317–24.

21  Xu X, Yang J, Chen C et al. Familial aggregation of pulmonary function in a rural Chinese community. *Am J Respir Crit Care Med* 1999; **160**: 1928–33.

22  McClearn GE, Svartengren M, Pedersen NL et al. Genetic and environmental influences on pulmonary function in aging Swedish twins. *J Gerontol* 1994; **49**: 264–8.

23  Lewitter FI, Tager IB, McGue M et al. Genetic and environmental determinants of level of pulmonary function. *Am J Epidemiol* 1984; **120**: 518–30.

24 Devor EJ, Crawford MH. Family resemblance for normal pulmonary function. *Ann Hum Biol* 1984; **11**: 439–48.

25 Cotch MF, Beaty TH, Cohen BH. Path analysis of familial resemblance of pulmonary function and cigarette smoking. *Am Rev Respir Dis* 1990; **142**: 1337–43.

26 Coultas DB, Hanis CL, Howard CA et al. Heritability of ventilatory function in smoking and nonsmoking New Mexico Hispanics. *Am Rev Respir Dis* 1991; **144**: 770–5.

27 Province MA. Linkage and association with structural relationships. In: Rao DC, Province MA (eds) *Genetic dissection of complex traits*. Boston: Academic Press, 2001: 183–90.

28 Astemborski JA, Beaty TH, Cohen BH. Variance components analysis of forced expiration in families. *Am J Med Genet* 1985; **21**: 741–53.

29 Beaty TH, Liang KY, Seerey S, Cohen BH. Robust inference for variance components models in families ascertained through probands: II. Analysis of spirometric measures. *Genet Epidemiol* 1987; **4**: 211–21.

30 Palmer LJ, Knuiman MW, Divitini ML et al. Familial aggregation and heritability of adult lung function: results from the Busselton Health Study. *Eur Respir J* 2001; **17**: 696–702.

31 Rybicki BA, Beaty TH, Cohen BH. Major genetic mechanisms in pulmonary function. *J Clin Epidemiol* 1990; **43**: 667–75.

32 Chen Y, Horne SL, Rennie DC, Dosman JA. Segregation analysis of two lung function indices in a random sample of young families: the Humboldt Family Study. *Genet Epidemiol* 1996; **13**: 35–47.

33 Givelber RJ, Couropmitree NN, Gottlieb DJ et al. Segregation analysis of pulmonary function among families in the Framingham Study. *Am J Respir Crit Care Med* 1998; **157**: 1445–51.

34 Holberg CJ, Morgan WJ, Wright AL, Martinez FD. Differences in familial segregation of FEV1 between asthmatic and nonasthmatic families. Role of a maternal component. *Am J Respir Crit Care Med* 1998; **158**: 162–9.

35 Kurzius-Spencer M, Holberg CJ, Martinez FD, Sherrill DL. Familial correlation and segregation analysis of forced expiratory volume in one second (FEV1), with and without smoking adjustments, in a Tucson population. *Ann Hum Biol* 2001; **28**: 222–34.

36 Wilk JB, Djousse L, Arnett DK et al. Evidence for major genes influencing pulmonary function in the NHLBI family heart study. *Genet Epidemiol* 2000; **19**: 81–94.

37 Chen Y, Rennie DC, Lockinger LA, Dosman JA. Major genetic effect on forced vital capacity: the Humboldt Family Study. *Genet Epidemiol* 1997; **14**: 63–76.

●38 Sandford AJ, Chagani T, Weir TD et al. Susceptibility genes for rapid decline of lung function in the Lung Health Study. *Am J Respir Crit Care Med* 2001; **163**: 469–73.

39 Silva GE, Sherrill DL, Guerra S, Barbee RA. A longitudinal study of alpha 1-antitrypsin phenotypes and decline in FEV1 in a community population. *Chest* 2003; **123**: 1435–40.

40 Kurzius-Spencer M, Sherrill DL, Holberg CJ et al. Familial correlation in the decline of forced expiratory volume in one second. *Am J Respir Crit Care Med* 2001; **164**: 1261–5.

41 Gottlieb DJ, Wilk JB, Harmon M et al. Heritability of longitudinal change in lung function. The Framingham study. *Am J Respir Crit Care Med* 2001; **164**: 1655–9.

42 Chen Y, Dosman JA, Rennie DC, Lockinger LA. Major genetic effects on airway-parenchymal dysanapsis of the lung: the Humboldt family study. *Genet Epidemiol* 1999; **16**: 95–110.

●43 Joost O, Wilk JB, Cupples LA et al. Genetic loci influencing lung function: a genome-wide scan in the Framingham Study. *Am J Respir Crit Care Med* 2002; **165**: 795–9.

44 Wilk JB, DeStefano AL, Joost O et al. Linkage and association with pulmonary function measures on chromosome 6q27 in the Framingham Heart Study. *Hum Mol Genet* 2003; **12**: 2745–51.

45 Wilk JB, DeStefano AL, Arnett DK et al. A genome-wide scan of pulmonary function measures in the National Heart, Lung, and Blood Institute Family Heart Study. *Am J Respir Crit Care Med* 2003; **167**: 1528–33.

46 Dausset J, Cann H, Cohen D et al. Centre d'etude du polymorphisme humain (CEPH): collaborative genetic mapping of the human genome. *Genomics* 1990; **6**: 575–7.

47 Malhotra A, Peiffer AP, Ryujin DT et al. Further evidence for the role of genes on chromosome 2 and chromosome 5 in the inheritance of pulmonary function. *Am J Respir Crit Care Med* 2003; **168**: 556–61.

48 Mathias RA, Freidhoff LR, Blumenthal MN et al. Genome-wide linkage analyses of total serum IgE using variance components analysis in asthmatic families. *Genet Epidemiol* 2001; **20**: 340–55.

49 Altmuller J, Palmer LJ, Fischer G et al. Genomewide scans of complex human diseases: true linkage is hard to find. *Am J Hum Genet* 2001; **69**: 936–50.

50 Mannino DM, Homa DM, Akinbami LJ et al. Chronic obstructive pulmonary disease surveillance – United States, 1971–2000. *MMWR Surveill Summ* 2002; **51**: 1–16.

51 *Morbidity and mortality: 2002 chart book on cardiovascular, lung, and blood diseases*. Bethesda, MD: National Institutes of Health: National Heart, Lung, and Blood Institute, 2002.

52 Sullivan SD, Ramsey SD, Lee TA. The economic burden of COPD. *Chest* 2000; **117**: 5S–9S.

✳53 Fabbri LM, Hurd SS. Global strategy for the diagnosis, management and prevention of COPD: 2003 update. *Eur Respir J* 2003; **22**: 1–2.

54 Vestbo J, Lange P. Can GOLD Stage 0 provide information of prognostic value in chronic obstructive pulmonary disease? *Am J Respir Crit Care Med* 2002; **166**: 329–32.

●55 Burrows B, Knudson RJ, Cline MG, Lebowitz MD. Quantitative relationships between cigarette smoking and ventilatory function. *Am Rev Respir Dis* 1977; **115**: 195–205.

◆56 Silverman EK, Speizer FE. Risk factors for the development of chronic obstructive pulmonary disease. *Med Clin North Am* 1996; **80**: 501–22.

57 Orie NGM, Sluiter HJ, DeVries K et al. The host factor in bronchitis. In: Orie NGM, Sluiter HJ (eds). *Bronchitis*. Assen: Royal von Gorcum, 1961.

58 Tager IB, Segal MR, Speizer FE, Weiss ST. The natural history of forced expiratory volumes. Effect of cigarette smoking and respiratory symptoms. *Am Rev Respir Dis* 1988; **138**: 837–49.

✳59 Standards for the diagnosis and care of patients with chronic obstructive pulmonary disease. American Thoracic Society. *Am J Respir Crit Care Med* 1995; **152**: S77–121.

✳60 Siafakas NM, Vermeire P, Pride NB et al. Optimal assessment and management of chronic obstructive pulmonary disease (COPD). The European Respiratory Society Task Force. *Eur Respir J* 1995; **8**: 1398–420.

✳61 BTS guidelines for the management of chronic obstructive pulmonary disease. The COPD Guidelines Group of the Standards of Care Committee of the BTS. *Thorax* 1997; **52** (Suppl. 5): S1–28.

62   Chronic bronchitis, asthma and pulmonary emphysema. A statement by the Committee on Diagnostic Standards for Nontuberculous Respiratory Diseases. *Am Rev Respir Dis* 1962; **85**: 762.

63   Vestbo J, Prescott E, Lange P. Association of chronic mucus hypersecretion with FEV1 decline and chronic obstructive pulmonary disease morbidity. Copenhagen City Heart Study Group. *Am J Respir Crit Care Med* 1996; **153**: 1530–5.

64   American Thoracic Society. Single-breath carbon monoxide diffusing capacity (transfer factor). Recommendations for a standard technique – 1995 update. *Am J Respir Crit Care Med* 1995; **152**: 2185–98.

65   Morrison NJ, Abboud RT, Ramadan F et al. Comparison of single breath carbon monoxide diffusing capacity and pressure-volume curves in detecting emphysema. *Am Rev Respir Dis* 1989; **139**: 1179–87.

◆66   Muller NL, Coxson H. Chronic obstructive pulmonary disease. 4: imaging the lungs in patients with chronic obstructive pulmonary disease. *Thorax* 2002; **57**: 982–5.

67   Madani A, Keyzer C, Gevenois PA. Quantitative computed tomography assessment of lung structure and function in pulmonary emphysema. *Eur Respir J* 2001; **18**: 720–30.

68   Newell JD Jr. CT of emphysema. *Radiol Clin North Am* 2002; **40**: 31–42.

69   Rationale and design of the National Emphysema Treatment Trial: a prospective randomized trial of lung volume reduction surgery. The National Emphysema Treatment Trial Research Group. *Chest* 1999; **116**: 1750–61.

●70   Fishman A, Martinez F, Naunheim K et al. A randomized trial comparing lung-volume-reduction surgery with medical therapy for severe emphysema. *New Engl J Med* 2003; **348**: 2059–73.

●71   Dirksen A, Dijkman JH, Madsen F et al. A randomized clinical trial of alpha 1-antitrypsin augmentation therapy. *Am J Respir Crit Care Med* 1999; **160**: 1468–72.

72   Kauczor HU, Chen XJ, van Beek EJ, Schreiber WG. Pulmonary ventilation imaged by magnetic resonance: at the doorstep of clinical application. *Eur Respir J* 2001; **17**: 1008–23.

73   de Lange EE, Mugler JP 3rd, Brookeman JR et al. Lung air spaces: MR imaging evaluation with hyperpolarized 3He gas. *Radiology* 1999; **210**: 851–7.

74   van Beurden WJ, Dekhuijzen PN, Smeenk FW. Exhaled biomarkers in COPD: their potential role in diagnosis, treatment and prognosis. *Monaldi Arch Chest Dis* 2002; **57**: 258–67.

75   Garey KW, Neuhauser MM, Robbins RA et al. Markers of inflammation in exhaled breath condensate of young healthy smokers. *Chest* 2004; **125**: 22–6.

76   Paredi P, Kharitonov SA, Barnes PJ. Analysis of expired air for oxidation products. *Am J Respir Crit Care Med* 2002; **166**: S31–7.

77   Jones HA, Marino PS, Shakur BH, Morrell NW. In vivo assessment of lung inflammatory cell activity in patients with COPD and asthma. *Eur Respir J* 2003; **21**: 567–73.

●78   Fletcher CM, Peto R, Tinker CM, Speizer FE. *The natural history of chronic bronchitis and emphysema.* Oxford: Oxford University Press, 1976.

79   Xu X, Dockery DW, Ware JH et al. Effects of cigarette smoking on rate of loss of pulmonary function in adults: a longitudinal assessment. *Am Rev Respir Dis* 1992; **146**: 1345–8.

80   Stone PJ, Bryan-Rhadfi J, Lucey EC et al. Measurement of urinary desmosine by isotope dilution and high performance liquid chromatography. Correlation between elastase-induced air-space enlargement in the hamster and elevation of urinary desmosine. *Am Rev Respir Dis* 1991; **144**: 284–90.

81   Stone PJ, Gottlieb DJ, O'Connor GT et al. Elastin and collagen degradation products in urine of smokers with and without chronic obstructive pulmonary disease. *Am J Respir Crit Care Med* 1995; **151**: 952–9.

82   Gottlieb DJ, Stone PJ, Sparrow D et al. Urinary desmosine excretion in smokers with and without rapid decline of lung function: the Normative Aging Study. *Am J Respir Crit Care Med* 1996; **154**: 1290–5.

83   Fiorenza D, Viglio S, Lupi A et al. Urinary desmosine excretion in acute exacerbations of COPD: a preliminary report. *Respir Med* 2002; **96**: 110–4.

84   Cantor JO, Shteyngart B. How a test for elastic fiber breakdown products in sputum could speed development of a treatment for pulmonary emphysema. *Med Sci Monit* 2004; **10**: RA1–4.

85   Ma S, Lieberman S, Turino GM, Lin YY. The detection and quantitation of free desmosine and isodesmosine in human urine and their peptide-bound forms in sputum. *Proc Natl Acad Sci USA* 2003; **100**: 12941–3.

◆86   US Department of Health and Human Services. *The health consequences of smoking: a report of the surgeon general.* Atlanta, GA: US Department of Health and Human Services, Centers for Disease Control and Prevention, National Center for Chronic Disease Prevention and Health Promotion, Office on Smoking and Health, 2004.

87   Gold DR, Wang X, Wypij D et al. Effects of cigarette smoking on lung function in adolescent boys and girls. *New Engl J Med* 1996; **335**: 931–7.

88   Sherrill DL, Lebowitz MD, Knudson RJ, Burrows B. Smoking and symptom effects on the curves of lung function growth and decline. *Am Rev Respir Dis* 1991; **144**: 17–22.

89   Stick SM, Burton PR, Gurrin L et al. Effects of maternal smoking during pregnancy and a family history of asthma on respiratory function in newborn infants. *Lancet* 1996; **348**: 1060–4.

90   Lodrup Carlsen KC, Jaakkola JJ, Nafstad P, Carlsen KH. In utero exposure to cigarette smoking influences lung function at birth. *Eur Respir J* 1997; **10**: 1774–9.

91   Hoo AF, Henschen M, Dezateux C et al. Respiratory function among preterm infants whose mothers smoked during pregnancy. *Am J Respir Crit Care Med* 1998; **158**: 700–5.

92   Guerassimov A, Hoshino Y, Takubo Y et al. The development of emphysema in cigarette smoke-exposed mice is strain dependent. *Am J Respir Crit Care Med* 2004; **170**: 974–80.

93   Savov JD, Whitehead GS, Wang J et al. Ozone-induced acute pulmonary injury in inbred mouse strains. *Am J Respir Cell Mol Biol* 2004; **31**: 69–77.

94   Kiraz K, Kart L, Demir R et al. Chronic pulmonary disease in rural women exposed to biomass fumes. *Clin Invest Med* 2003; **26**: 243–8.

95   Amoli K. Bronchopulmonary disease in Iranian housewives chronically exposed to indoor smoke. *Eur Respir J* 1998; **11**: 659–63.

96   Perez-Padilla R, Regalado J, Vedal S et al. Exposure to biomass smoke and chronic airway disease in Mexican women. A case-control study. *Am J Respir Crit Care Med* 1996; **154**: 701–6.

97   Dennis RJ, Maldonado D, Norman S et al. Woodsmoke exposure and risk for obstructive airways disease among women. *Chest* 1996; **109**: 115–9.

98   Dossing M, Khan J, al-Rabiah F. Risk factors for chronic obstructive lung disease in Saudi Arabia. *Respir Med* 1994; **88**: 519–22.

99   Behera D, Jindal SK. Respiratory symptoms in Indian women using domestic cooking fuels. *Chest* 1991; **100**: 385–8.

100  Samet JM, Marbury MC, Spengler JD. Health effects and sources of indoor air pollution. Part I. *Am Rev Respir Dis* 1987; **136**: 1486–508.

101  Samet JM, Marbury MC, Spengler JD. Respiratory effects of indoor air pollution. *J Allergy Clin Immunol* 1987; **79**: 685–700.

102  Heppleston AG. Prevalence and pathogenesis of pneumoconiosis in coal workers. *Environ Health Perspect* 1988; **78**: 159–70.

103  Armstrong BG, Kazantzis G. The mortality of cadmium workers. *Lancet* 1983; **1**: 1425–7.

104  Davison AG, Fayers PM, Taylor AJ et al. Cadmium fume inhalation and emphysema. *Lancet* 1988; **1**: 663–7.

105  Snider GL, Hayes JA, Korthy AL, Lewis GP. Centrilobular emphysema experimentally induced by cadmium chloride aerosol. *Am Rev Respir Dis* 1973; **108**: 40–8.

106  Paschal DC, Burt V, Caudill SP et al. Exposure of the US population aged 6 years and older to cadmium: 1988–1994. *Arch Environ Contam Toxicol* 2000; **38**: 377–83.

107  Elinder CG, Friberg L, Lind B, Jawaid M. Lead and cadmium levels in blood samples from the general population of Sweden. *Environ Res* 1983; **30**: 233–53.

108  Watanabe T, Koizumi A, Fujita H et al. Cadmium levels in the blood of inhabitants in nonpolluted areas in Japan with special references to aging and smoking. *Environ Res* 1983; **31**: 472–83.

109  Mannino DM, Holguin F, Greves HM et al. Urinary cadmium levels predict lower lung function in current and former smokers: data from the Third National Health and Nutrition Examination Survey. *Thorax* 2004; **59**: 194–8.

110  Bjorkman L, Vahter M, Pedersen NL. Both the environment and genes are important for concentrations of cadmium and lead in blood. *Environ Health Perspect* 2000; **108**: 719–22.

111  Takeda K, Ishizawa S, Sato M et al. Identification of a *cis*-acting element that is responsible for cadmium-mediated induction of the human heme oxygenase gene. *J Biol Chem* 1994; **269**: 22858–67.

112  Alam J, Shibahara S, Smith A. Transcriptional activation of the heme oxygenase gene by heme and cadmium in mouse hepatoma cells. *J Biol Chem* 1989; **264**: 6371–5.

113  Yamada N, Yamaya M, Okinaga S et al. Microsatellite polymorphism in the heme oxygenase-1 gene promoter is associated with susceptibility to emphysema. *Am J Hum Genet* 2000; **66**: 187–95.

114  Diaz PT, Clanton TL, Pacht ER. Emphysema-like pulmonary disease associated with human immunodeficiency virus infection. *Ann Intern Med* 1992; **116**: 124–8.

115  Wewers MD, Diaz PT, Wewers ME et al. Cigarette smoking in HIV infection induces a suppressive inflammatory environment in the lung. *Am J Respir Crit Care Med* 1998; **158**: 1543–9.

116  Weinberg JB, Matthews TJ, Cullen BR, Malim MH. Productive human immunodeficiency virus type 1 (HIV-1) infection of nonproliferating human monocytes. *J Exp Med* 1991; **174**: 1477–82.

117  Fagerhol MK, Laurell CB. The Pi system-inherited variants of serum alpha 1-antitrypsin. *Prog Med Genet* 1970; **7**: 96–111.

118  Fagerhol MK. Serum Pi types in Norwegians. *Acta Pathol Microbiol Scand* 1967; **70**: 421–8.

119  Hjalmarsson K. Distribution of alpha-1-antitrypsin phenotypes in Sweden. *Hum Hered* 1988; **38**: 27–30.

120  Arnaud P, Koistinen J, Wilson GB, Fudenberg HH. Alpha 1-antitrypsin (Pi) phenotypes in a Finnish population. *Scand J Clin Lab Invest* 1977; **37**: 339–43.

121  Arnaud P, Galbraith RM, Faulk WP, Black C. Pi phenotypes of alpha1-antitrypsin in southern England: identification of M subtypes and implications for genetic studies. *Clin Genet* 1979; **15**: 406–10.

122  Thymann M. Distribution of alpha-1-antitrypsin (Pi) phenotypes in Denmark determined by separator isoelectric focusing in agarose gel. *Hum Hered* 1986; **36**: 19–23.

123  Hoffmann JJ, van den Broek WG. Distribution of alpha-1-antitrypsin phenotypes in two Dutch population groups. *Hum Genet* 1976; **32**: 43–8.

124  Sesboue R, Charlionet R, Vercaigne D et al. Genetic variants of serum alpha-1-antitrypsin (Pi types) in Bretons. *Hum Hered* 1978; **28**: 280–4.

◆125  Luisetti M, Seersholm N. Alpha1-antitrypsin deficiency. 1: epidemiology of alpha1-antitrypsin deficiency. *Thorax* 2004; **59**: 164–9.

✳126  American Thoracic Society/European Respiratory Society Statement: Standards for the diagnosis and management of individuals with alpha-1 antitrypsin deficiency. *Am J Respir Crit Care Med* 2003; **168**: 818–900.

127  Crystal RG. Alpha 1-antitrypsin deficiency, emphysema, and liver disease. Genetic basis and strategies for therapy. *J Clin Invest* 1990; **85**: 1343–52.

128  Ogushi F, Fells GA, Hubbard RC et al. Z-type alpha 1-antitrypsin is less competent than M1-type alpha 1-antitrypsin as an inhibitor of neutrophil elastase. *J Clin Invest* 1987; **80**: 1366–74.

●129  Lomas DA, Evans DL, Finch JT, Carrell RW. The mechanism of Z alpha 1-antitrypsin accumulation in the liver. *Nature* 1992; **357**: 605–7.

130  Lee JH, Brantly M. Molecular mechanisms of alpha 1-antitrypsin null alleles. *Respir Med* 2000; **94** (Suppl. C): S7–11.

131  Sifers RN, Brashears-Macatee S, Kidd VJ et al. A frameshift mutation results in a truncated alpha 1-antitrypsin that is retained within the rough endoplasmic reticulum. *J Biol Chem* 1988; **263**: 7330–5.

132  Nukiwa T, Takahashi H, Brantly M et al. alpha 1-Antitrypsin nullGranite Falls, a nonexpressing alpha 1-antitrypsin gene associated with a frameshift to stop mutation in a coding exon. *J Biol Chem* 1987; **262**: 11999–2004.

133  Takahashi H, Nukiwa T, Satoh K et al. Characterization of the gene and protein of the alpha 1-antitrypsin 'deficiency' allele Mprocida. *J Biol Chem* 1988; **263**: 15528–34.

134  Hofker MH, Nukiwa T, van Paassen HM et al. A Pro-Leu substitution in codon 369 of the alpha-1-antitrypsin deficiency variant PI MHeerlen. *Hum Genet* 1989; **81**: 264–8.

135  Kalsheker N, Hayes K, Weidinger S, Graham A. What is Pi (proteinase inhibitor) null or PiQO?: a problem highlighted by the alpha 1-antitrypsin Mheerlen mutation. *J Med Genet* 1992; **29**: 27–9.

136  Curiel DT, Holmes MD, Okayama H et al. Molecular basis of the liver and lung disease associated with the alpha 1-antitrypsin deficiency allele Mmalton. *J Biol Chem* 1989; **264**: 13938–45.

137  Seyama K, Nukiwa T, Takabe K et al. Siiyama (serine 53 (TCC) to phenylalanine 53 (TTC)). A new alpha 1-antitrypsin-deficient

variant with mutation on a predicted conserved residue of the serpin backbone. *J Biol Chem* 1991; **266**: 12627–32.

138 Seyama K, Nukiwa T, Souma S et al. Alpha 1-antitrypsin-deficient variant Siiyama (Ser53[TCC] to Phe53[TTC]) is prevalent in Japan. Status of alpha 1-antitrypsin deficiency in Japan. *Am J Respir Crit Care Med* 1995; **152**: 2119–26.

139 Cox DW, Levison H. Emphysema of early onset associated with a complete deficiency of alpha-1-antitrypsin (null homozygotes). *Am Rev Respir Dis* 1988; **137**: 371–5.

140 Garver RI Jr, Mornex JF, Nukiwa T et al. Alpha 1-antitrypsin deficiency and emphysema caused by homozygous inheritance of non-expressing alpha 1-antitrypsin genes. *New Engl J Med* 1986; **314**: 762–6.

141 Martin NG, Clark P, Ofulue AF et al. Does the PI polymorphism alone control alpha-1-antitrypsin expression? *Am J Hum Genet* 1987; **40**: 267–77.

142 Silverman EK, Province MA, Campbell EJ et al. Family study of alpha 1-antitrypsin deficiency: effects of cigarette smoking, measured genotype, and their interaction on pulmonary function and biochemical traits. *Genet Epidemiol* 1992; **9**: 317–31.

◆143 Mahadeva R, Lomas DA. Genetics and respiratory disease. 2. Alpha 1-antitrypsin deficiency, cirrhosis and emphysema. *Thorax* 1998; **53**: 501–5.

144 Parmar JS, Mahadeva R, Reed BJ et al. Polymers of alpha 1-antitrypsin are chemotactic for human neutrophils: a new paradigm for the pathogenesis of emphysema. *Am J Respir Cell Mol Biol* 2002; **26**: 723–30.

145 Elliott PR, Bilton D, Lomas DA. Lung polymers in Z alpha 1-antitrypsin deficiency-related emphysema. *Am J Respir Cell Mol Biol* 1998; **18**: 670–4.

146 Beatty K, Bieth J, Travis J. Kinetics of association of serine proteinases with native and oxidized alpha-1-proteinase inhibitor and alpha 1-antichymotrypsin. *J Biol Chem* 1980; **255**: 3931–4.

147 Carrell RW. alpha 1-Antitrypsin: molecular pathology, leukocytes, and tissue damage. *J Clin Invest* 1986; **78**: 1427–31.

148 Lewis JH, Iammarino RM, Spero JA, Hasiba U. Antithrombin Pittsburgh: an alpha1-antitrypsin variant causing hemorrhagic disease. *Blood* 1978; **51**: 129–37.

149 Owen MC, Brennan SO, Lewis JH, Carrell RW. Mutation of antitrypsin to antithrombin. Alpha 1-antitrypsin Pittsburgh (358 Met leads to Arg), a fatal bleeding disorder. *New Engl J Med* 1983; **309**: 694–8.

150 Scott CF, Carrell RW, Glaser CB et al. Alpha 1-antitrypsin-Pittsburgh. A potent inhibitor of human plasma factor XIa, kallikrein, and factor XIIf. *J Clin Invest* 1986; **77**: 631–4.

151 McElvaney NG, Stoller JK, Buist AS et al. Baseline characteristics of enrollees in the National Heart, Lung and Blood Institute Registry of alpha 1-antitrypsin deficiency. Alpha 1-Antitrypsin Deficiency Registry Study Group. *Chest* 1997; **111**: 394–403.

●152 Silverman EK, Pierce JA, Province MA et al. Variability of pulmonary function in alpha-1-antitrypsin deficiency: clinical correlates. *Ann Intern Med* 1989; **111**: 982–91.

153 Larsson C. Natural history and life expectancy in severe alpha1-antitrypsin deficiency, Pi Z. *Acta Med Scand* 1978; **204**: 345–51.

154 Janus ED, Phillips NT, Carrell RW. Smoking, lung function, and alpha 1-antitrypsin deficiency. *Lancet* 1985; **1**: 152–4.

155 Tobin MJ, Cook PJ, Hutchison DC. Alpha 1-antitrypsin deficiency: the clinical and physiological features of pulmonary emphysema in subjects homozygous for Pi type Z. A survey by the British Thoracic Association. *Br J Dis Chest* 1983; **77**: 14–27.

156 Black LF, Kueppers F. Alpha1-Antitrypsin deficiency in nonsmokers. *Am Rev Respir Dis* 1978; **117**: 421–8.

157 Piitulainen E, Tornling G, Eriksson S. Effect of age and occupational exposure to airway irritants on lung function in non-smoking individuals with alpha 1-antitrypsin deficiency (Pi Z). *Thorax* 1997; **52**: 244–8.

158 Silverman EK, Province MA, Rao DC et al. A family study of the variability of pulmonary function in alpha 1-antitrypsin deficiency. Quantitative phenotypes. *Am Rev Respir Dis* 1990; **142**: 1015–21.

159 Silverman EK, Province MA, Campbell EJ et al. Variability of pulmonary function in alpha-1-antitrypsin deficiency: residual family resemblance beyond the effect of the Pi locus. *Hum Hered* 1990; **40**: 340–55.

160 Novoradovsky A, Brantly ML, Waclawiw MA et al. Endothelial nitric oxide synthase as a potential susceptibility gene in the pathogenesis of emphysema in alpha1-antitrypsin deficiency. *Am J Respir Cell Mol Biol* 1999; **20**: 441–7.

161 de Serres FJ. Worldwide racial and ethnic distribution of alpha1-antitrypsin deficiency: summary of an analysis of published genetic epidemiologic surveys. *Chest* 2002; **122**: 1818–29.

162 Barnett TB, Gottovi D, Johnson AM. Protease inhibitors in chronic obstructive pulmonary disease. *Am Rev Respir Dis* 1975; **111**: 587–93.

163 Bartmann K, Fooke-Achterrath M, Koch G et al. Heterozygosity in the Pi-system as a pathogenetic cofactor in chronic obstructive pulmonary disease (COPD). *Eur J Respir Dis* 1985; **66**: 284–96.

164 Cox DW, Hoeppner VH, Levison H. Protease inhibitors in patients with chronic obstructive pulmonary disease: the alpha 1-antitrypsin heterozygote controversy. *Am Rev Respir Dis* 1976; **113**: 601–6.

165 Kueppers F, Donhardt A. Obstructive lung disease in heterozygotes for alpha-1 antitrypsin deficiency. *Ann Intern Med* 1974; **80**: 209–12.

166 Kueppers F, Miller RD, Gordon H et al. Familial prevalence of chronic obstructive pulmonary disease in a matched pair study. *Am J Med* 1977; **63**: 336–42.

●167 Lieberman J, Winter B, Sastre A. Alpha 1-antitrypsin Pi-types in 965 COPD patients. *Chest* 1986; **89**: 370–3.

168 Poller W, Meisen C, Olek K. DNA polymorphisms of the alpha 1-antitrypsin gene region in patients with chronic obstructive pulmonary disease. *Eur J Clin Invest* 1990; **20**: 1–7.

169 Sandford AJ, Weir TD, Spinelli JJ, Pare PD. Z and S mutations of the alpha1-antitrypsin gene and the risk of chronic obstructive pulmonary disease. *Am J Respir Cell Mol Biol* 1999; **20**: 287–91.

170 Gulsvik A, Fagerhol MK. Alpha 1-antitrypsin phenotypes and obstructive lung disease in the city of Oslo. *Scand J Respir Dis* 1979; **60**: 267–74.

171 Klayton R, Fallat R, Cohen AB. Determinants of chronic obstructive pulmonary disease in patients with intermediate levels of alpha-antitrypsin. *Am Rev Respir Dis* 1975; **112**: 71–5.

172 Webb DR, Hyde RW, Schwartz RH et al. Serum alpha 1-antitrypsin variants. Prevalence and clinical spirometry. *Am Rev Respir Dis* 1973; **108**: 918–25.

173 Morse JO, Lebowitz MD, Knudson RJ, Burrows B. Relation of protease inhibitor phenotypes to obstructive lung diseases in a community. *New Engl J Med* 1977; **296**: 1190–4.

●174 Dahl M, Tybjaerg-Hansen A, Lange P et al. Change in lung function and morbidity from chronic obstructive pulmonary disease in alpha1-antitrypsin MZ heterozygotes: a longitudinal study of the general population. *Ann Intern Med* 2002; **136**: 270–9.

●175 Anthonisen NR, Connett JE, Kiley JP et al. Effects of smoking intervention and the use of an inhaled anticholinergic bronchodilator on the rate of decline of FEV1. The Lung Health Study. *J Am Med Assoc* 1994; **272**: 1497–505.

176 Hersh CP, Dahl M, Ly NP et al. Chronic obstructive pulmonary disease in alpha 1-antitrypsin PI MZ heterozygotes: a meta-analysis. *Thorax* 2004; **59**: 843–9.

●177 Larsson C, Dirksen H, Sundstrom G, Eriksson S. Lung function studies in asymptomatic individuals with moderately (Pi SZ) and severely (Pi Z) reduced levels of alpha1-antitrypsin. *Scand J Respir Dis* 1976; **57**: 267–80.

178 Gishen P, Saunders AJ, Tobin MJ, Hutchison DC. Alpha 1-antitrypsin deficiency: the radiological features of pulmonary emphysema in subjects of Pi type Z and Pi type SZ: a survey by the British Thoracic Association. *Clin Radiol* 1982; **33**: 371–7.

179 Hutchison DC, Tobin MJ, Cook PJ. Alpha 1 antitrypsin deficiency: clinical and physiological features in heterozygotes of Pi type SZ. A survey by the British Thoracic Association. *Br J Dis Chest* 1983; **77**: 28–34.

180 Turino GM, Barker AF, Brantly ML et al. Clinical features of individuals with PI*SZ phenotype of alpha 1-antitrypsin deficiency. alpha 1-Antitrypsin Deficiency Registry Study Group. *Am J Respir Crit Care Med* 1996; **154**: 1718–25.

181 Seersholm N, Kok-Jensen A. Intermediate alpha 1-antitrypsin deficiency PiSZ: a risk factor for pulmonary emphysema? *Respir Med* 1998; **92**: 241–5.

182 Hall WJ, Hyde RW, Schwartz RH et al. Pulmonary abnormalities in intermediate alpha-1-antitrypsin deficiency. *J Clin Invest* 1976; **58**: 1069–77.

183 Matzen RN, Bader PI, Block WD. alpha1-Antitrypsin deficiency in clinic patients. *Ann Clin Res* 1977; **9**: 88–92.

184 Kalsheker NA, Hodgson IJ, Watkins GL et al. Deoxyribonucleic acid (DNA) polymorphism of the alpha 1-antitrypsin gene in chronic lung disease. *Br Med J (Clin Res Ed)* 1987; **294**: 1511–4.

185 Kalsheker NA, Watkins GL, Hill S et al. Independent mutations in the flanking sequence of the alpha-1-antitrypsin gene are associated with chronic obstructive airways disease. *Dis Markers* 1990; **8**: 151–7.

186 Sandford AJ, Spinelli JJ, Weir TD, Pare PD. Mutation in the 3′ region of the alpha-1-antitrypsin gene and chronic obstructive pulmonary disease. *J Med Genet* 1997; **34**: 874–5.

187 Benetazzo MG, Gile LS, Bombieri C et al. Alpha 1-antitrypsin TAQ I polymorphism and alpha 1-antichymotrypsin mutations in patients with obstructive pulmonary disease. *Respir Med* 1999; **93**: 648–54.

188 Morgan K, Scobie G, Kalsheker N. The characterization of a mutation of the 3′ flanking sequence of the alpha 1-antitrypsin gene commonly associated with chronic obstructive airways disease. *Eur J Clin Invest* 1992; **22**: 134–7.

189 Morgan K, Scobie G, Marsters P, Kalsheker NA. Mutation in an alpha1-antitrypsin enhancer results in an interleukin-6 deficient acute-phase response due to loss of cooperativity between transcription factors. *Biochim Biophys Acta* 1997; **1362**: 67–76.

190 Sandford AJ, Chagani T, Spinelli JJ, Pare PD. Alpha1-antitrypsin genotypes and the acute-phase response to open heart surgery. *Am J Respir Crit Care Med* 1999; **159**: 1624–8.

191 Survival and FEV1 decline in individuals with severe deficiency of alpha1-antitrypsin. The Alpha-1-Antitrypsin Deficiency Registry Study Group. *Am J Respir Crit Care Med* 1998; **158**: 49–59.

192 Seersholm N, Wencker M, Banik N et al. Does alpha1-antitrypsin augmentation therapy slow the annual decline in FEV1 in patients with severe hereditary alpha1-antitrypsin deficiency? Wissenschaftliche Arbeitsgemeinschaft zur Therapie von Lungenerkrankungen (WATL) alpha1-AT study group. *Eur Respir J* 1997; **10**: 2260–3.

◆193 Stoller JK, Aboussouan LS. alpha1-Antitrypsin deficiency . 5: intravenous augmentation therapy: current understanding. *Thorax* 2004; **59**: 708–12.

194 Gardi C, Cavarra E, Calzoni P et al. Neutrophil lysosomal dysfunctions in mutant C57 Bl/6J mice: interstrain variations in content of lysosomal elastase, cathepsin G and their inhibitors. *Biochem J* 1994; **299** (Pt 1): 237–45.

195 Wenstrup R, Zhao H. Heritable disorders of connective tissue with skin changes. In: Freedberg IM, Eisen AZ, Wolff K et al. (eds) *Fitzpatrick's dermatology in general medicine.* New York: McGraw-Hill, 2003.

196 Online Mendelian Inheritance in Man, OMIM(TM). McKusick-Nathans Institute for Genetic Medicine, Johns Hopkins University, Baltimore, MD and National Center for Biotechnology Information, National Library of Medicine, Bethesda, MD, 2000.

197 Harris RB, Heaphy MR, Perry HO. Generalized elastolysis (cutis laxa). *Am J Med* 1978; **65**: 815–22.

198 Merten DF, Rooney R. Progressive pulmonary emphysema associated with congenital generalized elastolysis (cutis laxa). *Radiology* 1974; **113**: 691–2.

199 Mehregan AH, Lee SC, Nabai H. Cutis laxa (generalized elastolysis). A report of four cases with autopsy findings. *J Cutan Pathol* 1978; **5**: 116–26.

200 Ledoux-Corbusier M. Cutis laxa, congenital form with pulmonary emphysema: an ultrastructural study. *J Cutan Pathol* 1983; **10**: 340–9.

201 Turner-Stokes L, Turton C, Pope FM, Green M. Emphysema and cutis laxa. *Thorax* 1983; **38**: 790–2.

202 Van Maldergem L, Vamos E, Liebaers I et al. Severe congenital cutis laxa with pulmonary emphysema: a family with three affected sibs. *Am J Med Genet* 1988; **31**: 455–64.

203 Yanagisawa H, Davis EC, Starcher BC et al. Fibulin-5 is an elastin-binding protein essential for elastic fibre development in vivo. *Nature* 2002; **415**: 168–71.

204 Nakamura T, Lozano PR, Ikeda Y et al. Fibulin-5/DANCE is essential for elastogenesis in vivo. *Nature* 2002; **415**: 171–5.

205 Loeys B, Van Maldergem L, Mortier G et al. Homozygosity for a missense mutation in fibulin-5 (FBLN5) results in a severe form of cutis laxa. *Hum Mol Genet* 2002; **11**: 2113–8.

206 Corbett E, Glaisyer H, Chan C et al. Congenital cutis laxa with a dominant inheritance and early onset emphysema. *Thorax* 1994; **49**: 836–7.

207 Tassabehji M, Metcalfe K, Hurst J et al. An elastin gene mutation producing abnormal tropoelastin and abnormal

elastic fibres in a patient with autosomal dominant cutis laxa. *Hum Mol Genet* 1998; **7**: 1021–8.

208  Zhang MC, He L, Giro M et al. Cutis laxa arising from frameshift mutations in exon 30 of the elastin gene (ELN). *J Biol Chem* 1999; **274**: 981–6.

209  Markova D, Zou Y, Ringpfeil F et al. Genetic heterogeneity of cutis laxa: a heterozygous tandem duplication within the fibulin-5 (FBLN5) gene. *Am J Hum Genet* 2003; **72**: 998–1004.

210  Daish P, Wheeler EM, Roberts PF, Jones RD. Menkes's syndrome. Report of a patient treated from 21 days of age with parenteral copper. *Arch Dis Child* 1978; **53**: 956–8.

211  Peltonen L, Kuivaniemi H, Palotie A et al. Alterations in copper and collagen metabolism in the Menkes syndrome and a new subtype of the Ehlers–Danlos syndrome. *Biochemistry* 1983; **22**: 6156–63.

212  Beighton P, De Paepe A, Steinmann B et al. Ehlers–Danlos syndromes: revised nosology, Villefranche, 1997. Ehlers–Danlos National Foundation (USA) and Ehlers–Danlos Support Group (UK). *Am J Med Genet* 1998; **77**: 31–7.

213  Pepin M, Schwarze U, Superti-Furga A, Byers PH. Clinical and genetic features of Ehlers–Danlos syndrome type IV, the vascular type. *New Engl J Med* 2000; **342**: 673–80.

214  Dowton SB, Pincott S, Demmer L. Respiratory complications of Ehlers–Danlos syndrome type IV. *Clin Genet* 1996; **50**: 510–4.

215  Dietz HC, Pyeritz RE. Marfan syndrome and related disorders. In: Scriver CR, Beaudet AL, Sly WS, Valle D (eds) *The metabolic and molecular bases of inherited disease*. New York: McGraw-Hill, 2001: 5287–311.

216  Wood JR, Bellamy D, Child AH, Citron KM. Pulmonary disease in patients with Marfan syndrome. *Thorax* 1984; **39**: 780–4.

217  Day DL, Burke BA. Pulmonary emphysema in a neonate with Marfan syndrome. *Pediatr Radiol* 1986; **16**: 518–21.

218  Dominguez R, Weisgrau RA, Santamaria M. Pulmonary hyperinflation and emphysema in infants with the Marfan syndrome. *Pediatr Radiol* 1987; **17**: 365–9.

219  Turner JA, Stanley NN. Fragile lung in the Marfan syndrome. *Thorax* 1976; **31**: 771–5.

220  Dietz HC, Pyeritz RE. Mutations in the human gene for fibrillin-1 (FBN1) in the Marfan syndrome and related disorders. *Hum Mol Genet* 1995; **4** (Spec No): 1799–809.

221  Pereira L, Andrikopoulos K, Tian J et al. Targetting of the gene encoding fibrillin-1 recapitulates the vascular aspect of Marfan syndrome. *Nat Genet* 1997; **17**: 218–22.

222  Neptune ER, Frischmeyer PA, Arking DE et al. Dysregulation of TGF-beta activation contributes to pathogenesis in Marfan syndrome. *Nat Genet* 2003; **33**: 407–11.

223  Lubec B, Fang-Kircher S, Lubec T et al. Evidence for McKusick's hypothesis of deficient collagen cross-linking in patients with homocystinuria. *Biochim Biophys Acta* 1996; **1315**: 159–62.

224  Cochran FB, Sweetman L, Schmidt K et al. Pyridoxine-unresponsive homocystinuria with an unusual clinical course. *Am J Med Genet* 1990; **35**: 519–22.

225  Bass HN, LaGrave D, Mardach R et al. Spontaneous pneumothorax in association with pyridoxine-responsive homocystinuria. *J Inherit Metab Dis* 1997; **20**: 831–2.

226  Toro JR, Glenn G, Duray P et al. Birt–Hogg–Dube syndrome: a novel marker of kidney neoplasia. *Arch Dermatol* 1999; **135**: 1195–202.

227  Khoo SK, Giraud S, Kahnoski K et al. Clinical and genetic studies of Birt–Hogg–Dube syndrome. *J Med Genet* 2002; **39**: 906–12.

228  Zbar B, Alvord WG, Glenn G et al. Risk of renal and colonic neoplasms and spontaneous pneumothorax in the Birt–Hogg–Dube syndrome. *Cancer Epidemiol Biomark Prev* 2002; **11**: 393–400.

229  Nickerson ML, Warren MB, Toro JR et al. Mutations in a novel gene lead to kidney tumors, lung wall defects, and benign tumors of the hair follicle in patients with the Birt–Hogg–Dube syndrome. *Cancer Cell* 2002; **2**: 157–64.

230  Verheijen FW, Verbeek E, Aula N et al. A new gene, encoding an anion transporter, is mutated in sialic acid storage diseases. *Nat Genet* 1999; **23**: 462–5.

231  Paakko P, Ryhanen L, Rantala H, Autio-Harmainen H. Pulmonary emphysema in a nonsmoking patient with Salla disease. *Am Rev Respir Dis* 1987; **135**: 979–82.

232  Keppler OT, Hinderlich S, Langner J et al. UDP-GlcNAc 2-epimerase: a regulator of cell surface sialylation. *Science* 1999; **284**: 1372–6.

233  Enns GM, Seppala R, Musci TJ et al. Clinical course and biochemistry of sialuria. *J Inherit Metab Dis* 2001; **24**: 328–36.

234  Naureckiene S, Sleat DE, Lackland H et al. Identification of HE1 as the second gene of Niemann-Pick C disease. *Science* 2000; **290**: 2298–301.

235  Elleder M, Houstkova H, Zeman J et al. Pulmonary storage with emphysema as a sign of Niemann–Pick type C2 disease (second complementation group). Report of a case. *Virchows Arch* 2001; **439**: 206–11.

236  Yamaki S, Horiuchi T, Takahashi T. Pulmonary changes in congenital heart disease with Down's syndrome: their significance as a cause of postoperative respiratory failure. *Thorax* 1985; **40**: 380–6.

237  Joshi VV, Kasznica J, Ali Khan MA et al. Cystic lung disease in Down's syndrome: a report of two cases. *Pediatr Pathol* 1986; **5**: 79–86.

238  Gonzalez OR, Gomez IG, Recalde AL, Landing BH. Postnatal development of the cystic lung lesion of Down syndrome: suggestion that the cause is reduced formation of peripheral air spaces. *Pediatr Pathol* 1991; **11**: 623–33.

239  Gyves-Ray K, Kirchner S, Stein S et al. Cystic lung disease in Down syndrome. *Pediatr Radiol* 1994; **24**: 137–8.

240  Tyrrell VJ, Asher MI, Chan Y. Subpleural lung cysts in Down's syndrome. *Pediatr Pulmonol* 1999; **28**: 145–8.

241  Cooney TP, Thurlbeck WM. Pulmonary hypoplasia in Down's syndrome. *New Engl J Med* 1982; **307**: 1170–3.

◆242  Sahn SA, Heffner JE. Spontaneous pneumothorax. *New Engl J Med* 2000; **342**: 868–74.

243  Nickoladze GD. Surgical management of familial spontaneous pneumothorax. *Respir Med* 1990; **84**: 107–9.

244  Abolnik IZ, Lossos IS, Zlotogora J, Brauer R. On the inheritance of primary spontaneous pneumothorax. *Am J Med Genet* 1991; **40**: 155–8.

245  Morrison PJ, Lowry RC, Nevin NC. Familial primary spontaneous pneumothorax consistent with true autosomal dominant inheritance. *Thorax* 1998; **53**: 151–2.

246  Koivisto PA, Mustonen A. Primary spontaneous pneumothorax in two siblings suggests autosomal recessive inheritance. *Chest* 2001; **119**: 1610–2.

247  Sharpe IK, Ahmad M, Braun W. Familial spontaneous pneumothorax and HLA antigens. *Chest* 1980; **78**: 264–8.

248  Yamada A, Takeda Y, Hayashi S, Shimizu K. Familial spontaneous pneumothorax in three generations and its HLA. *Jpn J Thorac Cardiovasc Surg* 2003; **51**: 456–8.

249 Sugiyama Y, Maeda H, Yotsumoto H, Takaku F. Familial spontaneous pneumothorax. *Thorax* 1986; **41**: 969–70.

250 Lenler-Petersen P, Grunnet N, Jespersen TW, Jaeger P. Familial spontaneous pneumothorax. *Eur Respir J* 1990; **3**: 342–5.

251 Cheng YJ, Chou SH, Kao EL. Familial spontaneous pneumothorax – report of seven cases in two families. *Gaoxiong Yi Xue Ke Xue Za Zhi* 1992; **8**: 390–4.

252 Cardy CM, Maskell NA, Handford PA et al. Familial spontaneous pneumothorax and FBN1 mutations. *Am J Respir Crit Care Med* 2004; **169**: 1260–2.

252a Graham RB, Nolasco M, Peterlin B, Garcia CK. Nonsense mutations in folliculin presenting as isolated familial spontaneous pneumothorax in adults. *Am J Resp Crit Care Med* 2005 (in press).

253 Clements BS. Congenital malformations of the lungs and airways. In: Taussig LM, Laundau LI (eds) *Pediatric respiratory medicine*. St. Louis: Mosby, 1999: 1106–36.

254 Warner JO, Rubin S, Heard BE. Congenital lobar emphysema: a case with bronchial atresia and abnormal bronchial cartilages. *Br J Dis Chest* 1982; **76**: 177–84.

255 Sloan H. Lobar obstructive emphysema in infancy treated by lobectomy. *J Thorac Surg* 1953; **26**: 1–20.

256 Hendren WH, McKee DM. Lobar emphysema of infancy. *J Pediat Surg* 1966; **1**: 24–39.

257 Wall MA, Eisenberg JD, Campbell JR. Congenital lobar emphysema in a mother and daughter. *Pediatrics* 1982; **70**: 131–3.

258 Wisnieski JJ, Baer AN, Christensen J et al. Hypocomplementemic urticarial vasculitis syndrome. Clinical and serologic findings in 18 patients. *Medicine* (*Balt*) 1995; **74**: 24–41.

259 Schwartz HR, McDuffie FC, Black LF et al. Hypocomplementemic urticarial vasculitis: association with chronic obstructive pulmonary disease. *Mayo Clin Proc* 1982; **57**: 231–8.

260 Ghamra Z, Stoller JK. Basilar hyperlucency in a patient with emphysema due to hypocomplementemic urticarial vasculitis syndrome. *Respir Care* 2003; **48**: 697–9.

261 Wisnieski JJ, Emancipator SN, Korman NJ et al. Hypocomplementemic urticarial vasculitis syndrome in identical twins. *Arthritis Rheum* 1994; **37**: 1105–11.

262 Knudson RJ. James Jackson Jr, the young pulmonologist who described familial emphysema. An historical footnote. *Chest* 1985; **87**: 673–6.

263 Hurst A. Familial emphysema. *Am Rev Respir Dis* 1959; **80**: 179–80.

264 Wimpfheimer F, Schneider L. Familial emphysema. *Am Rev Respir Dis* 1961; **83**: 697–703.

265 Larson RK, Barman ML. The familial occurrence of chronic obstructive pulmonary disease. *Ann Intern Med* 1965; **63**: 1001–8.

266 Hole BV, Wasserman K. Familial emphysema. *Ann Intern Med* 1965; **63**: 1009–17.

267 Cederlof R, Friberg L, Jonsson E, Kaij L. Morbidity among monozygotic twins. *Arch Environ Health* 1965; **10**: 346–50.

268 Cederlof R, Edfors ML, Friberg L, Jonsson E. Hereditary factors, 'spontaneous cough' and 'smoker's cough'. A study on 7800 twin-pairs with the aid of mailed questionnaires. *Arch Environ Health* 1967; **14**: 401–6.

269 Nelson P, Kanner RE. Bullous emphysema in monozygotic twins. *Am Rev Respir Dis* 1989; **140**: 1796–9.

270 Speizer FE, Rosner B, Tager I. Familial aggregation of chronic respiratory disease: use of National Health Interview Survey data for specific hypothesis testing. *Int J Epidemiol* 1976; **5**: 167–72.

271 Tager I, Tishler PV, Rosner B et al. Studies of the familial aggregation of chronic bronchitis and obstructive airways disease. *Int J Epidemiol* 1978; **7**: 55–62.

272 Larson RK, Barman ML, Kueppers F, Fudenberg HH. Genetic and environmental determinants of chronic obstructive pulmonary disease. *Ann Intern Med* 1970; **72**: 627–32.

273 Cohen BH, Ball WC Jr, Bias WB et al. A genetic-epidemiologic study of chronic obstructive pulmonary disease. I. Study design and preliminary observations. *Johns Hopkins Med J* 1975; **137**: 95–104.

274 Cohen BH, Ball WC Jr, Brashears S et al. Risk factors in chronic obstructive pulmonary disease (COPD). *Am J Epidemiol* 1977; **105**: 223–32.

275 Cohen BH. Chronic obstructive pulmonary disease: a challenge in genetic epidemiology. *Am J Epidemiol* 1980; **112**: 274–88.

276 Khoury MJ, Beaty TH, Tockman MS et al. Familial aggregation in chronic obstructive pulmonary disease: use of the loglinear model to analyze intermediate environmental and genetic risk factors. *Genet Epidemiol* 1985; **2**: 155–66.

277 Khoury MJ, Beaty TH, Newill CA et al. Genetic–environmental interactions in chronic airways obstruction. *Int J Epidemiol* 1986; **15**: 65–72.

278 Montnemery P, Lanke J, Lindholm LH et al. Familial related risk-factors in the development of chronic bronchitis/emphysema as compared to asthma assessed in a postal survey. *Eur J Epidemiol* 2000; **16**: 1003–7.

●279 Silverman EK, Chapman HA, Drazen JM et al. Genetic epidemiology of severe, early-onset chronic obstructive pulmonary disease. Risk to relatives for airflow obstruction and chronic bronchitis. *Am J Respir Crit Care Med* 1998; **157**: 1770–8.

280 Celedón JC, Speizer FE, Drazen JM et al. Bronchodilator responsiveness and serum total IgE levels in families of probands with severe early-onset COPD. *Eur Respir J* 1999; **14**: 1009–14.

281 Silverman EK, Weiss ST, Drazen JM et al. Gender-related differences in severe, early-onset chronic obstructive pulmonary disease. *Am J Respir Crit Care Med* 2000; **162**: 2152–8.

282 DeMeo DL, Carey VJ, Chapman HA et al. Familial aggregation of FEF(25-75) and FEF(25-75)/FVC in families with severe, early onset COPD. *Thorax* 2004; **59**: 396–400.

283 McCloskey SC, Patel BD, Hinchliffe SJ et al. Siblings of patients with severe chronic obstructive pulmonary disease have a significant risk of airflow obstruction. *Am J Respir Crit Care Med* 2001; **164**: 1419–24.

●284 Silverman EK, Palmer LJ, Mosley JD et al. Genomewide linkage analysis of quantitative spirometric phenotypes in severe early-onset chronic obstructive pulmonary disease. *Am J Hum Genet* 2002; **70**: 1229–39.

285 Silverman EK, Mosley JD, Palmer LJ et al. Genome-wide linkage analysis of severe, early-onset chronic obstructive pulmonary disease: airflow obstruction and chronic bronchitis phenotypes. *Hum Mol Genet* 2002; **11**: 623–32.

286 Lander E, Kruglyak L. Genetic dissection of complex traits: guidelines for interpreting and reporting linkage results. *Nat Genet* 1995; **11**: 241–7.

287 Palmer LJ, Celedon JC, Chapman HA et al. Genome-wide linkage analysis of bronchodilator responsiveness and post-bronchodilator spirometric phenotypes in chronic obstructive pulmonary disease. *Hum Mol Genet* 2003; **12**: 1199–210.

288 Hakonarson H, Halapi E, Sigvaldason A et al. A linkage study in heavy smokers identifies both causative and protective genes for chronic obstructive pulmonary disease. *Am J Respir Crit Care Med* 2004; **169**: A506.

289 DeMeo DL, Celedon JC, Lange C et al. Genomewide linkage of forced mid-expiratory flow in chronic obstructive pulmonary disease. *Am J Respir Crit Care Med* 2004; **170**: 1294–301.

290 Celedon JC, Lange C, Raby BA et al. The transforming growth factor-β1 (TGFB1) gene is associated with chronic obstructive pulmonary disease (COPD). *Hum Mol Genet* 2004; **13**: 1649–1656.

291 Billingsley GD, Walter MA, Hammond GL, Cox DW. Physical mapping of four serpin genes: alpha 1-antitrypsin, alpha 1-antichymotrypsin, corticosteroid-binding globulin, and protein C inhibitor, within a 280-kb region on chromosome I4q32.1. *Am J Hum Genet* 1993; **52**: 343–53.

292 Eriksson S, Lindmark B, Lilja H. Familial alpha 1-antichymotrypsin deficiency. *Acta Med Scand* 1986; **220**: 447–53.

293 Lindmark BE, Arborelius M Jr, Eriksson SG. Pulmonary function in middle-aged women with heterozygous deficiency of the serine protease inhibitor alpha 1-antichymotrypsin. *Am Rev Respir Dis* 1990; **141**: 884–8.

294 Poller W, Faber JP, Scholz S et al. Mis-sense mutation of alpha 1-antichymotrypsin gene associated with chronic lung disease. *Lancet* 1992; **339**: 1538.

295 Samilchuk EI, Chuchalin AG. Mis-sense mutation of alpha 1-antichymotrypsin gene and chronic lung disease. *Lancet* 1993; **342**: 624.

296 Poller W, Faber JP, Weidinger S et al. A leucine-to-proline substitution causes a defective alpha 1-antichymotrypsin allele associated with familial obstructive lung disease. *Genomics* 1993; **17**: 740–3.

297 Sandford AJ, Chagani T, Weir TD, Pare PD. Alpha 1-antichymotrypsin mutations in patients with chronic obstructive pulmonary disease. *Dis Markers* 1998; **13**: 257–60.

298 Ishii T, Matsuse T, Teramoto S et al. Association between alpha-1-antichymotrypsin polymorphism and susceptibility to chronic obstructive pulmonary disease. *Eur J Clin Invest* 2000; **30**: 543–8.

299 White R, Janoff A, Godfrey HP. Secretion of alpha-2-macroglobulin by human alveolar macrophages. *Lung* 1980; **158**: 9–14.

300 Bergqvist D, Nilsson IM. Hereditary alpha 2-macroglobulin deficiency. *Scand J Haematol* 1979; **23**: 433–6.

301 Poller W, Barth J, Voss B. Detection of an alteration of the alpha 2-macroglobulin gene in a patient with chronic lung disease and serum alpha 2-macroglobulin deficiency. *Hum Genet* 1989; **83**: 93–6.

302 Poller W, Faber JP, Klobeck G, Olek K. Cloning of the human alpha 2-macroglobulin gene and detection of mutations in two functional domains: the bait region and the thiolester site. *Hum Genet* 1992; **88**: 313–9.

303 Shapiro SD. Elastolytic metalloproteinases produced by human mononuclear phagocytes. Potential roles in destructive lung disease. *Am J Respir Crit Care Med* 1994; **150**: S160–4.

304 Parks WC, Shapiro SD. Matrix metalloproteinases in lung biology. *Respir Res* 2001; **2**: 10–9.

●305 Hautamaki RD, Kobayashi DK, Senior RM, Shapiro SD. Requirement for macrophage elastase for cigarette smoke-induced emphysema in mice. *Science* 1997; **277**: 2002–4.

306 D'Armiento J, Dalal SS, Okada Y et al. Collagenase expression in the lungs of transgenic mice causes pulmonary emphysema. *Cell* 1992; **71**: 955–61.

307 Finlay GA, O'Driscoll LR, Russell KJ et al. Matrix metalloproteinase expression and production by alveolar macrophages in emphysema. *Am J Respir Crit Care Med* 1997; **156**: 240–7.

308 Zhang B, Ye S, Herrmann SM et al. Functional polymorphism in the regulatory region of gelatinase B gene in relation to severity of coronary atherosclerosis. *Circulation* 1999; **99**: 1788–94.

309 Minematsu N, Nakamura H, Tateno H et al. Genetic polymorphism in matrix metalloproteinase-9 and pulmonary emphysema. *Biochem Biophys Res Commun* 2001; **289**: 116–9.

310 Joos L, He JQ, Shepherdson MB et al. The role of matrix metalloproteinase polymorphisms in the rate of decline in lung function. *Hum Mol Genet* 2002; **11**: 569–76.

311 Hirano K, Sakamoto T, Uchida Y et al. Tissue inhibitor of metalloproteinases-2 gene polymorphisms in chronic obstructive pulmonary disease. *Eur Respir J* 2001; **18**: 748–52.

◆312 Barnes PJ. New concepts in chronic obstructive pulmonary disease. *Annu Rev Med* 2003; **54**: 113–29.

313 Rahman I, MacNee W. Role of oxidants/antioxidants in smoking-induced lung diseases. *Free Radic Biol Med* 1996; **21**: 669–81.

314 MacNee W. Oxidants/antioxidants and COPD. *Chest* 2000; **117**: 303S–17S.

315 Morse D, Choi AM. Heme oxygenase-1: the 'emerging molecule' has arrived. *Am J Respir Cell Mol Biol* 2002; **27**: 8–16.

316 Maestrelli P, El Messlemani AH, De Fina O et al. Increased expression of heme oxygenase (HO)-1 in alveolar spaces and HO-2 in alveolar walls of smokers. *Am J Respir Crit Care Med* 2001; **164**: 1508–13.

317 He JQ, Ruan J, Connett JE et al. Antioxidant gene polymorphisms and susceptibility to a rapid decline in lung function in smokers. *Am J Respir Crit Care Med* 2002; **166**: 323–8.

318 Hassett C, Aicher L, Sidhu JS, Omiecinski CJ. Human microsomal epoxide hydrolase: genetic polymorphism and functional expression in vitro of amino acid variants. *Hum Mol Genet* 1994; **3**: 421–8.

319 Paolini M, Chieco P. Polymorphism in gene for microsomal epoxide hydrolase and lung disease. *Lancet* 1997; **350**: 1554.

320 Smith CA, Harrison DJ. Association between polymorphism in gene for microsomal epoxide hydrolase and susceptibility to emphysema. *Lancet* 1997; **350**: 630–3.

321 Yoshikawa M, Hiyama K, Ishioka S et al. Microsomal epoxide hydrolase genotypes and chronic obstructive pulmonary disease in Japanese. *Int J Mol Med* 2000; **5**: 49–53.

322 Takeyabu K, Yamaguchi E, Suzuki I et al. Gene polymorphism for microsomal epoxide hydrolase and susceptibility to emphysema in a Japanese population. *Eur Respir J* 2000; **15**: 891–4.

323 Budhi A, Hiyama K, Isobe T et al. Genetic susceptibility for emphysematous changes of the lung in Japanese. *Int J Mol Med* 2003; **11**: 321–9.

324  Yim JJ, Park GY, Lee CT et al. Genetic susceptibility to chronic obstructive pulmonary disease in Koreans: combined analysis of polymorphic genotypes for microsomal epoxide hydrolase and glutathione S-transferase M1 and T1. *Thorax* 2000; **55**: 121–5.

325  Cheng SL, Yu CJ, Chen CJ, Yang PC. Genetic polymorphism of epoxide hydrolase and glutathione S-transferase in COPD. *Eur Respir J* 2004; **23**: 818–24.

326  Xiao D, Wang C, Du MJ et al. Relationship between polymorphisms of genes encoding microsomal epoxide hydrolase and glutathione S-transferase P1 and chronic obstructive pulmonary disease. *Chin Med J (Engl)* 2004; **117**: 661–7.

327  Zhang R, Zhang A, He Q, Lu B. [Microsomal epoxide hydrolase gene polymorphism and susceptibility to chronic obstructive pulmonary disease in Han nationality of North China]. *Zhonghua Nei Ke Za Zhi* 2002; **41**: 11–4.

328  Board P, Coggan M, Johnston P et al. Genetic heterogeneity of the human glutathione transferases: a complex of gene families. *Pharmacol Ther* 1990; **48**: 357–69.

329  Hengstler JG, Arand M, Herrero ME, Oesch F. Polymorphisms of N-acetyltransferases, glutathione S-transferases, microsomal epoxide hydrolase and sulfotransferases: influence on cancer susceptibility. *Rec Res Cancer Res* 1998; **154**: 47–85.

330  Engel LS, Taioli E, Pfeiffer R et al. Pooled analysis and meta-analysis of glutathione S-transferase M1 and bladder cancer: a HuGE review. *Am J Epidemiol* 2002; **156**: 95–109.

331  Harrison DJ, Cantlay AM, Rae F et al. Frequency of glutathione S-transferase M1 deletion in smokers with emphysema and lung cancer. *Hum Exp Toxicol* 1997; **16**: 356–60.

332  Baranova H, Perriot J, Albuisson E et al. Peculiarities of the GSTM1 0/0 genotype in French heavy smokers with various types of chronic bronchitis. *Hum Genet* 1997; **99**: 822–6.

333  Cantlay AM, Smith CA, Wallace WA et al. Heterogeneous expression and polymorphic genotype of glutathione S-transferases in human lung. *Thorax* 1994; **49**: 1010–4.

334  Sundberg K, Johansson AS, Stenberg G et al. Differences in the catalytic efficiencies of allelic variants of glutathione transferase P1-1 towards carcinogenic diol epoxides of polycyclic aromatic hydrocarbons. *Carcinogenesis* 1998; **19**: 433–6.

335  Ishii T, Matsuse T, Teramoto S et al. Glutathione S-transferase P1 (GSTP1) polymorphism in patients with chronic obstructive pulmonary disease. *Thorax* 1999; **54**: 693–6.

336  Yim JJ, Yoo CG, Lee CT et al. Lack of association between glutathione S-transferase P1 polymorphism and COPD in Koreans. *Lung* 2002; **180**: 119–25.

337  Lu B, He Q. [Correlation between exon5 polymorphism of glutathione S-transferase P1 gene and susceptibility to chronic obstructive pulmonary disease in northern Chinese population of Han nationality living in Beijing, China]. *Zhonghua Nei Ke Za Zhi* 2002; **41**: 678–81.

338  Cantlay AM, Lamb D, Gillooly M et al. Association between the CYP1A1 gene polymorphism and susceptibility to emphysema and lung cancer. *J Clin Pathol: Mol Pathol* 1995; **48**: 210M–4M.

339  Minematsu N, Nakamura H, Iwata M et al. Association of CYP2A6 deletion polymorphism with smoking habit and development of pulmonary emphysema. *Thorax* 2003; **58**: 623–8.

340  Ishii T, Keicho N, Teramoto S et al. [Genetic variation of NADPH/NADH oxidase and susceptibility to diffuse panbronchiolitis (DPB) and chronic obstructive pulmonary disease (COPD)]. *Nihon Kokyuki Gakkai Zasshi* 2001; **39**: 328–32.

341  Keatings VM, Collins PD, Scott DM, Barnes PJ. Differences in interleukin-8 and tumor necrosis factor-alpha in induced sputum from patients with chronic obstructive pulmonary disease or asthma. *Am J Respir Crit Care Med* 1996; **153**: 530–4.

342  Aaron SD, Angel JB, Lunau M et al. Granulocyte inflammatory markers and airway infection during acute exacerbation of chronic obstructive pulmonary disease. *Am J Respir Crit Care Med* 2001; **163**: 349–55.

343  Wilson AG, Symons JA, McDowell TL et al. Effects of a polymorphism in the human tumor necrosis factor alpha promoter on transcriptional activation. *Proc Natl Acad Sci USA* 1997; **94**: 3195–9.

344  Dunham I, Sargent CA, Trowsdale J, Campbell RD. Molecular mapping of the human major histocompatibility complex by pulsed-field gel electrophoresis. *Proc Natl Acad Sci USA* 1987; **84**: 7237–41.

345  Huang SL, Su CH, Chang SC. Tumor necrosis factor-alpha gene polymorphism in chronic bronchitis. *Am J Respir Crit Care Med* 1997; **156**: 1436–9.

346  Sakao S, Tatsumi K, Igari H et al. Association of tumor necrosis factor alpha gene promoter polymorphism with the presence of chronic obstructive pulmonary disease. *Am J Respir Crit Care Med* 2001; **163**: 420–2.

347  Sakao S, Tatsumi K, Igari H et al. Association of tumor necrosis factor-alpha gene promoter polymorphism with low attenuation areas on high-resolution CT in patients with COPD. *Chest* 2002; **122**: 416–20.

348  Higham MA, Pride NB, Alikhan A, Morrell NW. Tumour necrosis factor-alpha gene promoter polymorphism in chronic obstructive pulmonary disease. *Eur Respir J* 2000; **15**: 281–4.

349  Keatings VM, Cave SJ, Henry MJ et al. A polymorphism in the tumor necrosis factor-alpha gene promoter region may pre-dispose to a poor prognosis in COPD. *Chest* 2000; **118**: 971–5.

350  Patuzzo C, Gile LS, Zorzetto M et al. Tumor necrosis factor gene complex in COPD and disseminated bronchiectasis. *Chest* 2000; **117**: 1353–8.

351  Ferrarotti I, Zorzetto M, Beccaria M et al. Tumour necrosis factor family genes in a phenotype of COPD associated with emphysema. *Eur Respir J* 2003; **21**: 444–9.

352  Kucukaycan M, Van Krugten M, Pennings HJ et al. Tumor necrosis factor-alpha +489G/A gene polymorphism is associated with chronic obstructive pulmonary disease. *Respir Res* 2002; **3**: 29.

353  Ishii T, Matsuse T, Teramoto S et al. Neither IL-1beta, IL-1 receptor antagonist, nor TNF-alpha polymorphisms are associated with susceptibility to COPD. *Respir Med* 2000; **94**: 847–51.

354  Chung KF. Cytokines in chronic obstructive pulmonary disease. *Eur Respir J Suppl* 2001; **34**: 50s–9s.

355  Joos L, McIntyre L, Ruan J et al. Association of IL-1beta and IL-1 receptor antagonist haplotypes with rate of decline in lung function in smokers. *Thorax* 2001; **56**: 863–6.

356  McCormack FX, Whitsett JA. The pulmonary collectins, SP-A and SP-D, orchestrate innate immunity in the lung. *J Clin Invest* 2002; **109**: 707–12.

●357  Wert SE, Yoshida M, LeVine AM et al. Increased metalloproteinase activity, oxidant production, and emphysema in surfactant protein D gene-inactivated mice. *Proc Natl Acad Sci USA* 2000; **97**: 5972–7.

358  Guo X, Lin HM, Lin Z et al. Surfactant protein gene A, B, and D marker alleles in chronic obstructive pulmonary disease of a Mexican population. *Eur Respir J* 2001; **18**: 482–90.

359  Gabolde M, Guilloud-Bataille M, Feingold J, Besmond C. Association of variant alleles of mannose binding lectin with severity of pulmonary disease in cystic fibrosis: cohort study. *Br Med J* 1999; **319**: 1166–7.

360  Garred P, Madsen HO, Halberg P et al. Mannose-binding lectin polymorphisms and susceptibility to infection in systemic lupus erythematosus. *Arthritis Rheum* 1999; **42**: 2145–52.

361  Yang IA, Seeney SL, Wolter JM et al. Mannose-binding lectin gene polymorphism predicts hospital admissions for COPD infections. *Genes Immun* 2003; **4**: 269–74.

362  Schutte BC, McCray PB Jr. Beta-defensins in lung host defense. *Annu Rev Physiol* 2002; **64**: 709–48.

363  Matsushita I, Hasegawa K, Nakata K et al. Genetic variants of human beta-defensin-1 and chronic obstructive pulmonary disease. *Biochem Biophys Res Commun* 2002; **291**: 17–22.

364  Ballow M. Primary immunodeficiency disorders: antibody deficiency. *J Allergy Clin Immunol* 2002; **109**: 581–91.

365  Webb DR, Condemi JJ. Selective immunoglobulin A deficiency and chronic obstructive lung disease. A family study. *Ann Intern Med* 1974; **80**: 618–21.

366  Bjorkander J, Bake B, Oxelius VA, Hanson LA. Impaired lung function in patients with IgA deficiency and low levels of IgG2 or IgG3. *New Engl J Med* 1985; **313**: 720–4.

367  O'Keeffe S, Gzel A, Drury R et al. Immunoglobulin G subclasses and spirometry in patients with chronic obstructive pulmonary disease. *Eur Respir J* 1991; **4**: 932–6.

368  Kauffmann F, Kleisbauer JP, Cambon-De-Mouzon A et al. Genetic markers in chronic air-flow limitation. A genetic epidemiologic study. *Am Rev Respir Dis* 1983; **127**: 263–9.

369  Anagnostopoulou U, Toumbis M, Konstantopoulos K et al. HLA-A and -B antigens in chronic bronchitis. *J Clin Epidemiol* 1993; **46**: 1413–6.

370  Horne SL, Cockcroft DW, Dosman JA. Possible protective effect against chronic obstructive airways disease by the GC2 allele. *Hum Hered* 1990; **40**: 173–6.

371  Schellenberg D, Pare PD, Weir TD et al. Vitamin D binding protein variants and the risk of COPD. *Am J Respir Crit Care Med* 1998; **157**: 957–61.

372  Kasuga I, Pare PD, Ruan J et al. Lack of association of group specific component haplotypes with lung function in smokers. *Thorax* 2003; **58**: 790–3.

373  Ishii T, Keicho N, Teramoto S et al. Association of Gc-globulin variation with susceptibility to COPD and diffuse panbronchiolitis. *Eur Respir J* 2001; **18**: 753–7.

374  Ito I, Nagai S, Hoshino Y et al. Risk and severity of COPD is associated with the group-specific component of serum globulin 1F allele. *Chest* 2004; **125**: 63–70.

375  Laufs J, Andrason H, Sigvaldason A et al. Association of vitamin D binding protein variants with chronic mucus hypersecretion in Iceland. *Am J Pharmacogenomics* 2004; **4**: 63–8.

376  Sluiter HJ, Koeter GH, de Monchy JG et al. The Dutch hypothesis (chronic non-specific lung disease) revisited. *Eur Respir J* 1991; **4**: 479–89.

377  Vestbo J, Prescott E. Update on the 'Dutch hypothesis' for chronic respiratory disease. *Thorax* 1998; **53** (Suppl. 2): S15–9.

378  Boezen HM, Schouten JP, Weiss ST. The Dutch hypothesis on chronic nonspecific lung disease. In: Annesi-Maesano I, Gulsvik A, Viegi G (eds) *Respiratory epidemiology in Europe.* Sheffield, UK: European Respiratory Society, 2000: 37–47.

379  Raby BA, Weiss ST. Beta 2-adrenergic receptor genetics. *Curr Opin Mol Ther* 2001; **3**: 554–66.

380  Summerhill E, Leavitt SA, Gidley H et al. Beta 2-adrenergic receptor Arg16/Arg16 genotype is associated with reduced lung function, but not with asthma, in the Hutterites. *Am J Respir Crit Care Med* 2000; **162**: 599–602.

381  Ho LI, Harn HJ, Chen CJ, Tsai NM. Polymorphism of the beta 2-adrenoceptor in COPD in Chinese subjects. *Chest* 2001; **120**: 1493–9.

382  Joos L, Weir TD, Connett JE et al. Polymorphisms in the beta 2 adrenergic receptor and bronchodilator response, bronchial hyperresponsiveness, and rate of decline in lung function in smokers. *Thorax* 2003; **58**: 703–7.

383  Wills-Karp M. The gene encoding interleukin-13: a susceptibility locus for asthma and related traits. *Respir Res* 2000; **1**: 19–23.

384  He JQ, Connett JE, Anthonisen NR, Sandford AJ. Polymorphisms in the IL13, IL13RA1, and IL4RA genes and rate of decline in lung function in smokers. *Am J Respir Cell Mol Biol* 2003; **28**: 379–85.

385  van der Pouw Kraan TC, Kucukaycan M, Bakker AM et al. Chronic obstructive pulmonary disease is associated with the –1055 IL-13 promoter polymorphism. *Genes Immun* 2002; **3**: 436–9.

386  Ruse CE, Hill MC, Burton PR et al. Associations between polymorphisms of the high-affinity immunoglobulin E receptor and late-onset airflow obstruction in older populations. *J Am Geriatr Soc* 2003; **51**: 1265–9.

◆387  Welsh MJ, Ramsey BW, Accurso F, Cutting GR. Cystic fibrosis. In: Scriver CR, Beaudet AL, Sly WS, Valle D (eds) *The metabolic and molecular bases of inherited disease*, 8th edn. New York: McGraw-Hill, 2001: 5121–88.

388  Wood JA, Fishman AP, Reemtsma K et al. A comparison of sweat chlorides and intestinal fat absorption in chronic obstructive pulmonary emphysema and fibrocystic disease of the pancreas. *New Engl J Med* 1959; **260**: 951–7.

389  Anderson CM, Freeman M, Allan J, Hubbard L. Observations on (i) sweat sodium levels in relation to chronic respiratory disease in adults and (ii) the incidence of respiratory and other disease in parents and siblings of patients with fibrocystic disease of the pancreas. *Med J Aust* 1962; **49**: 965–9.

390  Batten J, Muir D, Simon G, Carter C. The prevalence of respiratory disease in heterozygotes for the gene for fibrocystic disease of the pancreas. *Lancet* 1963; **1**: 1348–50.

391  Hallett WY, Knudson AG Jr, Massey FJ Jr. Absence of detrimental effect of the carrier state for the cystic fibrosis gene. *Am Rev Respir Dis* 1965; **92**: 714–24.

392  Davis PB, Vargo K. Pulmonary abnormalities in obligate heterozygotes for cystic fibrosis. *Thorax* 1987; **42**: 120–5.

393  Dumur V, Lafitte JJ, Gervais R et al. Abnormal distribution of cystic fibrosis delta F508 allele in adults with chronic bronchial hypersecretion. *Lancet* 1990; **335**: 1340.

394  Kostuch M, Semczuk A, Szarewicz-Adamczyk W et al. Detection of CFTR gene mutations in patients suffering from chronic bronchitis. *Arch Med Res* 2000; **31**: 97–100.

395   Artlich A, Boysen A, Bunge S et al. Common CFTR mutations are not likely to predispose to chronic bronchitis in northern Germany. *Hum Genet* 1995; **95**: 226–8.

396   Gervais R, Lafitte JJ, Dumur V et al. Sweat chloride and delta F508 mutation in chronic bronchitis or bronchiectasis. *Lancet* 1993; **342**: 997.

397   Dahl M, Tybjaerg-Hansen A, Lange P, Nordestgaard BG. DeltaF508 heterozygosity in cystic fibrosis and susceptibility to asthma. *Lancet* 1998; **351**: 1911–3.

398   Dahl M, Nordestgaard BG, Lange P, Tybjaerg-Hansen A. Fifteen-year follow-up of pulmonary function in individuals heterozygous for the cystic fibrosis phenylalanine-508 deletion. *J Allergy Clin Immunol* 2001; **107**: 818–23.

399   Tzetis M, Efthymiadou A, Strofalis S et al. CFTR gene mutations – including three novel nucleotide substitutions – and haplotype background in patients with asthma, disseminated bronchiectasis and chronic obstructive pulmonary disease. *Hum Genet* 2001; **108**: 216–21.

400   Beaty TH, Menkes HA, Cohen BH, Newill CA. Risk factors associated with longitudinal change in pulmonary function. *Am Rev Respir Dis* 1984; **129**: 660–7.

401   Krzyzanowski M, Jedrychowski W, Wysocki M. Factors associated with the change in ventilatory function and the development of chronic obstructive pulmonary disease in a 13-year follow-up of the Cracow Study. Risk of chronic obstructive pulmonary disease. *Am Rev Respir Dis* 1986; **134**: 1011–9.

402   Higgins MW, Keller JB, Becker M et al. An index of risk for obstructive airways disease. *Am Rev Respir Dis* 1982; **125**: 144–51.

403   Horne SL, Cockcroft DW, Lovegrove A, Dosman JA. ABO, Lewis and secretor status and relative incidence of air flow obstruction. *Dis Markers* 1985; **3**: 55–62.

404   Vestbo J, Hein HO, Suadicani P et al. Genetic markers for chronic bronchitis and peak expiratory flow in the Copenhagen Male Study. *Dan Med Bull* 1993; **40**: 378–80.

405   Spitalnik PF, Spitalnik SL. Human blood group antigens and antibodies. In: Hoffman R, Benz EJJ, Shattil SJ et al. (eds) *Hematology: basic principles and practice*, 3rd edn. Philadelphia: Churchill Livingstone, 2000: 2188–205.

406   Cohen BH, Bias WB, Chase GA et al. Is ABH nonsecretor status a risk factor for obstructive lung disease? *Am J Epidemiol* 1980; **111**: 285–91.

407   Haines AP, Imeson JD, Meade TW. ABH secretor status and pulmonary function. *Am J Epidemiol* 1982; **115**: 367–70.

408   Kauffmann F, Frette C, Pham QT et al. Associations of blood group-related antigens to FEV1, wheezing, and asthma. *Am J Respir Crit Care Med* 1996; **153**: 76–82.

409   Abboud RT, Yu P, Chan-Yeung M, Tan F. Lack of relationship between ABH secretor status and lung function in pulp mill workers. *Am Rev Respir Dis* 1982; **126**: 1089–91.

410   Suadicani P, Hein HO, Meyer HW, Gyntelberg F. Exposure to cold and draught, alcohol consumption, and the NS-phenotype are associated with chronic bronchitis: an epidemiological investigation of 3387 men aged 53–75 years: the Copenhagen Male Study. *Occup Environ Med* 2001; **58**: 160–4.

411   Blobe GC, Schiemann WP, Lodish HF. Role of transforming growth factor beta in human disease. *New Engl J Med* 2000; **342**: 1350–8.

412   Bartram U, Speer CP. The role of transforming growth factor beta in lung development and disease. *Chest* 2004; **125**: 754–65.

413   Wu L, Chau J, Young RP et al. Transforming growth factor-beta 1 genotype and susceptibility to chronic obstructive pulmonary disease. *Thorax* 2004; **59**: 126–9.

414   Ioannidis JP, Ntzani EE, Trikalinos TA, Contopoulos-Ioannidis DG. Replication validity of genetic association studies. *Nat Genet* 2001; **29**: 306–9.

415   Hirschhorn JN, Lohmueller K, Byrne E, Hirschhorn K. A comprehensive review of genetic association studies. *Genet Med* 2002; **4**: 45–61.

416   Shapiro SD. Animal models for chronic obstructive pulmonary disease: age of klotho and marlboro mice. *Am J Respir Cell Mol Biol* 2000; **22**: 4–7.

◆417   Mahadeva R, Shapiro SD. Chronic obstructive pulmonary disease *3: Experimental animal models of pulmonary emphysema. *Thorax* 2002; **57**: 908–14.

418   Gross P, Pfitzer EA, Tolker E et al. Experimental emphysema: its production with papain in normal and silicotic rats. *Arch Environ Health* 1965; **11**: 50–8.

●419   Wright JL, Churg A. Cigarette smoke causes physiologic and morphologic changes of emphysema in the guinea pig. *Am Rev Respir Dis* 1990; **142**: 1422–8.

420   Kielty CM, Raghunath M, Siracusa LD et al. The tight skin mouse: demonstration of mutant fibrillin-1 production and assembly into abnormal microfibrils. *J Cell Biol* 1998; **140**: 1159–66.

421   Gordi C, Martorana PA, van Even P et al. Serum antielastase deficiency in tight-skin mice with genetic emphysema. *Exp Mol Pathol* 1990; **52**: 46–53.

422   Huang L, Kuo YM, Gitschier J. The pallid gene encodes a novel, syntaxin 13-interacting protein involved in platelet storage pool deficiency. *Nat Genet* 1999; **23**: 329–32.

423   Martorana PA, Brand T, Gardi C et al. The pallid mouse. A model of genetic alpha 1-antitrypsin deficiency. *Lab Invest* 1993; **68**: 233–41.

424   Keil M, Lungarella G, Cavarra E et al. A scanning electron microscopic investigation of genetic emphysema in tight-skin, pallid, and beige mice, three different C57 BL/6J mutants. *Lab Invest* 1996; **74**: 353–62.

425   Barbosa MD, Nguyen QA, Tchernev VT et al. Identification of the homologous beige and Chediak-Higashi syndrome genes. *Nature* 1996; **382**: 262–5.

426   Leco KJ, Waterhouse P, Sanchez OH et al. Spontaneous air space enlargement in the lungs of mice lacking tissue inhibitor of metalloproteinases-3 (TIMP-3). *J Clin Invest* 2001; **108**: 817–29.

●427   Morris DG, Huang X, Kaminski N et al. Loss of integrin alpha(v)beta6-mediated TGF-beta activation causes Mmp12-dependent emphysema. *Nature* 2003; **422**: 169–73.

●428   Zheng T, Zhu Z, Wang Z et al. Inducible targeting of IL-13 to the adult lung causes matrix metalloproteinase – and cathepsin-dependent emphysema. *J Clin Invest* 2000; **106**: 1081–93.

429   Wang Z, Zheng T, Zhu Z et al. Interferon gamma induction of pulmonary emphysema in the adult murine lung. *J Exp Med* 2000; **192**: 1587–600.

430   Alsaeedi A, Sin DD, McAlister FA. The effects of inhaled corticosteroids in chronic obstructive pulmonary disease: a systematic review of randomized placebo-controlled trials. *Am J Med* 2002; **113**: 59–65.

●431   Continuous or nocturnal oxygen therapy in hypoxemic chronic obstructive lung disease: a clinical trial. Nocturnal

Oxygen Therapy Trial Group. *Ann Intern Med* 1980;
**93**: 391–8.

●432   Long term domiciliary oxygen therapy in chronic hypoxic cor
pulmonale complicating chronic bronchitis and emphysema.
Report of the Medical Research Council Working Party.
*Lancet* 1981; **1**: 681–6.

◆433   Calverley PM, Walker P. Chronic obstructive pulmonary
disease. *Lancet* 2003; **362**: 1053–61.

434   Palmer LJ, Silverman ES, Weiss ST, Drazen JM.
Pharmacogenetics of asthma. *Am J Respir Crit Care Med*
2002; **165**: 861–6.

435   Hosenpud JD, Bennett LE, Keck BM et al. The Registry of the
International Society for Heart and Lung Transplantation:
eighteenth Official Report, 2001. *J Heart Lung Transplant*
2001; **20**: 805–15.

436   Hosenpud JD, Bennett LE, Keck BM et al. Effect of diagnosis
on survival benefit of lung transplantation for end-stage
lung disease. *Lancet* 1998; **351**: 24–7.

437   Charman SC, Sharples LD, McNeil KD, Wallwork J.
Assessment of survival benefit after lung transplantation by
patient diagnosis. *J Heart Lung Transplant* 2002; **21**: 226–32.

438   Ramsey SD, Berry K, Etzioni R et al. Cost effectiveness of
lung-volume-reduction surgery for patients with severe
emphysema. *New Engl J Med* 2003; **348**: 2092–102.

439   Spira A, Beane J, Pinto-Plata V et al. Gene expression
profiling of human lung tissue from smokers with severe
emphysema. *Am J Respir Cell Mol Biol* 2004; **31**: 601–10.

440   Hackett NR, Heguy A, Harvey BG et al. Variability of
antioxidant-related gene expression in the airway epithelium
of cigarette smokers. *Am J Respir Cell Mol Biol* 2003; **29**:
331–43.

441   Cigarette smoking among adults – United States, 2000. *Morb
Mortal Wkly Rep* 2002; ss**51**: 642–5.

442   Arinami T, Ishiguro H, Onaivi ES. Polymorphisms in genes
involved in neurotransmission in relation to smoking. *Eur J
Pharmacol* 2000; **410**: 215–26.

443   Benowitz NL. Drug therapy. Pharmacologic aspects of
cigarette smoking and nicotine addition. *New Engl J Med*
1988; **319**: 1318–30.

●444   Fagerstrom KO, Schneider NG. Measuring nicotine
dependence: a review of the Fagerstrom Tolerance
Questionnaire. *J Behav Med* 1989; **12**: 159–82.

445   Henningfield JE, Clayton R, Pollin W. Involvement of tobacco in
alcoholism and illicit drug use. *Br J Addict* 1990; **85**: 279–91.

446   Breslau N, Fenn N, Peterson EL. Early smoking initiation and
nicotine dependence in a cohort of young adults. *Drug
Alcohol Depend* 1993; **33**: 129–37.

447   Niu T, Chen C, Ni J et al. Nicotine dependence and its familial
aggregation in Chinese. *Int J Epidemiol* 2000; **29**: 248–52.

●448   Carmelli D, Swan GE, Robinette D, Fabsitz R. Genetic
influence on smoking – a study of male twins. *New Engl J
Med* 1992; **327**: 829–33.

449   Heath AC, Martin NG. Genetic models for the natural history
of smoking: evidence for a genetic influence on smoking
persistence. *Addict Behav* 1993; **18**: 19–34.

450   True WR, Heath AC, Scherrer JF et al. Genetic and
environmental contributions to smoking. *Addiction* 1997; **92**:
1277–87.

451   True WR, Xian H, Scherrer JF et al. Common genetic
vulnerability for nicotine and alcohol dependence in men.
*Arch Gen Psych* 1999; **56**: 655–61.

452   Kendler KS, Neale MC, Sullivan P et al. A population-based
twin study in women of smoking initiation and nicotine
dependence. *Psychol Med* 1999; **29**: 299–308.

453   Fisher RA. Lung cancer and cigarettes. *Nature* 1958; **182**:
108.

454   Fisher RA. Cancer and smoking. *Nature* 1958; **182**: 596.

455   Sullivan PF, Kendler KS. The genetic epidemiology of smoking.
*Nicotine Tob Res* 1999; **1** (Suppl. 2): S51–7; discussion
S69–70.

456   Kendler KS, Thornton LM, Pedersen NL. Tobacco consumption
in Swedish twins reared apart and reared together. *Arch Gen
Psych* 2000; **57**: 886–92.

◆457   Li MD. The genetics of smoking related behavior: a brief
review. *Am J Med Sci* 2003; **326**: 168–73.

◆458   Li MD, Cheng R, Ma JZ, Swan GE. A meta-analysis of
estimated genetic and environmental effects on smoking
behavior in male and female adult twins. *Addiction* 2003;
**98**: 23–31.

459   Straub RE, Sullivan PF, Ma Y et al. Susceptibility genes for
nicotine dependence: a genome scan and followup in an
independent sample suggest that regions on chromosomes 2,
4, 10, 16, 17 and 18 merit further study. *Mol Psychiatry*
1999; **4**: 129–44.

460   Duggirala R, Almasy L, Blangero J. Smoking behavior is under
the influence of a major quantitative trait locus on human
chromosome 5q. *Genet Epidemiol* 1999; **17** (Suppl. 1):
S139–44.

461   Bergen AW, Korczak JF, Weissbecker KA, Goldstein AM. A
genome-wide search for loci contributing to smoking and
alcoholism. *Genet Epidemiol* 1999; **17** (Suppl. 1): S55–60.

462   Bierut LJ, Rice JP, Goate A et al. A genomic scan for habitual
smoking in families of alcoholics: common and specific
genetic factors in substance dependence. *Am J Med Genet*
2004; **124A**: 19–27.

463   Li MD, Ma JZ, Cheng R et al. A genome-wide scan to identify
loci for smoking rate in the Framingham Heart Study
population. *BMC Genet* 2003; **4** (Suppl. 1): S103.

464   Walton R, Johnstone E, Munafo M et al. Genetic clues to the
molecular basis of tobacco addiction and progress towards
personalized therapy. *Trends Mol Med* 2001; **7**: 70–6.

465   Rossing MA. Genetic influences on smoking: candidate genes.
*Environ Health Perspect* 1998; **106**: 231–8.

466   Crabbe JC. Genetic contributions to addiction. *Annu Rev
Psychol* 2002; **53**: 435–62.

467   Cami J, Farre M. Drug addiction. *New Engl J Med* 2003; **349**:
975–86.

468   Wise RA, Bozarth MA. A psychomotor stimulant theory of
addiction. *Psychol Rev* 1987; **94**: 469–92.

469   Dani JA. Roles of dopamine signaling in nicotine addiction.
*Mol Psychiatry* 2003; **8**: 255–6.

470   Mihailescu S, Palomero-Rivero M, Meade-Huerta P et al.
Effects of nicotine and mecamylamine on rat dorsal raphe
neurons. *Eur J Pharmacol* 1998; **360**: 31–6.

471   Ribeiro EB, Bettiker RL, Bogdanov M, Wurtman RJ. Effects of
systemic nicotine on serotonin release in rat brain. *Brain Res*
1993; **621**: 311–8.

472   Raunio H, Rautio A, Gullsten H, Pelkonen O. Polymorphisms
of CYP2A6 and its practical consequences. *Br J Clin
Pharmacol* 2001; **52**: 357–63.

473   Pianezza ML, Sellers EM, Tyndale RF. Nicotine metabolism
defect reduces smoking. *Nature* 1998; **393**: 750.

474 Tyndale RF, Sellers EM. Variable CYP2A6-mediated nicotine metabolism alters smoking behavior and risk. *Drug Metab Dispos* 2001; **29**: 548–52.

475 Sellers EM, Tyndale RF, Fernandes LC. Decreasing smoking behavior and risk through CYP2A6 inhibition. *Drug Discov Today* 2003; **8**: 487–93.

476 Sellers EM, Kaplan HL, Tyndale RF. Inhibition of cytochrome P450 2A6 increases nicotine's oral bioavailability and decreases smoking. *Clin Pharmacol Ther* 2000; **68**: 35–43.

477 Tricker AR. Nicotine metabolism, human drug metabolism polymorphisms, and smoking behavior. *Toxicology* 2003; **183**: 151–73.

478 Carter B, Long T, Cinciripini P. A meta-analytic review of the CYP2A6 genotype and smoking behavior. *Nicotine Tob Res* 2004; **6**: 221–7.

479 London SJ, Idle JR, Daly AK, Coetzee GA. Genetic variation of CYP2A6, smoking, and risk of cancer. *Lancet* 1999; **353**: 898–9.

480 Daly AK, Fairbrother KS, Andreassen OA et al. Characterization and PCR-based detection of two different hybrid CYP2D7P/CYP2D6 alleles associated with the poor metabolizer phenotype. *Pharmacogenetics* 1996; **6**: 319–28.

481 Lovlie R, Daly AK, Molven A et al. Ultrarapid metabolizers of debrisoquine: characterization and PCR-based detection of alleles with duplication of the CYP2D6 gene. *FEBS Lett* 1996; **392**: 30–4.

482 Cholerton S, Boustead C, Taber H et al. CYP2D6 genotypes in cigarette smokers and non-tobacco users. *Pharmacogenetics* 1996; **6**: 261–3.

483 Boustead C, Taber H, Idle JR, Cholerton S. CYP2D6 genotype and smoking behavior in cigarette smokers. *Pharmacogenetics* 1997; **7**: 411–4.

484 Pontieri FE, Tanda G, Orzi F, Di Chiara G. Effects of nicotine on the nucleus accumbens and similarity to those of addictive drugs. *Nature* 1996; **382**: 255–7.

485 Blum K, Noble EP, Sheridan PJ et al. Allelic association of human dopamine D2 receptor gene in alcoholism. *J Am Med Assoc* 1990; **263**: 2055–60.

486 Thompson J, Thomas N, Singleton A et al. D2 dopamine receptor gene (DRD2) Taq1 A polymorphism: reduced dopamine D2 receptor binding in the human striatum associated with the A1 allele. *Pharmacogenetics* 1997; **7**: 479–84.

487 Jonsson EG, Nothen MM, Grunhage F et al. Polymorphisms in the dopamine D2 receptor gene and their relationships to striatal dopamine receptor density of healthy volunteers. *Mol Psychiatry* 1999; **4**: 290–6.

488 Noble EP. D2 dopamine receptor gene in psychiatric and neurologic disorders and its phenotypes. *Am J Med Genet* 2003; **116B**: 103–25.

489 Noble EP, St Jeor ST, Ritchie T et al. D2 dopamine receptor gene and cigarette smoking: a reward gene? *Med Hypotheses* 1994; **42**: 257–60.

490 Comings DE, Ferry L, Bradshaw-Robinson S et al. The dopamine D2 receptor (DRD2) gene: a genetic risk factor in smoking. *Pharmacogenetics* 1996; **6**: 73–9.

491 Anokhin AP, Todorov AA, Madden PA et al. Brain event-related potentials, dopamine D2 receptor gene polymorphism, and smoking. *Genet Epidemiol* 1999; **17** (Suppl. 1): S37–42.

492 Anokhin AP, Vedeniapin AB, Sirevaag EJ et al. The P300 brain potential is reduced in smokers. *Psychopharmacology (Berl)* 2000; **149**: 409–13.

493 Singleton AB, Thomson JH, Morris CM et al. Lack of association between the dopamine D2 receptor gene allele DRD2*A1 and cigarette smoking in a United Kingdom population. *Pharmacogenetics* 1998; **8**: 125–8.

494 Bierut LJ, Rice JP, Edenberg HJ et al. Family-based study of the association of the dopamine D2 receptor gene (DRD2) with habitual smoking. *Am J Med Genet* 2000; **90**: 299–302.

495 Comings DE, Gade R, Wu S et al. Studies of the potential role of the dopamine D1 receptor gene in addictive behaviors. *Mol Psychiatry* 1997; **2**: 44–56.

496 Shields PG, Lerman C, Audrain J et al. Dopamine D4 receptors and the risk of cigarette smoking in African-Americans and Caucasians. *Cancer Epidemiol Biomarker Prev* 1998; **7**: 453–8.

497 Lerman C, Caporaso N, Main D et al. Depression and self-medication with nicotine: the modifying influence of the dopamine D4 receptor gene. *Health Psychol* 1998; **17**: 56–62.

498 Gelernter J, Kranzler HR, Satel SL, Rao PA. Genetic association between dopamine transporter protein alleles and cocaine-induced paranoia. *Neuropsychopharmacology* 1994; **11**: 195–200.

499 Lerman C, Caporaso NE, Audrain J et al. Evidence suggesting the role of specific genetic factors in cigarette smoking. *Health Psychol* 1999; **18**: 14–20.

500 Sabol SZ, Nelson ML, Fisher C et al. A genetic association for cigarette smoking behavior. *Health Psychol* 1999; **18**: 7–13.

501 Ling D, Niu T, Feng Y et al. Association between polymorphism of the dopamine transporter gene and early smoking onset: an interaction risk on nicotine dependence. *J Hum Genet* 2004; **49**: 35–9.

502 Jorm AF, Henderson AS, Jacomb PA et al. Association of smoking and personality with a polymorphism of the dopamine transporter gene: results from a community survey. *Am J Med Genet* 2000; **96**: 331–4.

503 Vandenbergh DJ, Bennett CJ, Grant MD et al. Smoking status and the human dopamine transporter variable number of tandem repeats (VNTR) polymorphism: failure to replicate and finding that never-smokers may be different. *Nicotine Tob Res* 2002; **4**: 333–40.

504 Jonsson E, Sedvall G, Brene S et al. Dopamine-related genes and their relationships to monoamine metabolites in CSF. *Biol Psychiatry* 1996; **40**: 1032–43.

505 Lerman C, Shields PG, Main D et al. Lack of association of tyrosine hydroxylase genetic polymorphism with cigarette smoking. *Pharmacogenetics* 1997; **7**: 521–4.

506 Olsson C, Anney R, Forrest S et al. Association between dependent smoking and a polymorphism in the tyrosine hydroxylase gene in a prospective population-based study of adolescent health. *Behav Genet* 2004; **34**: 85–91.

507 Checkoway H, Franklin GM, Costa-Mallen P et al. A genetic polymorphism of MAO-B modifies the association of cigarette smoking and Parkinson's disease. *Neurology* 1998; **50**: 1458–61.

508 Costa-Mallen P, Costa LG, Smith-Weller T et al. Genetic polymorphism of dopamine D2 receptors in Parkinson's disease and interactions with cigarette smoking and MAO-B intron 13 polymorphism. *J Neurol Neurosurg Psychiatry* 2000; **69**: 535–7.

509 McKinney EF, Walton RT, Yudkin P et al. Association between polymorphisms in dopamine metabolic enzymes and tobacco consumption in smokers. *Pharmacogenetics* 2000; **10**: 483–91.

510 Kenny PJ, Markou A. Neurobiology of the nicotine withdrawal syndrome. *Pharmacol Biochem Behav* 2001; **70**: 531–49.

511 Nielsen DA, Virkkunen M, Lappalainen J et al. A tryptophan hydroxylase gene marker for suicidality and alcoholism. *Arch Gen Psychiatry* 1998; **55**: 593–602.

512 Sullivan PF, Jiang Y, Neale MC et al. Association of the tryptophan hydroxylase gene with smoking initiation but not progression to nicotine dependence. *Am J Med Genet* 2001; **105**: 479–84.

513 Lerman C, Caporaso NE, Bush A et al. Tryptophan hydroxylase gene variant and smoking behavior. *Am J Med Genet* 2001; **105**: 518–20.

514 Heils A, Teufel A, Petri S et al. Allelic variation of human serotonin transporter gene expression. *J Neurochem* 1996; **66**: 2621–4.

515 Lerman C, Shields PG, Audrain J et al. The role of the serotonin transporter gene in cigarette smoking. *Cancer Epidemiol Biomarker Prev* 1998; **7**: 253–5.

516 Ishikawa H, Ohtsuki T, Ishiguro H et al. Association between serotonin transporter gene polymorphism and smoking among Japanese males. *Cancer Epidemiol Biomarker Prev* 1999; **8**: 831–3.

517 do Prado-Lima PA, Chatkin JM, Taufer M et al. Polymorphism of 5HT2A serotonin receptor gene is implicated in smoking addiction. *Am J Med Genet* 2004; **128B**: 90–3.

518 Feng Y, Niu T, Xing H et al. A common haplotype of the nicotine acetylcholine receptor alpha 4-subunit gene is associated with vulnerability to nicotine addiction in men. *Am J Hum Genet* 2004; **75**: 112–21.

519 Lerman C, Niaura R. Applying genetic approaches to the treatment of nicotine dependence. *Oncogene* 2002; **21**: 7412–20.

520 Lancaster T, Stead L, Silagy C, Sowden A. Effectiveness of interventions to help people stop smoking: findings from the Cochrane Library. *Br Med J* 2000; **321**: 355–8.

521 Ascher JA, Cole JO, Colin JN et al. Bupropion: a review of its mechanism of antidepressant activity. *J Clin Psychiatry* 1995; **56**: 395–401.

522 Ball K, Turner R. Smoking and the heart. The basis for action. *Lancet* 1974; **2**: 822–6.

523 Faucette SR, Hawke RL, Lecluyse EL et al. Validation of bupropion hydroxylation as a selective marker of human cytochrome P450 2B6 catalytic activity. *Drug Metab Dispos* 2000; **28**: 1222–30.

524 Lerman C, Shields PG, Wileyto EP et al. Pharmacogenetic investigation of smoking cessation treatment. *Pharmacogenetics* 2002; **12**: 627–34.

525 Lerman C, Shields PG, Wileyto EP et al. Effects of dopamine transporter and receptor polymorphisms on smoking cessation in a bupropion clinical trial. *Health Psychol* 2003; **22**: 541–8.

526 Lerman C, Wileyto EP, Patterson F et al. The functional mu opioid receptor (OPRM1) Asn40Asp variant predicts short-term response to nicotine replacement therapy in a clinical trial. *Pharmacogenomics J* 2004; **4**: 184–92.

527 Konu O, Kane JK, Barrett T et al. Region-specific transcriptional response to chronic nicotine in rat brain. *Brain Res* 2001; **909**: 194–203.

528 Zhang S, Day IN, Ye S. Microarray analysis of nicotine-induced changes in gene expression in endothelial cells. *Physiol Genomics* 2001; **5**: 187–92.

529 Hu D, Cao K, Peterson-Wakeman R, Wang R. Altered profile of gene expression in rat hearts induced by chronic nicotine consumption. *Biochem Biophys Res Commun* 2002; **297**: 729–36.

●530 Sullivan PF, Neale BM, van den Oord E et al. Candidate genes for nicotine dependence via linkage, epistasis, and bioinformatics. *Am J Med Genet* 2004; **126B**: 23–36.

531 Stein EA, Pankiewicz J, Harsch HH et al. Nicotine-induced limbic cortical activation in the human brain: a functional MRI study. *Am J Psychiatry* 1998; **155**: 1009–15.

532 Salokangas RK, Vilkman H, Ilonen T et al. High levels of dopamine activity in the basal ganglia of cigarette smokers. *Am J Psychiatry* 2000; **157**: 632–4.

533 Swan GE, Hudmon KS, Jack LM et al. Environmental and genetic determinants of tobacco use: methodology for a multidisciplinary, longitudinal family-based investigation. *Cancer Epidemiol Biomarker Prev* 2003; **12**: 994–1005.

◆534 DeMeo DL, Silverman EK. Alpha1-antitrypsin deficiency. 2: genetic aspects of alpha 1-antitrypsin deficiency: phenotypes and genetic modifiers of emphysema risk. *Thorax* 2004; **59**: 259–64.

535 Klein W, Rohde G, Arinir U et al. A promotor polymorphism in the Interleukin 11 gene is associated with chronic obstructive pulmonary disease. *Electrophoresis* 2004; **25**: 804–8.

536 Hu RC, Xu YJ, Zhang ZX, Xie JG. [Polymorphism of interleukin-10 gene promoter and its association with susceptibility to chronic obstructive pulmonary disease in Chinese Han people]. *Zhonghua Yi Xue Yi Chuan Xue Za Zhi* 2003; **20**: 504–7.

537 Sakao S, Tatsumi K, Hashimoto T et al. Vascular endothelial growth factor and the risk of smoking-related COPD. *Chest* 2003; **124**: 323–7.

538 Hegab AE, Sakamoto T, Uchida Y et al. CLCA1 gene polymorphisms in chronic obstructive pulmonary disease. *J Med Genet* 2004; **41**: e27.

539 Lucey EC, Keane J, Kuang PP et al. Severity of elastase-induced emphysema is decreased in tumor necrosis factor-alpha and interleukin-1beta receptor-deficient mice. *Lab Invest* 2002; **82**: 79–85.

# 11

# Cystic fibrosis

JOSHUA GROMAN AND GARRY R. CUTTING

## INTRODUCTION

Cystic fibrosis (CF) is the most common autosomal recessive disorder that limits life span in Caucasians. The incidence of CF in Caucasians is approximately 1 in 3000 live births, and is less frequent in non-Caucasian populations.[1] Individuals with CF have obstructive and inflammatory disease affecting epithelial tissues of numerous organ systems typically including the pancreas, respiratory tract, male reproductive tract, and sweat gland[2] (Fig. 11.1). However, clinical severity can be quite variable among individuals, and in some cases organ system involvement can also vary. Significant advances in the diagnosis and treatment of CF have increased median survival in the past 20 years to approximately 33 years.[3]

Mutations in the cystic fibrosis transmembrane conductance regulator gene (*CFTR*) have been show to cause CF, and provide a molecular basis for the defective cAMP-mediated salt and water transport across epithelial tissues.[4–6]

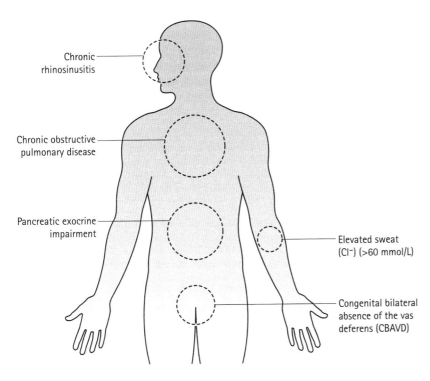

Chronic rhinosinusitis

Chronic obstructive pulmonary disease

Pancreatic exocrine impairment

Elevated sweat (Cl⁻) (>60 mmol/L)

Congenital bilateral absence of the vas deferens (CBAVD)

**Figure 11.1** *Organ systems affected in patients with CF. Patients with CF have disease manifestations in epithelial tissues of many organ systems. Individuals with classic CF have manifestations in each of the organ systems shown below, whereas patients with nonclassic CF have symptoms in a limited subset of these organ systems.*

Genotype–phenotype studies have revealed that disease in some organ systems is correlated with *CFTR* genotype (e.g., the pancreas), whereas in other organ systems (e.g., the respiratory tract) variability in severity seems to be influenced by factors other than *CFTR* genotype such as environmental exposure or genetic background.[7–10] These findings have fueled the search for additional genes that modify the severity of the CF phenotype.[11–13] In this chapter, we will summarize our current understanding of the molecular pathophysiology of CF.

## CLINICAL BACKGROUND

### Organ system involvement

#### RESPIRATORY TRACT

Lung disease is the primary factor leading to early mortality in CF.[2] Patients with CF develop chronic obstructive pulmonary disease manifesting as chronic cough and wheeze, excessive sputum production, abnormal radiographs revealing chronic dilatation of the airways (bronchiectasis) and inflammatory infiltrates, and digital clubbing. Lung pathology in CF is primarily limited to the large airways and submucosal glands, and affects the alveolar sacs in later stages of disease through expansion of fibrosis originating from the airways. Pathology specimens from the lungs of CF patients typically reveal bronchiectasis, airways plugged with mucus, and dilated submucosal glands with impacted mucus.[14,15] The persistent decline in pulmonary function ultimately results in hypoxia due to pulmonary insufficiency, bronchial artery hemorrhage, tension pneumothorax, and/or cardiac complications.[16]

Patients with CF have decreased mucociliary clearance rates and are highly susceptible to bacterial, mycobacterial, and fungal infections that influence the rate of pulmonary decline. Several unusual organisms are particularly able to infect and colonize the lungs of CF patients including: *Pseudomonas aeruginosa* (60 percent), *Staphylococcus aureus* (42 percent), *Haemophilus influenzae* (15 percent), *Strenotrophomonas maltophilia* (5 percent), and *Burkholderia cepacia* (4 percent).[3] In addition to these bacterial infections, approximately 7 percent of CF patients develop allergic bronchopulmonary aspergillosis[17,18] and approximately 13 percent of patients have nontuberculosis mycobacterial infections.[19] Typically, patients become infected early in life with *S. aureus* and/or *H. influenzae*, followed by infection with *P. aeruginosa*.[3,20] Colonization with *P. aeruginosa* is a significant event in the pathogenesis of CF lung disease, leading to a decrease in pulmonary function and an increase in pulmonary exacerbations.[21] Chronic infection with *P. aeruginosa* can lead to the formation of mucoid strains that are phenotypically and genetically different from normal strains and result in the formation of biofilms. Biofilms form through an aggregation of bacterial cells that are recalcitrant

to clearance by the host immune system, and are completely resistant to antibiotic therapy.[22,23]

While infection with one of the previously mentioned organisms has been shown to increase peribronchial inflammation and thickening,[24] several recent studies have suggested that inflammatory cells and cytokines are elevated prior to infection. This observation suggests that airway inflammation may be related to the primary defect in CF, rather than exclusively as a consequence of infection.[25–27] The progressive pulmonary disease seen in CF appears to be a consequence of heightened inflammatory status and chronic infection.

In addition to lung disease, CF patients also have abnormal mucus secretion, chronic inflammation, and infection of the nasal sinuses leading to radiographic changes and clinical symptoms.[28] Nearly 100 percent of patients have some detectable abnormality using paranasal sinus CT scans including maxillary opacification, absence of frontal and sphenoid sinuses, and medial bulging of the lateral nasal wall.[29,30] Despite the presence of definite radiographic abnormalities in almost all subjects, symptoms involving the sinuses are reported in only 60 percent of CF patients. These symptoms include nasal obstruction, rhinorrhea, nasal polyposis, mouth breathing, and broadening of the nasal bridge.[31] While sinus disease does not contribute to mortality in CF, it is a very common feature that contributes to the morbidity of the disease.

#### GASTROINTESTINAL TRACT

The term 'cystic fibrosis' was coined after pathologists observed fibrotic cysts throughout postmortem pancreas samples from infants with CF. The pathology observed in the pancreas usually results in complete loss of exocrine pancreatic function due to chronic dilatation of the small pancreatic ducts, and obstruction of the normal flow of pancreatic enzymes. The acinar cells of the pancreas continue to produce digestive enzymes that eventually digest the normal tissue of the pancreas, resulting in fibrosis and cyst formation. Approximately 85 percent of CF patients have pancreatic exocrine impairment causing malabsorption, fat soluble vitamin deficiency, hypoproteinemia, and failure to thrive.[32] Prior to the advent of pancreatic enzyme replacement therapy, pancreatic insufficiency was the primary cause of early mortality in CF. In approximately 5 percent of CF patients, fibrosis extends to involve the endocrine pancreas resulting in insulin-dependent diabetes mellitus.[33] Some patients retain pancreatic function and may experience transient blockage and inflammation resulting in painful episodes of pancreatitis.[34] In some cases, recurrent pancreatitis can result in complete destruction of the exocrine ducts and acini resulting in insufficiency.

Disease manifestations in the intestines occur much less frequently than pancreatic disease. Approximately 15–20 percent of infants born with CF have obstruction of the small bowel with meconium, termed meconium ileus (MI).[33]

If left untreated, MI may persist resulting in blockage and perforation of the bowel. Older children and adults may also have various intestinal symptoms including chronic constipation, distal intestinal obstruction syndrome, and rectal prolapse.

## HEPATOBILIARY DISEASE

Complications due to liver disease account for approximately 2 percent of mortality in CF, and are the second leading cause of mortality.[33] Similar to disease pathophysiology seen in other organ systems, disease in the liver is believed to be due to excessive mucus secretion, ductal obstruction, and dilatation resulting in fibrosis. The prevalence of liver disease increases with age and reaches a peak of nearly 9 percent in 16–20 year olds.[35] Almost 5 percent of adults with CF will have symptoms of hepatic cirrhosis or portal hypertension.[36] Disease manifestations can also be seen in the gall bladder, and in some cases require cholecystectomy. Subclinical liver disease evidenced by enzyme elevation has an estimated incidence of 1.8 cases per 100 patient years.[37] Pancreatic insufficiency, meconium ileus, male sex, and presence of severe CFTR mutations are associated with an increased incidence of liver disease.[37,38]

## MALE REPRODUCTIVE TRACT

Infertility due to congenital bilateral absence of the vas deferens (CBAVD) is a very common trait in male patients with CF, affecting 95 percent of men with the disease.[39] CBAVD is believed to occur due to abnormal development or atresia of Wolffian duct structures including the vas and the seminal vesicles. Absence of the vas deferens can be identified in prepubescent boys by palpation or transrectal ultrasonography. In men, absence of the vas can also be inferred through analysis of semen revealing low sperm count, low ejaculate volume, and abnormal semen chemistry. Interestingly, gametogenesis is completely normal in men with CF, and retrieval of sperm from sites proximal to the obstruction (epididymus) has been successfully used for in vitro fertilization.[40] The nearly uniform occurrence of male infertility suggests that development of the vas deferens is sensitive to defects in the CFTR gene.[41]

## SWEAT GLAND

Salty sweat distinguishes individuals with CF from those with failure to thrive or lung disease due to other causes. This observation reportedly dates back to the mid-1600s when a salty taste on the skin of a newborn would portend the infants impending death.[14] In 1951, Kessler and Anderson identified several CF patients with heat prostration during a heat wave in New York City,[42] and it was later shown that these patients indeed had elevated salt concentrations in their sweat.[43] In 1959, Gibson and Cooke developed the pilocarpine iontophoresis sweat test, which has evolved

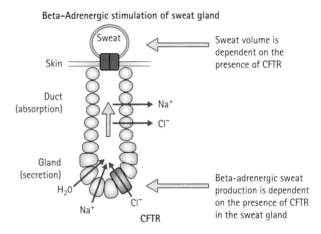

**Figure 11.2**  *Sweat gland function following cholinergic and beta-adrenergic stimulation. Sweat production can be activated by cholinergic or beta-adrenergic stimulation. Cholinergic stimulation is independent of CFTR function, and beta-adrenergic stimulation is dependent on CFTR function. In CF patients, cholinergic stimulation results in normal sweat volume, but abnormal sweat [Cl⁻], due to absence of CFrR-mediated Cl⁻ absorption in the sweat gland duct. Beta-agonist stimulation results in abnormally low sweat volume in CF patients, due to absence of CFTR-mediated Cl⁻ secretion into the lumen of the sweat gland.*

into the standard diagnostic test for CF.[44] This test involves stimulating sweat production through local iontophoresis of a cholinergic stimulant, pilocarpine, into the skin of the forearm. Sweat is collected from the site of iontophoresis and the chloride concentration is calculated (Fig. 11.2). Typically, patients with CF have sweat chloride concentrations ranging from 60–166 mmol/L, whereas normal individuals typically have levels below 40 mmol/L.[45] Subsequent studies have shown that patients with atypical forms of CF have borderline levels of sweat chloride concentration ranging from 40–60 mmol/L, and a small fraction of patients have been shown to have normal sweat levels, <40 mmo/L.[46–51] It is now known that the elevated sweat electrolytes seen in CF patients are due to a defect in re-absorption of Cl⁻ and Na⁺ from the sweat gland duct[52,53] (Fig. 11.2).

A defect in glandular secretion of sweat has also been seen in CF. Specifically, Sato and Sato discovered that CF patients have a defect in sweat production following stimulation with beta-agonists such as isoproterenol.[54] It is believed that cAMP-activation of the protein involved in CF is responsible for Cl⁻ secretion into the lumen of the gland, along with Na⁺ and water (Fig. 11.2). In the absence of the CF protein, Cl⁻ and therefore Na⁺ and water are not moved into the gland resulting in lower sweat production. Callen and colleagues have developed a cAMP-mediated sweat rate test that exploits this feature.[55] This test involves quantifying the amount of sweat produced over a 20-min period following intradermal injection of a solution containing a beta-agonist (isoproterenol), a phosphodiesterase inhibitor (theophylline), and a cholinergic inhibitor (atropine). Patients with CF produce a lower volume of sweat than normal individuals, and the technique has proven sensitive enough to identify an intermediate effect in CF carriers.

## Familial aggregation, linkage analysis, and identification of the *CFTR* gene

Familial recurrence of CF was recognized soon after the delineation of the disorder. The occurrence of disease in siblings, but not in parents, suggested an autosomal recessive mode of inheritance, and that a single gene most likely caused CF.[56,57] However, identification of the responsible gene proved elusive until the technique of positional cloning was available. The gene responsible for CF was first localized to chromosome 7q via an association with variation in the paraoxonase enzyme.[58] Linkage of the CF phenotype with DNA markers allowed further localization of the CF gene between the previously identified MET oncogene and the D7S8 marker.[59,60] At this point, carrier detection and prenatal diagnosis could be offered to patients using linkage analysis within families. The identification of additional DNA markers in this region allowed for more refined mapping of the gene and revealed that a single haplotype in this region was responsible for the majority of CF-associated alleles.[61] Using chromosome walking and jumping techniques, the genomic organization of the region containing the CF causing gene was determined.[4] Identification of the gene responsible for CF was achieved by matching sequences within the genomic clones to those found in a cDNA clone mapped to this region.[5] This effort eventually facilitated identification of all 27 exons of the gene. The gene was confirmed to be the CF-causing gene when mutations were identified that segregated with disease in many families.[6]

The 27 exon gene shown to be mutated in CF was named the cystic fibrosis transmembrane conductance regulator (*CFTR*). The *CFTR* gene encodes a ≈6.1 kb transcript that has been shown to be expressed in the organ systems involved in CF including the pancreas, lung, colon, male reproductive tract, as well as most other epithelial tissues.[5] *CFTR* encodes a 1480 amino acid glycoprotein that shows considerable homology with the ABC transporter

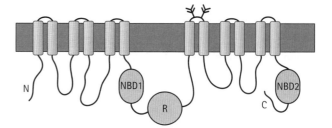

**Figure 11.3**   *The cystic fibrosis transmembrane conductance regulator (CFTR) is an integral membrane protein. CFTR is a member of the ABC transporter family and has two nucleotide binding domains (NBD1 and NDB2). Despite sequence similarities to ABC transporters, the CFTR protein has been shown to be a major chloride channel in epithelial tissues of numerous organ systems. Protein kinase A-mediated phosphorylation of the regulatory domain (R) is required for cAMP-mediated chloride transport.*

family.[5] Hydrophobicity analysis predicted, and experimental data have proven, that the protein has 12 transmembrane segments with a large cytoplasmic region.[62] Within the cytoplasmic region there are two ATP binding domains and a regulatory region which has been shown to be phosphorylated by protein kinase A (Fig. 11.3). The CFTR protein resides primarily in the apical membrane of epithelial cells and has been shown to be a major channel for chloride conductance following activation via the cAMP-protein kinase pathway.[63] The CFTR protein has also been shown to act as a conduit for other compounds such as bicarbonate and ATP. Several studies have suggested that the absence of proper transport of these compounds contributes to the pathology seen in patients with CF.[64–68] Surprisingly, 14 years following the identification of the *CFTR* gene and protein, there remains considerable controversy regarding its role in the pathogenesis of the CF phenotype.[69,70]

## Making a diagnosis of CF

Despite advances in our understanding of the molecular etiology of CF, the diagnosis of this disorder relies primarily on clinical evidence, and can be made in the absence of any abnormality in the CFTR gene.[71,72] For the most part, diagnosis of patients with classic CF is relatively straightforward and is made in the first year of life for the majority (approximately 71 percent) of patients.[33] However, genetic and physiologic testing have identified previously unrecognized, mild forms of CF.[47,48] To alleviate confusion around what constitutes a CF diagnosis, Rosenstein and Cutting outlined a consensus statement for the diagnosis of CF.[71] According to these criteria, the diagnosis for CF can be made if the patient has at least one clinical feature of CF or a history of CF in a sibling or a positive newborn screening test result, as well as laboratory evidence of CFTR dysfunction or identification of two CFTR mutations.

Several recent advances have improved the sensitivity and specificity of a CF diagnosis, particularly for patients with nonclassic forms of CF. Bioelectric assays aimed at

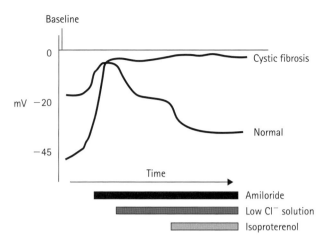

Baseline

Cystic fibrosis

Normal

Amiloride

Low Cl⁻ solution

Isoproterenol

**Figure 11.4** *Patients with CF have measurable bioelectric abnormalities of the nasal epithelium. This conceptual diagram illustrates the use of the nasal potential difference (NPD) test in identifying individuals with CF. In black is a typical NPD tracing from a normal individual, and in red is a reading from a patient with CF. Patients with CF have hyperabsorption of Na⁺ causing hyperpolarized baseline values. CF patients also fail to repolarize following perfusion with low Cl⁻ buffer and isoproterenol, due to the absence of normal Cl⁻ transport.*

identifying electrolyte transport defects indicative of CF have come into clinical practice.[73,74] The nasal potential difference (NPD) test measures electrical potential across epithelial cells of the inferior nasal turbinate. Due to hyperabsorption of sodium, patients with CF have a baseline potential difference that is substantially more negative than that seen in normal (Fig. 11.4). Administration of amiloride, an inhibitor of the epithelial sodium channel, produces an exaggerated depolarization in CF patients. Perfusion of a low chloride solution creates a gradient favorable to secretion of chloride from the nasal epithelia. Finally, CFTR function is tested directly by inclusion of a beta-agonist such as isoproterenol in a solution containing amiloride and low or zero chloride. The NPD of normal individuals exhibits depolarization in response to these maneuvers due to chloride secretion via activated CFTR channels. CF patients exhibit little or no depolarization due to the absence of functional CFTR. In Europe, measurements of chloride conductance from rectal biopsy samples has also come into clinical use, and this test demonstrates abnormalities similar to those seen in nonclassic CF.[75]

Several states have newborn screening programs to diagnose CF in the neonatal period. Most of these programs rely on the immunoreactive trypsinogen test (IRT) to identify newborns with elevated serum trypsinogen. Elevated IRT levels indicate the onset of pancreatic inflammation and, in many cases, insufficiency.[76] Because many unaffected babies have elevated IRT levels, most programs also perform a sweat and/or genetic test of babies that have a positive IRT.[77] Several studies have suggested that early interventions made possible through newborn screening can have a positive impact on clinical outcome.[78,79]

Genetic testing of the CFTR gene is sensitive and specific for patients with the classic form of CF. Analysis of the entire CFTR gene by sequencing can detect nearly 100 percent of mutations in classic CF patients.[80,81] Since sequencing of CFTR is a substantial undertaking, standard genetic testing for CF involves testing for about 30 of the most common mutations.[82,83] These assays can detect at least 80 percent of CF causing mutations in Caucasian populations. Population screening to identify individuals at risk of having an affected child has also become common practice in the USA following recent recommendations from the American College of Obstetrics and Gynecology.[84] In instances where both members of a couple are CF carriers, prenatal diagnosis can be used to determine the genotype of the fetus. More recently, preimplantation genetic diagnosis has become available that allows at risk couples to test for, and selectively transfer, embryos that are genetically confirmed to be unaffected.[40,85]

## The CF phenotypic spectrum

The vast majority of patients with CF have the classic form of disease that affects the pancreas, respiratory tract, sweat gland, and male reproductive tract.[2] Several decades after the delineation of CF as a distinct clinical entity, it was realized that a fraction of patients with CF have milder symptoms with limited organ system involvement.[86] Typically, these patients have later onset of pulmonary features, and do not have malabsorption due to pancreatic insufficiency. Since the advent of genetic testing, the CF spectrum has grown to include patients with normal sweat chloride concentration.[48,50,51,87,88] Originally, patients were grouped into two broad categories based on whether they were pancreatic insufficient or pancreatic sufficient. However, some patients with pancreatic sufficiency do not have consistent involvement of other organ systems usually affected in the classic form of CF (e.g., the sweat gland). Thus, patients with the presence of CF-like disease in two or more (but not all) of the aforementioned organ systems are termed nonclassic CF.

Following identification of the CFTR gene, it was realized that most patients with nonclassic forms of CF have at least one mutation in the *CFTR* gene that permits some residual CFTR function. While some of these partial function mutations are included in the screen for common CF mutations, most are rare and their detection requires complete scanning of the *CFTR* gene. In a recent study, Hughes et al. scanned the *CFTR* gene in 31 unrelated atypical CF patients from Northern Ireland and failed to find any *CFTR* mutations in 42 percent of patients.[49] Interestingly, in a separate study, Mekus et al.[89] presented a boy with clinical and laboratory evidence of CF in the absence of *CFTR* mutations, and with evidence against linkage to the *CFTR* gene. Other reports have described individual patients with atypical CF phenotypes in the absence of *CFTR* mutations.[50,90,91] Finally, Groman et al.[80] studied a large group of patients with nonclassic CF phenotypes, and found that 41 percent of the 74 patients did not have mutations identified after exhaustive scanning of the *CFTR* gene. Together, these observations bring into question the exclusive role of the *CFTR* gene in the etiology of nonclassic CF.

Within the CF phenotypic spectrum are patients who have CF-like disease in a single organ system and have one or two mutations in the *CFTR* gene. These phenotypes include isolated congenital bilateral absence of the vas deferens, idiopathic chronic pancreatitis, idiopathic bronchiectasis, allergic bronchopulmonary aspergillosis, primary sclerosing cholangitis, and isolated elevated sweat chloride concentration.[92–99] While many of these patients are initially diagnosed with disease in a single organ system, specific clinical investigations often reveal physiologic abnormalities and/or subclinical pathology in other organ systems that are usually involved in CF.[100,101]

## MUTATION ANALYSIS AND GENOTYPE–PHENOTYPE CORRELATIONS

As predicted from haplotype analyses during the cloning of *CFTR*, a single mutation, ΔF508, accounts for a large fraction (approximately 75 percent) of the mutant CF alleles.[6] This mutation is an in-frame three base pair deletion in exon 10 resulting in a deletion of a phenylalanine at codon 508. ΔF508 is found on a highly conserved haplotype, with an extended area of linkage disequilibrium suggesting that the mutation has occurred once in evolution. Approximately 50 percent of classic CF patients are homozygous for ΔF508. Another 23 mutations have been shown to account for an additional 5 percent of the CF causing alleles, and the remaining 20 percent of disease-associated alleles are due to rare mutations.[2] Thus far, there have been over 1000 mutations identified in the *CFTR* gene that have been associated with CF, or a variant CF phenotype.[102]

A functional classification system organized according to the molecular, cellular, and physiological consequences of *CFTR* mutations has been developed to help make a connection between the genetic defect and the phenotype in CF.[103,104] Class I mutations are those predicted to result in defective protein synthesis and these include nonsense, frameshift, and splice site mutations that result in nonsense-mediated decay due to the introduction of a premature termination codon. Class II mutations are those that affect abnormal processing and trafficking of the CFTR protein. These include mutations such as ΔF508 that produce proteins that are misfolded and degraded instead of trafficking to the apical membrane. Class III and IV mutations create proteins that are inserted into the apical membrane. However, the former class has defective regulation, whereas the latter class exhibits decreased chloride conductance. Class V mutations are generally mild mutations with reduced (but not complete loss of) synthesis and trafficking. Examples of mutations from this class included leaky splice site mutations

and missense mutations that diminish proper trafficking of the protein. A number of amino acid substitutions have been shown to have effects upon several functions of CFTR thus making it difficult to assign these alterations to a particular class.

The CF phenotype can vary according to the types of organ systems involved and in the severity of disease within an organ system.[2] After identification of the *CFTR* gene, numerous studies attempted to correlate *CFTR* mutations with particular CF phenotypes.[48,105–108] However, the large number of low frequency mutations in the *CFTR* gene, and the extreme variability of the CF phenotype, have hindered the ability to detect genotype–phenotype correlations for most of the specific mutations. Grouping mutations according to specific functional classes using the above system has revealed that only a subset of features that constitute the CF phenotype are correlated with CFTR function.

Phenotypes affecting the gastrointestinal tract are strongly correlated with the severity of the *CFTR* defect.[7,8] Approximately 85 percent of CF patients have pancreatic exocrine impairment. Nearly all of these patients have mutations in the *CFTR* gene that are predicted to result in complete loss of protein function.[2,109] Examples of these mutations are those found in class I, II, and III. In light of this observation, mutations that are definitively associated with pancreatic insufficiency have been classified as 'severe mutations,' even in the absence of empirical data regarding the molecular consequence of the mutation. Conversely, mutations that are associated with pancreatic sufficiency are typically regarded as 'mild' mutations. Ultimately, the correlation of pancreatic insufficiency with mutations that have severe loss of function suggests that the exocrine pancreas is relatively resilient to mild reductions in CFTR function. Furthermore, because pancreatic insufficiency requires such a drastic reduction in CFTR function, it is commonly associated with severe disease in many of the other organ systems.[7] Less common phenotypes of the GI tract including diabetes mellitus, meconium ileus, liver disease, and distal intestinal obstructive syndrome (DIOS) are also associated with severe loss of CFTR function.[2,109] However, it is unclear to what extent these mutations are directly due to a reduction in CFTR function, or simply a secondary product of pancreatic insufficiency.

By far the most important and variable phenotype in CF is the pulmonary phenotype. Factors such as age of infection with bacterial pathogens, degree of bronchiectasis, and rate of pulmonary decline are highly variable between patients.[105] In fact, it has been shown that the severity of pulmonary disease in CF can vary between individuals from the same family with the same *CFTR* mutations.[105,110] Thus, it is not surprising that there is no clear relationship between *CFTR* genotype and pulmonary disease. Comparisons of pulmonary disease status among patients homozygous for the most common and severe *CFTR* mutation, ΔF508, reveal significant variability that is apparently due to factors other than CFTR.[105,111] These observations have fueled many groups to begin searching for genetic (e.g., modifier genes) and environmental factors that influence the severity of pulmonary disease (e.g., infectious exposure, access to treatment, nutrition etc.).[112,113]

There are several examples of specific mutations being associated with less severe lung disease. For example, patients with the mutation A455E have better pulmonary function than age, center, and sex-matched $\Delta$F508 homozygotes.[114,115] Furthermore, the degree of pulmonary disease and obstruction as measured by $FEV_1$, and infection rates with *P. aeruginosa* are significantly lower in patients with mutations in class IV or V.[10,111,116] Nevertheless, mutations in class IV and V account for a small fraction of the total CF causing alleles, and thus cannot account for the majority of the variation in CF pulmonary disease seen in CF.

Sweat chloride concentrations have been shown to vary slightly between patients with class IV and V mutations versus other CF patients.[117] In addition, relationships between genotype and sweat gland pathology have been identified. Two mutations in the *CFTR* gene (D1152H and 3849 + 10KB C $\rightarrow$ T) have been found in individuals with CF lung disease and normal sweat chloride concentrations.[48,87] These examples provided the first evidence that indicators of sweat gland pathology are not always found in individuals with CF-lung disease due to CFTR dysfunction. These observations expanded the definition of the CF phenotype. Conversely, Mickle et al.[99] described a family with two members who were compound heterozygous for a classic CF-causing mutation and the novel nonsense mutation S1455X. These individuals were clinically healthy, but had diagnostically elevated sweat chloride concentration. Further studies of this mutation have revealed that the nonsense mutation resulted in a stable, truncated protein that lacks a critical C-terminal region required for specific trafficking to the apical membrane. Additional studies of CFTR containing the S1455X mutation have begun to elucidate the cellular mechanism underlying the highly specific trafficking of CFTR to the apical membrane.[118]

As mentioned previously, dysfunction of the *CFTR* gene has been cited as a cause of many disorders that are limited to a single organ system. The majority of mutations in these patients have been splice site and missense mutations in functional classes IV and V.[94,119] Interestingly, many mutations that have been first identified in patients with single organ system dysfunction, have also been seen in patients with nonclassic forms of CF and vice versa. The 5T is an example of a mutation that was initially identified to be disease associated in men with congenital absence of the vas,[92,93] and was later shown to also be associated with nonclassic forms of CF.[80,120,121] Currently, the factors that influence variable expressivity of these mild mutations remain unclear.

## ANIMAL MODELS

Cloning of the CFTR gene enabled the creation of mice with absent or dysfunctional CFTR as a means to better understand disease pathogenesis and to test new therapies for CF. Numerous mouse models have been created using knock-out technology that disrupt the coding sequence of *CFTR*,[122–124] and knock-in technology to introduce specific mutations that are known to cause disease in humans.[125–128] Both knock-out and knock-in mutation disease models mimic the physiologic defects seen in humans, as demonstrated by excessive sodium absorption and reduced chloride excretion across the luminal membranes of the intestines and the airways.[129] Thus, CF mice provide a useful model to test therapies aimed at correction of the electrolyte transport defect.[130]

While CF mouse models exhibit defects at the cellular level that are similar to human CF patients, the clinical phenotypes differ considerably. A common phenotype seen in the majority of mouse models for CF is severe obstruction of the distal intestine, leading to intestinal perforation and death (approximately 50–95 percent).[122] Survival can be improved by keeping mice on liquid diets that ultimately minimize the potential for lethal complications due to intestinal obstructions. CF mice do not exhibit the severe, life-limiting lung disease seen in humans with CF.[123,131] However, pathologic changes similar to that seen in humans with CF are observed in the lungs, GI tract, and vas deferens of older CF mice.[132] In addition, CF mice appear to have difficulties clearing bacterial infections after repeated exposure to bacteria isolated from human CF patients.[133–135] At this time, it is not clear to what extent experimental exposure to pathogens will lead to the destructive inflammation that ultimately leads to pulmonary insufficiency in humans with CF. Recent studies suggest that alternate approaches may produce chronic infection models that more accurately represent the human situation.[133,136] Finally, an entirely different molecular approach appears to have created an obstructive pulmonary phenotype that more convincingly mimics human CF pulmonary pathophysiology. Instead of altering CFTR expression, investigators overexpressed different subunits of the epithelial sodium channel (ENaC). Mice with increased expression of the beta subunit manifest sodium hyperabsorption in the airways that resulted in altered mucus viscosity and clearance leading to severe obstructive lung disease.[137] This study suggests that mice may have a different balance of chloride secretion to sodium absorption than humans, but that recreating the imbalance observed in humans with CF produces a similar clinical disease.

The differences in phenotypic outcome between mice and humans with absent functional CFTR are likely to be due to genetic and environmental differences. For example, CF mice have been shown to have alternative modes of chloride transport in the airways that are more active than in humans.[138] Identification and modulation of these alternate pathways may reveal viable therapeutic avenues in humans. Deciphering the factors underlying the differences in disease expression between strains of mice may also unveil genetic modifiers of disease pathogenesis. Variation in the survival of CF mice due to different levels of intestinal obstruction among strains have aided researchers in identifying a potential genetic factor on mouse chromosome 7 that ameliorates the intestinal phenotype.[11] Studies of differences in lung disease severity between different strains are ongoing[139,140] and may reveal unforeseen pathways that modulate disease. Ultimately, discovery of these pathways may lead to a better understanding of the phenotypic diversity seen in patients with CF.

## MODIFIER STUDIES IN HUMANS

The lack of complete correlation between CFTR genotype and severity of organ disease suggests a role for modifying factors. These factors may be genetic and consist of gene variants that manifest as functional differences in proteins involved, in some manner, with CF pathophysiology. Alternatively, factors in the environment can lead to considerable differences in outcome. Finally, stochastic effects can influence disease severity in a manner that is often very difficult to ascertain. Despite the challenges posed by searches for modifier effects, our understanding of CF at the molecular level and the sequencing of the human genome provide an infrastructure for evaluating genetic factors other than CFTR that contribute to phenotype variation. Furthermore, several observations indicate that disease severity, even the CF phenotype, can be attributed to factors separate from CFTR.[80,89,141]

The study of related affected individuals can provide insight into the relative impact of gene sharing upon disease outcome. In an analysis of a small number of affected twins and siblings, Santis and coworkers suggested that genetic factors were more important than nongenetic factors in determining lung and pancreatic disease severity.[142,143] The European CF Twin and Sibling Study concluded that dizygous (DZ) twins had greater differences in lung function as measured by $FEV_1$ percent predicted corrected for patient age than monozygous twins (MZ).[144] Since DZ twins share 50 percent of genes while MZ twins share 100 percent, this observation supported a role for genetic factors independent of CFTR in differences in lung disease severity. In addition, the European group has found evidence that a region near the CFTR gene may contribute to differences in nutritional status[145] and that the magnitude of chloride secretion was more similar in MZ compared to DZ twins.[9,146] Finally, investigators in Toronto utilized evolutionary similarity between human chromosome 19 and the region of mouse chromosome 7 that contains a modifier for intestinal obstruction in CF mice to demonstrate that the human chromosome appears to contain one or more genes that contribute to meconium ileus.[12] The precise genes involved have not yet been identified.

The availability of considerable information regarding CF pathophysiology has encouraged investigators to search for modifier effects among candidate genes. For the most part, these genes encode proteins that either interact with CFTR or are involved in innate immunity or inflammatory responses (see Table 11.1). However, most association studies have not been repeated in different populations. Exceptions include the $\alpha_1$-antitrypsin gene ($\alpha_1$-AT; also known as SERPINA1 in HUGO nomenclature) and mannose binding lectin (MBL2). The $\alpha_1$-AT gene encodes a serine proteinase inhibitor that regulates the activity of proteinases that are abundant in the CF lung. Since functional variants of $\alpha_1$-AT are relatively common in the Caucasian population, it was reasonable to postulate that this gene might alter pulmonary disease severity.[147] However, the results have been quite mixed with some reports concluding that $\alpha_1$-AT deficiency is associated with milder rather than more severe lung disease[148–150] while the study with the largest number of patients to date found no association with lung disease severity.[151]

On the other hand, there appears to be some consensus that a common variant in mannose binding lectin is associated with worse outcome for CF patients.[13,152,153] Three independent amino acid substitutions termed $B$ (glycine to aspartic acid at codon 54), $C$ (glycine to glutamic acid at codon 57), and $D$ (arginine to cysteine at codon 52) occur in exon 1 of MBL2 at considerably different frequencies among human populations.[154,155] These three variants have collectively been designated as $O$ alleles while the wildtype is termed $A$. Each of the three structural variants act in a dominant negative fashion to reduce the amount of functional MBL multimers in heterozygous ($A/O$) individuals, whereas primarily nonfunctional monomeric forms of MBL are found in the plasma of homozygous ($O/O$) individuals.[154,156–158] Single nucleotide variants in the promoter of MBL2 (e.g., $X$ and $Y$) have been identified that reduce the levels of structurally normal forms of MBL.[159,160] MBL is a member of the collectin protein family that share common structural features such as a collagenous N-terminal domain and a C-terminal region that can bind with carbohydrate shells of various infectious organisms.[154] MBL binding of bacteria and viruses facilitates activation of the complement pathway although the mechanism is unclear.[161] While low levels of functional forms of MBL may predispose some individuals to infections, it appears that a coexisting defect in host defense is necessary to expose compromised innate defense due to MBL deficiency.[154] Abnormal fluid and electrolyte transport in CF leads to a compromise of primary defense mechanisms in the lungs (e.g., ciliary clearance) that is believed to be the antecedent to chronic bacterial infection. Thus, deficiency of functional multimeric forms of MBL or excess of monomeric forms of MBL could affect disease severity in CF patients by altering the innate immunity or the inflammatory response. Various other components of inflammatory pathways important for the lungs have been implicated but not definitively confirmed as modifiers for CF (Table 11.1).

**Table 11.1** Modifier genes typed in CF patients

| Candidate gene | Variant(s) | Variant effect | Genotype groups compared and (n) | Phenotype association | Ref. |
|---|---|---|---|---|---|
| Alpha 1 AT | S, Z | Reduced serum alpha1 AT levels | MS(12), MZ(9), MM(137) | NS for $FEV_1$ | 147 |
| | | | MS(9), MZ(8), MM(102) | Earlier onset of Pseudomonas aeruginosa infection, higher total IgG and P.a. specific IgG antibodies for MS and MZ | 147 |
| | | | MS(16), SS(1), MZ(3), MM(127) | Higher $FEV_1$ for MS, SS and MZ; NS for Pa | 148 |
| | | | MS(4), MZ(2), MM(73) | No increase in variants in transplanted (72) or deceased (7) patients | 149 |
| | 1237A/G | Unknown | G/A(16), G/G(108) | Higher chest X-ray score; fewer colonized with Pa fro G/A; NS for $FEV_1$ | 150 |
| | S, Z, 1237G/A | As above | MS(69), SS(13), MZ(18), MM(616) G/A(95), A/A(7), G/G (610) | NS for $FEV_1$, frequency of P. aeruginosa colonization, age of P. aeruginosa colonization and vital status | 151 |
| Alpha 1-anti-chymotrypsin | | Reduced serum levels | 10 deficient versus 147 normal | Higher $FEV_1$ and fewer colonized with P. aeruginosa for deficient patients | 194 |
| Beta 2-adrenergic receptor | Arg16Gly | Gly16 allele confers enhanced down-regulation | CF: Arg16/Arg16 (32), Arg16/Gly16 or Gly16/Gly16 (55) | Lower $FEV_1$, FVC, $MEF_{50\%V/C}$, and greater 5 year decline in $FEV_1$ associated with at least one Gly16 allele | 195 |
| Glutathione S-transferase M1 | GSTM1-0 ($\approx$10 kb deletion) | Absent GSTM1 mRNA | CF children: 0/0 (26), normal/0 or normal/normal (27) | Higher chest Xray score (Chrispin-Norman) and lower Shwachman score associated with 0/0 | 196 |
| HLA class II | DR4, DR7 and DR7/DQA*0201 | Association with IgE response | Adult CF (97), Non-atopic controls (39) | Higher frequency of DR4, DR7 and DR7/DQA*0201 alleles in CF patients | 197 |
| | DR7 | | Adult CF: DR7+ (26), DR7− (60) | Higher IgE and higher rate of P. aeruginosa colonization associated with DR7+ | 197 |
| Mannose binding lectin | '0' alleles (B, C and D); X-A promoter variant | Reduced serum level of functional multimer, 0 alleles only: increased level of non-functional monomer | 0/0 (4), X-A/0 (15) A/0 (48), A/A (94) | Lower FEV1 and higher frequency of Burkholderia cepacia in 0/0 and X-A/0; reduced survival for A/0 and 0/0 | 13 |
| | | | A/A (11), A/0 or 0/0 (11); age-, sex- and center-matched A/A (60), A/0, X-A/0, X-A/X-A or 0/0 (53) | Lower $FEV_1$ for A/0 and 0/0 | 152 |
| Nitric oxide synthase 1 | (GT)n in 5'UT | >27 GT repeats associated with higher exhaled NO | 16 with none, 24 with one and 19 with both alleles >27 repeats | Fewer A/0 and 0/0 patients with $FEV_1$ > 90% | 153 |
| | (AAT)n in intron 20 | >12 AAT repeats associated with lower exhaled NO | 28 with at least one and 12 with two alleles ≥12 repeats | Lower annual rate of $FEV_1$ decline with both alleles >27 repeats | 198 |
| Nitric oxide synthase 3 | 894G/T | T allele associated with higher exhaled NO in females only | G/G (29), G/T (35), T/T (6) | Higher P. aeruginosa colonization rate with both alleles ≥ 12 repeats | 199 |
| Tumor necrosis factor-alpha | −308G/A | A allele associated with higher levels of transcription | CF children: G/G (33), G/A (20) | Lower P. aeruginosa colonization rate in females with T allele | 200 |
| Transforming growth factor beta 1 | 869T/C (L10P) | C allele associated with lower synthesis | Controls: T/T (44), C/T (51), C/C (12) CF: T/T(67), C/T (90), C/C (14) | Lower $FEV_1$ % predicted associated with G/A genotype | 196 |
| | | | Controls: G/G (87), G/G (19), C/C (1) | $FEV_1$ < 50% predicted and FVC < 70% predicted associated with 869T | 201 |
| | 915G/C (R25P) | C allele associated with lower synthesis | CF: G/G (149), G/C (21), C/C (1) | NS for $FEV_1$ % predicted and FVC | 201 |

## DISEASE MANAGEMENT/FUTURE DEVELOPMENTS

Therapy for CF continues to be aimed at the treatment of symptoms.[2] The identification of the *CFTR* gene raised the possibility that therapies could be devised to ameliorate or circumvent the disease process at the molecular level. Indeed, a number of approaches appeared feasible based upon in vitro or animal studies but have not proven to be efficacious at the clinical level. One example is the use of agonists of the adenylate cyclase/protein kinase A pathway to increase the activity of mutant CFTR.[162,163] Despite impressive effects in CF airway cell lines and nasal epithelium of CF mice, humans with CF did not generate appreciable chloride secretion in response to these agents.[164,165] One of the hurdles faced by molecular based therapy is the need to tailor treatment to the specific defect. Thus, misfolding of CFTR caused by the ΔF508 mutation may require a different approach than loss of CFTR synthesis due to a nonsense mutation.[166] Mutation-specific therapies are currently under development.[167,168]

Correction of the CFTR defect by providing a working copy of the protein has been an attractive yet elusive goal. Gene therapy using a variety of vectors, both viral and nonviral, has been extensively investigated for applications in CF.[169] Currently, the adeno-associated virus (AAV) has the most favorable attributes for gene transfer to pulmonary epithelia. While AAV appears safe, efficacy of gene expression is suboptimal.[170–172] Although the concept of gene replacement remains sound in principle, a number of technical and biological hurdles remain.[173] Eventually, correction of endogenous *CFTR* genes using short DNA sequences transferred to lung epithelia by nonbiologic vectors, may provide the highest safety and greatest efficacy.[174]

## OTHER GENETIC CAUSES OF BRONCHIECTASIS

Primary ciliary dyskinesia (PCD) is a genetically heterogeneous group of disorders, also known as immotile cilia syndrome, that manifest as abnormalities of motile cilia. The condition is estimated to affect 1 in 20 000 to 1 in 60 000 individuals.[175] Motile cilia are found on respiratory airway cells, ependymal cells lining the ventricles of the brain and spinal cord, and ciliated cells of the Fallopian tubes and spermatozoa. Loss of cilia function creates a clinical syndrome characterized by sinusitis, bronchiectasis, male fertility, and reduced female fertility.[176] Since motile cilia play a key role in left–right axis determination in early development, approximately 50 percent of patients with PCD have *situs inversus* (Kartagener syndrome) due to randomization of the left–right axis.[177] In the absence of *situs inversus*, PCD can be challenging to differentiate from other causes of bronchitis in childhood.[176] Persistence of a productive cough, chronic otitis media, and chronic rhinosinusitis in the absence of polyps, are suggestive clinical features. Since many cases of PCD appear to be due to recessive genetic defects,[178]

careful evaluation of siblings is warranted. Exclusion of a cystic fibrosis diagnosis may require extensive study of ion transport as CF patients who do not manifest pancreatic insufficiency can have a number of clinical features that overlap with PCD including familial recurrence. A sweat chloride concentration less than 40 mmol/L would reduce the likelihood of a CFTR defect. However, patients with repeated measurements in the borderline range (40–60 mmol/L) should be investigated further by nasal potential difference measurement and *CFTR* gene analysis. Cilia function can be assessed by the saccharine test in the compliant patient, while functional and structural studies of the cilia require expertise available in specialized laboratories.[176]

Proper function of motile cilia is believed to involve the function of over 250 proteins.[179] The identification of proteins involved in formation and function of the two flagella of the unicellular algae *Chylamydomonas reinhardtii* has provided numerous candidate genes for study in human cases of PCD.[179] However, only two genes have been identified as definitively causative of PCD so far. DNAI1 that encodes dynein intermediate chain type 1, was found to be mutated in a patient with PCD due to missing outer dynein arms.[180] Several other PCD patients have since been reported with mutations in this gene.[179] The second gene, DNAH5 encoding axonemal heavy chain 5, was implicated by linkage analysis followed by candidate gene sequencing.[181] Eight families segregating PCD were found to have mutations in each DNAH5 gene, while two families had a mutation identified in one DNAH5 gene. A third gene, DNAH11 encoding a heavy dynein chain β, has been implicated in a patient with CF and PCD.[182] The study of cilia function in murine models by selected elimination of proteins known to constitute cilia, or to contribute to cilia function, by gene knock-out is also providing considerable insight into role of specific components.[183,184] The availability of the complete human genome sequence will facilitate cross-species analysis that will likely lead to discovery of additional genes responsible for human forms of PCD.[179]

## YOUNG SYNDROME

The combination of chronic rhinosinusitis, pulmonary disease, and male infertility is common to CF and PCD. Young syndrome is a third inherited condition with similar clinical features that is distinguished from the other two based on the nature of the reproductive tract lesion and the absence of cilia abnormalities or CFTR dysfunction. The existence of a separate disorder involving obstructive azoospermia and sinopulmonary disease was first recognized by Young in 1970.[185] He noted that 54 percent of males with infertility due to a defect in the epididymis had evidence of pulmonary disease ranging from long-standing bronchitis to bronchiectasis requiring surgery. Subsequent reports indicated that this form of infertility was frequent among men with obstructive azoospermia. Furthermore, proven fertility of some males with Young syndrome led to the suggestion that the epididymal obstruction was progressive in nature rather than the result of a congenital malformation.[186] Lung disease manifests as persistent cough and sputum production with recurrent pulmonary infection in childhood. Symptoms decrease markedly in adulthood although radiologic evidence of bronchiectasis persists in most patients.[186] Pulmonary function in adults appears minimally impaired as does exercise tolerance.

The etiology of Young syndrome is unknown. Ultrastructural studies of cilia have not identified a specific defect, however, the reports of reduced inner dynein arms of respiratory cilia of identical twins, and a patient with Young syndrome and *situs inversus* suggests that cilia dysfunction may be involved.[187,188] Normal sperm motility and evidence of sperm transport beyond ciliated regions of the male reproductive tract usually differentiates Young syndrome from disorders of cilia motility.[186,189] Lack of progressive lung disease, exocrine pancreatic disease, and normal concentrations of sweat chloride distinguishes this condition clinically from cystic fibrosis. Furthermore, the presence of normally formed derivatives of the Wolffian duct (e.g., vas deferens) excludes atypical forms of CF and congenital bilateral absence of the vas deferens. Finally, genetic studies have failed to confirm an increased frequency of CF mutations among men with Young syndrome.[190,191]

A genetic origin for Young syndrome has been suggested on the basis of familial clustering. Two sets of affected twins (one identical, one fraternal) have been reported.[187,192] There have also been anecdotal reports of sinopulmonary problems among family members of a fraction of affected individuals. From these observations, an autosomal recessive form of inheritance has been proposed.[178] However, formal studies to examine inheritance patterns, and to evaluate the causes of sinopulmonary problems in siblings of patients with Young syndrome, have not been reported. The proposal that mercury poisoning from teething powders and worm medication may have played a role in Young syndrome raises the possibility of multiple etiologies.[193]

---

## Key learning points

- Cystic fibrosis (CF) is caused by mutations in the CF transmembrane conductance regulator (CFTR).

- CFTR resides at the apical membranes of epithelial cells lining the airways and pancreatic ducts, and functions as a cAMP-regulated chloride channel and as a regulator of other ion channels.

- Loss of CFTR function results in abnormal ion and fluid movement in the lungs and pancreas causing progressive destruction of both organs.

- CF is a highly variable disorder and variation in CFTR genotype correlates with severity of pancreatic disease but not severity of lung disease.

- Factors other than CFTR genotype play a major role in the progression of the pulmonary phenotype.

- Therapy of CF in the future will be directed at the underlying defect in CFTR and at non-CFTR factors (modifier genes, environment) shown to influence outcome.

## ACKNOWLEDGEMENT

This work was supported by grants from the National Heart, Lung and Blood Institute (HL 68927) and National Institutes of Diabetes, Digestive and Kidney Diseases (DK 44003).

## REFERENCES

1 Hamosh A, Fitzsimmons S, Macek M Jr et al. Comparison of the clinical manifestations of cystic fibrosis in black and white patients. *J Pediatr* 1998; **132**: 255–9.

◆2 Welsh MJ, Ramsey BW, Accurso FJ et al. (eds). *The metabolic and molecular bases of inherited disease.* New York: McGraw-Hill, Inc., 2001: 5121–88.

3 Cystic Fibrosis Foundation. Cystic Fibrosis Foundation Patient Registry Annual Data Report 2001. 9-1-2002.

●4 Rommens JM, Iannuzzi MC, Kerem B et al. Identification of the cystic fibrosis gene: chromosome walking and jumping. *Science* 1989; **245**: 1059–65.

●5 Riordan JR, Rommens JM, Kerem B et al. Identification of the cystic fibrosis gene: cloning and characterization of complementary DNA. *Science* 1989; **245**: 1066–73.

●6 Kerem B, Rommens JM, Buchanan JA et al. Identification of the cystic fibrosis gene: genetic analysis. *Science* 1989; **245**: 1073–80.

7 Kerem E, Corey M, Kerem B-S et al. The relation between genotype and phenotype in cystic fibrosis – analysis of the most common mutation (deltaF508). *N Engl J Med* 1990; **323**: 1517–22.

8 Kristidis P, Bozon D, Corey M et al. Genetic determination of exocrine pancreatic function in cystic fibrosis. *Am J Hum Genet* 1992; **50**: 1178–84.

9 Bronsveld I, Mekus F, Bijman J et al. Residual chloride secretion in intestinal tissue of deltaF508 homozygous twins and siblings with cystic fibrosis. The European CF Twin and Sibling Study Consortium. *Gastroenterology* 2000; **119**: 32–40.

10 McKone EF, Emerson SS, Edwards KL, Aitken ML. Effect of genotype on phenotype and mortality in cystic fibrosis: a retrospective cohort study. *Lancet* 2003; **361**: 1671–6.

●11 Rozmahel R, Wilschanski M, Matin A et al. Modulation of disease severity in cystic fibrosis transmembrane conductance regulator deficient mice by a secondary genetic factor. *Nature Genet* 1996; **12**: 280–7.

12 Zielenski J, Corey M, Rozmahel R et al. Detection of a cystic fibrosis modifier locus for meconium ileus on human chromosome 19q13. *Nature Genet* 1999; **22**: 128–9.

13 Garred P, Pressler T, Madsen HO et al. Association of mannose-binding lectin gene heterogeneity with severity

of lung disease and survival in cystic fibrosis. *J Clin Invest* 1999; **104**: 431–437.

14  Quinton PM. Physiological basis of cystic fibrosis: a historical perspective. *Physiol Rev* 1999; **79**(1 Suppl): S3–S22.

15  Gibson RL, Burns JL, Ramsey BW. Pathophysiology and management of pulmonary infections in cystic fibrosis. *Am J Respir Crit Care Med* 2003; **168**: 918–51.

◆16  Cutting GR. *Cystic fibrosis. Emery and Rimon's principles and practice of medical genetics*, 4th edn. London: Churchill-Livingstone, 2001.

17  Taccetti G, Procopio E, Marianelli L, Campana S. Allergic bronchopulmonary aspergillosis in Italian cystic fibrosis patients: prevalence and percentage of positive tests in the employed diagnostic criteria. *Eur J Epidemiol* 2000; **16**: 837–42.

18  Mastella G, Rainisio M, Harms HK et al. Allergic broncho-pulmonary aspergillosis in cystic fibrosis. A European epidemiological study. Epidemiologic Registry of Cystic Fibrosis. *Eur Respir J* 2000; **16**: 464–71.

19  Olivier KN, Weber DJ, Wallace RJ Jr et al. Nontuberculous mycobacteria. I: multicenter prevalence study in cystic fibrosis. *Am J Respir Crit Care Med* 2003; **167**: 828–34.

20  Abman SH, Ogle JW, Harbeck RJ et al. Early bacteriologic, immunologic, and clinical courses of young infants with cystic fibrosis identified by neonatal screening. *J Pediatr* 1991; **119**: 211–217.

21  Kerem E, Corey M, Gold R, Levison H. Pulmonary function and clinical course in patients with CF after pulmonary colonization with *Pseudomonas aeruginosa*. *J Pediatr* 1990; **116**: 714–19.

●22  Drenkard E, Ausubel FM. Pseudomonas biofilm formation and antibiotic resistance are linked to phenotypic variation. *Nature* 2002; **416**: 740–3.

●23  Mah TF, Pitts B, Pellock B et al. A genetic basis for *Pseudomonas aeruginosa* biofilm antibiotic resistance. *Nature* 2003; **426**: 306–10.

◆24  Pilewski JM, Frizzell RA. Role of CFTR in airway disease. *Physiol Rev* 1999; **79** (1 Suppl): S215–S255.

25  Rosenfeld M, Gibson RL, McNamara S et al. Early pulmonary infection, inflammation, and clinical outcomes in infants with cystic fibrosis. *Pediatr Pulmonol* 2001; **32**: 356–366.

26  Khan TZ, Wagener JS, Bost T. Early pulmonary inflammation in infants with cystic fibrosis. *Am J Respir Cell Mol Biol* 1995; **151**: 1075–1082.

27  Muhlebach MS, Stewart PW, Leigh MW, Noah TL. Quantitation of inflammatory responses to bacteria in young cystic fibrosis and control patients. *Am J Respir Crit Care Med* 1999; **160**: 186–191.

28  Cutting GR. Genetics of rhinosinusitis. In: Kennedy DW, Zinreich SJ (eds) *Diseases of the sinuses: diagnostic and endoscopic management*. Hamilton, ON: BC Decker, 2000.

29  Gysin C, Alothman GA, Papsin BC. Sinonasal disease in cystic fibrosis: clinical characteristics, diagnosis, and management. *Pediatr Pulmonol* 2000; **30**: 481–9.

30  Nishioka GJ, Cook PR, McKinsey JP, Rodriguez FJ. Paranasal sinus computed tomography scan findings in patients with cystic fibrosis. *Otolaryngol Head Neck Surg* 1996; **114**: 394–9.

31  Sullivan WB, Linehan AT, Hilman BC et al. Flexible fiberoptic rhinoscopy in the diagnosis of nasal polyps in cystic fibrosis. *Allergy Asthma Proc* 1996; **17**: 287–92.

32  Ahmed N, Corey M, Forstner G et al. Molecular consequences of cystic fibrosis transmembrane regulator (CFTR) gene mutations in the exocrine pancreas. *Gut* 2003; **52**: 1159–64.

33  Cystic Fibrosis Foundation. Cystic Fibrosis Foundation Patient Registry Annual Data Report – 1998.

34  Shwachman H, Lebenthal E, Khaw KT. Recurrent acute pancreatitis in patients with cystic fibrosis with normal pancreatic enzymes. *Pediatrics* 1975; **55**: 86.

35  Scott-Jupp R, Lama M, Tanner MS. Prevalence of liver disease in cystic fibrosis. *Arch Dis Child* 1991; **66**: 698–701.

36  di Sant 'Agnese PA, Hubbard VA. The hepatobiliary system. In: Taussig LM (ed.) *Cystic fibrosis*. New York: Thieme Stratton, 1984: 296–322.

37  Colombo C, Battezzati PM, Crosignani A et al. Liver disease in cystic fibrosis: A prospective study on incidence, risk factors, and outcome. *Hepatology* 2002; **36**: 1374–82.

38  Wilschanski M, Rivlin J, Cohen S et al. Clinical and genetic risk factors for cystic fibrosis-related liver disease. *Pediatrics* 1999; **103**: 52–7.

39  Dodge JA. Male fertility in cystic fibrosis. *Lancet* 1995; **346**: 587–8.

40  Liu J, Lissens W, Silber SJ et al. Birth after preimplantation diagnosis of the cystic fibrosis deltaF508 mutation by polymerase chain reaction in human embryos resulting from intracytoplasmic sperm injection with epididymal sperm. *J Am Med Assoc* 1994; **272**: 1858–60.

41  Mak V, Jarvi K, Zielenski J et al. Higher proportion of intact exon 9 CFTR MRNA in nasal epithelium compared with vas deferens. *Hum Mol Genet* 1997; **6**: 2099–107.

42  Kessler WR, Andersen DH. Heat prostration in fibrocystic disease of the pancreas and other condition. *Pediatrics* 1951; **8**: 648.

●43  di Sant 'Agnese PA, Darling RC, Perera GA, Shea E. Abnormal electrolyte composition of sweat in cystic fibrosis of the pancreas. *Pediatrics* 1953; **12**: 549–63.

✳44  Gibson LE, Cooke RE. A test for concentration of electrolytes in sweat in cystic fibrosis of the pancreas utilizing pilocarpine by iontophoresis. *Pediatrics* 1959; **23**: 545–9.

45  Farrell PM, Koscik RE. Sweat chloride concentrations in infants homozygous or heterozygous for $F_{508}$ cystic fibrosis. *Pediatrics* 1996; **97**: 524–8.

46  Augarten A, Kerem B-S, Yahav Y et al. Mild cystic fibrosis and normal or borderline sweat test in patients with the 3849 + 10 kb C → T mutation. *Lancet* 1993; **342**: 25–6.

47  Stewart B, Zabner J, Shuber AP et al. Normal sweat chloride values do not exclude the diagnosis of cystic fibrosis. *Am J Respir Crit Care Med* 1995; **151**: 899–903.

●48  Highsmith WE Jr, Burch LH, Zhou Z et al. A novel mutation in the cystic fibrosis gene in patients with pulmonary disease but normal sweat chloride concentrations. *N Engl J Med* 1994; **331**: 974–80.

49  Hughes D, Dork T, Stuhrmann M, Graham C. Mutation and haplotype analysis of the CFTR gene in atypically mild cystic fibrosis patients from Northern Ireland. *J Med Genet* 2001; **38**: 136–9.

50  Desmarquest P, Feldmann D, Tamalat A et al. Genotype analysis and phenotypic manifestations of children with intermediate sweat chloride test results. *Chest* 2000; **118**: 1591–7.

51  Feldmann D, Couderc R, Audrezet MP et al. CFTR genotypes in patients with normal or borderline sweat chloride levels. *Hum Mutat* 2003; **22**: 340.

●52   Quinton PM. Chloride impermeability in cystic fibrosis. *Nature (London)* 1983; **301**: 421–2.

●53   Quinton PM, Bijman J. Higher bioelectric potentials due to decreased chloride absorption in the sweat glands of patients with cystic fibrosis. *N Engl J Med* 1983; **308**: 1185–9.

●54   Sato K, Sato F. Defective beta-adrenergic response of cystic fibrosis sweat glands in vivo and in vitro. *J Clin Invest* 1984; **73**: 1763–71.

55   Callen A, Diener-West M, Zeitlin PL, Rubenstein RC. A simplified cyclic adenosine monophosphate-mediated sweat rate test for quantitative measure of cystic fibrosis transmembrane regulator (CFTR) function. *J Pediatr* 2000; **137**: 849–55.

●56   Andersen DH. Progress in pediatrics. *Am J Dis Child* 1936; **56**: 344–99.

57   Romeo G, Bianco M, Devoto M et al. Incidence in Italy, genetic heterogeneity and segregation analysis of cystic fibrosis. *Am J Hum Genet* 1985; **37**: 338–49.

58   Eiberg H, Mohr J, Schmiegelow K et al. Linkage relationships of paraoxonase (PON) with other markers: Indication of PON-cystic fibrosis synteny. *Clin Genet* 1985; **28**: 265–71.

59   Beaudet AL, Bowcock A, Buchwald M et al. Linkage of cystic fibrosis to two tightly linked DNA markers: Joint report from a collaborative study. *Am J Hum Genet* 1986; **39**: 681–93.

60   Lathrop GM, Farrall M, O'Connell P et al. Refined linkage map of chromosome 7 in the region of the cystic fibrosis gene. *Am J Hum Genet* 1988; **42**: 38–44.

61   Estivill X, Farrall M, Williamson R et al. Linkage disequilibrium between cystic fibrosis and linked DNA polymoorphisms in Italian families: A collaborative study. *Am J Med Genet* 1988; **43**: 23–8.

62   Chang X-B, Hou Y-X, Jensen TJ, Riordan JR. Mapping of cystic fibrosis transmembrane conductance regulator membrane topology by glycosylation site insertion. *J Biol Chem* 1994; **269**: 18572–5.

63   Drumm ML, Pope HA, Cliff WH et al. Correction of the cystic fibrosis defect in vitro by retrovirus-mediated gene transfer. *Cell* 1990; **62**: 1227–33.

64   Fulmer SB, Schwiebert EM, Morales MM et al. Two cystic fibrosis transmembrane conductance regulator mutations have different effects on both pulmonary phenotype and regulation of outwardly rectified chloride currents. *Proc Natl Acad Sci USA* 1995; **92**: 6832–6.

65   Wang XF, Zhou CX, Shi QX et al. Involvement of CFTR in uterine bicarbonate secretion and the fertilizing capacity of sperm. *Nat Cell Biol* 2003; **5**: 902–6.

66   Choi JY, Muallem D, Kiselyov K et al. Aberrant CFTR-dependent HCO3-transport in mutations associated with cystic fibrosis. *Nature* 2001; **410**: 94–7.

67   Tate S, MacGregor G, Davis M et al. Airways in cystic fibrosis are acidified: detection by exhaled breath condensate. *Thorax* 2002; **57**: 926–9.

68   Schwiebert EM, Egan ME, Hwang T-H et al. CFTR regulates outwardly rectifying chloride channels through an autocrine mechanism involving ATP. *Cell* 1995; **81**: 1–20.

◆69   Guggino WB. Cystic fibrosis and the salt controversy. *Cell* 1999; **96**: 607–10.

◆70   Wine JJ. The genesis of cystic fibrosis lung disease. *J Clin Invest* 1999; **103**: 309–12.

✳71   Rosenstein BJ, Cutting GR. The diagnosis of cystic fibrosis: A consensus statement. *J Pediatr* 1998; **132**: 589–95.

72   Rosenstein BJ. Cystic fibrosis diagnosis: new dilemmas for an old disorder. *Pediatr Pulmonol* 2002; **33**: 83–4.

✳73   Knowles MR, Paradiso AM, Boucher RC. In vivo nasal potential difference: Techniques and protocols for assessing efficacy of gene transfer in cystic fibrosis. *Hum Gene Therapy* 1995; **6**: 445–55.

74   Wilson DC, Ellis L, Zielenski J et al. Uncertainty in the diagnosis of cystic fibrosis: possible role of in vivo nasal potential difference measurements. *J Pediatr* 1998; **132**: 596–9.

75   Veeze HJ, Sinaasappel M, Bijman J et al. Ion transport abnormalities in rectal suction biopsies from children with cystic fibrosis. *Gastroenterology* 1991; **101**: 398–403.

76   Waters DL, Dorney SFA, Gaskin KJ et al. Pancreatic function in infants identified as having cystic fibrosis in a neonatal screening program. *N Engl J Med* 1990; **322**: 303–8.

77   Gregg RG, Simantel A, Farrell PM et al. Newborn screening for cystic fibrosis in Wisconsin: comparison of biochemical and molecular methods. *Pediatrics* 1997; **99**: 819–24.

78   Farrell PM, Kosorok MR, Rock MJ et al. Early Diagnosis of cystic fibrosis through neonatal screening prevents severe malnutrition and improves long-term growth. *Pediatrics* 2001; **107**: 1–13.

79   Waters DL, Wilcken B, Irwing L et al. Clinical outcomes of newborn screening for cystic fibrosis. *Arch Dis Child Fetal Neonatal Ed* 1999; **80**: F1–F7.

80   Groman JD, Meyer ME, Wilmott RW et al. Variant cystic fibrosis phenotypes in the absence of CFTR mutations. *N Engl J Med* 2002; **347**: 401–7.

81   Strom CM, Huang D, Chen C et al. Extensive sequencing of the cystic fibrosis transmembrane regulator gene: assay validation and unexpected benefits of developing a comprehensive test. *Genet Med* 2003; **5**: 9–14.

82   Wang X, Myers A, Saiki RK, Cutting GR. Development and evaluation of a PCR-based, line probe assay for the detection of 58 alleles in the Cystic Fibrosis Transmembrane Conductance Regulator (CFTR) gene. *Clin Chem* 2002; **48**: 1121–3.

83   Strom CM, Huang D, Buller A et al. Cystic fibrosis screening using the College panel: platform comparison and lessons learned from the first 20,000 samples. *Genet Med* 2002; **4**: 289–96.

✳84   Grody WW, Cutting GR, Klinger KW et al. Laboratory standards and guidelines for population-based cystic fibrosis carrier screening. *Genet Med* 2001; **3**: 149–54.

85   Ao A, Ray P, Harper J et al. Clinical experience with preimplantation genetic diagnosis of cystic fibrosis (deltaF508). *Prenat Diagn* 1996; **16**: 137–42.

86   Huff DS, Huang NN, Arey JB. Atypical cystic fibrosis of the pancreas with normal levels of sweat chloride and minimal pancreatic lesions. *J Pediatr* 1979; **94**: 237–9.

87   Lebecque P, Leal T, De Boeck C et al. Mutations of the cystic fibrosis gene and intermediate sweat chloride levels in children. *Am J Respir Crit Care Med* 2002; **165**: 757–61.

88   Padoan R, Bassotti A, Seia M, Corbetta C. Negative sweat test in hypertrypsinaemic infants with cystic fibrosis carrying rare CFTR mutations. *Eur J Pediatr* 2002; **161**: 212–15.

89   Mekus F, Ballmann M, Bronsveld I et al. Cystic fibrosis-like disease unrelated to the cystic fibrosis transmembrane conductance regulator. *Hum Genet* 1998; **102**: 582–6.

90   Wallis C. Atypical cystic fibrosis – diagnostic and management dilemmas. *J R Soc Med* 2003; **96** (Suppl 43): 2–10.

91   Wine JJ, Kuo E, Hurlock G, Moss RB. Comprehensive mutation screening in a cystic fibrosis center. *Pediatrics* 2001; **107**: 280–6.

92  Zielenski J, Patrizio P, Corey M et al. CFTR gene variant for patients with congenital absence of vas deferens. *Am J Hum Genet* 1995; **57**: 958–60.

●93  Chillón M, Casals T, Mercier B et al. Mutations in the cystic fibrosis gene in patients with congenital absence of the vas deferens. *N Engl J Med* 1995; **332**: 1475–80.

94  Cohn JA, Friedman KJ, Noone PG et al. Relation between mutations of the cystic fibrosis gene and idiopathic pancreatitis. *N Engl J Med* 1998; **339**: 653–8.

95  Pignatti PF, Bombieri C, Marigo C et al. Increased incidence of cystic fibrosis gene mutations in adults with disseminated bronchiectasis. *Hum Mol Genet* 1995; **4**: 635–9.

96  Miller PW, Hamosh A, Macek M Jr et al. Cystic fibrosis transmembrane conductance regulator (CFTR) gene mutations in allergic bronchopulmonary aspergillosis. *Am J Hum Genet* 1996; **59**: 45–51.

97  Marchand E, Verellen-Dumoulin C, Mairesse M et al. Frequency of cystic fibrosis transmembrane conductance regulator gene mutations and 5T allele in patients with allergic bronchopulmonary aspergillosis. *Chest* 2001; **119**: 762–7.

98  Sheth S, Shea JC, Bishop MD et al. Increased prevalence of CFTR mutations and variants and decreased chloride secretion in primary sclerosing cholangitis. *Hum Genet* 2003; **113**: 286–92.

99  Mickle J, Macek M Jr, Fulmer-Smentek SB et al. A mutation in the cystic fibrosis transmembrane conductance regulator gene associated with elevated sweat chloride concentrations in the absence of cystic fibrosis. *Hum Mol Genet* 1998; **7**: 729–35.

100  Gilljam M, Moltyaner Y, Downey GP et al. Airway inflammation and infection in congenital bilateral absence of the vas deferens. *Am J Respir Crit Care Med* 2004; **169**: 174–9.

101  Castellani C, Bonizzato A, Pradal U et al. Evidence of mild respiratory disease in men with congenital absence of the vas deferens. *Respir Med* 1999; **93**: 869–75.

102  Cystic Fibrosis Mutation Data Base. http://www.genet.sickkids.on.ca. Website. 2004.

103  Tsui LC. The spectrum of cystic fibrosis mutations. *Trends Genet* 1992; **8**: 392–8.

◆104  Welsh MJ, Smith AE. Molecular mechanisms of CFTR chloride channel dysfunction in cystic fibrosis. *Cell* 1993; **73**: 1251–4.

●105  The Cystic Fibrosis Genotype-Phenotype Consortium. Correlation between genotype and phenotype in patients with cystic fibrosis. *N Engl J Med* 1993; **329**: 1308.

106  Hamosh A, King TM, Rosenstein BJ et al. Cystic fibrosis patients bearing the common missense mutation Gly → Asp at codon 551 and the deltaF508 are indistinguishable from deltaF508 homozygotes except for decreased risk of meconium ileus. *Am J Hum Genet* 1992; **51**: 245–50.

●107  Kiesewetter S, Macek M Jr, Davis C et al. A mutation in the cystic fibrosis transmembrane conductance regulator gene produces different phenotypes depending on chromosomal background. *Nature Genet* 1993; **5**: 274–8.

108  Gan KH, Heijerman HGM, Bakker W. Correlation between genotype and phenotype in patients with cystic fibrosis. *N Engl J Med* 1994; **330**: 865–6.

109  Zielenski J. Genotype and phenotype in cystic fibrosis. *Respiration* 2000; **67**: 117–33.

110  Dean M, Santis G. Heterogeneity in the severity of cystic fibrosis and the role of CFTR gene mutations. *Hum Genet* 1994; **93**: 364–8.

111  Koch C, Cuppens H, Rainisio M et al. European Epidemiologic Registry of Cystic Fibrosis (ERCF): comparison of major disease manifestations between patients with different classes of mutations. *Pediatr Pulmonol* 2001; **31**: 1–12.

112  Merlo CA, Boyle MP. Modifier genes in cystic fibrosis lung disease. *J Lab Clin Med* 2003; **141**: 237–41.

◆113  Drumm M. Modifier genes and variation in cystic fibrosis. *Respir Res* 2001; **2**: 125–8.

114  Gan K-H, Veeze HJ, van den Ouweland AM et al. A cystic fibrosis mutation associated with mild lung disease. *N Engl J Med* 1995; **333**: 95–9.

115  De Braekeleer M, Allard C, Leblanc J-P et al. Genotype-phenotype correlation in cystic fibrosis patients compound heterozygous for the A455E mutation. *Hum Genet* 1997; **101**: 208–211.

116  Kubesch P, Dörk T, Wulbrand U et al. Genetic determinants of airways' colonization with *Pseudomonas aeruginosa* in cystic fibrosis. *Lancet* 1993; **341**: 189–93.

117  Wilschanski M, Zielenski J, Markiewicz D et al. Correlation of sweat chloride concentration with classes of the cystic fibrosis transmembrane conductance regulator gene mutations. *J Pediatr* 1995; **127**: 705–10.

118  Moyer BD, Denton J, Karlson KH et al. A PDZ-interacting domain in CFTR is an apical membrane polarization signal. *J Clin Invest* 1999; **104**: 1353–61.

119  Mak V, Zielenski J, Tsui LC et al. Proportion of cystic fibrosis gene mutations not detected by routine testing in men with obstructive azoospermia. *J Am Med Assoc* 1999; **281**: 2217–24.

120  Friedman K, Heim R, Knowles M, Silverman L. Rapid characterization of the variable length polythymidine tract in the cystic fibrosis (CFTR) gene: association of the 5T allele with selected CFTR mutations and its incidence in atypical sinopulmonary disease. *Hum Mutat* 1997; **10**: 108–15.

121  Noone PG, Pue CA, Zhou Z et al. Lung disease associated with the IVS8 5T allele of the CFTR gene. *Am J Respir Crit Care Med* 2000; **162**: 1919–24.

●122  Snouwaert JN, Brigman KK, Latour AM et al. An animal model for cystic fibrosis made by gene targeting. *Science* 1992; **257**: 1083–8.

●123  Dorin JR, Dickinson P, Alton EW et al. Cystic fibrosis in the mouse by targeted insertional mutagenesis. *Nature* 1992; **359**: 211–15.

124  O'Neal WK, Hasty P, McCray PB Jr et al. A severe phenotype in mice with a duplication of exon 3 in the cystic fibrosis locus. *Hum Mol Genet* 1993; **2**: 1561–9.

125  Zeiher BG, Eichwald E, Zabner J et al. A mouse model for the deltaF508 allele of cystic fibrosis. *Am Soc for Clin Invest* 1999; **96**: 2051–64.

126  Hikke van Doorninck J, French PJ, Verbeek E et al. A mouse model for the cystic fibrosis deltaF508 mutation. *EMBO J* 1995; **14**: 4403–11.

127  Colledge WH, Abella BS, Southern KW et al. Generation and characterization of a deltaF508 cystic fibrosis mouse model. *Nature Genet* 1995; **10**: 445–52.

128  Delaney SJ, Alton E, Smith S et al. Cystic fibrosis mice carrying the missense mutation G551D replicate human genotype-phenotype correlations. *EMBO J* 1996; **15**: 955–63.

129  Grubb BR, Boucher RC. Pathophysiology of gene-targeted mouse models for cystic fibrosis. *APS Conf* 1999; **79**: S193–S214.

130 Egan ME, Pearson M, Weiner SA et al. Curcumin, a major constituent of turmeric, corrects cystic fibrosis defects. *Science* 2004; **304**: 600–2.

131 Clarke LL, Grubb BR, Gabriel SE et al. Defective epithelial chloride transport in a gene-targeted mouse model of cystic fibrosis. *Science* 1992; **257**: 1125–8.

132 Durie PR, Kent G, Phillips MJ, Ackerley CA. Characteristic multiorgan pathology of cystic fibrosis in a long-living cystic fibrosis transmembrane regulator knockout murine model. *Am J Pathol* 2004; **164**: 1481–93.

133 Coleman FT, Mueschenborn S, Meluleni G et al. Hypersusceptibility of cystic fibrosis mice to chronic *Pseudomonas aeruginosa* oropharyngeal colonization and lung infection. *Proc Natl Acad Sci USA* 2003; **100**: 1949–54.

134 Davidson DJ, Dorin JR, McLachlan G et al. Lung disease in the cystic fibrosis mouse exposed to bacterial pathogens. *Nature Genet* 1995; **9**: 351–7.

135 Gosselin D, Stevenson MM, Cowley EA et al. Impaired ability of CFTR knockout mice to control lung infection with *Pseudomonas aeruginosa*. *Am J Resp Crit Care Med* 1998; **157**: 1253–62.

136 Sajjan U, Thanassoulis G, Cherapanov V et al. Enhanced susceptibility to pulmonary infection with *Burkholderia cepacia* in Cftr(−/−) mice. *Infect Immun* 2001; **69**: 5138–50.

●137 Mall M, Grubb BR, Harkema JR et al. Increased airway epithelial Na+ absorption produces cystic fibrosis-like lung disease in mice. *Nat Med* 2004; **10**: 487–93.

138 Clarke LB, Grubb BR, Yankaskas JR et al. Relationship of a non-cystic fibrosis transmembrane conductance regulator-mediated chloride conductance to organ-level disease in CFTR (−/−) mice. *Proc Natl Acad Sci USA* 1994; **91**: 479–83.

139 Haston CK, McKerlie C, Newbigging S et al. Detection of modifier loci influencing the lung phenotype of cystic fibrosis knockout mice. *Mamm Genome* 2002; **13**: 605–13.

140 Kent G, Hes R, Bear C et al. Lung disease in mice with cystic fibrosis. *J Clin Invest* 1997; **100**: 3060–9.

141 Veeze HJ, Halley JJ, de Jongste JC et al. Determinants of mild clinical symptoms in cystic fibrosis patients. *J Clin Invest* 1994; **93**: 461–6.

142 Santis G, Osborne L, Knight RA, Hodson ME. Independent genetic determinants of pancreatic and pulmonary status in cystic fibrosis. *Lancet* 1990; **336**: 1081–4.

143 Santis G, Osborne L, Knight R et al. Genotype–phenotype relationship in cystic fibrosis: results from the study of monozygotic and dizygotic twins with cystic fibrosis. *Ped Pulm* 1992; **8**: 239–40.

144 Mekus F, Ballmann M, Bronsveld I et al. Categories of deltaF508 homozygous cystic fibrosis twin and sibling pairs with distinct phenotypic characteristics. *Twin Res* 2000; **3**: 277–93.

145 Mekus F, Laabs U, Veeze H, Tummler B. Genes in the vicinity of CFTR modulate the cystic fibrosis phenotype in highly concordant or discordant F508del homozygous sib pairs. *Hum Genet* 2003; **112**: 1–11.

146 Bronsveld I, Mekus F, Bijman J et al. Chloride conductance and genetic background modulate the cystic fibrosis phenotype of deltaF508 homozygous twins and siblings. *J Clin Invest* 2001; **108**: 1705–15.

147 Doring G, Krogh-Johansen H, Weidinger S, Hoiby N. Allotypes of alpha 1-antitrypsin in patients with cystic fibrosis, homozygous and heterozygous for deltaF508. *Pediatr Pulmonol* 1994; **18**: 3–7.

148 Mahadeva R, Westerbeek RC, Perry DJ et al. Alpha1-antitrypsin deficiency alleles and the Taq-I G → >A allele in cystic fibrosis lung disease. *Eur Respir J* 1998; **11**: 873–9.

149 Mahadeva R, Stewart S, Bilton D, Lomas DA. Alpha-1 antitrypsin deficiency alleles and severe cystic fibrosis lung disease. *Thorax* 1998; **53**: 1022–4.

150 Henry MT, Cave S, Rendall J et al. An alpha(1)-antitrypsin enhancer polymorphism is a genetic modifier of pulmonary outcome in cystic fibrosis. *Eur J Hum Genet* 2001; **9**: 273–8.

151 Frangolias DD, Ruan J, Wilcox PJ et al. Alpha 1-antitrypsin deficiency alleles in cystic fibrosis lung disease. *Am J Respir Cell Mol Biol* 2003; **29** (3 Pt 1): 390–6.

152 Gabolde M, Guilloud-Bataille M, Feingold J, Besmond C. Association of variant alleles of mannose binding lectin with severity of pulmonary disease in cystic fibrosis: cohort study. *Br Med J* 1999; **319**: 1166–7.

153 Yarden J, Radojkovic D, De Boeck K et al. Polymorphisms in the mannose binding lectin gene affect the cystic fibrosis pulmonary phenotype. *J Med Genet* 2004; **41**: 629–33.

154 Turner MW, Hamvas RM. Mannose-binding lectin: structure, function, genetics and disease associations. *Rev Immunogenet* 2000; **2**: 305–22.

155 Kilpatrick DC. Mannan-binding lectin: clinical significance and applications. *Biochim Biophys Acta* 2002; **1572**: 401–13.

156 Wallis R, Cheng JYT. Molecular defects in variant forms of mannose-binding protein associated with immunodeficiency. *J Immunol* 1999; **163**: 4953–9.

157 Wallis R. Dominant effects of mutations in the collagenous domain of mannose-binding protein. *J Immunol* 2002; **168**: 4553–8.

158 Garred P, Larsen F, Madsen HO, Koch C. Mannose-binding lectin deficiency-revisited. *Mol Immunol* 2003; **40**: 73–84.

159 Madsen HO, Garred P, Thiel S et al. Interplay between promoter and structural gene variants control basal serum level of mannan-binding protein. *J Immunol* 1995; **155**: 3013–20.

160 Crosdale DJ, Ollier WE, Thomson W et al. Mannose binding lectin (MBL) genotype distributions with relation to serum levels in UK Caucasoids. *Eur J Immunogenet* 2000; **27**: 111–17.

161 Ezekowitz RA. Role of the mannose-binding lectin in innate immunity. *J Infect Dis* 2003; **187**(Suppl 2): S335–S339.

●162 Kelley TJ, Al Nakkash L, Cotton CU, Drumm ML. Activation of endogenous deltaF508 cystic fibrosis transmembrane conductance regulator by phosphodiesterase inhibition. *J Clin Invest* 1996; **98**: 513–20.

163 Kelley TJ, Thomas K, Milgram LJ, Drumm ML. In vivo activation of the cystic fibrosis transmembrane conductance regulator mutant deltaF508 in murine nasal epithelium. *Proc Natl Acad Sci USA* 1997; **94**: 2604–8.

164 Grubb B, Lazarowski E, Knowles M, Boucher R. Isobutylmethylxanthine fails to stimulate chloride secretion in cystic fibrosis airway epithelia. *Am J Respir Cell Mol Biol* 1993; **8**: 454–60.

165 Smith SN, Middleton PG, Chadwick S et al. The in vivo effects of milrinone on the airways of cystic fibrosis mice and human subjects. *Am J Respir Cell Mol Biol* 1999; **20**: 129–34.

◆166   Zeitlin PL. Novel pharmacologic therapies for cystic fibrosis. *J Clin Invest* 1999; **103**: 447–52.

167   Rubenstein RC, Zeitlin PL. A pilot clinical trial of oral sodium 4-phenylbutyrate (buphenyl) in deltaF508-homozygous cystic fibrosis patients. *Am J Resp Crit Care Med* 1998; **157**: 484–90.

168   Wilschanski M, Yahav Y, Yaacov Y et al. Gentamicin-induced correction of CFTR function in patients with cystic fibrosis and CFTR stop mutations. *N Engl J Med* 2003; **349**: 1433–41.

◆169   Driskell RA, Engelhardt JF. Current status of gene therapy for inherited lung diseases. *Annu Rev Physiol* 2003; **65**: 585–612.

170   Wagner JA, Messner AH, Moran ML et al. Safety and biological efficacy of an adeno-associated virus vector-cystic fibrosis transmembrane regulator (AAV-CFTR) in the cystic fibrosis maxillary sinus. *Laryngoscope* 1999; **109** (2 Pt 1): 266–74.

171   Flotte TR, Zeitlin PL, Reynolds TC et al. Phase I trial of intranasal and endobronchial administration of a recombinant adeno-associated virus serotype 2 (rAAV2)-CFTR vector in adult cystic fibrosis patients: a two-part clinical study. *Hum Gene Ther* 2003; **14**: 1079–88.

172   Moss RB, Rodman D, Spencer LT et al. Repeated adeno-associated virus serotype 2 aerosol-mediated cystic fibrosis transmembrane regulator gene transfer to the lungs of patients with cystic fibrosis: a multicenter, double-blind, placebo-controlled trial. *Chest* 2004; **125**: 509–21.

173   Boucher RC. Status of gene therapy for cystic fibrosis lung diesease. *J Clin Invest* 1999; **103**: 441–5.

174   Gruenert DC, Bruscia E, Novelli G et al. Sequence-specific modification of genomic DNA by small DNA fragments. *J Clin Invest* 2003; **112**: 637–41.

175   Afzelius BA, Mossberg B, Bergstrom SE. Immotile cilia syndrome (primary ciliary dyskinesia), including Kartagener syndrome. In: Scriver CR, Beaudet AL, Sly WS, Valle D (eds). *The metabolic and molecular basis of inherited disease.* New York: McGraw-Hill, 2001: 4817–27.

176   Bush A, Cole P, Hariri M et al. Primary ciliary dyskinesia: diagnosis and standards of care. *Eur Respir J* 1998; **12**: 982–8.

177   Moreno A, Murphy EA. Inheritance of Kartagener syndrome. *Am J Med Genet* 1981; **8**: 305–13.

178   McKusick VA. Online Mendelian inheritance in man. Website 2/18/1999. 2004. Johns Hopkins Institute for Genetic Medicine, Johns Hopkins University.

179   Geremek M, Witt M. Primary ciliary dyskinesia: genes, candidate genes and chromosomal regions. *J Appl Genet* 2004; **45**: 347–61.

●180   Pennarun G, Escudier E, Chapelin C et al. Loss-of-function mutations in a human gene related to *Chlamydomonas reinhardtii* dynein IC78 result in primary ciliary dyskinesia. *Am J Hum Genet* 1999; **65**: 1508–19.

181   Olbrich H, Haffner K, Kispert A et al. Mutations in DNAH5 cause primary ciliary dyskinesia and randomization of left–right asymmetry. *Nat Genet* 2002; **30**: 143–4.

182   Bartoloni L, Blouin JL, Pan Y et al. Mutations in the DNAH11 (axonemal heavy chain dynein type II) gene cause one form of situs inversus totalis and most likely primary ciliary dyskinesia. *Proc Natl Acad Sci USA* 2002; **99**: 10282–6.

183   Supp DM, Witte DP, Potter SS, Brueckner M. Mutation of an axonemal dynein affects left-right asymmetry in inversus viscerum mice. *Nature* 1997; **389**: 963–6.

184   Ibanez-Tallon I, Gorokhova S, Heintz N. Loss of function of axonemal dynein Mdnah5 causes primary ciliary dyskinesia and hydrocephalus. *Hum Mol Genet* 2002; **11**: 715–21.

185   Young D. Surgical treatment of male infertility. *J Reprod Fertil* 1970; **23**: 541–2.

186   Handelsman DJ, Conway AJ, Boylan LM, Turtle JR. Young's syndrome. Obstructive azoospermia and chronic sinopulmonary infections. *N Engl J Med* 1984; **310**: 3–9.

187   Teichtahl H, Temple Smith PD, Johnson JL et al. Obstructive azoospermia and chronic sinobronchial disease (Young's syndrome) in identical twins. *Fertil Steril* 1987; **47**: 879–81.

188   Shiraishi K, Ono N, Eguchi S et al. Young's syndrome associated with situs inversus totalis. *Arch Androl* 2004; **50**: 169–72.

189   Schanker HM, Rajfer J, Saxon A. Recurrent respiratory disease, azoospermia, and nasal polyposis. A syndrome that mimics cystic fibrosis and immotile cilia syndrome. *Arch Intern Med* 1985; **145**: 2201–3.

190   Le Lannou DS, Jezequel P, Blayau M et al. Obstructive azoospermia with agenesis of vas deferens or with bronchiectasia (Young's syndrome): a genetic approach. *Hum Repro* 1995; **10**: 338–41.

191   Friedman KJ, Teichtahl H, Dekretser DM et al. Screening Young syndrome patients for CFTR mutations. *Am J Respir Crit Care Med* 1995; **152**: 1353–7.

192   Krishna S, Cranston D. Sinusitis and obstructive azoospermia (Young's syndrome) in twins. *Br Med J* 1985; **290**: 30.

193   Hendry WF, A'Hern RP, Cole PJ. Was Young's syndrome caused by exposure to mercury in childhood? *Br Med J* 1993; **307**: 1579–82.

194   Mahadeva R, Sharples L, Ross-Russell RI et al. Association of alpha(1)-antichymotrypsin deficiency with milder lung disease in patients with cystic fibrosis. *Thorax* 2001; **56**: 53–8.

195   Buscher R, Eilmes KJ, Grasemann H et al. Beta2 adrenoceptor gene polymorphisms in cystic fibrosis lung disease. *Pharmacogenetics* 2002; **12**: 347–53.

196   Hull J, Thomson AH. Contribution of genetic factors other than CFTR to disease severity in cystic fibrosis. *Thorax* 1998; **53**: 1018–21.

197   Aron Y, Polla BS, Bienvenu T et al. HLA class II polymorphism in cystic fibrosis. *Am J Respir Crit Care Med* 1999; **159**: 1464–8.

198   Texereau J, Marullo S, Hubert D et al. Nitric oxide synthase 1 as a potential modifier gene of decline in lung function in patients with cystic fibrosis. *Thorax* 2004; **59**: 156–8.

199   Grasemann H, Knauer N, Buscher R et al. Airway nitric oxide levels in cystic fibrosis patients are related to a polymorphism in the neuronal nitric oxide synthase gene. *Am J Respir Crit Care Med* 2000; **162**: 2172–6.

200   Grasemann H, van's Gravesande KS, Buscher R et al. Endothelial nitric oxide synthase variants in cystic fibrosis lung disease. *Am J Respir Crit Care Med* 2003; **167**: 390–4.

201   Arkwright PD, Laurie S, Super M et al. TGF-beta(1) genotype and accelerated decline in lung function of patients with cystic fibrosis. *Thorax* 2000; **55**: 459–62.

# PART 3

# Interstitial lung diseases

# 12

# Idiopathic pulmonary fibrosis

KARL W. THOMAS AND GARY W. HUNNINGHAKE

## INTRODUCTION

Multiple clinical forms of pulmonary fibrosis have been described. In some, such as asbestosis, the cause is known while in others, such as idiopathic pulmonary fibrosis (IPF), the cause is unknown. It is of interest that a minority of individuals exposed to agents known to cause pulmonary fibrosis develops clinical disease. This is the case even when development of clinical disease is corrected for amounts of exposure. This incomplete link of exposure with disease, as well as other observations of familial clusters of pulmonary fibrosis, strongly suggests the existence of an underlying genetic predisposition and/or the presence of environmental cofactors that determine expression of these disorders. The primary focus of this review will be IPF, the most common type of pulmonary fibrosis of unknown etiology. It is a rather pure form of pulmonary fibrosis characterized by the accumulation of fibroblasts, abundant extracellular matrix, and sparse inflammatory cells within the lung interstitium. IPF is not associated with systemic disorders and has not been linked to known environmental exposures. To help understand potential genetic factors that may contribute to the development of IPF, we will discuss studies of other forms of pulmonary fibrosis to help understand how this disease might develop within the lung.

The initial definition of the IPF syndrome was rather imprecise. Initially, Hamman–Rich syndrome was equated with IPF. We now know that Hamman–Rich syndrome in its pure form is acute interstitial pneumonia (AIP). A further refinement of the definition occurred when it was recognized that there were at least two populations of patients that were included under the definition of IPF. One subgroup with a much better prognosis and a potential for improvement with anti-inflammatory therapy, is now defined as nonspecific interstitial pneumonia (NSIP). The other group, which is the focus of this discussion, is now more strictly defined as IPF. Other names for the latter disorder include cryptogenic fibrosing alveolitis and usual interstitial pneumonia. IPF is considered to be one the idiopathic interstitial pneumonias (Table 12.1).[1,2] Other members of this group include NSIP, AIP, cryptogenic organizing pneumonia (COP), desquamative interstitial pneumonia (DIP), and respiratory bronchiolitis-interstitial lung disease (RB-ILD). Some classification schemes also include lymphocytic interstitial pneumonia (LIP), although this disorder rarely occurs as an idiopathic disorder.

## CLINICAL FEATURES

Patients with IPF usually present with a clinical history that includes an insidious onset of dyspnea and cough. These symptoms are usually present for greater than 3 months and the cough often precedes the onset of dyspnea. Symptoms less than 3 months in duration suggest an alternative diagnosis. Systemic symptoms are rarely present. The cough is not productive of purulent sputum. Dyspnea at rest is not present until the disease is far advanced. Dyspnea with exertion is a hallmark of the disease and often limits physical activity for these patients. Velcro-type rales are usually found on the lung examination and clubbing of the digits is often present. A prominent second heart sound may be present if

**Table 12.1**  *Classification and distinguishing features of idiopathic interstitial pneumonias*[1,2]

| Clinical diagnosis | Histologic nomenclature and key histologic features | Patient and clinical features | Prognosis and treatment |
| --- | --- | --- | --- |
| Idiopathic pulmonary fibrosis/cryptogenic fibrosing alveolitis | Usual interstitial pneumonitis: Heterogeneous pattern of subpleural architectural destruction, fibroblast foci, and honeycomb change | Mean age >50; gradual, onset of dyspnea and cough, clubbing and Velcro rales are common, tobacco use is frequent | Median survival is 2–3 years after diagnosis or 4–5 years after onset of symptoms. Poor response to anti-inflammatory therapy |
| Desquamative interstitial pneumonia | Desquamative interstitial pneumonia: Uniform involvement of lung parenchyma with prominent accumulation of alveolar macrophages, usually with some fibrotic thickening of alveolar septa | Mean age 40–50; insidious onset of dyspnea, dry cough, clubbing may be present. M:F ratio 2:1. | Prognosis favorable with 70% survival. Favorable response to corticosteroids and smoking cessation, recovery possible |
| Acute interstitial pneumonia | Diffuse alveolar damage: Diffuse involvement with alveolar septal thickening, airspace organization, temporal appearance | Mean age 50; rapid onset of dyspnea, respiratory failure; diffuse crackles and hypoxemia common | Prognosis poor with 50% survival, poor response to corticosteroids, complete recovery possible |
| Nonspecific interstitial pneumonia | Nonspecific interstitial pneumonia: Uniform appearance of mild to moderate interstitial inflammation without temporal heterogeneity, variable presence of type II pneumocyte hyperplasia and interstitial fibrosis | Median age 40–50; may occur in children, variable onset of symptoms, no association with tobacco use | Prognosis favorable with 10–20% mortality, favorable response to corticosteroids and complete recovery possible |
| Respiratory bronchiolitis interstitial lung disease | Respiratory bronchiolitis: Bronchiolocentric accumulation of alveolar macrophages with associated bronchiolar fibrosis and chronic inflammation | Median age 40–50; strong association with tobacco use, mild to moderate dyspnea | Prognosis favorable if smoking cessation achieved, mortality and progression to death rare |
| Cryptogenic organizing pneumonia | Organizing pneumonia: Organizing pneumonia with intralumenal airspace fibrosis occurring in a patchy distribution but with uniform temporal appearance and preservation of underlying lung architecture | Median age at onset 55; subacute onset productive cough, dyspnea, systemic symptoms common, inverse association with tobacco use | Prognosis favorable with low mortality. Good response to corticosteroids, relapse may occur |
| Lymphocytic interstitial pneumonia | Lymphoid interstitial pneumonia: Diffuse interstitial infiltration in alveolar septal pattern by T-lymphocytes, plasma cells, and macrophages. Frequent finding of lymphoid hyperplasia | Typical age 50; female > male; systemic symptoms present; clinical overlap with multiple autoimmune diseases | Prognosis variable with one-third progressing to pulmonary fibrosis; favorable response to corticosteroids |

significant pulmonary hypertension is present at rest. An important component of the history that is necessary for diagnosis of the disorder is the absence of systemic illnesses that are associated with pulmonary fibrosis, absence of gastrointestinal or liver disease, no prior episode of acute lung injury requiring mechanical ventilation, and no exposure to irradiation or medications associated with the development of pulmonary fibrosis. An equally important component of the history is exclusion of other environmental exposures, including dusts and aerosols, that cause lung injury.

## FUNCTIONAL FEATURES

A hallmark of the disease is reduced lung volumes and diffusing capacity for carbon monoxide associated with a symmetrical reduction in forced expiratory volume in one second ($FEV_1$) and forced vital capacity (FVC). Hypoxemia may not be present at rest but usually develops with exercise. In a similar manner, pulmonary artery pressures may not be elevated with rest but often rise with exercise. The

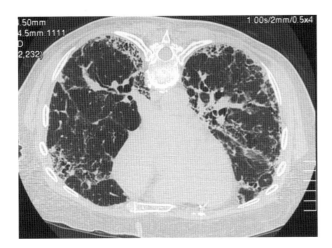

**Figure 12.1** *High resolution CT scan of IPF demonstrating subpleural honeycomb changes and traction bronchiectasis.*

latter two abnormalities often parallel the limitation of exercise in these patients. In some patients with a history of cigarette smoking, the presence of a second lung disorder, emphysema, may result in elevated lung volumes due to the opposing effects of fibrosis and emphysema.[3,4] In these patients, the ratio of $FEV_1/FVC$ is often normal and the DLCO, which is reduced by both the fibrosis and emphysema, is the best reflection of the combined effect of the two disorders on the lung.

## RADIOLOGICAL FEATURES

The initial screening test is often a chest X-ray. The typical findings are reticular nodular infiltrates that are more prominent in the lower lung zones. Often, the initial diagnosis is pneumonia or congestive heart failure. The failure of the patient's symptoms to improve or for the chest X-ray to clear is often the rationale to obtain a lung CT scan. For patients with IPF, the classic lung CT scan shows a patchy peripheral pattern of reticulation that is most prominent in the bases of the lung (Fig. 12.1).[5] Honeycombing and traction bronchiectasis are usually found in the lower lung zones. There is little if any ground glass change. For experienced clinicians, this classic lung CT pattern is diagnostic of IPF with a sensitivity and specificity that rivals that of the surgical lung biopsy.[6] Unfortunately, this classic lung CT pattern is present in only approximately half of the patients at the time of diagnosis. The other half of the patients have a lung CT pattern that is similar to that present in patients with NSIP. It is these latter patients who require a surgical lung biopsy for definitive diagnosis.

## HISTOPATHOLOGICAL FEATURES

Prior to surgical lung biopsy, a transbronchial biopsy is often performed to exclude the presence of other disorders

**Table 12.2** *Clinical criteria for diagnosis of idiopathic pulmonary fibrosis[2]*

| Criteria |
| --- |
| *Major criteria* |
| Exclusion of other known causes of ILD such as connective tissue disease, drug toxicities, environmental exposures |
| Abnormal pulmonary function studies that include evidence of restriction and impaired gas exchange |
| Bibasilar reticular abnormalities with minimal ground glass opacities on HRCT scans |
| Transbronchial lung biopsy or BAL showing no features to support an alternative diagnosis |
| *Minor criteria* |
| Age >50 years |
| Insidious onset of otherwise unexplained dyspnea on exertion |
| Duration of illness >3 months |
| Bibasilar, inspiratory crackles |
| *Histological criteria* |
| Architectural destruction of lung with a heterogeneous appearance including areas of normal lung, acute interstitial inflammation, interstitial fibrosis, and honeycomb change |
| Presence of scattered fibroblast foci |
| Peripheral and subpleural involvement which is patchy and not uniformly distributed |

such as chronic hypersensitivity pneumonitis that may mimic IPF. A pathological diagnosis of IPF cannot be made using a transbronchial lung biopsy. The histopathology of IPF can usually be differentiated from other idiopathic interstitial pneumonias by recognition of the patchy distribution of lung remodeling and fibrosis that is most prominent in subpleural areas (Table 12.1). There is temporal heterogeneity of the development of fibrosis characterized by areas with mature collagen deposition and other areas with newly injured lung recognized by the presence of fibroblast foci. Areas of normal lung are also present. Significant inflammation characterized by accumulation of neutrophils or lymphocytes is not a histologic feature of IPF.

## FAMILIAL IPF AND AGE OF ONSET

One clue to the genetics of IPF may be its association with age. The vast majority of patients with IPF are greater than 55 years of age and many are in their 6th and 7th decades of life. The exception to this observation is patients with a familial form of the disorder (termed familial pulmonary fibrosis (FPF)) who may present at a somewhat earlier age. Thus, when a patient less than 55 years of age presents with a lung disease resembling IPF, the following questions should be asked: (1) is the diagnosis of IPF correct, and (2) does the patient have a familial form of IPF? In addition to standard clinical criteria for the diagnosis of IPF (Table 12.2), familial IPF is defined as the presence of at least two members of a

**Table 12.3**  *Epidemiology of pulmonary fibrosis*

| Country | Year | Prevalence/ 100 000 | Incidence/ 100 000/year | Average age (yr) | M/F ratio | Ref. |
|---------|------|---------------------|--------------------------|------------------|-----------|------|
| Norway | 1998 | 23.9 | 4.3 | 59.2 | 0.5 / 1 | 7 |
| Finland | 1997 | 16–18 | – | 65.3 | equal | 8 |
| Japan | 1995–1999 | 10.6 | 2.03 | N/A | 2.3 / 1 | 9 |
| United States | 1990 | 20.2 male 13.2 female | 10.7 male 7.4 female | 69 | 1.5/1 | 10 |
| England | 1998–1989 | 6 | – | 66.9 | – | 11 |

biological family having both clinical features and histological features of the disease.[2] The medical history in any patient with clinical features of pulmonary fibrosis should include a complete review for the presence of biological relatives with breathing disorders. While no specific recommendations for genetic counseling can be made, family members with symptoms and findings suggestive of pulmonary fibrosis should be encouraged to have screening evaluations including pulmonary function testing and lung CT scanning as indicated.

## Older studies of IPF

In many instances, older studies of IPF did not utilize the uniform criteria for diagnosis. Thus, historical studies of IPF are limited by inclusion of patients who had idiopathic diseases other than IPF and diseases now known to have established etiologies. A recent expert consensus statement by major American and European respiratory societies has endorsed rigorous clinical case definition criteria not only as a method of coordinating research, but also to establish standardized clinical criteria (Table 12.2).[2]

## Epidemiology

IPF is found worldwide with no apparent influence of race or ethnicity on incidence or prevalence. However, the exact prevalence and incidence of IPF has not been clearly established because of variations in case definition as well as limitations in the sensitivity of population-based screening for the disease. Additionally, the low specificity of population-based screening techniques such as plain chest radiographs, pulmonary function tests, and medical record coding data limit the precision of the findings. With these limitations in mind, the following information is available.

Through a process of searching patient registries and screening medical records for coded diagnoses, three studies from Japan, Finland, and Norway have demonstrated a range in prevalence between 10.6 and 23.9 cases per 100 000 population.[7–9] These estimates are similar to earlier reports originating from southwestern USA, but higher than estimates developed from population studies in the UK.[10,11] Given the significant clinical overlap of IPF with other

chronic lung diseases and resulting classification errors, it is difficult to determine if these calculations under- or overestimate the true prevalence and incidence of the disease.

In these studies, the average age at diagnosis of IPF has been between 59 and 66 years. However, there is a consistent and significant increase of disease incidence with increasing age. It has been estimated that two-thirds of subjects are above 60 years at the time of diagnosis.[2] While a few cases of familial transmission have been described in children, the more common sporadic cases of IPF rarely, if ever, occur in children. Many studies have reported a predominance of male to female subjects with ratios as high as 2:1; however, this finding was not observed in a more recent population study in Norway (Table 12.3).[1,7]

Cigarette smoking is the most defined risk factor associated with the development of IPF. In a case–control study of 248 cases in the southwestern USA, the odds ratio for current or former tobacco smoking was 1.6.[12] In a recent large study of patients with familial IPF, cigarette smoking was strongly associated with expression of the disease (Schwartz DA, personal communication). Repeated observations have confirmed that cigarette smoking was a major risk factor for progression of the disease.[13,14] These findings are consistent with most large studies which reported that at least three-quarters of IPF patients are current or ex-cigarette smokers. The initial description of the association of pulmonary fibrosis and cigarette smoking was an early paper that also described the association between cigarette smoking and emphysema.[15] It is likely that cigarette smoking is an important cofactor, but not the primary environmental factor, that triggers the development of pulmonary fibrosis. In support of this hypothesis is the observation that cigarette smoking is a determinant for the expression of pulmonary fibrosis associated with many connective tissue disorders, asbestos, and silica exposure.[16–18] These observations suggest that cigarette smoking should be considered as a cofactor in genetic studies of IPF or other forms of pulmonary fibrosis.

In addition to cigarette smoking, several studies have suggested a link between viral infection, especially Epstein–Barr virus (EBV), and IPF. The evidence of this association between EBV and IPF was based on case–control studies and hence disease causality cannot be specifically established.[19,20] Other viruses reported to be associated with IPF have included influenza, cytomegalovirus, and hepatitis C.[2,21–24] Although viruses have been suggested as a cause of pulmonary fibrosis for some time, there is no consistent evidence to support this hypothesis.[25] Finally, several studies have also linked multiple respiratory disorders, including IPF, to gastro-esophageal reflux or chronic aspiration of gastric contents.[26,27] Although chronic aspiration can cause pulmonary fibrosis, it is not clear that it is a primary cause of IPF. It may, however, be a cofactor that determines its rate of progression.

## Natural history

In most recent studies, the mean time to death after diagnosis for patients with IPF ranged from 2.5 to 3.5 years.[1,2,28,29] This survival period is consistently shorter than the average survival for other forms of interstitial lung disease. An example of this survival difference is a cohort of 54 men and 50 women who had undergone open lung biopsy for diagnosis of a fibrotic lung disease. For the entire group, the median survival was 3.8 years with a 10-year survival rate of 27 percent. For the subset of these patients who had histological confirmation of IPF, the median survival was only 2.8 years from the time of diagnosis. The other subtypes of lung disease, including NSIP and COP, had significantly longer mean survival rates.[30] A study of English patients documented a median survival time of 5.6 years after onset of dyspnea in a cohort of patients with histologically defined disease.[31] This study is consistent with other studies which showed that the median survival of patients after onset of symptoms is 4–6 years. Taken together, these observations suggest that patients often have symptoms for several years prior to diagnosis.

In a Japanese autopsy series of subjects with clinical and pathological diagnosis of IPF, the mean subject age at time of death was 80.5 years and the leading causes of death were disease progression, bacterial pneumonia, severe respiratory failure, and lung cancer.[32] Numerous investigations have been conducted to identify factors that predict survival. Most studies have shown that lower lung function and advanced changes on radiographic studies predict a shortened survival.[13,14,33] The simplest explanation of these findings is that they reflect the stage of the disease, i.e., patients with disease of longer duration have more significant abnormalities on lung function and radiological tests. Other critical factors in the determination of disease survival include age, comorbid illness at the time of diagnosis, and subsequent development of cancer.

## Treatment

For many years, patients with IPF were treated with corticosteroids and/or cytotoxic agents, such as azathioprine or cyclophosphamide. The rationale for this therapy was observations from early studies of corticosteroid treatment for IPF. These studies suggested that 10–40 percent of patients improved or stabilized following the initiation of therapy. However, these studies included patients with other forms of pulmonary fibrosis, such as NSIP.[2,31,34] It is now clear that IPF does not respond to anti-inflammatory therapy.[13,14,34–38] Similarly, antifibrotic agents, including penicillamine and colchicine, which interfere with collagen synthesis and cross-linking, have not halted disease progression.[34,39,40] Recent studies utilizing interferon gamma also showed no effect.[41,42] Subgroup analysis after completion of the latter study suggests that patients with early disease might obtain benefit from the therapy; however, this has not been substantiated in a prospective study.[42] Numerous studies are now underway to determine if other medications offer some survival benefit. These include medications to increase levels of glutathione, inhibit mediators that regulate collagen production, decrease pulmonary artery pressure, inhibit specific inflammation cascades, and decrease angiogenesis. However, to date, no form of medical therapy has been shown to alter the natural history of the disease. Since essentially all patients will experience disease progression, the final treatment approach should include a consideration of pulmonary transplantation. Many IPF patients are not eligible for transplantation because of their age and comorbid conditions. Unfortunately, despite the possibility of this one effective treatment for pulmonary fibrosis, many eligible patients die while waiting for transplantation.

## Monogenic disorders associated with pulmonary fibrosis

The rationale for implicating a genetic basis for the development of IPF is outlined above. There are also several monogenic syndromes associated with pulmonary fibrosis which may shed some light on the potential mechanisms of disease. While none of these syndromes have consistent overlap with the clinical manifestations of IPF, they nevertheless provide useful information regarding the range of possible genetic mechanisms that might be associated with the development of pulmonary fibrosis.

An association of hypercalcemia and hypocalcuria with progressive pulmonary fibrosis was reported by Demedts and Auwrex in 1985.[43,44] They reported an autosomal dominant pattern of inheritance and found that 45 percent of contacted family members had a decreased diffusing capacity and interstitial lung disease. Additional findings in this extended family included an apparent increase in susceptibility to lower respiratory tract infections. Further evaluation suggested the existence of an intrinsic defect in granulocyte function in affected family members. Later work by Chou and Pollak[45,46] demonstrated the presence of a mutation in a calcium-sensing receptor gene (CASR) located on chromosome 3. This calcium-sensing gene is of particular importance in that members of this receptor gene superfamily appear to play a role in the function and activity of thrombin and angiotensin II, as well as the regulation of extra- and intracellular calcium levels. Treatment of the disorder includes control of hyper-calcemia, frequent antibiotic courses for respiratory infections, and supportive pulmonary care. The role for corticosteriods in the treatment of this disorder has not been defined.[47]

As discussed in more detail in Chapter 18C, the Hermansky–Pudlak syndrome is a genetically heterogeneous disorder characterized by the clinical triad of oculocutaneous albinism, platelet dysfunction, and lysosomal accumulation of ceroid lipofuscin.[48,49] Although significant variation exists, some patients with Hermansky–Pudlak syndrome also develop progressive pulmonary fibrosis and respiratory failure. Additional clinical manifestations of this disease include congenital nystagmus, decreased visual acuity, easy bruising, frequent epistaxis, and hypopigmentation of the skin and hair. Pathological findings include prolonged bleeding time and absent dense bodies on electron microscopic examination of platelets.[50,51] While this disease has been described worldwide, it appears to have the highest incidence in Puerto Rico and is inherited in an autosomal recessive pattern. At least seven genetically distinct forms of the disease have been described and linked to mutations in genes referred to as HPS-1 to HPS-7. HPS-1 has been mapped to the region on chromosome 10q23.1-23.3 by linkage analysis. At least 12 different mutations of HPS-1 have been identified in the Puerto Rican population.[50,52–57] While the specific function of HPS-1 protein has not been established, the remaining HPS genes appear to encode proteins closely involved in normal endocytic vesicle trafficking.[58] The incidence and severity of pulmonary fibrosis in patients with HPS appears to be variable, however the pulmonary manifestations may be more common in patients with HPS-1 and HPS-4 mutations.[50,58–60] HPS patients with pulmonary fibrosis appear to have disease onset at an earlier age compared to patients with IPF. In one series of patients with HPS-1 mutations, the average age for pulmonary disease onset was 35 years.[50] The disease in these patients appears to be slowly progressive and has no established cure or treatment. The specific molecular and/or cellular mechanisms of pulmonary fibrosis have not been elucidated.

In addition to mutations in calcium-sensing genes and HPS genes, more recent observations have implicated surfactant protein mutations in the development of pulmonary fibrosis. In 2001, Amin et al.[61] described an 11-year-old girl who had progressive lung disease and required supplemental oxygen. The patient's mother had been given the diagnosis of interstitial lung disease at age 26. The patient's half-sister (maternal) was born prematurely and had recurrent pulmonary infections and chronic respiratory insufficiency. Subsequent evaluation of these three patients revealed that amounts of surfactant protein C were below levels of detection in their bronchoalveolar lavage fluid while surfactant proteins A, B, and D were present in normal amounts.

Interestingly, sequence analysis of the SP-C gene did not reveal an apparent mutation. In the same year, another report detailed the cases of an infant girl with respiratory distress born to a mother who was known to have desquamative interstitial pneumonia. The child underwent lung biopsy, which revealed nonspecific interstitial pneumonia. DNA sequence analysis of the infant's SP-C gene revealed a heterozygous substitution of A for G at the first base of intron 4. Evaluation of the mother's genotype revealed similar changes. The finding that the SP-C mutation was identified in only one allele in both mother and child suggests an autosomal dominant effect. The precise mechanism by which this SP-C mutation produced the interstitial lung disease in these two subjects was postulated to include a dominant negative effect of the abnormal protein on normal intracellular transport and post-translational modification.[62] The findings of two different patterns of lung disease suggests that the genetic abnormality did not dictate the type of lung disease but more likely prevented normal lung repair. It is of interest that the lung disease in both mother and child followed an illness that appeared to be viral in origin.

The most compelling evidence supporting a potentially significant role for surfactant protein mutations arose from an investigation of a large kindred containing 11 adults and three children, many of whom had lung disease similar to IPF. The entire kindred included 97 family members who were studied through four generations covering a span of 60 years. Sequence determination of the SP-C gene in three affected family members revealed a heterozygous leucine to glutamine substitution in the c-terminal region of the protein. The authors again postulated that this region is critical for intracellular trafficking or folding the protein. In review of genotypes in 88 control patients without pulmonary disease, this mutation was not observed, suggesting that the aberration did not represent an inconsequential or common gene polymorphism. The mutation was identified in two unaffected family members from this kindred, suggesting incomplete penetrance.[63]

Unlike both the sporadic form of IPF and other reports of familial IPF, these cases of lung disease linked to mutations in SP-C experienced disease onset and death at a much earlier age. In some of the reported cases, the affected individuals had evidence of severe pulmonary disease in infancy. In each of the three cases which occurred in infants, the pathologic type was nonspecific interstitial pneumonia. Of the three adults who underwent autopsy or open lung biopsy, the reported pathologic type was usually interstitial pneumonia (the pathologic feature of IPF). These observations raise the possibility that, in some instances, NSIP and IPF may not be distinct disorders.[63] The average age at death for the 11 adults with mutations in SP-C was 33 years in comparison to 55 years for familial IPF and 65 for sporadic IPF.[64] It is clear that SP-C mutations do not explain all spontaneous IPF and other forms of familial IPF; however, these findings do provide important clues that may help define how this disorder may occur in the lung.

## Familial aggregation

The first recognition of familial IPF has generally been attributed to Sandoz[65] who first described a familial cluster of IPF in 1907. Multiple other authors have supported these findings and a general consensus exists that rare familial clusters do occur and in these families there is vertical transmission through successive generations. Although the precise number of kindreds with more than one member having IPF remains unknown, between 43 and 68 such families have been described throughout the world in recent reviews.[47,66–69]

Two important studies exist which examine the relative epidemiological prevalence of sporadic and familial cases of IPF. Marshall et al.[64] examined the prevalence of familial and sporadic cases of IPF in England and estimated that between 0.5 and 2.2 percent of all cases were likely to have a familial basis. The familial cases appeared to be younger (55 versus 67 years at time of diagnosis), but were otherwise indistinguishable. A more recent population-based study of medical record diagnostic categories identified 17 families in Finland with 2–5 members having IPF. This represents a much higher proportion (3.3–3.7 percent) of cases than in the British investigation.[8] Given the overall low incidence of familial IPF in relation to sporadic cases, the strength of inferences made from studies of these family clusters to the larger population with the disease will depend on assumptions that these two clinical forms of the disease are genetically similar.

The most suggestive evidence for an inherited component of IPF comes from case reports of monozygotic twins. In 1980, Javaheri[70] described a 50-year-old male who developed a progressive lung disease consistent with IPF. The patient's monozygotic twin brother developed a similar syndrome at age 57. The patients had not lived together since childhood. Additional descriptions of monozygotic twins have appeared, including the description of identical twin sisters, who died of pulmonary fibrosis at age 46 and 47. As in the first description, these and other twin cases had also lived apart for a significant period of time prior to onset of disease in these families.[69,71]

A large number of cases in a single family were first described by Bonanni[68] with results of continued follow-up reported by Marney.[69] This single kindred has now been followed for five generations and includes detailed evaluations for 84 family members. In this family, there are 15 affected family members and three probable cases. This family includes cases involving twin sisters, mother to son transmission, and father to son transmission. Based on inheritance patterns in this particular family, as well as results from at least 14 other families, it is most likely that the gene primarily responsible for the disease in these families is inherited in an autosomal dominant pattern with reduced penetrance.[47]

Despite the evidence for a genetic component in the development of IPF found in these families, as yet, no single gene or marker has been clearly identified and consistently linked to the expression of the disease. Javaheri[70] and

Musk[72] performed HLA typing and concluded that there was no clear association of HLA type with the disease. These results are consistent with the conclusions drawn from a study of 33 patients and 329 healthy controls which did not establish a link between IPF and HLA-A or HLA-B antigen genes on chromosome 6.[73] Additional investigations for linkage to the alpha-1-antitrypsin and immunoglobulin (GM) haplo-types on chromosome 14 are limited by studying a single family, but also do not provide convincing evidence for linkage.[72] Finally, a single report described increased alveolar macrophage activity and neutrophil counts in bronchoalveolar lavage fluid from both affected and unaffected family members in three kindreds with familial IPF.[74] While the finding of lung inflammation, but not fibrosis, in unaffected family members is of interest, it is not clear if these findings can be generalized to all groups with familial IPF or are related to the pathogenesis of the disorder.

## Animal models

Early observations showed that wildtype C57BL/6 mice are particularly sensitive to pulmonary fibrosis following bleomycin administration, while other wildtype strains including Balb/c, C3Hf/Kam, and the 129 strains, are less susceptible. These findings suggest that there is a genetic susceptibility to the development of pulmonary fibrosis. Most of the information related to pulmonary fibrosis in mice has been generated using a single intratracheal injection of bleomycin. There are two major limitations of these studies. The first of these is that this model initially produces severe acute lung injury that may then, in some species, progress to pulmonary fibrosis. In humans, the link between severe acute inflammation and alveolar damage with the subsequent development of IPF has not been firmly established. The predominant pathologic findings of pure IPF do not include severe acute inflammation or diffuse alveolar damage. Thus, the bleomycin-mouse model may reflect the acute inflammatory response as much as, or more than, the fibrotic response. The second limitation is that while the model reliably produces acute inflammation, the resulting degree of fibrotic disease is highly variable and not necessarily progressive. In contrast, IPF is characterized by slowly progressive disease which does not remit. Persistent lung disease may be triggered by bleomycin in some strains of mice (DBA); however, this requires repeated exposure to bleomycin.[75] Given these important limitations of the pulmonary fibrosis mouse model, it nevertheless appears that susceptibility to bleomycin-induced pulmonary fibrosis in mice is linked to at least two loci. The first of these loci is located on mouse chromosome 17 in the major histocompatibility complex. The second locus is on chromosome 11. While the specific mechanism through which the gene in the MHC complex affects disease phenotype has not been determined, the locus on mouse chromosome 11 appears to be a bleomycin hydrolase which may also function as an MHC class 1 epitope-processing protease.[76]

## GENOME DESTABILIZATION AND IDIOPATHIC PULMONARY FIBROSIS

Lung carcinoma and cigarette smoking are often found in association with IPF.[77] A large case–control study involving 890 subjects with IPF and almost 5900 controls in the UK demonstrated an increased risk of lung cancer in the IPF population. With and without adjustment for smoking, the relative risk for lung cancer in these patients was 7.3 and 8.2, respectively.[78] These observations raise the possibility that accumulation of acquired mutations may also determine the development of IPF. Supporting evidence for this hypothesis has been developed through investigations of loss of heterozygosity (LOH) and microsatellite instability (MSI) in patients with IPF. In a small case–control study of 10 highly polymorphic microsatellite markers comparing genotypes in sputum and peripheral blood, 50 percent of patients with IPF demonstrated acquired genetic defects compared with 0 percent of the controls.[79] The small number of study subjects, and the relatively small number of candidate genes, limits the strength of this conclusion. An additional study examining microsatellite instability of the TGF-β receptor type II (TGFBR2) gene in 11 subjects from Japan with IPF demonstrated an increased rate of deletion mutations in this gene.[80] Together, these studies introduce the possibility that acquired genetic alterations may be frequent in the lungs of patients with IPF and hence the disease may arise in the setting of multiple genetic defects or genome destabilization.

## GENETIC PREDISPOSITION TO IPF AND AUTOIMMUNE DISEASES

While the diagnosis of IPF cannot be established in patients with known autoimmune diseases, there are some similarities in the type of lung disease found in IPF and the connective tissue disorders. Both usual interstitial pneumonia (the pathologic pattern found in IPF) and nonspecific interstitial pneumonia occur in these latter diseases.[81–83] The predominant type of lung disease is nonspecific interstitial pneumonia. Ethnic background, particularly African-American race, is a strong risk factor for progression of pulmonary fibrosis in systemic sclerosis.[84–86] Additional investigations of fibronectin gene polymorphisms, HLA loci, and SPARC (secreted protein, acidic and rich in cysteine) polymorphisms in patients with systemic sclerosis have also been associated with pulmonary fibrosis and progression of disease.[87–89] Thus, while direct inferences cannot be made regarding IPF and these associations seen in systemic autoimmune diseases, the linkage of pulmonary disease with ethnic/racial background, as well as the identification of several candidate genes, support the hypothesis that similar genetic links may exist in IPF.

## CANDIDATE GENE ASSOCIATION STUDIES

A large number of relatively small, case–control studies have been carried out to examine the presence or absence of genetic alterations in selected candidate genes in patients with IPF. While these studies have the advantage of targeting a relatively small number of genes which are believed to be critical in the development of the lung disease, the major limitations of these investigations are the assumptions that the noted differences in allele frequencies are directly related to disease causality and that there are no unobserved confounding effects.[90] Many of these investigations have attempted to control for population stratification through matching on ethnicity. However, it remains possible that population stratification exists and accounts for at least several of the reported genotype–phenotype associations in IPF which are discussed below.

The complement receptor proteins are transmembrane glycoproteins located on the surface of many cells, including erythrocytes, and are responsible for the binding and transportation of immune complexes in the bloodstream. Phagocytic cells in the spleen and liver recognize immune complexes bound to complement receptor proteins and subsequently clear the circulating immune complexes. It has been postulated that decreases in the surface density or function of complement receptor 1 (CR-1 or CR1) may lead to prolonged immune stimulation and upregulation of inflammatory responses. Based on these observations, a small study to assess genetic association in 74 patients of Italian descent with IPF and 166 healthy controls was conducted. The major finding of this study was an increased frequency of a polymorphism involving a C to G substitution in exon 33 in patients with IPF. One possible explanation for this observation is that the C to G substitution found in these patients had produced a decrease in density and/or function of CR-1 resulting in decreased rate of clearance of immune complexes leading to repeated lung injury and eventually pulmonary fibrosis.[91]

A significant effort has occurred to evaluate associations between pulmonary fibrosis and cytokine or cytokine receptor polymorphisms. Polymorphisms of IL-1α (IL1A), IL-1β (IL1B), IL-1 receptor antagonist (IL1RN), IL-6 (IL6), IL-8 (IL8), CXC chemokine receptor 1 (IL8RA), and CXC chemokine receptor 2 (IL8RB), have been examined in a series of European and Australian cohorts.[92–96] In these candidate gene studies, only two positive associations have been demonstrated. A single study demonstrated an increased frequency of an IL-6 promoter intron 4 polymorphism in an English population with IPF.[95] In cohorts of English and Italian patients who had clinical evidence of IPF, the presence of single base variations at position +2018 in the IL-1 receptor antagonist gene conferred a significantly increased odds ratio for the presence of pulmonary fibrosis.[94] However, other studies of polymorphisms in this gene did not demonstrate an association with pulmonary fibrosis.[92,96] In summary, there have been no consistent or reproducible studies of associations of cytokine or cytokine receptor polymorphisms and IPF.

An early report by Geddes et al.[97] in 1977 suggested a strong correlation between the presence of the MZ phenotype of $\alpha$1-antitrypsin ($\alpha$1-AT or SERPINA1), with fibrosing alveolitis and rheumatoid arthritis. A subsequent evaluation in patients with rheumatoid arthritis and systemic sclerosis demonstrated an increase in frequency of variant phenotypes of $\alpha$1-AT within the subset of patients who also had radiographic evidence of pulmonary fibrosis.[98] An additional association between $\alpha$1-AT deficiency and IPF was described in a single family in the USA.[99] These investigations were limited by low numbers of subjects and use of nonspecific case definitions for pulmonary fibrosis. More recently, a case–control study examining the relationship of $\alpha$1-AT phenotypes and IPF did not confirm these prior findings and strongly challenged the earlier reports.[100] This larger study included 189 patients with IPF and 189 matched controls from England, and was powered sufficiently to detect a small increased odds ratio of fibrosis with any $\alpha$1-AT phenotype. Thus, there does not appear to be a link between $\alpha$1-AT genetic alterations and IPF.

Tumor necrosis factor has been an important candidate gene for evaluation in patients with IPF. The gene for TNF-$\alpha$ (TNF), is located on chromosome 6 within the major histocompatibility complex class III region. Two separate investigations have demonstrated an increased frequency of the polymorphism consisting of a guanine to adenine substitution at position $-308$ in the promoter region of the TNF-$\alpha$ gene. One study in Australia included 22 patients and 140 control subjects and a similar-sized investigation included a cohort of English and Italian subjects.[94,96] Both studies employed strict case definition criteria and included relatively large numbers of cases and controls. In contrast, in an English population of 72 IPF patients and 192 controls, the observed genotype frequency for this and two other TNF-$\alpha$ polymorphisms did not demonstrate significant differences in gene frequency.[95] Thus, it is not clear if alterations in the TNF gene are associated with IPF.

Transforming growth factor is a potent growth factor for fibroblasts and it promotes extracellular matrix synthesis. It also inhibits degradation of collagen through induction of protease inhibitors and reduction of metalloproteases.[101,102] The gene for TGF-$\beta$1 (TGFB1) is located on chromosome 19 and multiple distinct polymorphisms of this gene have been described.[103] TGF-$\beta$1 polymorphisms in codon 10 have been found to have a higher frequency in systemic sclerosis patients with pulmonary fibrosis in comparison to those with normal lung function.[104] However, a single study of 128 patients with IPF and 140 controls demonstrated no significant difference in frequencies of polymorphisms in codons 10 or 25 of this gene. This same group of investigators followed the cohort of patients for approximately 30 months. They found evidence that the presence of a T to C single base substitution in codon 10 was associated with a significant increase in alveolar arterial oxygen tension difference and reduced diffusion capacity. Thus, while this particular TGF-$\beta$ polymorphism has not been associated with the presence or absence of disease, it may be associated with disease severity or progression of disease.[105]

## CONCLUSIONS

There are many issues that will need to be considered for future genetic studies of IPF and other fibrotic lung diseases. One is the small numbers of informative patients that are available for study. This will necessitate cooperation of multiple centers to accumulate adequate numbers of patients. Another issue relates to the interaction of genetic and environmental factors as they relate to the development of these diseases. There is an effect of cigarette smoking that has only recently been recognized. Most likely, this is an environmental factor that modifies expression of the disease but is not the direct trigger for disease development. There may be many other cofactors like this that modify disease expression. In a similar fashion, the genetic predisposition to the disease might not be explained by a single genetic abnormality but by the combined effects of multiple genes. Thus, identification of the genetic components of the disease may be a daunting task in the setting of multiple possible genes and multiple probable environmental stimuli.

Another consideration is our current definition of the types of pulmonary fibrosis. A major unresolved question is whether NSIP and IPF are always distinct disorders, or in some instances, may be different stages of the same disorder. As noted above, these two disorders were initially considered different manifestations of the same disease. They were separated because of apparent differences in pathology, natural history, and response to therapy. However, a recent study by Flaherty et al.[106] showed that the pathological features of NSIP and IPF may be present in the same patient. The findings of both types of pathology in the same patient either suggests that the same patient may have two distinct types of lung disease, or more likely, that in some patients NSIP and IPF may be different pathological manifestations of the same disorder. Although it is unlikely that most patients with idiopathic NSIP will develop IPF, it is also likely that the lung disease in some patients with IPF has features of NSIP. This question has clear implications for the understanding of the genetics of IPF, since some large families with pulmonary fibrosis have individuals with pathology suggesting IPF and others have pathology suggesting NSIP. This was also observed in family studies where a single genetic defect in the SP-C gene was identified.

Overall, there is compelling circumstantial evidence for a genetic predisposition to develop IPF and other forms of pulmonary fibrosis. This is supported by clear evidence of IPF and other fibrotic lung diseases in families through several generations and identification of specific genetic abnormalities in small groups of patients. Efforts to identify specific genetic factors that relate to larger populations of patients have been hampered by the low incidence of disease and by the high degree of overlap of various types of pulmonary fibrosis. Future progress to define genetic abnormalities that relate to IPF and other fibrotic lung disease will require consistent and precise application of case definition and inclusion criteria. It is unlikely that a single genotype will be identified which leads to the development of IPF. Rather, it is more plausible that multiple genes with different levels of penetrance or expression, as well as multiple environmental triggering factors combine to produce the disease. Thus, a clear link of the genetic component for most patients with IPF will depend upon simultaneous recognition and careful control of environmental and other nongenetic factors.

## Key learning points

- The idiopathic interstitial pneumonias are a heterogenous group of disorders with closely related manifestations but distinct histologic findings and diagnostic criteria.

- Research of the genetic components of pulmonary fibrosis, and specifically idiopathic pulmonary fibrosis, has been limited by the inclusion of heterogenous patient populations and the low incidence of the disease.

- The clinical diagnosis of IPF depends on the rigorous application of clinical, radiographic, and histologic criteria.

- The only treatment that has been shown to alter the natural history of IPF is lung transplantation.

- Numerous studies in animal models have suggested genetic associations with the development of pulmonary fibrosis; however, none of these animal models related directly to idiopathic pulmonary fibrosis.

- Familial clusters of pulmonary fibrosis have been well described and clearly demonstrate vertical transmission of disease and establish the high likelihood of a genetic component of IPF.

- Mutations in surfactant protein C have been identified in association with pulmonary fibrosis and include the histologic types of usual interstitial pneumonia as well as nonspecific interstitial pneumonia.

- Although numerous candidate gene case–control association studies have been performed, none of these results have been consistently reproduced in large populations.

## REFERENCES

◆1  Katzenstein AL, Myers JL. Idiopathic pulmonary fibrosis: clinical relevance of pathologic classification. *Am J Respir Crit Care Med* 1998; **157**(4 Pt 1): 1301–15.

◆2  American Thoracic Society. Idiopathic pulmonary fibrosis: diagnosis and treatment. International consensus statement. American Thoracic Society (ATS), and the European Respiratory Society (ERS). *Am J Respir Crit Care Med* 2000; **161**(2 Pt 1): 646–64.

3  Schwartz DA, Merchant RK, Helmers RA et al. The influence of cigarette smoking on lung function in patients with idiopathic pulmonary fibrosis. *Am Rev Respir Dis* 1991; **144**(3 Pt 1): 504–6.

4  Wiggins J, Strickland B, Turner-Warwick M. Combined cryptogenic fibrosing alveolitis and emphysema: the value of high resolution computed tomography in assessment. *Respir Med* 1990; **84**: 365–9.

5  Hunninghake GW, Lynch DA, Galvin JR et al. Radiologic findings are strongly associated with a pathologic diagnosis of usual interstitial pneumonia. *Chest* 2003; **124**: 1215–23.

●6  Hunninghake GW, Zimmerman MB, Schwartz DA et al. Utility of a lung biopsy for the diagnosis of idiopathic pulmonary fibrosis. *Am J Respir Crit Care Med* 2001; **164**: 193–6.

7  von Plessen C, Grinde O, Gulsvik A. Incidence and prevalence of cryptogenic fibrosing alveolitis in a Norwegian community. *Respir Med* 2003; **97**: 428–35.

8  Hodgson U, Laitinen T, Tukiainen P. Nationwide prevalence of sporadic and familial idiopathic pulmonary fibrosis: evidence of founder effect among multiplex families in Finland. *Thorax* 2002; **57**: 338–42.

9  Kudo K, Takahashi H, Fujishima T et al. Epidemiological survey of idiopathic pulmonary fibrosis in a north region of Japan. *Am J Respir Crit Care Med* 2001; **163**: A710.

●10  Coultas DB, Zumwalt RE, Black WC, Sobonya RE. The epidemiology of interstitial lung diseases. *Am J Respir Crit Care Med* 1994; **150**: 967–72.

11  Scott J, Johnston I, Britton J. What causes cryptogenic fibrosing alveolitis? A case-control study of environmental exposure to dust. *Br Med J* 1990; **301**: 1015–7.

12  Baumgartner KB, Samet JM, Stidley CA et al. Cigarette smoking: a risk factor for idiopathic pulmonary fibrosis. *Am J Respir Crit Care Med* 1997; **155**: 242–8.

●13  Schwartz DA, Van Fossen DS, Davis CS et al. Determinants of progression in idiopathic pulmonary fibrosis. *Am J Respir Crit Care Med* 1994; **149**(2 Pt 1): 444–9.

●14  Schwartz DA, Helmers RA, Galvin JR et al. Determinants of survival in idiopathic pulmonary fibrosis. *Am J Respir Crit Care Med* 1994; **149**(2 Pt 1): 450–4.

●15  Auerbach O, Stout AP, Hammont EC. Smoking and age in relation to pulmonary changes. *N Engl J Med* 1963; **269**: 1045–54.

16  Lilis R, Miller A, Godbold J et al. Radiographic abnormalities in asbestos insulators: effects of duration from onset of exposure and smoking. Relationships of dyspnea with parenchymal and pleural fibrosis. *Am J Ind Med* 1991; **20**: 1–15.

17  Saag KG, Kolluri S, Koehnke RK et al. Rheumatoid arthritis lung disease. Determinants of radiographic and physiologic abnormalities. *Arthritis Rheum* 1996; **39**: 1711–9.

18  Schwartz DA, Galvin JR, Merchant RK et al. Influence of cigarette smoking on bronchoalveolar lavage cellularity in

asbestos-induced lung disease. *Am Rev Respir Dis* 1992;
**145**(2 Pt 1): 400–5.

19  Egan JJ, Woodcock AA, Stewart JP. Viruses and idiopathic
pulmonary fibrosis. *Eur Respir J* 1997; **10**: 1433–7.

20  Stewart JP, Egan JJ, Ross AJ et al. The detection of
Epstein–Barr virus DNA in lung tissue from patients with
idiopathic pulmonary fibrosis. *Am J Respir Crit Care Med* 1999;
**159**(4 Pt 1): 1336–41.

21  Jakab GJ. Sequential virus infections, bacterial superinfections,
and fibrogenesis. *Am Rev Respir Dis* 1990; **142**: 374–9.

22  Jiwa M, Steenbergen RD, Zwaan FE et al. Three sensitive
methods for the detection of cytomegalovirus in lung tissue of
patients with interstitial pneumonitis. *Am J Clin Pathol* 1990;
**93**: 491–4.

23  Ueda T, Ohta K, Suzuki N et al. Idiopathic pulmonary fibrosis
and high prevalence of serum antibodies to hepatitis C virus.
*Am Rev Respir Dis* 1992; **146**: 266–8.

24  Meliconi R, Andreone P, Fasano L et al. Incidence of hepatitis C
virus infection in Italian patients with idiopathic pulmonary
fibrosis. *Thorax* 1996; **51**: 315–7.

◆25  Geist LJ, Hunninghake GW. Role of viruses in the pathogenesis
of pulmonary fibrosis. In: Lynch JP (ed.) *Idiopathic pulmonary
fibrosis*. New York: Marcel Dekker, Inc. 2003.

26  Sladen A, Zanca P, Hadnott WH. Aspiration pneumonitis – the
sequelae. *Chest* 1971; **59**: 448–50.

27  Tobin RW, Pope CE 2nd, Pellegrini CA et al. Increased
prevalence of gastroesophageal reflux in patients with
idiopathic pulmonary fibrosis. *Am J Respir Crit Care Med* 1998;
**158**: 1804–8.

28  Katzenstein AL, Myers JL, Prophet WD et al. Bronchiolitis
obliterans and usual interstitial pneumonia. A comparative
clinicopathologic study. *Am J Surg Pathol* 1986; **10**: 373–81.

29  Nagai S, Kitaichi M, Hamada K et al. Hospital-based historical
cohort study of 234 histologically proven Japanese patients
with IPF. *Sarcoidosis Vasc Diffuse Lung Dis* 1999; **16**: 209–14.

30  Bjoraker JA, Ryu JH, Edwin MK et al. Prognostic significance of
histopathologic subsets in idiopathic pulmonary fibrosis.
*Am J Respir Crit Care Med* 1998; **157**: 199–203.

31  Carrington CB, Gaensler EA, Coutu RE et al. Natural history and
treated course of usual and desquamative interstitial
pneumonia. *N Engl J Med* 1978; **298**: 801–9.

32  Araki T, Katsura H, Sawabe M, Kida K. A clinical study of
idiopathic pulmonary fibrosis based on autopsy studies in
elderly patients. *Intern Med* 2003; **42**: 483–9.

33  King TE Jr, Tooze JA, Schwarz MI et al. Predicting survival in
idiopathic pulmonary fibrosis: scoring system and survival
model. *Am J Respir Crit Care Med* 2001; **164**: 1171–81.

◆34  Gross TJ, Hunninghake GW. Idiopathic pulmonary fibrosis.
*N Engl J Med* 2001; **345**: 517–25.

35  Collard HR, Ryu JH, Douglas WW et al. Combined corticosteroid
and cyclophosphamide therapy does not alter survival in
idiopathic pulmonary fibrosis. *Chest* 2004; **125**: 2169–74.

36  Kolb M, Kirschner J, Riedel W et al. Cyclophosphamide pulse
therapy in idiopathic pulmonary fibrosis. *Eur Respir J* 1998; **12**:
1409–14.

37  Dayton CS, Schwartz DA, Helmers RA et al. Outcome of
subjects with idiopathic pulmonary fibrosis who fail
corticosteroid therapy. Implications for further studies. *Chest*
1993; **103**: 69–73.

38  Zisman DA, Lynch JP 3rd, Toews GB et al. Cyclophosphamide in
the treatment of idiopathic pulmonary fibrosis: a prospective

study in patients who failed to respond to corticosteroids.
*Chest* 2000; **117**: 1619–26.

39  Selman M, Carrillo G, Salas J et al. Colchicine, D-penicillamine,
and prednisone in the treatment of idiopathic pulmonary
fibrosis: a controlled clinical trial. *Chest* 1998; **114**: 507–12.

40  Douglas WW, Ryu JH, Schroeder DR. Idiopathic pulmonary
fibrosis: Impact of oxygen and colchicine, prednisone, or no
therapy on survival. *Am J Respir Crit Care Med* 2000;
**161**(4 Pt 1): 1172–8.

41  Ziesche R, Hofbauer E, Wittmann K et al. A preliminary study
of long-term treatment with interferon gamma-1b and low-
dose prednisolone in patients with idiopathic pulmonary
fibrosis [erratum appears in *N Engl J Med* 2000; **342**: 524].
*N Engl J Med* 1999; **341**: 1264–9.

42  Raghu G, Brown KK, Bradford WZ et al. A placebo-controlled
trial of interferon gamma-1b in patients with idiopathic
pulmonary fibrosis. *N Engl J Med* 2004; **350**: 125–33.

43  Demedts M, Auwerx J, Goddeeris P et al. The inherited
association of interstitial lung disease, hypocalciuric
hypercalcemia, and defective granulocyte function.
*Am Rev Respir Dis* 1985; **131**: 470–5.

44  Auwerx J, Demedts M, Bouillon R, Desmet J. Coexistence of
hypocalciuric hypercalcaemia and interstitial lung disease in a
family: a cross-sectional study. *Eur J Clin Invest* 1985; **15**:
6–14.

45  Pollak MR, Brown EM, Chou YH et al. Mutations in the human
Ca(2+)-sensing receptor gene cause familial hypocalciuric
hypercalcemia and neonatal severe hyperparathyroidism.
*Cell* 1993; **75**: 1297–303.

46  Chou YH, Pollak MR, Brandi ML et al. Mutations in the human
Ca(2+)-sensing receptor gene that cause familial
hypocalciuric hypercalcemia. *Am J Hum Genet* 1995; **56**:
1075–9.

◆47  Marshall RP, McAnulty RJ, Laurent GJ. The pathogenesis of
pulmonary fibrosis: is there a fibrosis gene? *Int J Biochem Cell
Biol* 1997; **29**: 107–20.

48  Hermansky F, Pudlak P. Albinism associated with hemorrhagic
diathesis and unusual pigmented reticular cells in the bone
marrow: report of two cases with histochemical studies. *Blood*
1959; **14**: 162–9.

49  Hermos CR, Huizing M, Kaiser-Kupfer MI, Gahl WA.
Hermansky–Pudlak syndrome type 1: gene organization, novel
mutations, and clinical-molecular review of non-Puerto Rican
cases. *Hum Mutat* 2002; **20**: 482.

50  Brantly M, Avila NA, Shotelersuk V et al. Pulmonary function and
high-resolution CT findings in patients with an inherited form of
pulmonary fibrosis, Hermansky–Pudlak syndrome, due to
mutations in HPS-1. *Chest* 2000; **117**: 129–36.

51  Witkop CJ, Krumwiede M, Sedano H, White JG. Reliability of
absent platelet dense bodies as a diagnostic criterion for
Hermansky–Pudlak syndrome. *Am J Hematol* 1987; **26**:
305–11.

52  Wildenberg SC, Oetting WS, Almodovar C et al. A gene causing
Hermansky–Pudlak syndrome in a Puerto Rican population maps
to chromosome 10q2. *Am J Hum Genet* 1995; **57**: 755–65.

53  Fukai K, Oh J, Frenk E et al. Linkage disequilibrium mapping of
the gene for Hermansky–Pudlak syndrome to chromosome
10q23.1-q23.3. *Hum Mol Genet* 1995; **4**: 1665–9.

54  Shotelersuk V, Hazelwood S, Larson D et al. Three new
mutations in a gene causing Hermansky–Pudlak syndrome:
clinical correlations. *Mol Genet Metab* 1998; **64**: 99–107.

55 Oh J, Ho L, Ala-Mello S et al. Mutation analysis of patients with Hermansky–Pudlak syndrome: a frameshift hot spot in the HPS gene and apparent locus heterogeneity. *Am J Hum Genet* 1998; **62**: 593–8.

56 Spritz RA, Oh J. HPS gene mutations in Hermansky–Pudlak syndrome. *Am J Hum Genet* 1999; **64**: 658.

57 Oetting WS, King RA. Molecular basis of albinism: mutations and polymorphisms of pigmentation genes associated with albinism. *Hum Mutat* 1999; **13**: 99–115.

58 Lyerla TA, Rusiniak ME, Borchers M et al. Aberrant lung structure, composition, and function in a murine model of Hermansky–Pudlak syndrome. *Am J Physiol Lung Cell Mol Physiol* 2003; **285**: L643–53.

59 Avila NA, Brantly M, Premkumar A et al. Hermansky–Pudlak syndrome: radiography and CT of the chest compared with pulmonary function tests and genetic studies. *AJR Am J Roentgenol* 2002; **179**: 887–92.

60 Huizing M, Gahl WA. Disorders of vesicles of lysosomal lineage: the Hermansky–Pudlak syndromes. *Curr Mol Med* 2002; **2**: 451–67.

●61 Amin RS, Wert SE, Baughman RP et al. Surfactant protein deficiency in familial interstitial lung disease. *J Pediatr* 2001; **139**: 85–92.

●62 Nogee LM, Dunbar AE 3rd, Wert SE et al. A mutation in the surfactant protein C gene associated with familial interstitial lung disease. *N Engl J Med* 2001; **344**: 573–9.

●63 Thomas AQ, Lane K, Phillips J 3rd et al. Heterozygosity for a surfactant protein C gene mutation associated with usual interstitial pneumonitis and cellular nonspecific interstitial pneumonitis in one kindred. *Am J Respir Crit Care Med* 2002; **165**: 1322–8.

64 Marshall RP, Puddicombe A, Cookson WO, Laurent GJ. Adult familial cryptogenic fibrosing alveolitis in the United Kingdom. *Thorax* 2000; **55**: 143–6.

◆65 Mageto YN, Raghu G. Genetic predisposition of idiopathic pulmonary fibrosis. *Curr Opin Pulm Med* 1997; **3**: 336–40.

●66 Peabody JW, Peabody JWJ, Hayes EW, Hayes EWJ. Idiopathic pulmonary fibrosis; its occurrence in identical twin sisters. *Dis Chest* 1950; **18**: 330–43.

67 MacMillan JM. Familial pulmonary fibrosis. *Dis Chest* 1951; **20**: 426–36.

68 Bonanni PP, Frymoyer JW, Jacox RF. A family study of idiopathic pulmonary fibrosis. *Am J Med* 1965; **39**: 411–21.

69 Marney A, Lane KB, Phillips JA 3rd et al. Idiopathic pulmonary fibrosis can be an autosomal dominant trait in some families. *Chest* 2001; **120**(1 Suppl): 56S.

70 Javaheri S, Lederer DH, Pella JA et al. Idiopathic pulmonary fibrosis in monozygotic twins. The importance of genetic predisposition. *Chest* 1980; **78**: 591–4.

71 Swaye P, Van Ordstrand HS, McCormack LJ, Wolpaw SE. Familial Hamman–Rich syndrome. Report of eight cases. *Dis Chest* 1969; **55**: 7–12.

72 Musk AW, Zilko PJ, Manners P et al. Genetic studies in familial fibrosing alveolitis. Possible linkage with immunoglobulin allotypes (Gm). *Chest* 1986; **89**: 206–10.

73 Fulmer JD, Sposovska MS, von Gal ER et al. Distribution of HLA antigens in idiopathic pulmonary fibrosis. *Am Rev Respir Dis* 1978; **118**: 141–7.

74 Bitterman PB, Rennard SI, Keogh BA et al. Familial idiopathic pulmonary fibrosis. Evidence of lung inflammation in unaffected family members. *N Engl J Med* 1986; **314**: 1343–7.

75 Chung MP, Monick MM, Hamzeh NY et al. Role of repeated lung injury and genetic background in bleomycin-induced fibrosis. *Am J Respir Cell Mol Biol* 2003; **29**(3 Pt 1): 375–80.

76 Haston CK, Wang M, Dejournett RE et al. Bleomycin hydrolase and a genetic locus within the MHC affect risk for pulmonary fibrosis in mice. *Hum Mol Genet* 2002; **11**: 1855–63.

77 Turner-Warwick M, Lebowitz M, Burrows B, Johnson A. Cryptogenic fibrosing alveolitis and lung cancer. *Thorax* 1980; **35**: 496–9.

78 Hubbard R, Venn A, Lewis S, Britton J. Lung cancer and cryptogenic fibrosing alveolitis. A population-based cohort study. *Am J Respir Crit Care Med* 2000; **161**: 5–8.

79 Vassilakis DA, Sourvinos G, Spandidos DA et al. Frequent genetic alterations at the microsatellite level in cytologic sputum samples of patients with idiopathic pulmonary fibrosis. *Am J Respir Crit Care Med* 2000; **162**(3 Pt 1): 1115–9.

80 Mori M, Kida H, Morishita H et al. Microsatellite instability in transforming growth factor-beta 1 type II receptor gene in alveolar lining epithelial cells of idiopathic pulmonary fibrosis. *Am J Respir Cell Mol Biol* 2001; **24**: 398–404.

81 Bouros D, Wells AU, Nicholson AG et al. Histopathologic subsets of fibrosing alveolitis in patients with systemic sclerosis and their relationship to outcome. *Am J Respir Crit Care Med* 2002; **165**: 1581–6.

82 Kim DS, Yoo B, Lee JS et al. The major histopathologic pattern of pulmonary fibrosis in scleroderma is nonspecific interstitial pneumonia. *Sarcoidosis Vasc Diffuse Lung Dis* 2002; **19**: 121–7.

83 Schattner A, Aviel-Ronen S, Mark EJ. Accelerated usual interstitial pneumonitis, anti-DNA antibodies and hypocomplementemia. *J Intern Med* 2003; **254**: 193–6.

84 Kuwana M, Kaburaki J, Arnett FC et al. Influence of ethnic background on clinical and serologic features in patients with systemic sclerosis and anti-DNA topoisomerase I antibody. *Arthritis Rheum* 1999; **42**: 465–74.

85 Greidinger EL, Flaherty KT, White B et al. African-American race and antibodies to topoisomerase I are associated with increased severity of scleroderma lung disease. *Chest* 1998; **114**: 801–7.

86 Reveille JD. Ethnicity and race and systemic sclerosis: how it affects susceptibility, severity, antibody genetics, and clinical manifestations. *Curr Rheumatol Rep* 2003; **5**: 160–7.

87 Zhou X, Tan FK, Reveille JD et al. Association of novel polymorphisms with the expression of SPARC in normal fibroblasts and with susceptibility to scleroderma. *Arthritis Rheum* 2002; **46**: 2990–9.

88 Briggs DC, Vaughan RW, Welsh KI et al. Immunogenetic prediction of pulmonary fibrosis in systemic sclerosis. *Lancet* 1991; **338**: 661–2.

89 Avila JJ, Lympany PA, Pantelidis P et al. Fibronectin gene polymorphisms associated with fibrosing alveolitis in systemic sclerosis. *Am J Respir Cell Mol Biol* 1999; **20**: 106–12.

90 Cardon LR, Palmer LJ. Population stratification and spurious allelic association. *Lancet* 2003; **361**: 598–604.

91 Zorzetto M, Ferrarotti I, Trisolini R et al. Complement receptor 1 gene polymorphisms are associated with idiopathic pulmonary fibrosis. *Am J Respir Crit Care Med* 2003; **168**: 330–4.

92 Hutyrova B, Pantelidis P, Drabek J et al. Interleukin-1 gene cluster polymorphisms in sarcoidosis and idiopathic pulmonary fibrosis. *Am J Respir Crit Care Med* 2002; **165**: 148–51.

93 Renzoni E, Lympany P, Sestini P et al. Distribution of novel polymorphisms of the interleukin-8 and CXC receptor 1 and 2

genes in systemic sclerosis and cryptogenic fibrosing alveolitis. *Arthritis Rheum* 2000; **43**: 1633–40.

94 Whyte M, Hubbard R, Meliconi R et al. Increased risk of fibrosing alveolitis associated with interleukin-1 receptor antagonist and tumor necrosis factor-alpha gene polymorphisms. *Am J Respir Crit Care Med* 2000; **162**(2 Pt 1): 755–8.

95 Pantelidis P, Fanning GC, Wells AU et al. Analysis of tumor necrosis factor-alpha, lymphotoxin-alpha, tumor necrosis factor receptor II, and interleukin-6 polymorphisms in patients with idiopathic pulmonary fibrosis. *Am J Respir Crit Care Med* 2001; **163**: 1432–6.

96 Riha RL, Yang IA, Rabnott GC et al. Cytokine gene polymorphisms in idiopathic pulmonary fibrosis. *Intern Med J* 2004; **34**: 126–9.

97 Geddes DM, Webley M, Brewerton DA et al. Alpha 1-antitrypsin phenotypes in fibrosing alveolitis and rheumatoid arthritis. *Lancet* 1977; **2**: 1049–51.

98 Michalski JP, McCombs CC, Scopelitis E et al. Alpha 1-antitrypsin phenotypes, including M subtypes, in pulmonary disease associated with rheumatoid arthritis and systemic sclerosis. *Arthritis Rheum* 1986; **29**: 586–91.

99 Kim H, Lepler L, Daniels A, Phillips Y. Alpha 1-antitrypsin deficiency and idiopathic pulmonary fibrosis in a family. *South Med J* 1996; **89**: 1008–10.

100 Hubbard R, Baoku Y, Kalsheker N et al. Alpha1-antitrypsin phenotypes in patients with cryptogenic fibrosing alveolitis: a case-control study. *Eur Respir J* 1997; **10**: 2881–3.

101 Ward PA, Hunninghake GW. Lung inflammation and fibrosis. *Am J Respir Crit Care Med* 1998; **157**(4 Pt 2): S123–9.

102 Coker RK, Laurent GJ, Jeffery PK et al. Localisation of transforming growth factor beta1 and beta3 mRNA transcripts in normal and fibrotic human lung. *Thorax* 2001; **56**: 549–56.

103 Cambien F, Ricard S, Troesch A et al. Polymorphisms of the transforming growth factor-beta 1 gene in relation to myocardial infarction and blood pressure. The Etude Cas-Temoin de l'Infarctus du Myocarde (ECTIM) study. *Hypertension* 1996; **28**: 881–7.

104 Sugiura Y, Banno S, Matsumoto Y et al. Transforming growth factor beta1 gene polymorphism in patients with systemic sclerosis. *J Rheumatol* 2003; **30**: 1520–3.

105 Xaubet A, Marin-Arguedas A, Lario S et al. Transforming growth factor-beta1 gene polymorphisms are associated with disease progression in idiopathic pulmonary fibrosis. *Am J Respir Crit Care Med* 2003; **168**: 431–5.

●106 Flaherty KR, Travis WD, Colby TV et al. Histopathologic variability in usual and nonspecific interstitial pneumonias. *Am J Respir Crit Care Med* 2001; **164**: 1722–7.

# 13

# Sarcoidosis

PAUL A. BEIRNE, STAVROS E. ANEVLAVIS, AND ROLAND M. DU BOIS

## DEFINITION

The 1999 consensus statement by the American Thoracic Society (ATS), the European Respiratory Society (ERS), and the World Association of Sarcoidosis and Other Granulomatous Disorders (WASOG) defined sarcoidosis as a systemic disorder of unknown cause characterized by the presence of noncaseating epithelioid granulomas and the accumulation of T-lymphocytes and macrophages in multiple organs.[1] These granulomas can occur in any organ system but are more common in the lung and the lymph nodes. The characteristic granuloma found in sarcoidosis is made up of multinucleated giant cells, mononuclear phagocytes, and lymphocytes surrounded by tightly organized fibroblasts, mast cells, and an extracellular matrix.

Sarcoidosis most commonly affects young and middle-aged adults and frequently presents with bilateral hilar lymphadenopathy, pulmonary infiltration, and ocular and skin lesions. The liver, spleen, lymph nodes, salivary glands, heart, nervous system, muscles, bones, and other organs may also be involved.

### Clinical syndromes

Within the broad clinical definition of sarcoidosis, some distinct clinical subtypes are recognized. Lofgren's syndrome consists of fever, bilateral hilar lymphadenopathy, erythema nodosum, and arthralgia. Erythema nodosum is almost always the first manifestation of Lofgren's syndrome and usually remits within 6–8 weeks. Recurrence is unusual but may be experienced by about 10 percent of patients in the first 3 months.[1] Erythema nodosum is more common in white women of childbearing age. It is rare in African-American and Japanese patients, and uncommon in West Indian and Asian immigrants in the UK.

Ocular disease has been reported to occur in 11–83 percent of patients, with uveitis being the most common manifestation. Anterior uveitis usually runs a self-limiting course or responds to topical corticosteroid therapy.[1] Chronic uveitis may cause glaucoma, cataract, and blindness.

The combination of parotid gland enlargement, uveitis, fever, and cranial nerve palsies is known as Heerfordt's syndrome – an uncommon condition that presents acutely and runs a chronic course. Unilateral or bilateral parotitis with swollen, painful enlargement of the gland occurs in less than 6 percent of sarcoidosis patients. In about 40 percent of these patients, parotid enlargement resolves spontaneously.[2]

## EPIDEMIOLOGY

### Incidence and prevalence

Precise figures regarding the incidence of sarcoidosis are difficult to obtain, partly because many cases never come to clinical attention. There is variation in the reported incidence and prevalence of sarcoidosis in different countries and continents (see Table 13.1). This may be due to true differences in incidence, but may also be related to differences

**Table 13.1** *Prevalence of pulmonary sarcoidosis*

| Country | Prevalence per 100 000 | Reference |
|---|---|---|
| Sweden | 64 | 10 |
| USA | 39 African-American women | 12–14 |
| | 29.8 African-American men | |
| | 12.1 White women | |
| | 9.6 White men | |
| UK | 9–36 | 8 |
| Nordic countries | 27 | 9 |
| Cape Town | 27 Black South Africans | 17 |
| | 6 White South Africans | |
| Isle of Man | 14.7 | 18 |
| Japan | 1.3 | 19 |
| South America (Brazil, Uruguay) | 0.2 | 10 |

in local awareness of the disease, as well as a lack of sensitive and specific diagnostic tests.

Sarcoidosis occurs throughout the world, affecting both sexes and all races and ages. The disease most commonly affects adults less than 40 years of age, peaking in those 20–29 years old.[3] In a review of 1254 patients, 50 percent were in the 20–40 years age group with only 2 percent younger than 10 years, and only 4 percent older than 60. An 81-year-old woman in the UK is the oldest patient reported with the disease in the literature.[4] Sarcoidosis is more often associated with the development of chronic, progressive disease if it occurs in persons older than 40 years. In Scandinavian countries and Japan, there is a second peak incidence in women over the age of 50.[5–7] In the 1950s and 1960s, there were mass screening studies reporting radiographic abnormalities consistent with sarcoidosis in 9–36 per 100 000 of those screened.[8] In Scandinavia, similar studies over the same period reported a prevalence of 28 per 100 000 examined persons.[9] In a summary of 29 surveys in 24 countries published in 1964 by Bauer and Lofgren,[10] prevalence varied from 0.2 per 100 000 in Portugal, Brazil, and Uruguay to 64 per 100 000 in Sweden – the highest prevalence reported. The disease incidence is higher in African-American and in Scandinavian populations.[11] Most studies suggest a slightly higher disease rate for women. In a population-based incidence study of sarcoidosis in the USA, rates were 5.9 per 100 000 person-years for men and 6.3 per 100 000 person-years for women.[12] The lifetime risk of sarcoidosis is 0.85 percent for US whites and 2.4 percent for African-Americans.[13] The estimated prevalence of sarcoidosis ranges from less than one case to 40 cases per 100 000, with an age-adjusted annual incidence rate in the USA of 35.5 per 100 000 for African-Americans and 10.9 per 100 000 for whites.[12–14] In a review of newly diagnosed cases of sarcoidosis in patients belonging to a Detroit health maintenance organization between 1990 and 1994 and constituting about 5 percent of the metropolitan population in the ages studied, annual incidence rates were found to be 39.1 per 100 000 for African-American women, 29.8 for African-American men, 12.1 for white women, and 9.6 for white men.[13]

Sarcoidosis is reported to be very rare in Chinese people – in one mass community radiographic survey of 3.6 million people in Taiwan, no cases were indentified.[15] Reports from Spain, Portugal, India, Saudi Arabia, and South America suggest that sarcoidosis is a rarely reported disease.[11,16] Sarcoidosis was thought to be rare in Africa, but a prevalence study in 1992 in Cape Town reported prevalence rates of 27 per 100 000 in black South Africans and 6 per 100 000 in white South Africans.[17]

## Disease heterogeneity

Significant heterogeneity in disease presentation and severity occurs among different ethnic and racial groups. Blacks tend to have more severe musculoskeletal or constitutional symptoms on presentation and higher rates of liver, bone marrow, extrathoracic lymph node, and skin involvement (except erythema nodosum), while whites are more likely to present with asymptomatic disease.[13,20–25] Some of the extrathoracic manifestations are more common in certain populations, such as chronic uveitis in African-Americans, lupus pernio in Puerto Ricans, and erythema nodosum (EN) in Europeans. Erythema nodosum is uncommon in blacks and Japanese, although it is more common among Europeans.[26] Cardiac and ocular involvement in sarcoidosis is said to be more common in the Japanese population, where the most frequent cause of death for sarcoidosis patients is from myocardial involvement.[6,27,28] Elsewhere, mortality is due most commonly to respiratory failure.[22,29] Overall mortality from sarcoidosis is 1–5 percent.

## Disease clustering

There are several lines of epidemiological evidence that support the hypothesis that sarcoidosis may be triggered by an infective agent or agents. These include reports of spatial, seasonal, and occupational clustering of the disease. Reports of spatial clusters of illness have suggested person-to-person transmission or shared exposure to an environmental or infectious agent. One case–control study of residents in the Isle of Man observed that 40 percent of sarcoidosis cases reported prior contact with a person known to have the disease, compared with 1–2 percent of the controls.[30,31] Of these contacts, 14 pairs occurred in the same household, only nine of whom were blood relatives. Nine pairs came in contact with one another at work, two were neighbors, and 14 were non-cohabiting friends. All the individuals lived within 100 m of each other during an 'infective period' of 7 years (5 years before the diagnosis and 2 years after the diagnosis). Other clusters of sarcoidosis have been reported in northern Sweden and central Hokkaido in Japan.[33]

## Familial sarcoidosis

Familial cases of sarcoidosis have also been reported in most populations (see Table 13.2). The first reported cases

**Table 13.2**  *Familial risk in different populations*

| Population | Degree of familial aggregation | Reference |
|---|---|---|
| Finland | 3.6% | 34 |
| Japan | 4.3% | |
| Irish | 9.6% | 36 |
| African Americans | 10% | 37 |
| African Americans (siblings and parents) | 2.5-fold increase in the disease risk | 38 |
| UK Caucasians | Relative risk 36–73 | 39 |
| African Americans (parents and siblings) | Relative risk 3.1 | 40 |
| US whites (parents and siblings) | Relative risk 16.6 | |
| US African Americans | 19% | 41 |
| US whites | 5% | |

of familial sarcoidosis were in 1923, in two German sisters.[32] A survey from Pietinahlo and coworkers found a prevalence of familial sarcoidosis of 3.6 and 4.3 percent in Finnish and Japanese patients, respectively.[34] An increased prevalence of sarcoidosis has been described in the Furano district of northern Japan, with some evidence of familial clustering.[35]

The highest frequency of sarcoidosis among the immediate family of patients was found in an Irish population of 114 patients attending a specialist clinic; 9.6 percent of the patients were found to have one or more siblings with the same disease.[36] These findings are very similar to those from a study by Headings et al.[37] involving African-American patients in whom a sibling disease prevalence of 10 percent was reported. Rybicki and coworkers[38] studied 488 parents and siblings of 179 African-American sarcoidosis cases and found a 2.5-fold increased risk of history of sarcoidosis in case relatives over that in the general population. In the UK, McGrath et al.[39] reported a sarcoidosis risk ratio for siblings of between 36 and 73, indicating significant familial clustering of the disease. The population studied was mainly caucasian (62.5 percent). ACCESS (a case–control etiologic study of sarcoidosis) is the largest effort to date to quantify the familial aggregation of sarcoidosis.[40] It is a large case–control study consisting of 10 862 first-degree and 17 047 second-degree relatives identified by 706 sarcoidosis case–control pairs. The overall familial relative risk in siblings was larger than in parents (odds ratio (OR), 5.8 versus 3.8). For African-Americans, the familial relative risk for a sarcoidosis case was 2.8, whereas the familial relative risk for whites was markedly higher at 16.6. In summary, in the ACCESS study, cases were almost five times more likely than controls to report a sibling or a parent with a history of sarcoidosis.

## Seasonal variations

Some studies have observed a seasonal clustering of sarcoidosis cases in winter and early spring.[42,43] Seasonal

clustering has been reported in Greece, where 70 percent of the cases occurred between March and May every year between 1980 and 1989 and no diagnoses of asymptomatic stage I disease were made between July and November.[44] In Spain, almost 50 percent of the diagnoses of erythema nodosum and hilar lymphadenopathy are made between April and June.[42] In Japan, sarcoidosis is mainly diagnosed during June and July.[45] An outbreak of eight cases of acute sarcoidosis, accompanied by arthropathy, was reported in Norfolk, UK, in 1988.[46] All of the cases occurred during May.

## Environmental factors

Edmondstone's retrospective study[47] of patients with sarcoidosis revealed 7.5 times greater numbers of nurses with the condition than expected, results which are in keeping with reports from the USA.[48] In the Isle of Man study, 18.8 percent of sarcoidosis cases were healthcare workers (mainly nurses), compared with 4.2 percent of the controls.[18] There are also reports of increased frequency and significant association for increased risk of sarcoidosis in servicemen on US Navy aircraft carriers.[49] In 1993, Kern et al.[50] reported a cluster of three biopsy-proven cases of sarcoidosis in white male firefighters from Providence, RI.[50] This is not the only reported increased incidence of sarcoidosis in firefighters. A study contracted by the New York City Fire Department (FDNY) between 1985 and 1998 found increased annual incidence proportions and point prevalence in FDNY firefighters as compared to emergency medical services healthcare workers and historical controls.[51]

The increased frequency of the disease in the rural southern and eastern states of the USA has led to the hypothesis that geographic and environmental factors such as soil or pine tree pollen may play a role in the pathogenesis of sarcoidosis, but this has not been confirmed in further epidemiologic studies.[52,53]

Patients with sarcoidosis are less likely to smoke than people of similar age in the general population. In a study by Valeyre et al.[54] smoking was less common in patients with sarcoidosis (30 percent) than in control subjects (46 percent). There were no differences in clinical, radiographic, and functional abnormalities at presentation and at 1-year follow up between smokers and nonsmokers. The same results are also reported from Douglas[55] and Hance,[56] with 78 and 68 percent, respectively, of the patients with sarcoidosis being nonsmokers.

## NATURAL HISTORY

The symptoms and clinical findings of sarcoidosis have a tendency to wax and wane, either spontaneously or in response to therapy. However, determination of a general prognosis based on the patient's initial clinical presentation is possible.

Stage I disease, which is defined as the presence of hilar adenopathy without parenchymal infiltrates on radiography, remits spontaneously in 60–80 percent of cases; stage II (hilar adenopathy with infiltrates) remits spontaneously in 50–60 percent; stage III (infiltrates without adenopathy) remits spontaneously in less than 30 percent. More than 85 percent of spontaneous remissions occur within 2 years of presentation.[57]

Patients with Lofgren's syndrome have the best prognosis. The disease remits in more than 90 percent of cases. Erythema nodosum and fever usually remit spontaneously within 6 weeks; resolution of the hilar lymphadenopathy may be delayed for 1 year.[58]

Clinical variables associated with poorer prognosis include black race, onset of disease after the age of 40, symptoms that last for more than 6 months, the absence of erythema nodosum, splenomegaly, involvement of more than three organ systems, and stage III pulmonary disease.[20,59] Even in patients who respond to corticosteroids, up to 25 percent with stage II or III disease will relapse once therapy is discontinued.[60]

Asymptomatic disease with spontaneous remission of mediastinal adenopathy or pulmonary infiltration is the most common pattern. A significant number of entirely asymptomatic patients will be diagnosed by the incidental finding of hilar lymphadenopathy or interstitial infiltrates on routine chest radiography.[61] Two-thirds of a series of 505 cases of sarcoidosis in Sweden diagnosed by periodic health examinations were made by radiographic abnormalities in asymptomatic patients.[62] In a study by Mayock et al.,[20] 12 percent of the 145 patients were asymptomatic at presentation. However, only 5 percent of the 181 patients in Johns' series with subsequent chronic sarcoidosis (of greater than 5 years duration) were asymptomatic at the time of diagnosis.[63]

In a study by Zych et al.[64] involving 960 patients with sarcoidosis, complete or partial regression of the disease either spontaneously or after treatment was observed in 777 patients (80.9 percent). In 156 patients (16.3 percent) the disease remained stable and in 27 patients (2.8 percent) it progressed. Complete spontaneous regression was observed in 388 patients (40.8 percent); of these, 243 patients had stage I and 145 had stage II disease. Partial spontaneous regression was observed in 109 patients with stage I and in 100 patients with stage II. Combining complete and partial regression, a favorable spontaneous course of the disease was observed in 597 patients (62.2 percent). No spontaneous regression was observed in patients with stage III or IV disease. In the 214 patients who were treated, complete regression was observed in 60 of them, with partial regression in 120 patients. Overall, 84.1 percent of the treated patients had a favorable outcome.

Assessment of morbidity or mortality attributable to sarcoidosis is difficult. Fatalities occur in 1–5 percent of patients, typically owing to progressive respiratory insufficiency or central nervous system or cardiac involvement.[57,62,63]

Differing mortality rates reflect differences in severity of disease, referral bias, and diverse genetic and epidemiological factors. Studies from nonreferral centers report mortality rates less than 1 percent. In contrast, published series from referral centers (which include patients with severe and progressive disease) report higher mortality rates.[20,65,66] The causes of death vary in differing geographic regions (which may reflect genetic or environmental differences). In Japan, 77 percent of deaths from sarcoidosis were due to cardiac involvement.[6] In the USA, most deaths are due to pulmonary complications.[29]

There are reports of recurrence of sarcoidosis in patients who underwent lung or heart transplantation. The reported incidence is similar from two studies by Yeatman et al.[67] and Johnson and colleagues.[68] In the study by Yeatman et al., 11 patients underwent either lung or heart and lung transplantation and granulomata recurred in the lungs of two of the patients.

## PATHOGENESIS

Histologically, sarcoidosis is characterized by tissue infiltration by mononuclear phagocytes and lymphocytes with associated noncaseating granuloma formation. Granulomas have a protective role to play in many diseases of known etiology, principally those caused by microbial agents, such as mycobacteria. However, the role of the granuloma in diseases of unknown etiology is unclear. In pulmonary diseases such as sarcoidosis and Wegener's granulomatosis, and in nonpulmonary diseases such as Crohn's disease, the granulomatous inflammation accounts for much of the pathology, and the protective benefits, if any, are not known. Granulomatous inflammation is also the principal pathological lesion in hypersensitivity diseases of known etiology, such as chronic beryllium disease and extrinsic allergic alveolitis, in which the granulomatous inflammation appears to confer no protective benefit on the individual, but is primarily responsible for the tissue pathology.

Whatever the etiology, it is increasingly clear that granulomatous disease is the result of an interaction between environmental factors and host factors, and that many of the host factors are genetically determined. These genetic factors do not behave like the single gene disorders inherited in Mendelian fashion, such as cystic fibrosis, Huntington's chorea, or Duchenne muscular dystrophy. Rather, the granulomatous diseases are polygenic (or complex) diseases. They are the result of a complex interaction between many different genes and the environment. The importance of these genes is that elucidation of their roles will help us to explain disease etiology and pathogenesis. It could help us to explain mysteries such as why some people develop granulomatous diseases like sarcoidosis, and why some of them develop chronic intractable disease leading to disability and death. Answering these questions could help to direct future research, help identify patients with increased susceptibility to disease, and open up new avenues for novel therapies.

## Immunology of the granuloma

Granuloma formation is preceded by tissue infiltration by mononuclear inflammatory cells, mostly T cells and monocyte-macrophages. This occurs in response to the presence of antigen. When the antigen presentation is persistent, continuing activation of T cells leads to the accumulation of large numbers of macrophages. These give rise to epithelioid cells (large cells with a pale nucleus and abundant cytoplasm, that appear to have a secretory role) or fuse to form giant multinucleate cells. Giant cells and epithelioid cells are surrounded by a rim of T lymphocytes and a few B lymphocytes, with areas of fibrosis in the presence of fibroblasts and areas of necrosis. This characteristic aggregate of immune cells is the granuloma – a response to persistent antigen.[69]

Two cell types play mutually dependent roles in granuloma formation – cells of the monocyte–macrophage lineage and T lymphocytes (see Fig. 13.1). The antigen, in order to elicit the granulomatous response, must be processed by antigen presenting cells (such as alveolar or tissue macrophages) and presented in association with major histocompatibility complex (MHC) class II proteins. MHC class II protein and bound antigen is the ligand for the T-cell receptor (TCR). Recognition of antigen presented in association with an MHC class II protein leads to T cell activation, with upregulation of TCR mRNA, downregulation of cell-surface TCR numbers, and an increase in other cell-surface markers of activation such as HLA-DR. T cells release cytokines (proteins that act as the intercellular messengers of the immune system) that stimulate macrophages, leading to release of macrophage-derived cytokines, such as tumor necrosis factor-$\alpha$ (TNF-$\alpha$), interleukin-1 (IL-1), IL-6, IL-12, and IL-15. Macrophages also release chemokines (small peptides released by inflammatory cells that control the adhesion, chemotaxis, and activation of leukocytes) such as IL-8, 'regulated on activation, normal T-cell expressed and secreted' (RANTES), monocyte chemotactic protein (MCP-1), and macrophage inflammatory protein (MIP-1). Thus, macrophage stimulation is critical to granuloma formation, by contributing to a milieu of cytokines and chemokines with various actions. As well as actions on other inflammatory cells, they exert actions on other cells such as endothelial cells; for example, cytokines including IL-1, TNF-$\alpha$, and interferon-$\gamma$ (IFN-$\gamma$) increase the expression of adhesion molecules on endothelial cells, facilitating the recruitment of inflammatory cells to the site of inflammation.

The functions of individual cytokines are highly complex and often dependent upon the immunological context in which they are secreted. IL-1 is an accessory T cell growth factor, and is believed to be important for inflammatory

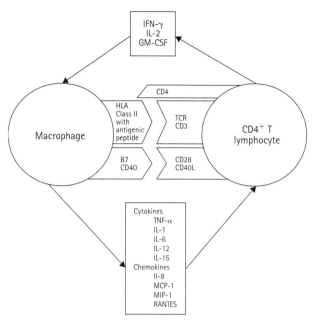

**Figure 13.1** *The stimulatory interactions between the antigen presenting cell (e.g., pulmonary macrophage) and T lymphocytes that drive the granulomatous reaction through cytokine and chemokine networks. IFN-$\gamma$, interferon-gamma; IL, interleukin; GM-CSF, granulocyte macrophage-colony stimulating factor; TNF-$\alpha$, tumor necrosis factor-alpha; MCP-1, monocyte chemotactic protein-1; MIP-1, macrophage inflammatory protein-1; RANTES, regulated on activation, normal T-cell expressed and secreted; HLA, human leukocyte antigen; TCR, T-cell receptor; CD40L, CD40 ligand*

cell recruitment and proliferation. TNF-$\alpha$ is believed to be important for maintenance and control of the inflammation. IL-12 promotes Th1 proliferation and specifically upregulates IFN-$\gamma$ secretion from T cells, and this IFN-$\gamma$ enhances macrophage accessory function, in a feedback loop.

T cell cytokine release is more variable. Two distinct profiles of T cell cytokine release have been recognized – T helper type 1 (Th1), dominated by IFN-$\gamma$ and IL-2, or Th2, dominated by IL-4 and IL-10. These two responses are mutually antagonistic – IFN-$\gamma$ inhibits Th2 proliferation, while IL-10 has been shown to inhibit the release of IL-2 and IFN-$\gamma$ from Th1 cells. In simplistic evolutionary terms, Th1 responses may be most important for cell-mediated immunity, whereas Th2 responses may mediate IgE and eosinophil-mediated immunity. In the granulomas of sarcoidosis, tuberculosis and most other granulomatous diseases, it is believed that Th1 responses predominate in most but not all patients.[70] However, in some granulomas, such as those initiated by parasitic infections, Th2 responses may predominate.[71] T-cell secretion of IL-2 and IFN-$\gamma$, as well as the colony-stimulatory factor GM-CSF, enhances the antigen-presenting capabilities of macrophages. IFN-$\gamma$ increases MHC expression on macrophages and increases TNF-$\alpha$ release from appropriately triggered macrophages. In this way, macrophages and lymphocytes interact with each other, and the resulting proliferation, activation, and cytokine release leads to the dynamic structure known as the granuloma.

Granulomatous inflammation is a reaction to ongoing antigen presentation, and the control of that granuloma will have a critical impact on tissue pathology and therefore the course of the disease. Cessation of the antigenic stimulation will lead to cessation of the inflammatory response, with cell apoptosis occurring passively in response to cytokine withdrawal. However, apoptosis can be active also, and these pathways have attracted attention as dysregulation of apoptosis could potentially contribute to pathological granulomatous inflammation. The TNF-receptor (TNF-R) and TNF-ligand (TNF-L) superfamilies may be dysregulated in certain fibrotic lung diseases, including sarcoidosis.[72] TNF-α is a member of the TNF-L superfamily, but there are conflicting reports over its exact role in granuloma control. As will be discussed later, certain genetic polymorphisms associated with increased TNF-α production have been associated with increased severity in certain granulomatous diseases. Oncogene products also regulate apoptosis. In sarcoidosis, the Bcl-2 oncogene protein product has been found to be elevated in T cells located within sarcoid granulomas. This protein has been shown to protect lymphoid cells against programmed cell death when IL-2 is withdrawn.[73]

The Th1/Th2 ratio is also pivotal in granuloma control. The Th1 cytokines IL-2 and IL-15 inhibit macrophage apoptosis, whereas the Th2 cytokines IL-4 and IL-10 appear to enhance macrophage apoptosis.[74] It has also been suggested that a shift from Th1 to Th2 cytokine release may favor progression from active granulomatous inflammation to resolution of granulomas, with or without fibrosis.[70] Fibrosis requires the recruitment and proliferation of fibroblasts, leading to the extracellular deposition of collagen matrix products. Both macrophages and T cells are involved in this process. Macrophages recruit fibroblasts through TNF-α release and then stimulate proliferation through numerous cytokines including IL-1, transforming growth factor-β (TGF-β), and platelet-derived growth factor (PDGF). Collagen matrix deposition is then stimulated by macrophage-derived products including PDGF and TGF-β, and by T cell-derived cytokines. There is some evidence that the Th2 cytokine IL-4 stimulates collagen production,[75] whereas the Th1 cytokine IFN-γ is inhibitory.

This overview of the immunological mechanisms involved in granuloma initiation, control, resolution, and progression to fibrosis, is by no means exhaustive. It is meant to provide an insight into the highly complex nature of the interactions between inflammatory cells, endothelial cells, and the numerous cytokines and chemokines they produce. It can be seen that a large number of genes will be involved in such a complex interaction, and it can be surmised that genetic polymorphisms in these genes could interact with environmental influences to explain individual variations in susceptibility, phenotype, and outcome of sarcoidosis.

## Immunology of sarcoidosis

The principal immune effector cells in sarcoidosis are macrophages and T cells.[70] Absolute levels of both cells are elevated in bronchoalveolar lavage (BAL) fluid, although a predominant lymphocytosis is characteristic. The evidence suggests that both cell populations are activated through normal physiological mechanisms and that a primary defect in cell-mediated immunity does not exist.

The alveolar macrophage is central in pulmonary sarcoidosis, and the respiratory system is involved in almost all cases of sarcoidosis, even when extrapulmonary disease predominates.[76] The absolute increase in BAL macrophages is due largely to the recruitment of peripheral blood monocytes as shown by the increased numbers of immunophenotypically immature macrophages, but there is also an increase in the percentage of cells undergoing local proliferation.[77] When cultured in vitro, these cells spontaneously release high levels of TNF-α and IL-1, indicating that they are activated.[78,79] Cytokine mRNA transcript levels are increased in macrophages taken from sites of disease activity only, and the pattern of cytokine upregulation is of a Th1 profile.

T cells also accumulate and proliferate at sites of disease activity. These cells are predominantly of the CD4 T helper cell type.[80] They are activated (they show downregulation of cell surface T-cell receptors (TCR) and upregulation of TCR mRNA transcripts compared to blood lymphocytes,[81] they spontaneously secrete cytokines including IL-2,[82] IFN-γ,[83] and lymphotoxin, and they express increased numbers of cell surface activation markers, such as HLA-DR and very late activation antigen-1 (VLA-1)).[84] As with macrophages, this activation is compartmentalized to sites of disease activity.[85] Analysis of TCRs has demonstrated overexpression of particular variable regions of the α and β chains (e.g. Vβ5, 8, 15, 16, 18, Vα2.3).[86] These restrictions in TCR expression are more marked in lung than blood lymphocytes and are accompanied by a background polyclonal expansion. A particular association between restricted AV2S3 gene usage by CD4 T cells and HLA-DR3 has been reported in sarcoidosis.[87,88] Similarly, a recent study of 121 Scandinavian sarcoidosis patients found an association between the presence of HLA-DRB1*0301 (i.e. DR17) or HLA-DRB3*0101 (i.e. DR52a) and the expansion of AV2S3+ T cells in BAL fluid, but not peripheral blood (i.e. lung-restricted expansion).[89] HLA-DRB1*0301 and HLA-DRB3*0101 have identical amino acid sequences in regions responsible for antigen binding, which may allow them to present similar antigenic peptides, stimulating the expansion of the same population of T cells. These studies would suggest that the T cells are responding to a persistent antigenic stimulus.

The Kveim–Siltzbach reagent was developed from sarcoid spleen tissue. It was noted that intradermal administration of this reagent would lead to granuloma formation in 80 percent of patients with sarcoidosis, but not other diseases.[90] This provides a human model allowing the study of the role of different cells and cytokines at each stage of granuloma formation. Following intradermal administration of the reagent, the first cells to accumulate are mononuclear phagocytes (equivalent to alveolar macrophages in the lung). Intradermal inoculation of autologous BAL cells triggers a reaction analogous to the Kveim reaction. This activity has been shown to lie in membrane fragments of alveolar macrophages, suggesting the presentation of a 'sarcoid antigen' by these cells in the lung.[91]

## The sarcoid antigen

The sarcoid antigen has proven to be elusive. There is a significant amount of evidence to support the theory that an infective agent may be the trigger antigen. Seasonal variation in incidence has been described in a number of studies, with peaks observed in the Spring months in both the northern and southern hemispheres.[92] Numerous cases of clustering have been described and it has been suggested that these represent outbreaks of sarcoidosis caused by a transmissible agent.

The histological similarity with mycobacterial infection has inspired many studies into a possible etiological role for mycobacteria.[92] However, histological, microbiological, antimycobacterial antibody, and molecular studies have failed to provide consistent evidence that these organisms are present in sarcoid tissues. Many molecular studies have examined sarcoidosis samples for mycobacterial DNA. In over half of the polymerase chain reaction (PCR)-based studies, evidence of mycobacterial DNA was found in less than 10 percent of subjects. Serological studies have associated sarcoidosis with antibodies to *Chlamydia pneumoniae* and *Borrelia burgdorferi*, but subsequent PCR studies have failed to find DNA from these bacteria in sarcoidosis samples, suggesting that the presence of the specific antibodies reflects generalized B-cell activation.[92] Human herpes viruses (HHV) are capable of inducing sarcoid-type granulomas and an increased prevalence of antibodies against herpes-like virus has been detected in sarcoidosis patients. One PCR study detected HHV-8 DNA in 38 of 39 sarcoid tissues versus seven of 113 controls.[93] However, two subsequent studies have failed to reproduce this result.[94,95] *Propionibacterium acnes* and *P. granulosum* are known to induce granulomatous reactions when injected into sensitized rabbits and rats.[96,97] They have been isolated by bacterial culture from sarcoidosis samples.[98] In a recent study, Eishi et al.[99] used PCR to look for propionibacterial and mycobacterial DNA in lymph nodes of patients with sarcoidosis. *P. acnes* or *P. granulosum* were identified in 106 of 108 sarcoidosis samples – significantly higher than in controls – and sarcoid samples contained significantly higher numbers of bacterial genomes than control samples. Furthermore, Ebe et al.[100] have reported that a recombinant protein from a *P. acnes* DNA expression library causes a proliferative response in peripheral blood mononuclear cells from some patients

with sarcoidosis, but not in controls without sarcoidosis. It would seem that propionibacteria are a leading candidate in the hunt for the sarcoid antigen.

## CLINICAL EVALUATION

### History and examination

Constitutional symptoms, such as fever, weight loss, and fatigue, may be the principal manifestation in approximately 25 percent of patients with sarcoidosis.[20] Patients may complain of dyspnea, dry cough, and chest pain. Crackles may be heard on auscultation of the chest. About one-third of patients may have palpable peripheral lymph glands and about 20 percent may exhibit hepatosplenomegaly on presentation. Cutaneous involvement occurs in about 25 percent of all patients with sarcoidosis and this can be in the form of skin lesions, such as erythema nodosum or lupus pernio. The joints most commonly affected are the knees, ankles, elbows, wrists, and small joints of the hands and feet. Less than 10 percent of patients with sarcoidosis have involvement of the nervous system, with facial palsies and hypothalamic and pituitary lesions being typical manifestations. Myocardial sarcoidosis can cause a range of problems, from benign arrhythmias to symptomatic paroxysmal arrhythmias or heart block, valvular abnormalities such as mitral insufficiency, angina-like pain due to small vessel involvement, or sudden death.

Serial clinical examinations including thorough history, chest radiography, pulmonary function testing, and assessment of the severity of disease in other affected organs, remain the best approach to assessing prognosis. The best general approach to monitoring the clinical course of sarcoidosis is to measure functional changes serially, using the most sensitive, least invasive, and least expensive tests first. Although there is some data from studies that have indicated three clinical tests that may reflect active disease (serum angiotensin-converting enzyme,[101,102] BAL cell differential count,[103] and gallium radionuclide scans ($^{67}$Ga)[104]), there are other data stating that these tests do not predict prognosis,[105] response to treatment[106–108] or presence or intensity of the inflammation in sarcoidosis.[109,110]

### Radiographic findings

The intrathoracic changes in sarcoidosis found on the plain chest X-ray are classified into stages 0 to IV (stage 0, normal chest radiograph; stage I, bilateral hilar lyphadenopathy (BHL); stage II, BHL plus pulmonary infiltrates; stage III, pulmonary infiltration without BHL; stage IV, pulmonary fibrosis). However, this system is of limited usefulness, as patients do not necessarily progress through these stages – some patients will present with a stage IV radiographic, but their disease will not progress, and radiographic stage at presentation cannot predict subsequent clinical course. Many patients with a stage IV radiograph may actually have milder disease than some patients with a stage II or stage III radiograph.

Computed tomography (CT) has therefore become widely used in the assessment of suspected and confirmed sarcoidosis. CT scanning is indicated when there are atypical clinical and radiological findings, to increase diagnostic certainty or to detect any complications of the lung disease, such as bronchiectasis, fibrosis, infection, or malignancy. The characteristic findings on CT scanning include (1) mediastinal and hilar lymphadenopathy; (2) disease predominant in the upper lobes; (3) widespread small nodules with distribution being predominantly subpleural and along bronchovascular bundles; (4) thickened interlobular septae. None of these findings are specific enough to be diagnostic for sarcoidosis, but a characteristic CT in a patient with pulmonary fibrosis can strongly suggest the correct diagnosis. High-resolution computed tomography of the thorax may help guide therapy. Findings of groundglass, nodular, and irregular linear opacities and interlobular septal thickening on computed tomography represent potentially reversible conditions, whereas findings of cystic air spaces and architectural distortion with honeycombing suggest irreversible pulmonary disease.[111]

Magnetic resonance imaging (MRI) has been used for the demonstration of evidence of neurological, muscular, or cardiac sarcoidosis; contrast enhancement with gadolinium allows improved resolution of bone, central nervous system, and meningeal disease.

## Electrocardiogram and echocardiography

Electrocardiogram (ECG) abnormalities are more common in sarcoidosis patients than in healthy controls and may include conduction defects, such as atrial or ventricular arrhythmias, atrioventricular (AV) nodal block, or bundle branch block.[112] Echocardiography may show increased right ventricular anterior wall thickness that is compatible with pulmonary hypertension, or in patients with myocardial sarcoidosis focal abnormalities of the wall motion in the absence of coronary artery disease.

## Thallium-201

Cardiac imaging with thallium-201 can be used for the diagnosis of heart involvement in a patient with sarcoidosis. It may reveal resting myocardial perfusion defects which decrease with exercise in contrast to the increase during exercise that is seen with coronary artery disease.[113,114]

## Gallium scan

Gallium scans ($^{67}$Ga) were used during the 1980s as a diagnostic and prognostic tool in sarcoidosis.[104,115] The findings

of characteristic 'lambda' gallium distribution (well circumscribed, uniform, symmetric uptake of gallium in both the parahilar and infrahilar lymph nodes and in the right paratracheal mediastinal lymph nodes), or a 'panda' image (abnormal bilateral, symmetric uptake by the lacrimal and parotid glands with or without submandibular gland uptake) together with bilateral symmetrical hilar lymphadenopathy or bilateral symmetric pulmonary fibrosis on plain radiography, have both been found to be highly specific for sarcoidosis.[116] Gallium 67 has been used as a marker of disease activity in a number of studies.[104,105,115,117] It is taken up mainly by macrophages and there is evidence that uptake reflects the presence of granulomata. The use of somatostatin receptor scintigraphy (SRS) may offer better evaluation of organ involvement in patients with sarcoidosis compared to gallium 67 scans, especially in patients having corticosteroid treatment.[118]

## DTPA scan

Technetium 99m-diethylenetriamine pentaacetate (DTPA) lung scanning is a measure of epithelial cell permeability and has been evaluated as a marker of disease activity, but is not valuable for the diagnosis of disease. Chinet and colleagues[119] concluded that DTPA clearance can identify those patients who are likely to remain stable (patients with normal DTPA clearance), and changes in DTPA clearance can identify those patients with sarcoidosis with changes in respiratory function tests. More studies are needed in order to clarify the use of DTPA in patients with sarcoidosis.

## Blood

There are no specific hematological features. Anemia occurs in 4–20 percent of patients with sarcoidosis. A moderate reduction in the peripheral blood leukocyte count occurs in as many as 40 percent of patients.[120] Thrombocytopenia and eosinophilia have been described, but are rare. The erythrocyte sedimentation rate (ESR) is commonly elevated.

Hypercalcemia is seen in about 2–10 percent of patients with sarcoidosis; hypercalciuria is seen in approximately a third of sarcoidosis patients. These abnormalities appear to be the result of dysregulated production of 1,25-$(OH)_2$-$D_3$ (calcitriol) by activated macrophages and granulomas.[121,122]

The base-line level of serum angiotensin-converting enzyme does not discriminate patients whose condition will deteriorate from those whose condition will improve, and it should therefore not be used alone as a reason to initiate therapy. The measurement of angiotensin converting enzyme activity or disease extent on gallium-67 scans do not add to the predictive value of serial chest X-rays and pulmonary function testing.[117]

## Kveim test

This test, evolved by Kveim,[123] revised by Siltzbach, and known as the Kveim–Siltzbach test, involves the injection of a test dose (0.15 mL) of finely particulate saline suspension of human sarcoid tissue prepared from the spleen of a patient with active sarcoidosis intracutaneously on the flexor surface of the forearm. The only reliable way of reading the result is by microscopic assessment after biopsy of the full thickness of the skin at the site of the test 4–6 weeks after the injection. The presence of granulomatous reaction is a positive result.

The sensitivity of the test depends on the stage of the disease. Acute sarcoidosis with fever, erythema nodosum, and bilateral hilar lymphadenopathy is associated with 85–90 percent positivity for the test, whereas only a third of the patients test positive in stage III and IV disease. Unfortunately, therefore, the test is more helpful in situations in which sarcoidosis is easy to diagnose. Furthermore, it has a false-positive rate of 0.7–2 percent in healthy control.[124] A negative test does not exclude the diagnosis. Kveim–Siltzbach test is not available worldwide and is no longer in routine use due to concerns over its biological safety.

## Bronchoalveolar lavage

Elevated lymphocytes with a specific increase in T-helper lymphocytes leading to an elevated CD4/CD8 ratio in the BAL fluid plus compatible clinical and radiological findings is regarded as a strong adjuvant to the diagnosis of sarcoidosis in the absence of biopsy.[125–129] The positive predictive value of a CD4/CD8 ratio of 4:1 is only 50 percent for distinguishing sarcoidosis from other pulmonary diseases, but this reaches 94 percent when only patients with interstitial lung disease are examined.[130] Different studies have investigated any link between the initial BAL fluid lymphocyte count and the progress or steroid-responsiveness of the disease. Studies from Laviolette et al.[107] and Drent et al.[131] have shown that neither the CD4/CD8 ratio nor the degree of lymphocytosis can predict the outcome or response to treatment. One study reported that a BAL fluid neutrophilia ($>0.2 \times 10^4$ neutrophils/mL) was associated with subsequent significant deterioration in chest radiographs and pulmonary function.[131] However, those patients with BAL neutrophilia had more fibrotic disease at time of lavage, so BAL neutrophilia could alternatively be interpreted as a marker of the degree of pulmonary fibrosis.

## Biopsy

In the absence of a history of exposure to antigens known to cause hypersensitivity pneumonitis and in the absence of acid-fast bacilli or fungi on staining, the presence of non-necrotizing granulomas is the histological hallmark of sarcoidosis.

The transbronchial biopsy is the most favored form of biopsy for the diagnosis of sarcoidosis. The sensitivity of transbronchial biopsy increases in the more advanced stages of the disease, ranging from 55 percent for stage I disease to 70 percent for stage II and III.[132] It has been shown that the biopsy number affects the diagnostic yield, with most investigators suggesting that four to six specimens are adequate for diagnosis.[133–136] When biopsies are taken from different lobes and from the areas most involved the diagnostic yield is higher.[133]

Endobronchial biopsies may also be performed and can be diagnostic in some patients despite the mucosa appearing normal, although the diagnostic yield is higher from abnormal mucosa.[137,138] Some investigators have shown an increase in the diagnostic yield of transbronchial biopsies when they were combined with endobronchial biopsies.[138–140]

Transbronchial needle aspiration in the presence of mediastinal or hilar lymphadenopathy may confirm a diagnosis of sarcoidosis, but studies to date have involved only small numbers of patients.[140]

When the results of the transbronchial or endobronchial biopsies are nondiagnostic, and diagnostic uncertainty about pulmonary disease seen on CT scans remains, then an open lung biopsy may need to be considered.

## Pulmonary function tests

Pulmonary function tests are essential for the baseline measurement of any lung impairment and as a reference for improvement or deterioration of the disease. The lung function impairment in sarcoidosis may appear as a restrictive pattern or as an obstructive pattern. In a recent study of 210 patients with sarcoidosis, 121 patients (57.6 percent) had impaired ventilatory function.[141] Of these, 98 had an obstructive pattern and 23 had a restrictive pattern. Most of the patients in the group with restrictive functional impairment had chronic, relapsing sarcoidosis. There were no differences between acute and chronic disease in the obstructive functional impairment group.

Serial pulmonary function tests are used to monitor disease progression in sarcoidosis and are the only way to evaluate progressive change in organ function.[142] Most investigators have shown an increasing prevalence of low DLCO with increasing radiographic stage.[143,144] In patients whose chest radiographs improved, both the vital capacity and the DLCO improved, although the pulmonary function tests did not return to normal when the chest radiograph showed complete resolution of the abnormalities.

## Sarcoidosis and malignancy

Chronic inflammation is often associated with an increased risk of malignancy in the affected tissue. One study of 2700 cases of sarcoidosis reported a higher incidence of lymphoma, but lower rates of lung cancer compared to that expected in the general population.[145] A second study concluded that patients with sarcoidosis appear to be at higher risk of developing malignancy in the lung, stomach, small intestine, liver, and skin, as well as non-Hodgkin's lymphoma and leukemia.[146] However, other studies have found no association between sarcoidosis and malignancy.[147,148] The exact incidence of malignancy complicating sarcoidosis and the reasons for any such association are not known. It is conceivable that a genetic variation predisposing patients to chronic inflammation (such as variations in candidate apoptosis-regulating genes) could also predispose those patients to malignancy, although no such association has been reported to date.

# TREATMENT

Sarcoidosis may remit or stabilize without treatment, so the decision whether or not to treat pulmonary sarcoidosis is often a dilemma. It is important to understand the natural course of pulmonary sarcoidosis when making a therapeutic decision.

Patients may present acutely with symptoms, chest X-ray abnormalities, and abnormalities in pulmonary function tests, or with established pulmonary fibrosis suggesting a more insidious chronic disease. The future course of acute pulmonary sarcoidosis cannot be predicted for an individual patient. Chronic pulmonary sarcoidosis has been defined as disease with persistence of symptoms for more than 2 years – such patients may have progressive or persistent pulmonary disease and require treatment.[149]

Thus the decision to prescribe treatment for a patient whose disease may remit spontaneously is difficult. Patients with erythema nodosum should not be treated with corticosteroids, as the toxic effects of the systemic corticosteroids exceed the benefits of treatment. Because many patients undergo spontaneous remission within 6 months of diagnosis, it is recommended that patients with mild to moderate pulmonary sarcoidosis be observed for 2–6 months.[150,151] The patients who have improved will have avoided the toxicity of corticosteroids, while those who deteriorate over the observation period should be treated. A patient whose condition neither improves nor deteriorates may be given a corticosteroid trial or otherwise be observed further.[150] Patients with severe impairment of pulmonary function or with pulmonary symptoms that cause significant reduction in quality of life should be treated with corticosteroids. Treatment for patients with chronic pulmonary sarcoidosis can continue for prolonged periods of time or even for life.

Judson[152] in 1999 proposed a six phase scheme of treatment with corticosteroids for patients with acute pulmonary sarcoidosis: initial dosing, taper to maintenance, maintenance dosing, corticosteroid taper, monitoring while not receiving therapy, and treatment of relapse. The dosing and the duration of the phases have not been standardized. The six phases must be individualized based on the severity of the disease and the response to therapy.

Inhaled corticosteroids are often prescribed as an adjunct to maintenance therapy in patients with an obstructive airways disease pattern on pulmonary function testing. Currently, however, there is insufficient trial data to recommend their routine use.

## Other immunosuppressants

In patients requiring persistent corticosteroid therapy, cytotoxic agents and antimalarial agents may be considered as second-line, steroid-sparing agents. There is limited evidence for a steroid-sparing effect of methotrexate in chronic steroid-dependent sarcoidosis, and Baughmann et al.[153] suggest a protocol for methotrexate treatment in such patients. There are conflicting reports on the efficacy of azathioprine in treating chronic sarcoidosis with or without concurrent prednisone;[154,155] the efficacy of the drug when used at a dose of 1–2 mg/kg per day appears to be similar to that of methotrexate.

Chloroquine and hydroxychloroquine have been used to treat intrathoracic or cutaneous lesions and hypercalcemia, although hydroxychloroquine is usually tolerated better.[156,157] Thalidomide at various doses has been reported to be useful for the disfiguring facial skin lesion lupus pernio.[158–160] It has a rapid onset of action and is well tolerated by most patients. Its effect on pulmonary sarcoidosis is not yet known.

Cyclophosphamide has been used in a limited number of patients.[161,162] Its higher toxicity, with side-effects including bone marrow suppression, hemorrhagic cystitis, bladder cancer, and nausea, has limited its use to refractory cases that have failed to respond to other treatments.

Cyclosporine, an immunophilin that has T-cell inhibitory effects, has been shown to have limited[163] to no effectiveness for pulmonary sarcoidosis.[164] Cyclosporine use must be restricted to the most serious cases of sarcoidosis that have failed other treatments, due to its high renal toxicity and the increased risk of malignancy with long-term use.

Two inhibitors of TNF-α have recently been trialed in sarcoidosis. Etanercept is a dimeric protein that binds specifically to TNF-α, blocking its interaction with cell surface TNF-α receptors. In one study, only five of 17 patients with stage II and III progressive pulmonary sarcoidosis clinically improved with etanercept as the only treatment.[165] Infliximab is a monoclonal antibody against human TNF-α, and early case reports in sarcoidosis are encouraging.[166–168] However, further studies are awaited before conclusions can be drawn on which patients could be treated with each drug.

Pentoxifylline is a phosphodiesterase inhibitor that has been shown to block the spontaneous release of TNF-α by alveolar macrophages from patients with sarcoidosis.[169] Given its overall safety profile, further studies are indicated in order to access its utility as a potential steroid sparing drug.

With all of these drugs, a recurrent theme is that response to treatment is unpredictable. A drug's interactions with host proteins will be affected by genetic polymorphisms in the genes encoding those proteins. It is possible that an individual's response to corticosteroids, cytotoxic agents, or new immunomodulatory drugs, such as TNF-α inhibitors, is genetically determined. The pharmacogenetics underlying these variable responses have not yet been elucidated in sarcoidosis. However, it is possible that in the future analysis of implicated genetic polymorphisms will predict response to treatment, allowing the physician to tailor the drug regimen to the individual patient.

## Organ transplantation

Lung and other organ transplantations have been performed for patients with end-stage sarcoidosis. The principle problem specific to sarcoidosis is the reported recurrence of sarcoid lesions in the donor organ. Post-transplantation immunosuppressant therapy seems to control the sarcoidosis.

## MONOGENIC COMPONENTS

There are no monogenic components to sarcoidosis or any of the clinical subtypes. Sarcoidosis in all its clinical phenotypes is a genetically complex disease.

## LINKAGE STUDIES

There is a paucity of linkage studies in sarcoidosis, partly due to the difficulties in gathering large numbers of familial cases. However, Schurmann et al. have completed two studies using microsatellite markers and multipoint nonparametric linkage (NPL) analysis. In an initial study, they genotyped 122 affected siblings from 55 families for seven DNA polymorphisms in the MHC region.[170] NPL analysis showed linkage for the entire MHC region, with the peak score identified at a marker locus in the class III region (D6S1666). They concluded that the MHC genes do affect susceptibility to sarcoidosis, with the greatest influence being exerted by genes in the class III region (the region carrying genes including TNF). A follow-up, genome-wide study using 225 microsatellite markers in 63 families with 138 affected siblings also found the most prominent peak at the MHC ($P = 0.001$), including the D6S1666 marker identified in the first study.[171] However, six additional minor peaks ($P < 0.05$) were found on chromosomes 1, 3 (close to the chemokine receptor genes CCR2 and CCR5), 7 (two peaks, one close to the T-cell receptor B gene), 9 (close to the gene for transforming growth factor-β receptor 1 (TGFBR1), and the X chromosome (close to the gene coding for the interleukin-2 receptor gamma chain (IL2RG)). The authors warned that with 225 markers, 11 similar minor peaks would be expected by chance alone. They also noted the lack of association with markers near other candidate genes such as ACE and NRAMP1, but again warned that for genes with minor effects on susceptibility, a greater marker density and a much larger sample of affected sibling pairs would be required. More linkage studies in different ethnic groups, employing larger samples and more microsatellite markers, are required to allow identification of other candidate genes exerting minor effects on susceptibility.

## ASSOCIATION STUDIES

### Major histocompatibility complex

#### HLA CLASS I

Early studies of candidate genes in sarcoidosis concentrated on HLA class I typing at the serological level by antigen detection, and are included in the summary of these studies in Table 13.3.

**Table 13.3** *Reported associations with HLA class I antigens*

| Population | Sample size (patients /controls) | Susceptibility associations | Protection associations | Phenotype associations | Ref. |
|---|---|---|---|---|---|
| UK | 65 patients | B8 | | | 173 |
| UK | 37 resolved disease/50 fibrosed disease/164 healthy | | | B8 acute self-limiting disease | 177 |
| American Caucasians | 174/97 | B8 | | | 174 |
| African American | 28/80 | B7 | | | 180 |
| Czech | 123/500 | A1, B8, B13 | | | 175, 178 |
| Italian | 107/510 | B8 | | | 178 |
| Japanese | 114/478 | | B7 | | 179 |
| Scandinavian | 166/210 | B*07, B*08 | | Haplotype A*03,B*07,DRB1*15 with chronic disease | 181 |

The earliest such study in 1974 failed to detect any association between sarcoidosis in 132 German patients and HLA locus A.[172] Subsequent studies reported associations with HLA-B8 (also known as HLA-B*08) in Caucasian patients,[173–175] but not in black patients.[176] One of these studies in Czech patients also found an association with HLA-B13, and B8 B13 heterozygotes had a relative risk of 8.5 for sarcoidosis.[175] When these results were compared with 127 Italian patients, the association with HLA-B8 was confirmed, as well as an association with HLA-A1.[178] HLA-B8 has been associated with disease of acute onset and short duration.[177] One study of 114 Japanese patients failed to find any association with class I antigens that could not be better explained by linkage disequilibrium with class II antigens, although they did find a reduction in HLA-B7 in patients compared to controls.[179] This is of interest because HLA-B7 has been found in increased frequency in African-American patients (a population with a high disease prevalence).[180] To conclude on the basis of these studies, the association with HLA-B8 seems to be the most commonly reported across racial boundaries, but it has not been found in all studies and other reported associations are even weaker. In any case, the immunology of sarcoidosis would suggest that HLA class II molecules are more likely to be involved in antigen presentation; any reported disease associations with class I genes may merely represent linkage with more relevant class II genes. However, a very recent study in Scandinavian patients again found that both HLA-B*07 and HLA-B*08 independently increased the risk of sarcoidosis.[181] Other class I associations were secondary to their linkages to class II alleles. The common allele combination A*03, B*07, DRB1*15 was most strongly associated with persistent disease and was found in 25.3 percent of such patients against 7.1 percent of healthy controls. The authors conclude that HLA class I alleles may have more influence on disease susceptibility and prognosis than has been recently thought.

## HLA CLASS II

Numerous studies have reported associations between various class II alleles and sarcoidosis. These associations appear to be population specific, and the major findings are summarised in Table 13.4.

Most of the earlier studies reported associations with HLA-DR-associated antigens. In Japanese patients, HLA-DR5, -DR6 and -DR8[182,183] and -DR8 and -DR9[179] have been associated with disease. In Germans, HLA-DR5 has been associated with chronic disease,[184] but HLA-DR3 has been associated with acute disease.[185] Similarly, in Scandinavia, certain alleles have been associated with chronic disease (HLA-DR14 and -DR15), while others have been associated with acute self-limiting disease (DR17(3)).[186] HLA-DR14 was also associated with chronic disease in a recent study of Asian Indians.[187] HLA-DR9 has been associated with disease risk in Japanese patients, but with disease protection in Scandinavians.[92] Some attempt to find

consensus from this confused picture has been made. HLA-DR1 and -DR4 have been found to be protective in Scandinavians, Japanese, Italians, and in a study of UK, Polish, and Czech patients.[188] This study showed position 11 of the HLA-DRB1 amino acid sequence to be the most variable, with three susceptibility alleles all coding for small hydrophilic amino acids, and two protective alleles coding for amino acids with bulky, hydrophobic, aliphatic side chains. As the position 11 amino acid is located at a crucial interface between the HLA-DR α and β chains, it is easy to imagine how these different alleles could affect HLA-DR heterodimer conformation and antigen binding. However, all the above studies were limited by the techniques used to identify HLA molecules – serological and low-resolution molecular typing. A recent study performed high resolution typing for the HLA-DPB1, HLA-DQB1, HLA-DRB1, and HLA-DRB3 loci in the first 474 ACCESS patients and case-matched controls.[189] They found a highly significant association between HLA-DPB1 alleles and disease in both blacks and whites. The HLA-DRB1*1101 allele was associated with sarcoidosis in both blacks and whites, with a population attributable risk of 16 percent in blacks and 9 percent in whites. The only class II allele differentially distributed between blacks and whites with respect to disease was HLA-DRB1*1501, being associated with controls in blacks and with sarcoidosis in whites. This caused the authors to speculate that broadly similar HLA class II alleles may be associated with sarcoidosis in both populations, and that the increased risk in blacks could be due to increased prevalence of susceptibility alleles in the black population.

The HLA-DP locus has attracted considerable interest due to the finding that chronic beryllium disease (a chronic multisystem granulomatous disease with many immunopathological similarities to sarcoidosis) is associated strongly with the presence of a glutamic acid residue at position 69 of the HLA-DP beta chain (see Disease models, page 347). However, this association has not been found in two studies in sarcoidosis,[190,191] although the latter study in African-Americans did find an increased risk of disease associated with Val36+ and Asp55+ alleles. Similarly, in the above-mentioned study on ACCESS patients, the HLA-DPB1 locus also contributed towards susceptibility, but with the HLA-DPB1*0101 allele conveying most of the risk.[189]

In another recent study in African-Americans, 225 sarcoidosis patients with family members as controls were genotyped for six microsatellite markers covering the MHC region.[192] An association was observed between disease and the marker closest to HLA-DQB1; further analysis of other markers at this locus confirmed that in this African-American cohort, it is HLA-DQB1 and not HLA-DRB1 that confers susceptibility to sarcoidosis. A follow-up study found that HLA-DQB1*0201 was transmitted to affected offspring only half as much as expected, whereas DQB1*0602 was transmitted to affected offspring about 20 percent more than expected, and was associated with radiographic

**Table 13.4** *Associations with HLA Class II antigens*

| Population | Sample size (patients/controls) | Susceptibility associations | Protection associations | Phenotype associations | Ref. |
|---|---|---|---|---|---|
| Asian Indians | 56/275 | DRB1*11 DRB1*14 | DRB1*07 DQB1*0201 | DRB1*14 severe disease | 187 |
| American Caucasians | 268/268 | DRB1*1101 DRB1*1501 DRB1*1401 DRB1*0402 | DQB1*0602 | DRB1*0401 eye DPB1*0101 hypercalcemia | 189 |
| African Americans | 193/193 | DRB1*1101 DRB1*1201 DPB1*0101 DQB1*0502 | | DRB1*0401 parotid/salivary glands DRB3 bone marrow | 189 |
| African Americans | 225/479 first-degree relatives | DQB1*0602 | DQB1*0201 | DQB1*0602 severe disease | 193 |
| Scandinavians | 122/250 | DR17(3) | | DR17(3) acute disease DR14, DR15 chronic disease | 186 |
| Japanese | 75/150 | DRB1*11 (DR5) DRB1*14 (DR6) DRB1*08 (DR8) | DRB1*0101 DQB1*0501 DPB*0402 | | 183 |
| Japanese | 40/110 | DRB1*12 DRB1*14 DRB1*08 | | | 182 |
| Japanese | 26/247 | | | DQB1*0601 cardiac | 197 |
| Japanese | 114/478 | DRw5 DRw8 DRw52 | | DR5 mild disease DR8 chronic disease | 179 |
| UK and Dutch Caucasians | 235/568 | | | DQB1*0201 mild disease including Lofgren's DQB1*0602 severe disease | 194 |
| Dutch Caucasians | 37 Lofgren's/88 | DQB1*0201-DRB1*03 (01) and Lofgren's | | DQB1*0201-DRB1*03(01) Lofgren's | 195 |
| Czech and Italian Caucasians | 233/1010 | DR3 | DR4 | DR3 mild disease | 178 |
| German | 78/50 | | | DR4 severe disease DR3 Lofgren's | 185 |
| German | 73/199 | | | DR5 chronic disease | 184 |
| UK Caucasians | 189/288 | DRB1*12 DRB1*14 DRB1*15 DQB1*0602 DQB1*0301/4 | DRB1*01 DRB1*04 DQB1*0603-9 | | 188 |
| Polish | 87/133 | DRB1*15 DQB1*0602 | DRB1*01 DQB1*05 DQB1*0603-9 | | 188 |
| Czech | 69/158 | DRB1*14 DQB1*02 DQB1*04 | DR7 | | 188 |

disease progression.[193] This contrasts with the study on ACCESS patients, in which the major association was with HLA-DRB1; however, that paper also reported an association of disease in blacks with HLA-DQB1*0502, albeit a weaker association than with HLA-DRB1.[189]

As well as being population-specific, it appears that some associations with class II alleles are specific to certain clinical phenotypes. In a study of the HLA-DQB1 locus in 235 Dutch and UK patients, the allele DQB1*0201 was found to be strongly protective against severe sarcoidosis (i.e. it was associated with stage I disease), whereas the DQB1*0602 allele tended to have the opposite effect.[194] Furthermore, the patient group included 15 patients with Lofgren's syndrome and 23 patients with erythema nodosum – carriage of the DQB1*0201 allele was greatly increased in these subgroups. In a follow-up study based on this finding and the previously reported associations between Lofgren's and the DRB1*0301 allele and the A allele at position −307 of the TNF-α gene (TNF),[185] 37 Dutch Lofgren's patients were genotyped for all three alleles.[195] The associations were confirmed, being strongest for DQB1*0201 (OR 8.6, versus 6.7 and 6.8 for DRB1*03 and TNF, respectively). In addition, there was 100 percent linkage disequilibrium between DQB1*0201 and DRB1*03, and 70 percent LD between these alleles and TNF. This paper, therefore, identified the DQB1*0201-DRB1*03(01)-TNF haplotype as an extended MHC haplotype that was present in 76 percent of Lofgren's (versus 24 percent of controls) and conferred the risk for Lofgren's syndrome in Dutch Caucasians (OR 9.9).

Lofgren's syndrome is extremely rare in Japanese patients, but cardiac sarcoidosis is more common than in Caucasians. One group reported an association between cardiac sarcoidosis and the TNFA2 allele,[196] but followed this up with more detailed genotyping of multiple candidate MHC alleles and microsatellite analysis around the TNF locus.[197] They concluded that the strongest association was in fact with the HLA-DQB1*0601 allele, with homozygosity for this allele conferring a relative risk of 29.5 compared to healthy controls. The TNFA2 allele was not in LD with the class II allele, so the authors concluded that this allele might confer an additional genetic risk for cardiac sarcoidosis.

The above-mentioned study on ACCESS patients also attempted to correlate HLA class II alleles with clinical phenotypes.[189] They found significant associations between DRB1*0401 and ocular sarcoidosis in blacks and whites, DRB3 and bone marrow sarcoidosis in blacks, and DPB1*0101 and hypercalcemia in whites.

## T–cell antigen receptor

Studies of the usage of TCR variable region genes in sarcoidosis have demonstrated an oligoclonal expansion of specific T cells, with a background polyclonal expansion.[86] However, there is little consistency in clonality between studies. Only one Scandinavian study has identified an association of a particular TCR with disease.[198] In patients with HLA-DR17(3), -DQ2, a strong association was demonstrated between the oligoclonal expansion of cells expressing the Vα2.3 TCR and acute disease. However, the repertoire of T cell receptor expression is determined by interaction with the triggering antigen. So these associations are likely to be secondary to the triggering antigen, rather than being primarily determined by genetic variations in the receptor genes and affecting disease susceptibility or phenotype.

## Cytokines

The cytokines involved in the granulomatous inflammation of sarcoidosis have been summarized above. They make attractive candidate genes, because it is easy to hypothesize that different alleles in these genes may affect cytokine levels, which may affect susceptibility to disease, and/or the clinical course of disease.[199] Many case–control studies have picked a candidate gene and speculatively genotyped for allelic variations – Table 13.5 details the positive reports to date.

### TUMOR NECROSIS FACTOR

The tumor necrosis factor gene complex is located within the MHC complex, and includes the TNF-α (TNF) and TNF-β (lymphotoxin α or LTA) genes. The pivotal role played by tumor necrosis factor in granulomatous inflammation in sarcoidosis and the many studies linking sarcoidosis to the MHC complex have aroused much interest in the genes of the tumor necrosis factor gene complex as candidate susceptibility genes.

Early studies focused on two biallelic markers in the TNFα gene (G to A at position −308, known as TNFA) and the TNFβ gene (in the first intron, known as TNFB). Both have been shown to affect cytokine production and the former has been linked to granulomatous disease caused by beryllium.[200] The less common TNFA2 allele (−308A), associated with high TNFα production, was first associated with Lofgren's syndrome in a study of 101 patients with pulmonary sarcoidosis (including 16 Lofgren's patients) compared to 216 healthy controls.[201] This same study found no association of either polymorphism with the sarcoidosis group as a whole. A study of 110 Japanese patients (in whom Lofgren's syndrome is extremely rare) and 161 controls also found no associations between either of these polymorphisms and susceptibility to sarcoidosis as a whole.[202] However, this study did find the TNFB1 allele to be associated with a prolonged clinical course, with carriage of this allele significantly prolonging the time to spontaneous disease resolution. It is important to distinguish prolonged disease from severe disease – this association was clear in patients who, despite a prolonged disease course, did not require corticosteroid therapy for severe symptoms or organ-threatening disease. The authors noted that TNFB1 has been associated with increased production of both TNF-β and TNF-α, so this polymorphism could have a functional role in affecting the process of disease remission.

The association between Lofgren's syndrome and TNFA2 has been confirmed in a more recent study of 196 UK and Dutch patients and 576 controls.[203] This study examined five biallelic TNF promoter polymorphisms, including the G to A allele at position −308 (now renumbered as position −307). As in the previous study, this less common TNFA2 allele was not associated with sarcoidosis susceptibility overall, but was significantly associated with the Lofgren's subgroup (n = 15). However, this study also

**Table 13.5**   *Reported associations with genes other than HLA class I and II*

| Gene | Population | Sample size (patients/controls) | Susceptibility associations | Protection associations | Phenotype associations | Ref. |
|------|-----------|-------------------------------|----------------------------|------------------------|----------------------|------|
| TNF-α | | 101/216 | | | TNFA2 (−308A) Lofgren's | 201 |
| | UK and Dutch | 196/576 | −857T | | TNFA2 Lofgren's | 203 |
| | UK and Dutch | 228 (46 Lofgren's) | | | TNFA2 Lofgren's −857T severe disease | 204 |
| TNF-β | Japanese | 110/161 | | | TNFB*1 prolonged disease | 202 |
| IL-1α | Czech | 95/199 | −889C/C homozygotes | | | 206[a] |
| IL-18 | Japanese | 119/130 | −607C | | | 208 |
| MIF | Spanish | 28 with EN/122 | | | −173C EN | 209 |
| IκB-α | UK and Dutch | 205/201 | −297T | | −826T mild disease | 210 |
| CCR2 | Japanese | 100/122 | | V64I | | 211[a] |
| | Dutch | 137 (47 Lofgren's)/167 | | | Haplotype 2 (−6752A, 3000A, 3547T, 4385T) Lofgren's | 213 |
| CCR5 | Czech | 66/386 | CCR5Δ32 | | CCR5Δ32 severe disease | 212 |
| RANTES | Japanese | 114/136 | | | −403A/A homozygotes severe disease | 214 |
| VDR | Japanese | | B allele intron 8 | | | 218 |
| NRAMP | African Americans | 157/111 | 5′(CA)n 120-bp allele | | | 228 |
| TAP2 | UK | 117/290 | | 565T 665A | | 230[a] |
| | Polish | 87/158 | | 379V | | 230[a] |
| CR1 | Italian | 91/94 | 5507G/G homozygotes | | | 232 |
| ACE | African Americans | 183/111 | Deletion polymorphism intron 16 | | | 235[a] |
| CFTR | Italian | 26/89 | CFTR mutations | | | 237[a] |

[a]Not replicated in subsequent studies, see text.

found a highly significant increase in the TNF-α −857T allele in the sarcoidosis patient group overall. Of the sarcoid patients, 25.5 percent carried the TNF −857T allele compared to 14.1 percent of controls; allele frequency was 13.5 percent in cases versus 7.3 percent in controls. This allele has been associated with higher transcriptional promoter activity.

Interestingly, this allele was not associated with Lofgren's patients – in fact there was a trend towards it being under-represented in this subgroup. In a follow-up study of 228 sarcoidosis patients including 46 Lofgren's, six haplotypes were constructed across the five polymorphisms studied in the TNF-α promoter.[204] The −307A allele associated with Lofgren's syndrome occurred exclusively in haplotype 2. The −857T allele associated with sarcoidosis susceptibility

but under-represented in the Lofgren's group occurred exclusively in haplotype 4. There was a very strong association between haplotype 2 and stage I disease with erythema nodosum, including Lofgren's patients ($p_c = 6.6 \times 10^{-11}$) and haplotype 2 carriage was associated with favorable radiological evolution over 4 years. By contrast, haplotype 4 was very strongly associated with stage I disease without erythema nodosum and with stages II–IV disease ($p_c < 0.01$) and haplotype 4 was associated with unfavorable radiological evolution over 4 years.

As discussed above, an early report of an association between cardiac sarcoidosis and the TNFA2 allele in Japanese was subsequently found to be due to linkage disequilibrium with the HLA-DQB1*0601 allele.[196,197] It remains unclear whether these other associations discussed above are functional polymorphisms, or whether one or both are in linkage disequilibrium with the causal site elsewhere in the MHC region.

## IL-1

A study by Rybicki et al.[205] in African-Americans of six polymorphic markers that are closely linked to certain candidate cytokine genes identified two alleles that may be associated with sarcoidosis. If both the IL-1α*137 and F13A*188 alleles were present, there was a six-fold increased risk of sarcoidosis, rising to a 15-fold increase in patients with a family history of sarcoidosis. The F13A marker is close to the gene for IRF-4 (a member of the interferon regulatory factor family – a transcription factor). The importance of IL-1 in granulomatous inflammation is well known; less is known about the role of IRF-4.

A Czech case–control study investigated the role in sarcoidosis of polymorphisms within the IL-1 gene cluster on chromosome 2q13–21.[206] They studied biallelic polymorphisms in the IL-1α (IL1A) and IL-1β (IL1B) genes, and an 86-bp variable number tandem repeat polymorphism in intron 2 of the interleukin-1 receptor antagonist (IL1RN) gene. They found an increase in the IL-1α-889 1.1 genotype (C/C homozygotes) in 95 patients with sarcoidosis compared to 199 controls (60.0 versus 44.2 percent, $P = 0.012$). There was a corresponding fall in the number of IL-1α-889 1.2 (C/T) heterozygotes (32.6 versus 47.7 percent, $P = 0.015$). The relative risk (OR) of disease for IL-1α-889 1.1 homozygotes compared to 1.2 heterozygotes or 2.2 homozygotes was 1.9. This finding was consistent with the study by Rybicki et al.[205] in African-Americans. However, a study of this same polymorphism in 147 UK patients with 101 UK controls and 102 Dutch patients with 166 controls failed to reproduce this association in either population.[207] This led the authors to surmise that the previously reported associations may have been due to linkage disequilibrium within the IL-1 gene cluster between the IL-1α-889C allele and the unidentified locus that actually confers the risk of sarcoidosis. So it could be the haplotype carrying this allele in African-American and Czech populations that confers the risk, and not a functional effect of this allele on IL-1α. Population-dependent differences in linkage could explain the failure to reproduce this finding in UK and Dutch populations.

## IL-18

Interleukin-18, encoded by the IL1B genes, is a cytokine known to act synergistically with IL-12 to induce IFN-γ production from Th1 cells. It is constitutively expressed in healthy airway epithelium and this expression is increased in sarcoidosis tissues. Serum and bronchoalveolar lavage levels of IL-18 are elevated in sarcoidosis patients. It is therefore an attractive candidate gene in sarcoidosis.

One Japanese study genotyped 119 patients with sarcoidosis and 130 controls for two polymorphisms in the gene promoter known to affect promoter activity after stimulation.[208] They found a significant increase in the percentage of patients carrying the C allele at position −607. This position may be a binding site for the cAMP-responsive element binding protein (CREB), and it is postulated that the A allele at this position may interfere with CREB binding, leading to a reduction in responsiveness with subsequent reduced IL-18 expression. The C allele could therefore be a genetic risk factor for susceptibility to sarcoidosis.

## MACROPHAGE MIGRATION INHIBITORY FACTOR (MIF)

Genetic polymorphism of this macrophage-derived pro-inflammatory cytokine, known to stimulate T cells and drive the delayed-type hypersensitivity reaction, has been studied in Spanish patients with erythema nodosum.[209] A single nucleotide polymorphism at position −173 (G to C) was genotyped in 28 patients with sarcoidosis-associated EN, 70 patients with EN of other etiologies, and 122 healthy controls. The C mutant allele was highly significantly over-represented in the sarcoidosis EN group compared to the non-sarcoid EN group and compared to the controls. Patients with EN carrying this allele were at increased risk of having sarcoidosis compared to EN patients without this allele. This G to C transition in the 5′-flanking region of the gene creates an AP-4 binding site and may therefore be of functional significance in controlling transcription of this key cytokine.

## INHIBITOR KAPPA B-ALPHA

Cytokine gene expression is influenced by several factors, of which the nuclear factor kappa B (NF-κB) transcription factor family is known to be crucial. Activation of this signalling pathway has been linked to the pathogenesis of sarcoidosis. In the resting cell, NF-κB is retained in the cell cytoplasm by the bound inhibitor protein inhibitor κB (IκB). This inhibitor protein degrades upon phosphorylation, unmasking the nuclear localization sequence of NFκ-B, allowing nuclear localization and initiation of transcription. IκB-α, an IκB protein that is essential for normal termination of the NF-κB response, has three single nucleotide polymorphisms in the promoter region of its gene (NFKBIA) on chromosome 14. Two hundred and five UK and Dutch sarcoidosis patients were genotyped for these polymorphisms and compared to 201 controls.[210] The T allele at position −297 was strongly associated with disease susceptibility ($P = 0.008$). By contrast, this allele was not associated with disease severity as measured by radiographic staging and pulmonary function test indices. However, the T allele at position −826 progressively and significantly declined in frequency across the stages of sarcoidosis from II to IV, suggesting that it could be protective against fibrotic disease in sarcoidosis. The functional effects of these polymorphisms are not known, but this study implicates them as potentially contributing both to disease susceptibility and disease phenotype.

## Chemokines

The importance of chemokines in the genesis of granulomatous disease has been outlined above. RANTES (regulated on activation, normal T lymphocyte expressed and secreted), monocyte chemoattractant protein (MCP-1), and macrophage inflammatory protein (MIP-1α) are known to be released by alveolar macrophages and increased levels may correlate with disease severity.[92] As with cytokines, chemokines and their receptors represent likely candidate genes (see also Table 13.5).

### CCR2

The C–C chemokine receptor CCR2 is a receptor for the MCP family. This receptor also acts as a coreceptor for human immunodeficiency virus (HIV) infection. A single nucleotide polymorphism in the CCR2 gene at position 64 substitutes isoleucine for valine (V64I). This polymorphism has a protective effect against progression of HIV infection to acquired immunodeficiency syndrome (AIDS). It was first studied in sarcoidosis in a Japanese population, and the V64I allele was found to be associated with a lower risk of sarcoidosis in 100 patients compared to 122 controls ($P < 0.001$).[211] This same polymorphism was studied in 65 Czech patients and 80 controls.[212] The allelic frequency of the polymorphism was again reduced in patients compared to controls, but did not reach statistical significance (6.9 versus 11.9 percent, $P = 0.17$).

Spagnolo et al.[213] investigated the CCR2 gene in more detail, genotyping 304 Dutch individuals (90 non-Lofgren's sarcoid, 47 Lofgren's syndrome, 167 controls) for eight single-nucleotide polymorphisms (including V64I) across the whole gene. When analyzing all sarcoidosis patients together, no statistically significant differences in any of the allele frequencies were found. However, analyzing the Lofgren's syndrome patients separately, strongly significant associations were found with five of these alleles when compared both to the healthy controls and also when compared to the non-Lofgren's sarcoidosis patients. The V64I polymorphism was not one of the alleles showing association with Lofgren's syndrome. They were able to construct nine haplotypes from the eight polymorphisms and found that four of the five alleles associated with Lofgren's syndrome were in 100 percent linkage, always occurring together and not occurring in any of the other haplotypes. This haplotype was strongly associated with Lofgren's syndrome (allele carriage 74 percent) when compared to either healthy controls (allele carriage 38 percent, $P < 0.0001$) or non-Lofgren's sarcoidosis (allele carriage 38 percent, $P < 0.0001$). The association remained strong after correcting for two other known associations with Lofgren's syndrome – female sex and carriage of HLA haplotype DRB1*0301-DQB1*0201. It remains unclear how this association should be interpreted – it is not yet known which of the polymorphisms has a functional effect which could explain the association, or whether the functional effect is due to an as yet unidentified polymorphism in the CCR2 gene or a neighboring gene that is in linkage disequilibrium with this CCR2 gene haplotype. It also remains unclear whether this CCR2 haplotype predisposes to Lofgren's in all carriers, or only in those positive for HLA DRB1*0301-DQB1*0201. In Lofgren's patients negative for HLA DRB1*0301-DQB1*0201, the CCR2 haplotype did not appear to be more common – but the number of subjects in this subgroup was too small for definitive statistical conclusions to be drawn.

### CCR5

CCR5 acts as a receptor for the chemokines RANTES and MIP-1α. A 32-bp deletion in the gene (CCR5Δ32) renders the surface receptor molecule nonfunctional. In a study of 66 Czech sarcoidosis patients and 386 controls, this allele was significantly more common in patients.[212] Furthermore, this allele was associated with clinically more apparent disease; it was present in 39.1 percent of patients requiring corticosteroids, but in only 16.7 percent of patients who needed no treatment. This study implicates the CCR5 gene as affecting both disease susceptibility and severity.

### RANTES (CC CHEMOKINE LIGAND 5 or CCL5)

This member of the C–C chemokine family is produced at sites of granulomatous reaction and is a potent chemoattractant for lymphocytes, monocytes, and eosinophils. One Japanese study genotyped 114 sarcoidosis patients and 136 healthy controls for an A/G single nucleotide polymorphism at position −403 in the promoter of the RANTES gene.[214] Although finding no association between alleles and disease, they did find the less common AA genotype was associated with disease in three or more organs. They also found that this genotype was associated with a higher CD4/8 T cell ratio in bronchoalveolar lavage cells than the GA or GG genotypes. They postulate that homozygosity for the A allele may be a risk factor for more extensive disease in Japanese patients.

## Infection susceptibility genes

The histopathological and immunological similarities between sarcoidosis and infectious granulomatous diseases, such as tuberculosis, have led to several studies attempting to associate sarcoidosis with allelic variations in genes necessary for innate immunity. These are discussed here and detailed in Table 13.5.

### MANNOSE BINDING LECTIN

Mannose binding lectin (MBL) is a serum protein encoded to the MBL2 gene that binds oligosaccharides on the surface of pathogens and triggers complement activation. It has generated interest in associations with susceptibility to infection and so has been investigated in sarcoidosis. Foley et al.[215] studied the MBL2 gene promoter and exon 1 variants known to decrease serum levels of MBL2 and increase susceptibility to infection. However, they found no associations in 167 UK patients and 164 controls between these MBL2 gene variants and susceptibility to sarcoidosis, age of disease onset, or severity of disease.

## VITAMIN D RECEPTOR

1,25-dihydroxycholecalciferol (1,25-DHCC) binds the nuclear vitamin D receptor (VDR). As well as its role in calcium homeostasis, it has an immunoregulatory effect, and polymorphisms within the VDR gene on chromosome 12 have been linked to susceptibility to infections such as tuberculosis and leprosy.[216] 1,25-DHCC is known to inhibit *M. tuberculosis* growth in human macrophages and monocytes. Pulmonary macrophages from sarcoidosis patients show an increased capacity to synthesize 1,25-DHCC and it then acts on other macrophages, inducing ICAM-1 expression, and reducing TNF-α release.[217] 1,25-DHCC is known to be produced at sites of granulomatous inflammation in sarcoidosis and this is responsible for the hypercalcemia seen in 10 percent of patients. Its role in granuloma formation is therefore pivotal and variations in the VDR gene could affect this pathway. A biallelic polymorphism in intron 8 accounts for three genotypes: bb, bB, and BB. The more common bb genotype is associated with reduced VDR mRNA expression. One Japanese study has found an association between susceptibility to sarcoidosis, and the presence of the bB genotype and B allele.[218] However, this study found no correlation of genotype with severity or spread of the disease. The authors postulated that over-representation of the B allele in the sarcoidosis patients suggests that the B allele, by promoting a more vigorous inflammatory response through increased VDR expression, could be a genetic risk factor for sarcoidosis. This remains to be tested in other ethnic groups.

## NATURAL RESISTANCE-ASSOCIATED MACROPHAGE PROTEIN (NRAMP)

The gene encoding for NRAMP was first identified in a murine model resistant to infection by the intracellular parasites leishmania, salmonella, and mycobacteria. A single nonconservative amino acid substitution of aspartate for glycine at position 169 (within the second predicted transmembrane domain) confers susceptibility to infection and *Nramp1* gene-disrupted mice are susceptible to all three pathogens.[219–221] Resistance is restored in transgenic mice when the *Nramp1*[G169] allele is transferred, proving that *Nramp1* is vital in mice to protect against mycobacteria and other intracellular pathogens.[222]

The human homolog of this gene is NRAMP1 (solute carrier family 11 (proton-coupled divalent metal ion transporters), member 1 (SLC11A1)). It has been cloned

and mapped to human chromosome 2q35.[223,224] Several polymorphisms of NRAMP1 have been described, but not the one responsible for immune deficiency in mice. The function of the NRAMP1 gene product remains uncertain, but the gene is expressed only in reticuloendothelial cells. The Nramp family is conserved from prokaryotes to eukaryotes. The Nramp2 protein is a divalent cation transporter,[225] and the Nramp1 protein is localized to the late endocytic compartment of resting macrophages.[226] After phagocytosis, it is recruited to the membrane of the phagosome, suggesting a role in controlling the phagolyposomal environment – possibly by regulating the concentration of divalent cations, such as iron or manganese.

Bellamy et al.[227] typed NRAMP1 polymorphisms in 410 patients with smear-positive pulmonary tuberculosis and 417 controls in West Africa. They found associations between smear-positive tuberculosis and heterozygosity for two NRAMP1 polymorphisms in intron 4 and the 3′ untranslated region (UTR).

The putative role of NRAMP1 in macrophage activation and the association of genetic polymorphisms with susceptibility to tuberculosis in humans, makes it an attractive candidate gene in sarcoidosis. Maliarik et al.[228] analyzed several NRAMP1 gene polymorphisms in 157 African Americans with sarcoidosis and 111 ethnically matched controls. They identified a statistically significant difference in allele frequency distribution of 5′(CA)$_n$ alleles between patients and controls. The most common 120-bp allele was over-represented in the sarcoidosis patients, suggesting that polymorphism at this site is protective against sarcoidosis. Interestingly, the two variants associated with susceptibility to tuberculosis did not affect susceptibility to sarcoidosis in this study. So this study implicates the NRAMP1 gene in sarcoidosis, but the mechanism of its effect in the studied population and other populations remain unclear.

## TRANSPORTER ASSOCIATED WITH ANTIGEN PROCESSING (TAP)

The TAP1 and TAP2 genes, located in the class II MHC region, encode subunits of a heterodimeric complex that functions in the endogenous antigen-processing pathway. TAP is inserted into the membrane of the endoplasmic reticulum, and facilitates the transport of proteasome-generated antigenic peptide fragments from the cytosol into the lumen of the endoplasmic reticulum, for subsequent presentation of the peptides in association with MHC class I molecules.[229] One study examined two single nucleotide dimorphisms in TAP1 and three single nucleotide dimorphisms in TAP2 in 117 UK Caucasoids with 290 UK controls and in 87 Polish Slavonic patients with 158 Polish controls.[230] They found different associations with different TAP2 variants in the two ethnically diverse populations studied. In the UK population, they found a threonine variant at position 565 and an alanine variant at position

665 to be significantly under-represented in the patient groups. By contrast, they failed to find these differences in the Polish population; rather they found that the valine variant at the third position studied (−379) was significantly under-represented in the patient group. The location of these genes in the MHC class II region suggests that these associations could be due to linkage disequilibrium, but they failed to find any significant linkage disequilibrium either between the TAP1 and TAP2 loci or between TAP variants and HLA-DPB1 variants. They suggested that the associations with sarcoidosis identified at the TAP loci occurred independently of HLA-DPB1 associations, and may influence susceptibility to disease. However, these influences must be population-specific; associations differed in the two ethnicities studied. This analysis would explain why another group's study in Japanese patients identified no effects of TAP1 or TAP2 polymorphisms on disease susceptibility in that population.[231] So whilst these studies leave the exact role of genetic variation in the antigen processing genes unclear, they do illustrate the critical importance of testing candidate gene associations across different ethnicities.

## COMPLEMENT RECEPTOR 1

One study has investigated polymorphisms in complement receptor 1 (CR1), also known as CD35 or C3b/C4b receptor.[232] CR1 is a membrane protein expressed on erythrocytes, phagocytes, lymphocytes, and dendritic cells which plays a number of roles in the complement system. CR1 on erythrocytes is also known to mediate the transport of immune complexes through the bloodstream to phagocytes in the liver and spleen. As sarcoidosis is accompanied by a polyclonal hypergammaglobulinemia, it could be hypothesized that interaction with the sarcoid antigen could lead to immune complex formation that may be involved in the pathogenesis of the disease. The CR1 gene on chromosome 1 is known to contain a number of single nucleotide polymorphisms that can be correlated with high or low expression of CR1 on erythrocytes. This study of 91 Italian sarcoidosis patients compared to ethnically matched controls demonstrated a significant association between the GG genotype at the C5507G polymorphism and sarcoidosis. This association was even stronger when the female subgroup was analyzed separately. This allele is known to be associated with low CR1 expression on erythrocytes and the authors postulated that reduced clearance of immune complexes could lead to deposition outside the reticuloendothelial system with the consequent granulomatous inflammation characteristic of sarcoidosis.

## Angiotensin converting enzyme

Elevated serum angiotensin converting enzyme (ACE) is found in about 60 percent of sarcoidosis patients. A 287-bp insertion/deletion (I/D) polymorphism in intron 16 of the ACE gene has attracted interest as a potential candidate gene. This I/D polymorphism has been reported to account for 47 percent of the phenotypic variation in serum ACE levels, such that the DD genotype is associated with the highest serum levels in patients and controls and the II genotype with the lowest.[233] However, no consistent correlation between ACE I/D polymorphisms and disease prevalence or severity have been demonstrated. In the most recent study, McGrath et al.[234] summarize the previous studies in this area. They also genotyped 118 UK and 56 Czech patients with sarcoidosis, and attempted to correlate ACE I/D polymorphisms with disease susceptibility and pulmonary disease severity or progression at 2 and 4 years from presentation. They found no such associations and concluded that this ACE gene polymorphism has no effect on disease susceptibility or progression in European whites.

The study that contrasts most strongly with this is in the African-American population.[235] An excess of D alleles was found in 183 cases compared to 111 controls and a gene dosage effect was seen causing an increased risk of sarcoidosis in DD homozygoyes that was even higher than the increased risk in ID heterozygotes. ACE genotype did not appear to influence disease severity or progression. This same study showed no difference in allele distribution between 60 Caucasian cases and 48 controls.

It may be concluded that there is no conclusive evidence to implicate the ACE I/D polymorphism in sarcoidosis susceptibility or phenotype in Caucasian or Japanese populations, but its role in other ethnic groups may require further investigation.

## CFTR

The cystic fibrosis transmembrane conductance regulator (CFTR) gene was first linked to sarcoidosis in an Italian study that screened the CFTR gene for mutations in 120 patients with pulmonary disease not due to cystic fibrosis.[236] Of the eight sarcoidosis patients studied, five had mutations in the CFTR gene. The same group then found eight mutations in 26 sarcoidosis cases in a follow-up study (nine mutations in 89 controls, $P = 0.014$).[237] However, a large German study of 63 families with two or more affected siblings found no association of the R75Q mutation with sarcoidosis and a further screening for 34 CFTR mutations in 54 patients from 25 families also failed to detect any increased prevalence of CFTR mutations.[238]

## DISEASE MODELS

Although animal models of granulomatous disease have been developed, no animal model of sarcoidosis exists. The animal models of granulomatous disease are sufficiently different from sarcoidosis to make extrapolation to the

human disease difficult. One such animal model is the murine schistosome soluble egg antigen (SEA) model. In this model, mice exposed to SEA develop a granulomatous reaction mediated by Th2 lymphocytes (in contrast to sarcoidosis, in which the granulomatous inflammation is mediated by predominantly Th1 lymphocytes). Models such as this have given us insights into the immunological mechanisms at play in determining the magnitude of the granulomatous reaction,[239] but have contributed little to our understanding of the genetic basis of sarcoidosis in humans. However, one interesting paper examined the role of TGF-β in determining the course of inflammation and fibrosis.[71] In the murine model, the degree of inflammation and hepatic fibrosis is highly variable, just as in sarcoidosis the clinical phenotype and degree of end-organ damage and fibrosis is highly variable. It is known that modulation of the Th1/Th2 cytokine balance in this model affects the outcome of the chronic inflammatory fibrotic disease. In this study, the TGF-β1 gene was targeted so that mice over-expressed, under-expressed, or failed to express TGF-β1. The expression of TGF-β1 was found to correlate with the degree of hepatic fibrosis. Extrapolating to humans, one could consider TGFB1 as a candidate gene in determining which patients suffer little fibrosis and which patients suffer progressive or severe fibrosis. To date, however, no such association in sarcoidosis has been reported.

The lack of good animal models of sarcoidosis has led to a search for alternative models of the disease. The Kveim–Siltzbach (KS) reagent has been used as an in vivo model of the granulomatous disease and has generated considerable data on the immunological mechanisms involved.[240] Unfortunately this model is not suitable for genetic manipulation or study, and the reagent is no longer widely administered due to concerns about it being potentially biohazardous.

The human diseases tuberculosis and leprosy have provided valuable clues to the genetic basis of infectious granulomatous diseases, which have been applied to studies of human sarcoidosis using the candidate gene approach. Some of these infection susceptibility genes are discussed above. However, the model that has provided the most exciting insight into the genetic basis of sarcoidosis is an occupational disease – chronic beryllium disease.

## Chronic beryllium disease

Chronic beryllium disease (CBD) is characterized histologically by noncaseating granulomata and interstitial mononuclear cell pneumonitis with fibrosis. It is characterized radiologically by bilateral hilar adenopathy in 50 percent and upper lobe interstitial changes.[241] CBD can also involve the liver, spleen, lymph nodes, kidneys, muscle, and skin. The similarities to sarcoidosis, a multisystem granulomatous disorder of unknown etiology, are striking.

Studies on proliferating BAL lymphocytes demonstrated that they were predominantly CD4$^+$ T helper (Th) cells, that they were activated (they exhibited increased expression of HLA-DR), that the beryllium response was blocked by antibodies to HLA class II molecules, that antibodies to the interleukin-2 (IL-2) receptor blocked the response (IL-2 is required for T cells to proliferate and IL-2 receptors are upregulated on activated T cells), and that the cells would respond specifically to beryllium and not to other substances including zirconium, nickel, or lithium.[242] Consistent with the disease process, it has been shown that beryllium induces IL-2 and interferon-γ (IFN-γ) in berylliosis, driving the granulomatous reaction.[243,244] The T cells are polyclonal, but are skewed by the expression of a limited set of T-cell antigen receptor variable region genes.[245,246] This is all consistent with normal immunological mechanisms being triggered by CD4$^+$ T cells recognizing beryllium as an MHC-restricted antigen/hapten.[247] Identical mechanisms are known to drive sarcoidosis – but the antigen is unknown.

Richeldi et al.[248] examined the association of the HLA-DP gene with CBD in a group of 33 CBD individuals and a group of 44 beryllium-exposed unaffected individuals, after a preliminary analysis of a small sample showed no strong associations with HLA-DR or HLA-DQ genes. They found the frequency of the HLA-DPB1*0201 allele was increased in the CBD group (CBD, 30 percent; unaffected, 10 percent; $P < 0.05$). In contrast, the frequency of the DPB1*0401 allele was reduced in the CBD group (CBD, 14 percent; unaffected, 48 percent; $P < 0.001$). Analysis of the phenotypic frequencies showed a similar bias, indicating that the expression of just one disease-associated allele is sufficient to confer susceptibility.

The HLA-DPB1 gene comprises six hypervariable regions, denoted as A, B, C, D, E, and F. The DPB1*0201 and DPB1*0401 alleles differ in three of these regions – B, C, and D. The strongest association was shown for region D, in which the HLA-DPB1*0201 allele codes Ile Leu Glu Glu Glu for Ile Leu Glu Glu Lys at positions 65 to 69. This was confirmed using a DNA amplification assay with direct sequencing of the HLA-DPB1 polymerase chain reaction-amplified DNA. The HLA-DPB1 Glu$^{69}$ epitope was found in 97 percent of patients with CBD and in 27 percent of controls ($P < 0.0002$). This strongly implicated HLA-DPB1 Glu$^{69}$ as an epitope that confers increased risk of developing CBD upon exposure to beryllium.

Three other studies subsequently confirmed this genetic association. Stubbs et al.[249] confirmed the association in the same laboratory, but also reported an association of CBD with certain HLA-DR alleles. A further study recognized that the risk of CBD is dependent upon the nature of the industrial exposure, with beryllium machinists known to be a high-risk group.[250] They therefore examined the prevalence of the HLA-DPB1 Glu$^{69}$ marker in machinists with or without CBD. They found a prevalence of CBD of 25 percent amongst HLA-DP Glu$^{69}$-positive machinists and of 3.2 percent amongst HLA-DP Glu$^{69}$-negative machinists

($P = 0.05$). Carriage of HLA-DP Glu[69] predicted CBD independent of machining history. In a third study, Wang et al.[251] again found a highly significant association between CBD and carriage of HLA-DPB Glu[69]. They found that carriage of two such alleles conferred even greater risk than one allele; however, other studies have not identified any association between allele frequency and risk of CBD. They also reported a possible association with certain HLA-DPA1 alleles.

Lombardi et al.[243] explored the association between DPB1 Glu[69] and CBD further. They raised 25 beryllium-specific clones from three individuals with CBD, all of which were restricted by HLA-DP alleles with Glu at DPB69. A single amino acid substitution at that position abolished the response, indicating that the proliferative responses to beryllium were absolutely dependent upon that epitope. Amicosante et al.[252] produced soluble HLA-DP with a Glu or a Lys at position 69 of the β chain. Beryllium binding assays using invariant chain peptide indicated a direct interaction of beryllium with the soluble HLA-DP Glu[69] molecule, but not with the soluble HLA-DP Lys[69] molecule. Similarly, beryllium decreased the binding of the monoclonal antibody (mAb) NFLD.M60 to L cells transfected with HLA-DP Glu[69], but not to L cells transfected with HLA-DP Lys[69]. These experiments show that beryllium affects peptide binding to HLA-DP Glu[69] in the absence of antigen processing.

Saltini et al.[253] looked not only at HLA class II molecules as described above, but in the same study they investigated the biallelic TNF-α (also known as TNF) polymorphism TNF-α-308. Both beryllium sensitization (BeS) and CBD were strongly associated with the TNF-α-308*2 marker (a G to A transition at position −308). This has been associated with the high TNF-α production in subjects carrying the HLA-A1, -B8, and -DR3 haplotype. Elevated production associated with the −308 polymorphism (in the TNF-α promoter region) may increase the risk of development of disease, and has been associated with sarcoidosis and silicosis. It is known that beryllium-antigen stimulates TNF-α from BAL cells in CBD.

Maier et al.[254] examined the implications of this polymorphism further in 20 CBD patients. They measured beryllium-stimulated BAL cell TNF-α production in these patients and classified patients into high or low TNF-α producers using an arbitrary cut-off. They identified 10 patients as being in each category. They sequenced the TNF-α promoter region in each patient and observed polymorphic variability at the −308 nucleotide position, with a TNF1 G allele frequency of 77.5 percent and a TNF2 A allele frequency of 22.5 percent. They observed a trend between the high TNF-α group and the presence of at least one TNF2 A allele (OR of 13.5, 95 percent CI 1.00–687.9, $P = 0.057$). They also observed significant associations between high TNF-α production and clinical parameters of more severe CBD (chest radiograph score, obstructive spirometry, and BAL beryllium lymphocyte proliferation).

They found a protective effect of the HLA-DR4 allele on beryllium-stimulated TNF-α production. They proposed a model in which the TNF-α −308 polymorphism, situated in the promoter region, may enhance TNF-α transcription. This would lead to elevated levels of TNF-α in response to beryllium stimulation. TNF-α increases the accumulation of macrophages, stimulates proliferation of activated T cells, increases its own production, and promotes the differentiation of noncaseating granulomas. This could lead to more severe disease.

This CBD model is clinically, histologically, and immunologically strikingly similar to sarcoidosis, and the highly successful studies into the genetic predisposition to CBD has dictated the direction of much of the research into the genetic basis of sarcoidosis in a way that no animal model has been able to do.

## FUTURE DIRECTIONS

Over the last decade, there has been rapid growth in the number of studies examining the genetic basis of sarcoidosis. A model has developed for the disease, in which an exogenous antigen such as pollen or a microbe interacts with HLA molecules in an ethnically dependent and possibly even individually dependent manner, to trigger a normal Th1 dominated granulomatous reaction – sarcoidosis. Numerous other genes encoding for proteins including chemokines, cytokines, and 'infection susceptibility proteins' also influence susceptibility; the subsequent course of the disease is probably a result of the interaction between the triggering antigen and numerous host genes.

Genetic susceptibility to the clinical subtype of sarcoidosis, known as Lofgren's syndrome, has been strongly associated with a particular extended MHC haplotype. It is likely that future research will identify genetic susceptibilities to other clinical subtypes such as uveitis. Such research may also correlate certain genetic variations with certain clinical phenotypes, to help explain the wide variation in clinical phenotypes within this disease.

It may be that a genetic susceptibility to granulomatous disease underlies all cases of sarcoidosis, with modifier genes acting to determine the clinical phenotype. It may become possible to predict the clinical phenotype based on genetic analysis of known effector genes. Achieving this will require tighter definition of clinical phenotypes and identification of other candidate genes. To date, most studies have used the candidate gene approach and case–control studies, and some of the associations described in the literature will need to be verified in other populations. However, the emergence of family cohorts and large databases such as ACCESS should allow better linkage studies, to identify all areas of the genome with even minor linkage to disease susceptibility or protection.

New technologies should also aid this process. The development of oligonucleotide arrays and the science of genomics will allow the rapid analysis of many thousands of polymorphisms in one experiment.[255] The study of differential gene expression in a disease, using these arrays, can lead to the identification of new candidate genes.[256,257] This approach has already been used to identify dysregulation of apoptosis-related genes in peripheral blood mononuclear cells in acute sarcoidosis compared to controls[258] and to examine differential gene expression in BAL cells from sarcoidosis compared to tuberculosis and extrinsic allergic alveolitis.[259] Future studies like these should provide insight into how the human genome interacts with the trigger to give rise to the disease, identifying new candidate genes for investigation.

It must be recognized that the study of genetic mechanisms alone will not provide all the answers to sarcoidosis. However, when used in conjunction with other molecular biological disciplines, the elucidation of the genetic background of sarcoidosis has great potential to expand our understanding of disease immunopathogenesis. With that greater understanding may come new opportunities for the prevention, amelioration, or cure of this relatively common disease.

## Key learning points

- Sarcoidosis is a multisystem granulomatous disease with clinical subtypes and varying phenotypes, in which an unknown antigen is persistently expressed on antigen presenting cells leading to Th1-mediated granulomatous inflammation.

- Although reported in almost all populations around the world, there are wide variations in the incidence and prevalence of the different subtypes and clinical phenotypes in different populations, suggesting genetic influence on disease susceptibility and phenotype.

- Further evidence for a genetic influence is provided by the familial cases of sarcoidosis that have been reported in most populations, and the collection of cohorts of familial sarcoidosis.

- Linkage studies in familial sarcoidosis have identified that some areas of the genome are linked to sarcoidosis, with the strongest linkage reported for the MHC genes.

- Many case–control studies have reported associations between sarcoidosis and allelic variations in the HLA genes responsble for antigen presentation, but these associations are ethnically dependent.

- Lofgren's syndrome has been strongly associated with an extended MHC haplotype encompassing alleles in HLA-DQ, HLA-DR, and TNF, suggesting that other clinical subtypes and phenotypes might be associated with different susceptibility genes.

- Other case–control studies using the candidate gene approach have reported associations with genes encoding for cytokines, chemokines, and infection susceptibility genes.

- The development of tighter definitions of clinical phenotypes and the emergence of larger cohort studies of sarcoidosis (including familial sarcoidosis) should combine with new technological advances to build a clear picture of the genetics of sarcoidosis susceptibility and phenotypes in the future.

## REFERENCES

❋1 Hunninghake GW, Costabel U, Ando M et al. ATS/ERS/WASOG statement on sarcoidosis. American Thoracic Society/European Respiratory Society/World Association of Sarcoidosis and other Granulomatous Disorders. *Sarcoidosis Vasc Diffuse Lung Dis* 1999; **16**:149–73.

2 Studdy PR. Sarcoidosis. In: Weatherall DJ, Ledingham JGG, Warrell DA (eds). *Oxford textbook of medicine*. Oxford: Oxford University Press, 1996; **28**: 17–32.

3 Cordis L. *Sarcoidosis: epidemiology of chronic lung diseases in children*. Baltimore: The John Hopkins University Press, 1973: 53–78.

4 Brown IG, Hamblin TJ, Mikhail JR. Oldest case of sarcoidosis in the world. *Br Med J (Clin Res Ed)* 1981; **283**: 190.

5 Alsbirk PH. Epidemiologic studies on sarcoidosis in Denmark based on a nation-wide central register. A preliminary report. *Acta Med Scand Suppl* 1964; **425**: 106–9.

6 Iwai K, Sekiguti M, Hosoda Y et al. Racial difference in cardiac sarcoidosis incidence observed at autopsy. *Sarcoidosis* 1994; 11: 26–31.

7 Milman N, Selroos O. Pulmonary sarcoidosis in the Nordic countries 1950–1982. Epidemiology and clinical picture. Sarcoidosis 1990; **7**: 50–57.

8 Anderson R, Brett GZ, James DG, Siltzbach LE. The prevalence of intrathoracic sarcoidosis. *Med Thorac* 1963; **20**: 152–62.

9 Forsen KO, Milman N, Pietinalho A, Selroos O. Sarcoidosis in the Nordic countries 1950–1987. *Sarcoidosis* 1992; **9**: 140–1.

10 Bauer HJ, Lofgren S. International study of pulmonary sarcoidosis in mass chest radiography. *Acta Med Scand* 1964; **176**: 103–5.

◆11 James GD. *Sarcoidosis and other granulomatous disorders*. New York: Marcel Dekker, 1994.

12 Henke CE, Henke G, Elveback LR et al. The epidemiology of sarcoidosis in Rochester, Minnesota: a population-based study of incidence and survival. *Am J Epidemiol* 1986; **123**: 840–5.

13 Rybicki BA, Major M, Popovich J Jr et al. Racial differences in sarcoidosis incidence: a 5-year study in a health maintenance organization. *Am J Epidemiol* 1997; **145**: 234–41.

◆14 Bresnitz EA, Strom BL. Epidemiology of sarcoidosis. *Epidemiol Rev* 1983; **5**: 124–56.

15 Hsing CT, Han FC, Liu HC, Chu BY. Sarcoidosis among Chinese. *Am Rev Respir Dis* 1964; **89**: 917–22.

16 Mana J, Badrinas J, Morera et al. Sarcoidosis in Spain. *Sarcoidosis* 1992; **9**: 118–22.

◆17  James DG. Epidemiology of sarcoidosis. *Sarcoidosis* 1992; **9**: 79–87.

18  Parkes SA, Baker SB, Bourdillon RE et al. Incidence of sarcoidosis in the Isle of Man. *Thorax* 1985; **40**: 284–7.

19  Hosoda Y, Yamaguchi M, Hiraga Y. Global epidemiology of sarcoidosis. What story do prevalence and incidence tell us? *Clin Chest Med* 1997; **18**: 681–94.

20  Maycock RI, Bertrand P, Morrison CE, Scott JH. Manifestations of sarcoidosis: analysis of 145 patients with review of nine series selected from the literature. *Am J Med* 1963; **35**: 67–89.

21  Siltzbach LE, James DG, Neville E et al. Course and prognosis of sarcoidosis around the world. *Am J Med* 1974; **57**: 847–52.

22  Keller AZ. Hospital, age, racial, occupational, geographical, clinical and survivorship characteristics in the epidemiology of sarcoidosis. *Am J Epidemiol* 1971; **94**: 222–30.

◆23  Mitchell DN, Scadding JG. Sarcoidosis. *Am Rev Respir Dis* 1974; **110**: 774–802.

24  McNicol MW, Luce PJ. Sarcoidosis in a racially mixed community. *J R Coll Phys Lond* 1985; **19**: 179–83.

25  Edmondstone WM, Wilson AG. Sarcoidosis in Caucasians, Blacks and Asians in London. *Br J Dis Chest* 1985; **79**: 27–36.

26  Pietinalho A, Ohmichi M, Hiraga Y et al. The mode of presentation of sarcoidosis in Finland and Hokkaido, Japan. A comparative analysis of 571 Finnish and 686 Japanese patients. *Sarcoidosis Vasc Diffuse Lung Dis* 1996; **13**: 159–66.

27  Iwai K, Tachibana T, Takemura T et al. Pathological studies on sarcoidosis autopsy. I. Epidemiological features of 320 cases in Japan. *Acta Pathol Jpn* 1993; **43**: 372–6.

28  Iwai K, Takemura T, Kitaichi M et al. Pathological studies on sarcoidosis autopsy. II. Early change, mode of progression and death pattern. *Acta Pathol Jpn* 1993; **43**: 377–85.

29  Gideon NM, Mannino DM. Sarcoidosis mortality in the United States 1979–1991: an analysis of multiple-cause mortality data. *Am J Med* 1996; **100**: 423–7.

●30  Parkes SA, Baker SB, Bourdillon RE et al. Epidemiology of sarcoidosis in the Isle of Man. **1**: A case controlled study. *Thorax* 1987; **42**: 420–6.

●31  Hills SE, Parkes SA, Baker SB. Epidemiology of sarcoidosis in the Isle of Man. 2: Evidence for space–time clustering. *Thorax* 1987; **42**: 427–30.

32  Martenstein H. Knochveranderungen bei Lupus pernio. *Zentralb Haut Geschlechtskrankh* 1923; **7**: 308.

33  Hiraga Y. [An epidemiological study of clustering of sarcoidosis cases]. *Nippon Rinsho* 1994; **52**: 1438–42.

●34  Pietinalho A, Ohmichi M, Hirasawa M et al. Familial sarcoidosis in Finland and Hokkaido, Japan. A comparative study. *Respir Med* 1999; **93**: 408–12.

35  Hiraga Y, Hosoda Y, Zenda I. A local outbreak of sarcoidosis in Northern Japan. *Z Erkr Atmungsorgane* 1977; **149**: 38–43.

36  Brennan NJ, Crean P, Long JP, Fitzgerald MX. High prevalence of familial sarcoidosis in an Irish population. *Thorax* 1984; **39**: 14–8.

37  Headings VE, Weston D, Young RC Jr, Hackney RL Jr. Familial sarcoidosis with multiple occurrences in eleven families: a possible mechanism of inheritance. *Ann NY Acad Sci* 1976; **278**: 377–85.

38  Rybicki BA, Kirkey KL, Major M et al. Familial risk ratio of sarcoidosis in African-American sibs and parents. *Am J Epidemiol* 2001; **153**: 188–93.

●39  McGrath DS, Daniil Z, Foley P et al. Epidemiology of familial sarcoidosis in the UK. *Thorax* 2000; **55**: 751–4.

40  Rybicki BA, Iannuzzi MC, Frederick MM et al. Familial aggregation of sarcoidosis. A case-control etiologic study of sarcoidosis (ACCESS). *Am J Respir Crit Care Med* 2001; **164**: 2085–91.

41  Harrington AC, Major M, Rybicki BA et al. Familial sarcoidosis: analysis of 91 families. *Sarcoidosis* 1994; **11**: 240–3.

42  Bardinas F, Morera J, Fite E, Plasencia A. Seasonal clustering of sarcoidosis. *Lancet* 1989; **2**: 455–6 (letter).

43  Glennas A, Kvien TK, Melby K et al. Acute sarcoid arthritis: occurrence, seasonal onset, clinical features and outcome. *Br J Rheumatol* 1995; **34**: 45–50.

44  Panayeas S, Theodorakopoulos P, Bouras A, Constantopoulos S. Seasonal occurrence of sarcoidosis in Greece. *Lancet* 1991; **338**: 510–1.

45  Hosoda Y, Hiraga Y, Odaka M et al. A cooperative study of sarcoidosis in Asia and Africa: analytic epidemiology. *Ann NY Acad Sci* 1976; **278**: 355–67.

46  Jawad AS, Hamour AA, Wenley WG, Scott DG. An outbreak of acute sarcoidosis with arthropathy in Norfolk. *Br J Rheumatol* 1989; **28**: 178.

●47  Edmondstone WM. Sarcoidosis in nurses: is there an association? *Thorax* 1988; **43**: 342–3.

48  Hennessy TW, Ballard DJ, DeRemee RA et al. The influence of diagnostic access bias on the epidemiology of sarcoidosis: a population-based study in Rochester, Minnesota, 1935–1984. *J Clin Epidemiol* 1988; **41**: 565–70.

●49  Sartwell PE, Edwards LB. Epidemiology of sarcoidosis in the US Navy. *Am J Epidemiol* 1974; **99**: 250–7.

50  Kern DG, Neill MA, Wrenn DS, Varone JC. Investigation of a unique time–space cluster of sarcoidosis in firefighters. *Am Rev Respir Dis* 1993; **148**: 974–80.

51  Prezant DJ, Dhala A, Goldstein A et al. The incidence, prevalence, and severity of sarcoidosis in New York City firefighters. *Chest* 1999; **116**: 1183–93.

52  Buck AA. Epidemiologic investigations of sarcoidosis: I. Introduction, material and methods. *Am J Hyg* 1961; **74**: 137–51.

53  Cummings MM. An evaluation of the possible relationship of pine pollen to sarcoidosis (a critical summary). *Acta Med Scand Suppl* 1964; **425**: 48–50.

●54  Valeyre D, Soler P, Clerici C et al. Smoking and pulmonary sarcoidosis: effect of cigarette smoking on prevalence, clinical manifestations, alveolitis, and evolution of the disease. *Thorax* 1988; **43**: 516–24.

55  Douglas JG, Middleton WG, Gaddie J et al. Sarcoidosis: a disorder commoner in non-smokers? *Thorax* 1986; **41**: 787–91.

56  Hance AJ, Basset F, Saumon G et al. Smoking and interstitial lung disease. The effect of cigarette smoking on the incidence of pulmonary histiocytosis X and sarcoidosis. *Ann NY Acad Sci* 1986; **465**: 643–56.

57  Romer FK. Presentation of sarcoidosis and outcome of pulmonary changes. *Dan Med Bull* 1982; **29**: 27–32.

◆58  Lynch JP III, Kazerooni EA, Gay SE. Pulmonary sarcoidosis. *Clin Chest Med* 1997; **18**: 755–85.

59  Mana J, Salazar A, Manresa F. Clinical factors predicting persistence of activity in sarcoidosis: a multivariate analysis of 193 cases. *Respiration* 1994; **61**: 219–25.

60  Takada K, Ina Y, Noda M et al. The clinical course and prognosis of patients with severe, moderate or mild sarcoidosis. *J Clin Epidemiol* 1993; **46**: 359–66.

◆61  DeRemee RA. Sarcoidosis. *Mayo Clin Proc* 1995; **70**: 177–81.

62 Hillerdal G, Nou E, Osterman K, Schmekel B. Sarcoidosis: epidemiology and prognosis. A 15-year European study. *Am Rev Respir Dis* 1984; **130**: 29–32.

63 Johns CJ, Schonfeld SA, Scott PP et al. Longitudinal study of chronic sarcoidosis with low-dose maintenance corticosteroid therapy. Outcome and complications. *Ann NY Acad Sci* 1986; **465**: 702–12.

64 Zych D, Krychniak W, Pawlicka L, Zielinski J. Sarcoidosis of the lung. Natural history and effects of treatment. *Sarcoidosis* 1987; **4**: 64–7.

65 Scadding JG. Prognosis of intrathoracic sarcoidosis in England. A review of 136 cases after five years' observation. *Br Med J* 1961; **5261**: 1165–72.

66 Gottlieb JE, Israel HL, Steiner RM et al. Outcome in sarcoidosis. The relationship of relapse to corticosteroid therapy. *Chest* 1997; **111**: 623–31.

67 Yeatman M, McNeil K, Smith JA et al. Lung transplantation in patients with systemic diseases: an eleven-year experience at Papworth Hospital. *J Heart Lung Transplant* 1996; **15**: 144–9.

68 Johnson BA, Duncan SR, Ohori NP et al. Recurrence of sarcoidosis in pulmonary allograft recipients. *Am Rev Respir Dis* 1993; **148**: 1373–7.

69 Roitt I. *Essential immunology*, 6th edn. Oxford: Blackwell Scientific, 1988.

◆70 Conron M, du Bois R. Immunological mechanisms in sarcoidosis. *Clin Exp Allergy* 2001; **31**: 543–54.

71 Wahl S, Frazier Jessen M, Jin W et al. Cytokine regulation of schistosome-induced granuloma and fibrosis. *Kidney Int* 1997; **51**: 1370–5.

72 Agostini C, Zambello R, Sancetta R et al. Expression of tumour necrosis factor-receptor superfamily members by lung T lymphocytes in interstitial lung disease. *Am J Respir Crit Care Med* 1996; **153**: 1359–67.

73 Gombert W, Borthwick N, Wallace D et al. Fibroblasts prevent apoptosis of IL-2 deprived T cells without inducing proliferation: a selective effect on Bcl-x$_L$ expression. *Immunology* 1996; **89**: 397–404.

74 Estaquier J, Ameisen J. A role for Th1 and Th2 cytokines in the regulation of human monocyte apoptosis. *Blood* 1997; **90**: 153–60.

75 Wallace W, Ramage E, Lamb D et al. A type 2 (Th-2 like) pattern of immune response predominates in the pulmonary interstitium of patients with cryptogenic fibrosing alveolitis. *Clin Exp Immunol* 1995; **101**: 436–41.

◆76 Mitchell D, Scadding J, Heard B et al. Sarcoidosis: histopathological definition and clinical diagnosis. *J Clin Pathol* 1977; **30**: 395–8.

77 Pforte A, Gerth C, Voss A et al. Proliferating alveolar macrophages in BAL and lung function changes in interstitial lung disease. *Eur Respir J* 1993; **6**: 951–5.

78 Muller-Quernheim J, Pfiefer S, Mannel D et al. Lung restricted activation of the alveolar macrophage/monocyte system in pulmonary sarcoidosis. *Am Rev Respir Med* 1992; **145**: 187–92.

79 Hunninghake G. Release of interleukin-1 by alveolar macrophages of patients with active pulmonary sarcoidosis. *Am Rev Respir Dis* 1984; **129**: 569–72.

80 Costabel U, Zaiss A, Guzman J. Sensitivity and specificity of BAL findings in sarcoidosis. In: Izumi T. (ed.) *Proceedings of the 1991 XII World Congress on Sarcoidosis*, Milan, **1992**: 211–4.

81 du Bois R, Kirby M, Balbi B et al. T-lymphocytes that accumulate in the lung in sarcoidosis have evidence of recent

stimulation of the T-cell antigen receptor. *Am Rev Respir Dis* 1992; **145**: 1205–11.

82 Pinkston P, Bitterman P, Crystal R. Spontaneous release of IL-2 by lung T-cells in active pulmonary sarcoidosis. *N Engl J Med* 1983; **308**: 793–800.

83 Robinson B, McLemore T, Crystal R. IFNγ is spontaneously released by alveolar macrophages and T-lymphocytes in patients with pulmonary sarcoidosis. *J Clin Invest* 1985; **75**: 1488–95.

84 Hunninghake G, Crystal R. Pulmonary sarcoidosis: a disorder mediated by excess helper T-lymphocyte activity at site of disease activity. *N Engl J Med* 1981; **305**: 429–34.

85 Muller-Quernheim J, Saltini C, Sondermeyer P et al. Compartmentalised activation of the IL-2 gene by lung T-lymphocytes in active pulmonary sarcoidosis. *J Immunol* 1986; **137**: 3475–83.

86 Jones C, Lake R, O'Hehir R et al. Oligoclonal V gene usage by T lymphocytes in BAL fluid from sarcoidosis patients. *Am J Respir Cell Mol Biol* 1996; **14**: 470–7.

87 Grunewald J, Hultman T, Bucht A et al. Restricted usage of TCR V alpha/J alpha gene segments with different nucleotide but identical amino acid sequences in HLA-DR3 +ve sarcoidosis. *Mol Med* 1995; **1**: 287–96.

88 Grunewald J, Shigematsu M, Nagai S. T cell receptor V gene expression in HLA typed Japanese patients with sarcoidosis. *Am J Respir Crit Care Med* 1995; **151**: 151–6.

89 Grunewald J, Wahlstrom J, Berlin M et al. Lung restricted T cell receptor AV2S3$^+$ CD4$^+$ T cell expansions in sarcoidosis patients with a shared HLA-DRbeta chain conformation. *Thorax* 2002; **57**: 348–52.

90 Siltzbach L. The Kveim test in sarcoidosis. *J Am Med Assoc* 1961; **178**: 476–82.

91 Holter J, Park H, Sloerdsma K et al. Non viable autologous bronchoalveolar lavage cell preparations induce intradermal epithelioid granulomas in sarcoidosis patients. *Am Rev Respir Dis* 1992; **145**: 864–71.

◆92 McGrath D, Goh N, Foley P et al. Sarcoidosis: genes and microbes – soil or seed? *Sarcoidosis Vasc Diffuse Lung Dis* 2001; **18**: 149–64.

93 Di Alberti L, Piattelli A, Artese L et al. Human herpes virus 8 variants in sarcoid tissues. *Lancet* 1997; **350**: 1655–61.

94 Belec L, Mohamed A, Lechapt-Zalcman E et al. Lack of HHV-8 DNA sequences in sarcoid tissues of French patients. *Chest* 1998; **114**: 948–9.

95 Lebbe C, Agbalika F, Flageul B et al. No evidence for a role of human herpesvirus type 8 in sarcoidosis: molecular and serological analysis. *Br J Dermatol* 1999; **141**: 492–6.

96 Yi E, Lee H, Suh Y et al. Experimental extrinsic allergic alveolitis and pulmonary angiitis induced by intratracheal or intravenous challenge with *Corynebacterium parvum* in sensitised rats. *Am J Pathol* 1996; **149**: 1303–12.

97 Ichiyasu H, Suga M, Matsukawa A et al. Functional roles of MCP-1 in *Propionibacterium acnes*-induced, T cell-mediated pulmonary granulomatosis in rabbits. *J Leukoc Biol* 1999; **65**: 482–91.

98 Abe C, Iwai K, Mikami R et al. Frequent isolation of *Propionibacterium acnes* from sarcoidosis lymph nodes. *Zentralbl Bakteriol Mikrobiol Hyg [A]* 1984; **256**: 541–7.

99 Eishi Y, Suga M, Ishige I et al. Quantitative analysis of mycobacterial and propionibacterial DNA in lymph nodes of Japanese and European patients with sarcoidosis. *J Clin Microbiol* 2002; **40**: 198–204.

100  Ebe Y, Ikushima S, Yamaguchi T et al. Proliferative response of peripheral blood mononuclear cells and levels of antibody to recombinant protein from *Propionibacterium acnes* DNA expression library in Japanese patients with sarcoidosis. *Sarcoidosis Vasc Diffuse Lung Dis* 2000; **17**: 256–65.

101  Rohatgi PK, Ryan JW, Lindeman P. Value of serial measurement of serum angiotensin converting enzyme in the management of sarcoidosis. *Am J Med* 1981; **70**: 44–50.

102  DeRemee RA, Rohrbach MS. Serum angiotensin-converting enzyme activity in evaluating the clinical course of sarcoidosis. *Ann Intern Med* 1980; **92**: 361–5.

103  Keogh BA, Hunninghake GW, Line BR, Crystal RG. The alveolitis of pulmonary sarcoidosis. Evaluation of natural history and alveolitis-dependent changes in lung function. *Am Rev Respir Dis* 1983; **128**: 256–65.

104  Klech H, Kohn H, Kummer F, Mostbeck A. Assessment of activity in sarcoidosis. Sensitivity and specificity of 67Gallium scintigraphy, serum ACE levels, chest roentgenography, and blood lymphocyte subpopulations. *Chest* 1982; **82**: 732–8.

105  Baughman RP, Fernandez M, Bosken CH et al. Comparison of gallium-67 scanning, bronchoalveolar lavage, and serum angiotensin-converting enzyme levels in pulmonary sarcoidosis. Predicting response to therapy. *Am Rev Respir Dis* 1984; **129**: 676–81.

106  Ward K, O'Connor C, Odlum C, FitzGerald MX. Prognostic value of bronchoalveolar lavage in sarcoidosis: the critical influence of disease presentation. *Thorax* 1989; **44**: 6–12.

107  Laviolette M, La Forge J, Tennina S, Boulet LP. Prognostic value of bronchoalveolar lavage lymphocyte count in recently diagnosed pulmonary sarcoidosis. *Chest* 1991; **100**: 380–4.

108  Buchalter S, App W, Jackson L et al. Bronchoalveolar lavage cell analysis in sarcoidosis. A comparison of lymphocyte counts and clinical course. *Ann NY Acad Sci* 1986; **465**: 678–84.

109  Wallaert B, Ramon P, Fournier E et al. Bronchoalveolar lavage, serum angiotensin-converting enzyme, and gallium-67 scanning in extrathoracic sarcoidosis. *Chest* 1982; **82**: 553–5.

110  Schoenberger CI, Line BR, Keogh BA et al. Lung inflammation in sarcoidosis: comparison of serum angiotensin-converting enzyme levels with bronchoalveolar lavage and gallium-67 scanning assessment of the T lymphocyte alveolitis. *Thorax* 1982; **37**: 19–25.

111  Murdoch J, Muller NL. Pulmonary sarcoidosis: changes on follow-up CT examination. *AJR Am J Roentgenol* 1992; **159**: 473–7.

112  Sekiguchi M, Yazaki Y, Isobe M, Hiroe M. Cardiac sarcoidosis: diagnostic, prognostic, and therapeutic considerations. *Cardiovasc Drugs Ther* 1996; **10**: 495–510.

113  Tellier P, Paycha F, Antony I et al. Reversibility by dipyridamole of thallium-201 myocardial scan defects in patients with sarcoidosis. *Am J Med* 1988; **85**: 189–93.

114  Tellier P, Valeyre D, Nitenberg A et al. Cardiac sarcoidosis: reversion of myocardial perfusion abnormalities by dipyridamole. *Eur J Nucl Med* 1985; **11**: 201–4.

115  Line BR, Hunninghake GW, Keogh BA et al. Gallium-67 scanning to stage the alveolitis of sarcoidosis: correlation with clinical studies, pulmonary function studies, and bronchoalveolar lavage. *Am Rev Respir Dis* 1981; **123**: 440–6.

116  Sulavik SB, Spencer RP, Palestro CJ et al. Specificity and sensitivity of distinctive chest radiographic and/or 67Ga images in the noninvasive diagnosis of sarcoidosis. *Chest* 1993; **103**: 403–9.

117  Turner-Warwick M, McAllister W, Lawrence R et al. Corticosteroid treatment in pulmonary sarcoidosis: do serial lavage lymphocyte counts, serum angiotensin converting enzyme measurements, and gallium-67 scans help management? *Thorax* 1986; **41**: 903–13.

118  Lebtahi R, Crestani B, Belmatoug N et al. Somatostatin receptor scintigraphy and gallium scintigraphy in patients with sarcoidosis. *J Nucl Med* 2001; **42**: 21–6.

119  Chinet T, Dusser D, Labrune S et al. Lung function declines in patients with pulmonary sarcoidosis and increased respiratory epithelial permeability to 99mTc-DTPA. *Am Rev Respir Dis* 1990; **141**: 445–9.

120  Lower EE, Smith JT, Martelo OJ, Baughman RP. The anemia of sarcoidosis. *Sarcoidosis* 1988; **5**: 51–5.

121  Goldstein RA, Israel HL, Becker KL, Moore CF. The infrequency of hypercalcemia in sarcoidosis. *Am J Med* 1971; **51**: 21–30.

122  Sharma OP. Vitamin D, calcium, and sarcoidosis. *Chest* 1996; **109**: 535–9.

●123  Kveim A. En ny og spesifikk kutan-reaksjon ved Boecks sarcoid. *Nord Med* 1941; **9**: 169–72.

124  Munro CS, Mitchell DN. The Kveim response: still useful, still a puzzle. *Thorax* 1987; **42**: 321–31.

125  Costabel U, Guzman J. Bronchoalveolar lavage in interstitial lung disease. *Curr Opin Pulm Med* 2001; **7**: 255–61.

126  Dent M, Jacobs JA, Cobben NA et al. Computer program supporting the diagnostic accuracy of cellular BALF analysis: a new release. *Respir Med* 2001; **95**: 781–6.

◆127  Costabel U. Sarcoidosis: clinical update. *Eur Respir J Suppl* 2001; **32**: 56s–68s.

●128  Costabel U. CD4/CD8 ratios in bronchoalveolar lavage fluid: of value for diagnosing sarcoidosis? *Eur Respir J* 1997; **10**: 2699–700.

129  Baughman RP, Drent M. Role of bronchoalveolar lavage in interstitial lung disease. *Clin Chest Med* 2001; **22**: 331–41.

130  Winterbauer RH, Lammert J, Selland M et al. Bronchoalveolar lavage cell populations in the diagnosis of sarcoidosis. *Chest* 1993; **104**: 352–61.

131  Drent M, Jacobs JA, De Vries J et al. Does the cellular bronchoalveolar lavage fluid profile reflect the severity of sarcoidosis? *Eur Respir J* 1999; **13**: 1338–44.

●132  Koonitz CH, Joyner LR, Nelson RA. Transbronchial lung biopsy via the fiberoptic bronchoscope in sarcoidosis. *Ann Intern Med* 1976; **85**: 64–6.

●133  Roethe RA, Fuller PB, Byrd RB, Hafermann DR. Transbronchoscopic lung biopsy in sarcoidosis. Optimal number and sites for diagnosis. *Chest* 1980; **77**: 400–2.

●134  Gilman MJ, Wang KP. Transbronchial lung biopsy in sarcoidosis. An approach to determine the optimal number of biopsies. *Am Rev Respir Dis* 1980; **122**: 721–4.

135  Descombes E, Gardiol D, Leuenberger P. Transbronchial lung biopsy: an analysis of 530 cases with reference to the number of samples. *Monaldi Arch Chest Dis* 1997; **52**: 324–9.

136  Torrington KG, Shorr AF, Parker JW. Endobronchial disease and racial differences in pulmonary sarcoidosis. *Chest* 1997; **111**: 619–22.

137  Armstrong JR, Radke JR, Kvale PA et al. Endoscopic findings in sarcoidosis. Characteristics and correlations with radiographic staging and bronchial mucosal biopsy yield. *Ann Otol Rhinol Laryngol* 1981; **90**: 339–43.

138  Gupta D, Mahendran C, Aggarwal AN et al. Endobronchial vis a vis transbronchial involvement on fiberoptic bronchoscopy

in sarcoidosis. *Sarcoidosis Vasc Diffuse Lung Dis* 2001; **18**: 91–2.

139 Shorr AF, Torrington KG, Hnatiuk OW. Endobronchial biopsy for sarcoidosis: a prospective study. *Chest* 2001; **120**: 109–14.

140 Chapman JT, Mehta AC. Bronchoscopy in sarcoidosis: diagnostic and therapeutic interventions. *Curr Opin Pulm Med* 2003; **9**: 402–7.

141 Mihailovic-Vucinic V, Zugic V, Videnovic-Ivanov J. New observations on pulmonary function changes in sarcoidosis. *Curr Opin Pulm Med* 2003; **9**: 436–41.

142 Winterbauer RH, Hutchinson JF. Use of pulmonary function tests in the management of sarcoidosis. *Chest* 1980; **78**: 640–7.

143 Sharma OP, Johnson R. Airway obstruction in sarcoidosis. A study of 123 nonsmoking black American patients with sarcoidosis. *Chest* 1988; **94**: 343–6.

144 Harrison BD, Shaylor JM, Stokes TC, Wilkes AR. Airflow limitation in sarcoidosis – a study of pulmonary function in 107 patients with newly diagnosed disease. *Respir Med* 1991; **85**: 59–64.

●145 Marschke R. Sarcoidosis and malignant neoplasm: the Mayo Clinic experience. *Sarcoidosis* 1986; 3: 149–50.

146 Askling J, Grunewald J, Eklund A et al. Increased risk for cancer following sarcoidosis. *Am J Respir Crit Care Med* 1999; **160**: 1668–72.

147 Romer FK, Hommelgaard P, Schou G. Sarcoidosis and cancer revisited: a long-term follow-up study of 555 Danish sarcoidosis patients. *Eur Respir J* 1998; **12**: 906–12.

148 Seersholm N, Vestbo J, Viskum K. Risk of malignant neoplasms in patients with pulmonary sarcoidosis. *Thorax* 1997; **52**: 892–4.

149 Neville E, Walker AN, James DG. Prognostic factors predicting the outcome of sarcoidosis: an analysis of 818 patients. *Q J Med* 1983; **52**: 525–33.

150 Gibson GJ, Prescott RJ, Muers MF et al. British Thoracic Society Sarcoidosis study: effects of long term corticosteroid treatment. *Thorax* 1996; **51**: 238–47.

151 Winterbauer RH, Kirtland SH, Corley DE. Treatment with corticosteroids. *Clin Chest Med* 1997; **18**: 843–51.

●152 Judson MA. An approach to the treatment of pulmonary sarcoidosis with corticosteroids: the six phases of treatment. *Chest* 1999; **115**: 1158–65.

●153 Baughman RP, Winget DB, Lower EE. Methotrexate is steroid sparing in acute sarcoidosis: results of a double blind, randomized trial. *Sarcoidosis Vasc Diffuse Lung Dis* 2000; **17**: 60–66.

154 Pacheco Y, Marechal C, Marechal F et al. Azathioprine treatment of chronic pulmonary sarcoidosis. *Sarcoidosis* 1985; **2**: 107–13.

155 Lewis SJ, Ainslie GM, Bateman ED. Efficacy of azathioprine as second-line treatment in pulmonary sarcoidosis. *Sarcoidosis Vasc Diffuse Lung Dis* 1999; **16**: 87–92.

156 Adams JS, Diz MM, Sharma OP. Effective reduction in the serum 1,25-dihydroxyvitamin D and calcium concentration in sarcoidosis-associated hypercalcemia with short-course chloroquine therapy. *Ann Intern Med* 1989; **111**: 437–8.

●157 Siltzbach LE, Teirstein AS. Chloroquine therapy in 43 patients with intrathoracic and cutaneous sarcoidosis. *Acta Med Scand Suppl* 1964; **425**: 302–8.

158 Carlesimo M, Giustini S, Rossi A et al. Treatment of cutaneous and pulmonary sarcoidosis with thalidomide. *J Am Acad Dermatol* 1995; **32** (5 Pt 2): 866–9.

159 Lee JB, Koblenzer PS. Disfiguring cutaneous manifestation of sarcoidosis treated with thalidomide: a case report. *J Am Acad Dermatol* 1998; **39**: 835–8.

160 Rousseau L, Beylot-Barry M, Doutre MS, Beylot C. Cutaneous sarcoidosis successfully treated with low doses of thalidomide. *Arch Dermatol* 1998; **134**: 1045–6.

161 Agbogu BN, Stern BJ, Sewell C, Yang G. Therapeutic considerations in patients with refractory neurosarcoidosis. *Arch Neurol* 1995; **52**: 875–9.

162 Demeter SL. Myocardial sarcoidosis unresponsive to steroids. Treatment with cyclophosphamide. *Chest* 1988; **94**: 202–3.

163 Pia G, Pascalis L, Aresu G et al. Evaluation of the efficacy and toxicity of the cyclosporine A-flucortolone-methotrexate combination in the treatment of sarcoidosis. *Sarcoidosis Vasc Diffuse Lung Dis* 1996; **13**: 146–52.

164 Wyser CP, van Schalkwyk EM, Alheit B et al. Treatment of progressive pulmonary sarcoidosis with cyclosporin A. A randomized controlled trial. *Am J Respir Crit Care Med* 1997; **156**: 1371–6.

●165 Utz JP, Limper AH, Kalra S et al. Etanercept for the treatment of stage II and III progressive pulmonary sarcoidosis. *Chest* 2003; **124**: 177–85.

●166 Baughman RP, Lower EE. Infliximab for refractory sarcoidosis. *Sarcoidosis Vasc Diffuse Lung Dis* 2001; **18**: 70–4.

●167 Yee AM, Pochapin MB. Treatment of complicated sarcoidosis with infliximab anti-tumor necrosis factor-alpha therapy. *Ann Intern Med* 2001; **135**: 27–31.

168 Keane J, Gershon S, Wise RP et al. Tuberculosis associated with infliximab, a tumor necrosis factor alpha-neutralizing agent. *N Engl J Med* 2001; **345**: 1098–104.

169 Marques LJ, Zheng L, Poulakis N et al. Pentoxifylline inhibits TNF-alpha production from human alveolar macrophages. *Am J Respir Crit Care Med* 1999; **159**: 508–11.

●170 Schurmann M, Lympany P, Reichel P et al. Familial sarcoidosis is linked to the major histocompatibility complex region. *Am J Respir Crit Care Med* 2000; **162**: 861–4.

●171 Schurmann M, Reichel P, Muller-Myhsok B et al. Results from a genome-wide search for predisposing genes in sarcoidosis. *Am J Respir Crit Care Med* 2001; **164**: 840–6.

172 Kueppers F, Mueller-Eckhardt C, Heinrich D et al. HL-A antigens of patients with sarcoidosis. *Tissue Antigens* 1974; **4**: 56–8.

173 Brewerton D, Cockburn C, James D et al. HLA antigens in sarcoidosis. *Clin Exp Immunol* 1977; **27**: 227–9.

174 Olenchock S, Heise E, Marz J et al. HLA-B8 in sarcoidosis. *Ann Allergy* 1981; **47**: 151–3.

175 Lenhart K, Kolek V, Bartova A. HLA antigens associated with sarcoidosis. *Dis Markers* 1990; **8**: 23–9.

176 Eisenberg H, Terasaki P, Sharma O, Mickey M. HLA association studies in black sarcoidosis patients. *Tissue Antigens* 1978; **11**: 484–6.

177 Smith M, Turton C, Mitchell D et al. Association of HLA-B8 with spontaneous resolution in sarcoidosis. *Thorax* 1981; **36**: 296–8.

178 Martinetti M, Tinelli C, Kolek V et al. 'The Sarcoidosis Map': a joint survey of clinical and immunogenetic findings in two European countries. *Am J Respir Crit Care Med* 1995; **152**: 557–64.

179 Ina Y, Takada K, Yamamoto M et al. HLA and sarcoidosis in the Japanese. *Chest* 1989; **95**: 1257–61.

180 McIntyre J, McKee K, Loadholt C et al. Increased HLA-B7 antigen frequency in South Carolina blacks in association with sarcoidosis. *Transplant Proc* 1977; **9**: 173–6.

181 Grunewald J, Eklund A, Olerup O. Human leukocyte antigen class I alleles and the disease course in sarcoidosis patients. *Am J Respir Crit Care Med* 2003 (Epub).

182 Ishihara M, Inoko H, Suzuki K et al. HLA class II genotyping of sarcoidosis patients in Hokkaido by PCR-RFLP. *Jpn J Ophthalmol* 1996; **40**: 540–3.

183 Ishihara M, Ishida T, Inoko H et al. HLA serological and class II genotyping in sarcoidosis patients in Japan. *Jpn J Ophthalmol* 1996; **40**: 86–94.

184 Nowack D, Goebel KM. Genetic aspects of sarcoidosis. Class II histocompatibility antigens and a family study. *Arch Intern Med* 1987; **147**: 481–3.

●185 Swider C, Schnittger L, Bogunia-Kubik K et al. TNF-alpha and HLA-DR genotyping as potential prognostic markers in pulmonary sarcoidosis. *Eur Cytokine Netw* 1999; **10**: 143–6.

186 Berlin M, Fogdell-Hahn A, Olerup O et al. HLA-DR predicts the prognosis in Scandinavian patients with pulmonary sarcoidosis. *Am J Respir Crit Care Med* 1997; **156**: 1601–5.

187 Sharma SK, Balamurugan A, Pandey RM et al. Human leukocyte antigen-DR alleles influence the clinical course of pulmonary sarcoidosis in Asian Indians. *Am J Respir Cell Mol Biol* 2003; **29**: 225–31.

●188 Foley P, McGrath D, Petrek M et al. HLA-DRB1 position 11 residues are a common protective marker for sarcoidosis. *Am J Respir Crit Care Med* 2001; **25**: 272–7.

●189 Rossman MD, Thompson B, Frederick M et al. HLA-DRB1*1101: a significant risk factor for sarcoidosis in blacks and whites. *Am J Hum Genet* 2003; **73**: 720–35.

190 Foley PJ, Lympany P, Puscinska E et al. HLA-DPB1 and TAP1 polymorphisms in sarcoidosis. *Chest* 1997; **111**: 73S.

191 Maliarik MJ, Chen KM, Major ML et al. Analysis of HLA-DPB1 polymorphisms in African-Americans with sarcoidosis. *Am J Respir Crit Care Med* 1998; **158**: 111–4.

192 Rybicki BA, Maliarik MJ, Poisson LM et al. The major histocompatibility complex gene region and sarcoidosis susceptibility in African Americans. *Am J Respir Crit Care Med* 2003; **167**: 444–9.

193 Iannuzzi MC, Maliarik MJ, Poisson LM, Rybicki BA. Sarcoidosis susceptibility and resistance HLA-DQB1 alleles in African Americans. *Am J Respir Crit Care Med* 2003; **167**: 1225–31.

●194 Sato H, Grutters JC, Pantelidis P et al. HLA-DQB1*0201: a marker for good prognosis in British and Dutch patients with sarcoidosis. *Am J Respir Cell Mol Biol* 2002; **27**: 406–12.

●195 Grutters JC, Ruven HJT, Sato H et al. MHC haplotype analysis in Dutch sarcoidosis patients presenting with Lofgren's syndrome. In: Grutters JC (ed.) *Genetic polymorphisms and phenotypes in sarcoidosis.* Utrecht: University Utrecht, 2003: 85–96 (thesis).

196 Takashige N, Naruse TK, Matsumori A et al. Genetic polymorphisms at the tumour necrosis factor loci (TNFA and TNFB) in cardiac sarcoidosis. *Tissue Antigens* 1999; **54**: 191–3.

197 Naruse TK, Matsuzawa Y, Ota M et al. HLA-DQB1*0601 is primarily associated with the susceptibility to cardiac sarcoidosis. *Tissue Antigens* 2000; **56**: 52–7.

198 Grunewald J, Janson C, Eklund A et al. Restricted V alpha 2.3 gene usage by CD4$^+$ T lymphocytes in bronchoalveolar lavage fluid from sarcoidosis patients correlates with HLA-DR3. *Eur J Immunol* 1992; **22**: 129–35.

199 Luisetti M, Beretta A, Casali L. Genetic aspects in sarcoidosis. *Eur Respir J* 2000; **16**: 768–80.

200 Somoskovi A, Zissel G, Seitzer U et al. Polymorphisms at position − 308 in the promoter region of the TNF-alpha and in the first intron of the TNF-beta genes and spontaneous and lipopolysaccharide-induced TNF-alpha release in sarcoidosis. *Cytokine* 1999; **11**: 882–7.

●201 Seitzer U, Swider C, Stuber F et al. Tumour necrosis factor alpha promoter gene polymorphism in sarcoidosis. *Cytokine* 1997; **9**: 787–90.

202 Yamaguchi E, Itoh A, Hizawa N, Kawakami Y. The gene polymorphism of tumor necrosis factor-beta, but not that of tumor necrosis factor-alpha, is associated with the prognosis of sarcoidosis. *Chest* 2001; **119**: 753–61.

●203 Grutters JC, Sato H, Pantelidis P et al. Increased frequency of the uncommon tumor necrosis factor −857T allele in British and Dutch patients with sarcoidosis. *Am J Respir Crit Care Med* 2002; **165**: 1119–24.

204 Grutters JC, Ruven HJT, Sato H et al. TNF promoter haplotypes associate with clinical phenotypes and prognosis in sarcoidosis. In: Grutters JC (ed.) *Genetic polymorphisms and phenotypes in sarcoidosis.* Utrecht: University Utrecht, 2003: 49–66 (thesis).

205 Rybicki B, Maliarik M, Malvitz E et al. The influence of T cell receptor and cytokine genes on sarcoidosis susceptibility in African Americans. *Hum Immunol* 1999; **60**: 867–74.

206 Hutyrova B, Pantelidis P, Drabek J et al. Interleukin-1 gene cluster polymorphisms in sarcoidosis and idiopathic pulmonary fibrosis. *Am J Respir Crit Care Med* 2002; **165**: 148–51.

207 Grutters JC, Sato H, Pantelidis P et al. Analysis of IL6 and IL1A gene polymorphisms in UK and Dutch patients with sarcoidosis. *Sarcoidosis Vasc Diffuse Lung Dis* 2003; **20**: 20–7.

208 Takada T, Suzuki E, Morohash K, Gejyo F. Association of single nucleotide polymorphisms in the IL-18 gene with sarcoidosis in a Japanese population. *Tissue Antigens* 2002; **60**: 36–42.

209 Amoli MM, Donn RP, Thomson W et al. Macrophage migration inhibitory factor gene polymorphism is associated with sarcoidosis in biopsy proven erythema nodosum. *J Rheumatol* 2002; **29**: 1671–3.

210 Abdallah A, Sato H, Grutters JC et al. Inhibitor kappa B-alpha (IkappaB-alpha) promoter polymorphisms in UK and Dutch sarcoidosis. *Genes Immunol* 2003; **4**: 450–4.

211 Hizawa N, Yamaguchi E, Furuya K et al. The role of the C-C chemokine receptor 2 gene polymorphism V64I (CCR2-64I) in sarcoidosis in a Japanese population. *Am J Respir Crit Care Med* 1999; **159**: 2021–3.

212 Petrek M, Drabek J, Kolek V et al. CC chemokine receptor gene polymorphisms in Czech patients with pulmonary sarcoidosis. *Am J Respir Crit Care Med* 2000; **162**: 1000–3.

●213 Spagnolo P, Renzoni EA, Wells AU et al. C-C chemokine receptor 2 and sarcoidosis: association with Lofgren's syndrome. *Am J Respir Crit Care Med* 2003; **168**: 1162–6.

214 Takada T, Suzuki E, Ishida T et al. Polymorphism in RANTES chemokine promoter affects extent of sarcoidosis in a Japanese population. *Tissue Antigens* 2001; **58**: 293–8.

215 Foley P, Mullighan C, McGrath D et al. Mannose-binding lectin promoter and structural gene variants in sarcoidosis. *Eur J Clin Invest* 2000; **30**: 549–52.

216   Fraser D. Vitamin D. *Lancet* 1995; **345**: 104–7.

217   Braun J, Dinkelacker C, Bohnet S et al. 1,25-dihydroxy-cholecalciferol stimulates ICAM-1 expression of human alveolar macrophages in healthy controls and patients with sarcoidosis. *Lung* 1999; **177**: 139–49.

218   Niimi T, Tomita H, Sato S et al. Vitamin D receptor gene polymorphism in patients with sarcoidosis. *Am J Respir Crit Care Med* 1999; **160**: 1107–9.

219   Vidal S, Malo D, Vogan K et al. Natural resistance to infection with intracellular parasites: isolation of a candidate for Bcg. *Cell* 1993; **73**: 469–85.

220   Malo D, Vogan K, Vidal S et al. Haplotype mapping and sequence analysis of the mouse Nramp gene predict susceptibility to infection with intracellular parasites. *Genomics* 1994; **23**: 51–61.

221   Vidal S, Tremblay M, Govoni G et al. The Ity/Lsh/Bcg locus: natural resistance to infection with intracellular parasites is abrogated by disruption of the Nramp1 gene. *J Exp Med* 1995; **182**: 655–66.

222   Govoni G, Vidal S, Gauthier S et al. The Bcg/Ity/Lsh locus: genetic transfer of resistance to infections in C57BL/6J mice transgenic for the Nramp1$^{Gly169}$ allele. *Infect Immun* 1996; **64**: 2923–9.

223   Cellier M, Govoni G, Vidal S et al. Human natural resistance-associated macrophage protein: cDNA cloning, chromosomal mapping, genomic organisation, and tissue-specific expresson. *J Exp Med* 1994; **180**: 1741–52.

224   Blackwell J, Barton C, White J et al. Genomic organisation and sequence of the human NRAMP gene: identification and mapping of a promoter region polymorphism. *Mol Med* 1995; **1**: 194–205.

225   Gunshin H, Mackenzie B, Berger UV et al. Cloning and characterisation of a mammalian proton-coupled metal-ion transporter. *Nature* 1997; **388**: 482–8.

226   Gruenheid S, Pinner E, Desjardins M et al. Natural resistance to infection with intracellular pathogens: the Nramp 1 protein is recruited to the membrane of the phagosome. *J Exp Med* 1997; **185**: 717–30.

227   Bellamy R, Ruwende C, Corrah T et al. Variations in the *NRAMP1* gene and susceptibility to tuberculosis in West Africans. *New Engl J Med* 1998; **338**: 640–4.

228   Maliarik MJ, Chen KM, Sheffer RG et al. The natural resistance-associated macrophage protein gene in African Americans with sarcoidosis. *Am J Respir Cell Mol Biol* 2000; **22**: 672–5.

229   Kelly A, Powis SH, Kerr LA et al. Assembly and function of the two ABC transporter proteins encoded in the human major histocompatibility complex. *Nature* 1992; **335**: 641–4.

230   Foley PJ, Lympany PA, Puscinska E et al. Analysis of MHC encoded antigen-processing genes TAP1 and TAP2 polymorphisms in sarcoidosis. *Am J Respir Crit Care Med* 1999; **160**: 1009–14.

231   Ishihara M, Ohno S, Mizuki N et al. Genetic polymorphisms of the major histocompatibility complex-encoded antigen-processing genes TAP and LMP in sarcoidosis. *Hum Immunol* 1996; **45**: 105–10.

232   Zorzetto M, Bombieri C, Ferrarotti I et al. Complement receptor 1 gene polymorphisms in sarcoidosis. *Am J Respir Cell Mol Biol* 2002; **27**: 17–23.

233   Arbustini E, Grasso M, Leo G et al. Polymorphism of angiotensin-converting enzyme gene in sarcoidosis. *Am J Respir Crit Care Med* 1996; **153**: 851–4.

◆234   McGrath DS, Foley PJ, Petrek M et al. Ace gene I/D polymorphism and sarcoidosis pulmonary disease severity. *Am J Respir Crit Care Med* 2001; **164**: 197–201.

235   Maliarik MJ, Rybicki BA, Malvitz E et al. Angiotensin-converting enzyme gene polymorphism and risk of sarcoidosis. *Am J Respir Crit Care Med* 1998; **158**: 1566–70.

236   Bombieri C, Benetazzo M, Saccomani A et al. Complete mutational screening of the CFTR gene in 120 patients with pulmonary disease. *Hum Genet* 1998; **103**: 718–22.

237   Bombieri C, Luisetti M, Belpinati F et al. Increased frequency of CFTR gene mutations in sarcoidosis: a case/control association study. *Eur J Hum Genet* 2000; **8**: 717–20.

238   Schurmann M, Albrecht M, Schwinger E, Stuhrmann M. CFTR gene mutations in sarcoidosis. *Eur J Hum Genet* 2002; **10**: 729–32.

239   Stradecker M. The development of granulomas in schistosomiasis: genetic backgrounds, regulatory pathways, and specific egg antigen responses that influence the magnitude of disease. *Microbes Infect* 1999; **1**: 505–10.

240   Teirstein AS. Kveim antigen: what does it tell us about causation of sarcoidosis? *Semin Respir Infect* 1998; **13**: 206–11.

241   Aronchick J, Rossman M, Miller W. Chronic beryllium disease: diagnosis, radiographic findings, and correlation with pulmonary function tests. *Radiology* 1987; **163**: 677–82.

●242   Saltini C, Winestock K, Kirby M et al. Maintenance of alveolitis in patients with chronic beryllium disease by beryllium-specific helper T cells. *New Engl J Med* 1989; **320**: 1103–9.

●243   Lombardi G, Germain C, Uren J et al. HLA-DP allele-specific T cell responses to beryllium account for DP-associated susceptibility to chronic beryllium disease. *J Immunol* 2001; **166**: 3549–55.

244   Tinkle S, Kittle L, Schumacher B et al. Beryllium induces IL-2 and IFN-gamma in berylliosis. *J Immunol* 1997; **158**: 518–26.

245   Fontenot A, Falta M, Freed B et al. Identification of pathogenic T cells in patients with beryllium-induced lung disease. *J Immunol* 1999; **163**: 1019–26.

246   Rossman M, Yang H-C, Murray R et al. Chronic beryllium disease: an immune response by restricted families of T cells. *Am Rev Respir Dis* 1992; **145**: A415.

◆247   Saltini C, Amicosante M, Franchi A et al. Immunogenetic basis of environmental lung disease: lessons from the berylliosis model. *Eur Respir J* 1998; **12**: 1463–75.

●248   Richeldi L, Sorrentino R, Saltini C. HLA-DPB1 glutamate 69: a marker of beryllium disease. *Science* 1993; **262**: 242–4.

249   Stubbs J, Argyris E, Lee C et al. Genetic markers in beryllium hypersensitivity. *Chest* 1996; **109**: 45s.

250   Richeldi L, Kreiss K, Mroz M et al. Interaction of genetic and exposure factors in the prevalence of berylliosis. *Am J Ind Med* 1997; **32**: 337–40.

251   Wang Z, White P, Petrovic M et al. Differential susceptibilities to chronic beryllium disease contributed by different Glu69 HLA-DPB1 and -DPA1 alleles. *J Immunol* 1999; **163**: 1647–53.

252   Amicosante M, Sanarico N, Berretta F et al. Beryllium binding to HLA-DP molecule carrying the marker of susceptibility to

berylliosis glutamate beta 69. *Hum Immunol* 2001; **62**: 686–93.

253 Saltini C, Richeldi L, Losi M et al. Major histocompatibility locus genetic markers of beryllium sensitisation and disease. *Eur Respir J* 2001; **18**: 677–84.

254 Maier L, Sawyer R, Bauer R et al. High beryllium-stimulated TNF-α is associated with the −308 TNF-α promoter polymorphism and with clinical severity in chronic beryllium disease. *Am J Respir Crit Care Med* 2001; **164**: 1192–9.

255 Chee M, Yang R, Hubbell E et al. Accessing genetic information with high-density DNA arrays. *Science* 1996; **274**: 610–4.

256 Meltzer P. Spotting the target: microarrays for disease gene discovery. *Curr Opin Genet Dev* 2001; **11**: 258–63.

257 Agostini C, Miorin M, Semenzato G. Gene expression profile analysis by DNA microarrays: a new approach to assess functional genomics in diseases. *Sarcoidosis Vasc Diffuse Lung Dis* 2002; **19**: 5–9.

258 Rutherford RM, Kehren J, Staedtler F et al. Functional genomics in sarcoidosis – reduced or increased apoptosis? *Swiss Med Wkly* 2001; **131**: 459–70.

259 Thonhofer R, Maercker C, Popper HH. Expression of sarcoidosis related genes in lung lavage cells. *Sarcoidosis Vasc Diffuse Lung Dis* 2002; **19**: 59–65.

PART **4**

# Miscellaneous pulmonary conditions

# 14

# Pulmonary hypertension

JAMES E. LOYD, JOHN H. NEWMAN, AND JOHN A. PHILLIPS III

## CLINICAL BACKGROUND

### Introduction

This chapter will concentrate on heritable forms of pulmonary hypertension, especially primary pulmonary hypertension (PPH). PPH is synonymous with the newly designated descriptor, idiopathic pulmonary arterial hypertension (IPAH), which has recently been adopted by a consensus conference of the WHO.[1,2] PPH can be sporadic or familial in presentation and these two disorders are clinically and histologically indistinguishable.[3,4] Familial primary pulmonary hypertension (FPPH) is linked to mutations in the bone morphogenetic protein receptor type 2 (BMPR2), which is a member of the TGFbeta superfamily of receptors.[5–8] Another less common hereditary predisposition to PPH occurs in some people with hereditary hemorrhagic telangiectasia (Osler–Weber–Rendu syndrome) where mutations in the gene encoding the activin-like kinase receptor (ACVRL1, or Alk-1) increase susceptibility to the development of PPH.[7] Like BMPR2, Alk-1 is a member of the TGFbeta superfamily of receptors;[9] insight into the pathogenesis of PPH should emerge from studies of the alterations in signal transduction of these genetically altered receptors, hopefully leading to therapies effective in reversal and perhaps prevention of this disease.[10,11]

The mean age at diagnosis of PPH in the 1987 NIH registry report was 36 ± 15 years with an approximate 2:1 female preponderance.[12] Age at diagnosis in PPH ranges from infancy to >80 years. Familial and sporadic forms have similar age and gender features. Mean age at death in FPPH was 33 ± 15 years. About 6 percent of all patients diagnosed with PPH are in families with two or more affected persons. When apparently sporadic PPH patients have been evaluated for BMPR2 mutations, the prevalence has been reported to be between 10 and 26 percent.[13] Some of these BMPR2 mutations appear to be new to the patient, referred to as de novo, and others have been found to be inherited, but without expression in other family members. Thus, the definition of sporadic versus familial PPH becomes uncertain unless the Alk-1 and BMPR2 status of the proband and parents is known. The true prevalence of TGFbeta family mutations in a large population of patients with PPH remains to be determined.

Other etiologies of pulmonary hypertension include mutations in genes primarily related to nonvascular function, such as inherited hypercoagulable states, hemoglobinopathies, ventilatory disorders, and lipid storage disease (Gaucher's disease). In addition, it seems likely that functional polymorphisms in genes that transcribe products that affect circulatory function will influence the onset and severity of pulmonary hypertension, both in primary and secondary disease. The search for these modifying genes is in its infancy.

### Clinical physiology of pulmonary hypertension

In order to understand the pathogenesis and clinical features of pulmonary hypertension, consideration of the genesis of pulmonary vascular pressures is warranted. Pulmonary hypertension is the presence of an elevated blood pressure in the lung circulation.[14] As such, it is a sign rather than a disease. Many situations, conditions, and diseases can cause pulmonary hypertension.[15] Pressure in the pulmonary circulation is generated by three related variables: blood flow, vascular resistance, and downstream pressure. Blood flow in the lung is normally the same as the cardiac output (CO), about 5 L/min at rest in normal adult man. The CO can rise to as high as 20–25 L/min during exhaustive exercise, and may be as high as 10 L/min at rest in high output states, such as cirrhosis or sepsis. Vascular resistance in the lung is normally quite low, almost 10-fold lower than that of the systemic circulation, about 1–2 Wood units at rest, and drops even lower during the vascular dilation that occurs with increased cardiac output. Downstream pressure is the emptying pressure of the lung, which is determined by the left atrial pressure ($Pla$), but is usually measured by the pulmonary arterial occlusion (wedge) pressure. The pulmonary arterial wedge pressure ($Pwedge$) is usually a few mmHg higher than the left atrial pressure. In normal man at rest, the mean pulmonary arterial pressure ($Ppa$) is about 15 mmHg, with systolic and diastolic pressures of 20 and 10 mmHg, the $Pw$ is about 5 mmHg and the cardiac output is 5 L/min. The calculated pulmonary vascular resistance (PVR) is ($Ppa$ − $Pwedge$)/CO, about 2 Wood units, or 160 dynes. This is in comparison to the systemic vascular resistance, which is normally about 1600 dynes.[16]

Consideration of the three components of pulmonary vascular pressure reveals the major mechanisms of pulmonary hypertension. The most common cause of pulmonary hypertension is left heart dysfunction.[14–16] In this situation, elevations in the left ventricular diastolic pressure or in left atrial pressure cause a passive rise in $Pwedge$, which increases the upstream pressure. The most common causes of passive pulmonary hypertension are overt left ventricular failure, diastolic dysfunction, and mitral valve stenosis or regurgitation, see Table 14.1. The mean pulmonary capillary pressure ($Pw$) is calculated as the $Pla$ + 0.4 ($Ppa$ − $Pla$). Thus, any rise in left-sided pressures, reflected in $Pw$, causes a simultaneous and similar rise in $Ppa$. Some people have an exaggerated pulmonary vascular response to back pressure, which induces pulmonary vasoconstriction and can result in persistent pulmonary hypertension even after resolution of the left-sided downstream hypertension.[17,18] The second component of pulmonary vascular pressure, flow, is not a frequent cause of pulmonary hypertension. The most common cause of mild pulmonary hypertension due to increased flow is liver disease, in which the cardiac output at rest may be double normal values.[19,20] Paget's disease, Beriberi, pheochromocytoma, and systemic arterio-venous shunts also cause high resting cardiac output and can also be associated with left ventricular failure.[21]

The third determinant of pulmonary vascular pressure is vascular resistance. Elevated vascular resistance is the major abnormality in most diseases where pulmonary

**Table 14.1**  *Mechanisms of pulmonary hypertension*

**Mechanisms**

*Alveolar hypoxia leading to hypoxic pulmonary vasoconstriction*
Chronic bronchitis and emphysema, cystic fibrosis
High-altitude dwelling and chronic mountain sickness (Monge's disease)
Chronic hypoventilation syndromes
  Obesity-hypoventilation
  Sleep apnea
  Neuromuscular diseases and post-polio syndrome
  Mechanical dysfunction of the chest wall (kyphoscoliosis)

*Obstruction of the pulmonary circulation*
Pulmonary arterial hypertension (PAH)
  Primary pulmonary hypertension (idiopathic PAH)
  Scleroderma spectrum of disease and lupus erythematosus
  Porto-pulmonary hypertension
  Related to HIV infection
Acute pulmonary thromboembolism
Chronic thrombotic pulmonary hypertension
Congenital heart disease (especially atrial septal defect)
Tumor emboli, parasitic ova, i.v. injection of foreign particles
Pulmonary veno-occlusive disease (PVOD)/pulmonary capillary hemangiomatosis
Sickle cell disease/sickle crisis/marrow embolism
Fibrosing mediastinitis, mediastinal tumor
Drug-induced lung disease (cocaine, tryptophan, toxic oil, fenfluramine)
Gaucher's disease
POEMS syndrome and amyloidosis
?Splenectomy
Hyper-reactive pulmonary vascular bed
Congenital platelet storage disease

*Vascular destruction due to parenchymal disease*
Bullous emphysema, alpha-1 antitrypsin deficiency
Diffuse bronchiectasis, cystic fibrosis
Diffuse interstitial diseases
Pneumoconiosis
Sarcoid, idiopathic pulmonary fibrosis
Langerhan's cell histiocytosis
Necrotising tuberculosis and chronic fungal infection
Collagen vascular disease (autoimmune lung disease)
Hypersensitivity pneumonitis

*Secondary to left heart dysfunction*
Left ventricular systolic failure
Left ventricular diastolic hypertension
Mitral stenosis or regurgitation
Pulmonary vascular hyper-reactivity to downstream pressure

hypertension is clinically significant. Pulmonary vascular resistance is an inverse function of cross-sectional area of the vascular bed. Increased resistance is usually due to pulmonary arterial vasoconstriction, or to obstruction of the vascular lumen by thromboembolism, obliterative vascular disease, or parenchymal destruction. Table 14.1 lists the diseases and conditions leading to pulmonary hypertension by mechanism of action, omitting conditions of the left heart.

The right ventricle is thin walled and asymmetric compared to the left ventricle, and is not normally exposed to high resistance. In situations of abrupt increases in PVR, leading to mean Ppa of greater than 40 mmHg, the RV dilates and becomes dysfunctional.[22,23] With chronic pulmonary hypertension, the RV is able to undergo hypertrophy and sustain mean pressures of greater than 60 mmHg for months to years, but ultimately dilates and fails, leading to reduced cardiac output and the signs and symptoms typical of clinical pulmonary hypertension. Traditionally, right heart failure due to lung disease is called cor pulmonale.[24]

## Clinical characteristics of PPH and diagnosis

The term, pulmonary arterial hypertension (PAH), has become the umbrella term for diseases that originate upstream of the pulmonary capillaries.[2] In practice, PPH is reserved for patients with the clinical diagnosis of pulmonary hypertension with all known etiologies excluded. The term PAH is used for diseases such as porto-pulmonary hypertension, HIV, and scleroderma-related pulmonary hypertension. The terms PPH and FPPH are likely to remain in common usage when no other etiology is found for the presentation of severe pulmonary hypertension.

The diagnosis of PPH requires a stepwise evaluation to establish the hemodynamic profile of the patient and to exclude other causes.[3,10] Because there is no diagnostic blood test and because lung biopsy is hazardous, this is a diagnosis that can be made with high accuracy only by careful exclusion of other causes of pulmonary hypertension. By the time affected people with PPH are symptomatic, their pulmonary hypertension is severe, the majority of the vascular bed is obstructed, and cardiac output is decreased. In the 1987 NIH Registry report, pulmonary pressures were: systolic 90 ± 22, diastolic 45 ± 17, mean Ppa 61 ± 21, Pw 9 ± 4 mmHg.[12] Cardiac index was 2.35 L/min/m$^2$, and PVR index 24 ± 11. The most common complaints are dyspnea on mild exertion, chronic loss of energy and easy fatigue, chest pain (perhaps RV ischemia), near fainting or true syncope, edema, cough, and, rarely, hemoptysis. None of these is unique to PPH, but the findings of dyspnea on exertion and loss of energy in an otherwise normal young female should alert a clinician to the possibility of this diagnosis.

The physical findings of PPH are primarily found in the cardiac examination.[1,2,10] Patients usually appear healthy at rest. Blood pressure is usually normal, although mild systemic hypertension is found in some patients, and if PPH is advanced there may be hypotension and resting tachycardia. The lungs are clear to auscultation and percussion. The heart may be hyperdynamic to palpation. On auscultation, S1 is normal but S2 is loud and sharp, and there may be a wide inspiratory split with an accentuated pulmonic component. Occasionally, there is a right ventricular heave with an S4 gallop and the murmur of tricuspid regurgitation. In some cases, we have also heard midsystolic clicks

and the murmur of pulmonic insufficiency. Occasionally, even with severe pulmonary hypertension, the cardiac examination is surprisingly normal, with only sharpening of S2. If right ventricular failure has developed, there may be jugular vein hypertension, variable liver engorgement, leg edema and, if failure is advanced, ascites. There are no peripheral signs of disease except for Raynaud's phenomenon in about 15 percent of patients and acral cyanosis if peripheral perfusion is impaired.

The evaluation of a patient with suspected pulmonary hypertension is summarized in Fig. 14.1. The causes of pulmonary hypertension listed in Table 14.1 can be diagnosed or eliminated by a series of studies. Two-dimensional echocardiography is used to assess pulmonary arterial systolic pressure by Doppler, to evaluate left and right ventricular size and function, to detect mitral valve stenosis or regurgitation, and to look for atrial septal defect.[3,16] Pulmonary function tests (PFT) are used to detect significant obstructive or restrictive disease that would point to a different diagnosis. The PFT in PPH on average reveal a normal TLC and low normal FVC and FEV$_1$ with mild to moderate reduction in DLCO (mean 60–70 percent predicted). Some patients present with marked reduction in DLCO, compatible with large reduction in perfused capillary surface area.[3,12] Complete blood count is usually normal in PPH, but can reveal secondary erythrocytosis related to hypoxemia in hypoventilation syndromes. Blood chemistries can reveal hypoventilation if the $CO_2$ content is elevated. The pursuit of other blood tests, such as serologic markers of collagen vascular disease, HIV viral load, hepatitis antigens and antibodies, anti-phospholipid antibodies,[25] and tests of hypercoagulability rely on an index of suspicion of disease. The chest radiograph usually shows cardiomegaly and enlarged main pulmonary arteries, with normal parenchyma or a rapid tapering of the pulmonary vasculature with paucity of peripheral markings (Fig. 14.2). The electrocardiogram may be nonspecific, but usually shows some evidence of right heart strain with right axis deviation, sharp p waves in lead II, $r > s$ in V1, incomplete or complete right bundle branch block, and sometimes S1, Q3, T3 (Fig. 14.3). The EKG rarely displays all of these features.[26]

Patients presenting with pulmonary hypertension should have radionuclide lung perfusion imaging to detect occult pulmonary embolism and the syndrome of chronic thrombotic pulmonary hypertension. In PPH, the perfusion scan is usually either normal or shows a nonspecific pattern of mottled perfusion, probably related to the multifocal obstructing lesions.[27,28] The presence of two or more segmental or a lobar defect should raise suspicion for chronic thrombotic disease which is diagnosed by pulmonary arteriography.[29–31] High resolution CT scanning with contrast can assist in detecting parenchymal lung diseases and can identify some central thrombi, but does not yet have the resolution or specificity to reliably diagnose chronic thromboembolic disease.[2] Future generations of scanners may provide studies of satisfactory sensitivity and specificity.

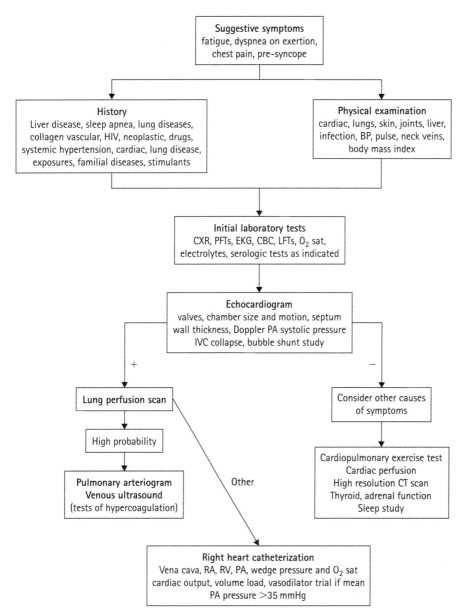

**Figure 14.1** *Algorithm for the diagnosis of pulmonary arterial hypertension (PAH). See text for details. Pulmonary arterial hypertension includes idiopathic PAH (primary pulmonary hypertension, PPH) and PAH resulting from conditions that cause similar pulmonary vascular lesions, pulmonary hypertension, and right heart failure (Table 14.2, page 379). Idiopathic PAH is diagnosed by the exclusion of other important causes of pulmonary hypertension, including chronic thrombotic pulmonary hypertension, congenital heart disease, scleroderma spectrum of disease, liver disease, HIV, and ingestion of anorectic drugs. Finally, noncompliance of the left ventricle should be sought by fluid challenge during right heart catheterization in patients with conditions that predispose to LV disease, especially hypertension.*

Right heart catheterization is important for both diagnostic and therapeutic reasons and should be done by a physician who has experience in the diagnosis of pulmonary hypertension.[2,3,10] Because a defect of the atrial septum may remain occult even after echocardiography, oxygen saturation increments should be sought to identify intracardiac left to right shunts. Pressures should be measured and recorded in all chambers, because RV diastolic and right atrial hypertension have prognostic value and dictate therapeutic urgency. Pulmonary diastolic pressure should be recorded to see what the pressure difference is compared to the measured Pw. A small gradient suggests passive pulmonary hypertension. The wedge pressure should be measured, because back pressure from left-sided dysfunction is still the most common cause of pulmonary hypertension. If the wedge pressure is borderline, above 12 mmHg, an

intravenous volume load of 500–1000 mL saline should be considered to stress LV function. If the Pw rises to >20 mmHg, the problem is likely to be in the left ventricle. All diastolic pressures should be compared to detect pericardial constriction, and x and y descents should be analyzed for four chamber filling abnormalities. CO should be measured by thermal dilution. If a septal defect is discovered, CO should be estimated by the Fick method. The CO may be the most important measure of cardiac function in PPH. Cardiac index of less than 2 L/min/m$^2$ correlates well with decreased functional capacity.[2,3,10,32]

Finally, cardiac catheterization allows testing for the presence of inducible vasodilation.[2,3,10,16] About 10–20 percent of patients with PPH have a significant response to any of a variety of vasodilator stimuli, including calcium blockers, inhaled nitric oxide (NO), sildenafil, adenosine, or

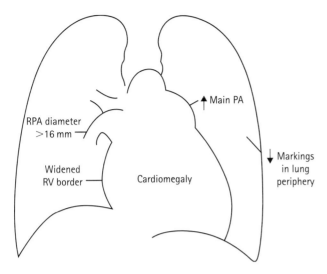

**Figure 14.2** *Schematic of the main findings on chest radiograph in pulmonary arterial hypertension. Findings are cardiomegaly, an RV and RA border that extends to the right of the vertebral column, dilated main PA, right descending PA diameter > 16 mm, and pruning of lung markings in the periphery. These findings are typical of idiopathic PAH. In collagen vascular diseases and HIV, there may be coincident parenchymal and pleural findings. In chronic thrombotic disease, there may be variable perfusion of the peripheral vessels.*

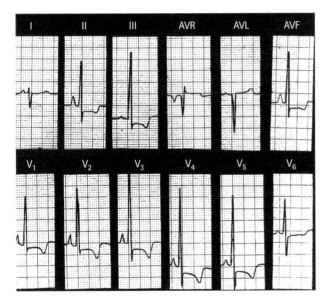

**Figure 14.3** *Electrocardiographic abnormalities in pulmonary hypertension with right heart strain. The electrical axis is rightward. R > S in V1 suggesting RV hypertrophy with increased anterior forces. P waves are large and peaked, denoting 'p' pulmonale. There are diffuse ST–T wave abnormalities that are nonspecific.*

prostacyclins.[2,3,10] Vasodilator testing may improve decisions about the use of oral vasodilators versus initiation of chronic intravenous or subcutaneous therapy. A positive vasodilator trial is empirically defined as a 25 percent decrease in PVR or a 20 percent decrease in Ppa.[2,3,10]

## Treatment and prognosis in PPH

Untreated, PPH has a 50 percent, 3-year survival and is almost always ultimately fatal.[32] No effective therapies were available until the advent of calcium channel blockers in the 1980s. However, only about 10–20 percent of patients have a sustained response to calcium channel blockers, but many patients in this small subset function well for years to decades.[33,34] Intravenous therapy with a prostacyclin formulation, epoprostenol, has markedly improved function and survival in PPH.[35,36] Intravenous epoprostenol must be given by continuous pump infusion through a central vein catheter, is technically demanding, has undesirable side-effects (acute withdrawal syndrome, diarrhea, weight loss, flushing), and costs about $80 000 per year. Although i.v. epoprostenol is the current best therapy for PPH, the 3-year mortality is still about 30 percent.[37] Other delivery systems include chronic subcutaneous,[38] oral,[39] and aerosol prostacyclin[40,41] formulations, but i.v. prostacyclin is currently the best studied and most reliable delivery system. Newer effective drugs include endothelin receptor antagonists[41,42] and phosphodiesterase 5 inhibitors,[43,44] and the search for drugs aimed specifically at pathogenetic abnormalities in PPH is a growing reality, now that some of the signaling mechanisms of PPH are better understood.[2,45]

Double lung transplantation is possible for some patients with end-stage PPH. Approximately 50 PPH patients per year receive lung or heart–lung transplants, out of a total of 1000 lung or heart–lung transplant operations.[46] The problems with transplantation include limited donor availability, difficulty in anticipating the time of decompensation and imminent death, and a poorer outcome than in other diseases treatable with transplantation (emphysema, cystic fibrosis, and interstitial lung disease). Bronchiolitis obliterans results in a 50 percent, 4-year survival after lung transplantation, with a slow linear decline in survival.[47]

## FAMILIAL PRIMARY PULMONARY HYPERTENSION: EVOLVING CONCEPTS

### Descriptions of familial PPH

Dresdale et al.[48] first reported hemodynamic variables and coined the name of the disease known as primary pulmonary hypertension in 1951. Because the disease did not have an accepted name before that report, review of old charts and literature on PPH before 1950 is unsatisfactory. In 1954, the same group reported two cases in a mother and son and suggested there might be a genetic basis.[49] From 1954 to 1983, there were 13 reports in the USA literature of families with two or more members with PPH. There was no consensus about whether there was an inherited form of the disease. In 1984, Loyd et al.[50] contacted 12 of the 13 previously reported families and reported new members in a fourteenth family that had six affected females. In the Vanderbilt Registry, families are listed numerically in order of discovery. There is no national registry and reports from other investigators do not use the Vanderbilt system. It is likely that some families are coreported.

A typical family scenario is shown in Fig. 14.4, showing previously reported patients and newly afflicted members in family 5 from the 1984 report.[50] A number of interesting features of the disease were confirmed or discovered. New cases occurred in about half of the known families, suggesting durability and true heritability of the disease. It was apparent that the disease could skip generations, where the mutation was transmitted through two generations before disease was manifest. Thus, FPPH demonstrates incomplete expression or reduced penetrance. We now know that disease expression occurs in about 20 percent of mutation carriers, although there is a great deal of variability among families and between genders.[51] In one family, disease was clearly transmitted from father to son, demonstrating that the abnormality was on an autosome rather than the X chromosome. Analysis of the age of onset suggested that disease occurred at an earlier age in subsequent generations, raising the possibility of the phenomenon of genetic anticipation. Survival after the onset of symptoms in FPPH was

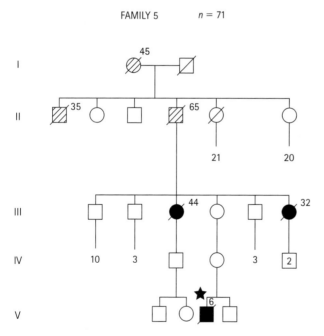

FAMILY 5      n = 71

**Figure 14.4**  *Pedigree of Family 5 of the Vanderbilt FPH Registry.[50] This family demonstrates several features typical of familial primary pulmonary hypertension (FPPH). Roman numerals denote generation. Hatched symbols represent probable PPH, with age at death. Black symbols denote documented PPH. The starred individual was a new case. The grandmother and mother of the 6-year-old in generation V were carriers, showing skipped generations. Without an accurate family pedigree, new cases are likely to be diagnosed as sporadic. There are a large number of people at risk in multiple generations.*

similar to reports in sporadic PPH, suggesting that sporadic and familial PPH had the same clinical manifestations. Finally, most families had no idea that they carried a heritable disease. This is because of geographical dispersion of families, failure to maintain communication, and failure of accurate medical diagnoses. We hypothesized that this disease might have a greater genetic basis than was recognized or expected. A careful, extended family history is crucial to detect the familial basis of this disease. This hypothesis has been confirmed by Elliott et al.[52] and in our own evaluation of BMPR2 mutations in apparently sporadic PPH, where familial disease was confirmed by family pedigree after identical BMPR2 mutations were discovered in several patients.[13]

In 1995, we reported data from 24 families, comprising 429 family members, 129 of whom were known to carry the mutation for PPH. In addition to confirming the gender ratio and penetrance, these data showed a skewed gender ratio at birth.[51] More females, 160, than males, 122, were born to people carrying the mutation. This observation suggests male fetal wastage or other alteration of the normal sex ratio. It is known that BMPR2 knockout mice are nonviable in embryo, but gender differences have not been investigated. The data also extended observations on the possibility of genetic anticipation.

## Genetic anticipation – an unresolved observation

Genetic anticipation is the phenomenon of younger age of onset, or greater penetrance or severity in subsequent generations in a heritable disease. It appears to be present in FPPH.[50,51] Until recently the sole molecular mechanism known to cause genetic anticipation was trinucleotide repeat expansion (TRE).[53,54] Recently, tetranucleotide repeat expansion was described as another cause in myotonic dystrophy[55] and pentanucleotide repeat expansion[56] was added as a cause of genetic anticipation in spinocerebellar ataxia.

Although the observation of genetic anticipation can be artefactual because of incomplete ascertainment of affected family members or other cohort bias, it is strikingly apparent in PPH families. TRE was first described in Fragile X syndrome in 1990, and is now believed to be the molecular mechanism of at least 14 neurologic diseases including Huntington's, myotonic dystrophy, and several of the spinocerebellar ataxias.[57,58] In these diseases, TRE is the molecular basis for incomplete penetrance, variable age of onset, and genetic anticipation. In spinocerebellar ataxia 10, there is an inverse correlation between the number of expanded pentanucleotide repeats and the time of onset of the disease.[59]

Exciting new information suggests that expanded repeats also may develop in cells that are not replicating, probably related to abnormalities of the mechanisms for repairing damaged DNA.[56] Recent investigations have also demonstrated the presence of microsatellite instability of DNA repair enzymes (MSH) in PPH lungs,[60] which further suggests this plausible mechanism for expansion of repeat sequences.

Genetic anticipation was first suspected in several PPH family reports early in the 1960s.[50] We confirmed this observation in the 1984 report, where the ages at death in successive generations were 45.6 versus 36.3 versus 24.2 years, $P < 0.05$.[51] The potential for bias of ascertainment was not excluded. One analytic approach to decrease bias of ascertainment is to test only affected parents who have affected children. In the 1994 report, we identified 60 affected parent–child pairs for analysis (Fig. 14.5). Age of onset in offspring was an average of 14.1 years earlier than in parents ($P = 0.0001$). Age of death was an average of 15.1 years earlier ($P = 0.0001$). To remove bias due to multiple parent–child pairs from families, we limited analysis to only one pair from each sibship, yielding 40 pairs. In families with multiple affected siblings, the tests were done by randomly choosing one sibling to make the parent–child pair. Analysis of the parent to child pairs suggested that onset was 14.8 years earlier on average in children ($P = 0.0001$).

Further, to consider the possibility of bias due to phenotypic variation and carrier status of unaffected parents, we also performed the analysis including unaffected parent and affected child pairs, yielding 91 pairs. This analysis gave further evidence for anticipation, with an average disease onset in children of 21.1 years earlier than their parent ($P = 0.0001$). Another source of potential bias could be introduced by improvement in diagnostic testing over recent generations to produce apparent genetic anticipation. To adjust for this we stratified the 60 affected-affected pairs by parental calendar decade of disease onset and then conducted the paired $T$-test within these strata. The overall trend remains positive. In all strata, the child's age of onset is earlier than the parent's, with increasingly earlier onset and higher significance ($P < 0.01$) in children in more recent decades.

The recent discovery of TRE as a molecular mechanism of a potential modifier gene, NOS1,[61] validates the concept that repeat expansion may be a molecular mechanism in a modifying gene, and has potential relevance to FPPH. Sullivan et al.[61] compared FENO (exhaled nitric oxide level), plasma nitric oxide metabolites, serum arginine and citrulline levels, and the number of AAT repeats in intron 20 of NOS1 in subjects with sickle cell disease (SCD) who had a history of at least one episode of ACS (ACS+), in subjects with SCD and no prior history of ACS, and in healthy children. The level of FENO was significantly associated with the sum of AAT repeats in intron 20 of NOS I gene alleles. FENO levels were significantly reduced in subjects who had a history of ACS and the FENO levels were significantly correlated with the number of AAT repeats in NOSI. The role of TRE in modifying ACS appears to be the first demonstration of a mechanistic role as a modifying gene, or of TRE functioning in a vascular disease.

Genetic anticipation remains an unsolved but intriguing observation in FPPH, but may hold clues to understanding the penetrance and phenotype of this disease.

## Histopathological abnormalities in PPH and FPPH

Lesions in small pulmonary arteries and arterioles are the hallmark of PPH.[62–64] Changes in the large pulmonary arteries are secondary to pulmonary hypertension and include dilatation, medial hypertrophy, and atherosclerotic plaques. Changes in the heart are related to the ventricular response to chronic pulmonary hypertension. The right ventricle is hypertrophied and usually dilated, and hypertrophy of the inferior apex of the heart and of the septum occur. The right atrium is dilated especially if RV decompensation occurs. Occasionally, the pulmonic valve is incompetent.

The classical histological findings in the pulmonary circulation are obliterative lesions in arterioles between 500–1000 microns in diameter. Medial hypertrophy, concentric intimal fibrosis, and plexiform lesions coexist in varying proportions in the pulmonary circulation of most cases of PPH (Fig. 14.6). Other lesions include eccentric intimal fibrosis, and recanalizing thrombotic occlusions in some cases. The vascular changes in PPH extend through the vessel wall and involve the aventitia, which is thickened and hyperplastic in many sections. Many lungs reveal what appears to be new growth of microvessels, called angiomatous (angioid) changes. The histopathological findings in the lungs of patients with FPPH are identical to those of sporadic PPH.[65]

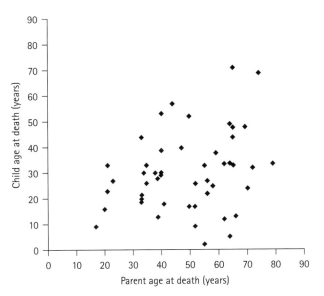

**Figure 14.5** *Graph comparing age at death within families with FPPH. Each point represents one group of a parent and child with FPPH, taken from multiple families in the Vanderbilt FPPH Registry without regard for gender of parent or child. No person was used more than once. In some cases, the parent was the first person diagnosed and the child in others. The distribution of ages should cluster around the line of age identity, but the age at death is lower for offspring. This is the most objective evidence that genetic anticipation may occur in FPPH.*

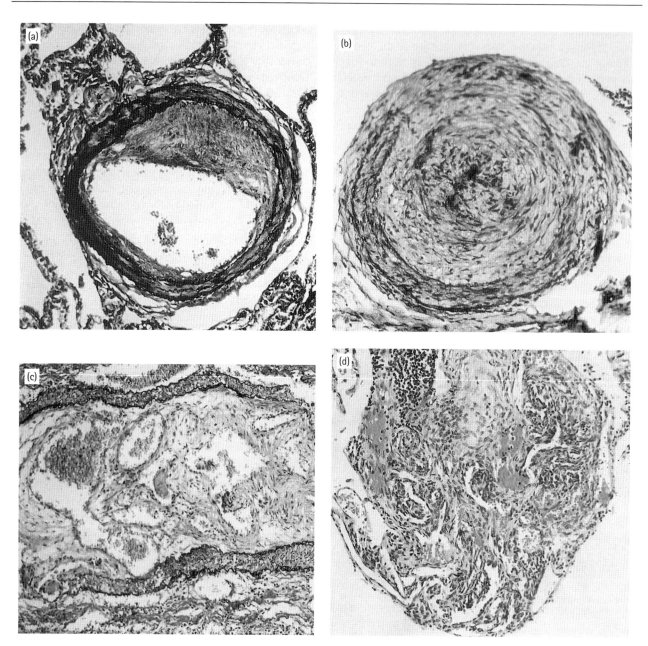

**Figure 14.6**   *Lesions of the small pulmonary arterioles found in all forms of PAH, including FPPH.[65] Lesion (a) demonstrates eccentric intimal fibrosis and medial hypertrophy (Verhoff van Gieson, magnification × 100). This lesion was originally thought to represent pulmonary microembolism, but is widespread in FPPH, denoting a differing mechanism. Lesion (b) shows concentric intimal fibrosis, an onion skin-like layering of fibrotic reaction (Movat stain, magnification × 100). Lesion (c) is a recanalized thrombus in a microvessel. Lesion (d) is a plexiform lesion, showing a neovascular response (hematoxylin and eosin, magnification × 100). It is unclear whether these lesions are a response to upstream obstruction or are a primary lesion in PAH. (See Plate 1 for colour version.)*

For many years, it was assumed that each of the several pathological changes seen in the pulmonary arterioles represented a pathogenic subset of PPH.[62,63] Histological analysis of lung tissue from multiple affected family members, both within and among families, revealed that all of the reported histological features were present both within and among families (Fig. 14.7). In familial PPH, the pathogenesis of disease should be unique and the same within each family, and therefore the histological features should reflect the pathogenetic sequence of disease. Because members within a family demonstrated multiple histological subtypes, it was concluded that the histological features did not represent differing causes of PPH.[65]

The histological features of PPH are the same among several etiologies of pulmonary arterial hypertension including sporadic PPH, familial PPH, HIV infection, portopulmonary hypertension, and the scleroderma spectrum of disease (excluding coincident interstitial fibrosis).[62–65] The

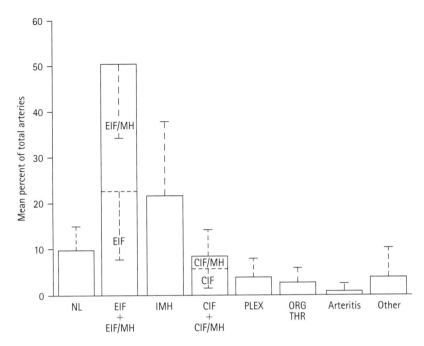

**Figure 14.7**  *Distribution of types of lesions in the lungs of 23 patients with familial primary pulmonary hypertension.[65] NL, normal vessel; EIF, eccentric intimal fibrosis; MH and IMH, medial hypertrophy and isolated MH; CIF, concentric intimal fibrosis; PLEX, plexiform lesions; ORG/THR, organized thrombus; OTHER, other lesion types. All vessels in each specimen were labeled and counted, a mean of 109 ± 62 per patient. Bars represent means and standard deviation. The broad distribution of lesions in a disease with a genetic basis strongly suggests that the histological lesions do not represent distinct pathogenetic processes.*

changes seen in Eisenmenger's syndrome are similar.[64] Despite histological similarities among the several conditions leading to pulmonary arterial hypertension, there are likely to be differences in the sequence or triggers of the process leading to vasculopathy. Geraci et al.[66] microdissected plexiform lesions from patients with sporadic and familial PPH and found differences in clusters of cDNA that could distinguish the two forms. In addition, somatic mutations in TGFBR2 occur in the endothelial cells of plexiform lesions, suggesting that the vasculopathic process is analogous to neoplastic tranformation that occurs in gut and other tissues.[60] The biologic meaning of these findings remains to be determined.

The vascular lesions seen in PPH are not shared by diseases leading to hypoxic pulmonary hypertension or by interstitial lung diseases. In hypoxic pulmonary hypertension, medial hypertrophy and extension of vascular smooth muscle downstream towards the precapillaries occurs.[67] In interstitial lung disesases, there is widespread disappearance of microvessels into the fibrotic milieu of the alveolar wall and interstitium.[67] Neither of these two major categories of pulmonary hypertension is associated with eccentric or concentric intimal fibrosis or plexiform lesions. Occasionally, these lesions are seen downstream to the vascular obstruction in chronic thrombotic pulmonary hypertension.[68]

## SEARCH FOR THE GENES IN FAMILIAL PRIMARY PULMONARY HYPERTENSION

### Linkage analysis in familial primary pulmonary hypertension

In the mid-1990s, sufficient numbers of families had been identified and DNA banked to embark on linkage analysis to determine the chromosomal location of the FPPH gene. A genome-wide microsatellite marker search was employed using a set of highly polymorphic short tandem repeat markers in 19 affected individuals from six PPH families. Initial evidence for linkage (Fig. 14.8) was obtained with two chromosome 2q markers.[69] Subsequently, patients and all available family members were analyzed for 19 additional markers spanning approximately 40 cM on the long arm of chromosome 2. We obtained a two-point LOD score of 6.97 at theta = 0 with the marker D2S389. Multipoint linkage analysis yielded a maximum LOD score of 7.86 with the marker D2S311. Haplotype analysis established a minimum candidate interval of approximately 25 cM. Subsequent studies narrowed the region of interest for the FPPH gene to a region of 6 cM. Linkage to chromosome 2q31–32 was simultaneously confirmed by Deng et al.[6] in families from the Columbia registry.

### Identification of mutations in BMPR2 in familial PPH

Because the human genome had not been sequenced in 1997 and the span known to contain the affected gene was 30 million base pairs, the search on chromosome 2 initially employed the candidate gene approach. Several genes, including an insulin-like growth factor and neuropilin, a VEGF receptor, were known to exist in the span, but no variations likely to cause PPH were found when DNAs of affected family members was sequenced. BMPR2 was the third candidate gene studied, chosen because of its membership in the TGFbeta family of receptors.

We amplified exonic segments of BMPR2 from individuals with FPPH by polymerase chain reaction (PCR) and screened these amplicons for alterations by dideoxy

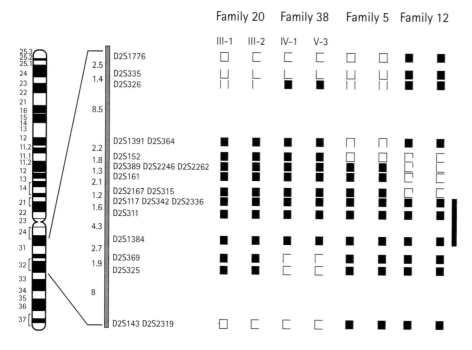

**Figure 14.8** *Original linkage data demonstrating location of common gene on chromosome 2q31–33, narrowed by analysis of affected and unaffected members of four families in the Vanderbilt FPPH Registry.[69] Analysis was made by microsatellite marker search; LOD score 7.4. The region of interest originally spanned over 20 million base pairs.*

fingerprinting (ddF), and found an altered pattern in a patient and one parent in family 55. This change was the first proof of BMPR2 mutations in PPH patients. By DNA sequencing we found that the change was a T deletion (2579–80 del T). This change removed the restriction site *Ase*I from this amplicon. We PCR-amplified the segment containing this mutation from DNAs of members of this family. These amplified segments were subjected to restriction endonuclease digestion and the result analyzed by agarose gel electrophoresis. These studies showed that in US family 55, the BMPR2 2579–80 del T mutation and the FPPH phenotype cosegregated. The 2579–80 del T mutation in US family 55 created an *Ase*I restriction endonuclease site that was used to confirm segregation of the mutation within the family and exclude the presence of the mutation in controls. This and a series of BMPR2 mutations in multiple families were reported by the international consortium and from Columbia in 2000.[5,6]

Figure 14.9 summarizes the process of discovery of the BMPR2 gene as the locus for mutations that result in familial PPH.

## Range of BMPR2 mutations

The gene encoding BMPR2 resides on chromosome 2q33 and has 13 exons.[70–72] It is a long gene, spanning 184 000 base pairs, of which 3000 comprise 13 exons. The receptor has an extracellular (exon 1–3), transmembrane (exon 4), an intracellular serine/threonine kinase domain (exons 5–11) and a large C-terminus (exons 12 and 13) of unknown function that is not shared by other TGFbeta receptors. Polymorphisms in the BMPR2 coding region in the normal population are unusual but have been found in exons

6, 8, and 12.[4,71] Mutations leading to familial PPH have been found in all exons except 13. In families, every affected member has the same mutation, and each of over 40 families has a mutation unique to that kindred. BMPR2 is highly conserved in nature. Each amino acid substitution that results from the point mutations found in FPPH is predicted to alter receptor function. Mutations are equally divided among frameshift, nonsense, and missense, all predicted to alter coding of the transcript and result in a dysfunctional receptor. None of the mutations associated with FPPH result in a receptor structure that would appear to be compatible with normal or increased function. The location of mutations in BMPR2 is shown in Fig. 14.10. Polymorphisms are found in BMPR2, especially in exon 12 at codon 937. Except for the possibility of altered penetrance among families, there are no apparent differences in gender, age of onset, or severity of disease based on the location of mutations. Vanderbilt family 14 has a T354G missense mutation in exon 3 that encodes an amino acid substitution of tryptophan for cysteine, and should eliminate function of the extracellular domain.[72] Theoretically, the receptor may have no response to BMP stimulation.

An initial screening of 50 patients with sporadic PPH revealed germline mutations in BMPR2 in 13, including three missense, three nonsense, and five frameshift mutations.[13] More recent unpublished surveys of small populations of sporadic PPH patients suggest that the prevalence may be less than the 26 percent in this first report.[4] At least two of the original patients classified as sporadic were later found to come from families with known disease. The true prevalence of BMPR2 mutations will require a study of at least 200 sporadic patients for whom family histories are well documented. In order to determine whether BMPR2 mutations are de novo in these patients or whether they are

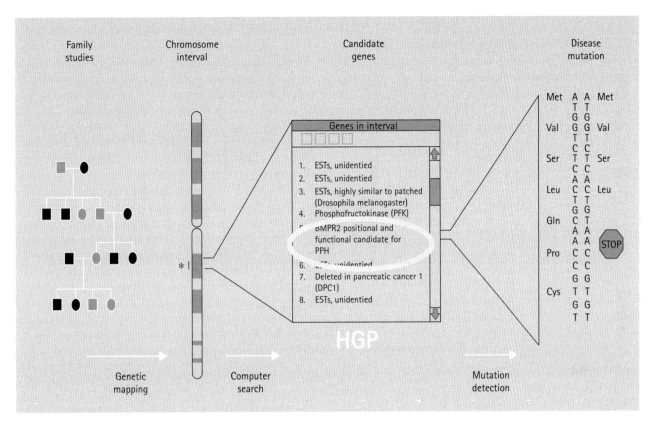

**Figure 14.9**  *Summary of the strategy used to discover mutations in BMPR2 as the autosomal dominant cause of PPH in most families with familial PPH. DNA was banked from families in a registry until there were sufficient numbers of affected and unaffected to detect differences by restriction length polymorphisms. The gene was linked to chromosome 2q31–33. Candidate genes were searched in the span, and BMPR2 was tested because of its role in TGFbeta family signaling. By DNA fingerprinting, a base pair deletion was detected in a family that caused a frameshift and was unique to affected members.*

inherited will require haplotype analysis of the parents and the affected person. Any new germline mutation that enters the gene pool may convert designation of a sporadic case to hereditary and, if expressed in other family members, familial disease. Because at least 75–90 percent of patients with sporadic PPH do not have mutations in BMPR2, there must be other genetic predispositions, gene–gene interactions, or environmental triggers that result in the development of PPH in these patients. It is unknown whether Alk-1 mutations cause sporadic PPH.

Other cohorts with pulmonary arterial hypertension have been tested for the presence of BMPR2 mutations. Three of 33 French patients with PPH related to fenfluramine ingestion had BMPR2 mutation; each mutation is predicted to alter receptor function.[73,74] BMPR2 mutations were not found in 24 patients with pulmonary arterial hypertension related to the scleroderma spectrum of disease.[75] One patient with CREST syndrome appeared to have a rare polymorphism in exon 13. No BMPR2 mutations were found in three studies of a total of 55 patients with HIV-related pulmonary arterial hypertension.[76] There is insufficient data to report the presence of BMPR2 mutations in Eisenmenger's syndrome or in portopulmonary hypertension. No BMPR2 mutations predicted to alter receptor function have been found in over 350 controls published to date.[4,71]

As noted earlier, mutations have only been identified in 50 percent of families studied and 10–25 percent of isolated cases.[13] There are several different potential causes that could explain these 'missing' mutations. First, the BMPR2 gene is >180 kb in size and previous studies have only examined about 4.5 kb which corresponds to the exons and exon–intron boundries. Second, the major portion of the BMPR2 gene has not been examined. Third, the promoter and the intronic regions of BMPR2 remain as logical areas that need to be examined for inherited PPH mutations in FPPH, as well as in sporadic PPH cases. Preliminary evidence suggests that intronic mutations in BMPR2 may be responsible for another 25 percent of familial cases that link to chromosome 2 q33.[77]

## Signal transduction of BMPs through BMPR2

Bone morphogenetic proteins (BMP) were first identified as cellular products found in normal bone that promote ectopic bone formation and the healing of fractures.[8,9]

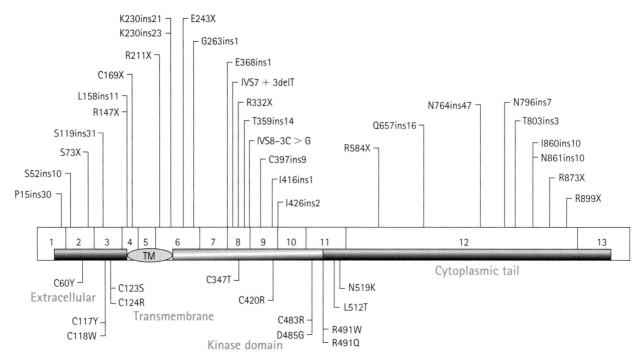

**Figure 14.10** *Known mutations in the BMPR2 gene. The gene has 180 000 base pairs, comprising 13 exons. Mutations have not been found in exon 13. The long cytoplasmic tail is of unknown functional significance. Polymorphisms in the coding region of the gene are extremely rare. Each mutation is unique to each known family. Intronic mutations, not shown, may be responsible for a large percentage of FPPH in which the gene links to chromosome 2q33, but no exonic mutations are found.*

These proteins are members of the transforming growth factor beta (TGF beta) superfamily of circulating proteins that regulate tissue growth and repair in all organs.[78] BMPs exert their effects through the activation of receptors 1 and 2, which are expressed adjacent to each other on cell surfaces and transduce intracellular signaling (Fig. 14.11). Ligand binding of BMP with the extracellular domain of BMPR2 leads to phosphorylation of BMPR1, and activation of the serine-threonine kinase intracellular domain of BMPR1. The activated type I receptor then phosphorylates response-Smad proteins which bind with Smad 4 in the cytosol and migrate to the nucleus where they regulate DNA transcription in concert with nuclear binding factors.[8,9,78] The effect of activation of BMP receptors depends on the cell and the circumstances, and can result either in growth promotion or inhibition. Because the likelihood of developing clinical PPH is only 10–20 percent in known carriers of BMPR2 mutations, we speculate that gene modifiers, such as environmental factors, estrogens, or second mutations in unknown regulatory genes may be necessary for clinical expression of disease. The BMPR2 mutations that have already been identified are likely to cause impairment in receptor function; thus, the normal function of BMPR2 in the pulmonary circulation may be antiproliferative. If two functioning alleles are necessary for this inhibitory function, then haplo-insufficiency related to the heterozygotic state may be the mechanism of vascular dysregulation leading to FPPH.[79]

## Functional effects: haploinsufficiency

BMP signaling is critical in lung development and high expression of BMPR2 in the adult lung suggests that it plays an ongoing role in lung homeostasis.[80–83] The signaling cascade of the BMP family has many similarities to those of the other TGFβ family ligands. The major differences are that BMP ligands are secreted in an active form and bind with low affinity to either the type 1 or type 2 receptor independently.[80,84] Type 1 and 2 receptors are cell surface membrane bound proteins, which are thought to act cooperatively to facilitate high affinity binding. Signal transduction after receptor ligation occurs through the serine/threonine kinase activities of the receptor complex.[80,85] In brief, the type 2 receptor phosporylates the type 1 receptor at specific serine residues.[80,84,86] This phosphorylation activates the type 1 receptor and allows the phosporylation of the second messengers, in this case SMAD1 and/or 5.[80,87] These phosphorylated response SMADs interact with the common SMAD4, translocate to the nucleus, and activate transcription.

BMPR2 is the only receptor that responds uniquely to BMP. BMPs interact with other TGFβ receptors, including activin type 1 receptors, but BMPR2 has only been associated with BMP ligand signaling.[84,88] BMPR2 is regulated in both a developmental and tissue specific manner.[80] The sequence 5′ to the reported BMPR2 transcriptional start site is available in the public database (NCBI, GenBank

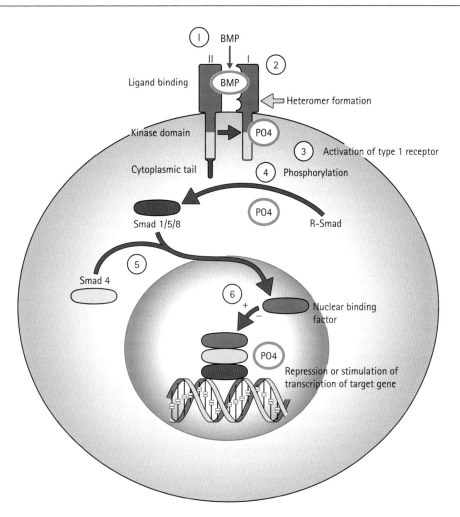

**Figure 14.11** *Schema of signal transduction of BMPR2. Bone morphogenetic receptors type II and I (BMPR II and I) sit adjacent on cell membranes.[72] BMP binds to the extracellular domain (ligand binding) of BMPRII (step 1) resulting in heteromeric formation with BMPRI (step 2). BMPRII then phosphorylates the transmembrane region of BMPRI, activating the kinase domain (step 3). The activated BMPRI phosphorylates one or more receptor-dependent cytoplasmic Smad proteins (step 4) which bind with Smad 4 and migrate to the nucleus (step 5). The phosphorylated Smad complex attaches to a nuclear binding factor in the nucleus and the resulting assembly either stimulates or represses gene transcription by interacting with DNA (step 6). In familial primary pulmonary hypertension, mutations have been found along the entire span of the BMPRII receptor. In the family of this report, there is a single point mutation in the kinase domain. The cells in which the mutation causes PPH have not been identified, although endothelial cells, smooth muscle cells, and fibroblasts are likely candidates.*

accession No. AC064836.6 position 142601–186626). This region shares many similarities with the promoter regions reported for other members of the TGFβ receptor family. Regulation of the TGFβ receptors is modulatable by pathway-specific as well as 'common' inducers of transcriptional regulation.[89–91] TGFβ receptors are differentially expressed in a temporally and tissue-specific pattern.[80,92–94] With the finding that BMPR2 mutations cause FPPH which has onset in most cases in adulthood but with reduced penetrance, it seems timely to define normal BMPR2 regulation so that the roles played by its perturbed regulation in FPPH can be determined.

The simplest genetic model to explain diverse mutations resulting in a single common outcome is haploinsufficiency.

The hypothesis of haploinsufficiency is that a threshold amount of gene product is needed for 'normal' function. This threshold amount, in the case of many genes, requires the combined expression of two alleles. If one allele is deleted or in some other way compromised, expression of the product may fall below the 'threshold' level and a disease phenotype is expressed. Haploinsufficiency is often seen in diseases with a dominant mode of transmission.[95–99]

A recent transgenic model of BMPR2 heterozygous mutation driven by a tetracycline-sensitive promoter showed the development of pulmonary hypertension during overexpression of the receptor, suggesting a dominant negative mode in that model.[100]

## Reduced penetrance in FPPH

There are several potential causes of variable phenotypes and reduced penetrance of autosomal dominant traits. These include alternative alleles (allelic heterogeneity), alternative loci (locus heterogeneity), modifier genes, and environmental factors. An example of a genetic modifier in humans is the decreased amount of sickle hemoglobin that is seen in patients with sickle trait who also are heterozygous for alpha thalassemia trait.[101,102] The lower sickle hemoglobin is caused by the globin not competing as well as the B globin for the limited globin molecules required to form a2B2 heterotetramers. Genetic modifiers can affect penetrance, expressivity, and pleiotropy. Depending on the nature of the phenotypic effect, modifiers might cause more or less extreme, novel or normal phenotypes. Modifier genes discovered in experimental species, such as mice, are often relevant to human diseases and genetic linkages discovered in other species can guide the search for linkage in humans.[102,103]

Studies of the estrogen-response elements in the BMPR2 promoter are needed to determine if they contribute to the penetrance of, as well as the female preponderance that is seen in FPPH. Second, promoters in the normal BMPR2 allele may subtlely affect its expression and thus may alter effects of the mutant BMPR2 product.[104] Third, variations in modifier genes that are encoded in the nuclear or mitochondrial chromosomes may affect the penetrance of FPPH.[104] Fourth, somatic mutations in the normal BMPR2 genes of those heterozygous for one BMPR2 mutation in lung tissue could cause loss of heterozygosity so that both BMPR2 alleles are defective. This could trigger changes that begin in one cell, but which could result in PPH. While mutational analysis of the promoter and other regions of BMPR2, analysis of modifier genes and/or somatic changes may be found, the functional importance of this allelic and non-allelic variation will have to be proven.

Familial PPH is a complex genetic disease. Except for gender, there are no known influences on penetrance. In nonfamilial PPH, there are clearcut environmental and biological triggers for the development of disease, including the well-known associations with appetite suppressants, HIV infection, portal hypertension, and collagen vascular disease. The best documented environmental associations are fenfluramine and stimulants such as amphetamines.[75] Studies to look at parity, cigarette smoke, depression, hormone therapy, childhood infections, hypertension, activity, altitude dwelling, diet, medicines, lifestyles, or other potential influences on development of disease studies are needed.

The search for modifying genes is in its infancy. Analysis of a number of genes with the potential to alter vascular function is underway. One approach is to pick candidate genes that both have a role in vascular structure and function, but also possess polymorphisms that confer differences in function of the product. A partial list includes the serotonin transporter, nitric oxide synthases, vasoactive intestinal polypeptide, the urea cycle enzyme carbamyl phosphate synthetase, endothelin receptors, and ion channels.[78,105,106] There are undoubtedly many others, including many intracellular signaling molecules. HIV has a well-documented association with PPH, and the recent finding of HHV8 in the lungs of patients with sporadic and familial PPH raises the possibility of chronic vascular damage related to cytokine stimulation resulting from permanent viral infections.[107] HHV8 is also present in the vascular tumor, Kaposi's sarcoma.[107] There are a number of ways that the disease and vascular lesions of PPH can be acquired. These include the major genes, modifying genes,

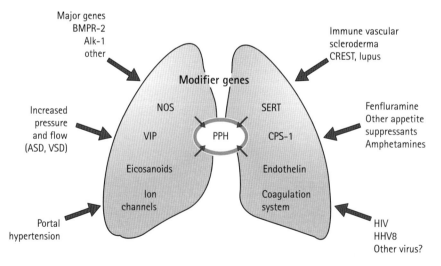

**Figure 14.12** *Primary pulmonary hypertension can be induced in susceptible individuals by a number of conditions or stimuli, shown in circumference around the cartoon of the lungs. These conditions elicit a response which is modulated by genetic susceptibility, in the form of functional polymorphisms of an unknown number of genes. Listed are some genes with functional polymorphisms known to influence vascular function, including NOS (nitric oxide synthases), SERT (serotonin transporter), VIP (vasoactive intestinal peptide), AII (angiotensin II), CPS (carbomyl phosphate synthetase), E-receptors (endothelin). The state of knowledge with regard to modifying genes is in its infancy.*

and other biological and external stimuli. A schematic summary of known and likely influences is shown in Fig. 14.12.

## PPH and FPPH: lessons from a superfamily

As we increased our Vanderbilt Registry and accrued both sporadic and familial PPH cases, we noted that many cases of apparently sporadic PPH were actually inherited, due to several features of the disease: (1) in FPPH, skipped generations related to low disease expression; (2) because family relationships were unknown due to loss of contact; and (3) misdiagnosis by the medical community of other affected family members.[50,51] We list 107 FPPH families currently in the registry and have longitudinal information on 81 families. Our registry has uncovered an FPPH superfamily spanning seven generations, arising from five family groups initially not known to be related.[72] This kindred includes 12 affected members who were initially thought to have sporadic PPH, and seven affected members who were first misdiagnosed with other cardiovascular diseases. This family is an extension of Family 14, the family group that initiated our first search in 1980. The mutation in BMPR2 from six affected members, revealed that all have a T354G missense mutation in exon 3 that encodes a cysteine to tryptophan amino substitution.[5,72]

The index case was a 30-year-old woman, who gave a history of unusual deaths in her extended family, including her mother, three aunts, and a cousin.[50] The cousin had been misdiagnosed with postpartum cardiomyopathy but was later diagnosed with PPH. Two aunts died suddenly at 23 and 24 years of age several days post-partum without obstetric complications. Her mother died of undiagnosed heart failure, and inspection of the lung sections 20 years later revealed classic concentric intimal fibrosis and plexiform lesions in the pulmonary arteries.

New families have been discovered by a number of methods, including referrals from clinicians and investigators from the USA and other countries, contacts from the NIH Prospective Registry, contacts through the Pulmonary Hypertension Association (PHA), and crossreferencing of extensive family histories. The search relied heavily on key individuals who keep family records and maintain family contacts and who are willing to share information crucial to make connections. As the pedigree database has expanded, we have been able to link hitherto unrelated families, usually by crosschecking common surnames.

The family pedigree is shown in Fig. 14.13. The husband (b. 1835) and wife (b. 1838) of generation I had seven children, two of whom parented all the currently known branches of this superfamily. We do not know which parent transmitted PPH and have no information on the

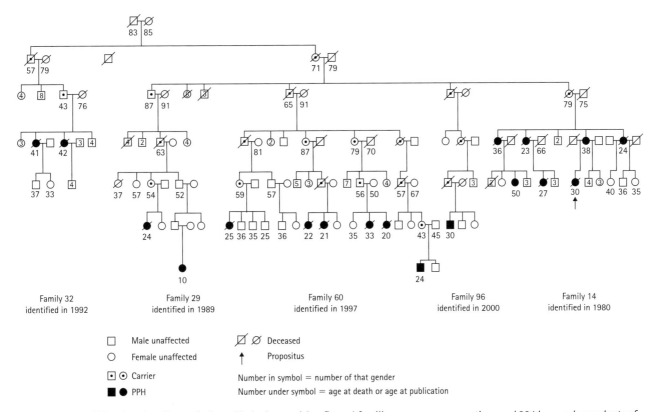

**Figure 14.13** *Abbreviated pedigree of a large kindred comprising five subfamilies over seven generations and 384 known descendants of generation I.[72] The propositus was the female in generation V of family 14 who died at age 30, diagnosed by one of us (JEL) in 1980. Details of the discovery and linkage of these families is described in the text. There are at least 200 descendants at varying risk of developing PPH. Eighteen members (16 female, 2 male) have been diagnosed with FPPH and at least 23 (12 female, 11 male) are known to carry the FPPH gene.*

mother's family. If the mother were the carrier, there is another potentially large branch of this kindred. There are 394 named descendants, over 200 of whom are alive and at risk of possessing the gene. There have been 23 unaffected mutation carriers, known because of having an affected descendant plus ancestor who was a carrier or was affected. Eighteen members have been diagnosed with FPPH, for a total of 41 members known to have the gene. Of the 18 with FPPH, 16 were female and two were male. Of the carriers, 11 were female and 12 were male. Seven of the 18 with FPPH (40 percent) were initially misdiagnosed and 12 (67 percent) were originally thought to have sporadic disease, until familial disease was uncovered. Misdiagnoses included postpartum cardiomyopathy, hypothyroid cardiomyopathy, pericardial tamponade, 'heart attack', atrial septal defect, ventricular septal defect, and pulmonic valve insufficiency. Because of the high prevalence of asymptomatic carriers at least 200 offspring are at risk for having inherited the BMPR2 mutation. The number of future descendants at risk should grow geometrically.

In this superfamily, five family branches were originally considered to be separate unrelated kindreds. The thread of evidence that connected them is instructive. In the early 1980s, we obtained an extended family history and examined public records to fully document family 14. Later, a patient was seen in consultation (family 29), and was thought to have sporadic PPH but had a dead grandparent with the same surname as an ancestor in family 14. Linking the two families was not possible because of lack of information due to migration of ancestors and geographical separation. Family 32 was discovered in 1992. A communication from family 60 in 1997 revealed that the family 14 ancestral name was also in family 60's lineage, and that family 60 also had a surname in common with generation I and family 32. The final family, 29, and the unnamed branch identified in 2000, were easily matched by family histories, which revealed the same great grandparents. The patient in generation VII of family 29 was recently referred for management of suspected congenital heart disease. The 30-year-old male in generation VI of the family found in 2000 was identified in the superfamily when he was asked to counsel a new patient about epoprostenol therapy at a time when, by chance, both were hospitalized. The new patient happened to be in one of our families and the two discovered that they had an ancestor with the same surname.

The discovery of this very large FPPH kindred confirms and extends the hypothesis that many cases of presumed sporadic PPH are in fact genetic. Two thirds (12/18) of the patients in this kindred were initially thought to have sporadic disease. A recent report suggests that PPH may even more frequently have a genetic basis. Gruenig et al.[108] studied 188 relatives of 32 PPH patients using Doppler echocardiography and right heart catheterization for estimation of pulmonary artery systolic pressure (PASP) during exercise. Linkage analysis was performed in 93 relatives within six families. Overt clinical PPH was detected in at least one relative ($n = 15$) of 28 percent of the index patients. 'Latent'

PPH with abnormal PASP-response to exercise ($>40$) was present in at least one relative ($n = 37$) of another 58 percent of the index patients. In the families examined genetically, all relatives with abnormal PASP response to exercise shared the 2q32-34 linkage pattern with the PPH patients. In total, 81 percent of all PPH patients had strong evidence of familial disease. The authors concluded that PPH is predominantly a genetic disease. The affected haplotypes link to a similar area in chromosome 2q33, where the BMPR2 gene resides.[109] To this point, haplotype analysis of large numbers of sporadic PPH patients has not been performed to determine the prevalence of this finding.

Genetic testing and genetic counseling will soon become important issues to address for PPH patients and their families, and some of the current uncertainties with regard to transmission and risk of disease will be resolved. Currently, there are few certified clinical laboratory protocols to test for the presence of BMPR2 mutations, but these will become available in the near future. Family history will become increasingly important as methods of ascertaining those at risk are developed. The family history should be extensively reviewed in all patients with presumed sporadic PPH and surnames of ancestors should be ascertained. It is only through documentation of pedigrees that these relationships will be discovered.

## Summary of FPPH

Surveillance for onset of disease in subjects who carry a BMPR2 mutation will become increasingly important as improved therapies are developed, such as oral or inhaled vasodilators and antiproliferative agents. Hopefully, presymptomatic diagnosis will lead to prevention of disease progression and prolonged survival. Personal and family counseling are dependent on accurate diagnosis. Although we know that approximately 10–20 percent of people carrying an FPPH gene will develop clinical disease in their lifetime, there is no current predictive functional test or biomarker to detect the presence of disease process or of who will develop disease. Investigations of potentially useful biomarkers are needed including endothelin, BMPs, thromboxanes, VEGF, angiopoeitin, and others, to develop information about sensitivity and specificity for disease.[11,110–114] Each of these endogenous mediators has been found to be elevated in patients with established PPH. Each is associated with vascular remodeling, and endothelin and thromboxanes also cause vasoconstriction, a feature in some cases of PPH.

Echocardiography with Doppler assessment of pulmonary arterial systolic pressure is currently the best noninvasive method to detect preclinical pulmonary hypertension.[108] In people known to carry an FPPH gene mutation, serial evaluations of selected circulating mediators and echocardiograms may eventually be the best tools to screen for the development of disease. Until we are better able to assess ongoing pathogenesis, it will be impossible to offer reliable guidance of carriers in lifestyle decisions, including exercise activities, birth control, and childbearing. Avoidance of smoking, diet drugs, and vasoconstrictor decongestant medicines is obviously wise.

Finally, genetic and family counseling have become issues of growing importance in this and other families, demanding better insights and information from medical scientists, so that these people can plan their lives with as much certainty as possible.

## PRIMARY PULMONARY HYPERTENSION AND HEREDITARY HEMORRHAGIC TELANGIECTASIA

Hereditary hemorrhagic telangiectasia is an autosomal dominant inherited disease characterized by mucocutaneous telangiectasias, causing recurrent epistaxis and gastrointestinal blood loss, and arteriovenous malformations of the pulmonary, hepatic, and cerebral circulations. Heterogeneous defects in components of the TGFβ receptor complex, including endoglin (ENG) and activin receptor-like kinase 1 (ALK1), have been implicated in the autosomal dominant vascular dysplasia of HHT.[115,116] Pulmonary arteriovenous malformations create significant right-to-left shunts causing systemic hypoxemia, paradoxical embolism, stroke, and cerebral abscesses, and typically cause decreased pulmonary vascular resistance. In contrast, pulmonary hypertension has also been reported to occur in individuals with hereditary hemorrhagic telangiectasia.[7,117]

Because members of the TGFβ signaling pathway are implicated in both hereditary hemorrhagic telangiectasia and PPH, we examined whether a common molecular mechanism could underlie the coexistence of these disorders. We identified five unique kindreds with different members affected by HHT and pulmonary hypertension. Our investigations reported new mutations of ALK1 in families with PPH and HHT.[7,118] A mutation in endoglin, part of the Alk-1 signaling complex, was recently reported in association with HHT and PPH in one family.[119]

## FAMILIAL PULMONARY VENO-OCCLUSIVE DISEASE

Pulmonary veno-occlusive disease (PVOD) is a distinctive histopathologic subset of PPH[64,120] characterized by widespread obliterative changes in postcapillary pulmonary venules. Because these obstructive lesions raise pressure in upstream capillaries and arterioles, there is medial thickening and other reactive changes in the precapillary bed. The broad distribution of abnormalities in the pulmonary vasculature in PVOD poses both diagnostic and management dilemmas.[121] Symptomatology is similar to that of PPH, as are noninvasive tests including electrocardiogram and echocardiogram. The rapid development of pulmonary edema, sometimes overwhelming and catastrophic, is a complication of vasodilator therapy in the treatment of PVOD, but not of classic PPH. The clinical, radiographic, and hemodynamic findings that provide clues to the diagnosis of PVOD include peripheral interstitial infiltrates or Kerley B lines, a markedly reduced DLCO and mediastinal adenopathy.[120] PVOD is the cause of pulmonary hypertension in about 5 percent of cases suspected of having PPH.[1,3,12]

There are four published reports of PVOD occurring in families.[122] Interestingly, each of these reports described PVOD in siblings only, and the disease of sibling cases occurred close in time to one another. This observation raises the possibility of a common inciting event such as ingestion, infection, toxin, or other environmental exposure.[121] We were referred a family that had the first evidence of vertical transmission of PVOD.[122] A 36-year-old woman was diagnosed in 1997 with pulmonary hypertension with pulmonary artery pressure of 85/37 mmHg. Surgical lung biopsy was performed because of interstitial lung changes and the biopsy revealed widespread occlusion of small vessels, including pulmonary veins, along with hemosiderin-laden macrophages, changes which are typical of PVOD. Unlike classic PPH, PVOD is known to be associated with pulmonary interstitial changes, which are often characteristic of desquamative interstitial pneumonitis. The patient's mother was diagnosed by cardiac catheterization with PPH at age 36, and the patient's maternal grandfather died at a young age of unknown cause. We discovered that the patient has an exon 1 mutation (44delC) of BMPR2, a frameshift predicted to cause termination 30 codons downstream. One of two siblings had the same mutation. Although no maternal tissue was available for study, it is highly likely that the mother had PVOD, inherited from a new germline mutation in a grandparent of the proband. In this family, there are also two cases of complex congenital heart disease in maternal cousins. Studies are underway in the DNA from large cohorts of PVOD to determine the prevalence of BMPR2 mutations in sporadic and familial PVOD. It seems clear that PPH and PVOD can now be linked mechanistically in some cases, as different sites of the same pathogenetic process.

## IMMUNOGENETIC ABNORMALITIES IN PULMONARY ARTERIAL HYPERTENSION

Low level positive titers for antinuclear antibodies were reported in early studies of PPH, but the sensitivity and specificity for PPH were not high enough to be useful.[1,12] Pulmonary hypertension is a complication of immune disorders, including the scleroderma spectrum of disease, especially the CREST variety, and in systemic lupus erythematosus.[1–3] Hypothyroidism is reported to be found in PPH in a higher prevalence than in the general population. As many as 22.5 percent of PPH patients in small studies have hypothyroidism, although epoprostenol therapy may exacerbate any tendency towards thyroid dysfunction.[3] PPH has been reported in the POEMS syndrome, a myeloma-like illness characterized by polyneuropathy, organomegaly, endocrinopathy, M proteinopathy, and skin changes, which is associated with increased circulating immune mediators.[123] In scleroderma, inflammatory cells are found in proximity to plexiform lesions, suggesting a pathogenic link. Increased IL-6, the production of CX3C-chemokine fractalkine, and anti-fibrillin antibodies are increased in PPH, all immune mediators.[124] Treatment of a small number of patients with active systemic lupus erythematosus with immunosuppressive therapy has been reported to be associated with reductions in pulmonary arterial pressure, but similar success has not been reported in the scleroderma spectrum of disease.[37] In general, patients with lupus respond better to epoprostenol therapy than do patients with scleroderma, with better functional status and longer survival.

Small studies in PPH have reported antibody/HLA-DR,-DQ correlations.[125] Whites with PPH have more anti-centromere antibodies and African-Americans more anti-U1-ribonucleoprotein and anti-fibrillarin, U3-RNP, antibodies. HLA-DQB1*0301 (DQ7) was associated with tissue plasminogen activator antibodies in sporadic PPH. Antibodies against the the nucleolar phosphoprotein, B23, were associated with SSc and PPH. Anti-topoisomerase IIa antibodies in association with PPH in patients with scleroderma and HLA-B35 were found in an Italian cohort.[126] To date, no direct HLA-DR,-DQ associations have been found in patients with PPH. The immunogenetic associations and inherited HLA types deserve further screening in large cohorts, but no early consistent patterns have emerged. Immunogenetic mechanisms may well be modifying factors, especially in patients with inflammatory, HIV, HHV8, and auto-immune etiologies of PPH.

## GENETIC TESTING AND COUNSELING IN FAMILIAL PULMONARY HYPERTENSION

Familial PPH is a devastating disease for affected persons and their families. Recent therapies have markedly improved quality of life and even survival, but it remains a tragic thread in afflicted families. Most poignant, the disease is sometimes manifest during pregnancy, a time when health and future parenting are so heavily invested. The young members of families with FPPH are confronted with very difficult decisions about the personal risk of pregnancy, the possibility that they might not survive as parents, and that they may pass on this fatal disease to their offspring. The possibility of genetic anticipation causes enhanced apprehension in FPPH families who fear for the health of their children.

General lifestyle counseling has been given to family members at risk of disease for a number of years, but the ability to be quantitative about risk has not existed until now

with the discovery of the BMPR2 mutations. We have published preliminary data from a questionnaire of 82 members of families at risk in our registry, undertaken before the BMPR2 mutation was identified.[127] With the advent of knowledge that a genetic test for risk of disease is now available, we are extending our study of people at risk to measure their understanding of the quantitative risks for inheriting and passing the mutation, assessing the risk of developing disease even if the mutation is present, anticipating the personal impact on life and health decisions, anticipating the impact of this knowledge on the family and on current and unborn children, and understanding the social, economic, and health insurance impact of this knowledge. We will determine how individuals who consider and/or have had genetic testing conceptualize risk and analyze how family members influence individuals' decision-making processes as well as their behavioral and emotional responses to the test results. It needs to be emphasized that the insights gained from these evaluations are not predictable. Huntington disease (HD) is a case in point.[128] Attitudes about genetic testing of people at risk of having an HD mutation altered radically after the gene was discovered and many who initially desired the certainty of this knowledge declined testing once it was available.

We have made a successful first step in measuring and understanding the psychosocial implications of FPPH.[129] Our first study was done before the mutation in BMPR2 was known and was well before any realistic hope of genetic testing existed. Eighty-two members of the Vanderbilt Registry (75 percent) agreed to take part in the first study. This high rate indicates the level of interest these individuals have and also the quality of their relationship with the interested medical community. Of the 82, 75 percent completed a telephone interview. The questionnaire included demographic information, family dynamics regarding the disease, numerous questions about attitudes towards genetic testing, understanding of the disease and its inheritance, and the impact of the disease on their lives. Participants were also given time to make comments about PPH and the research being done on PPH. The telephone interviews averaged about an hour. More than 66 percent of respondents stated that they probably or definitely would have genetic testing if it became available. There was a greater interest in testing if a definite answer could be provided ($P < 0.001$). The most important reason for wanting testing done was to learn about the risk to their children. Reasons given for not wanting testing included concern about the effects on family, ability to handle the results emotionally, and concern about insurance and insurability (although this factor was less prominent than in other studies). Nearly 20 percent of the respondents appeared to be confused about the difference between diagnostic testing and the donation of blood for research studies.

Numerous studies have revealed that the expressed interest in predictive genetic testing often exceeds follow through.[129] The case of Huntington disease reveals this most dramatically; before the gene was discovered, more than

80 percent of people at risk expressed interest in testing, but approximately 10 percent of these people have actually been tested in the last decade.[129] Uptake varies for different genetic tests. Approximately 50 percent of those at risk for having mutations in BRCA1 and HNPCC actually are tested, while as many as 80 percent are tested for mutations that cause familial adenomatous polyposis and Van Hippel Lindau syndrome.[130] The factors that affect individuals' decisions about testing vary and include perceived burden of disease, perceived risk to have the gene, gender (women are more likely to be tested), perceived risk, desire to decrease uncertainty, availability of effective and acceptable medical interventions, concern about their current and future children, and the presence of depressive symptoms.[131]

A study of genetic testing for PPH should add substantially to the literature in a number of ways. The mutations that have been studied to date have unusually high penetrance so that most people who have these mutations will develop disease if they live long enough. Understanding how people at risk for having a mutation with very low penetrance – 80 percent of those with the mutation will never develop PPH – make decisions about testing and how they respond to the results could provide important insights as modestly predictive tests for common complex disorders become more widely available. The fact that PPH is neither common (like cancer) nor stigmatizing (like HD) offers the possibility of new insights as well.

The best current quantitative information about genetic risk is summarized in Table 14.2. Familial PPH is autosomal dominant. Thus, on average, 50 percent of the offspring of a mutation carrier, affected or unaffected, will inherit the mutation. The disease has decreased penetrance and, on average, about 20 percent of carriers will develop primary pulmonary hypertension, although the penetrance varies among sibships. The risk is higher for females, about 2:1 over males. Thus, if a parent carries the mutation, each child has a 50 percent chance of inheriting the gene and a 20 percent chance of developing disease if the gene is inherited, for a pretest probability of 10 percent of developing PPH. The risk for disease from a grandparent if the parent is clinically normal is about 5 percent. The risk in a nephew or niece of an affected uncle or aunt through a clinically normal parent is about 5 percent.

The importance of individual and family genetic counseling is shown by the example in Fig. 14.14. A young woman was about to be married and contemplating having a family. Her family had several affected members, including her aunt, who died of PPH. Her father (the aunt's brother) was clinically normal. The young woman had siblings. Her desire for genetic testing had implications for her father and siblings. Her father did not want to know if he was a carrier, both for himself and because of the anxiety and guilt if he had transmitted the mutation. The siblings were at risk of learning that they were at defined risk of having the mutation without their consent. The decision, because her risk was reasonably low, was to undergo

**Table 14.2** *Genetic basis of PPH: current understanding*

**Genetic basis of PPH**

About 5–10% of PPH occurs in families with two or more affected persons

Linkage studies locate the gene for FPPH to chromosome 2q32–33

Exonic BMPR2 mutations are identified in about 50% of PPH families

Intronic BMPR2 mutations, promoter mutations, or closely linked genes may be responsible for the remaining 50% of mutations

The penetrance of BMPR2 mutations is about 20%

In sporadic PPH, BMPR2 mutations are found in 10–25% of cases. Some of these are new spontaneous germline mutations, others are inherited, but are the only observed case in a family

A small number of PPH cases are due to inherited mutations in Alk-1, related to hereditary hemorrhagic telangiectasia

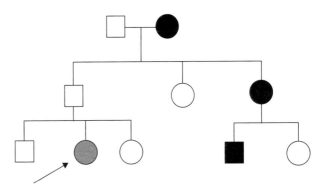

**Figure 14.14** *This pedigree shows the implications of genetic testing on family dynamics. The female in generation 3, denoted by the arrow, desired genetic testing to determine if she might pass the mutation to her children. Her grandmother, aunt, and a cousin died of PPH, but her father was clinically normal. The father did not want to know his genetic status. If the woman had genetic testing and discovered she had the mutation, then the father would be a carrier and the siblings would be known to be at risk. The decision to undergo genetic testing requires counseling to fully understand the implications of the information obtained.*

clinical screening at intervals and not to pursue haplotype testing of the family.

## GENETIC BASIS OF OTHER FORMS OF PULMONARY ARTERIAL HYPERTENSION

### Sickle cell anemia

In 1910, a practicing physician in Chicago, James Herrick, noted under the microscope that the red cells of an anemic patient from the West Indies were curved and sharp at the ends, and he described them as 'sickle shaped'.[132] By 1940, the correct inference was made that the hemoglobin in sickle cells polymerized in response to deoxygenation, resulting in deformation of the cells.[133] It was also noted that fetal hemoglobin did not allow sickling, explaining the paucity of sickle cells in the peripheral blood of newborns. In 1948, Pauling et al.[134] showed that the hemoglobin in sickle cell disease had electrophoretic differences from normal hemoglobin, and suggested that the protein structure was abnormal. Ingram[135] sequenced the amino acid structure of hemoglobin in 1956, and showed that sickle hemoglobin had a single substitution, valine for glutamic acid at position 6 of the beta chain. The abnormal hemoglobin was designated as HbS, and sickle cell anemia became the first disease with a known genetic mutation leading to an abnormal protein with well characterized molecular features. The homozygous form, HbSS, carries a high morbidity and mortality. The most common heterozygotic state is HbSA, sickle trait, in which sickling occurs rarely and only under severe hypoxic stress. Despite its unique place in the history of molecular medicine, sickle cell anemia has remained a very difficult illness, with no cure, with unsatisfactory therapies, and a great burden of suffering for those afflicted.[136,137] Hydroxyurea, by increasing fetal hemoglobin, has reduced sickle crises and improved quality of life, and newer therapies aimed at reducing sickling and improving blood flow in the microcirculation show promise.[138–140] Bone marrow transplantation has been effective in reducing HgbS production in some cases where there was a separate indication for transplantation.[141,142]

The highest prevalence of HbS in the world is in tropical central East Africa where HbS trait is as high as 45 percent, and in populations derived from migrations from West Africa.[141] The Mediterranean basin, India, and parts of Saudi Arabia have an intermediate prevalence. In the USA, Latin America, and the Caribbean, about 8 percent of blacks have sickle trait, and the expected incidence of sickle cell anemia is one in 650 births.[142] Extrapolation of these numbers suggests that almost 70 000 citizens of the USA are homozygous for HbS (HbSS) and most will develop consequences of sickle cell anemia. HbS is most often found in the heterozygous state with HbA. In combination with hemoglobin C or α-thalassemia, which do not impede sickling to the degree of HbA and HbF, sickle cell crises are less frequent but can be clinically disabling. Another modification of risk is associated with polymorphisms in the beta globin-like gene cluster and in polymorphisms in an X linked gene called the F-cell production locus, which influences the expression of HbF. Populations with HbSS but HbF levels of 15–30 percent, such as in Iran, India, and parts of Saudi Arabia, are highly protected from sickle cell anemia. Sickle cell anemia is no longer considered a single gene disorder because of the large number of pleiotropic and epistatic genes that have been identified.[143,144]

The clinical manifestations of sickle cell anemia are protean and relate to focal multiorgan ischemia and infarction.[145] Sickle cells occlude small vessels, reducing local oxygen tension which perpetuates and augments polymerization and sickling of red cells. The concomitant anemia accentuates tissue hypoxia, and organ damage increases susceptibility to subsequent crises. The most common clinical consequences of sickle cell anemia are painful bone crises, with infarction, splenic infarction and fibrosis, stroke, abdominal pain, acute chest syndrome, pulmonary hypertension, bone marrow failure, and susceptibility to infection especially *Streptococcus pneumoniae*, *Escherichia coli*, *Salmonella* osteomeylitis, and parvovirus B19.[145–148] The mortality from HbSS was nearly 100 percent before the age of 5 years in equatorial Africa when first measured. Morbidity and mortality have gradually improved with early detection and aggressive therapy. Currently, the median age at death is 42 years for men and 48 years for women.[145] Prognosis is highly related to HbF levels, the severity of anemia, and the presence of multisystem disease, especially chronic pulmonary complications, including pulmonary hypertension.[149]

The pulmonary complications of sickle cell anemia are common and account for about 20 percent of deaths.[150,151] The most common complications are asthma, thromboembolism, and the acute chest syndrome. Obstructive lung disease was found in 37 percent of 49 patients (FeV$_1$/FVC ratio <0.8) and 60 percent had increased airway reactivity. Restrictive disease is also found, presumably due to chronic repetitive airway insults related to the inflammatory chest syndrome and perhaps ischemia.[150,151] Thromboembolism is diagnosed clinically and at autopsy, but the true incidence is unknown. In addition to cell sickling, there may be a hypercoagulable state that develops during painful crises. There are no prospective studies to fully explain hypercoagulability. The acute chest syndrome is the most common cause of death and the second most frequent reason for hospitalization in adults with sickle cell anemia. The acute chest syndrome is characterized by new pulmonary infiltrate(s) on chest radiograph, fever, and chest pain, accompanied by cough, wheezing, and tachypnea.[152–154] It is unclear what or if there is a unifying etiology of the acute chest syndrome, but multiple factors including infection, pulmonary fat embolism from marrow infarction, fluid overload, intravascular pulmonary sickling, and thromboembolism have been implicated.[150–154] Unquestionably, an inflammatory milieu of cytokines, cyclooxygenase products, activated neutrophils, and fatty acids contribute to the lung injury. The acute chest syndrome frequently follows a vaso-occlusive crisis.

Pulmonary hypertension is increasingly recognized as a complication of sickle cell anemia.[155–158] Retrospective series of echocardiograms from a sickle cell disease center reveal increased pulmonary artery systolic pressure in up to 40 percent of cases. Clearly, this is a cohort with a high pretest probability of cardiopulmonary disease. Data on 34 patients with cardiopulmonary disease was recently obtained by right heart catheterization to correlate severity of pulmonary hypertension with survival.[159] Of the 20 patients with pulmonary hypertension, the pulmonary arterial pressures were: 54.3 systolic, 25.2 diastolic, and 36.0 mean mmHg, with a wedge pressure of 16.0 mmHg and cardiac output of 8.6 L/min. Pulmonary hypertension was not present in 14 patients. Of note, the mean wedge pressure in the pulmonary hypertensive group was clearly abnormal, and the mean cardiac output was almost double normal baseline value. Compared to PPH (see Clinical physiology of pulmonary hypertension), these patients with sickle cell anemia-related pulmonary hypertension had lower mean pressures, higher cardiac output, lower PVR, and evidence for left ventricular dysfunction. Each increase in mean pulmonary arterial pressure of 10 mmHg in this cohort of 34 patients was associated with a 1.7-fold increase in the rate of death (95 percent; CI, 1.1–2.7; $P = 0.028$). The median survival for patients with pulmonary hypertension was 25.6 months and over 70 percent of the non-hypertensive patients were alive at the end of the 119-month period of observation.

A recent prospective echocardiographic screening study of individuals with sickle cell anemia revealed a 30 percent prevalence of abnormal pulmonary arterial systolic pressure, ranging from mild to severe.[158]

The pathological features in the lungs of patients dying with sickle cell anemia reveal multiple mechanisms of injury.[158,160,161] Pulmonary artery intimal proliferation and organized and recanalized thromboemboli are found. There may be widespread occlusion of small- and medium-sized arteries. In acute crisis, the vasculature may be packed with marrow elements, fat and sickled red cells along with inflammatory cells. In some patients, plexiform lesions are found in small pulmonary arterioles, along with eccentric intimal fibrosis and fibrinoid necrosis. These findings point to both acute and chronic changes, with additive and progressive occlusion of vessels, a hypertensive phenotype of the media, acute and chronic thrombosis in situ, and thromboembolism. It should be noted that pulmonary hypertension is seen with increased frequency in other hematological diseases associated with hemolysis, including pyruvate kinase deficiency and thalassemia, and is also found in diseases resulting in splenectomy.[162–164] Thus, a role of free hemoglobin and iron may exist in the pathogenesis of chronic lung vascular injury and of platelet excess in situations where the spleen is dysfunctional. Both hemolysis and autosplenectomy are complications of sickle cell anemia.

The current treatment of sickle cell anemia is early detection, aggressive management of organ crisis and infection, transfusion, and chronic treatment with hydroxyurea.[165] Hydroxyurea increases fetal hemoglobin and is associated with a significant reduction in morbidity and mortality.[166a] Newer therapies with arginine supplementation to augment endogenous nitric oxide and of inhaled nitric oxide in acute chest syndrome show promise.[166] Of interest, polymorphisms in nitric oxide synthase 3 correlate with severity of the chest syndrome, where variants expected to reduce NO production are associated with worse crises.[161] Direct management of pulmonary hypertension in patients with pulmonary hypertension related to sickle cell anemia has not been studied in controlled trials.

## Gaucher's disease

Gaucher's disease (also known as Gaucher disease) is an autosomal recessive disease of the glucocerebrosidase (acid B-glucosidase) gene on chromosome 1q21, leading to defective clearance of glucocerebroside and its accumulation in the monocyte-macrophage system of multiple organs.[167,168] It is the most prevalent lysosomal storage disease, with a carrier frequency of one in 16 in Ashkenazai Jews and an incidence of one in 1000 births. The other two lysosomal storage diseases are Niemann–Pick and Fabry's diseases. Three clinical types of Gaucher's have been identified: type 1 is the adult, non-neuropathic form, in which lung disease occurs; type 2 is the infantile, neuropathic form; and type 3 is a juvenile form. Differences in phenotype are not fully understood, but four common mutations, of 35 known mutations, account for 90–95 percent of cases of Gaucher's disease.[169] Individuals homozygous for the N370S allele have less aggressive disease than those with mixed heterozygous mutations. Almost no enzymatic activity is expressed in Gaucher's tissue taken from individuals with the infantile form.[169] The large phenotypic differences in subjects with the Gaucher's genotype are not well understood. Some individuals with a Gaucher's mutation are completely normal, from families with affected members carrying the identical mutation.[170]

The most common presentations in Gaucher's disease are a combination of hepatosplenomegaly, anemia and thrombocytopenia, and bone pain.[170] Anemia and thrombocytopenia are related to bone marrow and splenic infiltration, and liver failure and pathological fractures can complicate infiltration of liver and bone. The age of presentation in type 1 disease ranges from early childhood to late adulthood, and the range and severity of manifestations varies greatly among patients. Some homozygotes are totally without symptoms or signs of disease. Radiographs of the bones may reveal lytic lesions, osteonecrosis, and the typical Ehrlenmyer flask deformity of the distal femur. Diagnosis is usually made by bone marrow biopsy, which shows brilliant macrophages on periodic acid Schiff staining, and can be confirmed either by B glucosidase enzyme assay or by DNA sequencing.[169]

Infiltration of the lung with Gaucher cells can involve the alveolar space and septum, peribronchial tissue, and the vessels themselves.[169] Occasionally, PAS-positive macrophages are seen lining the alveolar capillary luminal walls. In a prospective study, 68 percent of subjects with type I disease had some identified pulmonary function abnormality, but most were without clinical symptoms. In a referral cohort sent to a Gaucher's center, only eight of 411 (2 percent) subjects had symptomatic lung disease.[170] Three had prior splenectomy; all of the adults had bone involvement (four of four), but none of the children had evident bone disease. Thus, it appears that symptomatic pulmonary involvement is rare.

Pulmonary hypertension in Gaucher's disease has been reported in multiple small case studies. A recent clinical survey used Doppler echocardiography to measure pulmonary artery systolic pressure in a cohort of 134 patients, 90 of whom were being treated with enzyme replacement, and 40 were not treated.[171] Mild pulmonary hypertension (RV systolic pressure >35 and <50 mmHg) was detected in 30 percent of the 40 untreated patients and in 7.4 percent of the 94 treated patients. Only one patient of the 134 was symptomatic, with an RV systolic pressure greater than 55 mmHg. Of interest, the mean RV systolic pressure in untreated patients was significantly higher than those receiving enzyme therapy, $30 \pm 10$ mmHg versus $23 \pm 8$ mmHg. In a separate group of nine patients referred to these investigators for severe pulmonary hypertension, all were asplenic and had thrombocytosis. Responses to glucocerebrocidase therapy with or without vasodilator therapy were promising, with a reduction in RVSP from $92 \pm 27$ to $56 \pm 25$ mmHg. Other positive responses to intravenous epoprostenol and inhaled iloprost in patients with Gaucher's disease and severe pulmonary hypertension have been reported.[172,173] Glucocerebrosidase is effective in reducing radiographic pulmonary infiltration, increasing DLCO and $FEV_1$ and improving arterial oxygenation in a growing number of reports of Gaucher's patients with advanced pulmonary disease.

In summary, symptomatic pulmonary disease occurs in a minority of patients with Gaucher's disease, but subclinical lung infiltration is probably common, including pulmonary vascular obstruction. Severe pulmonary hypertension occurs in about 1 percent of cases, which is much more common than in the general population. The pulmonary hypertension is probably multifactorial, including obstruction of the vasculature by cerebroside-laden macrophages, chronic complications of splenectomy, and possible contributions of portopulmonary disease. It seems unlikely that enzyme replacement therapy causes the pulmonary hypertension, but pulmonary hypertension can worsen during therapy. The clinical approach to pulmonary hypertension in Gaucher's disease should probably be similar to that of idiopathic pulmonary arterial hypertension, with consideration of vasodilator therapy and anticoagulation, especially in splenectomized patients.[174] A trial of enzyme therapy in patients with advanced disease seems warranted.

## Inherited thrombophilia and pulmonary hypertension

Thrombophilia is a synonym for the hypercoagulable state, but is a preferable term because many people with thrombophilic diseases are not manifestly hypercoagulable and may completely avoid the thrombotic consequences of their predisposition.[175,176] The link between thrombophilia and pulmonary hypertension is venous thrombosis complicated by pulmonary embolism (VTE). The most common inherited disorders of coagulation are shown in Table 14.3.

**Table 14.3**   *Inherited thrombophilia and pulmonary embolism*

| Condition | Carrier state (%) | Risk of VTE (%) | Prevalence in VTE series (%) |
|---|---|---|---|
| Factor V Leiden | 4–7 | 13–20 | 25–50 |
| Prothrombin mutation | 1–3 | 10 | 6 |
| Protein C deficiency | 0.2–0.4 | 10–50 by age 40 | up to 4 |
| Protein S deficiency | 2 | 20 | 3 |
| Antithrombin deficiency | 0.02 | 80 by age 55 | <1 |
| Compound heterozygotes | <0.2% | >80 | 2 |

Factor V Leiden: autosomal dominant, mutation Arg506Gln in factor Va heavy chain, causing resistance to activated protein C cleavage. Homozygotes have an 80-fold increased risk of VTE. *Prothrombin mutation*: Point mutation G20210A in 3'UTR of prothrombin gene, autosomal dominant, causes increased prothrombin levels, a gain of function mutation. *Protein C deficiency*: Unclear whether autosomal recessive or requires mixed heterozygosity. Up to 160 mutations reported, associated with reduced Protein C levels. *Protein S deficiency*: Autosomal dominant, may require concomitant APC resistance in heterozygous state. *Anti-thrombin deficiency*: a serine protease inactivates thrombin, and factors Xa–X11a, autosomal dominant, major effect is deficient neutralization of factor Xa.

In general, each of these disorders carries an increased inherent risk for the development of VTE, which can be multiplied by a number of additional conditions including immobilization, trauma, surgery, pregnancy, use of birth control pills, neoplastic diseases, and the compound heterozygous state of carriage of two or more inherited risks. In addition, acquired conditions of antiphospholipid antibodies, hyperhomocysteinemia, and increased levels of factor VIII increase the risk of VTE, especially in the context of inherited thrombophilia.[177] Inherited fibrinolytic defects are rare in the general population and do not show up in most surveys. Fibrinolytic defects are associated with venous thrombosis, pulmonary embolism, and pulmonary arterial hypertension in case reports of families.[178]

As discussed in Clinical physiology of pulmonary hypertension, pulmonary hypertension usually occurs only when a majority of the pulmonary vascular bed is occluded. In acute pulmonary embolism, probably because of the release of vasoconstrictive mediators, a smaller occlusion can result in measurable increases in pulmonary vascular pressure. In pulmonary embolism, as little as 30 percent reduction of perfusion of the vascular bed as measured by perfusion lung scan is associated with significant right ventricular strain.[179] The position of the embolus partly determines its effect on right ventricular pressure; an embolus lodged in a main pulmonary artery has a greater impact on right ventricular outflow resistance and pressure than does a similar-sized clot distributed to peripheral branches. Thus, multiple small emboli, even those that result in distal lung infarction, may have a lesser impact on pulmonary pressures and right ventricular strain.

The true incidence of pulmonary hypertension after acute pulmonary thromboembolism is unknown, but Doppler echocardiography provides an index of the incidence and of impact on right ventricular performance.[180,181] A prospective study of 110 consecutive patients with suspected pulmonary embolism yielded 43 cases confirmed by pulmonary angiography.[180] The following echocardiographic criteria were used to detect pulmonary hypertension: right ventricular hypokinesis, RV end-diastolic diameter >27 mm, or tricuspid regurgitation velocity >2.7 m/s (corresponding to a RV to right atrial pressure gradient of about 30 mmHg). The echocardiogram was 56 percent sensitive and 90 percent specific for the presence of pulmonary embolism. Thus, about 56 percent of patients with acute pulmonary embolism have evidence of at least mild pulmonary hypertension. The cohort of patients included about 60 percent with known cardiovascular, pulmonary, or neoplastic disease, and the majority had known risks including surgery or fractures or other causes of immobilization. One might guess that echocardiograms would have erred towards overdiagnosis in a cohort with heart and lung disease, suggesting that the discovery of a 56 percent incidence of pulmonary hypertension was not an overestimate. As expected, higher RV systolic pressures, greater than 55 mmHg, were associated with greater RV dysfunction and morbidity. In one prospective study of 78 patients with documented PE, the regression of PA pressures was exponential, with the majority of patients achieving normal pressures within 10–21 days.[180] Longterm prognosis was related to right ventricular function and PA pressure. A right ventricular-to-left ventricular end diastolic diameter ratio greater than 1, an RV end diastolic diameter greater than 30 mm, or paradoxical RV septal systolic motion are the best predictors of outcome in acute pulmonary embolism (PE) associated with pulmonary hypertension.

Management of large pulmonary embolism with RV strain remains controversial.[182,183] Recommended therapies range from heparinization, to heparinization plus inferior vena caval filter, thrombolytic therapy, catheter-based fragmentation, or acute surgical thrombectomy. There is no clearly superior, evidence-based standard of care for acute massive pulmonary embolism with right heart failure.

A small number of patients with acute pulmonary embolism develop the syndrome, chronic thromboembolic pulmonary hypertension (CTEPH).[184] The reasons for the transformation are unclear, but may relate to the extent of embolism, failure to fully lyse the clot, the pulmonary vascular response to increased pressure, and interactions between the clot and the cells of the vascular intima. Prior splenectomy may be a risk.[185] CTEPH is estimated to occur in less than 0.5 percent of patients with acute pulmonary thromboembolism. Patients present with symptoms and signs typical of advanced pulmonary arterial hypertension with dyspnea, easy fatigue, cough, chest pain, and edema. In many cases, careful history will reveal a remote episode of thrombophlebitis or of an episode of an acute lung process

that was, in restrospect, misdiagnosed as pneumonia. The thromboembolic episode may predate the presentation of symptomatic CTEPH by 2–10 years.[184]

Management of CTEPH relies on accurate diagnosis, which is suspected by appropriate history and physical examination and confirmed by tests in the algorithm (Fig. 14.1, page 364). Curative management is pulmonary thromboendarterectomy. The world's largest experience is at the University of California, San Diego, where 1500 cases have been reported since 1990.[184] In the last 500 patients, 45 percent gave a prior history of deep venous thrombosis and 30 percent had no history suggestive of pulmonary embolism. The mean PA pressures were 46 ± 5 mmHg, mean systolic 77 ± 18, cardiac output 3.8 L/min and PVR 893 dynes/s/cm. Surgical survival was 95.6 percent. The majority of patients improve by at least one New York heart class, and most patients become clinically normal, residing in NYH class 1 or 2 post-endarterectomy. All patients receive inferior vena caval filters and are anticoagulated for life.

Most evaluations of patients with CTEPH for an increased prevalence of inherited thrombophilia have been surprisingly negative.[185,186] Approximately 15–30 percent of patients with CTEPH have an acquired or inherited hypercoagulable state.[186] Antiphospholipid antibodies are the most frequent finding, in 12 of one study of 24 patients, with hyperhomocysteinemia found in seven. Inherited thrombophilia was found only in one case each of protein C deficiency, protein S deficiency, antithrombin deficiency, and prothrombin gene mutation. Factor V Leiden, the most prevalent inherited thrombophilia, was not found. Five patients were compound heterozygotes. In other studies of CTEPH, Factor V Leiden was found in the same 5 percent prevalence as in the general population.[187] Search for fibrinolytic defects has been largely unrewarding, including plasminogen activator inhibitor (PAI-1) abnormalities.[186] Inherited thrombolytic defects have been reported in case studies of single families with CTEPH, but these diseases are too rare for a population effect. Thus, the pathogenesis of chronic thrombotic pulmonary hypertension does not appear to involve abnormalities of coagulation or lysis out of proportion to that seen in acute venous thrombosis and pulmonary embolism.

Testing for the presence of inherited or acquired thrombophilia depends on the pretest likelihood of disease, and on the therapeutic impact of seeking such information. Inherited thrombophilia should be considered in the circumstances listed in Table 14.4. Recurrent idiopathic VTE should engender a search, as should a single idiopathic VTE under the age of 45 years. A family history of VTE, especially in members under the age of 45, warrants evaluation.[188–190] A known familial cause of thrombophilia should generate a search because the intensity and duration of prophylaxis and therapy might be altered. Stroke, arterial thrombosis, or recurrent fetal loss during pregnancy should trigger a search, especially for acquired antiphospholipid antibodies.[189] Because immobilization, surgery, birth control pills,

**Table 14.4** *Indications for testing for inherited or acquired thrombophilia*

Idiopathic venous thromboembolism (VTE) (not secondary to known risks)
Thrombosis or embolism from unusual sites
Recurrent VTE or recurrent unexplained loss of pregnancy
VTE under the age of 45 years
Positive family history of VTE or of known inherited thrombophilia

and pregnancy are such multipliers of the risk of VTE in persons with inherited thrombophilia, up to 30-fold increased risk, knowledge of a hypercoagulable state can help prevent thrombotic occurrences.[189] Purpura fulminans in an infant should engender a search for heterozygous Protein C deficiency in the parents.[189] Warfarin skin necrosis is an indication for searching for Protein C or S deficiency.[189]

Accurate testing for thrombophilia requires knowledge of the basis of the test and the influence of clinical condition and anticoagulation on test results. DNA tests, including Factor V Leiden and the prothrombin G20210A mutation are feasible at any stage of disease or therapeutic intervention.[188] The most common Factor V mutation accounts for 92 percent of inherited cases of activated protein C resistance, so the recommended screening test is for activated protein C resistance, which should detect nearly 100 percent of cases.[191] If positive, DNA testing can detect the nature of the mutation. Protein C and S are both vitamin K-dependent and cannot be reliably done if the patient is receiving warfarin.[191] Protein C and S are also consumed during acute thrombosis and levels may be reduced at the time of acute VTE. Antithrombin is also depleted during acute thrombosis and levels are unreliable during heparin anticoagulation.[189] Antiphospholipid antibodies can be measured at any time during disease, however the activated partial thromboplastin time (aPTT) will be prolonged by heparin.[189] Homocysteine levels are dependent on dietary methionine but can be measured during acute thrombosis or anticoagulation.[191]

Other rare inherited causes of either thrombophilia, platelet dysfunction, or fibrinolytic defects include: heparin cofactor II deficiency, an autosomal dominant trait; hyperhomocysteinemia due to mutation in cystathionine B-synthase (which metabolizes homocysteine to cystathionine) in 0.3 to 1 percent of the population or in methylene tetrahydrofolate reductase (which remethylates homocysteine to methionine), a C677T polymorphism; increased factor VIII activity (of unclear genetic origin and an acute phase reactant); dysplasminogenemia (more common in Japan); thrombomodulin deficiency (rare, associated with arterial and venous thrombosis); and tissue plasminogen activator polymorphisms. Inherited platelet abnormalities are more associated with arterial thrombosis and coronary disease than with venous thrombosis and embolism.[191] These include polymorphisms for glycoprotein (gp) IIIa (ITGB3), gpIa (807T allele), and GP1BA.[191]

In summary, pulmonary hypertension is associated with inherited disorders of blood coagulation and lysis primarily by the complications of venous thrombosis and pulmonary embolism. Although disorders of coagulation are very common in cohorts of patients with pulmonary embolism, the presence of acute or chronic thrombotic pulmonary hypertension does not seem dependent on the mechanism of thrombophilia. Mild pulmonary hypertension, PA systolic pressure >30 mmHg and <55 mmHg, occurs in about 50 percent of acute pulmonary embolism, but resolves over days to weeks. Severe pulmonary hypertension, with RV strain and dysfunction, occurs in less than 5 percent of diagnosed pulmonary embolism. Management of acute pulmonary embolism is not altered by knowledge of the presence of inherited thrombophilia. The practice of full anticoagulation with a heparin formulation during the first 2 days of a vitamin K antagonist avoids the complication of skin necrosis in patients with undiagnosed protein C or S deficiency. Chronic thromboembolic pulmonary hypertension is best managed by surgical endarterectomy. The duration of anticoagulation after VTE may be extended in patients with known inherited thrombophilia. The antiphospholipid syndrome, highly associated both with thromboembolic pulmonary hypertension, as well as histological PPH, requires lifelong anticoagulation.[192,193]

## Hypoxic pulmonary hypertension

Hypoxic pulmonary vasoconstriction, followed by muscularization of the pulmonary arterioles and precapillary vessels, is the cause of pulmonary hypertension in a large number of conditions and diseases.[194,195] These range from hypoventilation syndromes,[196] to diseases of ventilation–perfusion mismatch, especially emphysema[197] to neuromuscular diseases[198] and to high altitude illnesses.[199] Independent of diseases that interfere with oxygenation and ventilation, the two major inherited characteristics that determine the pulmonary response to hypoxia are ventilatory drives and the hypoxic pressor response.[200,201]

Hypoxic pulmonary vasoconstriction was first discovered by von Euler and Liljestrand in 1946.[202] They correctly surmized that focal hypoxic vasoconstriction might function to improve oxygenation by diverting blood from poorly ventilated regions of lung, but that generalized hypoxic vasoconstriction could lead to elevated pulmonary arterial pressure. Despite over 50 years of effort, the exact mechanism of acute hypoxic vasoconstriction remains elusive, although much is known about modifying influences.[200] Pulmonary vasoconstriction is enhanced by acidosis, most often by retention of carbon dioxide, and the pulmonary vascular pressures are modified by the degree of secondary erthrocytosis and other determinants of viscosity. Hypoxic vasoconstriction relies on calcium entry into smooth muscle cells, and on activation of actin filaments.[201,202] Of interest, recent data show that the normal BMPR2 receptor inhibits

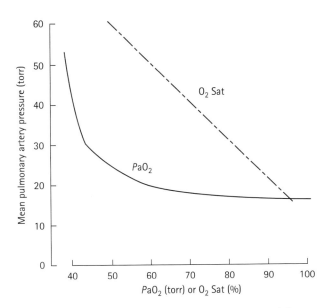

**Figure 14.15** *Graph of the effect of arterial pO₂ or arterial blood oxygen saturation on pulmonary arterial pressure in normal man. Pulmonary arterial pressure rises as the pO₂ decreases below 55 torr. The relationship reflects the shape of the oxyhemoglobin desaturation curve.*

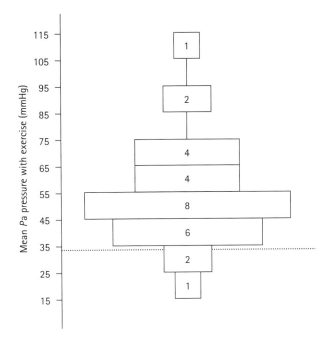

**Figure 14.16** *Pulmonary arterial pressure by right heart catheterization in 28 normal young adults residing chronically at high altitude (10 200 ft) during supine exercise.[208] All but three developed significant pulmonary hypertension. The dotted line represents the upper limit of normal during exercise at sea level. The width of the bars represents the frequency of distribution of pressures within a 5 mmHg range. Thus, pulmonary hypertension is normal and can be sustained by normal hearts at altitude.*

LIMK1, which normally regulates cofilin, an actin depolymerizing factor.[203] Thus, mutated BMPR2 might be associated with increased vasoreactivity, a potential new modifying effect in the development of pulmonary hypertension. Variations in K channel activity and NOS polymorphisms in hypoxia sensing genes are being studied.[200–202] Differences among individuals in the response of the pulmonary vascular bed to back pressure from left heart mechanics and to shear stress through alterations in pressure and flow may also have a genetic basis. No major genes in humans have been identified that determine the strength of the hypoxic pressor response. However, multiple observations have confirmed that inherited variation in ventilatory responses and the hypoxic pressor response have major effects on pulmonary artery dynamics.[201]

The pulmonary hypertensive response to chronic hypoxia in humans is shown in Fig. 14.15. Pulmonary hypertension does not occur until the *p*O₂ decreases into the range of 50–60 mmHg, consistent with the steep portion of the oxyhemoglobin dissociation curve. Of interest, the shape of the pulmonary pressor response to graded hypoxia is quite similar to the ventilatory response to hypoxia and that of secondary erythrocytosis. Pulmonary arterial pressures can be quite high in normal humans exposed to hypoxia for prolonged periods of time. Right heart catheterization at rest and exercise in 18 normal subjects in Leadville, CO, elevation 10 600 feet, is shown in Fig. 14.16.[204] The variance in pressure and the degree of pulmonary hypertension are striking in these normal high-altitude dwellers. A genetic basis of high altitude pulmonary hypertension

is best demonstrated in the cow.[205] Brisket disease is the development of edema secondary to right heart failure in cows that develop high altitude pulmonary hypertension. It is not present in all herds and some cows can live at 3000–4000 m without disease. The tendency to this complication is clearly inherited. Cows with the pre-exposure tendency to hypoxic pulmonary hypertension pass the trait to their offspring and cows that thrive at altitude breed resistant offspring.[205] The gene or genes controling this attribute are not known. Species differences in the pulmonary vascular response to acute and chronic hypoxia are well documented. Cattle and pigs have a high response, whereas sheep, llamas, and rabbits have a lesser response.[203] Humans have a mid-range acute pulmonary pressor response to hypoxia, but clearly are able to generate high degrees of pulmonary hypertension with chronic high altitude dwelling. It is not clear what predispositions determine the response. The basal degree of medial thickness roughly correlates with severity of chronic pulmonary hypertension in most species, as does the basal hypoxic pressor response, and collateral ventilation may have a protective effect in situations of regional alveolar hypoxia.

Racial differences may underly some of the responses to high altitude exposure.[201,206,207] Chronic high altitude pulmonary hypertension is rare in the Tibetan sherpa, but not uncommon in the Quechua of the Andes. Numerous studies have been unable to clearly separate high altitude responses in these two populations, but the weight of evidence is that the sherpa has more responsive ventilation to hypoxia and may be protected at high altitudes during exercise and perhaps during sleep.[201] The ventilatory response to hypoxia and to hypercarbia clearly varies among individuals and has a genetic component. Hypoventilation, especially during sleep when the stimulus response is downregulated, causes hypoxia and hypercapnia and may result in chronic pulmonary hypertension, the cause of which is not easily diagnosed when the subject is awake. The ventilatory response to chronic hypoxia is complicated and depends on the chronicity. Studies are underway in animals to determine genes responsible for control of ventilation, but genetic control of ventilation in humans is not known.

The genetic basis of variations in the hypoxic pressor response and in ventilatory responses in humans is unknown and will certainly come under active scrutiny. As with other inherited conditions, families with measurable, heritable disorders will need to be identified and have DNA banked for linkage studies and studies of candidate genes of interest. There may be no single, or even multiple, genes of major effect, but it is likely that sets of polymorphisms will predispose to pulmonary hypertension during acute and chronic hypoxic exposure.

## Key learning points

- Genes play a dominant role in some forms of pulmonary hypertension, especially pulmonary arterial hypertension, hereditary hemorrhagic telangiectasia, and sickle cell anemia.

- Multiple genes may modify pulmonary hypertension through functional polymorphisms, such as serotonin transport.

- Collections of genes may determine susceptibility to disease, such as with blunted ventilatory drives and the tendency to develop obesity or the metabolic syndrome.

- The study of the genetic basis of pulmonary hypertension is in its infancy.

- Understanding of the signaling abnormalities of TGFbeta receptors will lead to therapies to treat or prevent idiopathic pulmonary arterial hypertension.

## ACKNOWLEDGMENTS

This work was supported by grants NIH NHLBI PO1 HL 072058, Clinical Research Center RR 00095, VA TVHS GRECC.

## REFERENCES

1   Rich S. (ed.) Primary pulmonary hypertension. Executive Summary from the World Symposium on Cardiovascular Diseases. World Health Organization, 1998.

◆2   Rubin LJ, Galie N (eds). Third World Symposium on Pulmonary Hypertension, Venice, June 2003, 23–25. *J Am Coll Cardiol* 2004; 43S.

✳3   Rubin LJ. Primary pulmonary hypertension. *N Engl J Med* 1997; **336**: 111–7.

4   Newman JH, Trembath RC, Morse JA et al. Genetic basis of pulmonary arterial hypertension: current understanding and future directions. *J Am Coll Cardiol* 2004; **43**: 33–40S.

●5   Lane KB, Machado RD, Pauciulo MW et al. Heterozygous germline mutations in BMPR2, encoding a TGF-beta receptor, cause familial primary pulmonary hypertension. The International PPH Consortium. *Nat Genet* 2000; **26**: 81–4.

●6   Deng Z, Morse JH, Slager SL et al. Familial primary pulmonary hypertension (gene PPH1) is caused by mutations in the bone morphogenetic protein receptor-II gene. *Am J Hum Gen* 2000; **67**: 737–44.

●7   Trembath RC, Thomson JR, Machado RD et al. Clinical and molecular genetic features of pulmonary hypertension in patients with hereditary hemorrhagic telangiectasia. *N Engl J Med* 2001; **345**: 325–34.

8   Waite KA, Eng C. From developmental disorder to heritable cancer: it's all in the BMP/TGF-β family. *Nature Rev* 2003; **4**: 763–73.

9   de Caestecker M. The transforming growth factor-beta superfamily of receptors. *Cytokin Growth Factor Rev* 2004; **15**: 1–11.

10   Farber HW, Loscalzo J. Pulmonary arterial hypertension. *N Engl J Med* 2004; **351**: 1655–65.

11   Newman JH, Fanburg BL, Archer SL et al. Pulmonary arterial hypertension: future directions report of an NHLBI/ORD Workshop. *Circulation* 2004; **109**: 2947–54.

●12   Rich S, Dantzker DR, Ayres SM et al. Primary pulmonary hypertension. A national prospective study. *Ann Intern Med* 1987; **107**: 216–23.

●13   Thomson JR, Machado RD, Pauciulo MW et al. Sporadic primary pulmonary hypertension is associated with germline mutations of the gene encoding BMPR2, a receptor member of the TGF-beta family. *J Med Genet* 2000; **37**: 741–5.

14   Weir EK, Reeves JT. *Pulmonary vascular physiology and pathophysiology, lung biology in health and disease*, Vol. 38. New York: Marcel Dekker, 1989.

15   Fishman AP, Fisher AB, Geiger SR. *Section 3. The pulmonary circulation, in the respiratory system. Handbook of physiology*. Bethesda, MD: American Physiological Society, 1995: 93–165.

16   Chatterjee K, De Marco T, Alpert J. Pulmonary hypertension: hemodynamic diagnosis and management. *Arch Intern Med* 2002; **162**: 1925–33.

17   Janicki JS, Weber KT, Likoff MJ, Fishman AP. The pressure-flow response of the pulmonary circulation in patients with heart failure and pulmonary vascular disease. *Circulation* 1985; **6**: 1270–8.

18   Konstam MA, Levine HJ. Effects of afterload and preload on right ventricular systolic performance. In: *In the right heart*. New York: Martinus Nijhoff 1988: 17–35 (Chapter 2).

19  Yang YY, Lin HC, Lee WC et al. Portopulmonary hypertension: distinctive hemodynamic and clinical manifestations. *J Gastroenterol* 2001; **36**: 181–6.

20  Fallon MB. Portopulmonary hypertension: new clinical insights and more questions on pathogenesis. *Hepatology* 2003; **37**: 253–5.

21  Braunwald E, Colucci W, Grossman W. Clinical aspects of heart failure. In: Braunwald E. (ed.) *Heart disease,* Vol. 1, Philadelphia: WB Saunders, 1997; **15**: 443–67.

22  Guyton AC, Lindsey AW, Gilluly JJ. The limits of right ventricular compensation following acute increases in pulmonary circulatory resistance. *Circ Res* 1954; **2**: 326.

23  Brooks H, Kirk ES, Bokibasm PS et al. Performance of the right ventricle under stress: relation to right coronary flow. *J Clin Invest* 1971; **50**: 2176.

◆24  Fishman AP. State of the art: chronic cor pulmonale. *Am Rev Respir Dis* 1976; **114**: 775–94.

25  Asherson RA, Cervera R. Review: antiphospholipid antibodies and the lung. *J Rheumatol* 1995; **22**: 62–6.

26  Kanemoto N. Electrocardiogram in primary pulmonary hypertension – with special reference to prognosis. *Tokai J Exp Clin Med* 1987; **12**: 73–9.

27  Powell JE, Palevsky HI, McCarthy KE, Alavi A. Pulmonary arterial hypertension: value of perfusion scintigraphy. *Radiology* 1987; **164**: 727–30.

◆28  Fedullo PF, Auger WR, Channick RN et al. Chronic thromboembolic pulmonary hypertension. *Clin Chest Med* 2001; **22**: 561–81.

29  The PIOPED Investigators. Value of the ventilation/perfusion scan in acute pulmonary embolism: results of the prospective investigation of pulmonary embolism diagnosis (PIOPED). *J Am Med Assoc* 1993; **263**: 2753.

30  Auger WR, Fedullo PF, Moser KM et al. Chronic major-vessel thromboembolic pulmonary artery obstruction: appearance at angiography. *Radiology* 1992; **182**: 393–5.

✳31  Jamieson SW, Kapelanski DP, Sakakibara N et al. Pulmonary endarterectomy: experience and lessons learned in 1500 cases. *Ann Thorac Surg* 2003; **76**: 1457–64.

32  D'Alonzo GE, Robyn DO, Barst J et al. Survival in patients with primary pulmonary hypertension results from a national prosective registry. *Ann Int Med* 1991; **115**: 343–9.

●33  Rich S, Kaurmann EL. The effect of high doses of calcium channel blockers on survival in primary pulmonary hypertension. *N Engl J Med* 1992; **327**: 76–81.

34  Rich S, Brundage BH. High-dose calcium channel-blocking therapy for primary pulmonary hypertension: evidence for long-term reduction in pulmonary arterial pressure and regression of right ventricular hypertrophy. *Circulation* 1987; **76**: 135–41.

●35  Barst RJ, Rubin LJ, Long WA et al. A comparison of continuous intravenous epopostenol (prostacyclin) with conventional therapy for primary pulmonary hypertension. The Primary Pulmonary Hypertension Study Group. *N Engl J Med* 1996; **334**: 296–302.

36  McLaughlin VV, Genthnew DE, Panella MM, Rich S. Reduction in pulmonary vascular resistance with long-term epoprostenol (prostacylin) therapy in primary pulmonary hypertension. *N Engl J Med* 1998; **338**: 273–7.

37  Kuhn KP, Byrne DW, Arbogast PG et al. Outcome in 91 consecutive patients with pulmonary arterial hypertension receiving epoprostenol. *Am J Resp Crit Care Med* 2003; **167**: 580–6.

38  Simonneau G, Barst RJ, Galie N et al. Treprostinil Study Group. Continuous subcutaneous infusion of treprostinil, a prostacyclin analogue, in PAH. *Am J Respir Crit Care Med* 2002; **165**: 800–4.

39  Galie N, Humbert M, Vachiery JL et al. Arterial pulmonary hypertension and beraprost European Study Group. Effects of beraprost sodium, an oral prostacyclin analogue, in PAH. *J Am Coll Cardiol* 2002; **39**: 1496–502.

40  Olschewski H, Simonneau G, Galie N et al. Inhaled iloprost for severe pulmonary hypertension. *N Engl J Med* 2002; **347**: 332–9.

✳41  Hoeper MM, Galie N, Simonneau G, Rubin LJ. New treatments for pulmonary arterial hypertension. *Am J Resp Crit Care Med* 2002; **165**: 1209–16.

42  Rubin LJ, Badesch DB, Barst RJ et al. Bosentan in patients with pulmonary artery hypertension: a randomized, placebo controlled, multicenter strudy. *N Engl J Med* 2002; **346**: 896–903.

43  Michelakis E, Tymachak W, Lien D et al. Oral sildenafil is an effective and specific pulmonary vasodilator in patients with pulmonary arterial hypertension: comparison with inhaled nitric oxide. *Circulation* 2002; **105**: 2398–403.

44  Prasad S, Wilinson J, Gatzoulis MA. Sildenafil in primary pulmonary hypertension. *N Engl J Med* 2000; **343**: 1342.

45  Nishimura T, Faul JL, Berry GL et al. Simvastatin attenuates smooth muscle neointimal proliferation and pulmonary hypertension in rats. *Am J Resp Crit Care Med* 2002; **166**: 1403–8.

46  Reichart B, Gulbins M, Meiser BM et al. Improved results after heart–lung transplantation: a 17 year experience. *Transplantation* 2003; **75**: 127–32.

47  Edwards LB, Keck BM. Thoracic organ transplantation in the US. *Clin Transpl* 2002; 29–40.

●48  Dresdale DT, Shultz M, Michtom RJ. Primary pulmonary hypertension. Clinical and hemodynamic study. *Am J Med* 1951; **11**: 686–701.

49  Dresdale DT, Michtom RT, Shultz M. Recent studies in primary pulmonary hypertension, including observation on pulmonary vascular resistance. *Bull NY Acad Med* 1954; **30**: 195–207.

●50  Loyd JE, Primm RK, Newman JH. Familial primary pulmonary hypertension: clinical patterns. *Am Rev Resp Dis* 1984; **129**: 194–7.

●51  Loyd JE, Butler MG, Foroud TM et al. Genetic anticipation and abnormal gender ratio at birth in familial primary pulmonary hypertension. *Am J Resp Crit Care Med* 1995; **152**: 93–97.

52  Elliott G, Alexander G, Leppert M et al. Coancestry in apparently sporadic primary pulmonary hypertension. *Chest* 1995; **108**: 973–7.

●53  Thomson JR, Machado RD, Pauciulo MW et al. Sporadic primary pulmonary hypertension is associated wth germline mutations of the gene encoding BMPR-II, a receptor member of the TGF-beta family. *J Med Genet* 2000; **37**: 741–5.

54  Reddy PS, Housman DE. The complex pathology of trunucleotide repeats. *Curr Opin Cell Biol* 1997; **9**: 364–72.

55  Liquori CL, Ricker K, Moseley ML et al. Myotonic dystrophy type II caused by a CCTG expansion in intron 1 of ZNF9. *Science* 2001; **293**: 864–7.

56  Siden RR. Origins of instability. Neurodegenerative disease. *Nature* 2001; **411**: 757–8.

57  Ashley CT Jr, Warren ST. Trinucleotide repeat expansion and human disease. *Ann Rev Genet* 1995; **29**: 703–28.

58  Inaminshi T, Itoh T, Suzuki Y et al. Integrative annotation of 21,037 human genes validated by full-length cDNA clones. *PLOS Biol* 2004; **4** (Epub).

59  Matsuura T, Yamagata T, Burgess DL et al. Large expansion of the ATTCT pentanucleotide repeat in spinocerebellar ataxia type 10. *Nat Genet* 2000; **26**: 191–4.

●60  Yaeger ME, Halley GR, Golpon HA et al. Microsatellite instability of endothelial cell growth and apoptosis genes within plexiform lesions in primary pulmonary hypertension. *Circ Res* 2001; **88**: E2–E11.

●61  Sullivan KJ, Kissoon N, Duckworth LJ et al. NOS gene is associated with acute chest syndrome. *Am J Respir Crit. Care Med* 2001; **164**: 2186–90.

62  Wagenvoort CA, Wagenvoort N. Primary pulmonary hypertension: a pathological study of the lung vessels in 156 clinically diagnosed cases. *Circulation* 1970; **42**: 1163–82.

63  Edwards WD. Pathology of pulmonary hypertension. *Cardiovasc Clin* 1987; **18**: 321–59.

◆64  Pietra GG, Edwards WD, Kay JM et al. Histopathology of PPH. Study of 58 patients from the NIH Registry. *Circulation* 1989; **80**: 1198–1206.

65  Loyd JE, Atkinson JB, Pietra GG et al. Heterogeneity of pathological lesions in familial primary pulmonary hypertension. *Am Rev Resp Dis* 1988; **138**: 952–7.

●66  Geraci MW, Moore M, Gesell T et al. Gene expression patterns in the lungs of patients with primary pulmonary hypertension: a gene microarray analysis. *Circ Res* 2001; **88**: 555–62.

67  Wagenvoort CA. Lung biopsy findings in secondary pulmonary hypertension. *Heart Lung* 1986; **15**: 429–50.

68  Moser KM, Bloor CM. Pulmonary vascular lesions occurring in patients with chronic major vessel thromboembolic pulmonary hypertension. *Chest* 1993; **103**: 685–92.

69  Nichols WC, Koller DL, Slovis B et al. Localization of the gene for familial PPH to chromosome 2q31-32. *Nat Genet* 1997; **15**: 277–81.

70  Morse JH, Barst RJ, Fotino et al. Primary pulmonary hypertension, tissue plasminogen activator antibodies and HLA-DQ7. *Am J Resp Crit Care Med* 1997; **155**: 274–8.

71  Morse JH. Bone morphogenetic protein receptor 2 mutations in pulmonary hypertension. *Chest* 2002; **121**: 50–3S.

◆72  Newman JH, Wheeler L, Lane KB et al. Mutation in the gene for bone porphogenetic protein receptor II as a course of primary pulmonary hypertension in a large kindred. *N Engl J Med* 2001; **345**: 319–24.

73  Abenhaim L, Moride Y, Brenot F et al. Appetite-suppressant drugs and the risk of primary pulmonary hypertension. International Primary Pulmonary Hypertension Study Group. *N Engl J Med* 1996; **335**: 609–16.

74  Humbert M, Deng Z, Simonneau G et al. BMPR2 germline mutations in pulmonary hypertension associated with fenfluramine derivatives. *Eur Resp J* 2002; **20**: 518–23.

75  Morse J, Barst R, Horn E et al. Pulmonary hypertension in scleroderma spectrum of disease: lack of bone morphogenetic protein receptor 2 mutations. *J Rheumatol* 2002; **29**: 2379–81.

76  Nunes H, Humbert M, Sitbon O et al. Prognostic factors for survival in HIV-associated pulmonary arterial hypertension. *Am J Resp Crit Care Med* 2003; **167**: 1433–9.

77  Wheeler L, Newman JH, Phillips JA, Loyd JE. Update of the primary pulmonary hypertension family registry: new mutations, modifier genes and apparently sporadic cases. *Am J Resp Crit Care Med* 2005 (in press).

◆78  Blobe GC, Schiemann WP, Lodish HF. Mechanisms of disease: role of transforming growth factor (beta) in human disease. *N Engl J Med* 2000; **342**: 1350–8.

●79  Machado RD, Pauciulo MW, Thomson JR et al. BMPR2 haploinsufficiency as the inherited molecular mechanism for primary pulmonary hypertension. *Am J Hum Genet* 2001; **68**: 92–102.

80  Kawabata M, Chytil A, Moses HL. Cloning of a novel type II serine/threonine kinase receptor through interaction with the type I transforming growth factor-beta receptor. *J Biol Chem* 1995; **270**: 5625–30.

81  Nohno T, Ishikawa T, Saito T et al. Identification of a human type II receptor for bone morphogenetic protein-4 that forms differential heteromeric complexes with bone morphogenetic protein type I receptors. *J Biol Chem* 1995; **270**: 22522–6.

82  Bellusci S, Henderson G, Winnier G et al. Evidence from normal expression and targeted misexpression that bone morphogenetic protein (Bmp-4) plays a role in mouse embryonic lung morphogenesis. *Development* 1996; **122**: 1693–702.

◆83  Warburton D, Schwarz M, Tefft D et al. The molecular basis of lung morphogenesis. *Mech Dev* 2000; **92**: 55–81.

84  Ducy P, Karsenty G. The family of bone morphogenetic proteins. *Kidney Int* 2000; **57**: 2207–14.

85  Josso N, di Clemente N. Serine/threonine kinase receptors and ligands. *Curr Opin Genet Dev* 1997; **7**: 371–7.

◆86  Heldin CH, Miyazono K, ten Dijke P. TGF-beta signaling from cell membrane to nucleus through SMAD proteins. *Nature* 1997; **390**: 465–71.

87  Hild M, Dick A, Bauer H et al. The roles of BMP's, BMP antagonists, and the BMP signaling transucers Smad1 and Smad5 during dorsoventral patterning of the zebrafish embryo. *Ernst Schering Research Foundation Workshop* 2000; **29**: 81–106.

88  Ramsdell AF, Yost HJ. Cardiac looping and the vertebrate left-right axis: antagonism of left-sided Vg1 activity by a right-sided ALK2-dependent BMP pathway. *Development* 1999; **126**: 5195–205.

89  Ammanamanchi S, Kim SJ, Sun LZ, Brattain MG. Introduction of transforming growth factor-beta receptor type II expression in estrogen receptor-positive breast cancer cells through SP1 activation by 5-aza-2′-deoxycytidine. *J Biol Chem* 1998; **273**: 16527–34.

90  Bloom BB, Humphries DE, Kuang PP et al. Structure and expression of the promoter for the R4/ALK5 human type I transforming growth factor-beta receptor: regulation by TGF-beta. *Biochim Biophys Acta* 1996; **3**: 243–8.

91  Rius C, Smith JD, Almendro N et al. Cloning of the promoter region of human endoglin, the target gene for hereditary hemorrhagic telangiectasia type 1. *Blood* 1998; **92**: 4677–90.

92  Beppu H, Minowa O, Miyazono K, Kawabata M. cDNA cloning and genomic organization of the mouse BMP type II receptor. *Biochem Biophys Res Comm* 1997; **235**: 499–504.

93  Wozney JM. The bone morphogenetic protein family: multifunctional cellular regulators in the embryo and adult. *Eur J Oral Sci* 1998; **1**: 160–6.

94  Qu R, Silver MM, Letarte M. Distribution of endoglin in early human development reveals high levels on endocardial cushion tissue mesenchyme during valve formation. *Cell Tissue Res* 1998; **292**: 4878–84.

95 Celli JE, van Beusekom E, Hennekam RC et al. Familial syndromic esophageal atresia maps to 2p23-p24. *Am J Hum Gen* 2000; **66**: 436-44.

96 Dreyer SD, Morello R, German MS et al. LMXIB transactivation and expression in nail-patella syndrome. *Hum Mol Gene* 2000; **9**: 1067-74.

97 Flomen RH, Vatcheva R, Gorman PR et al. Construction and analysis of a sequence-ready map in 4q25: Rieger syndrome can be caused by haploinsufficiency of RIEG, but also by chromosome breaks approximately 90 kb upstream of this gene. *Genomics* 1998; **47**: 409-13.

98 Pilia G, Uda M, Macis D et al. Jagged-1 mutation analysis in Italian Alagille syndrome patients. *Hum Mutat* 1999; **14**: 394-400.

99 Sina M, Hinney A, Ziegler A et al. Phenotypes in three pedigrees with autosomal dominant obesity caused by haploinsufficiency mutations in the melanocortin-4 receptor gene. *Am J Hum Gen* 1999; **65**: 1501-7.

●100 West J, Fagan K, Steudel W et al. Pulmonary hypertension in transgenic mice expressing a dominant-negative BMPRII gene in smooth muscle. *Circ Res* 2004; **94**: 1-7.

101 Embury SH, Clark MR, Monroy G, Mohandas N. Concurrent sickle cell anemia and alpha-thalassemia. Effect on pathological properties of sickle erythrocytes. *J Clin Invest* 1994; **73**: 116-123.

102 Houlston RS, Tomlinson IP. Modifier genes in humans: strategies for identification. *Eur J Hum Gen* 1998; **6**: 80-8.

◆103 Nadeau JH. Modifier genes in mice and humans. *Nature Rev Genet* 2001; **28**: 165-74.

104 Ji C, Casinghino S, McCarthy TL, Centrella M. Cloning, characterization, and expression of the transforming growth factor-beta type I receptor prometer in fetal rat bone cells. *J Cell Biochem* 1996; **63**: 478-90.

105 Kato T, Kato N. Mitochondrial dysfunction in bipolar disorder. *Bipolar Disorder* 2000; **3**: 180-90.

◆106 Archer S, Rich S. Primary pulmonary hypertension: a vascular biology and translation research: work in progress. *Circulation* 2000; **102**: 2781-91.

107 Cool CD, Rai PR, Yeager ME et al. Expression of human herpesvirus 8 in primary pulmonary hypertension. *N Engl J Med* 2003; **349**: 1113-22.

108 Grunig E, Janssen B, Mereles D et al. Abnormal pulmonary artery pressure response in asymptomatic carriers of primary pulmonary hypertension gene. *Circulation* 2000; **102**: 1145-50.

●109 Petkov V, Mosgeoller W, Ziesche R et al. Vasoactive intestinal polypeptide as a new drug for treatment of primary pulmonary hypertension. *J Clin Invest* 2003; **111**: 1339-46.

110 Rindermann M, Grunig E, von Hippel A et al. Primary pulmonary hypertension may be a heterogeneous disease with a second locus on chromosome 2q31. *J Am Coll Card* 2003; **41**: 2237-44.

●111 Du L, Sullivan CC, Chy D et al. Signaling molecules in nonfamilial pulmonary hypertension. *N Engl J Med* 2003; **348**: 500-9.

●112 Christman BW, McPherson CD, Newman JH et al. An imbalance between the excretion of thromboxane and protacyclin metabolities in pulmonary hypertension. *N Engl J Med* 1992; **327**: 70-5.

113 Rich S, McLaughlin VV. Endothelin receptor blockers in cardiovascular disease. *Circulation* 2003; **108**: 2084-86.

114 Giaid A, Yanagisawa M, Langleben D et al. Expression of endothelin-1 in the lungs of patients with pulmonary hypertension. *N Engl J Med* 1993; **328**: 1732-9.

115 McAllister KA, Grogg KM, Johnson DW et al. Endoglin, a TGF-β binding protein of endothelial cells is the gene for hereditary haemorrhagic telangiectasia type 1. *Nat Genet* 1994; **8**: 345-51.

116 Johnson DW, Berg JN, Baldwin MA et al. Mutations in the activin like receptor kinase 1 gene in HHT type 2. *Nat Genet* 1996; **13**: 189-195.

117 Abdalla SA, Gallione CJ, Barst RJ et al. Primary pulmonary hypertension in families with hereditary haemorrhagic telangiectasia. *Eur Respir J* 2004; **23**: 373-7.

118 Harrison RE, Flanagan JA, Saneklo M et al. Molecular and functional anaylsis identifies ALK-1 as the predominant cause of pulmonary hypertension related to hereditary haemorrhagic talengiectasia. *J Med Gen* 2003; **40**: 865-71.

119 Chaouat A, Coulet G, Favre C et al. Endoglin germline mutation, hereditary hemorrhagic telangiectasia and dexfenfluramine-associated pulmonary arterial hypertension. *Thorax* 2004; **59**: 446-8.

120 Holcomb BW, Loyd JE, Ely EW et al. Pulmonary veno-occlusive disease: a case series and new observations. *Chest* 2000; **118**: 1671-9.

121 Mandel J, Mark EJ, Hales CA. Pulmonary veno-occlusive disease. *Am J Resp Crit Care Med* 2000; **162**: 1964-73.

●122 Runo JR, Vnencak-Jones CL, Prince M et al. Pulmonary veno-occlusive disease caused by an inherited mutation in bone morphogenetic protein receptor II. *Am J Respir Crit Care Med* 2003; **167**: 889-94.

123 Dorfmuller P, Perros F, Balabanian K, Humbert M. Inflammation in pulmonary arterial hypertension. *Eur Respir J* 2003; **22**: 358-63 (review).

124 Balabanian K, Foussat A, Dorfmuller P et al. CX(3) chemokine fractaline in pulmonary arterial hypertension. *Am J Respir Crit Care Med* 2002; **165**: 1350-1.

125 Ulanet DB, Wigley FM, Gilbert AC, Rosen A. Autoantibodies against B23, a nucleolar phosphoprotein, occur in scleroderma and are associated with pulmonary hypertension. *Arth Rheum* 2003; **49**: 85-92.

126 Grigolo B, Mazzetti I, Meliconi R et al. Anti-topoisomerase II autoantibodies in systemic sclerosis-association with pulmonary hypertension and HLA-B35. *Clin Exp Immunol* 2000; **121**: 539-43.

127 Lientz EA, Clayton EW. Psychosocial implications of primary pulmonary hypertension. *Am J Hum Gen* 2000; **259** (Suppl.): 209-11.

◆128 Hayden M. Predictive testing for Huntington's disease: the calm after the storm. *Lancet* 2000; **356**: 1944-5.

129 Wiggins S, Whyte P, Huggins M et al. The psychological consequences of testing for Huntington's Disease. *N Engl J Med* 1992; **237**: 1401-5.

130 Evans D, Gareth R, Eamonn R et al. Uptake of genetic testing for cancer predisposition. *J Med Gen* 1997; **34**: 746-8.

131 Marteau TM, Croyle RT. The new genetics: psychological responses to genetic testing. *Br Med J* 1999; **316**: 693-6.

132 Herrick JB. Peculiar elongated and sickle-shaped red corpuscles in a case of severe anemia. *Arch Intern Med* 1910; **6**: 517-21.

133  Sherman IJ. The sickling phenomenon, with special reference to the differentiation of sickle cell anemia from the sickle cell trait. *John Hopkins Med J* 1940; **67**: 309–24.

●134  Pauling L, Itano HA, Singer SJ et al. Sickle cell anemia, a molecular disease. *Science* 1949; **1110**: 543–8.

135  Ingram VA. A specific difference between the globins of normal human and sickle cell anemia hemoglobins. *Nature* 1956; **178**: 792–4.

136  Neel JV. Sickle cell disease: a worldwide problem. In: Abramson H, Bertles JF, Wethers DL (eds). *Sickle cell disease: diagnosis, management, education, and research.* St. Louis: Mosby, 1973 (Chapter 1).

137  Serjeant GR. The geography of sickle cell disease: opportunities for understanding its diversity. *Ann Saudi Med* 1994; **14**: 237–46.

✷138  Charache S, Terrin ML, Moore RD et al. Effect of hydroxyurea on the frequency of painful crises in sickle cell anemia. Investigators of the Multicenter Study of Hydroxyurea in Sickle Cell Anemia. *N Engl J Med* 1995; **332**: 1317–22.

139  Walters MC, Patience M, Leisenring W et al. Bone marrow transplantation for sickle cell disease. *N Engl J Med* 1996; **335**: 369–76.

140  Platt OS, Guinan EC. Bone marrow transplantation in sickle cell anemia – the dilemma of choice. *N Engl J Med* 1996; **335**: 426–8.

141  Livingstone FB. *Abnormal hemoglobins in human populations. A summary and interpretation.* Chicago: Aldine, 1967.

142  Pagnier J, Mears JG, Dunda-Belkhodja O et al. Evidence for the multicentric origin of the sickle cell hemoglobin gene in Africa. *Proc Natl Acad Sci USA* 1984; **81**: 1771–3.

143  Pierce HI, Kurachi S, Sofroniadou K et al. Frequencies of thalassemia in American blacks. *Blood* 1977; **49**: 981–6.

144  Motulsky AG. Frequency of sickling disorders in US blacks. *N Engl J Med* 1973; **288**: 31–3.

145  Wang W. Sickle cell anemia and other sickling syndromes. In: Greer J. (ed.) *Wintrobe's clinical hematology.* Philadelphia: Williams and Wilkins, 2004: 1263–311 (Chapter 40).

146  Hook EW, Campbell CG, Weens HS, Cooper GR. Salmonella osteomyelitis in patients with sickle cell anemia. *N Engl J Med* 1957; **257**: 403–7.

147  Wierenga KJ, Serjeant BE, Serjeant GR. Cerebrovascular complications and parvovirus infection in homozygous sickle cell disease. *J Pediatr* 2001; **139**: 438–42.

148  Wong WY, Overturf GD, Powars D et al. Infection caused by *Streptococcus pneumoniae* in children with sickle cell disease: epidemiology, immunologic mechanisms, prophylaxis, vaccination. *Clin Infect Dis* 1992; **14**: 1124–36.

●149  Gladwin MT, Sachdev V, Jison ML et al. Pulmonary hypertension as a risk factor for death in patients with sickle cell disease. *N Engl J Med* 2004; **350**: 886–95.

●150  Miller GJ, Serjeant GR. An assessment of lung volumes and gas transfer in sickle-cell anemia. *Thorax* 1971; **26**: 309–15.

●151  Bromberg P. The lung in sickle cell disease. *Arch Int Med* 1974; **133**: 652–5.

152  Castro O, Brambilla DJ, Thorington B et al. The acute chest syndrome in sickle cell disease: incidence and risk factors. The Cooperative Study of Sickle Cell Disease. *Blood* 1994; **84**: 643–9.

153  Vichinsky EP, Neumayr LD, Earles AN et al. Causes and outcomes of the acute chest syndrome in sickle cell disease.

National Acute Chest Syndrome Study Group. *N Engl J Med* 2000; **342**: 1855–65.

154  Sprinkle RH, Cole T, Smith S et al. Acute chest syndrome in children with sickle cell disease. A retrospective analysis of 100 hospitalized cases. *Am J Pediatr Hematol Oncol* 1986; **8**: 105–10.

155  Sutton LL, Castro O, Cross, DJ et al. Pulmonary hypertension in sickle cell disease. *Am J Cardiol* 1994; **74**: 626–8.

●156  Castro O, Hoque M, Brown BD. Pulmonary hypertension in sickle cell disease cardiac catherization results and survival. *Blood* 2003; **101**: 1257–61.

157  Haque AK, Gokhale S, Rampy BA et al. Pulmonary hypertension in sickle cell hemoglobinopahy: a clinicopathologic study of 20 cases. *Hum Pathol* 2002; **33**: 1037–43.

158  Minter KR, Gladwin MT. Pulmonary complications of sickle cell anemia: a need for increased recognition, treatment and research. *Am J Respir Crit Care Med* 2001; **164**: 2016–9.

159  Castro P, Haque M, Brown BD. Pulmonary hypertension in sickle cell disease: cardiac catheterization results and survival. *Blood* 2003; **101**: 1257–61.

160  Haque AK, Gokhale S, Rampy BA et al. Pulmonary hypertension in sickle cell hemoglobinopahy: a clinicopathologic study of 20 cases. *Hum Pathol* 2002, **33**: 1037–43.

161  Carlos T, Escoffery DM, Shirley SE. Autopsy findings in sickle cell disease. *Jasksonville Med* 2000; **6**: 1–7.

162  Chou R, DeLoughery TG. Recurrent thromboembolic disease following splenectomy for pyruvate kinase deficiency. *Am J Hematol* 2001; **67**: 197–9.

◆163  Humbert M, Nunes H, Sitbor N et al. Risk factors for pulmonary arterial hypertension. *Clin Chest Med* 2001; **3**: 459–75.

164  Hoeper MM, Niedermeyer J, Hoffmeyer F et al. Pulmonary hypertension after splenectomy. *Ann Intern Med* 1999; **130**: 506–9.

✷165  Steinberg MH, Barton F, Catstro O et al. Effect of hydroxyurea on mortality and morbidity in adult sickle cell anemia: risks and benefits up to 9 years of treatment. *J Am Med Assoc* 2003; **289**: 1645–51.

166  Morris CR, Morris SM, Hagar W et al. Arginine therapy. *Am J Resp Crit Care Med* 2003; **68**: 63–69.

166a  Sullivan KJ, Kissoon N, Duckworth LJ et al. Low exhaled nitric oxide and a polymorphism in the NOS1 gene is associated with acute chest syndrome. *Am J Resp Crit Care Med* 2001; 164: 2186–90.

167  Beutler E. Gaucher's disease. *N Engl J Med* 1991; **375**: 1354–60.

168  Zimran A, Kay A, Gelbart T et al. Clinical laboratory, radiologic, and genetic features of 53 patients. *Medicine* 1992; **71**: 337–53.

169  Eng CM, Schechter C, Robinowitz J et al. Prenatal genetic carrier testing using triple disease screening. *J Am Med Assoc* 1997; **278**: 1268–1272.

170  Goitein O, Elstein D, Abrahamov A et al. Lung involvement and enzyme replacement therapy in Gaucher's disease. *Q J Med* 2001; **94**: 407–415.

✷171  Mistry PK, Sirrs S, Chan A et al. Pulmonary hypertension in type I Gaucher's disease: genetic and epigenetic determinants of phenotype and response to therapy. *Mol Gen Metab* 2002; **77**: 91–98.

172  Pelini M, Boice D, O'Neil K, LaRocque J. Glucocerebrosidase treatment of type I Gaucher disease with severe pulmonary involvement. *Ann Int Med* 1994; **121**: 196–7.

173  Dawson A, Elias DJ, Rubenson D et al. Pulmonary hypertension developing after alglucerase therapy in two patients with type I Gaucher disease complicated by the hematopulmonary syndrome. *Ann Intern Med* 1996; **125**: 901–4.

174  Bakst AE, Gaine SP, Rubin LJ. Continuous intravenous epoprostenol therapy for pulmonary hypertension in Gaucher's disease. *Chest* 1999; **116**: 1127–30.

175  Seligsohn U, Lubetsky A. Genetic susceptibility to venous thrombosis. *N Engl J Med* 2001; **344**: 1222–31.

◆176  Martinelli I, Pier MM, DeStefano V et al. Different risks of thrombosis in four coagulation defects associated with inherited thrombopilia: a study of 150 families. *Blood* 1998; **92**: 2353–8.

177  Martinelli I. Risk factors in venous thromboembolism. *Thromb Haemos* 2001; **86**: 395–403.

178  Welsh CH, Hassell KL, Badesch DB et al. Coagulation and fibrinolytic profiles in patients with severe pulmonary hypertension. *Chest* 1996; **110**: 710–7.

179  Massimo M, Simonetta M, Lorenza P et al. Value of transthoracic echocardiography in the diagnosis of pulmonary embolism: results of a prospective study in unselected patients. *Am J Med* 2001; **110**: 528–35.

180  Ribeiro A, Lindmarker P, Johnsson H et al. Pulmonary embolism: one year follow-up with echocardiography doppler and five-year survival analysis. *Circulation* 1999; **99**: 1325–30.

181  Mansencal N, Joseph T, Vieillar-Baron A et al. Comparison of different echocardiographic indexes secondary to right ventricular obstruction in acute pulmonary embolism. *Am J Cardiol* 2003; **92**: 116–9.

◆182  Goldhaber S. Echocardiography in the management of pulmonary embolism. *Ann Intern Med* 2002; **136**: 691–700.

✳183  Konstantinides S, Geibel A, Heusel G et al. Management strategies and prognosis of pulmonary embolism-3 trial investigators. *N Engl J Med* 2002; **347**: 1143–50.

✳184  Jamieson SW, Kapelanski DP, Sakakibara N et al. Pulmonary endarterectomy: experience and lessons learned in 1,500 cases. *Ann Thorac Surg* 2003; **76**: 1457–62; discussion 1462–4.

185  Atichartakarn V, Likittanasombat K, Chuncharunee S et al. Pulmonary arterial hypertension in previously splenectomized patients with beta-thalassemic disorders. *Int J Hematol* 2003; **78**: 139–45.

◆186  Colorio CC, Martinuzzo ME, Forastiero RR et al. Thrombophilic factors in chronic thromboembolic pulmonary hypertension. *Blood Coagul Fibrinolysis* 2001; **12**: 427–32.

187  Miliauskas NA. Factor V Leiden and post thromboembolic pulmonary hypertension. *Medicina (Kaunas)* 2003; **39**: 1171–4.

188  Emmerich J, Rosendaal FR, Cattaneo M et al. Combined effect of factor V Leiden and prothrombin 20210A on the risk of venous thromboembolism – pooled analysis of 8 case control studies including 2310 cases and 3204 controls. Study group

for pooled-analysis in venous thromboembolism. *Thromb Haemostas* 2001; **86**: 809–16.

◆189  Colleges of American Pathologists Consensus Panel on Thrombophilia. *Arch Pathol Lab Med* 2001; **126**: 1277–1433.

190  Bauer KA. The thrombophilias: well defined risk factors with uncertain therapeutic implications. *Ann Intern Med* 2001; **135**: 367–73.

191  Deitcher SR, Rodgers GM. Thrombosis and antithrombotic therapy. In: Greer J (ed.) *Wintrobe's clinical hematology.* Philadelphia: Lippincott Williams Wilkins, 2004: 1713–58 (Chapter 61).

192  Casais P, Alberto MF, Gennari LC et al. Anticoagulation in the antiphospholipid syndrome. *Haematologica* 2004; **89**: 504–3.

193  Alarcon-Segovia D, Boffa MC, Bronda W et al. Prophylaxis of antiphospholipid syndrome: a consensus report. *Lupus* 2003; **12**: 499–503.

◆194  Palevsky HI, Fishman AP. Chronic cor pulmonale. *J Am Med Assoc* 1990; **263**: 2347–54.

◆195  MacNee W. Pathophysiology of cor pulmonale in chronic obstructive pulmonary disease. State of the art. *Am J Pulm Crit Care Med* 1994; **150**: 833–92, 1158–63.

196  Burwell CS, Robin Ed, Whaley RD et al. Extreme obesity associated with alveolar hypoventilation – a Pickwickian syndrome. *Am J Med* 1956; **21**: 811–18.

197  Burrows B. Arterial oxygenation and pulmonary hemodynamics in patients with chronic airways obstruction. *Am Rev Resp Dis* 1974; **110** (Suppl.): 64–70.

◆198  Fanburg BL, Sicilian L (eds). *Respiratory dysfunction in neuromuscular disease.* Philadelphia: WB Saunders,1994.

199  Glover RF. Pulmonary circulation in animals and man at high altitude. *Ann NY Acad Sci* 1965; **127**: 632–9.

●200  Sylvester JT. Hypoxic pulmonary vasoconstriction: a radical view. *Circ Res* 2001; **88**: 1228–9.

◆201  Fagan KA, Weil JV. Potential genetic contributions to control of the pulmonary circulation and ventilation at high altitude. *High Altitude Med* 2001; **2**: 165–71.

202  Richards DW. The right heart and the lung with some observations on teleology. The J. Burns Amberson Lecture. *Am Rev Resp Dis* 1966; **94**: 691–702.

203  Tucker A, McMurtry IF, Reeves JT et al. Lung vascular smooth muscle as a determinant of pulmonary hypertension at high altitude. *Am J Phys* 1975; **228**: 762–7.

204  Foletta VA, Lim MA, Soosairajah JK et al. Direct signaling by the BMP type II receptor via the cytoskeletal regulator LIMK1. *J Cell Biol* 2003; **162**: 1089–98.

205  Grover RF. Comparative physiology of hypoxic pulmonary hypertension. *Proc Int Sym Cardiovasc Resp: Effects of hypoxia.* Kingston, Ontario. 1965: 307–21.

◆206  Rupert JL, Hochachka PW. The evidence of hereditary factors contributing to high altitude adaptation in Andean natives; a review. *High Alt Med Biol* 2001; **2**: 235–6.

207  Mortimer H, Patel S, Peacock AJ. The genetic basis of high-altitude pulmonary oedema. *Pharmacol Ther* 2004; **101**: 183–92.

208  Grover RF. Pulmonary circulation in animals and man at high altitude. *Ann NY Acad Sci* 1965; **127**: 632–9.

# 15

# Genetics of lung cancer

## REBECCA SUK AND DAVID C. CHRISTIANI

## DISEASE DEFINITION AND EPIDEMIOLOGY/NATURAL HISTORY

Lung cancer is the leading cause of cancer mortality among both men and women in the USA, with over 170 000 new cases and over 150 000 deaths estimated in 2003.[1] Approximately 80 percent of cases diagnosed are nonsmall cell lung cancer, including the major subtypes of squamous cell, adenocarcinoma, and large cell, while 20 percent are small cell lung cancer.[2] Among the nonsmall cell lung cancers, the incidence of adenocarcinoma has risen over the past two decades to surpass that of squamous cell carcinoma in North America.

Survival for both nonsmall cell and small cell lung cancer is poor. Small cell lung cancer is typically categorized into limited stage, involving one hemithorax, and extensive stage, extending beyond the ipsilateral hemithorax. Median survival for limited stage small cell lung cancer is 14–20 months and for extensive stage, 8–13 months. Two-year survival in limited stage ranges from 20 to 40 percent, with 5-year survival of 10–20 percent. For extensive stage disease, 2-year survival is less than 5 percent.[3–5]

Nonsmall cell lung cancer comprises the majority of newly diagnosed lung cancer and is staged by the TNM system, where T stage describes the size and location of the primary tumor, N stage describes nodal involvement, and M stage describes distant metastatic disease. Stage and TNM classification is shown in Table 15.1. Five-year survival for stage IA disease (T1N0M0) is 61 percent, but drops sharply thereafter, with 5-year survival in stage IB of 38 percent, IIA 34 percent, IIB 24 percent, IIIA 13 percent, IIIB 5 percent, and IV 1 percent.[6] Over half of patients with nonsmall cell lung cancer present with stage III or IV disease.

Cigarette smoking is the leading cause of lung cancer and accounts for approximately 90 percent of all lung cancer cases in the USA. Both duration of smoking and number of cigarettes per day are directly correlated with lung cancer risk. Patients who quit smoking decrease their lung cancer risk, although not to never-smoking levels.[7] Cigarette smoking patterns vary by birth cohort, and lung cancer risk and mortality follow this trend.[8] Among white males, lung cancer mortality peaked for the 1925–30 birth cohort, and among white women, for the 1935–40 birth cohort, corresponding with prevalence of cigarette smoking.[9] Age-adjusted lung cancer incidence and mortality rates have decreased in men since 1990, reflecting the later birth cohorts' relative decline in smoking, while in women, for whom smoking behavior lagged a decade behind men, the rate is still increasing.[10–12] Environmental tobacco smoke, occupational exposures to tar and soot, asbestos, and metals such as arsenic, chromium, and nickel, have also been associated with increased lung cancer risk.[7]

## IDENTIFIED MONOGENIC COMPONENTS/SYNDROMES

### Genetic etiology

A single genetic abnormality leading to lung cancer has yet to be identified. Although diseases such as Li–Fraumeni syndrome are known to increase the risk of cancer overall, lung cancer is not one of the cancers most commonly associated with this syndrome, which typically involves an inherited mutation in p53 (TP53). Indeed, the most important cause of lung cancer is exposure to cigarette smoke. However, despite the clear causal connection between cigarette smoking and the vast majority of lung cancers, not all smokers develop lung cancer, and lung cancer is found in never-smokers. This suggests that genetic and epigenetic phenomena have a role

**Table 15.1** *Staging of lung cancer[6]*

| Lung cancer stage | |
| --- | --- |
| *Small cell* | |
| Limited stage | Disease confined to ipsilateral hemithorax and encompassed within one radiotherapy port |
| Extensive stage | Metastatic disease outside ipsilateral hemithorax |

*Nonsmall cell lung cancer*

*Primary tumor (T)*

T1: Tumor $\leq$ 3 cm diameter without invasion more proximal than lobar bronchus

T2: Tumor > 3 cm diameter, or tumor of any size with any of the following:
Invasion of visceral pleura
Atelectasis of less than entire lung
Proximal extent at least 2 cm from carina

T3: Tumor of any size with any of the following:
Invasion of chest wall
Involvement of diaphragm, mediastinal pleura, or pericardium
Atelectasis involving entire lung
Proximal extent within 2 cm of carina

T4: Tumor of any size with any of the following:
Invasion of mediastinum
Invasion of heart or great vessels
Invasion of trachea or esophagus
Invasion of vertebral body or carina
Presence of malignant pleural or pericardial effusion
Satellite tumor nodule(s) within same lobe as primary tumor

*Nodal involvement (N)*
N0: No regional nodal involvement
N1: Metastasis to ipsilateral hilar and/or ipsilateral peribronchial nodes
N2: Metastasis to ipsilateral mediastinal and/or subcarinal nodes
N3: Metastasis to contralateral mediastinal or hilar nodes, or ipsilateral or contralateral scalene or supraclavicular nodes

*Metastasis (M)*
M0: Distant metastasis absent
M1: Distant metastasis present (includes metastatic tumor nodules in a different lobe from the primary tumor)

| *Stage groupings of TNM subsets* | |
| --- | --- |
| IA | T1N0M0 |
| IB | T2N0M0 |
| IIA | T1N1M0 |
| IIB | T2N1M0 |
| IIIA | T3N1M0 |
| | T1-3N2M0 |
| IIIB | AnyT N3M0 |
| | T4 AnyN M0 |
| IV | AnyT AnyN M1 |
| | T3N0M0 |

in the pathogenesis of lung cancer, and efforts have focused on defining the elements that contribute to differential susceptibility to the carcinogens found in cigarette smoke.

Multiple lines of study are being pursued to elucidate the genetic basis of lung cancer. The search for a hereditary predisposition to lung cancer has focused on germline polymorphisms that confer differential ability to metabolize carcinogens. Particular interest has focused on polymorphisms in carcinogen metabolizing pathways and DNA repair pathways. Although these hereditary factors may define a predisposition to mutagenesis, they are generally insufficient for the development of malignancy in the absence of additional mutations. Thus, many investigators have attempted to enumerate the acquired somatic mutations that accumulate in tumor cells and over the course of decades lead to dysplasia, neoplasia, and metastasis. Rather than a defined monogenic syndrome, then, a dynamic interplay of multiple genetic, epigenetic, and environmental factors ultimately leads to lung cancer.

## Disease pathogenesis

Hanahan and Weinberg[13] outlined six essential changes in cell behavior that define the hallmarks of cancer: self sufficiency in growth signals, insensitivity to growth-inhibitory signals, evasion of programmed cell death (apoptosis), limitless replicative potential, sustained angiogenesis, and tissue invasion/metastasis. The acquisition of these capabilities defines the cancer cell and is necessary for carcinogenesis.

Genetic changes, both hereditary and acquired, drive these cellular changes from normal to cancerous capability. Carcinogenesis is a multistep process whereby a normal cell acquires malignant capability via a series of mutations that alter cell growth, proliferation, and interaction. Classically, these mutations have involved oncogenes, where gain of function exerts cell proliferative effects, and tumor suppressor genes, where loss of function removes a brake on cell proliferation.[14] Once bronchial cells start to acquire mutations, it is unclear whether these mutations must occur in a specific order or if there is any specific combination of mutations that is necessary and sufficient for carcinogenesis. In addition, inherited susceptibility to carcinogen-mediated damage may predispose certain individuals to have greater lung cancer risk. Interaction of genes and environment continues to play a role in tobacco-induced lung cancer. Figure 15.1 illustrates how germline and somatic mutations may interact with environment in the development of lung cancer.

## Clinical evaluation

A detailed history and physical examination are necessary for the evaluation of any newly diagnosed patient with lung cancer. Particular attention should be paid to smoking history, environmental exposures, and family history of lung cancer.

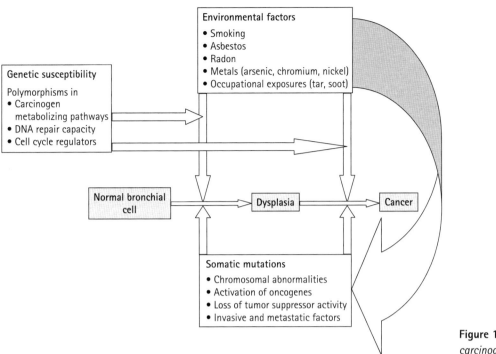

**Figure 15.1** *Model of lung carcinogenesis.*

Symptoms may be related to the growth of the primary tumor or metastatic disease. Common presenting symptoms include cough and shortness of breath. Patients should be evaluated for hemoptysis; although massive hemoptysis is rare, many patients may experience blood-streaked sputum. Obstruction of airways may lead to pneumonia, atelectasis, and worsening dyspnea. Invasion of adjacent structures may produce symptoms as well, and manifestations of chest wall involvement, superior vena cava (SVC) syndrome, and pericardial and pleural effusions, should be sought. In addition to these logoregional symptoms, patients may manifest signs of metastatic disease. Metastases to the bone may present with pain or pathologic fracture. Central nervous system (CNS) metastases may manifest themselves via neurologic sequelae. In addition to these organ-specific signs and symptoms, constitutional symptoms, such as fatigue and weight loss, are commonly seen.[15]

Once the diagnosis of lung cancer is made, a full staging evaluation should be completed to assess the extent of disease. This typically includes computed tomography (CT) of the chest, with liver and adrenal cuts, bone scan, and head imaging. Patients with suspicious mediastinal lymphadenopathy, defined as greater than 1 cm in short axis on CT, also undergo mediastinoscopy for surgical and pathological evaluation of the mediastinal nodes. Positron emission tomography (PET) scans are being used more frequently as part of the staging work up.[15] These studies enable the clinician to classify nonsmall cell lung cancer into the international staging system described above, and small cell lung cancer into limited or extensive stage disease. Treatment decisions hinge on the stage designation as defined by these studies. Response to treatment is evaluated with periodic restaging scans. Typically, tumor size measurements on CT are used to determine complete response, partial response, stable disease, or progressive disease. The use of PET avidity as a marker of response is under investigation.

## Treatment

### TREATMENT OF SMALL CELL AND NONSMALL CELL LUNG CANCER

The treatment of lung cancer depends on histology and stage. Limited stage small cell lung cancer is treated with a combination of chemotherapy and radiation. The addition of radiation during the first few cycles of platinum-based chemotherapy has been shown to have survival benefit in limited stage disease.[16–18] For extensive stage small cell lung cancer, chemotherapy alone is the standard. Again, chemotherapy regimens are typically platinum-based. A recent study demonstrated that the combination of cisplatin and irinotecan may have better survival than the older standard of cisplatin and etoposide;[19] confirmatory studies are ongoing.

For nonsmall cell lung cancer, treatment has typically revolved around a combination of surgery, radiation, and chemotherapy.[20,21] Early stage NSCLC (stage I and II) has traditionally been treated with surgery alone, and early studies failed to show a benefit with adjuvant chemotherapy. However, a 1995 meta-analysis suggested an approximately 5 percent absolute survival benefit from cisplatin-based chemotherapy at 5 years,[22] and several recent large randomized trials have demonstrated benefit from adjuvant chemotherapy. The largest trial to date, which randomized 1867 patients with resected stage I, II, and III non-small cell lung cancer to observation or adjuvant cisplatin-based chemotherapy, found a survival benefit in the adjuvantly treated arm (44.5 versus 40.4 percent at 5 years).[23] Other studies have corroborated this benefit in the early stage population, with one study showing an increase in 5-year survival from 54 to 69 percent with adjuvant chemotherapy in the stage IB/II resected population,[24] and another reporting an increase in 4-year survival from 59 to 71 percent in stage IB.[25]

The standard of care for stage IIIA nonsmall cell lung cancer remains debated. While a trimodality approach combining surgery, chemotherapy, and radiation is commonly used, the optimal regimen has yet to be defined. In addition, studies are ongoing to assess whether the addition of surgery to chemoradiation has survival benefit; a preliminary report has shown mixed results and long-term follow-up is needed.[26]

Advanced stage NSCLC is treated with a combination of chemotherapy and radiation for Stage IIIB disease, and chemotherapy alone for Stage IV disease. In Stage IV disease, platinum-based doublets form the backbone of most first-line chemotherapy regimens. Cisplatin has been combined with navelbine,[27] gemcitabine,[28-30] taxol,[31] and taxotere[32] with response rates in Phase III trials in the 20–40% range in first-line therapy. A randomized trial comparing four platinum-based chemotherapy regimens showed no difference in survival between the different regimens.[33] Numerous agents are available for second-line and beyond, including docetaxel, gefitinib, and pemetrexed.[34-38]

## TUMOR–SPECIFIC PREDICTORS OF RESPONSE: MOLECULAR PATHOLOGY

Given the narrow therapeutic window of most chemotherapy regimens, identifying predictors of response and toxicity would help clinicians make rational treatment decisions. Many investigators have sought to identify tumor-specific molecular markers of response. Some studies have suggested that intratumoral DNA repair capacity may be associated with response and survival. Lower levels of intratumoral ERCC1 mRNA, which is involved in nucleotide excision repair, has been associated with longer median survival among stage IV NSCLC patients treated with cisplatin and gemcitabine.[39] Low ERCC1 mRNA levels have also been shown to have a survival benefit in gastric,[40] colorectal,[41] and esophageal cancers.[42] A study in Europe is randomizing NSCLC patients to treatment based on ERCC1 levels in order to test these hypotheses prospectively.[43] Other potential markers of response may involve pathways of drug metabolism. Among patients treated with gemcitabine, low intratumoral RRM1 mRNA levels have been associated with longer median survival.[44,45] Researchers hope to one day provide targeted therapy, making rational chemotherapy choices guided by such molecular profiles.[46] Recently, investigators have identified mutations in the EGFR tyrosine kinase domain that may predict response to treatment with gefitinib. Gefitinib is an EGFR tyrosine kinase inhibitor which has been approved for use in the third-line setting for metastatic NSCLC. Phase II studies of single agent gefitinib in patients with advanced, chemorefractory NSCLC showed promising response rates and symptom improvement (RRs of 18.4 and 11.8 percent in IDEAL-1 and -2, respectively).[47,48] Despite these favorable results in the pretreated setting, however, the addition of gefitinib to first-line chemotherapy has not shown benefit. Two large randomized phase III trials comparing cisplatin/gemcitabine and carboplatin/taxol with or without gefitinib showed no difference in response rates, time to progression, or survival with the addition of gefitinib.[49,50] These trials have been criticized for failing to select patients based on likelihood of responding to gefitinib.[51] However, identifying this responsive subset has been difficult. While retrospective analyses have suggested some clinical correlates of response, such as Japanese ethnicity, female sex, adenocarcinoma and bronchoalveolar histology, and non-smoking history,[49,50,52,53] molecular markers have been difficult to pinpoint, as EGFR expression levels do not appear to correlate with response.[54,55]

Mutations in the EGFR gene have been discovered that may predict response to gefitinib. Lynch et al.[56] reported inframe deletions and missense mutations involving the EGFR tyrosine kinase domain in eight of nine patients responsive to gefitinib who had tumor tissue available. These mutations were not found in the matched normal tissue of the same patients, or in the tumor tissues of seven non-responding patients. Similarly, Paez et al.[57] found mutations in the EGFR tyrosine kinase domain in five of five tumor samples from responding patients and none of four tumor samples from non-responders. In vitro studies showed that in the presence of EGF the mutated EGFR had significantly increased and prolonged activation as compared to wildtype. The mutated receptors were also more sensitive to inhibition by gefitinib.

Notably, only a small percentage of all NSCLCs appear to carry this somatic mutation: Lynch et al.[56] found mutations in two of 25 non-gefitinib-treated NSCLC samples and Paez et al.[57] found mutations in 15 of 58 Japanese and one of 61 US samples. However, the discovery of specific EGFR mutations that predict responsiveness to gefitinib sets a paradigm for how it may be possible to identify patients who will respond to targeted therapy.

## PHARMACOGENOMICS

In addition to the somatic tumor-specific markers outlined above, germline polymorphisms may predict differential drug effect. As discussed in Chapter 8, pharmacogenomics is the study of how inherited differences in drug metabolism and disposition affect efficacy and toxicity. It has long been known that genetic variation in pathways of drug activity and metabolism can lead to differential drug effect.[58] Polymorphisms in genes coding for phase I and II enzymes have been noted to change the efficacy of a wide variety of drugs, ranging from antihypertensives and antibiotics to chemotherapeutic agents.[59] The application of pharmacogenomics to cancer therapy has been spurred by the goal of individualizing chemotherapy to maximize benefit while minimizing toxicity.

Polymorphisms in candidate genes may predict response to chemotherapy. Since platinum is the backbone for most chemotherapy regimens in lung cancer, many investigators have focused on polymorphisms that may confer differential response to platinum. Platinum agents form bulky intrastrand adducts and interstrand crosslinks, inhibiting DNA replication. Candidate genes in the nucleotide excision repair, base excision repair, mismatch repair, and double strand break repair pathways have been identified for study. Polymorphisms in XPD (ERCC2) and XRCC1 have been associated with differences in survival, with the variant alleles being associated with shorter overall survival.[60] The C/C genotype in codon 118 of ERCC1 was found in one study to be associated with longer survival in patients treated with cis-platin-based therapy,[61] although another study found no association.[62] Another group found a trend toward better response in patients with the XPD polymorphism in codon 312, which is thought to be associated with lower DNA repair capacity.[63] The Spanish Lung Cancer Group is conducting a trial examining the role of XPD and RRM polymorphisms among NSCLC patients treated with various chemotherapy combinations, including cisplatin- and gemcitabine-based therapy.[64–66] The functional significance of many of these polymorphisms will need to be further clarified in future studies.

Polymorphic variation may also predict severe toxicity. For example, polymorphisms leading to deficiencies in metabolic enzymes such as thiopurine methyltransferase and dihydropyrimidine dehydrogenase have been associated with severe toxicities with thiopurine and 5-FU therapy, respectively.[67] Recently, investigators have identified polymorphisms in UDP-glucuronosyl-transferase 1A1 that lead to reduced UGT1A1 expression and hence increased accumulation of the active SN-38 metabolite of irinotecan. A variant polymorphism has been associated with severe hematologic toxicity in advanced cancer patients treated with irinotecan.[68] In lung cancer, the UGT1A1 polymorphism has not been associated with toxicity among patients treated with irinotecan and docetaxel in the second-line setting.[69] Studies of other candidate genes are ongoing.

## COMPLEX DISEASE COMPONENTS

### Familial aggregation

In examining family history, it is important to control for tobacco and other environmental exposures, since these are often shared within a family. Several studies, some of which controled for smoking, demonstrate an increased risk of developing lung cancer within families with a history of lung cancer (Table 15.2).

**Table 15.2**   *Selected familial aggregation studies*

| Study | Comment | Estimated risk |
|---|---|---|
| *Risk of lung cancer among first-degree relatives of cases* | | |
| Tokuhata and Lilienfeld[70] | Smoking | 2–2.5 (mortality) |
| | Nonsmoking | 4 |
| Ooi et al.[71] | All | 2.4 (incidence) |
| *Odds ratio among cases for lung cancer in first-degree relative* | | |
| Shaw et al.[73] | All | 1.7–2.1 |
| Schwartz et al.[74] | Nonsmoking, age 40–59 | 7.2 |
| Kreuzer et al.[75] | Age =45 | 2.6 |
| Bromen et al.[76] | All | 1.67 |
| | Age ⩽50 | 4.75 |
| Poole et al.[79] | Women | 1.7 (mortality) |

Tokuhata and Lilienfeld[70] first reported in 1963 an increased lung cancer mortality among first-degree relatives of patients with lung cancer as compared to relatives of age-, race-, and sex-matched controls. Both smoking and nonsmoking relatives of cases were at higher risk of lung cancer than comparable relatives of controls. The familial association seemed particularly strong in female relatives.

More recently, Ooi et al.[71] studied the incidence of lung cancer among first-degree relatives of 336 deceased lung cancer cases and 307 controls (the cases' spouses) in Louisiana. After adjusting for age, sex, smoking, and occupational exposures, they found a 2.4-fold greater risk of lung cancer among relatives of cases. Among those over the age of 40 years, this risk was greater in women than men – the relative risk of lung cancer in male relatives of cases was 2.1 (P < 0.05); for female relatives, 7.2 (P < 0.05). Non-smoking female relatives of cases had four-fold the risk of lung cancer as compared to nonsmoking female relatives of controls. The relative risk of any type of cancer was also increased among case families (OR = 1.52).[72]

Similarly, Shaw et al.[73] found an increased lung cancer risk associated with reported lung cancer in first-degree relatives among cases in Texas. Cases with a parent with lung cancer were diagnosed at an earlier age than cases without a parent with lung cancer, and case siblings who developed lung cancer were diagnosed at an earlier age than control siblings. Whether this reflects an element of bias of early detection among case families or supports Knudson's hypothesis that genetically influenced forms of cancer should have earlier onset than sporadic forms remains unclear.[73]

In support of a genetic influence on early onset lung cancer, several studies have noted an increased risk among families of cases diagnosed at young age. Schwartz et al.[74] analyzed nonsmoking cases and controls in the Detroit metropolitan area and reported a six-fold increase in lung cancer risk among family members of the younger cases. In a study assessing lung cancer risk in a German population, Kreuzer et al.[75] reported that lung cancer in a first-degree relative was associated with a 2.6-fold increase in lung cancer risk among the younger, but not the older, age group. Bromen et al.[76] found a 4.75-fold increased risk of lung cancer among first-degree relatives of cases who were diagnosed before the age of 50 years. These data suggest that among those with early onset lung cancer, the genetic component may play a stronger role than environment.

Indeed, using the data from the Louisiana study, Sellers et al.[77] performed a segregation analysis to suggest that the results are compatible with a Mendelian codominant inheritance of a rare autosomal gene. With the model they fitted, they suggest that 69 percent of cases up to the age of 50 may be attributable to such a gene. By the age of 70, only 22 percent of cases may be attributable to the gene, suggesting that with increasing age, the effect of environmental and tobacco exposure may play a larger role.

Most recently, Etzel et al.[78] analyzed 806 cases with age, sex, ethnicity, and smoking matched controls. After adjusting for age and smoking history, in both the subjects and their families, they found a small but significant increased risk of lung cancer among first-degree relatives of the cases (RR, 1.33; 95 percent CI 1.03–1.72).

Several studies have utilized large cohorts of people to assess the association of family history with lung cancer risk. In a nested case–control study, Poole et al.[79] studied the incidence of cancer mortality among women enrolled in the American Cancer Society Prevention Study-1. Women were enrolled from 1959 and followed to 1972 for cancer mortality. Family history was defined as a history of cancer in any first-degree relative. Of 429 483 women who were cancer-free at baseline, 12 354 died of cancer during the period of follow-up. Looking at lung cancer specifically, 8785 of the women enrolled reported a family history of lung cancer. There were a total of 877 lung cancer deaths. A family history of lung cancer was significantly associated with mortality from lung cancer (odds ratio, 1.7; 95 percent CI 1.2–2.5). Logistic modeling took into account the smoking history of the study subject, but it is unclear how much smoking history of family members or other environmental history was obtained.

Similarly, others have used a Swedish nationwide cancer database to analyze the standardized incidence ratio (SIR) of lung cancer among offspring of lung cancer cases as compared to controls. SIR in offspring for lung cancer was increased to 1.87 (95 percent CI, 1.66–2.10) when a parent had lung cancer. The population attributable fraction of familial lung cancer was 2.97 percent.[80]

Taken together, these studies suggest that there may be an inherited susceptibility to lung cancer. Defining what this genetic susceptibility may be has been the pursuit of many molecular epidemiologic studies.

## Environmental factors

Cigarette smoking has been established as a major cause of lung cancer. Other environmental risk factors, including radon, asbestos, and occupational exposures, have been identified, but tobacco smoke is the major culprit, with attributable risk estimates in excess of 90 percent.[81] Multiple carcinogens have been found in cigarette smoke, with polycyclic aromatic hydrocarbons, aza-arenes, N-nitrosamines, aromatic amines, heterocyclic aromatic amines, and aldehydes forming the major classes of carcinogens.[82] At least 50 carcinogens in cigarette smoke have been identified that cause lung tumors in animals or humans.[83] Metabolic activation of these carcinogens leads to DNA adduct formation, whereby the active metabolite binds covalently to DNA. DNA repair systems will repair many DNA adducts; however, those that are not repaired can lead to aberrant coding. Multiple mutations can lead to loss of normal controls on cell growth.

The details of metabolic activation, adduct formation, and detoxification of tobacco carcinogens have been extensively studied. Phase I enzymes typically are involved in activation of carcinogenic substrates. The cytochrome P450 family of phase I enzymes, encoded by the CYP family of genes, is involved in the initial oxygenation of the carcinogenic substrate. Some of the metabolites produced by this reaction react with DNA to form covalent adducts. For example, benzo(a)pyrene, a polyaromatic hydrocarbon, is converted to 7,8-diol-9,10-epoxides (BPDE). One of the four enantiomers forms DNA adducts. Similar activation of one of the N-nitrosamines, 4-methylnitrosamino-1-3-pyridyl-1-butanone (NNK), by the P450 system leads to metabolites that form methyl and pyridyloxobutyl DNA adducts. Detoxification of the toxic metabolites occurs via the action of multiple phase II enzymes, most notably the glutathione-S-transferases. Repair of adducts by DNA repair mechanisms also protects the cell from further damage.[83] The balance between activation, detoxification, and repair is thought to affect cancer development. Genetic variability in these pathways has been of particular interest in studies of lung cancer risk.

## Linkage studies

Classical linkage studies identifying chromosomal regions that segregate with disease within affected family pedigrees are lacking in lung cancer. Linkage studies have been feasible in mouse models, and are described under Animal models below. In humans, although the segregation analysis performed by Sellers described above suggested a Mendelian inheritance pattern, most studies suggest that the genetic basis of lung cancer is complex, with a multitude of genetic variants conferring differential susceptibility to disease. With the advent of whole genome mapping techniques, the potential for applying linkage disequilibrium mapping to complex disease genes is being explored.[84,85] Studies in lung cancer are forthcoming.

## Association studies: lung cancer risk and genetic polymorphisms

Rare, highly penetrant mutations can significantly increase an individual's cancer risk, as evidenced by diseases such as Li–Fraumeni syndrome and xeroderma pigmentosum.

Inherited mutations in *CHEK2* and *p53* (*TP53*) in Li–Fraumeni syndrome lead to a cancer predisposition, particularly increasing the risk of developing certain soft-tissue sarcomas, osteosarcomas, breast and brain tumors, leukemia, and adrenocortical cancers. Similarly, inherited mutations in the xeroderma pigmentosum family of genes leads to increased risk of skin cancers.

Other more common genetic factors can be important determinants of population risk for cancers, particularly in relation to environmental and carcinogen exposure.[86] Gene–environment interactions are likely to play an important role in lung cancer. Although cigarette smoking is a major causative factor, not all smokers develop lung cancer, and lung cancer can arise in never-smokers. This variation has spurred interest in investigations of genetic polymorphisms, particularly in carcinogen-metabolizing pathways and DNA repair pathways, that may lead to different susceptibility to the carcinogens of tobacco smoke.

## POLYMORPHISMS IN METABOLIC GENES

Polymorphisms in phase I and II enzymes which are involved in activation and detoxification of carcinogens have been identified and may be associated with differential ability to process carcinogens (Table 15.3). Accumulation of active

**Table 15.3** *Selected genetic polymorphisms studied in lung cancer risk*

| | Nucleotide change | Amino acid change | Enzymatic activity |
|---|---|---|---|
| *Metabolic genes* | | | |
| CYP1A1 | T- → C (*Msp*I) | NA | Increased |
| | A- → G | Ile462Val | Increased |
| *CYP2E1* | T- → A (*Dra*I) | NA | Increased |
| | G- → C (*Rsa*I) | NA | Increased |
| CYP2A13 | C- → T | Arg257Cys | Decreased |
| GSTM1 | deletion | NA | None |
| GSTP1 | A- → G | Ile105Val | Decreased |
| GSTT1 | deletion | NA | None |
| NAT2 | T- → C | Ile114Thr | Decreased |
| | C- → T | Lys161Lys | Decreased |
| | A- → G | Lys268Arg | Decreased |
| | G- → A | Arg197Gln | Decreased |
| | C- → T | Tyr94Tyr | Decreased |
| | G- → A | Gly286Glu | Decreased |
| *mEH* | T- → C | Tyr113His | Decreased |
| | A- → G | His139Arg | Increased |
| *DNA repair genes* | | | |
| ERCC2 | A- → C | Lys751Gln | Inconclusive |
| | G- → A | Asp312Asn | Decreased |
| *XRCC1* | C- → T | Arg194Trp | Inconclusive |
| | G- → A | Arg280His | Inconclusive |
| | G- → A | Arg399Gln | Decreased |
| *Cell cycle regulators* | | | |
| *p53* | G- → C | Arg72Pro | Inconclusive |

Table adapted from Wu et al.[386]

carcinogen metabolites and hence increased DNA adduct formation is hypothesized to add to lung cancer risk. Studies in the lung tissue of cancer-free autopsy cases have demonstrated that polymorphisms in *CYP2D6*, *CYP2E1*, and *GSTM1* are associated with higher DNA adduct levels, suggesting that variations in metabolic pathways can play a role in how individuals respond to carcinogen exposure.[87] Numerous studies have extended this line of analysis, to investigate whether this differential ability to metabolize carcinogens leads to differential lung cancer risk. Overall, the data from the study of these polymorphisms have generated inconsistent results. These inconsistencies may be due to a combination of small sample size and the variable frequencies of the polymorphic alleles within different ethnic populations.

### CYP1A1

CYP1A1 is a member of the cytochrome P450 family, a class of phase I enzymes. It is hypothesized that interindividual variations in the ability to activate carcinogens, such as polyaromatic hydrocarbons, may lead to a differential carcinogenic effect. At least two variant polymorphisms have been described in the *CYP1A1* gene. The first is a $T^{3801}C$ base change in intron 6, which results in a new *Msp*I restriction site,[88] the second is an $A^{2455}G$ base change in exon 7, which results in an Ile to Val amino acid change.[89] These polymorphisms appear to be linked. Consistency in study results is lacking, with widely disparate results among different populations.

In Japanese populations, both of the *CYP1A1* variant polymorphisms have been associated with increased lung cancer risk. Nakachi et al.[90] were the first to report an association of the *Msp*I polymorphism with lung cancer risk. Patients with lung cancer had a more than two-fold higher frequency of having the homozygous variant genotype. Among patients with squamous cell carcinoma, the homozygous variant genotype was associated with increased risk of developing lung cancer, especially at a lower cumulative dose of cigarette smoke. At low levels of exposure to cigarette smoke, the odds ratio for developing lung cancer among those with the homozygous variant genotype was 7.31 (95 percent CI, 2.13–25.12). This increased risk was persistent, but of lesser magnitude, at higher dose levels of cigarette smoke (OR, 2.00 and 1.13). Okada et al.[91] reported similar findings.

The *Ile462Val* polymorphism of *CYP1A1* has also been associated with lung cancer risk in Japanese populations. Again, the homozygous variant *Val–Val* genotype was associated with lung cancer at lower cumulative doses of cigarette smoke.[92] One explanation posited for the relationship with low dose level has been that at high dose levels, the relevant enzyme is saturated, while at low doses it is not.[93] The effects of genetic variability and differential enzymatic activity are more apparent at the lower cigarette dose levels, when saturation has not yet been reached.

Outside Japan, consistent results have been more difficult to achieve. Individual studies may be underpowered,[94] since the *CYP1A1* polymorphisms, which are relatively common in Japan (30 percent of population),[92] are much less common in Europeans and North Americans (<10 percent of population).[95] While a study of African-Americans and Mexican-Americans showed a two-fold increased risk of lung cancer among light smokers with the *Msp*I variant genotype,[96] a Brazilian study showed increased risk with the *Ile–Val* polymorphism and not the *Msp*I polymorphism.[97] Reports from Norway and Finland show a lack of association of either of the *CYP1A1* polymorphisms with lung cancer risk.[98,99] A meta-analysis provided little support for the association of *CYP1A1* polymorphisms with lung cancer risk.[100]

Given the small sample sizes in these studies, Vineis et al.[101] conducted a pooled analysis using the international gene susceptibility to environmental carcinogenesis (GSEC) dataset. This dataset included raw data from 22 case–control studies, with a total of 2451 cases and 3358 controls; this comprised approximately half of the case–control studies published at that time. An association was found in Caucasians between the *CYP1A1* homozygous *Msp*I variant and lung cancer risk, when adjusted for age and gender (OR, 2.36; 95 percent CI, 1.16–4.81). The association held for both squamous cell carcinoma and adenocarcinoma.[101] Interestingly, among Asians in this pooled analysis, this association failed to meet statistical significance; of note, studies such as the Nakachi study were not included, making the Asian data difficult to interpret.

### CYP2E1

The shift in histology from squamous cell to adeno-carcinoma has been attributed to changes in cigarette content and smoking behavior. Filtered low tar cigarettes which became common after the 1950s permit deeper inhalation of smoke to compensate for the lesser nicotine content; as particulate matter deposits further along the bronchial tree, peripherally located adenocarcinomas become more common. In addition, the newer cigarettes contain less polycyclic aromatic hydrocarbons and more nitrosamines than older cigarettes. CYP2E1 is a member of the CYP phase I family that is involved in activation of nitrosamines. Le Marchand et al. performed a population-based case–control study among 341 lung cancer cases and 456 controls, and found that *CYP2E1* polymorphisms were associated with a decrease in adenocarcinoma risk. On the other hand, the presence of at least one variant *CYP1A1 Msp*I allele was associated with an increased risk of squamous cell carcinoma, both alone (2.4-fold increase in risk) and in combination with *GSTM1* deletion (3.1-fold increase in risk).[102] The authors suggest that the associations between *CYP1A1* and squamous cell carcinoma and *CYP2E1* and adenocarcinoma may indicate a specificity of PAHs for inducing SCC and NNKs for inducing adenocarcinoma.

### CYP2A13

CYP2A13 is expressed primarily in the respiratory tract and participates in the metabolic activation of N-nitrosamines such as 4-(methylnitrosamino)-1-(3-pyridyl)-1-butanone (NNK). A polymorphism in CYP2A13 has been identified where a C- $\rightarrow$ T transition leads to an Arg $\rightarrow$ Cys substitution at position 257. The variant 257Cys protein has a two- to three-fold reduced capacity to activate NNK compared to the 257Arg protein.[103,104] In a study of 724 lung cancer patients and 791 controls, Wang et al.[105] demonstrated that the variant *CYP2A13* genotype (*CT* or *TT*) was associated with reduced risk for lung cancer, particularly adenocarcinoma (OR, 0.41; 95 percent CI, 0.23–0.71). The reduction in risk did not reach statistical significance for squamous cell or other histolologies. The reduced risk for adenocarcinoma was apparent only in smokers, and in light smokers rather than heavy smokers,[105] again suggesting that genetic polymorphisms may play a greater role when the carcinogen dose is present, but does not saturate, enzymatic capacity. Interestingly, the frequency of this polymorphism varies, with reports in different ethnic populations from 2 to 14 percent, and a French group that screened for polymorphisms in *CYP2A13* among 102 Caucasians found none in their population, although six other polymorphisms were identified.[106]

### GSTM1

The glutathione-S-transferases are a class of phase II enzymes which protect DNA against damage and adduct formation by conjugating glutathiones to electrophilic substances, creating a hydrophilic less reactive metabolite that can be excreted. Different GST families exist (alpha, mu, pi, theta).[107] Large variations in enzymatic activity have been noted for several GSTs. About 50 percent of the population is homozygous for a deletion in the *GSTM1* gene which leads to null expression.[108] Since the GSTM1 enzyme is thought to be important in detoxifying carcinogens, numerous studies have investigated the possible association of the *GSTM1* null genotype with lung cancer risk.

Several studies have found an association between the *GSTM1* null mutation and lung cancer across many populations. In a Japanese population, the *GSTM1* null genotype was positively correlated with squamous cell carcinoma of the lung, although not with adenocarcinoma.[109] Similar analysis in a Finnish population again demonstrated a correlation of the *GSTM1* null genotype with squamous cell cancer,[110] as well as in Scottish,[111] Norwegian,[112] and Turkish populations.[113] However, data are not consistent and some studies have shown a lack of significant association between the *GSTM1* null genotype and lung cancer risk for both squamous cell carcinoma and overall lung cancer.[114–116] A meta-analysis of 12 case–control studies comprising 1593 cases and 2135 controls showed a moderate increase in risk of lung cancer across all histologies with the *GSTM1* null genotype, with an odds ratio of 1.41 (95 percent CI, 1.23–1.61).[117] A more recent meta-analysis of 43 studies including over 18 000 individuals shows a smaller, although still statistically significant, OR of 1.17 (95 percent CI, 1.07–1.27).[118]

Indeed, the risk conferred may be quite small in magnitude, but may be enhanced by interaction with smoking. Kihara and colleagues[119] analyzed 178 Japanese lung cancer patients and 201 healthy controls and found that the GSTM1 null genotype was associated with overall lung cancer risk (OR, 1.87; 95 percent CI, 1.21–2.87), with the strongest association for squamous cell carcinoma (OR, 2.13; 95 percent CI, 1.11–4.07). When stratified by amount of smoking, the proportion of GSTM1 null genotype increased progressively in the squamous cell carcinoma group from 50 percent in the lowest smoking group, to 72 percent in the highest smoking group.

The role of GSTM1 in second-hand smoke and lung cancer risk has also been studied. Bennett et al.[120] analyzed archival tumor tissue from 106 never-smoking women who developed lung cancer, and analyzed them based on exposure to environmental tobacco smoke. Analysis for germline polymorphisms in CYP1A1, GSTM1, and GSTT1 revealed a significant association of the GSTM1 polymorphism and lung cancer risk among those exposed to environmental smoke. When compared to the never-smoking lung cancer cases who had no environmental tobacco exposure, those who had exposure to environmental tobacco smoke were more likely to have the GSTM1 null mutation (OR, 2.6; 95 percent CI, 1.1–6.1). Increasing risk occurred with increasing environmental tobacco smoke exposure.[120] Similar results were found for the GSTM1 null genotype and high environmental tobacco smoke exposure among Japanese women.[121]

Thus, while the effect of GSTM1 by itself may be small, it may be magnified by the gene–environment interaction, with significantly larger effects seen with increasing exposure to cigarette smoke, including second-hand smoke. In addition, the relatively high frequency of GSTM1 polymorphism observed across all ethnicities may contribute to its importance.

### CYP1A1 and GSTM1 polymorphisms in combination

The combination of the CYP1A1 and GSTM1 variant genotypes has been of particular interest, since the combined phase I and II actions of increased activation and decreased metabolism of polyaromatic hydrocarbons in tobacco smoke has been hypothesized to lead to increased lung cancer risk. Numerous studies have explored this association; perhaps the strongest studies come from Japan, although limited in general by small sample size.

The combined genotype of the CYP1A1 variant genotype and the GSTM1 null genotype was shown to enhance the risk of smoking-related lung cancers in a Japanese population. This was demonstrated with the Ile–Val polymorphism by Hayashi and colleagues,[122] who showed an increased frequency of the homozygous Val–Val genotype combined with the GSTM1 null genotype in lung cancer patients compared to controls (8.5 versus 2.2 percent). Nakachi and colleagues[123] reported similar results with both the MspI and Ile–Val polymorphisms and GSTM1 null.

In a case–control study, they found either of the two CYP1A1 susceptible genotypes combined synergistically with the deficient GSTM1 genotype to create a high risk for lung cancer (OR, 16 and 41, respectively, with 95 percent CI, 3.76–68.02 and 8.68–193.61, respectively) at low cigarette dose levels. Eighty-seven percent of those who developed lung cancer in the low cigarette dose group had at least one of the three homozygous variant genotypes. The authors suggest that particularly when cigarette dose is low, CYP1A1 and GSTM1 may play important roles in defining susceptibility to lung cancer.[123]

The synergistic effect was again demonstrated by Kihara et al.[124] Individuals with the variant genotypes in both CYP1A1 and GSTM1 had a much higher risk of lung cancer than those with the variant CYP1A1 but wildtype GSTM1 (OR of 21.9 versus 3.2). Studies in Scandinavian populations,[125,126] as well as American populations,[127] support the increased risk of lung cancer with the combination of variant CYP1A1 and GSTM1 genotypes. A pooled analysis of 302 cases and 1631 controls among Caucasian nonsmokers showed an increased risk with the combined CYP1A1 Ile/Val polymorphism and GSTM1 null polymorphism.[128]

### GSTP1

GSTP1 is a member of the GST family of phase II enzymes that has high expression in the lung. Polymorphisms in GSTP1 have been reported, where an A → G base change leads to an isoleucine → valine substitution resulting in lower enzymatic activity and higher levels of PAH-DNA adducts.[129] Several studies showed no statistically significant association between GSTP1 polymorphisms and lung cancer risk.[116,130–133] However, a study with the largest sample size of 1042 cases and 1161 controls found that the GSTP1 homozygous variant genotype was associated with higher lung cancer risk at any level of smoking exposure when compared to wildtype, approximately doubling the risk associated with pack-years of smoking.[134] The same group analyzed the GSTP1 variant genotype in relation to environmental tobacco smoke exposure and lung cancer risk. Environmental tobacco smoke exposure was associated with higher lung cancer risk, and the presence of the homozygous variant (GG) genotype increased this risk even further.[135]

The combination of GSTM1 null and GSTP1 GG genotypes may confer increased lung cancer risk.[112,136,137] In a study of 1694 cases and controls, double variants in GSTM1 and GSTP1 as well as GSTP1 and p53 have been associated with increased lung cancer risk among individuals age 55 or younger (AOR 4.03, 95 percent CI 1.47–11.1 for the M1-P1 DV; AOR 5.10, 95 percent CI 1.42–18.30 for the P1-p53 DV).[138]

### GSTT1

GSTT1, another member of the GST family of phase II enzymes, is involved in the metabolism of monohalomethanes and ethylene oxide found in tobacco smoke. Results generally have not supported an association with lung cancer risk,[139–143] although one Danish study reported an increased risk of lung cancer with the GSTT1 null genotype.[144]

## NAT2

N-acetyltransferase 2 (NAT2) has dual actions; it inactivates aromatic amines through N-acetylation, but can also activate certain arylamine metabolites through N- and O-acetylation. There are several widely studied polymorphisms for the *NAT2* gene associated with decreased activity or stability of the enzyme. Phenotypically these polymorphisms result in slow or fast acetylation. Studies have been conflicting regarding the association with lung cancer risk. Most studies report no overall increase in risk with either the slow or fast acetylators,[145–148] whereas a few have reported increased risk with either the slow[149,150] or fast[151] acetylator genotype. In the largest study of 1115 lung cancer patients and 1250 controls, no association was found between the *NAT2* genotype and lung cancer risk. However, a significant interaction was found with smoking: among nonsmokers, the rapid acetylator genotype had a decreased lung cancer risk when compared to the slow acetylator genotype; among smokers this relationship reversed, and the rapid acetylators had a higher risk. The authors hypothesize that for nonsmokers, NAT2 may provide an alternative pathway to CYP-mediated activation, providing a means of N-acetylating and detoxifying the aromatic amines and protecting against cancer. However, in smokers, CYP oxidation is markedly induced by cigarette smoke and the production of reactive intermediates is increased. In this setting NAT2 may instead O-acetylate these metabolites and thereby produce more reactive metabolites, thus augmenting cancer risk.[152]

## mEH (also known as EPHX1)

Microsomal epoxide hydrolase has several functions and like NAT2 can act as both an activator and detoxifier of carcinogens. In its detoxifying role, mEH catalyzes the hydrolysis of highly reactive epoxide intermediates to less reactive dihydrodiols which are excretable. In its activating role, mEH can metabolize polyaromatic hydrocarbons into reactive diol-epoxides. Several polymorphisms have been identified, including a T → C base change in exon 3 leading to a tyrosine → histidine substitution at residue 113 which is associated with decreased activity of the enzyme, and a A → G base change in exon 4 leading to a histidine → arginine substitution at residue 139 which leads to increased enzymatic activity.[153]

Several studies have noted an increased risk of lung cancer among those carrying the polymorphisms associated with increased enzymatic activity. A study of Mexican-Americans and African-Americans found a greater risk of lung cancer among young Mexican-Americans with the exon 4 polymorphism, but not the exon 3 polymorphism. No association was observed for African-Americans.[154] The homozygous variant genotype at exon 4, conferring increased enzymatic activity, was again found to be associated with increased lung cancer risk in a study in Texas. The combination of exon 3 and 4 polymorphisms that confer high enzymatic activity also significantly increased risk.[155] In a Taiwanese population, high mEH activity, as defined by the corresponding combination of exon 3 and 4 polymorphisms, was associated with risk for squamous cell carcinoma,[156] and in a French population, high mEH activity was similarly associated with lung cancer risk.[157]

Interestingly, a study of 974 Caucasian lung cancer patients and 1142 controls found no relationship between *mEH* polymorphisms and lung cancer risk overall. However, there was evidence of gene–environment interaction, as having the low activity *mEH* genotypes was a risk factor for lung cancer among nonsmokers (OR, 1.89; 95 percent CI, 1.08–3.28), but protective among heavy smokers (OR, 0.65; 95 percent CI, 0.42–1.00).[158] This effect was stronger in squamous cell than adenocarcinoma. The authors hypothesize that this difference may be explained by the dual actions of mEH. In nonsmokers, having low mEH activity may lead to decreased ability to detoxify environmental pollutants, thus increasing lung cancer risk. In smokers, the polyaromatic hydrocarbons of cigarette smoke may be activated by mEH; hence having low activity is protective.

## Others

Many other enzymes involved in the metabolism of carcinogens have been studied. Examples include manganese superoxide dismutase (known as MnSOD or SOD2), which detoxifies oxygen radicals by catalyzing the conversion of superoxide radicals into hydrogen peroxide and oxygen. An alanine to valine substitution at codon 16 has been identified which may be associated with less efficient enzyme transport into mitochondria. The *Val/Val* genotype has been associated with increased risk of lung cancer as compared to wildtype (AOR, 1.67; 95 percent CI, 1.27–2.20), as was the heterozygous variant genotype (AOR, 1.34; 95 percent CI, 1.05–1.70).[159] Myeloperoxidase (MPO) is yet another metabolic enzyme which has been of interest. MPO is involved in activating an intermediate metabolite of benzo(a)pyrene into a more reactive form. A G → A polymorphism in the promoter region has been identified, where the A allele is thought to result in decreased transcription. Studies have been conflicting regarding lung cancer risk. Feyler et al.[160] found a decreased risk of lung cancer with the heterozygous variant *G/A* genotype; this decrease in risk was not statistically significant among the homozygous variants (*A/A*). In contrast, Xu et al.[161] found no association between either the heterozygous or homozygous variant genotypes and lung cancer risk.

## POLYMORPHISMS IN DNA REPAIR GENES

DNA repair and maintenance is important in protecting cells against damage from carcinogens. Reduced DNA repair capacity may permit accumulation of mutations which will eventually promote cancer development. Wei and colleagues measured DNA repair capacity (DRC) among lung cancer cases compared to controls. DRC was measured in peripheral blood lymphocytes by the host–cell reactivation assay, which measures cellular reactivation of a reporter gene damaged by a benzo(a)pyrene diol epoxide. Lung cancer cases had significantly lower levels of DRC compared to controls.[162,163] Using similar techniques, Shen et al.[164] also found decreased DRC among lung cancer cases as compared to controls. Interestingly, they also reported that smokers tended to have more proficient DRC than nonsmokers, suggesting that there may be an adaptive increase in ability to repair DNA damage from prolonged tobacco smoke exposure. Polymorphisms in several DNA repair genes have been identified and targeted for study.

## ERCC2

ERCC2 (or XPD) is involved in nucleotide excision repair. Spitz and colleagues[165] examined polymorphisms at *Lys751Gln* and *Asp312Asn* in 341 lung cancer cases and 360 controls. There was a trend toward increased lung cancer risk with the variant genotype at either allele; when combined, individuals homozygous for the variant genotype at either locus were at increased risk of lung cancer. In addition, the homozygous variant *Gln/Gln* and *Asn/Asn* genotypes were associated with less optimal DRC as measured by the host–cell reactivation assay. Conflicting results were noted by Lunn and colleagues,[166] who found the *Asp312Asn* polymorphism did not affect DNA repair, but that the *Lys/Lys* wildtype genotype led to more chromatid aberrations.

Butkiewicz and colleagues[167] studied 96 cases and 96 controls in Poland and found an increased risk of lung cancer with the *Asp/Asp* genotype, and suggested that the variant *Asn* allele was protective. The strongest association was in light smokers. Contrasting results were obtained in a US study which used a larger sample of 1092 cases and 1290 controls: Zhou et al.[168] found that the *Asn/Asn* genotype was associated with increased lung cancer risk (AOR, 1.47; 95 percent CI, 1.1–2.0, *Asn/Asn* versus *Asp/Asp*). However, while the variant *Asn* allele was a risk factor among non- and light smokers, it was a protective factor among heavy smokers. A similar modification by smoking was found when the combined genotypes were compared. In comparing individuals homozygous for the variant genotype in both polymorphisms compared to individuals homozygous for the wildtype in both, the fitted OR was 2.56 (95 percent CI, 1.3–5.0) among nonsmokers and 0.69 (95 percent CI, 0.4–1.2) among heavy smokers.[168] The authors hypothesize that among light smokers or nonsmokers, DNA damage induced by tobacco-related carcinogens may be differentially repaired by polymorphic variants of the *ERCC1* gene. However, among heavy smokers, the damage may be too great for these polymorphisms to have a significant effect.

The same study did not find a significant association between the *Lys751Gln* polymorphism and lung cancer risk (AOR, 1.06; 95 percent CI, 0.8–1.4, *Gln/Gln* versus *Lys/Lys*).[168] Several other studies corroborate this lack of association.[169–171]

## XRCC1

XRCC1 also has a role in repairing DNA damage.[172] Several polymorphisms have been identified, including *Arg194Trp*, *Arg280His*, and *Arg399Gln*. Duell et al.[173] examined human blood mononuclear cells of healthy subjects for DNA damage and found that damage as measured by both DNA adducts and sister chromatid exchange was increased among carriers of the *XRCC1 399Gln* allele. Matullo and colleagues[174] found similar results among nonsmokers only.

The association of the *Arg399Gln* polymorphism of *XRCC1* with lung cancer has been inconsistent across studies. Park and colleagues[175] found that the presence of at least one *Gln* allele was associated with an increased risk of squamous cell carcinoma (OR, 1.77; 95 percent CI, 1.06–2.93), with increasing risk as the number of *Gln* alleles increased. Similarly, Divine et al.[176] reported a significant association between the *Gln/Gln* homozygous variant genotype and adenocarcinoma risk. However, Ratnasinghe and colleagues[177] found no significant association between the *Arg399Gln* polymorphism and lung cancer risk. A small association was found with *Arg280His* (OR, 1.8; 95 percent CI, 1.0–3.4).[177,178] In the largest sample size of 1091 cases and 1240 controls, the *XRCC1 Arg399Gln* polymorphism had only a borderline association with lung cancer risk (AOR, 1.3; 95 percent CI, 1.0–1.8, *Gln/Gln* versus *Arg/Arg*). This risk was significantly higher among younger subjects. Among nonsmokers and light smokers, the *Gln/Gln* genotype was a risk factor for lung cancer, but among heavy smokers it was protective. When combined with the *ERCC2* polymorphisms, having more than three variant alleles were risk factors for nonsmokers, but protective factors for heavy smokers.[179]

## POLYMORPHISMS IN CELL CYCLE REGULATORS

### p53 (also known as TP53)

The *p53* tumor suppressor gene is one of the most frequently mutated genes in human cancer.[180] The p53 protein is involved in control of the cell cycle, DNA repair, cell differentiation, and apoptosis.[181] Both somatic and germline mutations in p53 have been studied and implicated in human cancers. A germline polymorphism in codon 72 has been studied (Arg → Pro substitution), with conflicting results. Weston et al.[182] initially reported a trend toward increased frequency of the variant allele in adenocarcinomas, but later studies by the same group did not find the same association.[183] Similarly, a Spanish study reported no difference between cases and controls for the *Pro* allele.[184]

In contrast, the homozygous *Pro/Pro* variant genotype was found to be associated with a 1.7-fold higher risk of lung cancer among Japanese study patients.[185] Among African-Americans this increased risk did not reach statistical significance, but individuals with the *Pro/Pro* genotype appeared to have an earlier age at diagnosis, as well as lower cumulative pack-years of smoking.[186] A large study of 482 cases and 510 controls showed presence of the variant *Pro* allele was associated with a 1.45-fold higher risk of adenocarcinoma compared with the wildtype genotype, with higher risk with heavier smoking.[187] Wu and colleagues[188] performed an analysis of three p53 polymorphisms (exon 4 codon 72, intron 3, intron 6) among 635 cases and controls and found that each of the variant polymorphisms, as well as the variant haplotypes, were associated with increased risk of lung cancer.

## ACQUIRED SOMATIC MUTATIONS

While genetic polymorphisms may increase the risk of carcinogenesis, the actual development of lung cancer requires a series of somatic mutations as normal bronchial epithelial cells acquire malignant capabilities. Numerous molecular abnormalities have been described in the course of lung cancer pathogenesis.[189–194] These include chromosomal abnormalities, loss of normal growth signal inhibition via activation of oncogenes or loss of tumor suppressor genes, epigenetic events such as aberrant methylation, and increased expression of tumor invasive, metastatic, and angiogenic factors. While a detailed sequence of mutational events, as has been described for colon cancer, has not been developed for lung cancer, some of the most common somatic changes have been characterized. The study of these somatic genetic changes reflects not only the search for a better understanding of lung cancer, but also a search for molecular markers that would help define tumor aggressiveness and prognosis, as well as identify potential targets for treatment.[195]

### Structural chromosomal abnormalities

Multiple structural abnormalities in chromosomes have been associated with lung cancer. These include chromosomal imbalances which are frequently observed in both SCLC and NSCLC, telomerase activity, and epigenetic events, such as aberrant promoter methylation.

### Chromosomal imbalances

Recurrent chromosomal imbalances have been described for both small cell and nonsmall cell lung cancer, with losses in chromosomes 1, 3, 5, 13, and 17 being common in SCLC, and losses in 1, 3, 5, 6, 7, 8, 9, 11, 13, 14, 15, and 17 in NSCLC (Table 15.4).[196,197] Loss of heterozygosity may be an early event in lung cancer pathogenesis, as LOH has been shown in the bronchial epithelium of smokers, as well as in preoplastic lung tissue.

Damage by carcinogens associated with smoking may promote a field cancerization effect. LOH at 3p, 9p, and 17p has been shown in the bronchial epithelial cells of chronic smokers who were cancer-free; the frequency of LOH tended to be lower in former smokers than current smokers (62 versus 82 percent).[198] LOH in 3p, 9p, and 17p is present even in the histologically normal tissue of smokers,

**Table 15.4** *Common somatic molecular changes in lung cancer*

|  | SCLC | NSCLC |
|---|---|---|
| Common chromosomal imbalances | 1, 3, 5, 13, 17 | 1, 3, 5, 6, 7, 8, 9, 11, 13, 14, 15, 17 |
| Loss of *3p* (%) | 90 | 50–80 |
| Telomerase activity (%) | 90–100 | 80–85 |
| *Ras* mutation (%) | <1 | 15–20 |
| *Myc* amplification (%) | 15–30 | 5–10 |
| Bcl-2 expression (%) | 75–95 | 10–35 |
| EGFR overexpression (%) | Rare | 40–80 |
| *p53* mutation (%) | 75–100 | 50 |
| p53 abnormal expression (%) | 40–70 | 40–60 |
| Rb absent expression (%) | 90 | 15–30 |
| *p16* mutation (%) | <1 | 10–40 |
| p16 absent expression (%) | 0–10 | 30–70 |

Table adapted from Sekido et al.[328]

while in nonsmokers the presence of LOH appears to be virtually nil.[199] Increasing pack-years of smoking has been associated with increasing frequency of LOH.[200] In actual tumor tissue, LOH patterns differ between the cancers of smokers and nonsmokers.[201,202]

Numerous studies have shown a variety of allelic deletions in pre- or perimalignant tissue. Examination of normal epithelium, preneoplastic lesions, carcinoma-in-situ, and invasive tumor from 12 cases of NSCLC showed a progressive increase in overall LOH frequency with increasing histologic abnormality; 3p21 was one of the earliest changes.[203] LOH at 3p and 9p has been demonstrated in preinvasive lesions of the lungs of patients with NSCLC,[204–206] with many cases demonstrating identical patterns of allelic loss in preneoplastic and neoplastic tissue.[207,208] Bronchial cells adjacent to tumor also demonstrate chromosomal abnormalities, including LOH at 5p, 3p, 9p, and 17p.[209]

### 3p LOSS

Allelic loss at 3p is most frequently described and occurs in approximately 90 percent of SCLC and 50–80 percent of NSCLC. Studies suggest 3p loss may be associated with smoking.[210] Deletion of 3p(14-23) by karyotypic analysis was first noted in 12 of 12 cell lines cultured from human small cell lung cancer tissue.[211] Molecular genetic approaches using restriction fragment length polymorphisms (RFLPs) subsequently confirmed these cytogenetic findings: loss of heterozygosity for 3p markers was demonstrated in nine of nine small cell lung cancer cases;[212] in a larger sample, LOH at 3p was demonstrated in 23 of 25 (92 percent) SCLC cases.[213] While loss of 3p has been consistently reportedly in over 90 percent of SCLC, the frequency of allelic loss on 3p in NSCLC is more variable, with reports ranging from 25 to over 80 percent.[214–217]

The areas of deletion have been focused to 3p14, 3p21, and 3p25.[218–220] Allele loss is highly suggestive of the presence of tumor suppressor genes,[221] and investigators have explored various candidate genes in this region that would elucidate the functional consequences of these chromosomal abnormalities. The von Hippel–Lindau gene located at 3p25 was an early candidate, but was found to be rarely mutated in lung cancer cell lines.[222] Other potential candidate tumor suppressor genes in the 3p region involved in lung cancer include beta-catenin and beta retinoic acid receptor, as well as the semaphorin IV and A (V) genes.[223–227]

Recently, much interest has centered on FHIT and RASSF1A as potential candidate tumor suppressor genes on 3p. FHIT (fragile histidine triad) on 3p14.2 encodes a protein that is involved in metabolizing diadenosine tetraphosphate into adenosine triphosphate and monophosphate; without its activity, diadenosine tetraphosphate accumulates and stimulates DNA synthesis and proliferation. Sozzi et al.[228] analyzed 59 tumors and found that in SCLC, 11 of 14 (79 percent) had abnormal RNA transcripts of FHIT by RT-PCR; in NSCLC, 18 of 45 (40 percent) had abnormal transcripts. Over three-quarters of informative cases had loss of one FHIT allele. LOH at loci in the FHIT gene was found to affect the cancers of smokers more than non-smokers (80 versus 22 percent).[229] Loss of FHIT expression correlated with LOH at 3p14.2, the locus of the FHIT gene, and may also be more associated with squamous histology.[230]

The RASSF1 gene has also been identified as a possible tumor suppressor gene in this region. Dammann et al.[231] found that the RASSF1A transcript was missing in all 17 SCLC cell lines examined. Extending this analysis, Burbee et al.[232] found that RASSF1A was expressed in all normal lung epithelial tissues examined, but not in 32 of 32 (100 percent) SCLC cell lines, and 17 of 26 (65 percent) NSCLC cell lines. Aberrant promoter methylation may be the means of silencing transcription of RASSF1A in both SCLC and NSCLC.[231,233]

## TELOMERASE ACTIVITY

Another chromosomal structural abnormality that appears to promote tumorigenesis involves telomerase activity. Telomerase is a reverse transcriptase that synthesizes telomeres, the nucleoprotein structures that normally cap the ends of human chromosomes, protecting the chromosome from damage. Telomerase activity and the maintenance of telomere length has been associated with persistent replicative, and hence malignant, potential. Kim et al.[234] found that 98 of 100 immortalized cell lines, most derived from tumor, displayed telomerase activity, whereas none of 22 actively proliferating normal somatic cell cultures had detectable levels of telomerase activity. A balance between telomere length and telomerase activity acts to suppress and facilitate cancer progression; persistent telomerase activity may mediate persistent replicative potential by maintaining telomere length beyond normal senescence. However, without adequate telomerase activity, telomere lengths that are too short may also be carcinogenic, as they render the genome more unstable and susceptible to damage.[235] Telomerase

activity alone may not be sufficient for immortalization of cells, but the combination of Rb/p16 inactivation and telomerase activity can immortalize cell lines effectively.[236]

High levels of telomerase activity have been documented in lung cancer. Telomerase activity was found in 78 percent of NSCLCs and 100 percent of SCLCs examined in one study.[237] Telomerase activity appears to localize to cancerous tissue rather than adjacent normal lung tissue: in one study, telomerase activity was detected in 84 of 99 resected lung cancers, but not in the adjacent normal lung tissue;[238] another found telomerase activity in 80 percent of 136 primary resected lung cancer tissues, and in only 4 percent of 68 normal adjacent lung tissues. High telomerase activity was observed in metastatic lesions as well.[237] Telomerase activity has been associated with advanced pathologic stage and high rates of cell proliferation as detected by Ki-67 immunostaining.[238]

Telomerase activity may portend a worse prognosis. Among 107 patients with primary resected stage I NSCLC, 62 percent demonstrated telomerase activity in the tumor sample; this was associated with worse disease-free and overall survival.[239] Telomerase activity has been associated with more advanced grade and stage of disease, as well as shorter overall survival.[240] Interestingly, in light of the suggestion that telomerase activity and Rb/p16 inactivation are needed for cell immortality, one group found an interaction between telomerase activity and p16 expression, with expression of p16 being a protective factor among early stage tumors that had telomerase activity.[241]

## EPIGENETIC EVENTS

### Aberrant methylation

Epigenetic events may be important in modulating gene expression and function. Methylation of CpG islands in promoter regions is one mechanism by which gene expression is decreased. In a study of 107 resected NSCLC compared to 104 corresponding nonmalignant lung tissue samples, Zochbauer-Muller et al.[242] detected methylation in multiple genes, including RARB, TIMP3, p16 (CDKN2A), MGMT, DAPK, CHD1, and GSTP1. Demethylation can lead to restoration of transcription: Virmani et al.[243] reported that methylation of the P2 promoter region of RARB corresponds to silencing of transcripts of RARB2 and RARB4 in both NSCLC and SCLC, and that chemical demethylation via aza-CDR restored transcription. Smoking may be associated with aberrant methylation, and has been reported in multiple studies.[244–246] Investigators have sought to elucidate the prognostic impact of methylation, and some studies have associated aberrant methylation of various genes with advanced stage and poor prognosis.[247–249]

## Loss of normal growth inhibition: oncogenes

Activation of protooncogenes to oncogenes leads to constitutive activation and gain of function that can lead to cellular hyperproliferation.[250] A number of oncogenes have been identified in lung cancer and efforts have been made to characterize their association with prognosis.

## RAS

The *RAS* family of genes was one of the first oncogenes identified and encodes plasma membrane proteins which play a key role in signal transduction. Activation can lead to inappropriate signaling and cell proliferation. Mutations in *K-ras* are reported for up to 50 percent of NSCLC, but rarely for SCLC.[251,152] Mutations are most commonly reported in codons 12, 13, and 61, with G to T transversions in codon 12 being most prevalent.[253,254] *K-ras* mutations appear to be more common in adenocarcinomas and smokers.[255–257] Numerous studies have reported worse survival outcomes in patients carrying *K-ras* mutations,[258–261] and a meta-analysis reported worse prognosis with *K-ras* mutations, but with the caveat that there was considerable heterogeneity across studies.[262] Indeed, the data are not completely consistent and others have reported no association with prognosis.[263] Interestingly, Siegfried et al.[264] examined 181 adenocarcinomas and found no difference in survival with *K-ras* mutations overall; however, they found that specific amino acid substitutions (i.e. cysteine, arginine, or aspartate) may correlate with survival, and suggest that studies that show association with survival have higher proportions of these mutations than those that do not.

## Bcl-2

The *bcl-2* proto-oncogene encodes a protein that is thought to protect cells from apoptosis; overexpression of bcl-2 leads to downregulation of programmed cell death. The precise cause of the overexpression of bcl-2 in lung cancer is unknown; the characteristic (14;18) translocation that causes overexpression in hematologic malignancy has not been seen in lung cancer. However, expression of bcl-2 protein has been detected in 75 to 95 percent of SCLC,[265] and 10 to 25 percent of NSCLC.[266] Studies have been conflicting as to the relationship of *bcl-2* and prognosis. Several studies report that bcl-2 expression is associated with better prognosis,[267,268] and some have suggested that this improved survival may be limited to older and squamous histology subgroups.[269,270] However, shortened survival has also been reported with bcl-2 expression.[271–274] A meta-analysis suggested a trend towards improved survival with bcl-2 expression in NSCLC; data were insufficient to analyze SCLC.[275]

## Myc

Myc proteins belong to the basic helix–loop–helix leucine zipper class of transcription factors and participate in transcriptional activation of genes. Gene amplification of the *myc* family of oncogenes (*c-myc*, *n-myc*, *l-myc*) has been described for lung cancer[276–278] and is more common in SCLC than NSCLC.[279,280] Amplification of *myc* has been more frequently observed after treatment with chemotherapy in SCLC and may be associated with worse survival.[281–283]

DNA amplification of *myc* is thought to confer a growth advantage to the transformed cell, enhancing its capacity for further proliferation.[280]

## ErbB

The erbB family of tyrosine kinase receptor proteins plays an important role in signal transduction. On ligand binding, erbB receptors form homo- or heterodimers and initiate a signal transduction cascade that is important in growth stimulation. *EGFR* encodes the epidermal growth factor receptor (EGFR) and *ERBB2* encodes the her2/neu receptor.

Expression of EGFR is a frequent finding in cell lines of NSCLC, but not SCLC.[284] EGFR has been shown to be overexpressed in metaplastic and neoplastic lung tissue compared to normal bronchial epithelium.[285–287] EGFR protein overexpression as measured by immunohistochemistry correlates with increased gene copy numbers by FISH.[288] Data are conflicting as to the prognostic role of EGFR overexpression. Several studies have found no association with prognosis,[289–293] while a few studies have found worse prognosis with EGFR overexpression.[294,295] As described above, mutations in the tyrosine kinase domain of EGFR have been found in the tumor tissue of patients who respond to gefinitib. These mutations have been typically missense mutations or in-frame deletions that appear to localize to the tyrosine kinase domain.[56,57] This discovery has significant import for targeting therapy.

In the same family of tyrosine kinase receptors, her2/neu overexpression has also been reported in lung cancer, particularly adenocarcinoma.[296–298] Again, data on prognosis is conflicting with some studies reporting no association[290,291] and others reporting worse survival with her2/neu overexpression in lung cancer.[299,300]

## Loss of normal growth inhibition: tumor suppressor genes

The loss of tumor suppressor genes which normally act to inhibit cell growth and proliferation is critical in the stepwise progression to cancer. Multiple tumor suppressor genes have been studied, including the candidate genes hypothesized at the 3p locus. Other commonly mutated genes which play a role in lung cancer pathogenesis include *p53*, *Rb*, and *p16*.

### p53

The *p53* gene, located at chromosome 17p13.1, is involved in cell cycle regulation, induction of apoptosis, and stabilization of the genome, and is mutated in over half of all human cancers. Over 90 percent of SCLC and 50 percent of NSCLC have mutations in *p53*.[301] Studies have used variable means of assaying *p53* abnormalities, and run the gamut from immunohistochemical studies for p53 protein expression to detection of mutations by PCR or direct DNA sequencing. Measures of protein expression are based on the assumption that missense mutations lead to stabilization of *p53* protein, whereas wildtype protein would not be detectable;[302] concordance between the two assays is reported to be between 60 and 70 percent.[303]

Numerous abnormalities in *p53* have been described. Homozygous deletions and rearrangements of DNA, absent or abnormally sized mRNA, suggestive of abnormal splicing, initiation, and termination, as well as point mutations have been found.[304] Most mutations along p53 are concentrated within the relatively small DNA-binding domain, with missense mutations accumulating along these 'mutational hotspots.'[305]

Acquired abnormalities in *p53* may be an early event in lung cancer pathogenesis. Evidence of mutations in *p53* has been found in preneoplastic, dysplastic bronchial epithelium. Sozzi and colleagues[306] reported presence of mutant *p53* protein, loss of 17p, and missense mutation within the *p53* gene in both dysplastic and neoplastic bronchial epithelium from the same subjects. Bennett et al.[307] demonstrated increasing levels of *p53* protein, which is stabilized by missense mutations in *p53*, with increasing dysplasia.

*p53* mutations may be more associated with squamous and large cell carcinomas than adenocarcinomas, as well as higher T, N, and overall stage.[308] Smoking is thought to play a role in *p53* mutations, and the higher prevalence of *p53* abnormalities in smoking-related histologies (squamous cell, large cell versus adenocarcinoma) lends indirect support to this hypothesis. Interestingly, G:C → T:A transversions are common mutations in *p53* among squamous, large cell, and small cell carcinomas, but rarer in adenocarcinoma. These transversions are generally thought to result from PAH-adduct formation from tobacco smoke carcinogens.[309–312]

The prognostic impact of *p53* has been debated. Several meta-analyses have suggested that *p53* abnormalities are associated with worse survival; some suggest a significant negative prognostic effect in adenocarcinoma but not squamous cell carcinoma,[313] while others report worse survival in both histologies.[314] *p53* alterations have been associated with involvement of hilar and mediastinal lymph nodes among patients with primary resected NSCLC, suggesting an association with tumor aggressiveness.[315] In a recent prospective study, analysis of tumor samples from 188 patients with operable stage I–IIIA NSCLC for abnormalities in *p53* demonstrated an increased risk of death among stage I, but not stage II or III patients.[316] However, improved survival[317,318] or no association with survival has also been reported[319] and a definitive prognostic role for *p53* remains controversial.

## Rb (ALSO KNOWN AS Rb1)/p16 (ALSO KNOWN AS CDKN2A)

Progression through the cell cycle is a key component of cell growth and differentiation. The G1 to S phase transition of the cell cycle is mediated by a complex of proteins, including p16, cyclin D1, CDK4, and Rb. When the cell is in late G1, Rb protein becomes hypophosphorylated. This hypophosphorylated Rb complexes to E2F, a transcription factor that normally acts to upregulate the cell cycle. E2F becomes inactivated when Rb is bound to it, and hence the cell cycle arrests at G1. Phosphorylation of Rb leads to dissociation from E2F and progression of the cell cycle; this phosphorylation is mediated by CDK4. p16 inhibits CDK activity and thus serves as a mediator of cell cycle arrest.[320–322]

The *Rb* gene is inactivated in over 90 percent of small cell lung cancers,[323,324] but only a minority (15 to 30 percent) of nonsmall cell lung cancers.[325,326] Conversely, p16 is typically expressed in SCLC, but absent or low in NSCLC,[327] and abnormalities of p16 are found in 30–70 percent of NSCLC.[328] A variety of mechanisms for suppression of p16 expression has been found, including allele loss, point mutations, and hypermethylation of CpG islands in the promoter region.[329]

A reciprocal relationship between Rb inactivation and p16 expression has been noted in multiple studies.[330,331] It has been suggested that cell cycle arrest via inhibition of this pathway is mediated primarily via inactivation of Rb for SCLC, and p16 for NSCLC.[327]

The effect of altered Rb and p16 expression on survival has been controversial. Some studies demonstrate an association with worse prognosis,[332,333] perhaps limited to early stage[334] or squamous histology.[335] However, other studies show no effect on survival. Several studies have analyzed p16, Rb, and p53 abnormalities in combination and found no significant association with prognosis, either individually or in combination.[336,337]

## Increased expression of invasive and metastatic factors

Multiple steps are required for tumor cells to spread beyond their primary site. Degradation of extracellular matrix, penetration of basement membrane, entry into the lymphatic and vascular beds, and transit via these systems to distant sites are all part of the metastatic process. Multiple enzymes have been associated with these abilities, including MMP, VEGF, COX, and PAI. Altered levels of expression of these enzymes have been studied as surrogate markers for somatic genetic alterations that induce invasive and metastatic capabilities. Thus most of the studies described below measure levels of protein expression, and attempt to correlate this with tumor biology.

### MMP

The matrix metalloproteinases are a group of proteolytic enzymes that can degrade extracellular matrix and facilitate invasion through the basement membrane. In the MMP family, both MMP-2 and MMP-9 have been studied in lung cancer. Elevated levels of MMP-2 and MMP-9 have been demonstrated in tumor and stromal cells of resected lung cancers,[338,339] as well as elevated plasma MMP-9 levels.[340]

The MMPs (MMP-2 and MMP-9) have been associated with invasion and spread in NSCLC,[341] via their ability to remodel and degrade extracellular matrix, and mediate cell–cell adhesions.[342] MMP-2 overexpression was found in one study of resected NSCLC to be associated with worse prognosis among stage N0 patients, with a 2.6-fold increased risk of cancer-related death.[343]

### uPA (PLAU)

Urokinase-type plasminogen activator (uPA) facilitates the conversion of plasminogen to plasmin. Plasmin degrades extracellular matrix, either directly or indirectly via activation of metalloproteinases. Plasminogen inhibitors (PAI-1, -2; SERPINE1, 2) can inhibit uPA activity. UPA, the uPA-receptor (uPAR, PLAUR), and PAIs have been found to be overexpressed in lung cancer.[344] Levels of uPA may be positively correlated with tumor size[345] and nodal stage.[346] PAI-2 concentrations appear to be significantly higher in lymph node negative rather than positive cases.[345,347] Interestingly, PAI-1 expression has been associated with nodal metastasis, suggesting that although a plasminogen inhibitor, PAI-1 may play a role in mediating tumor aggressiveness.[347] Other studies have not found an association between uPA and PAI levels and tumor stage.[348] Studies have been conflicting as to the prognostic importance of this family of enzymes. Salden et al.[344] reported no association of levels of uPA, uPAR, PAI-1, and PAI-2 with overall survival. Pedersen et al.[348,349] found worse survival with low levels of PAI-1 and high levels of uPAR.

### VEGF

Angiogenesis is thought to play an important role in maintaining tumor growth, as new blood vessels are needed to supply the spreading cancer. Increasing vascularity of tumors, as measured by microvessel count, has been associated with worse prognosis in NSCLC.[350] Alternate splicing of mRNA leads to four different isoforms of VEGF, with 121, 165, 189, and 206 amino acids. VEGF expression has been correlated with high microvessel counts and poor prognosis in NSCLC.[351–353] Interestingly, higher vascularization of tumors may be associated with more sensitivity to chemotherapeutic agents. Volm and colleagues hypothesized that hypoxia may lead to drug resistance as chemotherapies require oxygen to be cytotoxic, and demonstrated resistance to doxorubicin in tumors that had poor microvessel density and VEGF expression.[354] Of note, some studies report no association between microvessel density and prognosis.[355,356]

### OTHERS

Numerous other molecular markers have been investigated with regard to their role in tumor progression and metastasis. Among these are cadherins, transmembrane glycoproteins that play an important role in cell to cell adhesion. Reduced E-cadherin (CDH1) expression has been associated with local invasion, metastasis, and reduced survival.[357] The cyclooxygenases, involved in the conversion of arachidonic acid to prostanoids, have also been studied. Expression of Cox-2 (PTGS2) has been shown in adenocarcinomas and squamous cell carcinomas, with a suggestion of more involvement in adenocarcinoma.[358,359] Elevated Cox-2 levels have been associated with worse prognosis in surgically resected early stage NSCLC, among both adenocarcinomas and squamous cell carcinomas.[360,361]

## Gene expression profiling

While the studies described above have all focused on single genes or molecular markers, microarray technology allows analysis of gene expression on a large scale.[362] As discussed in Chapter 5B, microarrays can provide a wealth of data and various analytic methods have been described to allow clustering, finding of relevant genes, and handling of multiple comparisons.[363] Investigators have used microarrays to classify lung cancers by characteristic gene expression signatures. Bhattacharjee et al. used hierarchical and probabilistic clustering to analyze mRNA expression patterns among 186 lung tumor samples; they were able to classify tumors into established histologies – carcinoid, SCLC, squamous, and adenocarcinoma, and also identified subclasses within adenocarcinoma.[364] Similarly, Garber et al.[365] found distinct cDNA expression patterns between squamous, large cell, small cell and adenocarcinomas, as well as subclasses of adenocarcinoma. Both these studies reported differential survival outcomes associated with the subclasses of adenocarcinoma. The clusters identified by microarray can be further analyzed to generate candidate genes that may be associated with differential outcomes. Beer et al.[366] classified 86 cases of primary adenocarcinoma into three groups based on expression profiling; these groups showed significant differences in terms of prognosis, regardless of histologic stage. Using both training and testing sets and a crossvalidation approach, the authors identified a group of 50 genes which reliably distinguished between poor and good prognosis.[366] Others have used microarrays to differentiate adenocarcinomas of smokers versus nonsmokers.[367,368] The potential for microarrays to help in classifying tumors, in predicting outcomes, and in generating hypotheses for identifying molecular markers of lung cancer, is still being actively explored.

## ANIMAL MODELS

As discussed in Chapter 7, animal models provide a means of performing genetic studies that would not be feasible in the human population. Murine mouse models are among the most prevalent animal systems used to study lung cancer. Several molecular changes noted in murine lung cancers seem to be similar to those found in human lung

cancer. Investigators have reported *K-ras* activating mutations in the majority of murine lung cancers, as well as loss
of heterozygosity in chromosomes 4, 11, and 14, known to
harbor *p16*, *p53*, and *Rb*, respectively.[369] However, most
murine lung cancers are early stage lesions, and are typically adenomas or adenocarcinomas, and hence do not
recapitulate the range of histologies found in human lung
cancer.[370] Despite these limitations, murine models provide a powerful tool for exploring molecular pathways of
lung cancer development.

## Spontaneous and chemically induced mouse models of lung cancer

Mouse strains that are susceptible to spontaneous lung cancer have been identified. A range of susceptibility is reported,
with some strains (A/J and SWR) being most susceptible,
while others have intermediate (BALB/c, O20) or low (DBA,
C57Bl/6) susceptibility.[369] Mice that are at risk for developing spontaneous lung cancers are also susceptible to chemically induced lung cancer. Chemicals such as urethane,
metals, aflatoxin, polyaromatic hydrocarbons, and nitrosamines have been reported to induce lung cancer in the
sensitive strains of mice.[371] Studies of susceptible mouse
strains and tobacco smoke have been performed to develop
an animal model of smoking-induced carcinogenesis.[372,373]

## Linkage studies

Linkage analyses using whole genome crosses have been performed to find loci of lung cancer susceptibility. Several
pulmonary adenoma susceptibility (*Pas*) loci have been identified by crosses between the sensitive and resistant strains
of mice.[374] Crosses between the A/J (sensitive) and C57BL/6J
(resistant) strains have shown that one of these *Pas* loci
appears to be tightly linked to *K-ras*;[375–377] and other susceptibility loci have been mapped to chromosomes 9, 17, and
19.[378] In addition to mapping single loci, investigators have
also used multilocus mapping methods to identify multiple
loci that might be involved in lung cancer development. F2
mice generated from recombinant congenic strains have been
used to identify *Sluc* (susceptibility to lung cancer) loci that
appear to be involved in complex polygenic interactions.[378,379]

## Transgenic mouse models of lung cancer

Transgenic mouse models have allowed investigators to
study specific genes in relation to lung cancer development.
Conventionally, a transgene DNA product is constructed
by fusing a cell-specific promoter to the gene being studied.
Once expressed in the mouse, the cell-specific promoter
directs transcription of the gene. Promoters for the surfactant
protein C (*SP-C*) and Clara cell secretory protein (known
as CLSP, CC10, or Scgb1a1) genes have been most widely

used, and enable targeted gene expression in alveolar type
II cells and nonciliated secretory cells of the bronchi,
respectively.[380] For example, investigators have demonstrated that transgenic mice overexpressing *c-myc* develop
bronchoalveolar hyperplasias, adenomas, and carcinomas,
while mice overexpressing *EGF* develop hyperplasias.[381]
Further studies have shown that in transgenic mice overexpressing *c-myc*, administration of NNK leads to accelera-
tion of carcinogenesis.[382]

A major limitation of the conventional transgenic model
is the lack of control over the timing of gene expression. *SP-C*
promoter regulated transcription occurs around embryonic
day 10 and *CCSP* promoter regulated expression occurs
around embryonic day 17. Many genes cannot be effectively
studied by this model as such early expression would lead
to an early lethal phenotype. In addition, such early oncogenic activation or tumor suppressor silencing is unlikely to
faithfully mimic the pathogenesis of human lung cancer.[380]

Conditional transgenic mouse models have been developed to address some of the limitations of the conventional models. Ligand-inducible binary transgenic systems
have been developed that utilize a regulator transgene and
a target transgene, to allow tighter control of expression of
the candidate gene. The regulator transgene is driven by
one of the cell-specific promoters such as the *CCSP* or *SP-C*
promoter. In the presence of ligand, the regulator induces
expression of the target transgene, allowing on/off switching of gene expression.[380] The tetracycline transactivator-
inducible system is commonly used in lung cancer. One
model uses the reverse *tet* transactivator, which binds to
the *tet* operon and activates gene expression upon administration of ligand (doxycycline). This model has been used
to regulate the expression of various oncogenes. Most
notably, activation of *K-ras* via this model resulted in
hyperplasia of type II pneumocytes, which subsequently
progressed to adenomas or adenocarcinomas. These
tumors regressed when the ligand was withdrawn and *K-
ras* expression declined. In mice that were also lacking
either *p53* or *INK4A/Arf*, *K-ras* expression led to more
rapid lung cancer development.[383]

## Knock-out/knock-in mouse models

The use of conventional knock-out mice has been limited
by the early lethal phenotype and the inability to limit extent
of expression of the candidate gene. However, 'hit and run'
gene targeting has been used to build strains where latent
oncogenes are somatically activated. Mice strains where
one allele is mutated and the other is wildtype have been
generated where somatic recombination leads to activation
and expression of the mutant oncogene.[380] This may better
reflect human lung cancer pathogenesis. Using this strategy,
investigators have shown development of adenocarcinoma
with targeted *K-ras* mutation.[384] Carcinogenesis seemed
to recapitulate human nonsmall cell development, with

morphologic stages from dysplasia to carcinoma observed. Crossing studies with a strain containing a *p53* germline deletion showed that double mutant mice had reduced survival and more malignant tumors.[384]

Attempts have been made to modify the timing and extent of gene expression. Investigators have used Cre recombinase to direct recombination between LoxP sites which flank the gene of interest. Removal of the flanked element (floxed gene) leads to ablation of that gene's expression. Investigators have reported using a floxed stop element to control expression of *K-ras*. *K-ras* expression led to the formation of atypical adenomatous hyperplasia, epithelial hyperplasia, and adenomas. With increasing *K-ras* expression, more lesions were found.[385]

These models hold great promise in allowing investigators to control gene expression and better understand human lung cancer. The ability to manipulate and study genes in a way that would not be possible in the human population gives animal models a powerful insight into the molecular pathways of disease pathogenesis.

## FUTURE DIRECTIONS

The genetic basis of lung cancer is complex, as inherited and somatic mutations interface in multiple ways with each other and with environmental factors, such as cigarette smoking. Some investigators have focused on the germline polymorphisms in metabolizing and DNA repair pathways that confer differential ability to process carcinogens, and hence differential lung cancer risk. Others have sought to elucidate the somatic alterations that transform a normal bronchial cell into one with malignant potential. Understanding the genetic and molecular changes that characterize lung cancer has important clinical applications. Molecular markers of lung cancer may allow for early detection and follow-up of disease. Potential serum markers of disease being investigated include circulating DNA levels of genes such as human telomerase reverse transcriptase (*TERT*), methylation status of various genes such as *p16*, *RASSF1*, and *DAPK*, mutations in specific oncogenes such as *K-ras*, and microsatellite alterations. A reliable serum marker would revolutionize screening for lung cancer, as most early stage curable disease is found incidentally, and radiologic screening studies have not demonstrated clear efficacy. In addition, the study of somatic mutations that alter normal cell behavior has enabled scientists to develop targeted therapies. EGFR and VEGF inhibitors are already in clinical use and the search for more molecular targets is ongoing. Finally, individuals' molecular and genetic profiles may help predict response to therapy. To date, some progress has been made in elucidating how both somatic mutations and genetic polymorphisms can affect the effectiveness and toxicity of certain chemotherapies. In the future, clinicians may be able to tailor chemotherapies based on an individual's known profile, choosing the regimens that are likely to be most effective and least toxic. Gene expression profiles using microarray technology are already providing new insights into lung cancer biology, providing a more panoramic view than that obtained from the investigation of single nucleotide polymorphisms alone. Ultimately, a clear understanding of the genetics of lung cancer, both in terms of inherited risk and somatic mutations, will allow for better risk assessment, prevention, and treatment for this deadly disease.

### Key learning points

- Although 80 percent of lung cancer is attributable to smoking, only 10 percent of smokers develop lung cancer.

- Familial studies, controled for environmental factors such as smoking, suggest that an inherited component to lung cancer exists.

- Germline polymorphisms in metabolic enzyme pathways that activate and detoxify carcinogens and in DNA repair pathways can lead to differential ability to handle carcinogen exposure, and hence differential lung cancer risk.

- Germline polymorphisms in metabolic enzyme pathways that activate and detoxify carcinogens and in DNA repair pathways can lead to differential ability to handle carcinogen exposure, and hence differential lung cancer risk.

- Multiple somatic changes are needed for the normal bronchial cell to transform into a cancerous cell.

- Structural chromosomal abnormalities, oncogenes, growth factors, tumor suppressor genes, as well as multiple molecular markers of tumor invasiveness and metastasis have been studied and characterize lung cancer cells.

- A complex interplay between inherited and somatic mutations and environment leads to the development of lung cancer.

- Future directions include the application of genetic and molecular markers of lung cancer to enhance prevention and treatment strategies.

## REFERENCES

1   American Cancer Society. Cancer facts and figures 2003, http://www.cancer.org/docroot/ STT/stt_0.asp

2   Osann KE, Anton-Culver H, Kurosaki T, Taylor T. Sex differences in lung cancer risk associated with cigarette smoking. *Int J Cancer* 1993; **54**: 44–8.

3  Osterlind K, Hansen HH, Hansen M et al. Long-term disease-free survival in small cell carcinoma of the lung: a study of clinical determinants. *J Clin Oncol* 1986; **4**: 1307–13.

4  Janne PA, Freidlin B, Saxman S et al. Twenty-five years of clinical research for patients with limited-stage small cell lung carcinoma in North America. *Cancer* 2002; **95**: 1528–38.

5  Tai P, Tonita J, Yu E, Skarsgard D. Twenty-year follow-up study of limited-stage small cell lung cancer and overview of prognostic and treatment factors. *Int J Radiat Oncol Biol Phys* 2003; **56**: 626–33.

●6  Mountain CF. Revisions in the International System for Staging Lung Cancer. *Chest* 1997; **111**: 1710–17.

◆7  Alberg AJ, Samet JM. Epidemiology of lung cancer. *Chest* 2003; **123**: 21S–49S.

8  Jemal A, Chu KC, Tarone RE. Recent trends in lung cancer mortality in the United States. *J Natl Cancer Inst* 2001; **93**: 277–83.

9  Devesa SS, Blott WJ, Fraumeni JF. Declining lung cancer rates among young men and women in the United States: a cohort analysis. *J Natl Cancer Inst* 1989; **81**: 1568–71.

●10  Wingo PA, Ries LA, Giovino GA et al. Annual report to the nation on the status of cancer, 1973–1996, with a special section on lung cancer and smoking. *J Natl Cancer Inst* 1999; **91**: 675–90.

11  Chu KC, Baker SG, Tarone RE. A method for identifying abrupt changes in US cancer mortality trends. *Cancer* 1999; **86**: 157–69.

●12  Weir HK, Thun MJ, Hankey BF et al. Annual report to the nation on the status of cancer, 1975–2000, featuring the uses of surveillance data for cancer prevention and control. *J Natl Cancer Inst* 2003; **95**: 1276–99.

◆13  Hanahan D, Weinberg RA. The hallmarks of cancer. *Cell* 2000; **100**: 57–70.

14  Bale AE, Brown SJ. Etiology of cancer: cancer genetics. In: DeVita VT (ed.) *Cancer, principles and practice of oncology*. Philadelphia: Lippincott Williams and Wilkins, 2001: 207–17.

15  Ginsberg RJ, Vokes EE, Rosensweig K. Non-small cell lung cancer. In: DeVita VT (ed.) *Cancer, principles and practice of oncology*. Philadelphia: Lippincott Williams and Wilkins, 2001: 925–51.

●16  Murray N, Coy P, Pater JL et al. Importance of timing of thoracic irradiation in the combined modality treatment of limited stage small cell lung cancer. *J Clin Oncol* 1993; **11**: 336–44.

●17  Takada M, Fukuoka M, Kawahara M et al. Phase III study of concurrent versus sequential thoracic radiotherapy in combination with cisplatin and etoposide for limited stage small cell lung cancer: results of the Japan Clinical Oncology Group Study 9104. *J Clin Oncol* 2002; **20**: 3054–60.

18  Pignon JP, Arriagada R, Ihde DC et al. A meta-analysis of thoracic radiotherapy for small cell lung cancer. *New Engl J Med* 1992; **327**: 1618–24.

●19  Noda K, Nishiwaki Y, Kawahara M et al. Irinotecan plus cisplatin compared with etoposide plus cisplatin for extensive stage small cell lung cancer. *New Engl J Med* 2002; **346**: 85–91.

20  Waller D, Fairlamb DJ, Gower N et al. The Big Lung Trial: determining the value of cisplatin-based chemotherapy for all patients with non-small cell lung cancer. Preliminary results in the surgical setting. *Proc ASCO* 2003; Abstr. 2543.

●21  Scagliotti GV, Fossati R, Torri V et al. Randomized study of adjuvant chemotherapy for completed resected Stage I, II or IIIA non-small cell lung cancer. *J Natl Cancer Inst* 2003; **95**: 1453–61.

22  Non-small Cell Lung Cancer Collaborative Group. Chemotherapy in non-small cell lung cancer: a meta-analysis using updated data on individual patients from 52 randomized clinical trials. *Br Med J* 1995; **311**: 899–909.

●23  The International Adjuvant Lung Cancer Trial Collaborative Group. Cisplatin-based adjuvant chemotherapy in patients with completely resected non-small cell lung cancer. *N Engl J Med* 2004; **350**: 351–60.

●24  Winton TL, Livingston R, Johnson D et al. A prospective randomized trial of adjuvant vinorelbine and cisplatin in completely resected stage IB and II non small cell lung cancer. Intergroup JBR.10. *Proc ASCO* 2004; Abstr. 7018.

●25  Strauss GM, Herndon J, Maddaus MA et al. Randomized clinical trial of adjuvant chemotherapy with paclitaxel and carboplatin following resection in Stage IB non small cell lung cancer: report of Cancer and Leukemia Group B Protocol 9633. *Proc ASCO* 2004; Abstr. 7019.

26  Albain KS, Scott CB, Rusch VR et al. Phase III comparison of concurrent chemotherapy plus radiotherapy (CT/RT) and CT/RT followed by surgical resection for Stage IIIA (N2) non-small cell lung cancer: initial results from Intergroup Trial 0139. *Proc ASCO* 2003; Abstr. 2497.

27  LeChevalier T, Brisgand D, Douillard JY et al. Randomized study of vinorelbine and cisplatin versus vindesine and cisplatin versus vinorelbine alone in advanced non-small cell lung cancer: results of a European multicenter trial including 612 patients. *J Clin Oncol* 1994; **12**: 360–7.

28  Cardenal F, Lopez-Cabrerizo MP, Anton A et al. Randomized phase III study of gemcitabine-cisplatin versus etoposide-cisplatin in the treatment of locally advanced or metastatic non-small cell lung cancer. *J Clin Oncol* 1999; **17**: 12–18.

29  Crino L, Scagliotti GV, Ricc S et al. Gemcitabine and cisplatin versus mitomycin, ifosfamide, and cisplatin in advanced non-small cell lung cancer: a randomized phase III study of the Italian Lung Cancer project. *J Clin Oncol* 1999; **17**: 3522–30.

30  Sandler AB, Nemuaitis J, Denham C et al. Phase III study of gemcitabine plus cisplatin versus cisplatin alone in patients with locally advanced or metastatic non-small cell lung cancer. *J Clin Oncol* 2000; **18**: 122–30.

31  Bonomi P, Kim KM, Fairclough D et al. Comparison of survival and quality of life in advanced non-small cell lung cancer patients treated with two dose levels of paclitaxel combined with cisplatin versus etoposide with cisplatin: results of an Eastern Cooperative Oncology Group trial. *J Clin Oncol* 2000; **18**: 623–31.

32  Fosella F, Pereira JR, von Pawel J et al. Randomized, multinational phase III study of docetaxel and platinum combinations versus vinorelbine and cisplatin for advanced non-small cell lung cancer: the TAX 326 study group. *J Clin Oncol* 2003; **21**: 3016–24.

●33  Schiller JH, Harrington D, Belani CP et al. Comparison of four chemotherapy regimens for advanced non-small cell lung cancer. *New Engl J Med* 2002; **346**: 92–8.

34  Sheperd FA, Dancey J, Ramlau R et al. Prospective randomized trial of docetaxel versus best supportive care in patients with non-small cell lung cancer previously treated with platinum-based therapy. *J Clin Oncol* 2000; **19**: 2095–103.

35  Fosella FV, DeVore R, Kerr RN et al. Randomized phase III trial of docetaxel versus vinorelbine or ifosfamide in patients with advanced non-small cell lung cancer previously treated with platinum-containing regimens. *J Clin Oncol* 2000; **18**: 2354–62.

36  Fukuoka M, Yano S, Giaccone G et al. Multi-institutional randomized phase II trial of gefitinib for previously treated patients with advanced non-small cell lung cancer. *J Clin Oncol* 2003; **21**: 2237–46.

37  Kris M, Natale R, Herbst RS et al. A phase II trial of ZD1839 (Iressa) in advanced non-small cell lung cancer patients who had failed platinum- and taxotere-based regimens (IDEAL 2). *Proc ASCO* 2002; Abstr. 1166.

38  Hanna N, Sheperd FA, Fossella FV et al. Randomized phase III trial of pemetrexed versus docetaxel in patients with non-small cell lung cancer previously treated with chemotherapy. *J Clin Oncol* 2004; **22**: 1589–97.

39  Lord RV, Brabender J, Gandara D et al. Low ERCC1 expression correlates with prolonged survival after cisplatin plus gemcitabine chemotherapy in non-small cell lung cancer. *Clin Cancer Res* 2002; **8**: 2286–91.

40  Metzger R, Leichman CG, Danenberg KD et al. ERCC1 mRNA levels complement thymidylate synthase mRNA levels in predicting response and survival for gastric cancer patients receiving combination cisplatin and fluorouracil chemotherapy. *J Clin Oncol* 1998; **16**: 309–16.

41  Shirota Y, Stoehlmacher J, Brabender J et al. ERCC1 and thymidylate synthase mRNA levels predict survival for colorectal cancer patients receiving combination oxaliplatin and fluorouracil chemotherapy. *J Clin Oncol* 2001; **19**: 4298–304.

42  Moore-Joshi M, Danenberg K, Lord R et al. Low thymidylate synthase and ERCC1 gene expressions are associated with increased survival after neoadjuvant 5FU/cisplatin/radiotherapy for esophageal adenocarcinoma. *Proc ASCO* 2000; Abstr. 944.

◆43  Rosell R, Taron M, Alberola V et al. Genetic testing for chemotherapy in non-small cell lung cancer. *Lung Cancer* 2003; **41** (Suppl. 1): S97–102.

44  Rosell R, Danenberg K, Alberola V et al. Ribonucleotide reductase messenger RNA expression and survival in gemcitabine/cisplatin-treated advanced non-small cell lung cancer patients. *Clin Cancer Res* 2004; **10**: 1318–25.

45  Rosell-Costa R, Danenberg K, Alberola V et al. ERCC1 and RRM1 expression predicts survival: a genetic analysis of a Spanish Lung Cancer Group trial of gemcitabine/cisplatin vs gem/cis/vinorelbine v sequential doublets of gem/vrb and vrb/ifosfamide in stage IV non-small cell lung cancer. *Proc ASCO* 2003; Abstr. 2590.

46  Rosell R, Crino L, Danenberg K et al. Targeted therapy in combination with gemcitabine in non-small cell lung cancer. *Semin Oncol* 2003; **30** (Suppl. 4): 19–25.

●47  Fukuoka M, Yano S, Giaccone G et al. Multi-institutional randomized phase II trial of gefitinib for previously treated patients with advanced non-small cell lung cancer. *J Clin Oncol* 2003; **21**: 2237–46.

●48  Kris MG, Natale RB, Herbst RS et al. Efficacy of gefitinib, an inhibitor of the epidermal growth factor tyrosine kinase, in symptomatic patients with non-small cell lung cancer. *J Am Med Assoc* 2003; **290**: 2149–58.

●49  Giaccone G, Herbst RS, Manegold C et al. Gefitinib in combination with gemcitabine and cisplatin in advanced non-small cell lung cancer: a phase III trial – INTACT 1. *J Clin Oncol* 2004; **22**: 777–84.

●50  Herbst RS, Giaccone G, Schiller JH et al. Gefitinib in combination with paclitaxel and carboplatin in advanced non-small cell lung cancer: a phase III trial – INTACT 2. *J Clin Oncol* 2004; **22**: 785–94.

51  Baselga J. Combining the anti-EGFR agent gefitinib with chemotherapy in non-small cell lung cancer: how do we go from INTACT to impact? *J Clin Oncol* 2004; **22**: 759–61.

52  Miller VA, Kris MG, Shah N et al. Bronchoalveolar pathologic subtype and smoking history predict sensitivity to gefitinib in advanced non-small cell lung cancer. *J Clin Oncol* 2004; **22**: 1103–9.

53  Janne PA, Gurubhagavatula S, Yeap BY et al. Outcomes of patients with advanced non-small cell lung cancer treated with gefitinib on an expanded access study. *Lung Cancer* 2004; **44**: 221–30.

◆54  Mendelsohn J, Baselga J. Status of epidermal growth factor receptor antagonists in the biology and treatment of cancer. *J Clin Oncol* 2003; **21**: 2787–99.

55  Bailey LR, Kris MG, Wolf M et al. Tumor EGFR membrane staining is not clinically relevant for predicting response in patients receiving gefitinib monotherapy for pretreated advanced non-small cell lung cancer: IDEAL 1 and 2. *Proc AACR* 2003; Abstr. LB-170.

●56  Lynch TJ, Bell DW, Sordella R et al. Activating mutations in the epidermal growth factor receptor underlying responsiveness of non-small cell lung cancer to gefitinib. *New Engl J Med* 2004; **350**: 2129–39.

●57  Paez JG, Janne PA, Lee JC et al. EGFR mutations in lung cancer: correlation with clinical response to gefitinib therapy. *Science* 2004; **304**: 1497–500.

◆58  Evans WE, Relling MV. Pharmacogenomics: translating functional genomics into rational therapeutics. *Science* 1999; **286**: 487–91.

◆59  Weinshilboum R. Inheritance and drug response. *New Engl J Med* 2003; **348**: 529–37.

●60  Gurubhagavatula S, Liu G, Park S et al. *XPD* and *XRCC1* genetic polymorphisms are prognostic factors in advanced non-small cell lung cancer patients treated with platinum chemotherapy. *J Clin Oncol* 2004; **22**: 2594–601.

61  Ryu JS, Hong YC, Han HS et al. Association between polymorphisms of ERCC1 and XPD and survival in non-small cell lung cancer patients treated with cisplatin combination chemotherapy. *Lung Cancer* 2004; **44**: 311–16.

62  Sarries C, Alberola V, Mendez P et al. Single nucleotide polymorphisms in DNA repair genes predict survival in gemcitabine/cisplatin treated non-small cell lung cancer patients. *Proc ASCO* 2003; Abstr. 3450.

63  Camps C, Sarries C, Roig B et al. Assessment of nucleotide excision repair XPD polymorphisms in the peripheral blood of gemcitabine/cisplatin-treated advanced non-small cell lung cancer patients. *Clin Lung Cancer* 2003; **4**: 237–41.

64  Cardenal F, Ramirez JL, Astudillo J et al. XPD and RRM1 gene polymorphisms predict gem/cis/doc outcome in stage III non-small cell lung cancer: a genetic analysis of the Spanish Lung Cancer Group phase II trial 9901. *Proc ASCO* 2003; Abstr. 2612.

65  Aron M, Alberola V, Sanchez JJ et al. Transcription-coupled repair XPD and RRM1 gene polymorphisms predict gem/cis outcome in non-small cell lung cancer. *Proc ASCO* 2003; Abstr. 2579.

66  Reguart N, Roig B, Vinyolas N et al. XPD polymorphisms in cis/vrb-treated stage IV non-small cell lung cancer patients: genetic analysis of a Spanish Lung Cancer Group phase II trial. *Proc ASCO* 2003; Abstr. 3528.

◆67  Watters JW, McLeod HL. Cancer pharmacogenomics: current and future applications. *Biochem Biophys Acta* 2003; **1603**: 99–111.

●68  Innocenti F, Undevia SD, Iyer L et al. Genetic variants in the UDP-glucuronosyltransferase 1A1 gene predict the risk of severe neutropenia of irinotecan. *J Clin Oncol* 2004; **22**: 1382–8.

69  Font A, Sanchez JM, Taron M et al. Weekly regimen of irinotecan/docetaxel in previously treated non-small cell lung cancer patients and correlation with uridine diphosphate glucuronosyltransferase 1A1 polymorphism. *Invest New Drugs* 2003; **21**: 435–43.

●70  Tokuhata GK, Lillienfeld AM. Familial aggregation of lung cancer in humans. *J Natl Cancer Inst* 1963; **30**: 289–312.

●71  Ooi WL, Elston RC, Chen VW et al. Increased familial risk for lung cancer. *J Natl Cancer Inst* 1986; **2**: 217–22.

72  Sellers TA, Ooi WL, Elston RC et al. Increased familial risk for non-lung cancer among relatives of lung cancer patients. *Am J Epidemiol* 1987; **126**: 237–46.

73  Shaw GL, Falk RT, Pickle LW et al. Lung cancer risk associated with cancer in relatives. *J Clin Epidemiology* 1991; **44**: 429–37.

74  Schwartz AG, Yang P, Swanson GM. Familial aggregation of lung cancer among nonsmokers and their relatives. *Am J Epidemiol* 1996; **144**: 554–62.

75  Kreuzer M, Kreienbrock L, Gerken M et al. Risk factors for lung cancer among young adults. *Am J Epidemiol* 1998; **147**: 1028–37.

76  Bromen K, Pohlabeln H, Ingeborg J et al. Aggregation of lung cancer in families: results from a population-based case-control study in Germany. *Am J Epidemiol* 2000; **152**: 497–505.

77  Sellers TA, Bailey-Wilson JE, Elston RC et al. Evidence for Mendelian inheritance in the pathogenesis of lung cancer. *J Natl Cancer Inst* 1990; **82**: 1272–9.

78  Etzel CJ, Amos CI, Spitz MR. Risk for smoking-related cancer among relatives of lung cancer patients. *Cancer Res* 2003; **63**: 8531–5.

79  Poole CA, Byers T, Calle EE et al. Influence of a family history of cancer within and across multiple sites on patterns of cancer mortality risk for women. *Am J Epidemiol* 1999; **149**: 454–62.

80  Li X, Hemminki K. Familial and second lung cancers: a nation-wide epidemiologic study from Sweden. *Lung Cancer* 2003; **39**: 255–63.

81  Samet JM. Environmental causes of lung cancer: what do we know in 2003? *Chest* 2004; **125**: 80S–3S.

◆82  Hecht S. Tobacco smoke carcinogens and lung cancer. *J Natl Cancer Inst* 1999; **91**: 1194–210.

◆83  Hoffman D, Hoffman I. The changing cigarette, 1950–1995. *J Toxicol Environ Health* 1997; **50**: 307–64.

◆84  Kruglyak L. Prospects for whole-genome linkage disequilibrium mapping of common disease genes. *Nature Genet* 1999; **222**: 139–44.

85  Jorde LB. Linkage disequilibrium and the search for complex disease genes. *Genome Res* 2000; **10**: 1435–44.

◆86  Perera FP. Environment and cancer: who are susceptible? *Science* 1997; **278**: 1068–73.

●87  Kato S, Bowman EF, Harrington A et al. Human lung carcinogen-DNA adduct levels mediated by genetic polymorphisms in vivo. *J Natl Cancer Inst* 1995; **87**: 902–7.

88  Kawajiri K, Nakachi K, Imai K et al. Identification of genetically high risk individuals to lung cancer by DNA polymorphisms of the cytochrome P450 gene. *FEBS Lett* 1990; **263**: 131–3.

89  Hayashi SI, Watanabe J, Nakachi K, Kawajiri K. Genetic linkage of lung cancer associated MspI polymorphisms with amino acid replacement in the heme binding region of the human cytochrome P4501A1 gene. *J Biochem* 1991; **110**: 407–11.

●90  Nakachi K, Imai K, Hayashi S et al. Genetic susceptibility to squamous cell carcinoma of the lung in relation to cigarette smoking dose. *Cancer Res* 1991; **51**: 5177–80.

91  Okada T, Kawashima K, Fukushi S et al. Association between a cytochrome P450 CYPIA1 genotype and incidence of lung cancer. *Pharmacogen* 1995; **4**: 333–40.

●92  Nakachi K, Imai K, Hayashi SI, Kawajiri K. Polymorphisms of the CYP1A1 and glutathione-S-transferase genes associated with susceptibility to lung cancer in relation to cigarette dose in a Japanese population. *Cancer Res* 1993; **53**: 2994–9.

◆93  Vineis P. Molecular epidemiology: Low-dose carcinogens and genetic susceptibility. *Int J Cancer* 1997; **71**: 1–3.

◆94  Shields PG, Harris CG. Cancer risk and low-penetrance susceptibility genes in gene-environment interactions. *J Clin Oncol* 2000; **18**: 2309–15.

◆95  Warren AJ, Shields PG. Molecular epidemiology: carcinogen–DNA adducts and genetic susceptibility. *Proc Soc Exp Biol Med* 1997; **216**: 172–80.

96  Ishibe N, Wiencke JK, Zuo ZF et al. Susceptibility to lung cancer in light smokers associated with CYP1A1 polymorphisms in Mexican- and African-Americans. *Cancer Epidemiol Biomarkers Prev* 1997; **6**: 1075–80.

97  Hamada GS, Sugimura H, Suzuki I et al. The heme-binding region polymorphism of cytochrome P4501A1 rather than the RsaI polymorphisms of IIE1 is associated with lung cancer in Rio de Janeiro. *Cancer Epidemiol Biomarkers Prev* 1995; **4**: 63–7.

98  Tefre T, Rybert D, Haugen A et al. Human CYP1A1 gene: lack of association between the MspI restriction fragment length polymorphism and incidence of lung cancer in a Norwegian population. *Pharmacogenetics* 1991; **1**: 20–5.

99  Hirvonen A, Husgafvel-Pursiainen K, Karjalainen A et al. Point mutational Msp and Ile-Val polymorphisms closely linked to the CYP1A1 gene: lack of association with susceptibility to lung cancer in a Finnish study population. *Cancer Epidemiol Biomarkers Prev* 1992; **1**: 485–9.

●100  Houlston RS. CYP1A1 polymorphisms and lung cancer risk: a meta-analysis. *Pharmacogenetics* 2000; **10**: 105–14.

●101  Vineis P, Fabrizio V, Benhamou S et al. CYP1A1 T3801 C polymorphism and lung cancer: a pooled analysis of 2451 cases and 3358 controls. *Int J Cancer* 2003; **104**: 650–7.

102  LeMarchand L, Sivaraman L, Pierce L et al. Associations of CYP1A1, GSTM1, and CYP2E1 polymorphisms with lung cancer suggest cell type specificities to tobacco carcinogens. *Cancer Res* 1998; **58**: 4858–63.

103  Su T, Bao Z, Zhang QY et al. Human cytochrome P450 CYP2A13: predominant expression in the respiratory tract and its high efficiency metabolic activation of a tobacco-specific carcinogen, 4-(methylnitrosamino)-1-(3-pyridyl)-1-butanone. *Cancer Res* 2000; **60**: 5074–9.

104   Zhang X, Su T, Zhang QY et al. Genetic polymorphisms of the human CYP2A13 gene: identification of single nucleotide polymorphisms and functional characterization of the Arg257Cys variant. *J Pharmacol Exp Ther* 2002; **302**: 416–23.

●105   Wang H, Tan W, Hao B et al. Substantial reduction in risk of lung adenocarcinoma associated with genetic polymorphism in CYP2A13, the most active cytochrome P450 for the metabolic activation of tobacco specific carcinogen NNK. *Cancer Res* 2003; **63**: 8057–61.

106   Cuffiez C, Lo-Guidice JM, Quaranta S et al. Genetic polymorphism of the human cytochrome CYP2A13 in a French population: implication in lung cancer susceptibility. *Biochem Biophys Res Commun* 2004; **317**: 662–9.

●107   Hayes JD, Pulford DJ. The glutathione-S-transferase supergene family: regulation of GST and the contribution of the isoenzymes to cancer chemoprevention and drug resistance. *Crit Rev Biochem Mol Biol* 1995; **30**: 445–600.

●108   Seidegard J, Vorachek WR, Pero RW, Pearson WR. Hereditary differences in the expression of the human glutathione transferase active in trans-stilbene oxide are due to a gene deletion. *Proc Natl Acad Sci USA* 1988; **85**: 7293–7.

●109   Kihara M, Kihara M, Noda K, Okamoto N. Increased risk for lung cancer in Japanese smokers with mu class glutathione-S-transferase gene deficiency. *Cancer Lett* 1993; **71**: 151–5.

110   Hirvonen A, Husgafvel-Pursiainen K, Anttila S, Vainio H. The GSTM1 null genotype as a potential risk modifier for squamous cell carcinoma of the lung. *Carcinogenesis* 1993; **14**: 1479–81.

111   Zhong S, Howie AF, Ketterer B et al. Glutathione-S-transferase mu locus: use of genotyping and phenotyping assays to assess association with lung cancer susceptibility. *Carcinogenesis* 1991; **12**: 1533–7.

112   Ryberg D, Skaug V, Hewer A et al. Genotypes of glutathione transferase M1 and P1 and their significance for lung DNA adduct levels and cancer risk. *Carcinogenesis* 1997; **18**: 1285–9.

113   Pinarbasi H, Silig Y, Cetinkaya O et al. Strong association between the GSTM1-null genotype and lung cancer in a Turkish population. *Cancer Genetics and Cytogenetics* 2003; **146**: 125–9.

114   London SJ, Daly AK, Cooper J et al. Polymorphism of glutathione-S-transferase M1 and lung cancer risk among African-Americans and Caucasians in Los Angeles County, California. *J Natl Cancer Inst* 1995 **87**; 1246–53.

115   Rebbeck TR. Molecular epidemiology of the human glutathione S-transferase genotypes GSTM1 and GSTT1 in cancer susceptibility. *Cancer Epidemiol Biomark Prev* 1997; **6**: 733–43.

116   Schneider J, Bernges U, Philipp M, Woitowitz HJ. *GSTM1, GSTT1,* and *GSTP1* polymorphism and lung cancer risk in relation to tobacco smoking. *Cancer Lett* 2004; **208**: 65–74.

●117   McWilliams JE, Sanderson BJS, Harris EL et al. Glutathione-S-transferase M1 deficiency and lung cancer risk. *Cancer Epidemiol Biomarkers Prev* 1995; **4**: 589–94.

●118   Benhamou S, Lee WJ, Alexandrie AK et al. Meta- and pooled analyses of the effects of glutathione-S-transferase M1 polymorphisms and smoking on lung cancer risk. *Carcinogenesis* 2002; **23**: 1343–50.

119   Kihara M, Kihara M, Noda K. Lung cancer risk of GSTM1 null genotype is dependent on the extent of tobacco smoke exposure. *Carcinogenesis* 1994; **15**: 415–8.

120   Bennett WP, Alavanja MCR, Blomeke B et al. Environmental tobacco smoke, genetic susceptibility, and risk of lung cancer in never-smoking women. *J Natl Cancer Inst* 1999; **91**: 2009–14.

121   Kiyohara C, Wakai K, Mikami H et al. Risk modification by CYP1A1 and GSTM1 polymorphisms in the association of environmental tobacco smoke and lung cancer: a case–control study in Japanese nonsmoking women. *Int J Cancer* 2003; **107**: 139–44.

●122   Hayashi SI, Watanabe J, Kawajiri K. High susceptibility to lung cancer analyzed in terms of combined genotypes of P4501A1 and mu-class glutathione-S-transferase genes. *Jpn J Cancer Res* 1992; **83**: 866–70.

123   Nakachi K, Imai K, Hayahis SI, Kawajiri K. Polymorphisms in the CYP1A1 and glutathione-S-transferase genes associated with susceptibility to lung cancer in relation to cigarette dose in a Japanese population. *Cancer Res* 1991; **53**: 2994–9.

124   Kihara M, Kihara M, Noda K. Risk of smoking for squamous and small cell carcinomas of the lung modulated by combinations of CYP1A1 and GSTM1 gene polymorphisms in a Japanese population. *Carcinogenesis* 1995; **16**: 2331–6.

125   Anttila S, Hirvonen A, Husgafvel-Pursiainen K et al. Combined effect of CYP1A1 inducibility and GSTM1 polymorphism on histologic type of lung cancer. *Carcinogenesis* 1994; **15**: 1133–335.

126   Alexandrie AK, Sundgerg MI, Seidegard J et al. Genetic susceptibility to lung cancer with special emphasis on CYP1A1 and GSTM1: a study on host factors in relation to age at onset, gender and histological cancer types. *Carcinogenesis* 1994; **15**: 1785–90.

127   Garcia-Closas M, Kelsey KT, Wiencke JK et al. A case–control study of cytochrome P4501A1, glutathione-S-transferase M1, cigarette smoking and lung cancer susceptibility. *Cancer Causes Control* 1997; **8**: 544–53.

●128   Hung RJ, Boffetta P, Brockmoller J et al. CYP1A1 and GSTM1 genetic polymorphisms and lung cancer risk in Caucasian non-smokers: a pooled analysis. *Carcinogenesis* 2003; **24**: 875–82.

●129   Watson MA, Stewart RK, Smith GB et al. Human glutathione-S-transferase P1 polymorphisms: relationship to lung tissue enzyme activity and population frequency distribution. *Carcinogenesis* 1998; **19**: 275–80.

130   To-Figueras J, Gene M, Gomez-Catalan J et al. Genetic polymorphism of glutathione-S-transferase P1 gene and lung cancer risk. *Cancer Causes Control* 1999; **10**: 65–70.

131   Harris MJ, Coggan M, Langton L et al. Polymorphism of the pi class glutathione-S-transferase in normal populations and cancer patients. *Pharmacogenetics* 1998; **8**: 27–31.

132   Katoh T, Kaneko S, Takasawa S et al. Human glutathione-S-transferase P1 polymorphism and susceptibility to smoking related epithelial cancer; oral, lung, gastric, colorectal and urothelial cancer. *Pharmacogenetics* 1999; **9**: 165–9.

133   Nazar-Stewart V, Vaugh TL, Stapleton P et al. A population-based study of glutathione-S-transferase M1, T1 and P1 genotypes and risk for lung cancer. *Lung Cancer* 2003; **40**: 247–58.

●134   Miller DP, Neuberg D, DeVivo I et al. Smoking and the risk of lung cancer: susceptibility with GSTP1 polymorphisms. *Epidemiology* 2003; **14**: 545–51.

135   Miller DP, De Vivo I, Neuberg D et al. Association between self-reported environmental tobacco smoke exposure and

lung cancer: modification by GSTP1 polymorphism. *Int J Cancer* 2003; **104**: 758–63.

136  Kihara M, Kihara M, Noda K. Lung cancer risk of the GSTM1 null genotype is enhanced in the presence of the GSTP1 mutated genotype in male Japanese smokers. *Cancer Lett* 1999; **137**: 53–60.

137  Perera FP, Mooney LA, Stampfer M et al. Associations between carcinogen-DNA damage, glutathione S-transferase genotypes, and risk of lung cancer in the prospective Physicians' Health Cohort Study. *Carcinogenesis* 2002; **23**: 1641–6.

138  Miller DP, Liu G, De Vivo I et al. Combinations of the variant genotypes of GSTP1, GSTM1 and p53 are associated with an increased lung cancer risk. *Cancer Res* 2002; **62**: 2819–23.

139  Stucker I, Hirvonen A, de Waziers I et al. Genetic polymorphisms of glutathione-S-transferases as modulators of lung cancer susceptibility. *Carcinogenesis* 2002; **9**: 1475–81.

140  Malats N, Camus-Radon AM, Nyberg F et al. Lung cancer risk in nonsmokers and GSTM1 and GSTT1 genetic polymorphism. *Cancer Epidemiol Biomark Prev* 2000; **9**: 827–33.

141  To-Figueras J, Gene M, Gomez-Catalan J et al. Glutathione-S-transferase M1 and T1 polymorphism and lung cancer risk among northwestern Mediterraneans. *Carcinogenesis* 1997; **18**: 1529–33.

142  Wang J, Deng Y, Cheng J et al. GST genetic polymorphisms and lung adenocarcinoma susceptibility in a Chinese population. *Cancer Lett* 2003; **201**: 185–93.

143  Ruano-Ravina A, Figueiras A, Loidi L, Barros-Dios JM. GSTM1 and GSTT1 polymorphisms, tobacco and risk of lung cancer: a case–control study from Galicia, Spain. *Anticancer Res* 2003; **23**: 4333–7.

144  Sorensen M, Autrup H, Tjonneland A et al. Glutathione S-Transferase T1 null genotype is associated with an increased risk of lung cancer. *Int J Cancer* 2004; **110**: 219–24.

145  Philip PA, Fitzgerald DL, Cartwright RA et al. Polymorphic N-acetylation capacity in lung cancer. *Carcinogenesis* 1988; **9**: 491–3.

146  Martinez C, Agundez JAG, Olivera M et al. Lung cancer and mutations at the polymorphic NAT2 locus. *Pharmacogenetics* 1995; **5**: 207–14.

147  Bouchardy C, Mitrunen K, Wikman H et al. N-acetyltransferase NAT1 and NAT2 genotypes and lung cancer risk. *Pharmacogenetics* 1998; **8**: 291–8.

148  Saarikoski ST, Reinikainen M, Antilla S et al. Role of NAT2 deficiency in susceptibility to lung cancer among asbestos-exposed individuals. *Pharmacogenetics* 2000; **10**: 183–5.

149  Oyama T, Kawamoto T, Mizoue T et al. N-acetylation polymorphism in patients with lung cancer and its association with p53 gene mutation. *Anticancer Res* 1997; **17**: 577–82.

150  Seow A, Zhao B, Poh WT et al. NAT2 slow acetylator genotype is associated with increased risk of lung cancer among non-smoking Chinese women in Singapore. *Carcinogenesis* 1999; **20**: 1877–81.

151  Cascorbi I, Brockmoller J, Mrozikiewicz PM et al. Homozygous rapid arylamine N-acetyltransferase (NAT2) genotype as a susceptibility factor for lung cancer. *Cancer Res* 1996; **56**: 3961–6.

●152  Zhou W, Liu G, Thurston SW et al. Genetic polymorphisms in N-acetyltransferase-2 and microsomal epoxide hydrolase, cumulative cigarette smoking, and lung cancer. *Cancer Epidemiol Biomark Prev* 2002; **11**: 15–21.

●153  Hassett C, Aicher L, Sidhu JS, Omiecinski CJ. Human microsomal epoxide hydrolase: genetic polymorphism and functional expression in vitro of amino acid variants. *Human Mol Genet* 1994; **3**: 421–8.

154  Wu X, Gwyn K, Lamos C et al. The association of microsomal epoxide hydrolase polymorphisms and lung cancer risk in African-Americans and Mexican-Americans. *Carcinogenesis* 2001; **22**: 923–8.

155  Cajas-Salazar N, Au WW, Zwischenberger JB et al. Effect of epoxide hydrolase polymorphisms on chromosome aberrations and risk for lung cancer. *Cancer Genet Cytogenet* 2003; **145**: 97–102.

156  Lin P, Wang SL, Wang HJ et al. Association of CYP1A1 and mEH polymorphisms with lung squamous cell carcinoma. *Br J Cancer* 2000; **82**: 852–7.

157  Benhamou S, Reinikainen M, Bouchardy C et al. Association between lung cancer and microsomal epoxide hydrolase genotypes. *Cancer Res* 1998; **58**: 5291–3.

158  Zhou W, Thurston SW, Liu G et al. The interaction between microsomal epoxide hydrolase polymorphisms and cumulative cigarette smoking in different histologic subtypes of lung cancer. *Cancer Epidemiol Biomark Prev* 2001; **10**: 461–6.

●159  Wang LI, Miller DP, Sai Y et al. Manganese superoxide dismutase alanine-to-valine polymorphism at codon 16 and lung cancer risk. *J Natl Cancer Inst* 2001; **93**: 1818–21.

●160  Feyler A, Voho A, Bouchardy C et al. Point: myeloperoxidase-463 G->A polymorphism and lung cancer risk. *Cancer Epidemiol Biomark Prev* 2002; **11**: 1550–4.

●161  Xu LL, Liu G, Miller DP et al. Counterpoint: the myeloperoxidase-463 G->A polymorphism does not decrease lung cancer susceptibility in Caucasians. *Cancer Epidemiol Biomarkers Prev* 2002; **11**: 1555–9.

●162  Wei Q, Cheng L, Hong WK, Spitz MR. Reduced DNA repair capacity in lung cancer patients. *Cancer Res* 1996; **56**: 4103–7.

●163  Wei Q, Cheng L, Amos C et al. Repair of tobacco carcinogen-induced DNA adducts and lung cancer risk: a molecular epidemiologic study. *J Natl Cancer Inst* 2000; **92**: 1764–72.

164  Shen H, Spitz MR, Qiao Y et al. Smoking, DNA repair capacity and risk of nonsmall cell lung cancer. *Int J Cancer* 2003; **107**: 84–8.

●165  Spitz MR, Wu X, Wang Y et al. Modulation of nucleotide excision repair capacity by XPD polymorphisms in lung cancer patients. *Cancer Res* 2001; **61**: 1354–7.

166  Lunn RM, Helzlsouer KJ, Parshad R et al. XPD polymorphisms: effects on DNA repair proficiency. *Carcinogenesis* 2000; **21**: 551–5.

167  Butkiewicz D, Rusin M, Enewold L et al. Genetic polymorphisms in DNA repair genes and risk of lung cancer. *Carcinogenesis* 2001; **22**: 593–7.

●168  Zhou W, Liu G, Miller DP et al. Gene–environment interaction for the ERCC2 polymorphisms and cumulative cigarette smoking exposure in lung cancer. *Cancer Res* 2002; **62**: 1377–81.

169  Wu X, Amos CI, Wang M et al. Association of a polymorphism in exon 23 of the DNA repair gene, XPD, and lung cancer risk. *Proc AACR* 1999; **40**: 89.

170  Escobar P, Modugno F, Kanbour-Shakir A et al. Analysis of the DNA repair enzyme XPD exon 23 polymorphism and cancer risk. *Proc AACR* 1999; **40**: 213.

171  David-Beabes GL, Lunn RM, London SJ. No association between the XPD (Lys751Gln) polymorphism or the XRCC3

(Thr241Met) polymorphism and lung cancer risk. *Cancer Epidemiol Biomark Prev* 2001; **10**: 911–12.

●172   Thompson LH, West MG. XRCC1 keeps DNA from getting stranded. *Mutat Res* 2000; **459**: 1–18.

●173   Duell EJ, Wiencke JK, Cheng TJ et al. Polymorphisms in the DNA repair genes XRCC1 and ERCC2 and biomarkers of DNA damage in human blood mononuclear cells. *Carcinogenesis* 2000; **21**: 965–71.

174   Matullo G, Palli D, Peluso M et al. XRCC1, XRCC3, XPD gene polymorphisms, smoking, and 32P-DNA adducts in a sample of healthy subjects. *Carcinogenesis* 2001; **22**: 1437–45.

175   Park JY, Lee SY, Jeoh HS et al. Polymorphism of the DNA repair gene XRCC1 and risk of primary lung cancer. *Cancer Epidemiol Biomark Prev* 2002; **11**: 23–7.

176   Divine KK, Gilliland F, Crowell RE et al. The XRCC1 399 glutamine allele is a risk factor for adenocarcinoma of the lung. *Mutat Res* 2001; **461**: 273–8.

177   Ratnasinghe D, Yao SX, Tangrea JA et al. Polymorphisms of the DNA repair gene XRCC1 and lung cancer risk. *Cancer Epidemiol Biomark Prev* 2001; **10**: 119–23.

178   David-Beabes GL, London SJ. Genetic polymorphisms of XRCC1 and lung cancer risk among African-Americans and Caucasians. *Lung Cancer* 2001; **34**: 333–9.

179   Zhou W, Liu G, Miller DP et al. Polymorphisms in the DNA repair genes XRCC1 and ERCC2, smoking, and lung cancer risk. *Cancer Epidemiol Biomark Prev* 2003; **12**: 359–65.

◆180   Hollstein M, Sidransky D, Vogelstein B, Harris CC. p53 mutations in human cancers. *Science* 1991; **253**: 49–53.

◆181   Harris CC, Hollstein M. Clinical implications of the p53 tumor suppressor gene. *New Engl J Med* 1993; **329**: 1318–27.

182   Weston A, Perrin LS, Forrester K et al. Allelic frequency of a p53 polymorphism in human lung cancer. *Cancer Epidemiol Biomark Prev* 1992; **1**: 481–3.

183   Weston A, Ling-Cawley HM, Caporaso NE et al. Determination of the allele frequencies of an L-myc and a p53 polymorphism in human lung cancer. *Carcinogenesis* 1994; **15**: 583–7.

184   To-Figueras J, Gene M, Gomez-Catalan JG et al. Glutathione-S-transferase M1 and codon 72 p53 polymorphism in a northwestern Mediterranean population and their relation to lung cancer susceptibility. *Cancer Epidemiol Biomark Prev* 1996; **5**: 337–42.

185   Kawajiri K, Nakachi K, Imai K et al. Germ line polymorphism of p53 and CYP1A1 genes involved in human lung cancer. *Carcinogenesis* 1993; **14**: 1085–9.

186   Jin X, Wu X, Roth JA et al. Higher lung cancer risk for younger African-Americans with the Pro/Pro p53 genotype. *Carcinogenesis* 1995; **16**: 2205–8.

187   Fan R, Wu MT, Miller D et al. The p53 codon 72 polymorphism and lung cancer risk. *Cancer Epidemiol Biomarker Prev* 2000; **9**: 1037–42.

188   Wu X, Zhao H, Amos CI et al. p53 genotypes and haplotypes associated with lung cancer susceptibility and ethnicity. *J Natl Cancer Inst* 2002; **94**: 681–90.

◆189   Forgacs E, Zochbauer-Muller S, Olah E, Minna JD. Molecular genetic abnormalities in the pathogenesis of human lung cancer. *Pathol Oncol Res* 2001; **7**: 6–13.

◆190   Salgia R, Skarin AT. Molecular abnormalities in lung cancer. *J Clin Oncol* 1998; **16**: 1207–17.

◆191   Fong KM, Sekido Y, Gazdar AF, Minna JD. Molecular biology of lung cancer: clinical implications. *Thorax* 2003; **58**: 892–900.

◆192   Sekido Y, Fong KM, Minna JD. Molecular genetics of lung cancer. *Annu Rev Med* 2003; **54**: 73–87.

◆193   Rom WN, Hay JG, Lee TC et al. Molecular and genetic aspects of lung cancer. *Am J Respir Crit Care Med* 2000; **161**: 1355–67.

◆194   Mitsuuchi Y, Testa JR. Cytogenetics and molecular genetics of lung cancer. *Am J Med Genet* 2002; **115**: 183–8.

◆195   Strauss GM, Kwiatkowski DJ, Harpole DH et al. Molecular and pathologic markers in stage I non-small cell carcinoma of the lung. *J Clin Oncol* 1995; **13**: 1265–79.

●196   Balsara BR, Testa JR. Chromosomal imbalances in human lung cancer. *Oncogene* 2002; **21**: 6877–83.

●197   Balsara BR, Sonoda G, du Manoir S et al. Comparative genomic hybridization analysis detects frequent, often high-level over-representation of DNA sequences at 3p, 5p, 7p, and 8q in human non-small cell lung carcinomas. *Cancer Res* 1997; **57**: 2116–20.

198   Mao L, Lee JS, Kurie JM et al. Clonal genetic alterations in the lungs of current and former smokers. *J Natl Cancer Inst* 1997; **89**: 857–62.

199   Wistuba II, Lam S, Behrens C et al. Molecular damage in the bronchial epithelium of current and former smokers. *J Natl Cancer Inst* 1997; **89**: 1366–73.

200   Yoshino I, Fukuyama S, Kameyama T et al. Detection of loss of heterozygosity by high-resolution fluorescent system in non-small cell lung cancer. *Chest* 2003; **123**: 545–50.

201   Sanchez-Cespedes M, Ahrendt SA, Piantadosi S et al. Chromosomal alterations in lung adenocarcinoma from smokers and nonsmokers. *Cancer Res* 2001; **61**: 1309–13.

202   Wong MP, Fung LF, Wang E et al. Chromosomal aberrations of primary lung adenocarcinomas in nonsmokers. *Cancer* 2003; **97**: 1263–70.

203   Wistuba II, Behrens C, Milchgrub S et al. Sequential molecular abnormalities are involved in the multistage development of squamous cell carcinoma. *Oncogene* 1999; **18**: 643–50.

204   Sundaresan V, Ganly P, Hasleton P et al. p53 and chromosome 3 abnormalities, characteristic of malignant lung tumours, are detectable in preinvasive lesions of the bronchus. *Oncogene* 1992; **7**: 1989–97.

205   Thiberville L, Payne P, Vielkinds J et al. Evidence of cumulative gene losses with progression of premalignant epithelial lesions to carcinoma of the bronchus. *Cancer Res* 1995; **55**: 5133–9.

206   Kohno H, Hiroshima K, Toyozaki T et al. p53 mutations and allelic loss of chromosome 3p, 9p of preneoplastic lesions in patients with non-small cell lung carcinoma. *Cancer* 1999; **85**: 341–7.

207   Hung J, Kishimoto Y, Sugio K et al. Allele-specific chromosome 3p deletions occur at an early stage in the pathogenesis of lung carcinoma. *J Am Med Assoc* 1995; **273**: 558–63.

208   Kishimoto Y, Sugio K, Hung JY et al. Allele-specific loss in chromosome 9p loci in preneoplastic lesions accompanying non-small cell lung cancers. *J Natl Cancer Inst* 1995; **87**: 1224–9.

209   Sanz-Ortega J, Saez MC, Sierra E et al. 3p21, 5q21, and 9p21 allelic deletions are frequently found in bronchial cells adjacent to non-small cell lung cancer, while they are unusual in patients with no evidence of malignancy. *J Pathol* 2001; **195**: 429–34.

210   Hirao T, Nelson HH, Ashok TDS et al. Tobacco smoke-induced DNA damage and early age of smoking initiation induce

chromosome loss at 3p21 in lung cancer. *Cancer Res* 2001; **61**: 612–5.

●211 Whang-Peng J, Kao-Shan CS, Lee EC. Specific chromosome defect associated with human small cell lung cancer; deletion 3p(14–23). *Science* 1982; **215**: 181–2.

●212 Naylor SL, Johnson BE, Minna JD, Sakaguchi AY. Loss of heterozygosity of chromosome 3p markers in small-cell lung cancer. *Nature* 1987; **329**: 451–4.

●213 Johnson BE, Sakaguchi AY, Gazdar AF et al. Restriction fragment length polymorphism studies show consistent loss of chromosome 3p alleles in small cell lung cancer patients' tumors. *J Cancer Inst* 1988; **82**: 502–7.

●214 Brauch H, Johnson B, Hovis J et al. Molecular analysis of the short arm of chromosome 3 in small-cell and non-small-cell carcinoma of the lung. *N Engl J Med* 1987; **317**: 1109–13.

215 Yokota J, Wada M, Shimosato Y et al. Loss of heterozygosity on chromosomes 3, 13, 17 in small cell carcinoma and on chromosome 3 in adenocarcinoma of the lung. *Proc Natl Acad Sci USA* 1987; **84**: 9252–6.

216 Rabbitts P, Douglas J, Daly M et al. Frequency and extent of allelic loss in the short arm of chromosome 3 in non small cell lung cancer. *Genes Chromosom Cancer* 1989; **1**: 95–105.

217 Horio Y, Takahashi T, Kuroishi T et al. Prognostic significance of p53 mutations and 3p deletions in primary resected non-small cell lung cancer. *Cancer Res* 1993; **53**: 1–4.

●218 Kok K, Osinga J, Carritt B et al. Deletion of a DNA sequence at the chromosomal region 3p21 in all major types of lung cancer. *Nature* 1987; **330**: 578–81.

219 Hibi K, Takahashi T, Yamakawa K et al. Three distinct regions involved in 3p deletions in human lung cancer. *Oncogene* 1992; **7**: 445–9.

220 Yokoyama S, Yamakawa K, Tsuchiya E et al. Deletion mapping on the short arm of chromosome 3 in squamous cell carcinoma and adenocarcinoma of the lung. *Cancer Res* 1992; **52**: 873–7.

◆221 Ponder B. Cancer: gene loss in human tumours. *Nature* 1988; **335**: 400–2.

222 Sekido Y, Bader S, Latif F et al. Molecular analysis of the von Hippel-Lindau disease tumor suppressor gene in human lung cancer lines. *Oncogene* 1994; **9**: 1599–604.

223 Shigemitsu K, Sekido Y, Usami N et al. Genetic alteration of the B-catenin gene in human lung cancer and malignant mesothelioma and identification of a new homozygous deletion. *Oncogene* 2001; **20**: 4249–57.

224 Zochbuer-Muller S, Fong M, Virmani K. Aberrant promoter methylation of multiple genes in non-small cell lung cancers. *Cancer Res* 2001; **61**: 249–55.

225 Virmani A, Rathi A, Zochbauer-Muller S. Promoter methylation and silencing of the retinoic acid receptor-B gene in lung carcinomas. *J Natl Cancer Inst* 2000; **92**: 1303–7.

226 Roche J, Boldog F, Robinson M et al. Distinct 3p21.3 deletions in lung cancer and identification of a new human semaphorin. *Oncogene* 1996; **12**: 1289–97.

227 Sekido Y, Bader S, Latif F et al. Human semaphorins A(V) and IV reside in the 3p21.3 small cell lung cancer deletion region and demonstrate distinct expression patterns. *Proc Natl Acad Sci USA* 1996; **93**: 4120–5.

228 Sozzi G, Veronese ML, Negrini M et al. The *FHIT* gene at 3p14.2 is abnormal in lung cancer. *Cell* 1996; **85**: 17–26.

229 Sozzi G, Sard L, de Gregorio L et al. Association between cigarette smoking and *FHIT* gene alterations in lung cancer. *Cancer Res* 1997; **57**: 2121–3.

230 Geradts J, Fong KM, Zimmerman PV, Minna JD. Loss of FHIT expression in non-small cell lung cancer: correlation with molecular genetic abnormalities and clinicopathologic features. *Br J Cancer* 2000; **82**: 1191–7.

231 Dammann R, Li C, Yoon JH et al. Epigenetic inactivation of a RAS association domain family protein from the lung tumour suppressor locus 3p21.3. *Nature Genet* 2000; **25**: 315–9.

232 Burbee DG, Forgacs E, Zochbauer-Muller S et al. Epigenetic inactivation of RASSF1A in lung and breast cancers and malignant phenotype suppression. *J Natl Cancer Inst* 2001; **93**: 691–9.

233 Endoh H, Yatabe Y, Shimizu S et al. RASSF1A gene inactivation in non-small cell lung cancer and its clinical implication. *Int J Cancer* 2003; **106**: 45–51.

●234 Kim NW, Piatyszek MA, Prowse KR et al. Specific association of human telomerase activity with immortal cells and cancer. *Science* 1994; **266**: 2011–5.

235 Hahn WC. Role of telomere and telomerase in the pathogenesis of human cancer. *J Clin Oncol* 2003; **21**: 2034–43.

●236 Kiyono T, Foster SA, Koop JI et al. Both Rb/p16INK4a inactivation and telomerase activity are required to immortalize human epithelial cells. *Nature* 1998; **396**: 84–8.

●237 Hiyama K, Hiaya E, Ishioka S et al. Telomerase activity in small-cell and non-small cell lung cancers. *J Natl Cancer Inst* 1995; **87**: 895–902.

●238 Albanell J, Lonardo F, Rusch V et al. High telomerase activity in primary lung cancers: association with increased cell proliferation rates and advanced pathologic stage. *J Natl Cancer Inst* 1997; **89**: 1609–15.

239 Marchetti A, Bertacca G, Buttitta F et al. Telomerase activity as a prognostic indicator in Stage I non-small cell lung cancer. *Clin Cancer Res* 1999; **5**: 2077–81.

240 Taga S, Osaki T, Ohgami A et al. Prognostic impact of telomerase activity in non-small cell lung cancers. *Ann Surg* 1999; **230**: 715–20.

241 Gonzalez-Quevedo R, Iniesta P, Moran A et al. Cooperative role of telomerase activity and p16 expression in the prognosis of non-small cell lung cancer. *J Clin Oncol* 2002; **20**: 254–62.

●242 Zochbauer-Muller S, Fong KM, Virmani AK et al. Aberrant promoter methylation of multiple genes in non-small cell lung cancers. *Cancer Res* 2001; **61**: 249–55.

243 Virmani AK, Rathi A, Zochbauer-Muller S et al. Promoter methylation and silencing of the retinoic acid receptor-B gene in lung carcinomas. *J Natl Cancer Inst* 2000; **92**: 1303–7.

244 Kim DH, Nelson HH, Wiencke JK et al. p16INK4a and histology-specific methylation of CpG islands by exposure to tobacco smoke in non-small cell lung cancer. *Cancer Res* 2001; **61**: 3419–24.

245 Eguchi K, Kanai Y, Kobayashi K, Hirohashi S. DNA hypermethylation at the D17S5 locus in non-small cell lung cancers: its association with smoking history. *Cancer Res* 1997; **57**: 4913–5.

246 Belinsky SA, Palmisano WA, Gilliland FD et al. Aberrant promoter methylation in bronchial epithelium and sputum from current and former smokers. *Cancer Res* 2002; **62**: 2370–7.

247  Kim DH, Nelson HH, Wiencke JK et al. Promoter methylation of DAP-kinase: association with advanced stage in non-small cell lung cancer. *Oncogene* 2001; **20**: 1765–70.

248  Brabender J, Usadel H, Metzger R et al. Quantitative O6-methylguanine DNA methyltransferase methylation analysis in curatively resected non-small cell lung cancer: associations with clinical outcome. *Clin Cancer Res* 2003; **9**: 223–7.

249  Kim DH, Kim JS, Ji YI et al. Hypermethylation of *RASSF1A* promoter is associated with the age at starting smoking and a poor prognosis in primary non-small cell lung cancer. *Cancer Res* 2003; **63**: 3743–6.

250  Varmus HE. The molecular genetics of cellular oncogenes. *Ann Rev Genet* 1984; **18**: 553.

●251  Mills NE, Fishman CL, Rom WN et al. Increased prevalence of K-ras oncogene mutations in lung adenocarcinoma. *Cancer Res* 1995; **55**: 1444–7.

●252  Slebos RJC, Rodenhuis S. The ras gene family in human non-small cell lung cancer. *J Natl Cancer Inst Monogr* 1992; **13**: 23–9.

253  De Gregorio L, Manenti G, Incarbone M et al. Prognostic value of loss of heterozygosity and Kras2 mutations in lung adenocarcinoma. *Int J Cancer* 1998; **79**: 269–72.

254  Sugio K, Ishida T, Yokoyama H et al. ras gene mutations as a prognostic marker in adenocarcinoma of the human lung without lymph node metastasis. *Cancer Res* 1992; **52**: 2903–6.

255  Rodenhuis S, Slebos RJC, Boot AJM et al. Incidence and possible clinical significance of K-ras oncogene activation in adenocarcinoma of the human lung. *Cancer Res* 1988; **48**: 5738–41.

256  Rodenhuis S, Slebos RJC. Clinical significance of ras oncogene activation in human lung cancer. *Cancer Res* 1992; **52**: 2665s–9s.

257  Ahrendt, SA, Decker, PA, Alawi EA et al. Cigarette smoking is strongly associated with mutation of the K-ras gene in patients with primary adenocarcinoma of the lung. *Cancer* 2001; **92**: 1525–30.

258  Slebos RJC, Kibbelaar RE, Dalesio O et al. K-ras oncogene activation as a prognostic marker in adenocarcinoma of the lung. *New Engl J Med* 1990; **323**: 561–5.

259  Sugio K, Ishida T, Yokoyama H et al. ras gene mutations as a prognostic marker in adenocarcinoma of the human lung without lymph node metastasis. *Cancer Res* 1992; **52**: 2903–6.

260  Nelson HH, Christiani DC, Mark EJ et al. Implications and prognostic value of K-ras mutation for early stage lung cancer in women. *J Natl Cancer Inst* 1999; **91**: 2032–8.

261  Mitsudomi T, Steinberg SM, Oie HK et al. Ras gene mutations in non-small cell lung cancers are associated with shortened survival irrespective of treatment. *Cancer Res* 1991; **51**: 4999–5002.

262  Huncharek M, Muscat J, Geschwind JF. Kras oncogene mutation as a prognostic marker in non-small cell lung cancer: a combined analysis of 881 cases. *Carcinogenesis* 1999; **20**: 1507–10.

●263  Schiller JH, Adak S, Feins RH et al. Lack of prognostic significance of p53 and K-ras mutations in primary resected non-small cell lung cancer on E4592: A laboratory ancillary study on an Eastern Cooperative Oncology Group prospective randomized trial of postoperative adjuvant therapy. *J Clin Oncol* 2001; **19**: 448–57.

264  Siegfried JM, Gillespie AT, Mera R et al. Prognostic value of specific k-ras mutations in lung adenocarcinoma. *Cancer Epidemiol Biomark Prev* 1997; **6**: 841–7.

●265  Kaiser U, Schilli M, Haag U. Expression of bcl-2 protein in small cell lung cancer. *Lung Cancer* 1996; **15**: 31–40.

●266  Pezzella F, Turley H, Kuzu I et al. bcl-2 protein in non-small cell lung carcinoma. *New Engl J Med* 1993; **329**: 690–4.

267  Fontanini G, Vignati S, Bigini D et al. bcl-2 protein: a prognostic factor inversely correlated to p53 in non-small cell lung cancer. *Br J Cancer* 1995; **71**: 1003–7.

268  Laudanski J, Chyczewski L, Niklinska WE et al. Expression of bcl-2 protein in non-small cell lung cancer: correlation with clinicopathology and patient survival. *Neoplasma* 1999; **46**: 25–30.

269  Pezzella F, Turley H, Kuzu I et al. bcl-2 protein in non-small cell lung carcinoma. *New Engl J Med* 1993; **329**: 690–4.

270  Higashiyama M, Doi O, Kodama K et al. Bcl-2 oncoprotein in surgically resected non-small cell lung cancer: possibly favorable prognostic factor in association with low incidence of distant metastasis. *J Surg Oncol* 1997; **64**: 48–54.

271  Takayama K, Ogata K, Nakanishi Y et al. Bcl-2 expression as a predictor of chemosensitivities and survival in small cell lung cancer. *Cancer J Sci Am* 1996; **2**: 212.

272  Borner MM, Brousset P, Pfanner-Meyer B et al. Expression of apoptosis regulatory proteins of the Bcl-2 family and p53 in primary resected non-small cell lung cancer. *Br J Cancer* 1999; **79**: 952–8.

273  Hwang JH, Lim SC, Kim YC et al. Apoptosis and bcl-2 expression as predictors of survival in radiation-treated non-small-cell lung cancer. *Int J Radiat Oncol Biol Phys* 2001; **50**: 13–18.

274  Huang CI, Neuberg D, Johnson BE et al. Expression of bcl-2 protein is associated with shorter survival in nonsmall cell lung carcinoma. *Cancer* 2003; **98**: 135–43.

275  Martin B, Paesmans M, Berghmans T et al. Role of bcl-2 as a prognostic factor for survival in lung cancer: a systematic review of the literature with meta-analysis. *Br J Cancer* 2003; **89**: 55–64.

●276  Little CD, Nau MM, Carney DN et al. Amplification and expression of the c-myc oncogene in human lung cancer lines. *Nature* 1983; **306**: 194–6.

●277  Wong AJ, Ruppert JM, Eggleston J et al. Gene amplification of c-myc and n-myc in small cell carcinoma of the lung. *Science* 1986; **233**: 461–4.

●278  Nau MM, Brooks BJ, Battey J et al. L-myc, a new myc-related gene amplified and expressed in human small cell lung cancer. *Nature* 1985; **318**: 69–73.

●279  Slebos R, Evers S, Wagenaar S et al. Cellular proto-oncogenes are infrequently amplified in untreated non-small cell lung cancer. *Br J Cancer* 1989; **59**: 76–80.

◆280  Richardson GE, Johnson BE. The biology of lung cancer. *Semin Oncol* 1993; **20**: 105–27.

281  Johnson BE, Ihde D, Makuch R et al. myc family oncogene amplification in tumor cell lines established from small cell lung cancer patients and its relationship to clinical status and course. *J Natl Cancer Inst* 1987; **79**: 1629–34.

282  Brennan J, O'Connor T, Makuch R et al. myc family DNA amplification in 107 tumors and tumor cell lines from patients with small cell lung cancer treated with different combination chemotherapy regimens. *Cancer Res* 1991; **51**: 1708–12.

283  Noguchi M, Hirohasi S, Hara F et al. Heterogenous amplification of myc family oncogenes in small cell lung carcinoma. *Cancer* 1990; **66**: 2053–8.

●284  Haeder M, Rotsch M, Bepler G et al. Epidermal growth factor expression in human lung cancer cell lines. *Cancer Res* 1988; **48**: 1132–6.

285  Rusch V, Baselga J, Cordon-Cardo C et al. Differential expression of an epidermal growth factor receptor and its ligands in primary non-small cell lung cancer and adjacent benign lung. *Cancer Res* 1993; **53**: 2379–85.

286  Piyathilake CJ, Frost AR, Manne U et al. Differential expression of growth factors in squamous cell carcinoma and precancerous lesions of the lung. *Clin Cancer Res* 2002; **8**: 734–44.

287  Kurie JM, Sjon HJC, Lee JS et al. Increased epidermal growth factor receptor expression in metaplastic bronchial epithelium. *Clin Cancer Res* 1996; **2**: 1787–93.

288  Hirsch FR, Varella-Garcia M, Bunn PA et al. Epidermal growth factor receptor in non-small cell lung carcinomas: correlation between gene copy number and protein expression and impact on prognosis. *J Clin Oncol* 2003; **21**: 3798–807.

289  Rusch V, Klimstra D, Venkatraman E et al. Overexpression of the epidermal growth factor receptor and its ligand transforming growth factor alpha is frequent in resectable non-small cell lung cancer but does not predict tumor progression. *Clin Cancer Res* 1997; **3**: 515–22.

290  Pfeiffer P, Clausen PP, Andersen K et al. Lack of prognostic significance of epidermal growth factor receptor and the oncoprotein p185HER-2 in patients with systemically untreated non-small cell lung cancer: an immunohistochemical study on cryosections. *Br J Cancer* 1996; **74**: 86–91.

291  Fontanini G, DeLaurentis M, Vignati S et al. Evaluation of epidermal growth factor-related growth factors and receptors and of neoangiogenesis in completely resected stage I-IIIA non-small cell lung cancer. *Clin Cancer Res* 1998; **4**: 241–9.

●292  D'Amico TA, Massey M, Herndon JE et al. A biologic risk model for stage I lung cancer: immunohistochemical analysis of 408 patients with the use of ten molecular markers. *J Thorac Cardiovasc Surg* 1999; **117**: 736–43.

●293  Pastorino U, Andreola S, Tagliabue E et al. Immunocytochemical markers in stage I lung cancers: relevance to prognosis. *J Clin Oncol* 1997; **15**: 2858–65.

294  Volm M, Rittgen W, Drings P et al. Prognostic value of ERBB-1, VEGF, cyclin A, FOS, JUN, and MYC in patients with squamous lung carcinomas. *Br J Cancer* 1998; **77**: 663–9.

295  Cox G, Jones JL, O'Byrne KJ. Matrix metalloproteinase 9 and the epidermal growth factor signal pathway in operable non-small cell lung cancer. *Clin Cancer Res* 2000; **6**: 2349–55.

296  Schneider PM, Hung MC, Chiocca SM et al. Differential expression of the c-erbB-2 gene in human small cell and non-small cell lung cancer. *Cancer Res* 1989; **49**: 4968–71.

297  Kern JA, Schwarts DA, Nordberg JE et al. P185neu expression in lung adenocarcinoma predicts shortened survival. *Cancer Res* 1990; **50**: 5184–91.

298  Weiner DM, Nordberg J, Robinson R et al. Expression of the neu gene-encoded protein p185 neu in human non-small cell carcinomas of the lung. *Cancer Res* 1990; **50**: 421–5.

299  Hsieh CC, Chow KC, Fahn HJ et al. Prognostic significance of her2/neu overexpression in stage I adenocarcinoma of the lung. *Ann Thorac Surg* 1998; **66**: 1159–64.

300  Brabender J, Danenberg KD, Metzger R et al. Epidermal growth factor receptor and her2/neu mRNA expression in non-small cell lung cancer is correlated with survival. *Clin Cancer Res* 2001; **7**: 1850–5.

◆301  Wistuba II, Gazdar AF, Minna JD. Molecular genetics of small cell lung carcinoma. *Semin Oncol* 2001; **28** (2 Suppl 4): 3–13.

●302  Gannon JV, Greaves R, Iggo R, Lane DP. Activating mutations in p53 produce a common conformational effect: A monoclonal antibody specific for the mutant form. *EMBO J* 1990; **9**: 1595–1602.

303  Mitsudomi T, Oyama T, Nishida K et al. p53 nuclear immunostaining and gene mutations in non-small cell lung cancer and their effects on patient survival. *Ann Oncol* 1995; **6**: S9–13.

◆304  Takahasi T, Nau MM, Chiba I et al. p53: a frequent target for genetic abnormalities in lung cancer. *Science* 1989; **246**: 491–4.

◆305  Robles AI, Linke SP, Harris CC. The p53 network in lung carcinogenesis. *Oncogene* 2002; **21**: 6898–907.

306  Sozzi G, Miozzo M, Donghi R et al. Deletions of 17p and p53 mutations in preneoplastic lesions of the lung. *Cancer Res* 1992; **52**: 6079–82.

307  Bennett WP, Colby TV, Vahakangas KH et al. p53 protein accumulates frequently in early bronchial neoplasia. *Cancer Res* 1993; **53**: 4817–22.

308  Tammemagi MC, McLaughlin JR, Bull SB. Meta-analyses of p53 tumor suppressor gene alterations and clinico-pathological features in resected lung cancers. *Cancer Epidemiol Biomark Prev* 1999; **8**: 625–34.

●309  Greenblatt MS, Bennett WP, Hollstein M, Harris CC. Mutations in the p53 tumor suppressor gene: clues to cancer etiology and molecular pathogenesis. *Cancer Res* 1994; **54**: 4855–78.

●310  Hainaut P, Pfeifer GP. Patterns of p53 G->T transversions in lung cancers reflect the primary mutagenic signature of DNA damage by tobacco smoke. *Carcinogenesis* 2001; **22**: 367–74.

◆311  Denissenko MF, Pao A, Tang GP et al. Preferential formation of benzo[a]pyrene adducts at lung cancer mutational hot spots in p53. *Science* 1996; **274**: 430–2.

312  Smith LE, Denissenko MF, Bennett WP et al. Targeting of lung cancer mutational hot spots by polycyclic aromatic hydrocarbons. *J Natl Cancer Inst* 2000; **92**: 803–11.

313  Mitsudomi T, Hamajima N, Ogawa M, Takahasi T. Prognostic significance of p53 alterations in patients with non-small cell lung cancer: a meta-analysis. *Clin Cancer Res* 2000; **6**: 4055–63.

314  Steels E, Paesmans M, Berghmans T et al. Role of p53 as a prognostic factor for survival in lung cancer: a systematic review of the literature with a meta-analysis. *Eur Resp J* 2001; **18**: 705–19.

315  Marchetti A, Buttitta F, Merlo G et al. p53 alterations in non-small cell lung cancers correlate with metastatic involvement of hilar and mediastinal lymph nodes. *Cancer Res* 1993; **53**: 2846–51.

316  Ahrendt SA, Hu Y, Buta M et al. p53 mutations and survival in Stage I non-small cell lung cancer: results of a prospective study. *J Natl Cancer Inst* 2003; **95**: 961–70.

317  Tan DF, Li Q, Rammath N et al. Prognostic significance of expression of p53 oncoprotein in primary (stage I-IIIA) non-small cell lung cancer. *Anticancer Res* 2003; **23**: 1665–72.

318  Top B, Mooi W, Klave S et al. Comparative analysis of p53 gene mutations and protein accumulation in human non-small cell lung cancer. *Int J Cancer* 1995; **64**: 83–91.

319  Schiller JH, Adak S, Feins RH et al. Lack of prognostic significance of p53 and K-ras mutations in primary resected non-small cell lung cancer on E4592: a laboratory ancillary study on an Eastern Cooperative Oncology Group prospective randomized trial of postoperative adjuvant therapy. *J Clin Oncol* 2001; **19**: 448–57.

●320  Shirodkar S, Ewen M, DeCaprio J et al. The transcription factor E2F interacts with the retinoblastoma product and a p107 cyclin A complex in a cell cycle regulated manner. *Cell* 1992; **68**: 157–66.

●321  Nevins J. E2F: a link between Rb tumor suppressor protein and viral oncoproteins. *Science* 1992; **258**: 424–9.

322  Kaye FJ. Rb and cyclin dependent kinase pathways: defining a distinction between Rb and p16 loss in lung cancer. *Oncogene* 2002; **21**: 6908–14.

●323  Harbour JW, Lai SL, Whang-Peng J et al. Abnormalities in structure and expression of the human retinoblastoma gene in SCLC. *Science* 1988; **241**: 353–7.

324  Yokota J, Akiyama T, Fung YK et al. Altered expression of the retinoblastoma gene in small cell carcinoma of the lung. *Oncogene* 1988; **3**: 471–5.

325  Reissman PT, Koga H, Takahasi R et al. Inactivation of the retinoblastoma susceptibility gene in non-small cell lung cancer. *Oncogene* 1993; **8**: 1913–9.

326  Shimizu E, Coxon A, Otterson GA et al. RB protein status and clinical correlation from 171 cell lines representing lung cancer, extrapulmonary small cell carcinoma, and mesothelioma. *Oncogene* 1994; **9**: 2441–8.

327  Shapiro GI, Edwards CD, Kobzik L et al. Reciprocal Rb inactivation and p16INK4 expression in primary lung cancers and cell lines. *Cancer Res* 1995; **55**: 505–9.

◆328  Sekido Y, Fong KM, Minna JD. Progress in understanding the molecular pathogenesis of human lung cancer. *Biochim Biophys Acta* 1998; **1378**: F21–59.

329  Shapiro GI, Park JE, Edwards CD et al. Multiple mechanisms of p16INK4A inactivation in non-small cell lung cancer cell lines. *Cancer Res* 1995; **55**: 6200–9.

330  Sakaguchi M, Fujii Y, Hirabayashi H et al. Inversely correlated expression of p16 and Rb protein in non-small cell lung cancers: an immunohistochemical study. *Int J Cancer* 1996; **65**: 442–5.

331  Otterson GA, Kratzke RA, Coxon A et al. Absence of p16INK4A protein is restricted to the subset of lung cancer lines that retain wildtype Rb. *Oncogene* 1994; **9**: 3375–8.

332  Xu HJ, Quinlan DC, Davidson AG et al. Altered retinoblastoma protein expression and prognosis in early stage non small cell lung cancer. *J Natl Cancer Inst* 1994; **86**: 695–9.

333  Kratzke RA, Greatens TM, Rubins JB et al. Rb and p16INK4a expression in resected non-small cell lung tumors. *Cancer Res* 1996; **56**: 3415–20.

334  Taga S, Osaki T, Ohgami A et al. Prognostic value of the immunohistochemical detection of p16INK4 expression in non-small cell lung carcinoma. *Cancer* 1997; **80**: 389–95.

335  Huang CI, Taki T, Higashiyama M et al. p16 protein expression is associated with a poor prognosis in squamous cell carcinoma of the lung. *Br J Cancer* 2000; **82**: 374–80.

336  Hommura F, Dosaka-Akita H, Kinoshita I et al. Predictive value of expression of p16INK4A, retinoblastoma and p53 proteins for the prognosis of non-small cell lung cancers. *Br J Cancer* 1999; **81**: 696–701.

337  Geradts J, Fong KM, Zimmerman PV et al. Correlation of abnormal Rb, p16INK4A, and p53 expression with 3p loss of heterozygosity, other genetic abnormalities, and clinical features in 103 primary non-small cell lung cancers. *Clin Cancer Res* 1999; **5**: 791–800.

338  Urbanski SJ, Edwards DR, Maitland A et al. Expression of metalloproteinases and their inhibitors in primary pulmonary carcinomas. *Br J Cancer* 1992; **66**: 1188–94.

●339  Brown PD, Bloxidge RE, Stuart NSA et al. Association between expression of activated 72-kilodalton gelatinase and tumor spread in non-small cell lung carcinoma. *J Natl Cancer Inst* 1993; **85**: 574–8.

●340  Iizasa T, Fujisawa T, Suzuki M et al. Elevated levels of circulating plasma matrix metalloproteinase 9 in non-small cell lung cancer patients. *Clin Cancer Res* 1999; **5**: 149–53.

341  Stetler-Stevenson WG. Progelatinase A activation during tumor cell invasion. *Invas Metast* 1994; **14**: 259–68.

◆342  Kleiner DE, Stetler-Stevenson WG. Matrix metalloproteinases and metastasis. *Cancer Chemother Pharmacol* 1999; **43** (Suppl): S42–51.

343  Passlick B, Sienel W, Seen-Hibler R et al. Overexpression of matrix metalloproteinase 2 predicts unfavorable outcome in early-stage non-small cell lung cancer. *Clin Cancer Res* 2000; **6**: 3944–8.

344  Salden M, Splinter TAW, Peters HA et al. The urokinase-type plasminogen activator system in resected non-small-cell lung cancer. Rotterdam Oncology Thoracic Study Group. *Ann Oncol* 2000; **11**: 327–32.

345  Nagayama M, Sato A, Hayakawa H et al. Plasminogen activators and their inhibitors in non-small cell lung cancer. *Cancer* 1994; **73**: 1398–405.

346  Oka T, Ishida T, Nishino T et al. Immunohistochemical evidence for urokinase plasminogen activator in primary and metastatic tumors of pulmonary carcinoma. *Cancer Res* 1991; **51**: 3522–5.

347  Robert C, Bolon I, Gazzeri S et al. Expression of plasminogen activator inhibitors 1 and 2 in lung cancer and their role in tumor progression. *Clin Cancer Res* 1999; **5**: 2094–102.

348  Pedersen H, Grondahl-Hansen J, Francis D et al. Urokinase and plasminogen activator inhibitor type 1 in pulmonary adenocarcinoma. *Cancer Res* 1994; **54**: 120–3.

349  Pedersen H, Brunner N, Francis D et al. Prognostic impact of urokinase, urokinase receptor, and type I plasminogen activator inhibitor in squamous and large cell lung cancer tissue. *Cancer Res* 1994; **54**: 4671–5.

●350  Fontanini G, Lucchi M, Vignati S et al. Angiogenesis as a prognostic indicator of survival in non-small cell lung carcinoma: a prospective study. *J Natl Cancer Inst* 1997; **89**: 881–6.

351  Oshika Y, Nakamura M, Tokunaga T et al. Expression of cell-associated isoform of vascular endothelial growth factor 189 and its prognostic relevance in non-small cell lung cancer. *Int J Oncol* 1998; **12**: 541–4.

352  Fontanini G, Boldrini L, Chine S et al. Expression of vascular endothelial growth factor mRNA in non-small cell lung carcinomas. *Br J Cancer* 1999; **79**: 363–9.

353  Giatromanolaki A, Koukourakis MI, Kakolyris S et al. Vascular endothelial growth factor, wild-type p53 and angiogenesis in early operable non-small cell lung cancer. *Clin Cancer Res* 1998; **4**: 3017–24.

●354  Volm M, Koomagi R, Mattern J. Interrelationships between microvessel density, expression of VEGF and resistance of non-small cell lung carcinoma. *Anticancer Res* 1996; **16**: 213–8.

355 Apolinario RM, van der Valk P, de Jong JS et al. Prognostic value of the expression of p53, bcl-2, and bax oncoproteins, and neovascularization in patients with radically resected non-small cell lung cancer. *J Clin Oncol* 1997; **15**: 2456–66.

356 Chandrachud LM, Pendelton N, Chisholm DM et al. Relationship between vascularity, age and survival in non-small cell lung cancer. *Br J Cancer* 1997; **76**: 1367–75.

357 Bremnes RM, Veve R, Gabrielson E et al. High-throughput tissue microarray analysis used to evaluate biology and prognostic significance of the E-cadherin pathway in non-small cell lung cancer. *J Clin Oncol* 2002; **20**: 2417–28.

358 Wolff H, Saukkonen K, Anttila S et al. Expression of cyclooxygenase-2 in human lung carcinoma. *Cancer Res* 1998; **58**: 4997–5001.

359 Hida T, Yatabe Y, Achiwa H et al. Increased expression of cyclooxygenase 2 occurs frequently in human lung cancers, specifically in adenocarcinomas. *Cancer Res* 1988; **58**: 3761–4.

360 Achiwa H, Yatabe Y, Hida Y et al. Prognostic significance of elevated cyclooxygenase 2 expression in primary resected lung adenocarcinoma. *Clin Cancer Res* 1999; **5**: 1001–5.

361 Khuri FR, Wu H, Lee JJ et al. Cyclooxygenase-2 overexpression is a marker of poor prognosis in stage I non-small cell lung cancer. *Clin Cancer Res* 2001; **7**: 861–7.

◆362 Lockhart DJ, Winzeler EA. Genomics, gene expression and DNA arrays. *Nature* 2000; **405**: 827–36.

◆363 Kaminski N, Friedman N. Practical approaches to analyzing results of microarray experiments. *Am J Respir Cell Mol Biol* 2002; **27**: 125–32.

●364 Bhattacharjee A, Richards WG, Staunton J et al. Classification of human lung carcinomas by mRNA expression profiling reveals distinct adenocarcinoma subclasses. *Proc Natl Acad Sci USA* 2001; **98**: 13 790–5.

●365 Garber ME, Troyanskaya OG, Schluens K et al. Diversity in gene expression in adenocarcinoma of the lung. *Proc Natl Acad Sci USA* 2001; **98**: 13 784–9.

366 Beer DG, Kardia SLR, Huang CC et al. Gene-expression profiles predict survival of patients with lung adenocarcinoma. *Nature Med* 2002; **8**: 816–24.

367 Miura K, Bowman ED, Simon R et al. Laser capture microdissection and microarray expression analysis of lung adenocarcinoma reveals tobacco-smoking and prognosis-related molecular profiles. *Cancer Res* 2002; **62**: 3244–50.

368 Powell CA, Spira A, Derti A et al. Gene expression in lung adenocarcinomas of smokers and nonsmokers. *Am J Resp Cell Mol Biol* 2003; **29**: 157–62.

◆369 Tuveson DA, Jacks T. Modeling human lung cancer in mice: similarities and shortcomings. *Oncogene* 1999; **18**: 5318–24.

370 Thaete LG, Malkinson AM. Cells of origin of primary pulmonary neoplasms in mice: morphologic and histochemical studies. *Exp Lung Res* 1991; **17**: 219–28.

●371 Stoner GD. Introduction to mouse lung tumorigenesis. *Exp Lung Res* 1998; **24**: 375–83.

372 Bogen KT, Witschi H. Lung tumors in A/J mice exposed to environmental tobacco smoke: estimated potency and implied human risk. *Carcinogenesis* 2002; **23**: 511–9.

373 DeFlora S, Balansky RM, D'Agostini F et al. Molecular alterations and lung tumors in p53 mutant mice exposed to cigarette smoke. *Cancer Res* 2003; **63**: 793–800.

374 Malkinson AM, Nesbitt MN, Skamene E. Susceptibility to urethan-induced pulmonary adenomas between A/J and C57BL/6J mice: use of AXB and BXA recombinant inbred lines indicating a three-locus genetic model. *J Natl Cancer Inst* 1985; **75**: 971–4.

375 Ryan J, Barker PE, Nesbitt MN, Ruddle FH. K-Ras-2 as a genetic marker for lung tumor susceptibility in inbred mice. *J Natl Cancer Inst* 1987; **79**: 1351–7.

376 Gariboldi M, Manenti G, Canzian F et al. A major susceptibility locus to murine lung carcinogenesis maps on chromosome 6. *Nat Genet* 1993; **3**: 132–6.

377 Lin L, Festing MF, Devereux TR et al. Additional evidence that the K-ras protooncogene is a candidate for the major mouse pulmonary adenoma susceptibility (Pas-1) gene. *Exp Lung Res* 1998; **24**: 481–97.

◆378 Jackson EL, Kim CFB, Jacks T. Murine lung cancer models. http://emice/nci/nih.gov/ mouse_models/organ_models/ lung _models/

379 Fijneman RJA, van der Valk MA, Demant P. Genetics of quantitative and qualitative aspects of lung tumorigenesis in the mouse: multiple interacting Susceptibility to lung cancer (Sluc) genes with large effects. *Exp Lung Res* 1998; **24**: 419–36.

◆380 Kwak I, Tsai SY, DeMayo FJ. Genetically engineered mouse models for lung cancer. *Annu Rev Physiol* 2004; **66**: 647–63.

381 Ehrhardt A, Bartels T, Geick A et al. Development of pulmonary bronchiolo-alveolar adenocarcinomas in transgenic mice overexpressing murine c-myc and epidermal growth factor in alveolar type II pneumocytes. *Br J Cancer* 2001; **84**: 813–8.

382 Ehrhardt A, Bartels T, Klocke R et al. Increased susceptibility to tobacco carcinogen 4-methylnitrosamino-1-3-pyridyl-1-butanone in transgenic mice overexpressing c-myc and epidermal growth factor in alveolar type II cells. *J Cancer Res Clin Oncol* 2003; **129**: 71–5.

383 Fisher GH, Wellen SL, Klimstra D et al. Induction and apoptotic regression of lung adenocarcinomas by regulation of a K-ras transgene in the presence and absence of tumor suppressor genes. *Genes Dev* 2001; **15**: 3249–62.

384 Johnson L, Mercer K, Greenbaum D et al. Somatic activation of the K-ras oncogene causes early onset lung cancer in mice. *Nature* 2001; **410**: 1111–16.

385 Jackson EL, Willis N, Mercer K et al. Analysis of lung tumor initiation and progression using conditional expression of oncogenic K-ras. *Genes Dev* 2001; **24**: 3243–48.

386 Wu X, Zhao H, Suk R, Christiani DC. Genetic susceptibility to tobacco-related cancer. *Oncogene* 2004; **23**: 6500–23.

# 16

# Respiratory infections

MICHAEL F. MURRAY AND PETER V. TISHLER

## INTRODUCTION

Human infection occurs at the interface of three distinct forces: the environment, the microbial genome, and the human genome. In a very broad manner, the importance of the human genome at this interface has been supported for decades by family studies of risk for infectious diseases. This is perhaps best exemplified in the study by Sorensen and colleagues who found in a large cohort of adults that the inherited risk for premature death by infection was stronger than the inherited risk for premature death by either vascular or oncologic causes.[1] Studies over many years, particularly in the mouse, have also established that host genetic susceptibility can be pathogen-specific and is not necessarily associated with broad susceptibility to microbial pathogens.[2] Increasingly, these types of observations are being furthered and more fully illuminated by studies linking specific human gene mutations and polymorphisms to alterations in susceptibility to all types of human infectious diseases, including those of the respiratory tract.

Ultimately, there is a definable set of human genes that interact with each microbial pathogen (Fig. 16.1a). Overlap in pathogen–gene sets can derive from either microbial or host factors. For example, a shared intracellular life cycle requirement of *Mycobacterium tuberculosis* and HIV-1 appears to result in a common interaction with the human SLC11A1 gene product (Fig. 16.1b).[3,4] On the other hand, modulation in the host gamma-interferon response, a response that is common to both *Mycobacterium tuberculosis* and *Listeria monocytogenes* infection, joins these pathogen–gene sets via a host-driven mechanism (Fig. 16.1c).[5] Some microbe–gene pairs do seem highly specific, however, and may in fact prove to be unique (e.g., the gene for $P^K$ synthase (A4GALT), which acts as an erythrocyte cell surface receptor for parvovirus B19).[6]

The relative influence of evolutionary forces, such as genetic drift or natural selection, on polymorphisms associated with altered susceptibility to pulmonary infection remains an open question.[7] It should be borne in mind, however, that respiratory infection causes approximately 10 percent of deaths worldwide (and proportionately more historically).[8] Thus, it seems likely that a selective advantage for some human polymorphisms may well have evolved, for reasons similar to the protection against *Plasmodium falciparum*-induced malaria that is afforded by hemoglobin S.[9] For example, there has long been speculation (and corroboration in animal models) that the modern frequency of CFTR mutations in Caucasian populations came about as a result of heterozygous advantage against gastrointestinal infection.[10–12] The case of *Mycobacterium tuberculosis* may prove to be particularly revealing in this regard, since this bacterium alone caused up to 25 percent of all deaths in Western Europe in the first half of the nineteenth century and has been a leading cause of early death from time immemorial.[13] *M. tuberculosis* should be viewed as having as great a potential for polymorphism selection within certain human populations as malaria has had in other populations.[14]

The genes associated with altered host susceptibility to infection can be divided into genes associated with altered

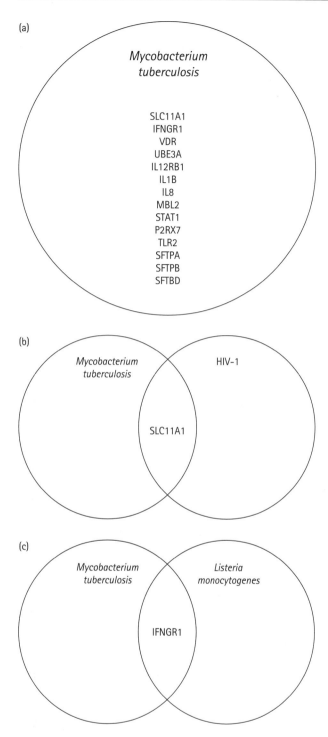

**Figure 16.1**  *(a) Model of pathogen–human gene set for*
Mycobacterium tuberculosis. *Although the complete set of human
genes with importance to any given infection is not known, the
current list for* M. tuberculosis *gives insight into the complexity of
the pathogen host–gene interaction. (b) Microbial life cycle driven
overlap: this potential example of overlap in pathogen–human
gene sets is based on limited data, however it is used to illustrate
the underlying principle. (c) Host response driven overlap: this
potential example of overlap in pathogen–human gene sets is
based on limited data, however it is used to illustrate the
underlying principle.*

host barriers against infection and genes associated with
altered host response to infection. To date, the majority of
human gene associations with pulmonary infections are
related to altered host responses once infected, and therefore are linked to susceptibility to varied outcomes rather
than susceptibility to initial infection. We shall review our
current knowledge.

## RESPIRATORY INFECTION IN MAN ASSOCIATED WITH GENE POLYMORPHISMS

Polymorphisms are exceedingly common throughout the
genome. Some of these appear to affect the host response
to infectious agents in a manner that might influence susceptibility to (but not of themselves cause) disease. Two
instructive polymorphisms are discussed herein; others are
presented subsequently, in the discussion of specific diseases.

### Mannose-binding lectin gene (MBL2) polymorphisms

The mannose-binding lectin is a well-characterized serum
protein that binds to mannose or *N*-acetyl-glucosamine
sugars present on bacteria, yeast, and some viruses. This
process activates the complement system, effecting opsonization of the microbes. The human MBL gene (MBL2), consisting of four exons, has three widely studied sites of
polymorphic variation (codons 52, 54, 57 in exon one), all
of which encode both decreased serum concentrations of
the protein and decreased opsonic function. Not surprisingly, a number of studies have addressed the possibility of
an association of MBL2 polymorphisms, which are relatively common, with infectious disease. Much of this literature is descriptive and based on reports of small numbers
of subjects. More controlled investigations of populations
suggest that homozygosity for MBL2 variant alleles may
be associated with meningococcal disease, and with risk
of developing or dying from sepsis.[15,16] Two studies have
addressed the association of MBL2 variants with respiratory illness. In one study from Japan, the frequency of
the MBL2 codon 54 variant was significantly higher in 62
patients with unexplained recurrent respiratory infections
and in 49 subjects with diffuse panbronchiolitis (55 and 51
percent, respectively) than in healthy control subjects (33
percent). Significant differences were not seen in groups with
nontuberculous mycobacteria or chronic aspergillus infections.[17] In a study of children from Denmark, MBL2 variants (in either homozygous or heterozygous state) were
associated with acute respiratory illness in children below the
age of 18 months, and particularly those aged 6–17 months
(relative risk, 2.9).[18] On the other hand, in another Danish
study, Dahl et al.[19] found no evidence for significant differences in infectious disease or mortality in mannose-binding lectin-deficient patients in a population of 9245 adults

(58 percent wild type, 37 percent heterozygotes, 5 percent homozygotes for the variant alleles). Clearly our understanding of the role of MBL2 is in evolution. The possible role of MBL2 in the lung disease of cystic fibrosis and in tuberculosis is considered in the discussions of these diseases.

## Surfactant protein gene polymorphisms

The surfactant proteins A, B, C, and D (SP-A, -B, -C, -D) are the major proteins of airway surfactant. SP-A is encoded by genes SFTPA1 and SFTPA2 (two highly homologous genes) and SP-D is encoded by SFTPD. All three genes reside in a cluster of related lectin genes on chromosome 10. Both surfactant proteins bind to various viral and bacterial pathogens and may enhance phagocytosis and microbial killing. SP-B and SP-C, small and highly hydrophobic proteins encoded by genes SFTPB and SFTPC on chromosomes 2 and 8, respectively, enhance the rate of spreading and stability of phospholipids during respiration, lowering surface tension and maintaining the patency of the distal airways and alveoli.[20,21] Details of these proteins and their physiologic function, as well as a description of noninfectious syndromes that result from defects in their genes, can be found in Chapter 18A.

Polymorphisms of SFTPB appear to be associated with the liability for acute respiratory distress syndrome (ARDS) that may result from overwhelming respiratory infection. Lin et al.[22] assessed the association of 19 polymorphisms of the genes for SP-A, -B and -D with ARDS from all causes and found a difference only for a C/T polymorphism at nucleotide 1580 of SFTPB. This is a missense mutation at the end of exon 4 that changes amino acid 131 from threonine to isoleucine, blocking N-glycosylation at this site. In the subgroup of 23 subjects with ARDS associated with pneumonia (20 subjects) or other unclear factors, this association persisted (odds ratio conferring susceptibility, 5.6; CI > 1). Quasney et al.[23] studied this same SFTPB polymorphism in a cohort of adults with community acquired pneumonia and found a significant association of homozygosity for the C allele with the development of ARDS, need for mechanical ventilation, and septic shock. Similar findings were reported by Gong et al.[24] in a study of an intron 4 polymorphism of SFTPB: females with this polymorphism and a direct pulmonary injury such as pneumonia (most subjects) and/or aspiration were significantly more liable for the development of ARDS. Thus, polymorphisms in certain areas of SFTPB appear to predispose to particularly severe infection and/or the development of ARDS. Perhaps the liability for infection or a deleterious inflammatory reaction in response to infection, is what drives the liability ultimately for ARDS.

A few additional studies hint at the importance of surfactant protein in the protection from (or liability for) infection. Polymorphisms in both SFTPD and SFTPA2 have been associated with the development of respiratory

syncytial virus bronchiolitis in infants. For SFTPD, the association was with homozygosity for an allele changing methionine at the amino terminal position 11 to threonine.[25] For SFTPA2, the association was with a minor allele (1A³) characterized by a substitution (of lysine) in the carbohydrate recognition domain that might affect binding to the virus.[26] Floros et al.[27] have also demonstrated both susceptibility and protective polymorphisms of SFTPA1, SFTPA2, SFTPB, and SFTPD in subjects with active pulmonary tuberculosis.

# RESPIRATORY INFECTION IN MAN ASSOCIATED WITH SINGLE GENE MUTATIONS

## Severe combined immunodeficiency syndromes

There are a number of monogenic causes of severe combined immunodeficiency in humans and they exist as both X-linked and autosomal recessive conditions. Each of these diseases is characterized by a combination of both humoral and cellular immune defects. They all leave the individual host with impaired response to, and thus increased risk for, respiratory (and other) infections, involving both common and unusual pulmonary pathogens. The pulmonary pathogens include those causing disease in typical hosts, as well as *Pneumocystis jiroveci (P. carinii)* and mycobacterium species, which are usually considered to be of lesser pathogenic potential.

In the case of X-linked severe combined immunodeficiency, mutations occur in the IL2RG gene encoding the common gamma chain γc found in receptors for a number of interleukins.[28] Mutations span all eight exons and frequently involve point mutations within CpG dinucleotides.[29] The net result is a loss of the normal receptor interaction with certain tyrosine kinases (JAK1 and JAK3) that play essential roles in cytokine receptor signal transduction and, ultimately, T-cell growth and maturation. This syndrome is the most common form of severe combined immunodeficiency and is estimated to occur in 1/50 000 to 1/100 000 births. The CpG 'hotspots' appear to predispose to new mutations, which constitute a significant proportion of cases which exist in equal frequency across all ethnic groups. The other forms of severe combined immunodeficiency disease also involving cytokine economy and signaling, are all autosomal recessive, and are associated with defects in the JAK3, IL7RA, CD45, ADA, RAG1, and RAG2 genes.[28]

## Interferon-gamma receptor defects

The interferon gamma receptor is a tetramer composed of two interferon-gamma receptor alpha chains and two interferon-gamma receptor beta chains. Defects in either of these proteins are associated with altered susceptibility to mycobacterial infection (see discussion of pulmonary tuberculosis).[30] Mutations in their corresponding genes (IFNGR1 and IFNGR2) are inherited as either autosomal dominant or autosomal recessive traits. In IFNGR1, a small deletion-prone hotspot results in a dominantly inherited mutation in which a truncated receptor acts as a dominant negative to interrupt interferon gamma signaling.[31] Recessively inherited IFNGR1 mutations are associated with susceptibility to mycobacterial infection (including BCG).[32,33]

Associations, which are less well characterized, also exist between interferon gamma receptor defects and nonmycobacterial infection. Dorman and colleagues[34] reported symptomatic and often severe viral respiratory infections in four patients with interferon gamma receptor deficiency; the viruses reported by this group included the human herpes viruses (cytomegalovirus, varicella-zoster virus, and herpes simplex virus), parainfluenza virus, and respiratory syncytial virus. A receptor defect has also been linked to human nonpulmonary bacterial infection in at least one case (i.e. *Listeria monocytogenes* infection).[5]

## Cystic fibrosis

Cystic fibrosis (CF) is an autosomal recessive, multisystem disease that results from the loss of functional cystic fibrosis transmembrane conductance regulator (CFTR) activity (for a general discussion, see Chapter 11). Although multiple organ systems are involved, only the respiratory tract is susceptible to infection. The chronic pulmonary infection and associated airways inflammation are linked to the progressive respiratory failure that is the cause of death in 80–95 percent of patients.[35] Interestingly, this susceptibility to sinopulmonary infection is not spontaneously recapitulated in the CFTR negative mouse model of the disease.

The increase in susceptibility to pulmonary infection in human patients is limited to a small group of bacteria, including *Haemophilus influenzae*, *Staphylococcus aureus*, *Pseudomonas aeruginosa*, *Burkholderia cepacia*, *Stenotrophomonas maltophilia*, and *Alcaligenes xylosoxidans*.[36] Early in life, patients with cystic fibrosis are predisposed to pulmonary infection with *S. aureus* and *H. influenzae*. Persistent colonization accompanied by repeated infection, usually with *P. aeruginosa* but sometimes with a member of the *B. cepacia* complex, follows later.[37]

Of the bacterial pathogens, *P. aeruginosa* is central to respiratory morbidity in most patients with CF. Its presence in the lower respiratory tract is associated with decreased survival. Once established, respiratory tract colonization with this bacterium is never fully cleared. The wildtype CFTR protein functions as a cell surface receptor for *P. aeruginosa*, permitting bacterial clearance. The most common delta F508 mutant CFTR protein cannot bind to this bacterium, a phenomenon associated with significantly delayed epithelial cell

apoptosis,[37] resulting in an increased intrapulmonary bacterial load and liability for infection.[38] While altered clearance is a critical factor in chronic colonization, it does not explain the entire clinical picture. The local inflammatory response is also altered and this may contribute to this chronic cycle of colonization and infection.[38]

Modifying genes and gene products, acting in concert with CFTR to alter susceptibility to infection, may also play a significant role in modulating the pulmonary phenotype in CF. One such protein is mannose-binding lectin, which binds to carbohydrates on the surface of microorganisms, leading to the activation of complement and phagocytosis.[39] Genes encoding variants in mannose-binding lectin (MBL2), which depress serum levels of functional protein, appear to be associated with increased liability for infection, decreased pulmonary function, and decreased survival time.[40,41]

## HUMAN RESPIRATORY INFECTIONS VIEWED AS COMPLEX HUMAN TRAITS

### Tuberculosis

Approximately one-third of the world's human population is chronically infected with *Mycobacterium tuberculosis*. It is presumed, mostly on the basis of (1) animal studies; (2) microbiological principles; and (3) a paucity of evidence to the contrary, that initial infection with *M. tuberculosis* is principally a matter of whether there is significant exposure to the aerosolized bacteria. Epidemiological data suggest, however, that even at the stage of initial infection host genetic factors are in play.[42] The study by Stead and colleagues[42] stands out for its capacity to convincingly differentiate people with new infection from those with latent infection in a controlled institutional environment. Specific genes that alter host barriers and facilitate the development of the initial infection with *M. tuberculosis* have not been identified.

Given the inherent difficulties in clinically dating an individual patient's initial infection with *M. tuberculosis*, collecting data on the phenotypic differences associated with established infection has proven to be a more ready endeavor. Once infection is established, the course of *M. tuberculosis* infection is known to be highly variable. A minority of patients develops acute disease, while the majority develops latent disease. A patient with chronic latent *M. tuberculosis* infection has a one in 10 lifetime risk of developing active disease.[43] In the category of acquired risk for active *M. tuberculosis* disease, advancing age is an inevitable risk factor. While we may speculate that host genes influence this risk for age-related reactivation disease, there are no available data bearing on this. Other acquired risk factors for reactivation disease are human immunodeficiency virus (HIV) infection, diabetes mellitus, smoking, malnutrition, and iatrogenic immunodeficiency.[44] In addition to the pharmacologic agents long known to be associated with reactivation (e.g., corticosteroids and chemotherapy), newer drugs such as TNF-alpha antagonists are also capable of inducing reactivation disease.[45,46]

Prior to the availability of effective chemotherapy, practicing twentieth-century clinicians assumed that tuberculosis risk was determined by both environment and heredity.[47] While it is unfortunate that enthusiasts of the eugenics movement exploited this belief, clinical observations supported the notion that a biological basis to susceptibility existed. For example, when in 1926 some 250 babies in Lubeck, Germany, were mistakenly immunized with an excessive titer of living, virulent human tubercle bacilli, the results were not entirely disastrous: 76 individuals died of acute tuberculous disease, 47 children did not develop discernible disease, and the remainder developed only minor, transient lesions.[48,49] A number of twin studies have supported the notion of familial risk,[2,50] with some of the best data on tuberculosis risk in twins coming from a study conducted by Simmonds from 1952–6 in London and later re-analyzed with more sophisticated statistical methods by Comstock.[51] This study defined tuberculosis in clinical terms and did not attempt to identify latent disease; so while it does not shed light on initial infection, there were significant findings regarding the development of active tuberculosis. In 202 twin pairs analyzed, the adjusted risk of active tuberculosis in the second twin was two-fold higher in monozygotic twins than in dizygotic twins (31 versus 15 percent; $P < 0.05$).[51]

In view of these observations, one may reasonably hypothesize that tuberculosis behaves like other complex human traits: multiple genetic and acquired factors conspire to result in a variable phenotype. In recent years, several candidate genes that may affect the host response to mycobacterial infection have in fact been identified. Perhaps the foremost of these is the SLC11A1 gene, formerly known as NRAMP1. A growing body of research, which will be summarized in the section on animal models, has accumulated compelling evidence of a role for this gene and its polymorphic variants in resistance or susceptibility to M. tuberculosis in experimental animals. The human homolog has been mapped to chromosome region 2q35 and several sequence variants have been delineated.[52] Studies assessing the relationship of SLC11A1 polymorphisms to the presence of clinical tuberculosis in humans have focused on four polymorphisms: INT4 (a single nucleotide change in intron 4; 469 + 14 G/C), D543N (a single-base substitution at codon 543, changing arginine to aspartic acid), 3'UTR (a TGTG deletion in the 3' untranslated region; 1729 + 55 del4); and $(CA)_n$ (a microsatellite in the immediate 5' region of the gene). The results are inconsistent. Studies from Asia have shown a distinct association of some or all of these polymorphisms with tuberculosis,[53–56] association only with cavitary pulmonary disease,[57] no association with disease,[58] and protection from disease.[59] Linkage analysis in a large aboriginal

Canadian family with epidemic pulmonary tuberculosis established a LOD score of 3.8 at marker D2S424, 'just distal to NRAMP1'.[60] Three studies from West Africa (two from Gambia and one from Guinea-Conakry) associated these polymorphisms with disease,[3,61,62] while a study from Morocco found no association with disease.[63] A single study of a Danish population demonstrated a relationship between INT4 and smear positive tuberculosis.[64] In northern Brazil, Shaw et al.[65] were unable to establish any relation of NRAMP1 to pulmonary tuberculosis in a candidate–gene linkage study of 98 pedigrees with disease. They did find evidence, from segregation analysis, for oligogenic inheritance of susceptibility to tuberculosis, however. A study of nuclear families of varying ethnicity in Harris County, Texas, published in abstract form, did show a significant relationship of two polymorphisms and disease in children.[66] Finding a common ground among these studies is difficult. Further studies should detail the background characteristics of both the experimental and control populations in greater detail, and strive for numbers that will permit detailed multivariate analyses of potentially confounding ethnic and other factors. Family studies (including twin studies) may be ideal in dealing with these background complexities.

Observations extending as far back as the eighteenth century have associated sunlight and/or increased vitamin D with improved outcomes in tuberculosis.[67–69] The active metabolite, 1,25-dihydroxyvitamin D3, has a number of immune functions, including activating monocytes and enhancing their ability to restrict the growth of M. tuberculosis in vitro. It also suppresses lymphocyte proliferation, immunoglobulin production, and cytokine synthesis.[70] Thus, studies in humans have focused on vitamin D receptor (VDR) polymorphisms, which, by influencing the bioavailability of vitamin D, may affect susceptibility to tuberculosis. Bellamy et al. sampled a population of 408 sputum smear-positive adult pulmonary tuberculosis patients and a similar number of controls in western Gambia for two single base polymorphisms (at codon 352 and within intron 8) of the gene VDR, finding that homozygosity for the codon 352 polymorphism was associated with a decreased frequency of disease (RR = 0.53; $P = 0.01$).[71] This allele is associated with increased serum concentrations of active hormone. A study from India purports to show that homozygosity for the codon 352 polymorphism is associated with a lower frequency of tuberculosis in males and a higher frequency in females, but this study is flawed by the nature of the control subjects.[72] Wilkinson et al.[73] studied this relationship in subjects with clinical tuberculosis who were immigrants to London from India. For the codon 352 polymorphism, they observed a decreased frequency of homozygosity in affected subjects (6 versus 11 percent in control subjects, but this difference was not statistically significant). The combination of vitamin D deficiency and one or two copies of the wild-type allele was significantly associated with clinical tuberculosis

(OR = 2.8; CI > 1). Similarly, significant results were obtained for the association of vitamin D deficiency plus homozygosity for the (non-wild type) Folk1 polymorphism and clinical disease (OR = 5.1; CI > 1). Vitamin D deficiency alone was also associated with disease, but these VDR alleles were an additive association. In the aforementioned family study from Harris County, Texas, an association of a vitamin D receptor polymorphism with pediatric tuberculosis was also observed.[66] To complete the confusing picture, Delgado et al.[59] found no association of this polymorphism with pulmonary disease in a Cambodian population. Bellamy[70] has proposed that a placebo-controlled trial of vitamin D therapy be carried out to resolve this issue.

The mannose-binding lectin gene (MBL2) has also been considered as a possible host response gene in tuberculosis. In Gambia, the frequency of the MBL2 codon 57 mutation was lower in 397 adults with smear-positive pulmonary tuberculosis than in controls (28 versus 33 percent, $P = 0.04$).[74] This potentially protective effect of an MBL2 polymorphism was also demonstrated for the G54D mutation in a South African population with pulmonary tuberculosis: the G54D allele was found in 12 of 91 affected subjects (13 percent) and in 22 of 79 TB-negative controls (28 percent; $P < 0.02$).[75] A reverse effect was demonstrated in a study in India, in which nearly 11 percent of the 202 subjects with pulmonary tuberculosis but only 2 percent of 109 controls were homozygous for one of the three functional polymorphisms ($P = 0.008$; OR = 6.5).[76] The frequency of all three variant alleles, particularly the G54D allele, was also greater in the subjects with tuberculosis than in the normal controls. These results, conflicting as they are, may well be confounded by factors related to the comparability of the controls, in societies with considerable ethnic/racial differences and admixturing.

Association analyses and case reports have linked a number of immune-response genes to the host response to tuberculosis. These candidates include genes of the HLA complex,[77,78] TNF and LTA (in association with HLA genes),[79] IFNG,[80,81] IFNGR1,[32,33] IFNGR2,[82] IL1B,[83,84] IL1RN[83,84] IL8,[85] IL12RB1,[86,87] IL12P40,[88] STAT1,[89] P2RX7,[90] TLR2,[91] SFTPA1, SFTPA2,[92] SFTPB, and SFTPD.[27] In general, each of these is supported by limited numbers of studies. As Malik and Schurr[93] have argued, these observations should be followed by 'population- and family-based studies … using common genetic polymorphisms for these genes'. Linkage analyses have also established a relationship of several chromosomal regions to infection: 15q,[94] Xq,[94] 17q11-21,[95] 10q26.13,[96] 11q12.3,[96] and 20p12.1.[96] Corroborative studies support the association at 15q11-13 with the gene UBE3A.[97] UBE3A (a gene encoding a ubiquitin ligase protein that has been associated with Angelman syndrome) is known to specifically interact with human papilloma virus proteins, but how it interacts with M. tuberculosis is unclear.[97] The genetic variants in UBE3A may simply be in linkage disequilibrium with the actual genetic variants of interest.

## Pneumococcal pneumonia

Most healthy individuals are repeatedly exposed to *Streptococcus pneumoniae* throughout life without infection. While the majority of children will experience at least one middle ear infection due to *S. pneumoniae*, infection with this bacterium in healthy adults is uncommon. The repeated 'exposure' in the case of this microbe consists of mucosal colonization and carriage, i.e. bacterial growth and replication on the surface of the host's tissue without tissue invasion, inflammatory reaction, or associated disease. Carriage without infection by *S. pneumoniae* stands in contrast to the relationship of *M. tuberculosis* with its human host, in which colonization without infection is believed to be uncommon. *S. pneumoniae* is estimated to reside in the nasopharynx of healthy adults about 5 percent of the time, but the incidence of pneumonia is only 20 cases per 100 000 young adults per year.[98] There are clearly bacterial strain differences that account for some differences in human disease and the story of the variability in virulence associated with *S. pneumoniae*'s polysaccharide capsule importantly illustrates the role of variable microbial genetics in the development of human disease.[99] Additionally, there are clearly defined 'acquired' factors that alter outcomes, including advancing age, smoking,[100] HIV infection, viral upper respiratory infection, diabetes, chronic lung disease, congestive heart failure, and immunosuppressive therapies.

While some of the host genes associated with susceptibility to *S. pneumoniae* have been described, other conditions are not yet understood at the level of a specific gene alteration. Human genes in which specific polymorphisms are linked to *S. pneumoniae* infection are mannose binding lectin (MBL2),[101] FCGR2A (also known as CD32),[102,103] fucosyltransferase 2 (FUT2; the 'nonsecretor status' mutation),[104] and beta hemoglobin (HBB; hemoglobin S).[105] The relatively common syndrome of familial 'IgA deficiency' is a risk for infection but has not yet been associated with specific genes or gene variations.[106]

## Coccidiodomycosis

*Coccidioides immitis* causes an estimated 100 000 infections annually in the USA, the majority of which are asymptomatic and limited to the respiratory tract.[107] Only 0.5 percent of infected individuals progress to extrapulmonary disease. The acquired risks for extrapulmonary disease include cancer, pregnancy, HIV infection, and immunosuppressive therapy. Clinical observations for over 50 years that 'non-white people' are at increased risk for such dissemination suggest that genetic factors are also operative.[108] The fact that people of both Filipino and African descent have a five- to 10-fold higher rate of disseminated coccidioidomycosis than Caucasians could be related to either increased resistance in Caucasians or increased susceptibility in non-whites.[109]

Specific genetic associations have not yet shed light on these epidemiological findings.

## ANIMAL MODELS OF HUMAN SUSCEPTIBILITY TO RESPIRATORY INFECTIOUS AGENTS

### Mycobacterium tuberculosis

Fifty years ago, in studies that may well have comprised the development of the first mammalian model system of host genetic resistance to infection, Lurie and colleagues[110] carried out experiments using inbred rabbit strains and demonstrated variable host resistance to *M. tuberculosis*. As would be expected given the era in which these studies took place, no specific genes were linked to these variable responses. These particular rabbit strains ultimately died out because of infertility.[111]

The mouse has since served as the predominant model of variable host resistance in the study of tuberculosis. The pursuit of evidence of variable susceptibility of inbred mouse strains to mycobacterial species has laid the groundwork for most of our current understanding of the role of Slc11a1 (formerly known as Nramp1) in these diseases. Initial studies established the importance of a single gene (variously called Bcg, Lsh, Ity, before their identity was recognized) in regulating susceptibility or resistance to a number of mycobacteria (Bacille Calmette–Guerin, BCG), *M. bovis, M. tuberculosis, M. lepraemurium, M. intracellulare, M. avium*), *Leishmania donovani*, and *Salmonella typhimurium*.[112,113] The common denominator in these and other susceptible microorganisms is the intracellular nature of their parasitism, and the common effect of the Slc11a1 gene and gene product is to regulate the activation of the host macrophage.[113] The gene, which was fine-mapped to the murine proximal chromosome 1,[114] is expressed almost exclusively in mature tissue macrophages, where it encodes a protein that is ultimately incorporated into the membrane of the phagosome.[115,116] Recently, the Slc11a1 gene was recognized to be a member of a gene family (Slc11) of metal-ion transporters that are energized by the electrochemical gradient generated by hydrogen ions.[117] The mechanism by which the Nramp1 protein functions in macrophage activation and host defense has not been established. It may operate either by extruding metal ions ($Fe^{++}$, $Mn^{++}$) from phagosomes, thereby minimizing ions that are essential for bacterial growth, or by concentrating these metal ions in phagosomes, thereby increasing the generation of toxic oxygen free radicals.[117] The relevance of the SLC11A1 to human disease, summarized previously, is under active investigation.

A number of genes encoding proteins that are important in various aspects of the immune response may play a role in modulating experimental tuberculosis in the mouse. Some of these genes, whose actions may ultimately affect host resistance or susceptibility via active oxygen species and nitric oxide,[118] are summarized in Table 16.1. The interactions among these genes and gene products are exceedingly complex. For example, whereas single gene-knockout mice deficient in either Il12b or Il18 were more liable for mycobacterial infection, double-knockout mice were protected from infection.[119] A hypothesis-generating review of these confusing data would be helpful in pointing the way

**Table 16.1** *Immune response genes associated with altered development of tuberculosis in the mouse*

| Gene | Gene product | Deficiency phenotype[a,b] | Reference |
|---|---|---|---|
| B2m | $\beta_2$-microglobulin | ↑ | 139 |
| Ifng | Interferon-γ | ↑ | 140 |
| Ifngr1 | Interferon-γ receptor | ↑ | 141 |
| Irf1 | Interferon regulatory factor 1 | ↑ | 142 |
| Il1r1 | Interleukin 1 receptor type 1 | ↑ | 143 |
| Tnf | Tumor necrosis factor-α | ↑ | 144 |
| Il4 | Interleukin 4 | ↓ | 145 |
| Il6 | Interleukin 6 | ↑ | 146 |
| Il10 | Interleukin 10 | ↓ | 147 |
| Il12b | Interleukin 12b | ↑ | 148 |
| Il18 | Interleukin 18 | ↑ | 149 |
| Cebpb[c] | CCAAT/enhancer binding protein, β | ↑ | 150 |
| Tlr2 | Toll-like receptor 2 | ↑ | 151 |
| Myd88 | Myeloid differentiation factor 88 | ↑ | 152 |
| Hc | Complement component 5 | ↑ | 153 |
| Nos2 | Inducible nitric oxide synthase | ↑ | 118 |

[a]Deficiency produced primarily by targeted gene disruption or knock out technologies.
[b]Deficiency phenotype is some measure of the development of tuberculous infection.
[c]Formerly known as Nfil6 (nuclear factor-interleukin-6).
↑, increased infection; ↓, decreased infection.

for future studies. New and different tuberculosis susceptibility loci have recently been described,[120–122] and further studies of these genes are awaited with interest.

## Legionella pneumophila

More than a decade ago, ex vivo macrophages from two different inbred mouse strains (A/J and C57BL/6J) were shown to differ in their permissiveness for intracellular *Legionella* replication.[123] This variation was later shown to segregate in a Mendelian fashion and the gene responsible for the macrophage permissiveness difference was mapped to a locus called *Lgn1* on mouse chromosome 13.[124,125] Recently, polymorphisms in the Birc1e gene at this locus were shown to be involved in the differences in permissiveness of mouse macrophages for intracellular *Legionella* replication.[126,127] The human homolog, BIRC1 has not yet been directly linked to altered susceptibility to *L. pneumophila*.

## Models with other organisms

Fierer and colleagues found a difference in resistance to *Coccidioides immitis* infection among inbred mouse strains.[128] They later extended their findings by mapping altered resistance to regions near the *Lv* locus on chromosome 4 and the *Tnfr1* locus on chromosome 6.[109,129] Specific genes within these chromosomal regions that confer altered susceptibility remain to be identified. Experimental *Pneumocystis jiroveci* (*P. carinii*) lung infection in Sftpd knockout mice (deficient for surfactant protein d) was characterized by an increased inflammatory response, delayed early clearance of organisms, and altered nitric oxide metabolism.[130] In a murine model of intranasal infection with *Streptococcus pneumoniae*, Sftpd deficiency knockout mice were significantly more susceptible to infection in the first 24 h following installation of bacteria. Absence of Sp-d resulted in reduced

pulmonary clearance of pneumococci and time to onset of bacteremia, and increased intrapulmonary inflammation and intravascular concentration of microorganisms.[131] In a murine model of nonfatal *Streptococcus pneumoniae* pneumonia, the degree of inflammatory response differed by strain. BALB/C mice cleared the inoculum, with high levels of phagocytosis and oxidative burst. C57BL/6 mice cleared the inoculum with a reduced immune response and were not able to contain or combat large inocula. The mechanisms and/or genes underlying these differential responses are not known.[132] In studies in mice with several inherited deficiencies of components of the complement system, Brown et al.[133] demonstrated that homozygous factor C1q- and factor B-deficient mice had greater susceptibility to intranasal pneumococcal infection than wild-type mice. In the C1qa−/− mice, the clearance of pneumococci from systemic circulation was reduced and macrophage activation was impaired, as would be expected with a defective complement opsonization system. Thus, their data demonstrated the vital role of the classical complement pathway in the immune response to this bacterial pathogen.

## FUTURE RESEARCH DIRECTIONS

In the coming years, a steady increase in the identification of genes associated with variable susceptibility to common pulmonary pathogens can be anticipated, leading to a more complete set of human susceptibility genes associated with each microbe (see Table 16.2, which summarizes the current state of our knowledge). As this research becomes increasingly powered by tools such as microarrays, it will move past simple candidate gene approaches, and the newly discovered gene associations will forge new understandings about microbial pathogenesis which will ultimately lead to new targets for rationally designed therapies.

**Table 16.2**   *Host genetic links to some common human respiratory pathogens*[a]

| Type of microbe | Organism | Animal model of altered susceptibility | Animal susceptibility loci or genes identified | Human evidence of familial susceptibility | Human susceptibility genes implicated |
|---|---|---|---|---|---|
| Bacteria | *Mycobacterium tuberculosis* | Yes[110,112] | Yes[113–116] | Yes[30,51] | Yes[3,5,71–92] |
| | *Streptococcus pneumoniae* | Yes[132] | Yes[154] | Yes[106] | Yes[104,105] |
| | *Legionella pneumophila* | Yes[123] | Yes[124,125] | No data | No data |
| | *Haemophilus influenzae* | No data | No data | No data | Yes[155] |
| Virus | Influenza | Yes[156] | Yes[157,158] | No data | No data |
| | Respiratory syncytial virus | Yes[159] | No data | No data | Yes[25,26,160] |
| Fungus | *Coccidioides immitis* | Yes[128] | Yes[109,129] | Yes[107,109] | No data |
| | *Histoplasma capsulatum* | Yes[161] | Yes[162] | No data | No data |
| | *Blastomyces dermatitidis* | Yes[163] | No data | No data | No data |

[a]Currently no data exist which link host genotype to susceptibility to the common pathogens *Staphylococcus aureus*, *Streptococcus agalactiae* (β-hemolytic streptocci), *Chlamydia pneumoniae*, *Mycoplasma pneumonia*, *Moraxella catarrhalis*, cytomegalovirus, measles virus, adenovirus, varicella-zoster virus, hantavirus.

In addition to the development of new therapies aimed at new targets, the expansion of the pharmacogenetic knowledge base will lead to better targeting of known therapies based on anticipation of an individual patient's specific responses. Better targeting of both antimicrobial agents and vaccines has the potential to result in improved patient outcomes by categorizing risks and predicting benefits.

One can anticipate that new infectious agents will be discovered and linked to pulmonary diseases that were once thought to have noninfectious etiologies. It is easy to forget the incredible paradigm shift that occurred with the linking of peptic ulcer disease to *Helicobacter pylori*, yet that type of paradigm shift may now be poised to occur with primary pulmonary hypertension and its recent association with KS-HV.[134] Like *H. pylori* and peptic ulcer disease,[135] the association of primary pulmonary hypertension and KS-HV is likely to also involve host gene variations that influence clinical course. One may speculate that other long suspected diseases, such as sarcoidosis, may finally be linked to infectious agents that differentially interact with polymorphic human gene products.

Lastly, the events of 11 September 2001 and the ongoing threat of bioterrorism have changed the biomedical research agenda, and this will likely change our knowledge base in relation to host genetic susceptibility to potential agents of terror. Three specific microorganisms that are potential bioweapons will primarily cause pulmonary infection: *Bacillus anthracis*,[136] *Yersinia pestis*,[137] and *Francisella tularensis*.[138] These three bacteria are generally relatively uncommon respiratory pathogens. However, they can cause deadly respiratory tract infections if weaponized and the increased research on the pathogenesis of these infections will likely identify new host gene–pathogen associations.

## Key learning points

- *Mycobacterium tuberculosis* may be a paradigm for the environmental pressures that impinge on the genotype to shape human evolution.

- Genes associated with altered host susceptibility to infection may include those associated with altered host barriers against infection, and those associated with altered host response to infection.

- Mutations in the genes for gamma chain γc interleukin receptor (IL2RG), interferon gamma receptor (IFNGR1, IFNGR2) and the cystic fibrosis transmembrane conductance regulator predispose to respiratory infection by various organisms, including (respectively) opportunistic organisms, *Mycobacterium tuberculosis* and *Pseudomonas aeruginosa*. Autosomal dominant and recessive and X-linked patterns of inheritance of these defects are operative.

- A number of gene polymorphisms may play important roles in the promotion of susceptibility or resistance to such respiratory infections as tuberculosis, pneumococcal pneumonia, and cystic fibrosis sinopulmonary disease. These include the genes for mannose-binding lectin (MBL2), surfactant proteins (SFTPA1, SFTPA2, SFTPB, SFTPC, SFTPD, and the corresponding mouse genes), natural resistance-associated macrophage protein (SLC11A1), and the vitamin D receptor. Evidence for the importance of these and other polymorphisms in humans is currently inconclusive, but studies in animal models are instructive.

- Despite the failure so far to conclusively associate specific genes with disease, the epidemiological evidence for the existence of host determinants of the risk for pulmonary tuberculosis is compelling.

## REFERENCES

●1  Sorensen TI, Nielsen GG, Andersen PK, Teasdale TW. Genetic and environmental influences on premature death in adult adoptees. *N Eng J Med* 1988; **318**: 727–32.

2  Puffer RR. *Familial susceptibility to tuberculosis.* Cambridge, MA: Harvard University Press, 1944: 22–3.

●3  Bellamy R, Ruwende C, Corrah T et al. Variations in the NRAMP1 gene and susceptibility to tuberculosis in West Africans. *N Eng J Med* 1998; **338**: 640–4.

4  Marquet S, Sanchez FO, Arias M et al. Variants of the human NRAMP1 gene and altered human immunodeficiency virus infection susceptibility. *J Infect Dis* 1999; **180**: 1521–5.

5  Roesler J, Kofink B, Wendisch J et al. *Listeria monocytogenes* and recurrent mycobacterial infections in a child with complete interferon-gamma-receptor (IFNγR1) deficiency: mutational analysis and evaluation of therapeutic options. *Exp Hematol* 1999; **27**: 1368–74.

6  Brown KE, Hibbs JR, Gallinella G et al. Resistance to parvovirus B19 infection due to lack of virus receptor (erythrocyte P antigen). *N Eng J Med* 1994; **330**: 1192–6.

7  Tishkoff SA, Verrelli BC. Patterns of human genetic diversity: implications for human evolutionary history and disease. *Annu Rev Genomics Hum Genet* 2003; **4**: 293–340.

8  World Health Organization. *WHO mortality database.* www3.who.int/whosis/menu.cfm (accessed 13 October 2004).

9  Hill AV, Allsopp CE, Kwiatkowski D et al. Common west African HLA antigens are associated with protection from severe malaria. *Nature* 1991; **352**: 595–600.

10  Knudson AG, Wayne L, Hallett WY. On the selective advantage of cystic fibrosis heterozygotes. *Am J Hum Genet* 1967; **19**: 388–92.

●11  Gabriel SE, Brigman KN, Koller BH et al. Cystic fibrosis heterozygote resistance to cholera toxin in the cystic fibrosis mouse model. *Science* 1994; **266**: 107–9.

●12  Pier GB, Grout M, Zaidi T et al. *Salmonella typhi* uses CFTR to enter intestinal epithelial cells. *Nature* 1998; **393**: 79–82.

◆13  Bellamy R. Susceptibility to mycobacterial infections: the importance of host genetics. *Genes Immun* 2003; **4**: 4–11.

14  Bellamy R, Hill AV. Genetic susceptibility to mycobacteria and other infectious pathogens in humans. *Curr Opin Immunol* 1998; **10**: 483–7.

15  Hibberd ML, Sumiya M, Summerfield JA. Association of variants of the gene for mannose-binding lectin with susceptibility to meningococcal disease. *Lancet* 1999; **353**: 1049–53.

16  Garred P, Strom JJ, Quist L. Association of mannose-binding lectin polymorphisms with sepsis and fatal outcome, in patients with systemic inflammatory response syndrome. *J Infect Dis* 2003; **188**: 1394–403.

17  Gomi K, Tokue Y, Kobayashi T. Mannose-binding lectin gene polymorphism is a modulating factor in repeated respiratory infections. *Chest* 2004; **126**: 95–9.

18  Koch A, Melbye M, Sorensen P. Acute respiratory tract infections and mannose-binding lectin insufficiency during early childhood. *J Am Med Assoc* 2001; **285**: 1316–21.

19  Dahl M, Tybjaerg-Hansen A, Schnohr P, Nordestgaard BG. A population-based study of morbidity and mortality in mannose-binding lectin deficiency. *J Exp Med* 2004; **199**: 1391–9.

◆20  Hawgood S, Poulain FR. The pulmonary collectins and surfactant metabolism. *Annu Rev Physiol* 2001; **63**: 495–519.

21  Whitsett JA, Nogee LM. Hereditary surfactant protein B deficiency. In: Scriver CR, Beaudet AL, Sly WS, Valle D (eds). *The metabolic and molecular bases of inherited disease*, 8th edn. New York: McGraw-Hill, 2001: 5553–8.

22  Lin Z, Pearson C, Chinchilli V et al. Polymorphisms of human SP-A, SP-B, and SP-D genes: association of SP-B Thr131Ile with ARDS. *Clin Genet* 2000; **58**: 181–91.

23  Quasney MW, Waterer GW, Dahmer MK. Association between surfactant protein B + 1580 polymorphism and the risk of respiratory failure in adults with community-acquired pneumonia. *Crit Care Med* 2004; **32**: 1115–9.

24  Gong MN, Wei Z, Xu L-L et al. Polymorphism in the surfactant protein-B gene, gender, and the risk of direct pulmonary injury and ARDS. *Chest* 2004; **125**: 203–11.

25  Lahti M, Lofgren J, Marttila R et al. Surfactant protein D gene polymorphism associated with severe respiratory syncytial virus infection. *Pediatr Res* 2002; **51**: 696–9.

26  Lofgren J, Ramet M, Renko M et al. Association between surfactant protein A gene locus and severe respiratory syncytial virus infection in infants. *J Infect Dis* 2002; **185**: 283–9.

27  Floros J, Lin H-M, Garcia A. Surfactant protein genetic marker alleles identify a subgroup of tuberculosis in a Mexican population. *J Infect Dis* 2000; **182**: 1473–8.

◆28  Belmont JW, Puck JM. T cell and combined immunodeficiency disorders. In: Scriver CR, Beaudet AL, Sly WS, Valle D (eds). *The metabolic and molecular bases of inherited disease*, 8th edn. New York: McGraw-Hill, 2001: 4751–83.

●29  Pepper AE, Buckley RH, Small TN, Puck JM. Two mutational hotspots in the interleukin-2 receptor gamma chain gene causing human X-linked severe combined immunodeficiency. *Am J Hum Genet* 1995; **57**: 564–71.

30  Dorman SE, Holland SM. Interferon-gamma and interleukin-12 pathway defects and human disease. *Cytokine Growth Factor Rev* 2000; **11**: 321–33.

●31  Jouanguy E, Lamhamedi-Cherradi S, Lammas D et al. A human IFNGR1 small deletion hotspot associated with dominant susceptibility to mycobacterial infection. *Nat Genet* 1999; **21**: 370–8.

32  Newport MJ, Huxley CM, Huston S et al. A mutation in the interferon gamma receptor gene and susceptibility to mycobacterial infection. *N Engl J Med* 1996; **335**: 1941–9.

33  Jouanguy E, Altare F, Lamhamedi S et al. Interferon gamma receptor deficiency in an infant with fatal bacille calmette guerin infection. *N Engl J Med* 1996; **335**: 1956–61.

34  Dorman SE, Uzel G, Roesler J et al. Viral infections in interferon-gamma receptor deficiency. *J Pediatr* 1999; **135**: 640–3.

◆35  Lyczak JB, Cannon CL, Pier GB. Lung infections associated with cystic fibrosis. *Clin Microbiol Rev* 2002; **15**: 194–222.

◆36  Chmiel JF, Davis PB. State of the art: Why do the lungs of patients with cystic fibrosis become infected and why can't they clear the infection? *Respir Res* 2003; **4**: 1–12.

37  Cannon CL, Kowalski MP, Stopak KS, Pier GB. *Pseudomonas aeruginosa*-induced apoptosis is defective in respiratory epithelial cells expressing mutant cystic fibrosis transmembrane conductance regulator. *Am J Respir Cell Mol Biol* 2003; **29**: 188–97.

38  Pier GB. Role of the cystic fibrosis transmembrane conductance regulator in innate immunity to *Pseudomonas aeruginosa* infections. *Proc Natl Acad Sci USA* 2000; **97**: 8822–8.

39  Davies J, Neth O, Alton E. Differential binding of mannose-binding lectin to respiratory pathogens in cystic fibrosis. *Lancet* 2000; **355**: 1885–6.

40  Garred P, Pressler T, Ho M. Association of mannose-binding lectin gene heterogeneity with severity of lung disease and survival in cystic fibrosis. *J Clin Invest* 1999; **104**: 431–7.

41  Gabolde M, Guilloud-Bataille M, Feingold J, Besmond C. Association of variant alleles of mannose binding lectin with severity of pulmonary disease in cystic fibrosis: cohort study. *Br Med J* 1999; **319**: 1166–7.

●42  Stead WW, Senner JW, Reddick WT, Lofgren JP. Racial differences in susceptibility to infection by *Mycobacterium tuberculosis*. *N Engl J Med* 1990; **322**: 422–7.

43  Tufariello JM, Chan J, Flynn JL. Latent tuberculosis: mechanisms of host and bacillus that contribute to persistent infection. *Lancet Infect Dis* 2003; **3**: 578–90.

44  Gajalakshmi V, Peto R, Kanaka TS, Jha P. Smoking and mortality from tuberculosis and other diseases in India: retrospective study of 43 000 adult male deaths and 35 000 controls. *Lancet* 2003; **362**: 507–15.

45  Keane J, Gershon S, Wise RP et al. Tuberculosis associated with infliximab, a tumor necrosis factor alpha-neutralizing agent. *N Engl J Med* 2001; **345**: 1098–104.

46  Gardam M, Iverson K. Rheumatoid arthritis and tuberculosis: time to take notice. *J Rheumatol* 2003; **30**: 1397–9.

47  McCrae T. *The principles and practice of medicine, designed for the use of practitioners and students of medicine, originally written by the late Sir William Osler*, 10th edn. New York: D. Appleton, 1925: 159–62.

48  Dubos R, Dubos J. *The white plague*. New Brunswick: Rutgers University Press, 1952: 122–3,162.

49  Newport MJ, Blackwell JM. Genetic susceptibility to tuberculosis. *Bailliere's Clin Infect Dis* 1997; **4**: 207–29.

50  Kallman FJ, Reisner D. Twin Studies on the significance of genetic factors in tuberculosis. *Am Rev Tuberculosis* 1943; **47**: 549–74.

●51  Comstock GW. Tuberculosis in twins: a re-analysis of the Prophit survey. *Am Rev Respir Dis* 1978; **117**: 621–4.

52  Liu J, Fujiwara TM, Buu NT et al. Identification of polymorphisms and sequence variants in the human homologue of the mouse natural resistance-associated

macrophage protein gene. *Am J Hum Genet* 1995; **56**: 845–53.

53 Liu W, Cao WC, Zhang CY et al. VDR and NRAMP1 gene polymorphisms in susceptibility to pulmonary tuberculosis among the Chinese Han population: a case-control study. *Int J Tuberc Lung Dis* 2004; **8**: 428–34.

54 Duan HF, Zhou XH, Ma Y, Li CY. [A study on the association of 3′UTR polymorphisms of NRAMP1 gene with susceptibility to tuberculosis in Han.] *Zhonghua Jie He He Hu Xi Za Zhi* 2003; **26**: 286–9. [Article in Chinese]. Abstract [online]: www.ncbi.nlm.nih.gov (accessed 11 October 2004).

55 Gao P-S, Fujishima S, Mao X-Q, Remus N. Genetic variants of NRAMP1 and active tuberculosis in Japanese populations. *Clin Genet* 2000; **58**: 74–6.

56 Ryu S, Park YK, Bai GH et al. 3′UTR polymorphisms in the NRAMP1 gene are associated with susceptibility to tuberculosis in Koreans. *Int J Tuberc Lung Dis* 2000; **4**: 577–80.

57 Abe T, Iinuma Y, Ando M. NRAMP1 polymorphisms, susceptibility and clinical features of tuberculosis. *J Infect* 2003; **46**: 215–20.

58 Liaw YS, Tsai-Wu JJ, Wu CH et al. Variations in the NRAMP1 gene and susceptibility of tuberculosis in Taiwanese. *Int J Tuberc Lung Dis* 2002; **6**: 454–60.

59 Delgado JC, Baena A, Thim S, Goldfeld AE. Ethnic-specific genetic associations with pulmonary tuberculosis. *J Infect Dis* 2002; **186**: 1463–8.

●60 Greenwood CM, Fujiwara TM, Boothroyd LJ et al. Linkage of tuberculosis to chromosome 2q35 loci, including NRAMP1, in a large aboriginal Canadian family. *Am J Hum Genet* 2000; **67**: 405–16.

61 Cervino ACL, Lakisss S, Sow O, Hill AVS. Allelic association between the NRAMP1 gene and susceptibility to tuberculosis in Guinea-Conakry. *Ann Hum Genet* 2000; **64**: 507–12.

62 Awomoyi AA, Marchant A, Howson JMM et al. Interleukin-10, polymorphism in SLC11A1 (formerly NRAMP1), and susceptibility to tuberculosis. *J Infect Dis* 2002; **186**: 1808–14.

63 El Baghdadi J, Remus N, Benslimane A. Variants of the human NRAMP1 gene and susceptibility to tuberculosis in Morocco. *Int J Tuberc Lung Dis* 2003; **7**: 599–602.

64 Soberg C, Andersen AB, Madsen HO. Natural resistance-associated macrophage protein 1 polymorphisms are associated with microscopy-positive tuberculosis. *J Infect Dis* 2002; **186**: 517–21.

65 Shaw MA, Collins A, Peacock CS. Evidence that genetic susceptibility to *Mycobacterium tuberculosis* in a Brazilian population is under oligogenic control: linkage study of the candidate genes NRAMP1 and TNFA. *Tuber Lung Dis* 1997; **78**: 35–45.

66 Malik S, Abel L, Tooker H. Genetic risk factors for pediatric tuberculosis disease. *Am J Hum Genet* 2002; **71**: Abstr. 1100.

67 Rook GA. The role of vitamin D in tuberculosis. *Am Rev Respir Dis* 1988; **138**: 768–70.

68 Davies PD. A possible link between vitamin D deficiency and impaired host defence to *Mycobacterium tuberculosis*. *Tubercle* 1985; **66**: 301–6.

69 Rockett KA, Brookes R, Udalova I et al. 1,25-Dihydroxyvitamin D3 induces nitric oxide synthase and suppresses growth of *Mycobacterium tuberculosis* in a human macrophage-like cell line. *Infect Immun* 1998; **66**: 5314–21.

◆70 Bellamy R. Evidence of gene-environment interaction in development of tuberculosis. *Lancet* 2000; **355**: 588–9.

71 Bellamy R, Ruwende C, Corrah T et al. Tuberculosis and chronic hepatitis B virus infection in Africans and variation in the vitamin D receptor gene. *J Infect Dis* 1999; **179**: 721–4.

72 Selvaraj P, Narayanan PRW, Reetha AM. Association of vitamin D receptor genotypes with the susceptibility to pulmonary tuberculosis in female patients and resistance in female contacts. *Indian J Med Res* 2000; **111**: 172–9.

●73 Wilkinson RJ, Llewelyn M, Toossi Z et al. Influence of vitamin D deficiency and vitamin D receptor polymorphisms on tuberculosis among Gujarati Asians in west London: a case-control study. *Lancet* 2000; **355**: 618–21.

74 Bellamy R, Ruwende C, McAdam KP et al. Mannose binding protein deficiency is not associated with malaria, hepatitis B carriage nor tuberculosis in Africans. *Q J Med* 1998; **91**: 13–8.

75 Hoal-Van Helden EG, Epstein J, Victor TC. Mannose-binding protein B allele confers protection against tuberculous meningitis. *Ped Res* 1999; **45**: 459–64.

76 Selvaraj P, Narayanan PR, Reetha AM. Association of functional mutant homozygotes of the mannose binding protein gene with susceptibility to pulmonary tuberculosis in India. *Tuber Lung Dis* 1999; **79**: 221–7.

77 Goldfeld AE, Delgado JC, Thim S. Association of an HLA-DQ allele with clinical tuberculosis. *J Am Med Assoc* 1996; **279**: 226–8.

78 Amirzargar AA, Yalda A, Hajabolbaghi M. The association of HLA-DRB, DQA1, DQB1 alleles and haplotype frequency in Iranian patients with pulmonary tuberculosis. *Int J Tuberc Lung Dis* 2004; **8**: 1017–21.

79 Selvaraj P, Sriram U, Kurian SM et al. Tumour necrosis factor alpha (−238 and −308) and beta gene polymorphisms in pulmonary tuberculosis: haplotype analysis with HLA-A, B and DR genes. *Tuberculosis* 2001; **81**: 335–41.

80 Rossouw M, Nel HJ, Cooke GS. Association between tuberculosis and a polymorphic NFKB binding site in the interferon gamma gene. *Lancet* 2003; **361**: 1871–2.

81 Lopez-Maderuelo D, Arnalich F, Serantes R et al. Interferon-γ and interleukin-10 gene polymorphisms in pulmonary tuberculosis. *Am J Respir Crit Care Med* 2003; **167**: 970–5.

82 Dorman SE, Holland SM. Mutation in the signal-transducing chain of the interferon-gamma receptor and susceptibility to mycobacterial infection. *J Clin Invest* 1998; **101**: 2364–9.

83 Bellamy R, Ruwende C, Corrah T et al. Assessment of the interleukin 1 gene cluster and other candidate gene polymorphisms in host susceptibility to tuberculosis. *Tuber Lung Dis* 1998; **79**: 83–9.

84 Wilkinson RJ, Patel P, Llewelyn M et al. Influence of polymorphism in the genes for the interleukin (IL)-1 receptor antagonist and IL-1β on tuberculosis. *J Exp Med* 1999; **189**: 1863–73.

85 Ma X, Reich RA, Wright JA. Association between interleukin-8 gene alleles and human susceptibility to tuberculosis disease. *J Infect Dis* 2003; **188**: 349–55.

●86 Altare F, Durandy A, Lammas D et al. Impairment of mycobacterial immunity in human interleukin-12 receptor deficiency. *Science* 1998; **280**: 1432–5.

87 Remus N, El Baghdadi J, Fieschi C. Association of IL12RB1 polymorphisms with pulmonary tuberculosis in adults in Morocco. *J Infect Dis* 2004; **190**: 580–7.

88 Altare F, Lammas D, Revy P et al. Inherited interleukin 12 deficiency in a child with bacille Calmette–Guerin and *Salmonella enteritidis* disseminated infection. *J Clin Invest* 1998; **102**: 2035–40.

89   Dupuis S, Dargemont C, Fieschi C et al. Impairment of mycobacterial but not viral immunity by a germline human STAT1 mutation. *Science* 2001; **293**: 300–3.

90   Li CM, Campbell SJ, Kumararatne DS et al. Association of a polymorphism in the P2X7 gene with tuberculosis in a Gambian population. *J Infect Dis* 2002; **186**: 1458–62.

91   Ogus AC, Yoldas B, Ozdemir T. The Arg753Gln polymorphism of the human toll-like receptor 2 gene in tuberculosis disease. *Eur Respir J* 2004; **23**: 219–23.

●92   Madan T, Saxena S, Murthy KJ et al. Association of polymorphisms in the collagen region of human SP-A1 and SP-A2 genes with pulmonary tuberculosis in Indian population. *Clin Chem Lab Med* 2002; **40**: 1002–8.

◆93   Malik S, Schurr E. Genetic susceptibility to tuberculosis. *Clin Chem Lab Med* 2002; **40**: 863–8.

94   Bellamy R, Beyers N, McAdam KP et al. Genetic susceptibility to tuberculosis in Africans: a genome-wide scan. *Proc Natl Acad Sci USA* 2000; **97**: 8005–9.

95   Jamieson SE, Miller EN, Black GF et al. Evidence for a cluster of genes on chromosome 17q11-q21 controlling susceptibility to tuberculosis and leprosy in Brazilians. *Genes Immun* 2004; **5**: 46–57.

96   Miller EN, Jamieson SE, Joberty C et al. Genome-wide scans for leprosy and tuberculosis susceptibility genes in Brazilians. *Genes Immun* 2004; **5**: 63–7.

97   Cervino AC, Lakiss S, Sow O et al. Fine mapping of a putative tuberculosis-susceptibility locus on chromosome 15q11-13 in African families. *Hum Mol Genet* 2002; **11**: 1599–603.

98   Garcia-Rodriguez JA, Fresnadillo Martinez MJ. Dynamics of nasopharyngeal colonization by potential respiratory pathogens. *J Antimicrob Chemother* 2002; **50** (Suppl. S2): 59–73.

99   Garcia E, Lopez R. Molecular biology of the capsular genes of *Streptococcus pneumoniae*. *FEMS Microbiol Lett* 1997; **149**: 1–10.

100   Marrie TJ. Pneumococcal pneumonia: epidemiology and clinical features. *Semin Respir Infect* 1999; **14**: 227–36.

101   Roy S, Knox K, Segal S et al. MBL genotype and risk of invasive pneumococcal disease: a case-control study. *Lancet* 2002; **359**: 1569–73.

102   Sanders LA, van de Winkel JG, Rijkers GT et al. Fc gamma receptor IIa (CD32) heterogeneity in patients with recurrent bacterial respiratory tract infections. *J Infect Dis* 1994; **170**: 854–61.

103   Sanders LA, Feldman RG, Voorhorst-Ogink MM et al. Human immunoglobulin G (IgG) Fc receptor IIA (CD32) polymorphism and IgG2-mediated bacterial phagocytosis by neutrophils. *Infect Immun* 1995; **63**: 73–81.

104   Blackwell CC, Jonsdottir K, Hanson M et al. Non-secretion of ABO antigens predisposing to infection by *Neisseria meningitidis* and *Streptococcus pneumoniae*. *Lancet* 1986; **2**: 284–5.

105   Bjornson AB, Gaston MH, Zellner CL. Decreased opsonization for *Streptococcus pneumoniae* in sickle cell disease: studies on selected complement components and immunoglobulins. *J Pediatr* 1977; **91**: 371–8.

106   Braconier JH, Nilsson B, Oxelius VA, Karup-Pedersen F. Recurrent pneumococcal infections in a patient with lack of specific IgG and IgM pneumococcal antibodies and deficiency of serum IgA, IgG2 and IgG4. *Scand J Infect Dis* 1984; **16**: 407–10.

107   Stevens DA. Coccidioidomycosis. *N Engl J Med* 1995; **332**: 1077–82.

108   Rosenstein NE, Emery KW, Werner SB et al. Risk factors for severe pulmonary and disseminated coccidioidomycosis: Kern County, California, 1995–1996. *Clin Infect Dis* 2001; **32**: 708–15.

109   Fierer J, Walls L, Wright F, Kirkland TN. Genes influencing resistance to *Coccidioides immitis* and the interleukin-10 response map to chromosomes 4 and 6 in mice. *Infect Immun* 1999; **67**: 2916–9.

●110   Lurie MB, Zappasodi P, Dannenberg AM, Weiss GH. On the mechanism of genetic resistance to tuberculosis and its mode of inheritance. *Am J Hum Genet* 1952; **4**: 302–14.

111   Dorman SE, Hatem CL, Tyagi S et al. Susceptibility to tuberculosis: clues from studies with inbred and outbred New Zealand White rabbits. *Infect Immun* 2004; **72**: 1700–5.

◆112   Gros P, Skamene E, Forget A. Genetic control of natural resistance to *Mycobacterium bovis* (BCG) in mice. *J Immunol* 1981; **127**: 2417–21.

113   Schurr E, Malo D, Radzioch D et al. Genetic control of innate resistance to mycobacterial infections. *Immunol Today* 1991; **12**: A42–5.

114   Malo D, Vidal SM, Hu J et al. High-resolution linkage map in the vicinity of the host resistance locus Bcg. *Genomics* 1993; **16**: 655–63.

115   Vidal SM, Malo D, Vogan K et al. Natural resistance to infection with intracellular parasites: isolation of a candidate for Bcg. *Cell* 1993; **73**: 469–85.

116   Gruenheid S, Pinner E, Desjardins M, Gros P. Natural resistance to infection with intracellular pathogens: the Nramp1 protein is recruited to the membrane of the phagosome. *J Exp Med* 1997; **185**: 717–30.

117   Mackenzie B, Hediger MA. SLC11 family of H+-coupled metal-ion transporters NRAMP1 and DMT1. *Pflugers Arch* 2004; **447**: 571–9.

118   MacMicking JD, North RJ, LaCourse R et al. Identification of nitric oxide synthase as a protective locus against tuberculosis. *Proc Natl Acad Sci USA* 1997; **94**: 5243–8.

119   Kawakami K, Kinjo Y, Uezu K et al. Interferon-γ production and host protective response against *Mycobacterium tuberculosis* in mice lacking both IL-12p40 and IL-18. *Microb Infect* 2004; **6**: 339–49.

120   Kramnik I, Dietrich WF, Demant P, Bloom BR. Genetic control of resistance to experimental infection with virulent *Mycobacterium tuberculosis*. *Proc Natl Acad Sci USA* 2000; **97**: 8560–5.

121   Sanchez F, Radaeva V, Nikonenko BV et al. Multigenic control of disease severity after virulent *Mycobacterium tuberculosis* infection in mice. *Infect Immun* 2003; **71**: 126–31.

122   Mitsos L-M, Cardon LR, Ryan L et al. Susceptibility to tuberculosis: a locus on mouse chromosome 19 (Trl-4) regulates *Mycobacterium tuberculosis* replication in the lungs. *Proc Natl Acad Sci USA* 2003; **100**: 6610–5.

●123   Yamamoto Y, Klein TW, Newton CA, Friedman H. Interaction of *Legionella pneumophila* with peritoneal macrophages from various mouse strains. *Adv Exp Med Biol* 1988; **239**: 89–98.

124   Beckers MC, Yoshida S, Morgan K et al. Natural resistance to infection with *Legionella pneumophila*: chromosomal localization of the Lgn1 susceptibility gene. *Mammal Genome* 1995; **6**: 540–5.

125  Dietrich WF, Damron DM, Isberg RR et al. Lgn1, a gene that determines susceptibility to *Legionella pneumophila*, maps to mouse chromosome 13. *Genomics* 1995; **26**: 443–50.

126  Wright EK, Goodart SA, Growney JD et al. Naip5 affects host susceptibility to the intracellular pathogen *Legionella pneumophila*. *Curr Biol* 2003; **13**: 27–36.

127  Diez E, Lee SH, Gauthier S et al. Birc1e is the gene within the Lgn1 locus associated with resistance to *Legionella pneumophila*. *Nat Genet* 2003; **33**: 55–60.

128  Kirkland TN, Fierer J. Inbred mouse strains differ in resistance to lethal *Coccidioides immitis* infection. *Infect Immun* 1983; **40**: 912–6.

129  Fierer J, Walls L, Kirkland TN. Genetic evidence for the role of the Lv locus in early susceptibility but not IL-10 synthesis in experimental coccidioidomycosis in C57BL mice. *J Infect Dis* 2000; **181**: 681–5.

130  Atochina EN, Gow AJ, Beck JM et al. Delayed clearance of *Pneumocystis carinii* infection, increased inflammation, and altered nitric oxide metabolism in lungs of surfactant protein-D knockout mice. *J Infect Dis* 2004; **189**: 1528–39.

131  Kadioglu A, Andrew PW. The innate immune response to pneumococcal lung infection: the untold story. *Trends Immunol* 2004; **25**: 143–9.

132  Preston JA, Beagley KW, Gibson PG, Hansbro PM. Genetic background affects susceptibility in nonfatal pneumococcal bronchopneumonia. *Eur Respir J* 2004; **23**: 224–31.

133  Brown JS, Hussell T, Gilliland SM et al. The classical pathway is the dominant complement pathway required for innate immunity to *Streptococcus pneumoniae* infection in mice. *Proc Natl Acad Sci USA* 2002; **99**: 16 969–74.

134  Cool CD, Rai PR, Yeager ME et al. Expression of human herpesvirus 8 in primary pulmonary hypertension. *N Engl J Med* 2003; **349**: 1113–22.

135  Malaty HM, Engstrand L, Pedersen NL, Graham DY. *Helicobacter pylori* infection: genetic and environmental influences. A study of twins. *Ann Intern Med* 1994; **120**: 982–6.

136  Inglesby TV, Henderson DA, Bartlett JG et al. Anthrax as a biological weapon: medical and public health management. *J Am Med Assoc* 1999; **281**: 1735–45.

137  Inglesby TV, Dennis DT, Henderson DA et al. Plague as a biological weapon: medical and public health management. *J Am Med Assoc* 2000; **283**: 2281–90.

138  Dennis DT, Inglesby TV, Henderson DA et al. Tularemia as a biological weapon: medical and public health management. *J Am Med Assoc* 2001; **285**: 2763–73.

139  Ladel CH, Daugelat S, Kaufmann SH. Immune response to *Mycobacterium bovis* bacille Calmette Guerin infection in major histocompatibility complex class I- and II-deficient knock-out mice: contribution of CD4 and CD8 T cells to acquired resistance. *Eur J Immunol* 1995; **25**: 377–84.

140  Cooper AM, Dalton DK, Stewart TA et al. Disseminated tuberculosis in interferon gamma gene-disrupted mice. *J Exp Med* 1993; **178**: 2243–7.

141  Kamijo R, Le J, Shapiro D et al. Mice that lack the interferon-gamma receptor have profoundly altered responses to infection with Bacillus Calmette–Guerin and subsequent challenge with lipopolysaccharide. *J Exp Med* 1993; **178**: 1435–40.

142  Yamada H, Mizuno S, Sugawara I. Interferon regulatory factor 1 in mycobacterial infection. *Microbiol Immunol* 2002; **46**: 751–60.

143  Sugawara I, Yamada H, Hua S, Mizuno S. Role of interleukin (IL)-1 type 1 receptor in mycobacterial infection. *Microbiol Immunol* 2001; **45**: 743–50.

144  Kaneko H, Yamada H, Mizuno S. Role of tumor necrosis factor-$\alpha$ in *Mycobacterium*-induced granuloma formation in tumor necrosis factor-$\alpha$-deficient mice. *Lab Invest* 1999; **79**: 379–86.

145  Rook GAW, Hernandez-Pando R, Dheda K, Seah GT. IL-4 in tuberculosis: implications for vaccine design. *Trends Immunol* 2004; **25**: 483–8.

146  Ladel CH, Blum C, Dreher A et al. Lethal tuberculosis in interleukin-6-deficient mutant mice. *Infect Immun* 1997; **65**: 4843–9.

147  Murray PJ, Young RA. Increased antimycobacterial immunity in interleukin-10-deficient mice. *Infect Immun* 1999; **67**: 3087–95.

148  Cooper AM, Magram J, Ferrante J, Orme IM. Interleukin 12 (IL-12) is crucial to the development of protective immunity in mice intravenously infected with mycobacterium tuberculosis. *J Exp Med* 1997; **186**: 39–45.

149  Kinjo Y, Kawakami K, Uezu K et al. Contribution of IL-18 to Th1 response and host defense against infection by *Mycobacterium tuberculosis*: a comparative study with IL-12p40. *J Immunol* 2002; **169**: 323–9.

150  Sugawara I, Mizuno S, Yamada H et al. Disruption of nuclear factor-interleukin-6, a transcription factor, results in severe mycobacterial infection. *Am J Pathol* 2001; **158**: 361–6.

151  Drennan MB, Nicolle D, Quesniaux VJF et al. Toll-like receptor 2 deficient mice succumb to *Mycobacterium tuberculosis* infection. *Am J Pathol* 2004; **164**: 49–57.

152  Feng CG, Scanga CA, Collazo-Custodio CM et al. Mice lacking myeloid differentiation factor 88 display profound defects in host resistance and immune responses to *Mycobacterium avium* infection not exhibited by toll-like receptor 2 (TLT2)- and TLR4-deficient animals. *J Immunol* 2003; **171**: 4758–64.

153  Jagannath C, Hoffman H, Sepulveda E et al. Hypersusceptibility of A/J mice to tuberculosis is in part due to a deficiency of the fifth complement component (C5). *Scand J Immunol* 2000; **52**: 369–79.

154  Denny P, Hopes E, Gingles N et al. A major locus conferring susceptibility to infection by *Streptococcus pneumoniae* in mice. *Mamm Genome* 2003; **14**: 448–53.

155  Blackwell CC, Jonsdottir K, Hanson MF, Weir DM. Non-secretion of ABO blood group antigens predisposing to infection by *Haemophilus influenzae*. *Lancet* 1986; **20**: 687.

156  Haller O, Acklin M, Staeheli P. Genetic resistance to influenza virus in wild mice. *Curr Top Microbiol Immunol* 1986; **127**: 331–7.

157  Arulanandam BP, Raeder RH, Nedrud JG et al. IgA immunodeficiency leads to inadequate T cell priming and increased susceptibility to influenza virus infection. *J Immunol* 2001; **166**: 226–31.

158  Staeheli P, Grob R, Meier E et al. Influenza virus-susceptible mice carry Mx genes with a large deletion or a nonsense mutation. *Mol Cell Biol* 1988; **8**: 4518–23.

159  Stark JM, McDowell SA, Koenigsknecht V et al. Genetic susceptibility to respiratory syncytial virus infection in inbred mice. *J Med Virol* 2002; **67**: 92–100.

160  Hacking D, Knight JC, Rockett K et al. Increased in vivo transcription of an IL-8 haplotype associated with respiratory

syncytial virus disease-susceptibility. *Genes Immun* 2004; **5**: 274–82.

161  Patton RM, Riggs AR, Compton SB, Chick EW. Histoplasmosis in purebred mice: influence of genetic susceptibility and immune depression on treatment. *Mycopathologia* 1976; **60**: 39–43.

162  Deepe GS. *Histoplasma capsulatum* and V beta a mice: cellular immune responses and susceptibility patterns. *J Med Vet Mycol* 1993; **31**: 181–8.

163  Morozumi PA, Halpern JW, Stevens DA. Susceptibility differences of inbred strains of mice to blastomycosis. *Infect Immun* 1981; **32**: 160–8.

# 17

# Congenital, metabolic, and neuromuscular diseases

NATASHA Y. FRANK AND PETER V. TISHLER

## INTRODUCTION

This chapter includes a discussion of a number of genetic diseases, of varying but lesser prevalence than many other diseases reviewed in this book, that have major (but usually not only) pulmonary manifestations. We have selected for our discussion representative diseases that impinge on pulmonary function by four differing and important mechanisms: a disturbance in anatomic development of the chest wall and diaphragm, change in alveolar and/or distal bronchiolar structure, modification of the neural or muscular mechanisms of respiratory control, and change in the pulmonary vasculature. Some diseases included in these areas of discussion are also associated with sleep apnea, through mechanisms involving either abnormalities of upper airways or central dysregulation of breathing. The list of diseases covered herein is not all-inclusive. In an attempt to approximate a complete listing, we have included in Table 17.1 a brief tabulation of other relevant diseases, with current references.

## DISEASES OF THE CHEST WALL AND DIAPHRAGM

A number of structural genetic diseases affect the respiratory system secondarily, usually as a result of the dysmorphology inherent in the syndrome.

## Osteogenesis imperfecta

The osteogenesis imperfecta (OI) syndromes are a group of genetic disorders of collagen and possibly other proteins affecting primarily bone mass, architecture, and strength. As other structures are also affected, these syndromes are generalized connective tissue disorders. Typical clinical characteristics of OI include fragile, fracture-prone bones, joint hypermobility, blue sclerae, skin hyperlaxity, dentinogenesis imperfecta, and hearing loss. Skeletal deformities resulting from fractures and abnormal bone size and shape, with resultant decreased height, are common.[1] Based on the severity of the clinical manifestations and rate of disease progression, OI is subdivided into six types.[2,3] Types I–IV appear to be the most prevalent. Patients with the mildest type of OI, type I (Online Mendelian Inheritance in Man (OMIM) 166200), have fractures of long bones particularly during childhood, blue sclerae, and little or no growth impairment or deformity. Type II OI (OMIM 166210), the most severe, is characterized by multiple intrauterine rib and other bony fractures, small chest, and severe skeletal deformity. This is almost always lethal perinatally. Patients with type III OI (OMIM 259420) have frequent fractures, severe progressive and global skeletal deformity that includes the chest, and abnormal impingement of the skull on vertebral column (platybasia) that can cause loss of neurologic function. Affected individuals usually survive into late childhood or adulthood, but may ultimately be confined to a wheelchair. Type IV OI (OMIM 166220) represents the

**Table 17.1** *Additional inherited syndromes with a significant pulmonary component*

| Syndrome (OMIM No.) | Respiratory defect | Inheritance | Key references |
|---|---|---|---|
| *Dwarfism syndromes* | | | |
| Thanatophoric dysplasia (187600) | Narrow thorax, short ribs, severely restricted rib cage, spinal cord compression → resp. failure | D | 150,151 |
| *Achondrogenesis* | | | |
| I (200600) | Narrow thorax, thin and very short ribs | R | 151,152 |
| II Hypochondrogenesis (200610) | Small thorax, thin and short ribs | D | 151,153 |
| Fibrochondrogenesis (228520) | Very short, narrow thorax and thin ribs | R | 150 |
| Metatropic dysplasia (250600) | Very small, ossified thorax, deformed ribs, kyphoscoliosis; hyperplasia of tracheobronchial cartilage, pulmonary hypoplasia | R | 150,154 |
| Short rib, polydactyly syndromes (263510–30; 269860) | Hypoplastic thorax and lungs; short ribs with poor cartilage maturation and endochondral bone formation | R | 155 |
| Asphyxiating thoracic dystrophy (208500) | Constricted chest wall, small thorax, respiratory failure | R | 150 |
| Diastrophic dysplasia (222600) | Tracheobronchomalacia → ↑ airway resistance, impaired expansion, airway collapse | R | 151,156 |
| Campomelic dysplasia (114290) | Small thorax with 11 slender ribs, tracheomalacia, recurrent apneas, stridor → respiratory failure; recurrent infections, kyphosis, scoliosis | D | 151,157,158 |
| *Infiltrative/storage diseases* | | | |
| Farber lipogranulomatosis (228000) | Infiltration of esophagus, lungs with ceramide laden cells → disturbed swallowing → aspiration, bronchospasm, infection, consolidation → respiratory failure | R | 163 |
| Fabry disease (301500) | In minority of patients: chronic cough, wheeze; dyspnea; obstructive airways disease with ↓FEV1, probably related to glycosphingolipid accumulation | X | 164,165 |
| *Gaucher disease* | | | |
| I (Nonneuronopathic, 'mild')[a] (230800) | In minority: dyspnea, cough, diffuse lower-zone infiltrates, ↓ FVC and DLCO, VO₂ max; pulmonary hypertension; hepatopulmonary syndrome; related to Gaucher cell infiltration | R | 166,167 |
| II (Acute neuronopathic) (230900) | Hypoplastic lungs; bulbar paralysis, Gaucher cell infiltration of lungs → apnea, resp. arrests, aspiration pneumonia | R | 168,169 |
| Glycogen storage disease type II (Pompe dis.; Acid maltase def.) (232300) | Infantile form: early respiratory muscle weakness, macroglossia → respiratory failure. Adult: respiratory muscle weakness → ↓ VC → sleep apnea, hypoxemia → pulmonary hypertension, respiratory failure | R | 170 |
| *Niemann–Pick disease* | | | |
| A (257200) | Diffuse reticular-nodular lung infiltrates | R | 171 |
| B (607616) | Foam cell infiltration → reticular-nodular infiltrates → ↓ DLCO, pO₂; pneumonias | R | 171,172 |
| C₂ (607625) | Storage macrophage infiltration → infiltrates, consolidation → hypoxia → respiratory failure; emphysema | R | 173 |

*Neuromuscular Diseases*

*Spinal muscular atrophies*

| Disease (OMIM) | Description | Inheritance | Ref. |
|---|---|---|---|
| I Werdnig Hoffman (253300) | Intercostal muscle paralysis, bulbar dysfunction → ↓ lung volumes and no. alveoli; aspiration, resp. failure | R | 96 |
| II (253550) | As above but lesser, scoliosis → ↓ vital capacity, impaired cough, aspiration, recurrent pneumonias, resp. failure | R | 96 |
| Infantile spinal muscular atrophy with respiratory distress (SMARD 1) (604320) | Diaphragmatic paralysis, inspiratory stridor, respiratory distress → respiratory failure | R | 176 |
| X-linked myotubular myopathy (310400) | Extreme respiratory muscle weakness at birth → respiratory failure, death/ventilator dependency | X | 177 |
| Congenital myasthenic syndromes (254200, 254210, 601462) | Respiratory, upper airway muscle weakness → aspiration, respiratory failure 'crises.' Periodic apneic episodes in one form. Hypersensitive to anesthesia. | R, D | 178,179 |
| Nemaline myopathy (161800, 256030) | Neonatal respiratory muscle weakness → early respiratory failure; many childhood infections, chest deformity, scoliosis, impaired central ventilatory drive → hypoventilation → hypoxemia, hypercarbia → respiratory failure | R, D | 179,180 |
| Myotonic dystrophy (160900, 602668) | Neonatal/infancy: atrophic respiratory muscles, pulmonary hypoplasia, central control defect → aspiration, respiratory failure. Adult: weak/myotonic respiratory muscles,→ aspiration → respiratory failure; central and peripheral sleep apnea | D | 180,182,183 |

*Miscellaneous diseases*

| Disease (OMIM) | Description | Inheritance | Ref. |
|---|---|---|---|
| Familial Mediterranean fever (249100) | Polyserositis, including pleuritis | R | 174 |
| Lysinuric protein intolerance (222700) | Interstitial lung disease, pulmonary fibrosis, pulmonary alveolar proteinosis, bronchiolitis obliterans, cholesterol granulomas, pulmonary hemorrhage, hypoxia, respiratory insufficiency | R | 175 |
| VATER/VACTERL association (192350) | Laryngeal stenosis, tracheoesophageal fistula, total anomalous pulmonary venous return, tracheal agenesis | D | 159,160 |
| Familial congenital bronchiectasis (Williams–Campbell syndrome) (211450) | Bronchial cartilage deficiency → distal airway collapse, cystic bronchiectasis, paracicatricial emphysema → restrictive and obstructive disease | ?D | 151 |
| Hereditary mucoepithelial dysplasia (158310) | Pneumonias, hemoptysis → restrictive disease → cor pulmonale; or frequent bronchitis, mild obstructive disease | D | 161,162 |
| Smith–Lemli–Opitz syndrome (270400) | Tracheal cartilage anomalies → tracheal narrowing, obstructive sleep apnea, pneumonias; abnormal lung lobation, pulmonary hypoplasia, accessory pulmonary arteries | R | 184 |
| Keutel syndrome (245150) | Peripheral pulmonic stenosis; calcifications of tracheal, bronchial rings | R | 185 |
| Marfan syndrome (154700) | Craniofacial abnormalities, obstructive sleep apnea | D | 186 |
| Down syndrome (190685) | Upper airway, craniofacial abnormalities, ?central nervous system abnormalities → mostly obstructive, some central sleep apnea | C | 187,188 |

aFor more details, see Chapter 14, Pulmonary hypertension. Type III Gaucher disease has been described but does not appear to have pulmonary complications.
OMIM, Online Mendelian Inheritance in Man; D, autosomal dominant; R, autosomal recessive; X, X-linked; C, chromosome defect (trisomy 21).

most diverse group, in whom the effect on bones, leading potentially to deformities, short stature, or neurologic impairment, can vary from severe to mild.

## RESPIRATORY MANIFESTATIONS

Respiratory compromise is the leading cause of death in adults with OI. McAllion and Peterson[4] have demonstrated that nearly 60 percent of affected individuals succumb to either a respiratory infection or respiratory failure. Respiratory death occurred at a young age (<30, in their experience) in individuals with type III OI, whereas respiratory death occurred at much later ages in types I and IV OI. A primary mechanism for the respiratory sequellae of OI is the deformity of the chest, restricting normal lung expansion with inspiration. Falvo et al.'s study of 11 subjects with OI demonstrated a decrease in vital capacity and increase in residual volume that were found only in subjects with kyphoscoliosis.[5] Widmann et al.[6] have demonstrated a strong correlation between thoracic scoliosis and decreased vital capacity, such that a vital capacity below 50 percent occurred at a curve magnitude of 60 degrees. Thus, individuals may have marginal respiratory reserve with which to respond to increased oxygen requirements (e.g., the febrile state). This is further compromised by loss of normal gas exchange in areas of an infiltrate (e.g., pneumonia, atelectasis), creating the potential for respiratory failure. A secondary mechanism may be the loss of the central control of respiration by brainstem compression from platybasia either acutely (e.g., as the result of coughing or trauma) or chronically and progressively. Some individuals may become ventilator dependent if they survive the acute insult. Pulmonary hypoplasia (reduction in lung growth) has also been reported, in OI type II.[7,8]

## GENETIC ETIOLOGY

Collagens are responsible for tensile strength and structural integrity of connective tissues.[9] A biochemical defect altering the amount or structure of type I collagen is responsible for most cases of OI.[10] At present, a few hundred mutations in the collagen genes COL1A1 (on chromosome 17q21.31-q22) and COL1A2 (on chromosome 7q22.1) have been described,[11] providing the basis for biochemical[12] and genetic[13] testing. OI types I–IV are generally inherited in an autosomal dominant fashion. New mutations are common, however, and an occasional family with type II or III disease appears to manifest an autosomal recessive pattern.

## DIAGNOSIS

The clinical manifestations of OI types II and III are usually sufficient to lead to the appropriate diagnosis. This is also the case in some patients with types I and IV, particularly if blue sclerae (type I) and/or dentinogenesis imperfecta (type IV) are present. Nonetheless, the clinical manifestations are highly variable. Family history may be helpful if

others are affected, but the high rate of mutation can confound this. Thus, biochemical/gene testing has some clinical relevance. Unfortunately, the procedures are laborious and expensive. Screening for a defect in collagen biosynthesis is recommended if the diagnosis of OI is not absolute. These studies are performed on cultured fibroblasts: collagens are labeled and analyzed by polyacrylamide gel electrophoresis.[14] This method identifies a biochemical abnormality in about 90 percent of patients known to have OI.[12] If gene mutation analysis is indicated, mutation screening techniques are used to both minimize the effort of dealing with these very large genes and maximize the yield. These techniques include chemical cleavage of DNA mismatches (CCM)[15] and conformation-sensitive gel electrophoresis (CSGE).[16,17] These approaches identify about 90 percent of OI cases.[18] Sequencing the entire coding region can also be done at some laboratories. More information about genetic testing can be obtained from www.genetests.org or www.gendia.net. Genetic testing for OI may be of value in genetic counseling and prenatal diagnosis, and in excluding child abuse.

## THERAPY

Periodic pulmonary function and neurologic studies to document liability for respiratory compromise is essential. Prompt attention to the pulmonary manifestations of OI during an intercurrent illness is equally important. Individuals should be monitored closely by critical care specialists, who should have a low threshold for intubation/tracheostomy and ventilatory assistance. Results of studies of the use of bisphosphonates to prevent the orthopedic complications of OI are promising, but what relevance this will have to the respiratory aspects of OI is not certain.

# Achondroplasia

Achondroplasia (OMIM 100800), a genetic disorder of bone growth, is characterized by short stature, rhizomelic (proximal limb) shortening of the extremities, and large head. It is caused by gain of function mutations of the FGFR3 gene and has unique genetic and phenotypic homogeneity. Infants with achondroplasia present neonatally with hypotonia, short limbs, redundant skin, and large head. Although their motor development is usually delayed, their muscle tone and function are usually normal by age 1–2 years. Sudden death, usually later than 6 months of age, may result from inability to support the heavy head, with resultant cervical-medullary compression of the spinal cord. Obesity may become a major problem beginning in childhood.[19] Adults with achondroplasia may develop symptomatic lumbar stenosis at the L1–L4 level.[20]

## RESPIRATORY MANIFESTATIONS

A large proportion of children with achondroplasia develop sleep apnea, cyanotic episodes, and chronic respiratory insufficiency.[21–26] Major contributing anatomical defects include those that predispose to obstructive events (choanal stenosis; small nasopharynx, trachea, and chest; and upper airway obstruction with soft tissue), those that may lead to central dysregulation of breathing (dysplasia of the basiocciput and craniovertebral junction, with foramen magnum stenosis and cervicomedullary cord compression), and thoracic cage restriction.[27] Central sleep apnea may also contribute to the high prevalence of sudden death in children with achondroplasia.[28] In adults, major respiratory problems are unusual, although one would expect the liability for obstructive sleep apnea to persist.[29,30]

## GENETIC ETIOLOGY

Achondroplasia is an autosomal dominant syndrome. A large proportion of individuals have no affected relatives; some 80–90 percent of cases appear to be due to new mutations.[31] A paternal age effect on the rate of mutation of this gene has been well documented. Achondroplasia is caused by a mutation in a transmembrane domain of the gene for fibroblast growth factor receptor 3 (FGFR3). FGFR3, located on chromosome 4p16.3, encodes an 840 amino acid protein that belongs to the family of fibroblast growth factor receptors.[32] Most cases identified to date are caused by activating mutations at nucleotide 1138, codon 380 (gly380arg [G380R]).[31,33] The G380R substitution causes constitutive activation of the FGF receptor. In mice, targeted disruption of FGFR3 gene enhances growth of long bones and vertebrae, suggesting that it (or FGF) has a role in negative regulation of bone growth.[34,35] Thus, an activating mutation of FGFR3 would be expected to over-regulate bone growth, leading to decreased bone growth and possibly abnormal skeletal development. Infants homozygous for this condition have severe disease and typically die in infancy from respiratory failure (either central or peripheral).

## DIAGNOSIS

The clinical diagnosis of achondroplasia is based on short stature, rhizomelic shortening of the arms and legs, limitation of elbow extension, large head with frontal bossing, mid-face hypoplasia, exaggerated lumbar lordosis, and genu varum.[36] A family history is helpful but is often absent.

## GENETIC TESTING

Clinical genetic testing is available for diagnostic confirmation and prenatal diagnosis. It is done by mutation analysis of the FGFR3 gene. About 98 percent of patients have the aforementioned G to A point mutation at nucleotide 1138 of the FGFR3 gene causing a Gly380Arg substitution.[31,37,38] About 1 percent of patients have a G to C point mutation at nucleotide 1138.[36] A number of diagnostic facilities offer this testing (see www.genetests.org and www.gendia.net).

## THERAPY

Patients should be monitored for the presence or development of symptoms of sleep apnea, with a low threshold for carrying out diagnostic polysomnography and initiating CPAP treatment. Similarly, imaging studies of the base of the skull should be carried out in infants and children before signs of cord compression are manifest. Neurosurgical relief of acute cervicomedullary compression is essential.

## Congenital diaphragmatic hernia

Congenital diaphragmatic hernia (CDH; OMIM 142340) is characterized by a defect in the diaphragm. Abdominal organs (stomach, small bowel, colon, liver, spleen) are herniated into the communicating hemithorax. This leads via mechanisms that are poorly understood to generalized pulmonary hypoplasia and pulmonary hypertension that may be life-threatening.

Four types of CDH, defined by the failure of development of certain components of the diaphragm during embryogenesis, are recognized.[39] They are the anterolateral hernia, posterolateral hernia, pars sternalis hernia, and Morgagni hernia.[40] Some 85 percent of CDH are left sided; and among them, posterolateral or Bochdalek hernia is the most common.[41] CDH occurs in 1:3000 newborns, but is found frequently in stillbirths. Despite advances in treatment, mortality worldwide remains on the order of 30 percent.[39]

## RESPIRATORY MANIFESTATIONS

The diagnosis of CDH is made either prenatally, via imaging studies, or perinatally, on the basis of respiratory distress that usually requires intubation. In earlier times, the respiratory manifestations were viewed as an impingement defect demanding instant surgical repair. This is clearly simplistic; rather, the physiologic behavior of the lungs of children with CDH is altered, and this is the most limiting factor in survival. The lungs of the newborn (primarily but not exclusively the lung on the side of the hernia) have a decreased number of both airways (including the number of alveoli per terminal airway) and vascular generations, and increased smooth muscle in the arterial walls. Fetal lung development appears to be both delayed (as exemplified by the airway and vascular development) and abnormal (i.e., arteriolar smooth muscle hypertrophy, presumably leading to pulmonary hypertension).[39] Surfactant production is said to be reduced.[39] The combination of pulmonary hypoplasia and pulmonary hypertension may result in respiratory failure that is lethal in the newborn period. The molecular mechanisms underlying these changes, although poorly understood presently, probably involve the dysregulation of transcriptional and other regulatory factors that are essential to normal anatomic development.[39]

Pulmonary function abnormalities persist in a significant minority of individuals who survive into childhood or adulthood.[42] Perfusion to the affected lung may be reduced. Pulmonary function testing usually reveals restrictive lung disease, but obstructive pathology can also be found. Whether these changes can be attributed to the severity of neonatal respiratory distress or to the nature of the therapy in the newborn period is not certain. No studies of lung function and health in aging affected adults have been reported.

### GENETIC ETIOLOGY

Investigators agree only that the etiology of CDH is complex. Generally, its etiology is said to be 'multifactorial,' probably involving both genetic and environmental determinants, but this term is really a shield to hide our ignorance of these determinants. In fact, Hitch et al.[43] have presented evidence for an autosomal recessive genetic etiology in at least some families. CDH is found in association with chromosomal abnormalities (e.g., trisomies 13, 18, 21; Turner syndrome). A number of recent reports suggest that chromosome region 15q24-26 may contain a gene or genes that lead, when abnormal, to CDH.[44] Genetic testing and prenatal diagnosis are not possible.

### THERAPY

As pointed out by Chinoy,[39] current treatments address the underlying pathophysiology of CDH (e.g., gas exchange, pulmonary hypertension). Surgical correction of the diaphragmatic defect in the neonatal period is of secondary importance. The most promising therapy appears to be gentle ventilation at low ventilator pressures with permissive hypercarbia, assuring by this means that iatrogenic long-term pulmonary damage is minimized.[45] Therapies that include inhaled nitric oxide and extracorporeal membrane oxygenation are also under consideration.

## DISEASES OF THE ALVEOLAE AND AIRWAYS

## Mucopolysaccharidoses

The mucopolysaccharidoses (MPS) are a group of genetic disorders caused by deficiencies in lysosomal enzymes involved in degradation of glycosaminoglycans (mucopolysaccharides). The impairment in the catabolism of these molecules leads to the intralysosomal accumulation of partially degraded products.[46] Manifestations of the MPS are generally related to cell and tissue dysfunction as the result of the accumulation of these metabolites. Common clinical features of MPS include a progressive course, facial coarseness, skeletal dysplasias, hepatosplenomegaly, and neurological abnormalities. The severity of the phenotype depends on residual enzyme activity.

Several MPS have been described, and MPS I–IV have important pulmonary manifestations. MPS type I, characterized by the accumulation and urinary excretion of dermatan and heparan sulfates, includes three types, based on the severity. Hurler syndrome (I-H; OMIM 607014), the most severe type, is manifested by a progressive delay in growth and development. Skeletal dysplasia leads to dwarfism and skeletal deformities, such as large skull and shortened tubular bones. Psychomotor development ultimately plateaus, with subsequent loss of even limited skills. Corneal clouding is a hallmark. Hepatomegaly, cardiac disease (cardiomyopathy, coronary artery disease), a communicating hydrocephalus, and recurrent infections are usual. Death occurs in childhood, primarily from infectious, cardiac, or pulmonary complications. At the other extreme, patients with Scheie syndrome (I-S; the mildest, adult form; OMIM 607016) have normal height, intelligence, and (potentially) lifespan. They may exhibit joint deformities, nerve entrapment syndromes, and progressive aortic or mitral valve disease that is amenable to valve replacement. The phenotype of the Hurler–Scheie syndrome (I-H/S; OMIM 607015) is of intermediate severity. The features of MPS II (Hunter syndrome; OMIM 309900), also characterized by accumulation of dermatan and heparan sulfates, are similar to those of the analogous MPS I subtypes, but affected individuals lack corneal clouding. Individuals with the severe form usually die at between 10 and 15 years. MPS III (Sanfillipo syndrome), types A–D (OMIM 252900–252940), a disease of heparan sulfate accumulation and excretion, is characterized by progressive neurologic deterioration, commencing usually between ages 2 and 6, often with behavioral changes. Severe neurologic degeneration, with loss of social and adaptive skills, occurs by 6–10 years of age. Major skeletal abnormalities do not occur. MPS IV (Morquio syndrome) type A (OMIM 253000) is characterized by a severe spondyloepiphyseal dysplasia and short-trunk dwarfism. Odontoid hypoplasia, a universal finding, predisposes subjects to atlantoaxial subluxations, cervical myelopathy, and premature death. Affected individuals have normal intelligence. Type B (GM1-gangliosidosis; OMIM 253010) includes a neurologic degeneration that ranges from total psychomotor regression in infants to a slowly progressive illness primarily involving the extrapyramidal system in adults. Skeletal abnormalities also range from mild to as severe as those of the type A syndrome. Keratan and chondroitin 6-sulfate accumulate in type A, while keratan sulfate alone accumulates in type B.

### RESPIRATORY MANIFESTATIONS

Severe and life-limiting respiratory complications can occur in all of these four MPS, although the prevalence and severity will vary directly with the overall severity of the MPS. A majority of patients who die succumb to the respiratory complications. The underlying pathology is complex, involving several factors:[47,48] truncal skeletal abnormalities (scoliosis, kyphosis, barrel-shaped chest, short rib cage); nervous system abnormalities (cervical spine subluxation, infiltration of respiratory control center with glycosaminoglycans), and progressive deposition of glycosaminoglycans in the tissues (walls and surrounding tissue) of both upper and lower airways. The infiltrative respiratory disease is progressive: it involves more of the airways with age, commencing with the uppermost (nasopharyngeal) and progressing to the lowermost (small bronchiolar) aspects.[49,50] Thus, successful treatment at one stage of disease may be inadequate at a later stage of disease.

The specific manifestations of respiratory dysfunction relate to airway obstruction,[47] with occasional superimposition of abnormalities in central respiratory control. Upper airway narrowing results from enlargement of the tongue, tonsils and adenoids, and infiltration of the pharynx and nasopharynx. Profuse nasal secretions also contribute to upper airway obstruction. Pulmonary involvement includes atelectasis (either persistent or recurrent), aspiration contributing to recurrent pneumonias, and persistent hypoxemia. On pulmonary function testing, both a restrictive and an obstructive pattern may be demonstrated, with gas diffusion abnormalities represented by a reduced DLCO. Subjects are very liable to develop sleep disturbed breathing, primarily obstructive sleep apnea, but also occasionally central sleep apnea or abnormal breathing patterns such as Cheyne–Stokes respiration.[49,51,52] The net effect of persistent sleep disturbed breathing coupled with daytime hypoxemia may be the development of cor pulmonale.[53]

Sedation or anesthesia pose a special risk for these patients, since the further relaxation of respiratory musculature may trigger airway collapse, leading to respiratory arrest. Intubation is exceedingly difficult because of the narrowed nature of the upper airways.

## GENETIC ETIOLOGY

With the exception of MPS II, which is X-linked, the MPS are all inherited as autosomal recessive illnesses. Although both MPS I and MPS II have similar patterns of urinary glycosaminoglycans excretion, this common intermediate phenotype is not the result of a unique enzyme deficiency. All forms of MPS I are caused by defects in the gene for the enzyme α-L-iduronidase (IDUA) on chromosome 4p16.3. Those leading to MPS IH produce no functional enzyme, while those leading to IS (often missense mutations) may lead to small amounts of residual enzyme activity.[54] MPS I H/S is the result of a single allele of both a type IH gene and a type IS gene (compound heterozygosity). Type II MPS results from defects in the gene at Xq28 for iduronate sulfatase (IDS). A rough correlation exists between severity of phenotype and extent of gene distortion, with rearrangements and large deletions associated with a more severe phenotype and point mutations, of which there are many, associated with a milder clinical course. Three different genes

in the path of glycosaminoglycan degradation are involved in the genesis of MPS III: SGSH at chromosome 17q25.3, encoding the enzyme heparan N-sulfatase (type IIIA); NAGLU at17q.21, encoding α-N-acetylglucosamine 6-sulfatase deficiency (IIIB); a gene (not yet mapped or characterized) that codes for acetyl-CoA:α-glucosaminide acetyltransferase (IIIC); and GNS at 12q14, encoding N-acetyl glucosamine 6-sulfatase (IIID). Deficiencies in the enzymes responsible for the metabolism of keratan sulfate underlie MPS IV: IVA, the gene coding for N-acetyl-galactosamine-6-sulfatase (GALNS) at 16q24.3; and GLB1 at 3p21.33, the gene for β-galactosidase. Other sources can be consulted for a more detailed discussion of the gene defects.[54] Enzyme assays remain the usual basis for establishing a diagnosis of an MPS, and a number of sources for these assays are available (www.genetests.org).

## GENETIC TESTING

Gene testing is complicated by the large number of mutations and the high prevalence of compound heterozygosity in affected individuals. Clinical gene testing is available only on a limited basis (www.genetests.org).

## THERAPY

Several approaches to the therapy of MPS I-H have as their common denominator the provision of replacement enzyme (α-L-iduronidase) in a form that can enter cells. The mature enzyme contains a mannose-6 phosphate residue which, by binding to its receptor in the clathrin-coated pit on the cell surface, facilitates its endocytosis and ultimate incorporation into lysosomes.[55] Bone marrow transplantation has had variable degrees of success in ameliorating the course of disease, and a recent paper has reported promising results with cord blood transplants (a source of hematopoietic stem cells) from unrelated donors.[56] Enzyme released from these stem cells is taken up by the affected cells of the recipient, with the resultant correction of the glycosaminoglycan storage defect. Indeed, hematopoietic stem-cell transplantation is considered the treatment of choice for affected individuals of age <2 years without central nervous system disease.[55] A commercial preparation of recombinant α-L-iduronidase has also been licenced for replacement therapy. Because this therapy is safer than transplantation, it is recommended particularly for patients with either milder forms or neurologic impairment (an irreversible complication of the disease). None of these treatments is curative and none of them has been studied in relation to the pulmonary manifestations of the MPS syndromes. In view of the progressive, obstructive nature of much of the pulmonary disease, clinicians must at least be prepared to offer one or several alternative therapies. These include tonsillectomy and/or adenoidectomy, cervical vertebral fusion, tracheostomy and/or bronchial stenting, CPAP for sleep apnea, chronic oxygen therapy, and medications, such as antibiotics.

# Autosomal recessive polycystic kidney disease

The manifestations of autosomal recessive kidney disease (ARPKD; OMIM 263200) usually begin in childhood. ARPKD is characterized by multiple cysts of the kidney and fibrosis of the liver, often in inverse proportions. A major manifestation of the neonatal disease is pulmonary hypoplasia, which is often life limiting.[57]

Guay-Woodford et al.[57] who have analyzed the clinical outcome of 254 patients with ARPKD, and others have commented on the high degree of variability of clinical manifestations of the disease.[58,59] Generally, patients ascertained as newborns or infants have severe renal dysfunction. Oligohydramnios is common, as is the typical (and probably etiologically related) 'Potter's facies,' thus creating early suspicion of this or a similar renal disease. Older patients may also have renal dysfunction, but their renal function is at least sufficient to sustain them through early development and even into adulthood. Ultimately, secondary effects of progressive renal failure, including azotemia, systemic hypertension, and secondary hyperparathyroidism, will likely intervene. Individuals may have significant hepatic cystic disease, with ascending cholangitis, progressive hepatic fibrosis, hepatocellular insufficiency, and portal hypertension. Thus, many individuals with ARPKD ultimately succumb because of respiratory, renal, or hepatic failure.

## RESPIRATORY MANIFESTATIONS

In severe cases of ARPKD, patients present neonatally with hypoxemia and respiratory failure. This is ascribed in large part to pulmonary hypoplasia, the definition of which differs somewhat among observers. In the pulmonary hypoplasia of ARPKD, the lungs are clearly reduced in weight and volume, and the size and usually the number of alveoli are also reduced. Whether the distal bronchioles are also maldeveloped or delayed is controversial,[60,61] but the final lung architecture does consist primarily of primitive tubular structures similar to those found in early gestation. The pulmonary hypoplasia is related to and may be the result of oligohydramnios, reflecting fetal oliguria, although the mechanism by which this occurs is unclear.[62] Hislop et al.[61] have also pointed out that the pulmonary developmental abnormalities may begin sufficiently early in gestation that amniotic fluid volume is irrelevant, but others would dispute such an early origin of the maldevelopment.[63] The massively enlarged kidneys that are often found in affected neonates may also inhibit normal lung development, in the same manner as does the ectopic abdominal viscera in individuals with congenital diaphragmatic hernia.[60] Additionally, affected individuals readily develop pneumothoraces or pneumomediastinum and, if they survive, atelectasis, pneumonia, and biventricular congestive heart failure.[64] As therapies of the respiratory insufficiency of the perinatal period have improved, the prevalence of

chronic lung disease in the survivors has increased.[57] The final word regarding chronic lung disease in ARPKD has not yet been written.

## DIAGNOSIS

Echogenic kidneys with or without large renal cysts are seen in the vast majority of patients, particularly symptomatic infants. Palpable flank masses, representing very enlarged kidneys, may be appreciated. The liver is normal by clinical, laboratory, and imaging assessment in more than half of infants, but liver dysfunction and portal hypertension are appreciated clinically with age. Both renal and liver biopsy are diagnostic, but are often unnecessary. The following diagnostic criteria for ARPKD of infancy, developed by Zerres et al.[58] are generally accepted: enlarged, echogenic kidneys with poor corticomedullary differentiation; and one or more of the following:

- absence of renal cysts in both parents on ultrasound;
- clinical/laboratory signs of hepatic fibrosis;
- characteristic hepatic pathology;
- pathoanatomical proof of ARPKD in an affected sibling;
- parental consanguinity suggesting autosomal recessive inheritance.

## GENETIC ETIOLOGY

The gene that is responsible for ARPKD (PKHD1), has been recently cloned by two independent groups.[65,66] PKHD1 is located on chromosome 6p21.1-p12. Its longest open reading frame contains 67 exons, yielding a 4072 amino acid protein.[67] This large protein with receptor-like properties is localized to kidney, bile ducts, and pancreas, and is expressed in primary cilia of renal tubular epithelium.[65] Multiple different disease-causing mutations have been identified. Some relationship exists between the clinical severity and type of mutation: severe disease is associated with truncating mutations, while less severe phenotypes are found in association with mutations giving rise to single amino acid substitutions.[66]

## GENETIC TESTING

Clinical genetic testing is available for confirmation of diagnosis, carrier detection, and prenatal diagnosis. Performed by mutation scanning or linkage analysis, the test is available from a limited number of laboratories (www.Genetests.org).

## THERAPY

Appropriate and intensive treatment of respiratory failure in the infant is the key to survival. Ensuring total expansion of the lungs by means of chest tubes to relieve a pneumothorax and mechanical ventilation to oppose massively enlarged abdominal viscera is essential. The requirement for mechanical ventilation in the neonatal period is a major predictor of mortality.[67] Nonetheless, such individuals are now often surviving, a phenomenon that was unknown several decades ago. Survival of these infants is directly attributable to the efforts of critical care specialists. What therapies will be required to cope with chronic lung disease in these survivors is uncertain at this time. The role of treatments for renal failure and its secondary phenomena (e.g., hypertension), hepatic dysfunction, and growth retardation have become significantly more important as these children survive and age.

# PULMONARY DISEASES RESULTING FROM DEFECTS IN NEUROMUSCULAR CONTROL OF RESPIRATION

The disorders discussed below have diverse genetic etiologies and manifestations, but result in pulmonary failure by affecting either respiratory musculature or central control of breathing. They include amyotrophic lateral sclerosis, muscular dystrophies, Prader–Willi syndrome, Ondine's curse, the spinocerebellar ataxias, and Rett syndrome.

## Amyotrophic lateral sclerosis

Amyotrophic lateral sclerosis (ALS; OMIM 105 400) is a progressive paralytic neurodegenerative disorder affecting the motor nervous system. The typical presenting symptoms are weakness, fatigue, muscle cramping, and fasciculations. When upper motor neurons are affected, clumsiness, stiffness, and fatigue are more pronounced. Lower motor neuron degeneration is associated with weakness or atrophy and fasciculations. Hoarseness and aspiration become apparent with bulbar involvement. The disease progresses inexorably to virtually total motor paralysis, requiring support for most bodily functions, including respiration. Although significant variation in disease duration and progression has been reported, the average life expectancy after diagnosis is about 3 years.[68]

### RESPIRATORY MANIFESTATIONS

The most serious complication of ALS is respiratory failure, which accounts for the majority of deaths.[69] Respiratory symptoms (dyspnea, air hunger) usually occur late in the course of disease, but can be a presenting symptom. Respiratory failure is thought to result from inspiratory compromise from the loss of respiratory muscle (including diaphragmatic) function, as motor units (nerve and muscle) atrophy. Affected individuals demonstrate both chronically restricted ventilation, with reduced total lung capacity and vital capacity and elevated residual volume (and a normal ratio of $FEV_1/FVC$), and easy fatigability of respiratory muscles upon exertion.[70] In addition, individuals may

develop sleep apnea, involving at least an obstructive component from upper airway muscle weakness. All pulmonary function abnormalities worsen as the disease progresses.

### GENETIC ETIOLOGY

About 10 percent of cases are familial,[71,72] usually as a result of mutations in the gene for superoxide dismutase 1 (SOD1, on chromosome 21q22.1). Five percent of sporadic ALS cases also have SOD1 mutations, presumably newly arisen. All SOD1 mutations behave as autosomal dominants, except for the mutation leading to a substitution of alanine for aspartate at position 90 (D90A), which may be either recessive[73] or dominant.[74] The most common SOD1 mutation substitutes a valine for alanine at position 4 (A4V).[68] Distinct syndromes, differing in age of onset (usually after age 40), length of survival (1–20 years after diagnosis), and clinical and histopathologic manifestations have been associated with different SOD1 mutations.[75,76] Rare mutations of other genes (e.g., the gene for *alsin* [ALS2] on chromosome 2q33) appear to be causal in some of the remaining familial cases.[77]

### PATHOGENESIS

Degeneration and loss of motor neurons with astrocytic gliosis are histopathologic features of ALS.[78,79] The exact molecular pathways leading to this selective motor neuron death have not been elucidated. Proposed mechanisms include a toxic effect of mutant SOD1, resulting in abnormal protein aggregation; abnormal tyrosine nitration and peroxidation; disorganization of intermediate filaments; and glutamate-mediated excitotoxicity resulting in mitochondrial damage, increased intracellular calcium concentration and apoptosis.[80–82]

### DIAGNOSIS

There is no specific test that is diagnostic of ALS, which makes it sometimes difficult to rule out other motor neuron diseases. In 1994, the El Escorial criteria were developed to standardize the diagnosis. These criteria, based on clinical, electrophysiological, or neuropathological data, include lower motor neuron degeneration, upper motor neuron degeneration, the progressive spread of dysfunction within a region or to other regions of the body, and the absence of evidence of other disease processes.[83]

### GENETIC TESTING

For the patients who have positive family history, molecular genetic testing of a blood sample for SOD1 gene abnormalities can be performed in several US and international laboratories (www.genetests.org or www.gendia.net). This information may be of value for personal and family planning, but is currently not relevant to treatment. Prenatal diagnosis via amniocentesis or chorionic villus sampling is also available.

## THERAPY

Maximizing the quality of life is important in the approach to dealing with this invariably fatal syndrome. If sleep apnea develops early on in the disease, the use of CPAP therapy may be remarkably beneficial. As affected individuals near total paralysis, only mechanical ventilation offers the possibility of prolonging life.

# Dystrophinopathies

Of the various muscular dystrophies, only the Duchenne/Becker form (OMIM 301200/300376) is regularly associated with respiratory complications. These two allelic syndromes constitute the largest portion of the dystrophinopathies, which result from mutations in the dystrophin gene on the X chromosome. Their cardinal manifestations are skeletal myopathy and dilated cardiomyopathy. Duchenne muscular dystrophy usually presents in early childhood with motor delay, waddling gait, and difficulty climbing. Proximal muscle weakness and pseudohypertrophy of the calves are apparent by the age 6 years. The steady decline of limb and torso muscle strength continues from ages 6 to 11 years. Affected children are usually wheelchair bound by age 12 and develop dilated cardiomyopathy by age 18 years. During the second decade of life, patients develop scoliosis from weakened paraspinal muscles, and hypoventilation from weakened respiratory muscles. Few patients survive beyond the third decade of life. Death is from respiratory or cardiac failure. Becker muscular dystrophy usually takes a milder although similar course. Its age at onset ranges from 1–20 years, with 90 percent of individuals manifesting the disease by age 20. Patients become wheelchair bound by age 40. The age at death, although variable, averages 42 years.[84]

## RESPIRATORY MANIFESTATIONS

Fifty-five to 90 percent of Duchenne patients die of respiratory failure,[85] in the majority of cases due to respiratory muscle weakness. The onset is often abrupt, precipitated by an acute respiratory infection. This may be followed rapidly by signs of respiratory failure (weakness and fatigue, tachypnea, and somnolence). A study of 25 boys with Duchenne dystrophy[86] showed that lung function is closely correlated with upper limb function. The respiratory compromise is restrictive, as assessed by pulmonary function testing. Similar findings would be expected in nonsmoking adults with Becker muscular dystrophy.

## GENETIC ETIOLOGY AND PATHOGENESIS

The dystrophin gene (DMD), located at Xp21.2, spans 2.4 Mb and has 79 exons. At least four promoters have been found. DMD encodes a membrane-associated protein that functions as a part of a protein complex linking cytoplasmic actin filaments (via its N-terminus) to complexes with proteins and glycoproteins (via its C-terminus). The intricacies of these associations suggest that dystrophin has multiple essential roles in cellular physiology, perhaps varying according to cell type.[87] Mutations in DMD are causal of both Duchenne and Becker muscular dystrophy. Multiple disease causing alleles have been identified to date; they include variable-size deletions (approximately 60 percent of mutations) and duplications (approximately 5 percent), insertions and single base changes (the remainder). There are two mutational hot spots: at the 5' end, exons 2–20 (30 percent); and at a more distal site, exons 44–53 (70 percent).[88] The deletions or duplications associated with Duchenne dystrophy generally cause a frameshift and no detectable gene product (dystrophin). Those associated with Becker dystrophy are nonframeshift mutations, leading to a reduced amount of (presumably partly functional) gene product. For example, a frameshift mutation can produce a truncated protein missing the carboxy terminus, which is unable to bind dystrophin-associated membrane proteins, resulting in the Duchenne phenotype. On the other hand, a nonframeshift mutation with a preserved carboxy terminus results in the milder Becker form.

## DIAGNOSIS

The clinical diagnosis of Duchenne muscular dystrophy is based on a positive family history suggestive of X-linked recessive inheritance, progressive symmetrical muscular weakness, calf hypertrophy, onset of symptoms before the age of 5 years, cardiomyopathy, and wheelchair dependency before 13 years. Similar but usually milder signs and symptoms (e.g., a later onset) accompany Becker dystrophy. All patients have markedly increased serum concentrations of creatine phosphokinase, and these tend to increase with time.[89,90] Electromyography is not specific for these dystrophies, but it does distinguish a myopathic from a neurogenic disorder.

## GENETIC TESTING

Gene testing is now used routinely for confirmation of the diagnosis, as well as for carrier and prenatal testing (www.genetests.org). Different methods are employed. Analysis of large deletions (approximately 60 percent of patients) is performed by multiplex polymerase chain reaction (PCR),[91] Southern blotting,[92] and chromosomal fluorescence in situ hybridization (FISH). Duplications (approximately 5 percent of patients) are detected by Southern blotting and quantitative PCR analysis. For detecting small insertions, deletions, point and splicing mutations (30 percent of cases), sequence analysis is also available.[93–95]

## THERAPY

Pulmonary function is the limiting factor in the quality and length of life in individuals with the muscular dystrophies.

The keystones of the respiratory management of patients with the spinal muscular atrophies have been summarized recently,[96] and most recommendations apply to the muscular dystrophies as well. These include management of acute and/or recurrent infections, and the prevention of pulmonary morbidity and chronic respiratory failure. Assisted ventilation prolongs life significantly in patients with DMD.[97,98] Medical treatment of the cardiomyopathy will also minimize secondary respiratory dysfunction, and is thus of great importance.

## Prader–Willi syndrome

The Prader–Willi syndrome (PWS; OMIM 176270) is a genetic disorder characterized by severe hypotonia, hyperphagia and obesity, short stature, small hands and feet, mental retardation, and hypogonadotrophic hypogonadism.[99] The fetal and early postnatal hypotonia results in decreased fetal movement, abnormal fetal position, poor suck in the newborn period, poor reflexes, and weak cry. At least 90 percent of patients have delayed motor and language development, and mild mental retardation (mean IQ, 60–70). Short stature and growth hormone deficiency (from hypothalamic dysfunction) are common and probably linked features.[100] Hyperphagia and obesity begin at ages 1–6 years, and are thought to be due to another hypothalamic abnormality resulting in a lack of satiety. In early childhood 70–90 percent of patients develop temper tantrums, obsessive-compulsive behavior, and difficulty with change in routine.

### RESPIRATORY MANIFESTATIONS

Pulmonary function has been studied intensively in 35 children and adults (mostly obese; 1/3 with kyphosis or scoliosis) with PWS. The mean $FEV_1$ and FVC were about 72 and 65 percent predicted, respectively.[101] Mean residual volume (RV) was elevated (189 percent predicted for males and 154 percent predicted for females), with a low normal total lung capacity (TLC) and an increased RV/TLC (approximately 0.40). Maximum expiratory and especially inspiratory pressures were reduced and were related directly to $FEV_1$ and FVC and indirectly to RV. These data have been interpreted to suggest that individuals with PWS have restrictive lung impairment, resulting from respiratory muscle weakness.[101] Excessive daytime sleepiness and abnormal daytime breathing are common features of PWS.[102] In general, these manifestations are poorly correlated with weight. Quantitative characteristics of sleep apnea (an increased apnea-hypopnea index; nocturnal oxygen desaturation) that were at least partially ameliorated by weight loss have been noted in several studies but not in others.[103] Children and adult patients (both obese and nonobese) appear also to have disturbed central respiratory control, as evidenced by a blunted ventilatory response to isocapnic hypoxia and/or hyperoxic hypercapnea.[104,105]

In babies and young children with Prader–Willi syndrome, acute respiratory illness that may be life-threatening is a common cause of both morbidity and mortality. Schrander-Stumpel et al.[106] recently reported that the major causes of death in affected individuals below the age of 5 years involve the respiratory system, and are infectious in etiology. They point out the unexpected, fulminant nature of even upper respiratory infections in affected individuals, and urge heightened concern and close monitoring of infected individuals. The superimposition of infection on possible hypothalamic dysregulation (with hypoventilation) may explain the excessively morbid response. Aspiration is also common in these children.

### GENETIC ETIOLOGY AND PATHOGENESIS

PWS is caused by deletions or gene disruption on the proximal long arm of the paternal chromosome 15 (15q11.2-13), or maternal uniparental disomy of chromosome 15. This area of chromosome 15 is influenced by imprinting, causing maternal genes to be inactive. Both the deletions and the maternal uniparental disomy result in the absence of the normally operative paternal genes. Two different deletions have been described. The more common is a 3–4 Mb deletion in a region containing several imprinted genes, some of which (e.g., NDN) have been implicated in the causation of PWS. The second is a microdeletion of the putative imprinting control center upstream from and including the first exon of the SNURF-SNRPN bicistronic gene, resulting in a maternal-specific methylation pattern and downstream gene inactivity. Currently, no consensus exists as to which of the several genes in this area of chromosome 15 play essential roles in the genesis of the phenotype of PWS.[107]

### DIAGNOSIS

Clinical diagnostic criteria for PWS were developed in 1993, and were summarized recently.[108] They include major (one point) and minor (one-half point) criteria. For children under 3 years of age, five points are required for diagnosis, four of which must be major criteria. For older patients, eight points are required for diagnosis, at least five of which must be major criteria.[108]

### GENETIC TESTING

Ninety-nine percent of PWS patients have a methylation abnormality, which is detected using methylation analysis: Southern blot analysis is carried out with a methylation-sensitive probe (of genes SNRPN or PW71B). Alternatively, PCR with parent-specific methylation-sensitive PCR primers can be exploited. If the methylation pattern is characteristic of maternal inheritance only, the diagnosis of PWS is confirmed. Deletions involving bands 15q11.2-12, present in 70 percent of PWS patients, can be detected by high-resolution chromosome studies at the 650 band level and fluorescence in situ hybridization. Uniparental disomy, responsible for 25 percent of PWS cases, is recognized by analysis of microsatellite markers.[109] An imprinting defect, observed in less than 5 percent of PWS patients, can be identified by mutation analysis. Details may be found in www.genests.org and www.gendia.net.

## THERAPY

The overall, long-term treatment of PWS, which is summarized by Goldstone,[108] is exceedingly complex because of the multisystem nature of the syndrome. With regard to the pulmonary manifestations, extreme vigilance in the care of children with PWS, so that acute respiratory infections can be discovered and treated and aspiration prevented early, is critical.[106] Hypoventilation/respiratory insufficiency must also be recognized early and treated (e.g., with intermittent positive pressure ventilation). Treating the sleep apnea, usually with CPAP, may improve behavior. Obesity should be prevented if possible.

# Congenital central hypoventilation syndrome

Congenital central hypoventilation syndrome (CCHS; Ondine's curse; OMIM 209880) is included because of its uniqueness among respiratory diseases. Although exceedingly rare, one may speculate that research on the pathophysiology and genetics of this disease will shed significant light on mechanisms underlying the central controls of both normal respiratory physiology and more common respiratory diseases.

## GENERAL AND RESPIRATORY MANIFESTATIONS

CCHS most likely has its onset in the newborn period and is a lifelong disease, although long-term studies to substantiate this are nonexistent. During sleep, affected individuals exhibit alveolar hypoventilation, diminished tidal volume, and progressive hypercapnea and hypoxemia, and have no arousal response to these stimuli. When awake these individuals will usually (but not always) have adequate ventilation. This may not be the case during exercise, when they may again develop hypercarbia and hypoxemia without any perception of dyspnea. The primary problem underlying these abnormal responses is a central insensitivity to both hypercarbia and especially hypoxia,[110] overcome in part during the waking state by conscious respiratory control. Without a prompt, early diagnosis and appropriate ventilatory support, the prognosis for many affected individuals is poor.

CCHS may represent a generalized autonomic dysfunction syndrome, since it includes such extrarespiratory manifestations as decreased heart rate beat-to-beat variability, diminished heart rate response to exercise, severe constipation, mild hypothermia ($<37°C$), episodic and profuse hyperhidrosis, esophageal dysmotility, and pupillary abnormalities.[111,112] Its major association (up to 50 percent) with Hirschsprung disease (Haddad syndrome), a congenital malformation characterized by the absence of

parasympathetic intrinsic ganglion cells of the hindgut, is further evidence of this association.[113] Some central autonomic functions appear to be preserved, however, suggesting that the mechanisms underlying the defects in CCHS are complex.[110]

## GENETIC ETIOLOGY

A segregation analysis of CCHS in families, and a case–control family study of the autonomic dysfunction syndrome that included CCHS in some individuals, established the familial nature of this syndrome.[112,114] The familial aggregation appeared to involve a gene of large effect that acts in a codominant manner.[111] Recently, Amiel et al.[115,116] described alterations in the homeobox gene PHOX2B on chromosome 4p12. In a series of 29 individuals with CCHS, these researchers observed heterozygous PHOX2B variations in 18 individuals. In 16 of these cases, the nucleotide variation was a triplet expansion of the normal sequence for polyalanine, from the usual of 20 to 25–29 (nucleotides (nt) 721–780). This expansion was not present in the PHOX2B gene of the 125 control subjects or the parents, supporting the causal relation of this expansion to CCHS. The gene in the other two cases contained a de novo cytosine insertion in a stretch of four cytosines and a deletion of 37 nucleotides (618–619insC and 722–759del37nt), predicting a mutant protein with no known function.[115] Weese-Mayer et al.[117] documented the same polyalanine expansion mutation in 65 of 67 subjects with CCHS, and a nonsense mutation leading to a truncated protein in one other. The expansion mutation was not present in their 67 control subjects. Matera et al.[118] found the same polyalanine expansion mutation in 22 of 27 affected subjects, and frameshift mutations in three additional subjects. Sasaki et al.[119] found expansion and frameshift mutations in four subjects and one subject, respectively. Both Weese-Mayer et al.[117] and Matera et al.[118] demonstrated parent to child transmission of the expansion mutation, but also found the mutation in a few phenotypically normal parents. Nonetheless, the weight of evidence strongly supports a causal relation between dominantly inherited PHOX2B mutations and CCHS in most affected individuals.[120] Isolated cases of CCHS have been associated with mutations in several other genes, such as those for endothelin 3 (EDN3), the RET proto-oncogene (RET), the glial cell line-derived neurotrophic factor (GDNF), the human aschaete-scute-homolog-1 (HASH1), and the brain-derived neurotrophic factor (BDNF).[119,121,122] In some of these instances, however, the PHOX2B mutation was also present.[120] Moreover, the mutated gene was also found in an unaffected parent in a number of these pedigrees,[116] casting uncertainty on the relevance of the genotype to the disease phenotype. Nonetheless, all of these proteins, as well as PHOX2, appear to be involved in neural crest stem cell development. Acting through the endothelin and RET signaling pathways, they may regulate brainstem neuronal progenitor proliferation and migration, and neuronal survival.[116,120]

## DIAGNOSIS

Currently, the diagnosis is made in large part by ruling out other conditions (primary neuromuscular, lung or cardiac disease, inborn metabolic disease, or a brainstem lesion). If Hirschsprung disease is also under consideration, a rectal biopsy should be obtained. An evaluation in a respiratory physiology laboratory is critical, to evaluate spontaneous breathing during sleep and wakefulness, and the ventilatory response to hypercarbia or hypoxia. Detailed recommendations were presented in 1999 in an official statement of the American Thoracic Society.[123] Genetic diagnosis is not available at this time.

## THERAPY

Mechanical ventilation is the basis of both short- and long-term therapy of infants, children, and adults with CCHS. The problems and issues in dealing with the needs of these patients, which range from the inexperience of many pulmonologists with this syndrome to ventilation needs that may be either constant or intermittent, are formidable. The recent statement from the American Thoracic Society[123] is the best summary of current treatment recommendations. The statement recommends the performance of a tracheostomy in all patients after the diagnosis is confirmed. Others have suggested that some newborns with CCHS can be switched directly to nasal mask bilateral positive airway pressure (BiPAP) from mechanical ventilation via endotracheal tube after the first few weeks of life.[124] Thus, tracheostomy may be avoided. The fact that 'published data show prolonged survival of children with CCHS as well as overall good quality of life'[123] is encouraging.

## Rett syndrome

This is a recently described X-linked syndrome (OMIM 312750) in which respiratory manifestations are only a part of a protean loss-of-function disorder. Because its genetic basis is known, Rett syndrome also offers the promise of explaining aspects of respiration that transcend those affected with this rare syndrome.

Virtually all affected individuals are female. Individuals develop normally until approximately 6 months of age. Thereafter, development proceeds at a markedly reduced rate, in four stages: I (6–18 months): decelerated head growth, reduced communication and eye contact, and hypotonia; II (approximately 1–3 years): loss of function, with severe dementia, loss of hand skills and frequent hand wringing, autistic features, loss of expressive language and possible onset of seizures; III (approximately 3–12 years): stabilization of manifestations, with even some amelioration of autistic manifestations but now with respiratory features; and IV (beginning in teen age): ultimately, further deterioration, with progressive scoliosis, upper and lower motor neuron signs, trophic disturbance of the feet but improved eye contact and reduced seizure frequency.[125] The details

of this staging, adopted by an international Rett syndrome diagnostic criteria work group, are presented by Jellinger.[126] In the UK, the prevalence of this disorder in females is 1:10 000–1:15 000;[125,127] it is said to be second only to Down syndrome as a cause of mental retardation in females.[126]

## RESPIRATORY MANIFESTATIONS

Overall, individuals with Rett syndrome have altered patterns of respiration that include periodic apnea during wakefulness, intermittent hyperventilation, breath-holding spells, and forced expulsions of air.[126] In a detailed study of these respiratory abnormalities in 56 females, Julu et al.[127] described a number of relatively consistent abnormalities in breathing patterns while awake, including apneustic breathing (e.g., a single fast full inspiration followed by a delayed fast expiration; breath holding; a prolonged and continuous inspiration followed abruptly by a fast, forceful full expiration), forceful breathing (e.g., exaggerated inspirations followed immediately by exaggerated expirations; tachypnea with exaggerated inspirations; exaggerated inspirations and expirations followed by a central apnea), inadequate breathing (shallow inspiration and expiration, either rapid or not; or shallow breathing followed by central apnea), valsalva breathing style (breath holds or protracted inspiration, with concomitant secondary effects on heart rate and blood pressure of reduced venous return), Cheyne–Stokes respiration, and Biot breathing (abrupt apnea followed by abrupt regular breathing, each of variable duration). Certain abnormal breathing patterns varied with age: apneustic breathing was most common in the youngest subjects (ages 2–9 years), forced breathing in children below age 18 years, and inadequate/valsalva breathing in older subjects (age >10 years). Concomitant changes in $pO_2$ and $pCO_2$ were noted with these abnormal patterns. Breathing patterns were invariably normal during sleep. Affected subjects had reduced brainstem autonomic function (cardiac vagal tone or sensitivity to baroreflex). The authors concluded that their evidence plus that of others 'points to a prenatal brain defect with early brain stem involvement . . . [with subsequent] brain stem immaturity and a lack of integrative inhibition, with consequent failure to respond normally to physiological demands . . . Rett disorder is a congenital dysantonomia.' Detailed neurophysiologic studies in patients with Rett syndrome (e.g., polysomnography) provide additional support for a pervasive developmental derangement in brainstem and midbrain monoaminergic (serotonin and catecholamine) systems.[128]

## GENETIC ETIOLOGY

The primary genetic defect, detected in 87 percent of British patients[127] is in the gene for the methyl-CpG-binding protein 2 (MECP), located at Xp28.[129] This protein selectively binds CpG dinucleotides in the mammalian genome and mediates transcriptional repression through interaction with other regulatory proteins. Mutations, which are predicted to lead to loss of function, presumably disrupt the normal modulation of gene activity by methylation, leading to overexpression of genes at inappropriate times during development. The mutations in MECP2, of which there are many, include missense mutations and truncations (nonsense mutations or insertions/deletions) resulting from frame shifts and premature stop codons.[125] There is no correlation between type of mutation and phenotype. A very high proportion of affected females derive the abnormal gene from a paternal chromosome, suggesting the existence of parental imprinting and explaining why affected males are infrequent.[130]

## DIAGNOSIS AND GENETIC TESTING

Clinical diagnostic criteria have been established by the Rett Syndrome Diagnostic Criteria Work Group.[131,132] Careful studies of the respiratory manifestations can also provide important supportive evidence. Many laboratories already offer testing for the mutant MeCP2 gene (www.genetests.org).

## THERAPY

Current therapy is largely supportive, but several studies of pharmacologic treatment of Rett syndrome are under consideration.

# GENETIC DISORDERS AFFECTING PULMONARY VASCULATURE

## Hereditary hemorrhagic telangiectasia

Hereditary hemorrhagic telangiectasia (HHT; OMIM 187300), also known as Rendu–Osler–Weber syndrome, is an autosomal dominant disease characterized by multiple arteriovenous malformations (AVMs) and telangiectasias of skin, mucous membrane, and viscera. Recent prevalence estimates (1:8350 in France and 1:7250 in Denmark) suggest that HHT is among the more common monogenic vascular diseases of man.

The earliest and most common general manifestation of HHT, epistaxis, occurs in the majority of affected individuals.[133] Recurrent epistaxes begin by the age of 10 years and become more severe, requiring blood transfusions and iron supplementation later in life. Oral and cutaneous telangiectasias develop later than epistaxis[134] and are usually found on the lips, tongue, palate, fingers, face, conjunctivas, trunk, arms, and nail beds. Bleeding from cutaneous telangiectasias is rarely clinically important. Cerebral arteriovenous malformations (AVMs) may cause migraine headaches, intracerebral and subarachnoid hemorrhage.[135] Gastrointestinal bleeding, from AVMs throughout the gastrointestinal tract, occurs in a significant minority of patients during the fifth or sixth decade of life, and may require multiple (chronic) blood transfusions.

## RESPIRATORY MANIFESTATIONS

Pulmonary involvement is said to be the most serious aspect of HHT.[136] Pulmonary AVMs are present in about 33 percent of patients.[137] They are often multiple and appear preferentially in the lower lobes. A minority of AVMs shunt blood from the left to the right circulation, involving the aorta via the bronchial, internal mammary or intercostal arteries.[138] The majority of shunts are right-to-left, from the pulmonary artery. If sufficiently large, they can shunt as much as 50 percent of the cardiac output. This shunting results in cyanosis, hypoxemia, and secondary polycythemia (unless counterbalanced by bleeding elsewhere), exertional dyspnea, and clubbing.[136,137,139–141] Paradoxical embolization, usually to the brain, may lead to a transient ischemic attack or stroke via a bland embolism or infection (abscess) from a mycotic embolism. The AVMs may also rupture and bleed, sometimes life-threatening amounts. Pulmonary hypertension has been described in a minority of patients, as discussed in Chapter 14.

## GENETIC ETIOLOGY

HHT is a heterogeneous disease with two underlying genes identified to date: the ENG gene, encoding the protein endoglin and leading to the more common HHT 1, and the activin receptor-like kinase 1 gene ACVRL1 (or ALK1) that is involved in HHT2. ENG, located on 9q34.1, has 14 exons and spans approximately 40 kb of genomic DNA. ALK1 is located on 12q11-14, contains 10 exons and spans approximately 14 kb of genomic DNA. ALK1 and ENG are both expressed predominantly in vascular endothelium and are part of the transforming growth factor beta (TGF-β) signaling pathway. TGF-β signaling affects both vascular differentiation and proliferation, and overexpression of the TGF-β1 ligand (as the result of nonfunctional mutations of either ENG or ALK1) promotes unregulated intimal/vascular growth and apoptosis.[142] The TGF-β signaling pathway appears to play an important role in the pathogenesis of primary pulmonary hypertension:[143] the BMPR2 gene, abnormalities of which cause a form of primary pulmonary hypertension that is indistinguishable from that associated with HHT, is also a member of this family of signaling pathway genes. The majority of disease-causing mutations of either ENG or ALK1 result in truncated proteins that may be expressed transiently if at all, leading to haploinsufficiency.[144] Generally, no correlations have been identified between clinical HHT phenotypes and the types of ALK1/ENG mutations. Individuals with ALK1 mutations may be less prone to pulmonary AVMs, but have also developed pulmonary hypertension.[143]

## DIAGNOSIS

The clinical diagnosis of HHT is based on the family history and findings of AVMs.[145] The HHT Foundation International recently published the diagnostic criteria for HHT, with a focus on epistaxes, mucocutaneous telangiectasias, visceral AVMs, and family history.[146] The diagnosis of HHT is considered to be definite if at least three criteria are present. All patients with HHT should be screened for pulmonary AVMs. On the basis of their retrospective study of 105 subjects, Cottin et al.[147] have proposed a screening algorithm involving, initially, a contrast echocardiogram plus an anteroposterior chest X-ray, followed if either is positive by computerized tomography (noncontrast at first, followed by a contrast study if an opacity is seen).[147] In an accompanying editorial, Morrell[148] has suggested sequential studies, beginning with chest radiography. If this suggests the presence of an AVM, it should be followed directly by CT; if it is negative, it should be followed by contrast echocardiography and then, if this is positive, by CT.[148]

## GENETIC TESTING

Clinical genetic testing is available for the purpose of diagnostic confirmation, prenatal and predictive testing. It is performed by direct sequencing of ENG and ALK1 for detection of missense and nonsense mutations, small insertions, deletions, and splice mutations. Quantitative PCR analysis is used to identify larger deletions.[149] A number of diagnostic facilities offer this testing (see www.genetests.org and www.gendia.net).

## THERAPY

The general therapy of HHT involves both preventing circumstances that might encourage hemorrhage (e.g., avoiding anticoagulants), and replacing iron and blood as necessary. Pulmonary AVMs that are of sufficient size to promote hypoxia and impair exercise capacity, or are involved in paradoxical embolization, are approached when possible by transcatheter coil embolization. Individuals with pulmonary AVMs should receive prophylactic antibiotics before surgical or dental procedures.

## COMMENT

The diseases discussed in this chapter are for the most part systemic diseases that also include pulmonary manifestations. These may or may not be of major clinical significance and/or potentially contributory to the morbidity and mortality of the disease. For most of the diseases presented in detail in this chapter, much of the basic biochemistry and molecular genetics is understood. Gaps do remain in linking these to clinical phenomena, and particularly in relating our knowledge to an effective treatment. Currently, treatment remains one that either addresses phenotypic manifestations (e.g., use of ventilators) or provides a replacement for the protein that is the absent or inactive gene product (e.g., enzyme replacement therapy of Gaucher or Fabry disease). The former type of therapy is problematic in many of the

diseases described herein (e.g., the ultimate efficacy of phenotypic therapies in patients with Duchenne dystrophy) and replacement therapies can be considered in only a limited selection of diseases (e.g., those in which the administration of gene product leads to its appropriate function in the right intra- or extracellular compartment and at the right time, or some approximation thereof). At the time of writing, gene therapy remains a 'glimmer in the eye' of the research beholder, and is unlikely to be of any major therapeutic significance in the present decade. We can take some satisfaction in the efficacy that current therapies have had in prolonging life and maximizing quality of life in many of the diseases discussed herein. Nonetheless, our current successes are both finite and inadequate.

> ## Key learning points
>
> - Many inherited diseases involve the lungs and respiratory mechanics in a deleterious manner. Both the end organs and the central neural respiratory processes may be affected, resulting in a multifactorial etiology of pulmonary dysfunction.
>
> - Certain diseases, such as dwarfing syndromes, osteogenesis imperfecta, and congenital diaphragmatic hernia affect respiratory mechanics primarily because of attendant chest deformity, which may also predispose to pulmonary hypoplasia.
>
> - Diseases of the alveolae and airways occur in infiltrative storage diseases (e.g., mucopolysaccharidoses) or by predisposing to pulmonary hypoplasia (e.g., autosomal recessive polycystic kidney disease).
>
> - Neuromuscular diseases may include life-limiting central respiratory dysregulation (in congenital central hypoventilation syndrome, Prader–Willi syndrome) with or without failure of respiratory musculature (amyotrophic lateral sclerosis, dystrophinopathies, Rett syndrome).
>
> - Diseases of the pulmonary vasculature (e.g., hereditary hemorrhagic telangiectasia) may result in shunting of blood with resultant a–v mismatch and paradoxical embolization.
>
> - The genetic basis of many of these syndromes is known and gene testing is available. Currently, specific treatments that will minimize pulmonary pathology are not available for most syndromes. Nonetheless, prompt attention to acute respiratory problems (e.g., acute infections in patients with Prader–Willi syndrome) or to the potential for respiratory failure (e.g., in Duchenne muscular dystrophy) may ensure a longer life with an improved quality.

# REFERENCES

1   Roughley PJ, Rauch F, Glorieux FH. Osteogenesis imperfecta – clinical and molecular diversity. *Eur Cell Mater* 2003; **5**: 41–7.

2   Sillence DO, Senn A, Danks DM. Genetic heterogeneity in osteogenesis imperfecta. *J Med Genet* 1979; **16**: 101–16.

3   Byers P. *Guidelines for laboratory testing for osteogenesis imperfecta*. University of Washington Department of Pathology website, 2003, www.pathology.washington.edu/clinical/collagen/guidelines/osteogenesis.php2003.

4   McAllion SJ, Paterson CR. Causes of death in osteogenesis imperfecta. *J Clin Pathol* 1996; **49**: 627–30.

5   Falvo KA, Klain DB, Krauss AN et al. Pulmonary function studies in osteogenesis imperfecta. *Am Rev Respir Dis* 1973; **108**: 1258–60.

6   Widmann RF, Bitan FD, Laplaza FJ et al. Spinal deformity, pulmonary compromise, and quality of life in osteogenesis imperfecta. *Spine* 1999; **24**: 1673–8.

7   Thibeault DW, Pettett G, Mabry SM, Rezaiekhaligh MM. Osteogenesis imperfecta type IIA and pulmonary hypoplasia with normal alveolar development. *Pediatr Pulmonol* 1995; **20**: 301–6.

8   Shapiro JR, Burn VE, Chipman SD et al. Pulmonary hypoplasia and osteogenesis imperfecta type II with defective synthesis of alpha I(1) procollagen. *Bone* 1989; **10**: 165–71.

9   Prockop DJ, Kivirikko KI. Collagens: molecular biology, diseases, and potentials for therapy. *Annu Rev Biochem* 1995; **64**: 403–34.

10  Penttinen RP, Lichtenstein JR, Martin GR, McKusick VA. Abnormal collagen metabolism in cultured cells in osteogenesis imperfecta. *Proc Natl Acad Sci USA* 1975; **72**: 586–9.

◆11  Byers P. Osteogenesis imperfecta. In: Royce PSB (ed.) *Connective tissue and its heritable disorders: molecular, genetic and medical aspects*, 2nd edn. New York: Wiley-Liss, 2002: 385–430.

12  Wenstrup RJ, Willing MC, Starman BJ, Byers PH. Distinct biochemical phenotypes predict clinical severity in nonlethal variants of osteogenesis imperfecta. *Am J Hum Genet* 1990; **46**: 975–82.

13  Korkko J, Ala-Kokko L, De Paepe A et al. Analysis of the COL1A1 and COL1A2 genes by PCR amplification and scanning by conformation-sensitive gel electrophoresis identifies only COL1A1 mutations in 15 patients with osteogenesis imperfecta type I: identification of common sequences of null-allele mutations. *Am J Hum Genet* 1998; **62**: 98–110.

14  Bonadio J, Holbrook KA, Gelinas RE et al. Altered triple helical structure of type I procollagen in lethal perinatal osteogenesis imperfecta. *J Biol Chem* 1985; **260**: 1734–42.

15  Bateman JF, Lamande SR, Hannagan M et al. Chemical cleavage method for the detection of RNA base changes: experience in the application to collagen mutations in osteogenesis imperfecta. *Am J Med Genet* 1993; **45**: 233–40.

16  Ganguly A, Rock MJ, Prockop DJ. Conformation-sensitive gel electrophoresis for rapid detection of single-base differences in double-stranded PCR products and DNA fragments: evidence for solvent-induced bends in DNA heteroduplexes. *Proc Natl Acad Sci USA* 1993; **90**: 10 325–9.

17  Korkko J, Annunen S, Pihlajamaa T et al. Conformation sensitive gel electrophoresis for simple and accurate detection of mutations: comparison with denaturing gradient gel electrophoresis and nucleotide sequencing. *Proc Natl Acad Sci USA* 1998; **95**: 1681–5.

18  Korkko J, Milunsky J, Prockop DJ, Ala-Kokko L. Use of conformation sensitive gel electrophoresis to detect single-base changes in the gene for COL10A1. *Hum Mutat* 1998; (Suppl 1): S201–3.

19  Hunter AG, Hecht JT, Scott CI Jr. Standard weight for height curves in achondroplasia. *Am J Med Genet* 1996; **62**: 255–61.

20  Thomeer RT, van Dijk JM. Surgical treatment of lumbar stenosis in achondroplasia. *J Neurosurg* 2002; **96** (Suppl. 3): 292–7.

21  Stokes DC, Phillips JA, Leonard CO et al. Respiratory complications of achondroplasia. *J Pediatr* 1983; **102**: 534–41.

22  Pauli RM, Scott CI, Wassman ER Jr et al. Apnea and sudden unexpected death in infants with achondroplasia. *J Pediatr* 1984; **104**: 342–8.

23  Reid CS, Pyeritz RE, Kopits SE et al. Cervicomedullary compression in young patients with achondroplasia: value of comprehensive neurologic and respiratory evaluation. *J Pediatr* 1987; **110**: 522–30.

24  Nelson FW, Hecht JT, Horton WA et al. Neurological basis of respiratory complications in achondroplasia. *Ann Neurol* 1988; **24**: 89–93.

25  Waters KA, Everett F, Sillence DO et al. Treatment of obstructive sleep apnea in achondroplasia: evaluation of sleep, breathing, and somatosensory-evoked potentials. *Am J Med Genet* 1995; **59**: 460–6.

26  Waters KA, Everett F, Sillence D et al. Breathing abnormalities in sleep in achondroplasia. *Arch Dis Child* 1993; **69**: 191–6.

27  Tasker RC, Dundas I, Laverty A et al. Distinct patterns of respiratory difficulty in young children with achondroplasia: a clinical, sleep, and lung function study. *Arch Dis Child* 1998; **79**: 99–108.

28  Hecht JT, Francomano CA, Horton WA, Annegers JF. Mortality in achondroplasia. *Am J Hum Genet* 1987; **41**: 454–64.

29  Stokes DC, Pyeritz RE, Wise RA et al. Spirometry and chest wall dimensions in achondroplasia. *Chest* 1988; **93**: 364–9.

30  Stokes DC, Wohl ME, Wise RA et al. The lungs and airways in achondroplasia. Do little people have little lungs? *Chest* 1990; **98**: 145–52.

31  Shiang R, Thompson LM, Zhu YZ et al. Mutations in the transmembrane domain of FGFR3 cause the most common genetic form of dwarfism, achondroplasia. *Cell* 1994; **78**: 335–42.

32  Green PJ, Walsh FS, Doherty P. Promiscuity of fibroblast growth factor receptors. *Bioessays* 1996; **18**: 639–46.

33  Vajo Z, Francomano CA, Wilkin DJ. The molecular and genetic basis of fibroblast growth factor receptor 3 disorders: the achondroplasia family of skeletal dysplasias, Muenke craniosynostosis, and Crouzon syndrome with acanthosis nigricans. *Endocr Rev* 2000; **21**: 23–39.

34  Colvin JS, Bohne BA, Harding GW et al. Skeletal overgrowth and deafness in mice lacking fibroblast growth factor receptor 3. *Nat Genet* 1996; **12**: 390–7.

35  Deng C, Wynshaw-Boris A, Zhou F et al. Fibroblast growth factor receptor 3 is a negative regulator of bone growth. *Cell* 1996; **84**: 911–21.

◆36  Francomano C. Achondroplasia. www.genereviews.org, 2003.

37  Bellus GA, McIntosh I, Smith EA et al. A recurrent mutation in the tyrosine kinase domain of fibroblast growth factor receptor 3 causes hypochondroplasia. *Nat Genet* 1995; **10**: 357–9.

38  Rousseau F, el Ghouzzi V, Delezoide AL et al. Missense FGFR3 mutations create cysteine residues in thanatophoric dwarfism type I (TD1). *Hum Mol Genet* 1996; **5**: 509–12.

◆39  Chinoy MR. Pulmonary hypoplasia and congenital diaphragmatic hernia: advances in the pathogenetics and regulation of lung development. *J Surg Res* 2002; **106**: 209–23.

40  Torfs CP, Curry CJ, Bateson TF, Honore LH. A population-based study of congenital diaphragmatic hernia. *Teratology* 1992; **46**: 555–65.

41  Bohn D. Congenital diaphragmatic hernia. *Am J Respir Crit Care Med* 2002; **166**: 911–5.

42  Stefanutti G, Filippone M, Tommasoni N et al. Cardiopulmonary anatomy and function in long-term survivors of mild to moderate congenital diaphragmatic hernia. *J Pediatr Surg* 2004; 39: 526–31.

43  Hitch DC, Carson JA, Smith EI et al. Familial congenital diaphragmatic hernia is an autosomal recessive variant. *J Pediatr Surg* 1989; 24: 860–4.

44  Biggio JR Jr, Descartes MD, Carroll AJ, Holt RL. Congenital diaphragmatic hernia: is 15q26.1–26.2 a candidate locus? *Am J Med Genet* 2004; **126A**: 183–5.

45  Bagolan P, Casaccia G, Crescenzi F et al. Impact of a current treatment protocol on outcome of high-risk congenital diaphragmatic hernia. *J Pediatr Surg* 2004; **39**: 313–8.

46  Beck M. Mucopolysaccharidoses and Oligosaccharidoses. In: J Fernandez JS, G van den Berghe (eds). *Inborn metabolic disorders*, 3rd edn. Berlin: Springer-Verlag, 2000: 415–21.

47  Semenza GL, Pyeritz RE. Respiratory complications of mucopolysaccharide storage disorders. *Medicine (Balt)* 1988; **67**: 209–19.

48  Walker PP, Rose E, Williams JG. Upper airways abnormalities and tracheal problems in Morquio's disease. *Thorax* 2003; **58**: 458–9.

49  Orliaguet O, Pepin JL, Veale D et al. Hunter's syndrome and associated sleep apnoea cured by CPAP and surgery. *Eur Respir J* 1999; **13**: 1195–7.

50  Davitt SM, Hatrick A, Sabharwal T et al. Tracheobronchial stent insertions in the management of major airway obstruction in a patient with Hunter syndrome (type-II mucopolysaccharidosis). *Eur Radiol* 2002; **12**: 458–62.

51  Leighton SE, Papsin B, Vellodi A et al. Disordered breathing during sleep in patients with mucopolysaccharidoses. *Int J Pediatr Otorhinolaryngol* 2001; **58**: 127–38.

52  Kurihara M, Kumagai K, Goto K et al. Severe type Hunter's syndrome. Polysomnographic and neuropathological study. *Neuropediatrics* 1992; **23**: 248–56.

53  Chan D, Li AM, Yam MC et al. Hurler's syndrome with cor pulmonale secondary to obstructive sleep apnoea treated by continuous positive airway pressure. *J Paediatr Child Health* 2003; **39**: 558–9.

◆ 54  Neufeld EF, Muenzer J. The mucopolysaccharidoses. In: Scriver CR, Beaudet AL, Sly WS, Valle D (eds). *The metabolic and molecular basis of inherited disease*, 8th edn. New York: McGraw-Hill, 2001: 3421–52.

55  Muenzer J, Fisher A. Advances in the treatment of mucopolysaccharidosis type I. *N Engl J Med* 2004; **350**: 1932–4.

56  Staba SL, Escolar ML, Poe M et al. Cord-blood transplants from unrelated donors in patients with Hurler's syndrome. *N Engl J Med* 2004; **350**: 1960–9.

●57  Guay-Woodford LM, Desmond RA. Autosomal recessive polycystic kidney disease: the clinical experience in North America. *Pediatrics* 2003; **111** (5 Pt 1): 1072–80.

58  Zerres K, Rudnik-Schoneborn S, Deget F et al. Autosomal recessive polycystic kidney disease in 115 children: clinical presentation, course and influence of gender. Arbeitsgemeinschaft fur Padiatrische, Nephrologie. *Acta Paediatr* 1996; **85**: 437–45.

59  Blyth H, Ockenden BG. Polycystic disease of kidney and liver presenting in childhood. *J Med Genet* 1971; **8**: 257–84.

60  Thomas IT, Smith DW. Oligohydramnios, cause of the nonrenal features of Potter's syndrome, including pulmonary hypoplasia. *J Pediatr* 1974; **84**: 811–5.

61  Hislop A, Hey E, Reid L. The lungs in congenital bilateral renal agenesis and dysplasia. *Arch Dis Child* 1979; **54**: 32–8.

62  Bain AD, Scott JS. Renal agenesis and severe urinary tract dysplasia: a review of 50 cases, with particular reference to the associated anomalies. *Br Med J* 1960; **5176**: 841–6.

63  Corrin B. *Pathology of the lungs*. London: Churchill-Livingstone, 2000: 46–7.

64  Lieberman E, Salinas-Madrigal L, Gwinn JL et al. Infantile polycystic disease of the kidneys and liver: clinical, pathological and radiological correlations and comparison with congenital hepatic fibrosis. *Medicine (Balt)* 1971; **50**: 277–318.

65  Ward CJ, Yuan D, Masyuk TV et al. Cellular and subcellular localization of the ARPKD protein; fibrocystin is expressed on primary cilia. *Hum Mol Genet* 2003; **12**: 2703–10.

66  Dell KM, Nemo R, Sweeney WE Jr, Avner ED. EGF-related growth factors in the pathogenesis of murine ARPKD. *Kidney Int* 2004; **65**: 2018–29.

67  Guay-Woodford LM. Autosomal recessive polycystic kidney disease (ARPKD): new insights from the identification of the ARPKD gene, PKHD1. *Pediatr Res* 2002; **52**: 830–1.

◆68  Rowland LP, Shneider NA. Amyotrophic lateral sclerosis. *N Engl J Med* 2001; **344**: 1688–700.

69  Braun SR. Respiratory system in amyotrophic lateral sclerosis. *Neurol Clin* 1987; **5**: 9–31.

70  Braun NM, Arora NS, Rochester DF. Respiratory muscle and pulmonary function in polymyositis and other proximal myopathies. *Thorax* 1983; **38**: 616–23.

71  Horton WA, Eldridge R, Brody JA. Familial motor neuron disease. Evidence for at least three different types. *Neurology* 1976; **26**: 460–5.

72  Rosen DR, Siddique T, Patterson D et al. Mutations in Cu/Zn superoxide dismutase gene are associated with familial amyotrophic lateral sclerosis. *Nature* 1993; **362**: 59–62.

73  Andersen PM, Nilsson P, Keranen ML et al. Phenotypic heterogeneity in motor neuron disease patients with CuZn-superoxide dismutase mutations in Scandinavia. *Brain* 1997; **120** (Pt 10): 1723–37.

74  Al-Chalabi A, Andersen PM, Chioza B et al. Recessive amyotrophic lateral sclerosis families with the D90A SOD1 mutation share a common founder: evidence for a linked protective factor. *Hum Mol Genet* 1998; **7**: 2045–50.

75 Cudkowicz ME, McKenna-Yasek D, Chen C et al. Limited corticospinal tract involvement in amyotrophic lateral sclerosis subjects with the A4V mutation in the copper/zinc superoxide dismutase gene. *Ann Neurol* 1998; **43**: 703–10.

76 Rowland LP. Molecular basis of genetic heterogeneity: role of the clinical neurologist. *J Child Neurol* 1998; **13**: 122–32.

77 Yang Y, Hentati A, Deng HX et al. The gene encoding alsin, a protein with three guanine-nucleotide exchange factor domains, is mutated in a form of recessive amyotrophic lateral sclerosis. *Nat Genet* 2001; **29**: 160–5.

78 Kikuchi S, Ogata A, Shinpo K et al. Detection of an Amadori product, 1-hexitol-lysine, in the anterior horn of the amyotrophic lateral sclerosis and spinobulbar muscular atrophy spinal cord: evidence for early involvement of glycation in motoneuron diseases. *Acta Neuropathol (Berl)* 2000; **99**: 63–6.

79 Chou SM, Wang HS, Taniguchi A, Bucala R. Advanced glycation endproducts in neurofilament conglomeration of motoneurons in familial and sporadic amyotrophic lateral sclerosis. *Mol Med* 1998; **4**: 324–32.

80 Cleveland DW. From Charcot to SOD1: mechanisms of selective motor neuron death in ALS. *Neuron* 1999; **24**: 515–20.

81 Wong PC, Rothstein JD, Price DL. The genetic and molecular mechanisms of motor neuron disease. *Curr Opin Neurobiol* 1998; **8**: 791–9.

82 Xiong ZQ, McNamara JO. Fas(t) balls and Lou Gehrig disease. A clue to selective vulnerability of motor neurons? *Neuron* 2002; **35**: 1011–3.

83 Brooks BR. El Escorial World Federation of Neurology criteria for the diagnosis of amyotrophic lateral sclerosis. Subcommittee on Motor Neuron Diseases/Amyotrophic Lateral Sclerosis of the World Federation of Neurology Research Group on Neuromuscular Diseases and the El Escorial 'Clinical Limits of Amyotrophic Lateral Sclerosis' Workshop contributors. *J Neurol Sci* 1994; **124** (Suppl.): 96–107.

◆84 Korf BD, Urion D. Dystophinopathies. www.genereviews.org, 2003.

85 Brooke MH, Fenichel GM, Griggs RC et al. Duchenne muscular dystrophy: patterns of clinical progression and effects of supportive therapy. *Neurology* 1989; **39**: 475–81.

86 Tangsrud S, Petersen IL, Lodrup Carlsen KC, Carlsen KH. Lung function in children with Duchenne's muscular dystrophy. *Respir Med* 2001; **95**: 898–903.

87 Ahn AH, Kunkel LM. The structural and functional diversity of dystrophin. *Nat Genet* 1993; **3**: 283–91.

88 Den Dunnen JT, Grootscholten PM, Bakker E et al. Topography of the Duchenne muscular dystrophy (DMD) gene: FIGE and cDNA analysis of 194 cases reveals 115 deletions and 13 duplications. *Am J Hum Genet* 1989; **45**: 835–47.

89 Hoffman EP, Fischbeck KH, Brown RH et al. Characterization of dystrophin in muscle-biopsy specimens from patients with Duchenne's or Becker's muscular dystrophy. *N Engl J Med* 1988; **318**: 1363–8.

90 Zatz M, Rapaport D, Vainzof M et al. Serum creatine-kinase (CK) and pyruvate-kinase (PK) activities in Duchenne (DMD) as compared with Becker (BMD) muscular dystrophy. *J Neurol Sci* 1991; **102**: 190–6.

91 van Essen AJ, Kneppers AL, van der Hout AH et al. The clinical and molecular genetic approach to Duchenne and Becker muscular dystrophy: an updated protocol. *J Med Genet* 1997; **34**: 805–12.

92 Koenig M, Hoffman EP, Bertelson CJ et al. Complete cloning of the Duchenne muscular dystrophy (DMD) cDNA and preliminary genomic organization of the DMD gene in normal and affected individuals. *Cell* 1987; **50**: 509–17.

93 Bennett RR, den Dunnen J, O'Brien KF et al. Detection of mutations in the dystrophin gene via automated DHPLC screening and direct sequencing. *BMC Genet* 2001; **2**: 17.

94 Dolinsky LC, de Moura-Neto RS, Falcao-Conceicao DN. DGGE analysis as a tool to identify point mutations, de novo mutations and carriers of the dystrophin gene. *Neuromuscul Disord* 2002; **12**: 845–8.

95 Gardner RJ, Bobrow M, Roberts RG. The identification of point mutations in Duchenne muscular dystrophy patients by using reverse-transcription PCR and the protein truncation test. *Am J Hum Genet* 1995; **57**: 311–20.

✣96 Manzur AY, Muntoni F, Simonds A. Muscular Dystrophy Campaign-sponsored workshop: recommendation for respiratory care of children with spinal muscular atrophy type II and III. 13 February 2002, London, UK. *Neuromuscul Disord* 2003; **13**: 184–9.

97 Fukunaga H, Okubo R, Moritoyo T et al. Long-term follow-up of patients with Duchenne muscular dystrophy receiving ventilatory support. *Muscle Nerve* 1993; **16**: 554–8.

98 Jeppesen J, Green A, Steffensen BF, Rahbek J. The Duchenne muscular dystrophy population in Denmark, 1977–2001: prevalence, incidence and survival in relation to the introduction of ventilator use. *Neuromuscul Disord* 2003; **13**: 804–12.

99 Cassidy SB. Prader–Willi syndrome. *J Med Genet* 1997; **34**: 917–23.

100 Burman P, Ritzen EM, Lindgren AC. Endocrine dysfunction in Prader–Willi syndrome: a review with special reference to GH. *Endocr Rev* 2001; **22**: 787–99.

●101 Hakonarson H, Moskovitz J, Daigle KL et al. Pulmonary function abnormalities in Prader-Willi syndrome. *J Pediatr* 1995; **126**: 565–70.

102 Nixon GM, Brouillette RT. Sleep and breathing in Prader–Willi syndrome. *Pediatr Pulmonol* 2002; **34**: 209–17.

103 Vgontzas AN, Kales A, Seip J et al. Relationship of sleep abnormalities to patient genotypes in Prader-Willi syndrome. *Am J Med Genet* 1996; **67**: 478–82.

104 Arens R, Gozal D, Omlin KJ et al. Hypoxic and hypercapnic ventilatory responses in Prader–Willi syndrome. *J Appl Physiol* 1994; **77**: 2224–30.

105 Schluter B, Buschatz D, Trowitzsch E et al. Respiratory control in children with Prader-Willi syndrome. *Eur J Pediatr* 1997; **156**: 65–8.

106 Schrander-Stumpel CT, Curfs LM, Sastrowijoto P et al. Prader-Willi syndrome: causes of death in an international series of 27 cases. *Am J Med Genet* 2004; **124A**: 333–8.

107 Saitoh S, Buiting K, Cassidy SB et al. Clinical spectrum and molecular diagnosis of Angelman and Prader–Willi syndrome patients with an imprinting mutation. *Am J Med Genet* 1997; **68**: 195–206.

108 Goldstone AP. Prader-Willi syndrome: advances in genetics, pathophysiology and treatment. *Trends Endocrinol Metab* 2004; **15**: 12–20.

109   Ledbetter DH, Engel E. Uniparental disomy in humans: development of an imprinting map and its implications for prenatal diagnosis. *Hum Mol Genet* 1995; **4**: 1757–64.

110   Macey PM, Valderama C, Kim AH et al. Temporal trends of cardiac and respiratory responses to ventilatory challenges in congenital central hypoventilation syndrome. *Pediatr Res* 2004; **55**: 953–9.

111   Marazita ML, Maher BS, Cooper ME et al. Genetic segregation analysis of autonomic nervous system dysfunction in families of probands with idiopathic congenital central hypoventilation syndrome. *Am J Med Genet* 2001; **100**: 229–36.

112   Weese-Mayer DE, Silvestri JM, Huffman AD et al. Case/control family study of autonomic nervous system dysfunction in idiopathic congenital central hypoventilation syndrome. *Am J Med Genet* 2001; **100**: 237–45.

113   Croaker GD, Shi E, Simpson E et al. Congenital central hypoventilation syndrome and Hirschsprung's disease. *Arch Dis Child* 1998; **78**: 316–22.

114   Weese-Mayer DE, Silvestri JM, Marazita ML, Hoo JJ. Congenital central hypoventilation syndrome: inheritance and relation to sudden infant death syndrome. *Am J Med Genet* 1993; **47**: 360–7.

115   Amiel J, Laudier B, Attie-Bitach T et al. Polyalanine expansion and frameshift mutations of the paired-like homeobox gene PHOX2B in congenital central hypoventilation syndrome. *Nat Genet* 2003; **33**: 459–61.

116   Gaultier C, Amiel J, Dauger S et al. Genetics and early disturbances of breathing control. *Pediatr Res* 2004; **55**: 729–33.

117   Weese-Mayer DE, Berry-Kravis EM, Zhou L et al. Idiopathic congenital central hypoventilation syndrome: analysis of genes pertinent to early autonomic nervous system embryologic development and identification of mutations in PHOX2b. *Am J Med Genet* 2003; **123A**: 267–78.

118   Matera I, Bachetti T, Puppo F et al. PHOX2B mutations and polyalanine expansions correlate with the severity of the respiratory phenotype and associated symptoms in both congenital and late onset central hypoventilation syndrome. *J Med Genet* 2004; **41**: 373–80.

119   Sasaki A, Kanai M, Kijima K et al. Molecular analysis of congenital central hypoventilation syndrome. *Hum Genet* 2003; **114**: 22–6.

◆120   Weese-Mayer DE, Berry-Kravis EM. Genetics of congenital central hypoventilation syndrome: lessons from a seemingly orphan disease. *Am J Respir Crit Care Med* 2004; **170**: 16–21.

121   Amiel J, Salomon R, Attie T et al. Mutations of the RET-GDNF signaling pathway in Ondine's curse. *Am J Hum Genet* 1998; **62**: 715–7.

122   Bolk S, Angrist M, Xie J et al. Endothelin-3 frameshift mutation in congenital central hypoventilation syndrome. *Nat Genet* 1996; **13**: 395–6.

123   American Thoracic Society. Idiopathic congenital central hypoventilation syndrome: diagnosis and management. *Am J Respir Crit Care Med* 1999; **160**: 368–73.

124   Tibballs J, Henning RD. Noninvasive ventilatory strategies in the management of a newborn infant and three children with congenital central hypoventilation syndrome. *Pediatr Pulmonol* 2003; **36**: 544–8.

125   Dunn HG, MacLeod PM. Rett syndrome: review of biological abnormalities. *Can J Neurol Sci* 2001; **28**: 16–29.

◆126   Jellinger KA. Rett syndrome – an update. *J Neural Transm* 2003; **110**: 681–701.

127   Julu PO, Kerr AM, Apartopoulos F et al. Characterisation of breathing and associated central autonomic dysfunction in the Rett disorder. *Arch Dis Child* 2001; **85**: 29–37.

128   Nomura Y. Neurophysiology of Rett syndrome. *Brain Dev* 2001; **23** (Suppl. 1): S50–7.

129   Amir RE, Van den Veyver IB, Wan M et al. Rett syndrome is caused by mutations in X-linked MECP2, encoding methyl-CpG-binding protein 2. *Nat Genet* 1999; **23**: 185–8.

130   Schanen C. Rethinking the fate of males with mutations in the gene that causes Rett syndrome. *Brain Dev* 2001; **23** (Suppl. 1): S144–6.

131   The Rett Syndrome Diagnostic Criteria Work Group. Diagnostic criteria for Rett syndrome. *Ann Neurol* 1988; **23**: 425–8.

132   Naidu S. Rett syndrome: a disorder affecting early brain growth. *Ann Neurol* 1997; **42**: 3–10.

133   AAssar OS, Friedman CM, White RI Jr. The natural history of epistaxis in hereditary hemorrhagic telangiectasia. *Laryngoscope* 1991; **101**: 977–80.

134   Plauchu H, de Chadarevian JP, Bideau A, Robert JM. Age-related clinical profile of hereditary hemorrhagic telangiectasia in an epidemiologically recruited population. *Am J Med Genet* 1989; **32**: 291–7.

135   Willinsky RA, Lasjaunias P, Terbrugge K, Burrows P. Multiple cerebral arteriovenous malformations (AVMs). Review of our experience from 203 patients with cerebral vascular lesions. *Neuroradiology* 1990; **32**: 207–10.

136   Porteous ME, Burn J, Proctor SJ. Hereditary haemorrhagic telangiectasia: a clinical analysis. *J Med Genet* 1992; **29**: 527–30.

137   Haitjema T, Westermann CJ, Overtoom TT et al. Hereditary hemorrhagic telangiectasia (Osler–Weber–Rendu disease): new insights in pathogenesis, complications, and treatment. *Arch Intern Med* 1996; **156**: 714–9.

138   Peery WH. Clinical spectrum of hereditary hemorrhagic telangiectasia (Osler–Weber–Rendu disease). *Am J Med* 1987; **82**: 989–97.

139   Kjeldsen AD, Oxhoj H, Andersen PE et al. Prevalence of pulmonary arteriovenous malformations (PAVMs) and occurrence of neurological symptoms in patients with hereditary haemorrhagic telangiectasia (HHT). *J Intern Med* 2000; **248**: 255–62.

140   Shovlin CL, Letarte M. Hereditary haemorrhagic telangiectasia and pulmonary arteriovenous malformations: issues in clinical management and review of pathogenic mechanisms. *Thorax* 1999; **54**: 714–29.

141   Guttmacher AE, Marchuk DA, White RI Jr. Hereditary hemorrhagic telangiectasia. *N Engl J Med* 1995; **333**: 918–24.

142   Schulick AH, Taylor AJ, Zuo W et al. Overexpression of transforming growth factor beta1 in arterial endothelium causes hyperplasia, apoptosis, and cartilaginous metaplasia. *Proc Natl Acad Sci USA* 1998; **95**: 6983–8.

143   Trembath RC. Mutations in the TGF-beta type 1 receptor, ALK1, in combined primary pulmonary hypertension and hereditary haemorrhagic telangiectasia, implies pathway specificity. *J Heart Lung Transplant* 2001; **20**: 175.

144   Pece N, Vera S, Cymerman U et al. Mutant endoglin in hereditary hemorrhagic telangiectasia type 1 is transiently

expressed intracellularly and is not a dominant negative. *J Clin Invest* 1997; **100**: 2568–79.

145   Marchuk DA, Guttmacher AE, Penner JA, Ganguly P. Report on the workshop on Hereditary Hemorrhagic Telangiectasia, 10–11 July 1997. *Am J Med Genet* 1998; **76**: 269–73.

146   Shovlin CL, Guttmacher AE, Buscarini E et al. Diagnostic criteria for hereditary hemorrhagic telangiectasia (Rendu–Osler–Weber syndrome). *Am J Med Genet* 2000; **91**: 66–7.

●147   Cottin V, Plauchu H, Bayle JY et al. Pulmonary arteriovenous malformations in patients with hereditary hemorrhagic telangiectasia. *Am J Respir Crit Care Med* 2004; **169**: 994–1000.

148   Morrell NW. Screening for pulmonary arteriovenous malformations. *Am J Respir Crit Care Med* 2004; **169**: 978–9.

149   Cymerman U, Vera S, Karabegovic A et al. Characterization of 17 novel endoglin mutations associated with hereditary hemorrhagic telangiectasia. *Hum Mutat* 2003; **21**: 482–92.

150   Rimoin LR, Lachman RS. Genetic disorders of the osseous skeleton. In: Beighton P (ed.) *McKusick's heritable disorders of connective tissue*, 5th edn. St Louis: Mosby, 1993: 557–689.

151   Baitner AC, Maurer SG, Gruen MB, Di Cesare PE. The genetic basis of the osteochondrodysplasias. *J Pediatr Orthop* 2000; **20**: 594–605.

152   Superti-Furga A. Achondrogenesis type 1B. *J Med Genet* 1996; **33**: 957–61.

153   Borochowitz Z, Ornoy A, Lachman R, Rimoin DL. Achondrogenesis II-hypochondrogenesis: variability versus heterogeneity. *Am J Med Genet* 1986; **24**: 273–88.

154   O'Sullivan MJ, McAllister WH, Ball RH et al. Morphologic observations in a case of lethal variant (type I) metatropic dysplasia with atypical features: morphology of lethal metatropic dysplasia. *Pediatr Dev Pathol* 1998; **1**: 405–12.

155   Sarafoglou K, Funai EF, Fefferman N et al. Short rib-polydactyly syndrome: more evidence of a continuous spectrum. *Clin Genet* 1999; **56**: 145–8.

156   Remes V, Helenius I, Peltonen J et al. Lung function in diastrophic dysplasia. *Pediatr Pulmonol* 2002; **33**: 277–82.

157   Mansour S, Hall CM, Pembrey ME, Young ID. A clinical and genetic study of campomelic dysplasia. *J Med Genet* 1995; **32**: 415–20.

158   Mansour S, Offiah AC, McDowall S et al. The phenotype of survivors of campomelic dysplasia. *J Med Genet* 2002; **39**: 597–602.

159   Corsello G, Maresi E, Corrao AM et al. VATER/VACTERL association: clinical variability and expanding phenotype including laryngeal stenosis. *Am J Med Genet* 1992; **44**: 813–5.

160   Wei JL, Rodeberg D, Thompson DM. Tracheal agenesis with anomalies found in both VACTERL and TACRD associations. *Int J Pediatr Otorhinolaryngol* 2003; **67**: 1013–7.

161   Palmer SM Jr, Layish DT, Kussin PS et al. Lung transplantation for Williams–Campbell syndrome. *Chest* 1998; **113**: 534–7.

162   Urban MD, Schosser R, Spohn W et al. New clinical aspects of hereditary mucoepithelial dysplasia. *Am J Med Genet* 1991; **39**: 338–41.

◆163   Moser HW, Linke T, Fensom AH et al. Acid ceramidase deficiency: Farber lipogranulomatosis. In: Scriver CR, Beaudet AL, Sly WS, Valle D (eds) *The metabolic and molecular bases of*

*inherited disease*, 8th edn. New York: McGraw-Hill, 2001: 3573–88.

164   Brown LK, Miller A, Bhuptani A et al. Pulmonary involvement in Fabry disease. *Am J Respir Crit Care Med* 1997; **155**: 1004–10.

◆165   Desnick R, Ioannou YA, Eng CM. Alpha-galactosidase A deficiency: Fabry disease. In: Scriver CR, Beaudet AL, Sly WS, Valle D (eds) *The metabolic and molecular basis of inherited disease*, 8th edn. New York: McGraw-Hill, 2001: 3733–74.

166   Kerem E, Elstein D, Abrahamov A et al. Pulmonary function abnormalities in type I Gaucher disease. *Eur Respir J* 1996; **9**: 340–5.

167   Miller A, Brown LK, Pastores GM, Desnick RJ. Pulmonary involvement in type 1 Gaucher disease: functional and exercise findings in patients with and without clinical interstitial lung disease. *Clin Genet* 2003; **63**: 368–76.

168   Finn LS, Zhang M, Chen SH, Scott CR. Severe type II Gaucher disease with ichthyosis, arthrogryposis and neuronal apoptosis: molecular and pathological analyses. *Am J Med Genet* 2000; **91**: 222–6.

169   Amir G, Ron N. Pulmonary pathology in Gaucher's disease. *Hum Pathol* 1999; **30**: 666–70.

◆170   Hirschhorn R, Reuser AJJ. Glycogen storage disease type II: acid a-glucosidase (acid maltase) deficiency. In: Scriver CR, Beaudet AL, Sly WS, Valle D (eds) *The metabolic and molecular bases of inherited disease*, 8th edn. New York: McGraw-Hill, 2001: 3389–420.

171   Minai OA, Sullivan EJ, Stoller JK. Pulmonary involvement in Niemann–Pick disease: case report and literature review. *Respir Med* 2000; **94**: 1241–51.

172   Gonzalez-Reimers E, Sanchez-Perez MJ, Bonilla-Arjona A et al. Case report. Pulmonary involvement in an adult male affected by type B Niemann–Pick disease. *Br J Radiol* 2003; **76**: 838–40.

173   Elleder M, Houstkova H, Zeman J et al. Pulmonary storage with emphysema as a sign of Niemann–Pick type C2 disease (second complementation group). Report of a case. *Virchows Arch* 2001; **439**: 206–11.

174   Grateau G. Clinical and genetic aspects of the hereditary periodic fever syndromes. *Rheumatology* 2004; **43**: 410–5.

175   Parto K, Svedstrom E, Majurin ML et al. Pulmonary manifestations in lysinuric protein intolerance. *Chest* 1993; **104**: 1176–82.

176   Grohmann K, Varon R, Stolz P et al. Infantile spinal muscular atrophy with respiratory distress type 1 (SMARD1). *Ann Neurol* 2003; **54**: 719–24.

177   Herman GE, Finegold M, Zhao W et al. Medical complications in long-term survivors with X-linked myotubular myopathy. *J Pediatr* 1999; **134**: 206–14.

178   Keesey JC. Clinical evaluation and management of myasthenia gravis. *Muscle Nerve* 2004; **29**: 484–505.

179   Engel AE. 73rd ENMC International Workshop: congenital myasthenic syndromes, 22–23 October 1999, Naarden, The Netherlands. *Neuromuscul Disord* 2001; **11**: 315–21.

✳180   Wallgren-Pettersson C, Bushby K, Mellies U, Simonds A. 117th ENMC workshop: ventilatory support in congenital neuromuscular disorders – congenital myopathies, congenital muscular dystrophies, congenital myotonic dystrophy and SMA (II), 4–6 April 2003, Naarden, The Netherlands. *Neuromuscul Disord* 2004; **14**: 56–69.

181 Schweitzer C, Danet V, Polu E et al. Nemaline myopathy and early respiratory failure. *Eur J Pediatr* 2003; **162**: 216–7.

182 Campbell C, Sherlock R, Jacob P, Blayney M. Congenital myotonic dystrophy: assisted ventilation duration and outcome. *Pediatrics* 2004; **113**: 811–6.

183 Harper PS. *Myotonic dystrophy*, 3rd edn. London: WB Saunders, 2001.

184 Kelley RI, Hennekam RC. The Smith–Lemli–Opitz syndrome. *J Med Genet* 2000; **37**: 321–35.

185 Teebi AS, Lambert DM, Kaye GM et al. Keutel syndrome: further characterization and review. *Am J Med Genet* 1998; **78**: 182–7.

186 Cistulli PA, Gotsopoulos H, Sullivan CE. Relationship between craniofacial abnormalities and sleep-disordered breathing in Marfan's syndrome. *Chest* 2001; **120**: 1455–60.

187 Resta O, Barbaro MP, Giliberti T et al. Sleep related breathing disorders in adults with Down syndrome. *Downs Syndr Res Pract* 2003; **8**: 115–9.

188 de Miguel-Diez J, Villa-Asensi JR, Alvarez-Sala JL. Prevalence of sleep-disordered breathing in children with Down syndrome: polygraphic findings in 108 children. *Sleep* 2003; **26**: 1006–9.

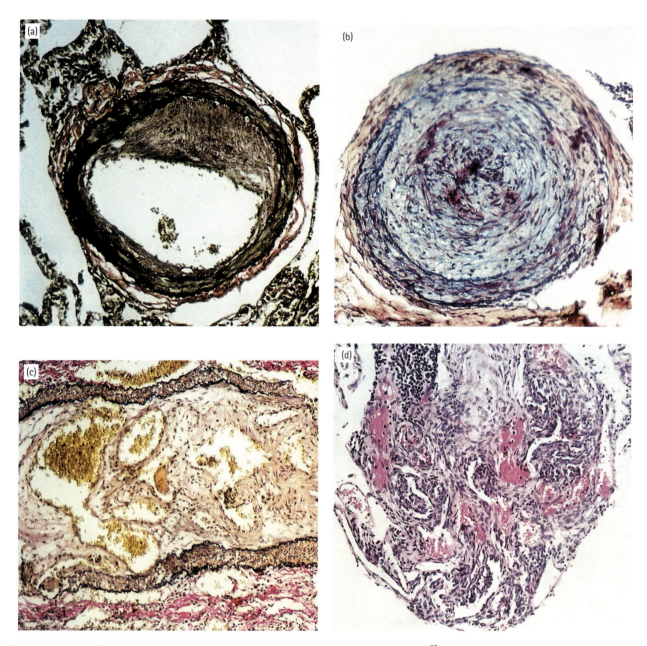

**Plate 1** *Lesions of the small pulmonary arterioles found in all forms of PAH, including FPPH.[65] Lesion one demonstrates eccentric intimal fibrosis and medial hypertrophy (Verhoff van Gieson, magnification × 100). This lesion was originally thought to represent pulmonary microembolism, but is widespread in FPPH, denoting a differing mechanism. Lesion 2 shows concentric intimal fibrosis, an onion skin-like layering of fibrotic reaction (Movat stain, magnification × 100). Lesion 3 is a plexiform lesion, showing a neovascular response (hematoxylin and eosin, magnification × 100). It is unclear whether these lesions are a response to upstream obstruction or are a primary lesion in PAH.* *(See p. 368.)*

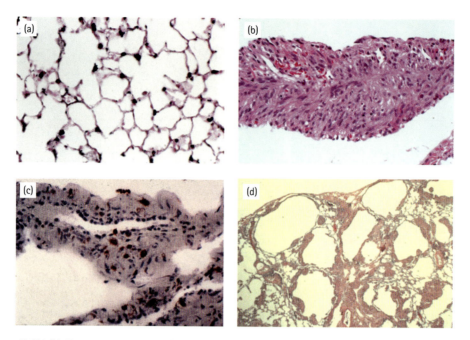

**Plate 6** *Pathology of LAM. (a) Normal lung histology; (b) Alveolar septum expanded by spindles shaped smooth muscle; (c) HMB-045 staining of smooth muscle in LAM; (d) Smooth muscle infiltration, cyst formation; tissue destruction in LAM. (See p. 485.)*

# 18

# Other rare lung diseases

# Disorders of surfactant homeostasis

RALPH J. PANOS AND BRUCE C. TRAPNELL

## INTRODUCTION

In Chapters 18A, 18B, and 18C, we will cover several rare lung diseases for which recent research has vastly improved our understanding of disease pathogenesis, opened the doors to new therapeutic interventions, and taught us important lessons about lung biology in health and disease. This group of rare diseases, defined by the Office of Rare Diseases at the National Institutes of Health as disorders affecting fewer than 200 000 individuals in the USA, includes a heterogeneous group of lung diseases affecting surfactant homeostasis. Recent observations from basic science, clinical medicine, and translational research have raised each of these diseases from obscurity to clarity in less than a decade.

## DISORDERS OF DISRUPTED SURFACTANT HOMEOSTASIS

Surfactant is a complex mixture of phospholipids and proteins produced by alveolar epithelial lining cells that is required to diminish alveolar surface tension and prevent end expiratory alveolar collapse. Surfactant lipids, predominantly phosphatidylcholine and phosphatidylglycerol, and the hydrophobic surfactant proteins, SP-B and SP-C, are synthesized and processed in alveolar type II cells. Surfactant is stored within cytoplasmic organelles called lamellar bodies that are secreted into the alveolar space and unravel to form tubular myelin which spreads creating mono- and multi-layers. This lipid and protein film dramatically reduces surface tension at the alveolar air–liquid interface and prevents alveolar collapse at the end of expiration. The alveolar structure is thereby stabilized maintaining an efficient ventilation perfusion relationship. The cellular and molecular mechanisms regulating surfactant production, composition, and homeostasis are highly regulated.

Surfactant is composed of 90 percent lipids and 10 percent proteins by weight. The proteins include the hydrophilic surfactant proteins A and D and the hydrophobic surfactant proteins B and C. SP-A and SP-D are members of the collectin protein family and have essential roles in the opsonization, killing, and clearance of bacteria within the alveolar space as well as immunomodulation of inflammatory cell recruitment and activation.[1]

SP-A-deficient mice have normal lung structure and surfactant metabolism and biophysical properties. However, these mice do lack tubular myelin.[2] In contrast, SP-D-deficient mice develop dilated alveoli with increased amounts of protein and lipid and accumulation of intraalveolar foamy, multinucleated macrophages and hyperplastic type II cells containing giant lamellar bodies[3] and progressive emphysema with aging (as discussed in Chapter 10).[4] No mutations in the genes encoding SP-A (SFTPA1, SFTPA2) or SP-D (SFTPD) have yet been proven to cause pulmonary disease in humans.

SP-B and SP-C are hydrophobic surfactant proteins that are necessary for surfactant homeostasis and to maintain normal pulmonary function.[5] SP-C is a 35 amino-acid protein that is extremely hydrophobic and enhances the formation of multilayer surfactant films in the alveolar lining layer as well as surfactant metabolism and homeostasis. Disorders of altered SP-C production are discussed in Chapter 12. SP-B is an amphipathic peptide that is synthesized as a much larger precursor protein called pro-SP-B and then proteolytically processed to yield mature, biologically active SP-B. SP-B is critical for lamellar body formation, regulates major steps in surfactant metabolism and homeostasis, and is essential for the transition to breathing air at birth.[5,6] Genetic disorders of SP-B and another critical regulator of surfactant metabolism, ABCA3, will be discussed in this section.

## DISORDERS OF ALTERED SURFACTANT PRODUCTION

### Surfactant protein B deficiency

#### DEFINITION

Mutations in the gene encoding SP-B (SFTPB) cause severe, usually fatal respiratory insufficiency in neonates. The clinical and histopathologic manifestations of SFTPB mutations are very similar to the syndromes described as congenital alveolar proteinosis or congenital desquamative interstitial pneumonitis: progressive, fulminant respiratory insufficiency associated with the histopathologic finding of dense, lipid-rich, eosinophilic, proteinaceous material within the alveolar spaces. SP-B protein is usually undetectable and SP-C is usually present as an aberrant, not fully processed propeptide. Genetic analysis has revealed multiple mutations within the *SFTPB* gene. Therefore, hereditary SP-B deficiency is the preferred term for this disorder.

## GENETIC ETIOLOGY

SP-B deficiency is caused by autosomal recessive mutations in SPTPB. Over 30 mutations have been identified to date in less than 100 infants with SP-B deficiency.[6–8] The predicted incidence of SP-B deficiency is estimated to be approximately 1 per 1.5 million births. Approximately two-thirds have an insertional frameshift mutation caused by the replacement of a single base pair by three base pairs in the SFTPB transcript corresponding to codon 121 of exon 4. This mutation has been designated 121ins2. In infants with hereditary SP-B deficiency, the 121ins2 mutation is present on both alleles in approximately 60 percent and on one allele in 25 percent.[9] Using two different populations, Cole and colleagues[10] estimated the gene frequency of the 121ins2 mutation to be approximately one per 1000–3000 individuals. The 121ins2 mutation has been identified predominantly in individuals of northern European descent whereas other less frequent mutations, 122delT, c.1043ins3, c.479g > T, and R295X, have been associated with individuals of Middle Eastern, Asian, French-Canadian, and Hispanic origin, respectively.[7,11–13]

## NATURAL HISTORY

Infants with SP-B deficiency are usually born at or near term without antecedent gestational difficulties. Within hours to days of birth they develop severe progressive respiratory failure with diffuse parenchymal lung disease usually requiring mechanical ventilatory support. Evidence of infection or congenital heart disease is usually not present, but there may be a history of siblings who died in infancy of respiratory failure of unknown cause. Wallot and coworkers[14] described a novel SFTPB mutation, 122delT, that was associated with misalignment of lung vessels in a large Kurdish kindred with several consanguineous marriages. Treatment with corticosteroids, surfactant replacement, and extracorporeal membrane oxygenation have been tried unsuccessfully to treat SP-B deficiency. Most infants die within 6–12 months, unless they undergo lung transplantation.[15]

In addition to absolute SP-B deficiency, partial and transient SP-B deficiencies have been described which appear to have a less fulminant course. Dunbar and colleagues[13] described two unrelated French-Canadian children with

a G to T transversion at genomic nucleotide 2479. Lung histopathology from both patients demonstrated eosinophilic material, foamy macrophages, and desquamated alveolar type II cells within the alveolar spaces. Ultrastructural studies of lung tissue from one patient showed structurally deranged lamellar bodies that appeared as noncompact irregularly spaced membranous whorls. No definite tubular myelin was present. Immunohistochemical staining using antigen retrieval techniques demonstrated proSP-B and mature SP-B in both patients. One infant had progressive respiratory failure and required double lung transplantation, whereas the other survived to early childhood with the use of supplemental oxygen. Ballard and coworkers[16] described an infant with severe respiratory insufficiency due to heterozygosity for two SFTPB mutations. One allele contained the 121ins2 mutation and the other contained a T for C substitution in codon 236. Lung tissue contained low but detectable levels of SP-B and normal SFTPB mRNA content. Klein and colleagues[17] described an infant with respiratory failure due to a G to A substitution at codon 417 in exon 5 of one allele of the *SFTPB* gene. Initial analysis of tracheal fluid demonstrated the absence of SP-B and the presence of SP-A. However, an open lung biopsy performed 34 days after the tracheal aspirate showed abundant staining for both SP-A and SP-B. Electron microscopy showed normal appearing lamellar bodies within alveolar type II cells. This child survived infancy with chronic lung disease and persistent need for supplemental oxygen. Interestingly, the mother who was also heterozygous for this mutation had no history of respiratory insufficiency.

Yusen and colleagues[18] studied the pulmonary function of nine individuals who ranged from 16 to 44 years of age and were heterozygous for 121ins2. None had a history of respiratory problems. One individual had an increased residual volume but all other measurements of air flow, compliance, and gas exchange were normal.

Although respiratory failure in neonates is the best characterized disorder due to mutations in the *SFTPB* gene, SFTPB polymorphisms have been associated with other pulmonary processes. Presence of the C/C or C/T polymorphism at the SFTPB + 1580 site in adults with community-acquired pneumonia was associated with need for mechanical ventilatory support, septic shock, and acute respiratory distress syndrome.[19] The 1580 T/C polymorphism causes the insertion of an isoleucine instead of threonine at amino acid position 131 which is within a functional glycosylation sequence. Variations in glycosylation may alter protein configuration and processing, as well as biologic function. This Ile131Thr polymorphism may determine susceptibility or resistance to neonatal respiratory distress syndrome in individuals with certain SFTPA alleles.[20,21] In addition, polymorphisms in intron 4 of the *SFTPB* gene are associated with acute respiratory distress syndrome,[22–24] neonatal respiratory distress syndrome,[25] and acute respiratory failure in patients with chronic obstructive pulmonary disease.[26] The SFTPB allele, B1580_C, has been shown to

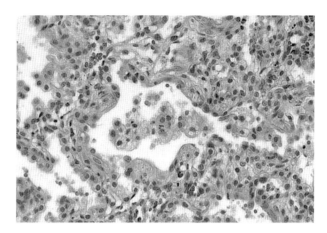

**Figure 18A.1** *Lung histopathology of an infant with SP-B deficiency. The interstitium is thickened and alveolar type II cells are prominent. There are macrophages and desquamated epithelial cells mixed with eosinophilic granular material within the alveolar space. (See Plate 2 for colour version.)*

occur with increased frequency in patients with idiopathic pulmonary fibrosis who smoke.[27] The C allele creates a potential N-linked threonine glycosylation site which might interfere with protein processing and function.

## PATHOGENESIS

The pulmonary histopathologic appearance in infants with *SFTPB* gene mutations is suggestive of pulmonary alveolar proteinosis and has been called congenital alveolar proteinosis.[28] The alveoli are filled with eosinophilic proteinaceous material mixed with macrophages and desquamated alveolar epithelial cells (Fig. 18A.1). The alveolar type II cells are hyperplastic and the intraalveolar septae are thickened and fibrotic.[29] Immunohistochemical staining reveals an absence of SP-B but abundant SP-C within alveolar type II cells, as well as the alveolar spaces. However, this SP-C protein is aberrantly large and appears to be due to a block in the proteolytic processing of pro-SP-C to the mature protein.[30] SP-A is present in the intraalveolar proteinaceous material and cells, but minimally present in type II cells lining the alveolus. Ultrastructural studies demonstrate numerous membranous vesicles and few lamellar bodies and multilamellar structures within the alveolar space, but tubular myelin is not present (Fig. 18A.2).[29] Alveolar type II cells contain rare lamellar bodies, but are filled with membranous vesicles and multivesicular bodies. These inclusions are present throughout the cell as well as between the cell and the basement membrane.

In vitro nuclear run-on studies utilizing lung tissue obtained from infants with hereditary SP-B deficiency demonstrated that SFTPA, SFTPB, and SFTPC transcription rates were similar to the levels of gene expression in normal lung tissue.[31] However, SFTPB transcripts were absent or minimally present suggesting that the SFTPB mutations caused decreased mRNA stability.[31] Phosphatidylglycerol

(a)

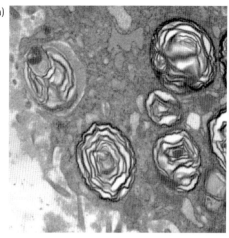

(b)

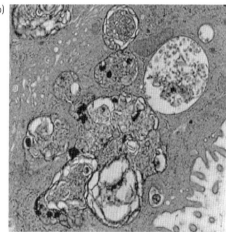

(c)

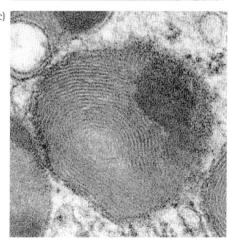

**Figure 18A.2** *Electron micrographs of lamellar bodies from normal lung (a). These lamellar bodies demonstrate organized compact laminated structure. (b) An infant with SP-B deficiency. These deranged lamellar bodies appear as noncompact, irregularly spaced membranous whorls. (c) An infant with ABCA3 deficiency. These lamellar bodies are smaller than observed in normal lung and have very densely compacted membranous structures within uniformly spaced linear whorls and peripheral, dense inclusions.*

levels in lavage and tissue from lungs of individuals with SP-B deficiency were reduced compared to levels from normals even though rates of synthesis of phospholipids, including phosphatidylglycerol, were similar.[31]

Although SP-C is present in the lungs and lavage fluid of infants with SP-B deficiency, it is usually present as an aberrantly large misprocessed protein.[30] Mature SP-C is a 4.2 kDa protein that is derived from a 21 kDa precursor by a multistep proteolytic processing of both the C-terminal and N-terminal domains of the propeptide. It appears that the final N-terminal cleavage of both the SP-B and SP-C propeptides occurs in the lamellar body and may be mediated by cathepsin H, napsin, and other proteases.[32,33] In hereditary SP-B deficiency, there is accumulation of a unique 12-kDa form of SP-C (SP-$C_i$) which contains the amino-terminal region of pro-SP-C.[30,34] Guttentag and colleagues[32] have proposed a sequential processing of SP-B followed by SP-C to permit proteases access to the N-terminus of the propeptides within small vesicles. If SP-B is not present, the protease is sterically inhibited from gaining access to the pro-SP-C, and SP-C processing cannot be completed. SP-$C_i$ associates with phospholipids but does not enhance phospholipid adsorption, reduce surface tension, or bind lipopolysaccharide.[34] Thus, SP-$C_i$ lacks significant biological activity.

Mature fully processed SP-C has been detected in the bronchoalveolar lavage fluid of an infant with SP-B deficiency due to the presence of compound heterozygous SFTPB mutations 1549CtoGAA and 457delC mutations.[35] SP-D was present at normal levels, SP-A levels were reduced, and SP-B was not detectable. Lung tissue was not available for histopathology and ultrastructural analysis to detect lamellar bodies. Therefore, most but not all SFTPB mutations are associated with aberrant processing of SP-C protein.

## CLINICAL EVALUATION

Hereditary SP-B deficiency should be considered in infants who develop respiratory insufficiency within the first 12–24 h after birth. A history of affected family members especially siblings or consanguinity may be elicited. There is usually no evidence of other congenital abnormalities or infection. Chest X-rays generally show a diffuse alveolar filling process, reduced lung volumes, and air bronchograms (Fig. 18A.3).[36] High resolution chest CT scans demonstrate ground-glass opacification and geometric interlobular septal thickening.[37] Although the absence of SP-B protein in tracheal aspirates suggests SP-B deficiency, it is not diagnostic. Definitive confirmation of hereditary SP-B deficiency is established by the demonstration of mutations in both alleles of the *SFTPB* gene. Prenatal diagnosis of surfactant protein B deficiency has been achieved by chorionic villus sampling and absence of SP-B protein in amniotic fluid.[38,39]

## TREATMENT

Neonates with SP-B deficiency have been treated with corticosteroids, surfactant replacement therapy, and

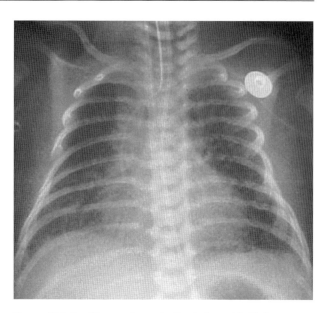

**Figure 18A.3** *Chest radiograph of an infant with SP-B deficiency. There is a diffuse alveolar filling process with ground-glass opacification.*

cardiopulmonary bypass, but none of these therapies have been shown to alter the clinical course and most infants die within 6 months. Lung transplantation is the only therapy that extends life beyond infancy. Study of three infants after lung transplantation for SP-B deficiency showed that cognitive development as well as somatic and lung growth are comparable to other infants who have undergone lung transplantation.[15] However, motor and auditory development are delayed. In addition, two of three transplant recipients developed serum antibody to SP-B which did not appear to be clinically, physiologically, or pathologically significant.

## DISEASE MODELS

Targeted deletion of SFTPB causes lethal respiratory failure within 20 min of birth in mice.[40] Histopathologic examination of these animals' lungs demonstrated normal morphogenesis of the conducting airways and no evidence of inflammation or epithelial desquamation. SP-B protein was not detected by immunohistochemistry or Western blot. SP-C protein was markedly reduced, whereas abundant pro-SP-C was detected. Electron microscopy revealed no lamellar bodies but large, irregular membranous inclusions within the respiratory epithelium. Within the alveolar space, small vesicles and electron-dense proteinaceous material were present and tubular myelin was absent. Pulmonary phosphatidylcholine and incorporation of precursors into phosphatidylcholine were similar in the SFTPB-deficient mice compared to wildtype mice.[41] Lung compliance was reduced in the *SFTPB* gene-targeted mice. Creation of compound transgenic mice in which SFTPB was conditionally expressed under the control of exogenous doxycycline demonstrated that reduction of SP-B levels to <25 percent of normal induced respiratory failure.[42] SP-B deficiency was associated with diminished lung compliance, increased intraalveolar protein, presence of misprocessed pro-SP-C protein, and reduced surfactant activity.[42] To reduce SFTPB expression, Foster and colleagues[43] created an adenovirus vector expressing antisense SFTPB that they used to infect human fetal lung explants. Antisense SFTPB expression caused reductions in SP-B and SP-C protein levels, and decreased numbers of lamellar bodies similar to SFTPB gene targeted mice.

Heterozygous SFTPB gene targeted mice demonstrate normal lung development and postpartum oxygenation and survival.[41] These animals have slightly reduced lung compliance and minimal air trapping.[41,44] Exposure of these mice to hyperoxia results in a more profound reduction in lung compliance and more severe pulmonary edema, hemorrhage, inflammation, and protein leak into the alveolar space compared with similarly exposed wildtype mice.[45]

Selective restoration of SFTPB expression in alveolar type II cells, but not in Clara cells of SFTPB gene targeted mice reverts lung structure and function to normal.[46] Mature SP-B protein was not detected in SFTPB gene targeted mice expressing SFTPB only in Clara cells suggesting that these cells lack the proteolytic enzymes necessary for the posttranslational processing of SP-B preprotein. In addition, no lamellar bodies were detected in the alveolar type II cells of these animals indicating that the immature SP-B protein found in the alveolar space was not taken up and processed by alveolar type II cells to reconstitute lamellar body formation.

## FUTURE DIRECTIONS

Identification of the environmental factors that modulate phenotypic expression of some of the SFTPB mutations may provide therapeutic options for the supportive care of patients with respiratory insufficiency due to mutated SFTPB. Replacement therapy with exogenous surfactant containing SP-B has not altered the natural history of SP-B deficiency. Currently, the only treatment offering long-term survival is lung replacement by transplantation. Future options may include gene therapy to increase intracellular as well as intraalveolar levels of SP-B. In addition, genetic screening may identify families at risk for hereditary SP-B deficiency.

## ABCA3 deficiency

ATP-binding cassette (ABC) transporters are proteins that hydrolyze ATP to drive the transport of substrates across cell membranes. The ABCA subfamily is a subset of the human ABC superfamily that includes lipid transporters, multidrug resistance/transmembrane-associated proteins, adrenoleukodystrophy proteins, and the cystic fibrosis transmembrane conductance regulator.[47] These transmembrane proteins transport numerous substrates including lipids, ions, amino acids, peptides, sugars, vitamins, steroid hormones, and toxic compounds.[47] Mutations in the ABC genes have been associated with several unique human genetic

diseases: ABCA1 with Tangier disease, ABCA4 with recessive disorders of retinal degeneration, ABCG5 and ABCG8 with sitosterolemia, ABCA12 with lamellar ichthyosis type 2, and, most recently, ABCA3 with fatal fetal surfactant deficiency.[48,49]

The ABCA3 gene is highly expressed in lung and encodes a 150 kDa protein that localizes to lamellar body membranes within alveolar type II cells.[50,51] ABCA3 transcript expression is developmentally regulated and is increased by glucocorticoids.[50,52] The ABCA3 protein is believed to transport lipid across the cell or lamellar body limiting membrane.[50] Cells transfected with the ABCA3 gene developed multilamellar vesicular structures suggesting that ABCA3 may play an important role in lamellar body formation.[53]

Shulenin and colleagues[49] identified homozygous or compound heterozygous mutations in the gene encoding ABCA3 in 16 of 21 patients who died of respiratory failure within 3 months of birth. These infants developed rapidly progressive respiratory insufficiency soon after birth. Chest radiographic studies demonstrated diffuse alveolar filling processes with ground-glass opacification, reduced lung volumes, and air bronchograms (Fig. 18A.4). These mutations included seven missense substitutions in conserved amino acids, homozygous nonsense mutations, a homozygous frameshift mutation, a heterozygous insertion mutation, and splice-site mutations. Lung tissue from nine patients with ABCA3 mutations demonstrated alveolar type II cell hyperplasia, interstitial widening, and accumulation of macrophages and proteinaceous material within alveolar spaces (Fig. 18A.5). Ultrastructural analysis showed either absent or highly abnormal lamellar bodies with tightly packed membranes and dense eccentric inclusion bodies (Fig. 18A.2).

The epidemiology and natural history of ABCA3 mutations are not known currently, but are the subject of intensive study. No animal models of this disorder have yet been described.

## DISORDERS OF ALTERED SURFACTANT CLEARANCE

Pulmonary alveolar proteinosis (PAP) (also referred to as alveolar proteinosis, alveolar phospholipidosis, pulmonary alveolar lipoproteinosis, and pulmonary alveolar phospholipoproteinosis) was first recognized in 1958[54] as a disorder of increased accumulation of lipoproteinaceous material in the alveoli and terminal airways. The accumulated material was quickly identified as pulmonary surfactant, composed of both lipids and proteins. However, for three decades after its initial description, the mechanism of accumulation could not be distinguished between increased production or decreased clearance of otherwise normal surfactant or production of an abnormal surfactant. Although hampered by the low incidence and prevalence of this disorder, clinical observations eventually identified three distinct forms of PAP: congenital, secondary, and idiopathic. The results of clinical, basic, and translational research have

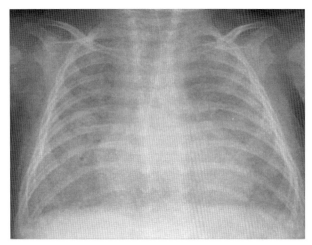

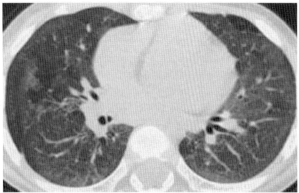

**Figure 18A.4** *Plain radiograph (top) and high resolution computerized tomogram (HRCT) (bottom) of the chest of an infant with ABCA3 deficiency. Both imaging studies demonstrate diffuse, ground-glass opacification due to an alveolar filling process.*

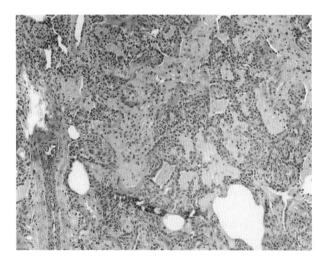

**Figure 18A.5** *Lung section from an infant with ABCA3 deficiency. The alveolar spaces are filled with macrophages, desquamated epithelial cells, and proteinaceous material. There is alveolar type II cell hypertrophy and widening of the interstitium. (See Plate 3 for colour version.)*

now demonstrated these three forms to be pathogenically distinct and the diagnostic and therapeutic approaches are quite specific to each form. Careful histopathological analysis and detailed molecular investigations demonstrated that congenital PAP is actually a heterogeneous collection of disorders that includes SP-B deficiency, ABCA3 deficiency (see above), GM-CSF receptor deficiency, and probably other disorders. Secondary PAP, while less well-studied, occurs in the setting of either decreased numbers or function of alveolar macrophages. Idiopathic PAP represents more than 90 percent of cases, although the exact incidence of each form has not been well established. Recent studies have identified idiopathic PAP as an autoimmune disease targeted at GM-CSF. This had important pathobiological and therapeutic consequences, namely, the development and testing of novel therapeutic approaches for PAP and the recognition that GM-CSF has a critical role in lung homeostasis. Consequently, the remainder of this section will focus primarily on idiopathic PAP.

## Idiopathic pulmonary alveolar proteinosis

### DEFINITION

Idiopathic PAP is a disorder characterized by accumulation of pulmonary surfactant in the alveoli and terminal airways, a variable clinical course ranging from respiratory failure to spontaneous resolution and a predilection for secondary opportunistic infections.

### EPIDEMIOLOGY

PAP is reported to occur in a worldwide distribution with an incidence of 0.36 cases per million individuals[55] and a prevalence of 3.7 per million individuals.[56] Idiopathic PAP occurs in previously healthy individuals and represents over 90 percent of PAP cases. While it occurs in individuals of all ages, the median age at the time of diagnosis is 39 years. No ethnic predominance has been reported.[57] African-American patients account for 17 percent of the reported cases in North America.[58]

### NATURAL HISTORY

#### Presentation

Recent analysis of PAP case reports and case series including one analysis of 410 separate PAP cases by Seymour, accounting for most if not all of the published cases has established the common clinical features of patients with PAP.[55,59–62] Acquired PAP presents in previously healthy individuals as progressive exertional dyspnea of insidious onset of approximately 7 months duration in about 75 percent of cases. However, in some cases, patients are symptomatic for much longer periods prior to diagnosis, while other individuals appear to present with more minimal symptoms. When present, cough is usually nonproductive or associated with scant whitish sputum. Less commonly, fever, chest pain, or hemoptysis may also occur, especially if secondary infection is present (see below). In most cases, the history does not reveal evidence of significant prior exposure to pulmonary toxins, e.g., metal dusts. The physical examination can be unremarkable, but reveals mild inspiratory crackles in 50 percent of cases, cyanosis in 25 percent of cases, and digital clubbing less frequently.

### Clinical course
The natural history of idiopathic PAP is variable with patients falling into three categories: stable persistent symptoms, progressive deterioration, or spontaneous improvement.[54] In the former, persistent symptoms may vary in intensity over time and respond to therapeutic whole lung lavage (see below), but subsequently recur. In others, the intensity of the disease is greater and patients progressively decline in pulmonary function despite treatment. A meta-analysis of 303 separate PAP cases for which individual patient records were available[55] showed that significant spontaneous improvement occurred in 8 percent.

### Survival
Based on a retrospective analysis of 343 PAP cases, the 5-year survival in individuals not undergoing whole lung lavage therapy is $85 \pm 5$ percent.[55] Of the deaths in this group, 72 percent were directly due to respiratory failure from PAP and 20 percent were indirectly due to PAP and uncontrolled infection.

### Secondary infections
Individuals with acquired PAP are at risk for secondary infections from a variety of microbial pathogens.[55,61,63] Although organisms that are commonly seen in community- and hospital-acquired respiratory infections have been reported, such organisms do not predominate. Thus, while *Streptococcus*, *Klebsiella*, *Hemophilus*, *Staphylococcus*, *Pseudomonas*, *Serratia*, *Proteus*, and *Escherichia coli* have been reported in PAP patients, a number of reports have identified 'unusual' organisms including opportunistic pathogens, such as *Mycobacteria*, *Aspergillus* spp., *Nocardia* and others.[55,61,64] While such infections are reported in the lungs, notably, a number of infections among PAP patients occur at sites outside the lung, particularly within the central nervous system.[55,65–67] This suggests that the predisposition to infection among patients with idiopathic PAP may represent a defect in systemic host defense rather than a consequence of local abnormalities within the lungs. In a comprehensive retrospective analysis, no disease- or patient-related factors were identified in association with the occurrence of opportunistic infection in patients with idiopathic PAP. Specifically, no abnormality of the numbers of circulating neutrophils has been reported in PAP patients who develop secondary infections. Similarly, such infections could not be linked to more frequent use of corticosteroids or smoking status. Interestingly, patients with opportunistic infections had a shorter duration of symptoms before

the diagnosis of PAP was made and were more likely to be diagnosed at autopsy than PAP patients who did not have secondary infection. The frequency of opportunistic infections in published cases has not changed over time.[55] Although the cellular or molecular basis underlying the propensity for secondary infections is unknown, the observation that anti-GM-CSF autoantibodies (see below) effectively eliminate GM-CSF bioactivity, systemically, in these individuals implies a potential role for this cytokine.

### CLINICAL EVALUATION

The diagnosis of PAP, often initially difficult due to the non-specific clinical presentation and insidious onset, is suggested by characteristic clinical and radiographic findings.[54,68,69] The differential diagnosis of the adult with PAP is broad because the disorder may simulate a broad range of conditions. The diagnostic evaluation includes a detailed pulmonary history and physical examination that focuses on exercise limitation and exclusion of other common cardiopulmonary conditions; chest radiograph and CT scan, pulmonary function tests; bronchoscopy with bronchoalveolar lavage (BAL) and transbronchial biopsy combined with special analysis of the BAL fluid and biopsies. These studies can usually establish a diagnosis in 75 percent of clinically suspected cases.[68] Open lung biopsy remains the gold standard for diagnosis of PAP, but is not always required and can be complicated by false negatives due to sampling error.[54,68,70] Recently, a serologic test has been developed for diagnosis of acquired PAP (see below) and is reported to have high sensitivity (100 percent) and specificity (98 percent).[71] A number of biological serum markers (see below) have been evaluated for the diagnosis of PAP that may be useful in following the clinical course of disease.[58]

### Radiographic findings
The plain chest radiograph reveals a patchy bilateral air-space disease often similar in appearance to pulmonary edema but without other radiographic signs of left heart failure (Fig. 18A.6).[54,68,72] High-resolution computed tomography shows patchy ground-glass opacifications with superimposed interlobular septal and intralobular thickening, which are typical but not diagnostic of PAP (Fig. 18A.6).[73,74] Notably, the extent of the radiographic abnormalities can be disproportionately greater than expected based on the associated symptoms and physical findings. While not specific for PAP,[74] the extent and severity of these radiographic findings correlate with degree of impairment in pulmonary function quantified by spirometry or arterial blood gas measurements.[73]

### Laboratory tests
In idiopathic PAP, routine hematological indices, blood chemistries, and urinalysis are frequently within the normal range.[61,68,75] More than 80 percent of patients have a slight to moderate elevation of serum lactate dehydrogenase, which

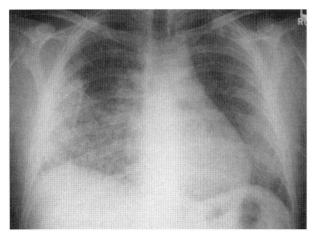

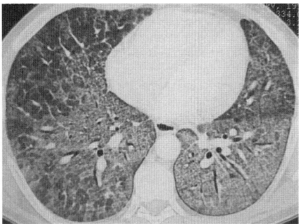

**Figure 18A.6** *Plain radiograph (top) and HRCT (bottom) of the chest of a 32-year-old male with idiopathic PAP. Patchy bilateral air-space disease is evident in the plain radiograph and appears as patchy ground-glass opacification with interstitial thickening on HRCT.*

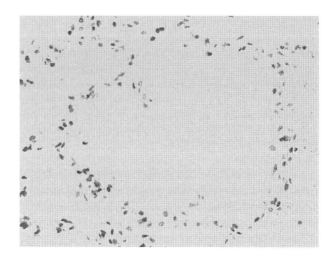

**Figure 18A.7** *Lung histopathology of an individual with idiopathic PAP. Note the fine granular eosinophilic material that completely fills the alveoli space and the normal appearance of the alveolar interstitium. (See Plate 4 for colour version.)*

can be a useful marker of disease severity or exacerbation.[55,76] Other serum markers include carcinoembryonic antigen,[77] cytokeratin 19,[78] KL-6,[79] monocyte chemotactic protein 1 (MCP-1), SP-A, and SP-D.[58,80,81] Of these, KL-6 has the highest specificity and sensitivity,[58] while SP-A and SP-D are not specific because elevated levels of these proteins occur in a variety of respiratory diseases. In more severe and untreated patients, PAP can result in elevated hemoglobin and hematocrit from chronic hypoxia.

### Arterial oxygen pressure

Hypoxemia caused by ventilation–perfusion inequality and intrapulmonary shunt results in a widened alveolar-arteriolar diffusion gradient ([A-a]DO$_2$) in nearly all symptomatic patients.[55,82] Retrospective analysis of arterial blood gas analysis in 410 cases of PAP revealed a $p_aO_2$ of 58.6 ± 15.8 mmHg at the time of diagnosis.[55]

### Pulmonary function

Spirometric evaluation can be normal, but typically shows a restrictive ventilatory defect with mild impairment of the forced vital capacity (FVC), total lung capacity (TLC), and a disproportionate, severe reduction of the diffusing capacity (DLCO).[55,83] This restrictive defect is partially reversible with symptomatic resolution either following whole lung lavage or spontaneous resolution.[55,58,59]

### Bronchoscopy and bronchoalveolar lavage

The diagnosis of PAP can frequently be made in clinically suspected cases by examination of the macroscopic and microscopic appearance of the bronchoalveolar lavage (BAL) fluid. The BAL fluid in PAP is milky in appearance and forms a waxy sediment upon standing. Microscopically, it is acellular with relatively few inflammatory cells. Alveolar macrophages are morphologically abnormal, ranging from small, monocyte-like cells to large foamy cells that are fragile and are destroyed during cytocentrifugation leaving large acellular eosinophilic bodies in a diffuse background of granular basophilic material. The extracellular lipoproteinaceous material and the material within alveolar macrophages stain positively with periodic acid Schiff (PAS) reagent and surfactant protein immunohistochemical stains.[68,84] Increased numbers of lymphocytes may be present, but relatively few other inflammatory cells are typically present.[84,85]

### Lung histopathology

The pulmonary parenchymal architecture is typically preserved in idiopathic PAP unless secondary infection is present. The walls of transitional airways and alveoli are usually normal, but are occasionally thickened by lymphocytic infiltration or less commonly fibrosis. Alveoli are filled with granular eosinophilic material (Fig. 18A.7) that stains pink to light purple with PAS stain. Intact, large foamy alveolar macrophages and apparently degenerating macrophages are usually evident within the granular material. Immunohistochemical staining reveals abnormally abundant accumulation of surfactant protein. Ultrastructural analysis shows that the intraalveolar material consists of amorphous granular debris containing numerous membranous structures resembling lamellar bodies and tubular myelin similar to normal surfactant preparations.

### Anti–GM-CSF antibody level

In 1999, the identification of neutralizing autoantibodies against GM-CSF in the BAL fluid from a small number of Japanese patients with idiopathic PAP was first reported by the laboratory of Koh Nakata.[86,87] Subsequent studies in larger series of patients from multiple countries demonstrated that this antibody is present in all patients with idiopathic PAP, but not in individuals with congenital or secondary PAP (see below), individuals with a variety of other lung disorders or normal individuals.[71,87–89] Anti-GM-CSF autoantibodies have been extensively characterized and consist of polyclonal IgG directed to various epitopes on the GM-CSF molecule with a high proportion of patients possessing antibodies directed at epitopes in the region of amino acids 78 to 94 of the mature peptide.[90] Various assays have been utilized to detect the antibody including Western blotting, latex agglutination, enzyme-linked immunoabsorbent assay (ELISA), and a bioassay using the GM-CSF-dependent cell line, TF-1, to determine the neutralizing anti-GM-CSF autoantibody titer.[71,87,90] The latex agglutination assay had a sensitivity of 100 percent and a specificity of 98 percent when tested on cohorts consisting of 24 idiopathic, four secondary, and two congenital PAP cases; 40 individuals with other lung diseases and 40 normal individuals.[71] The ELISA utilizes standards that permit an accurate determination of the amount of anti-GM-CSF autoantibody in affected individuals. This assay has now been tested on larger numbers of subjects and has a sensitivity and specificity approaching 100 percent and can be used with BAL fluid and serum from test subjects.[58,71,90] Interestingly, the total anti-GM-CSF autoantibody level does not correlate with DLCO while both serum KL-6 and serum CEA correlate fairly well.[58] One possible explanation derives from the fact that not all of the polyclonal anti-GM-CSF autoantibody present in PAP patients is capable of neutralizing GM-CSF. Future studies will be needed to determine if a correlation exists between the level of neutralizing anti-GM-CSF autoantibody and other biomarkers of disease severity.

## DISEASE MODELS

Murine models of idiopathic PAP, while discovered serendipitously, have had an important guiding effect on studies that have ultimately led to our current understanding of the disease as an autoimmune disease directed at GM-CSF. Since much of what we know of the pathogenesis of idiopathic PAP is directly or indirectly based on murine models that develop PAP, these animal models will be discussed prior to consideration of the pathogenesis of human idiopathic PAP.

### GM–CSF and GM-CSF receptor knockout mice
#### Surfactant homeostasis

GM-CSF, a 23-kDa cytokine expressed similarly in humans and mice, was purified in the 1970s, cloned in 1984, studied intensely over the following several decades and, prior to 1994, was thought to function primarily as a regulator of the growth of hematopoietic cells in the bone marrow.[91–93] Serendipitously and simultaneously, a critical role for GM-CSF in both surfactant homeostasis and in the pathogenesis of idiopathic PAP came in 1994 with the discovery that mice deficient in GM-CSF due to gene ablation (GM-CSF−/− mice) developed a pulmonary phenotype histologically similar to idiopathic PAP in humans.[94,95] While the absence of gross hematological abnormalities in these mice suggested that GM-CSF was not critical for normal hematopoiesis, the lung abnormalities linked GM-CSF with the lung and the pathogenesis of PAP because biochemically, histologically, and ultrastructurally, the murine PAP material was similar to that derived from acquired PAP in humans.[96] Surfactant accumulation in these mice was due to impaired pulmonary surfactant clearance due to decreased surfactant catabolism by alveolar macrophages.[94] The inability of alveolar macrophages to catabolize both surfactant lipids and surfactant proteins was also responsible for their abnormal foamy appearance.[97] Studies with mice in which systemic GM-CSF was deficient due to targeted gene deletion and where pulmonary GM-CSF expression was restored by a pulmonary airway-specific transgene, established the lung as the site of action for GM-CSF-mediated regulation of surfactant homeostasis.[98] However, these studies did not precisely identify the cellular target of GM-CSF, i.e., was the critical pulmonary GM-CSF regulation directed at alveolar macrophages or alveolar type II epithelial cells? This question was answered using another murine model of PAP caused by GM-CSF receptor gene ablation.[99,100] Transplantation of bone marrow from normal mice into GM-CSF Rβc−/− mice reversed the PAP phenotype thus indicating the site of action of GM-CSF to be regulation of alveolar macrophages.[101]

#### Role of pulmonary GM-CSF in innate immune lung host defense

Prompted by the clinical observation of unexpectedly frequent secondary infections in idiopathic PAP, pulmonary host defense was evaluated in GM-CSF−/− mice. Results demonstrated an increased susceptibility to pulmonary infection by bacterial[102] and fungal[103] pathogens and impaired pulmonary clearance of bacterial, fungal, and viral pathogens.[102–104] Alveolar macrophages from GM-CSF−/− mice were found to have a number of abnormalities in host defense functions, including impairment in cell adhesion, cell-surface pathogen recognition receptor expression, nonspecific and receptor-mediated phagocytosis, superoxide production, microbial killing, and proinflammatory cytokine secretion.[102–107] Expression of GM-CSF specifically in the lungs of these mice from a lung-specific transgene (SPC-GM-CSF+/+/GM-CSF−/− mice) prevented the defects in microbial susceptibility, pulmonary clearance, as well as the abnormalities of alveolar macrophage function demonstrating that GM-CSF plays a critical role in lung host defense.

### Alveolar macrophage terminal differentiation

The diverse nature of the alveolar macrophage abnormalities in GM-CSF−/− mice suggested the possibility that maturation of these cells may be arrested in the absence of GM-CSF. This hypothesis was supported by the observation that pulmonary GM-CSF regulates expression of the macrophage differentiation-inducing transcription factor, PU.1,[108] in alveolar macrophages.[107] Further support came from studies in which retroviral expression of PU.1 in cultured alveolar macrophages from GM-CSF−/− mice was able to restore all of the abnormal alveolar macrophage immune functions described above, as well as the defective surfactant catabolism.[104,105,107,109] In summary, the numerous and diverse defects observed in alveolar macrophages from GM-CSF−/− mice, all of which are coordinately corrected by either pulmonary GM-CSF expression in vivo or PU.1 expression (in the absence of GM-CSF) in vitro, strongly suggest that GM-CSF, via PU.1, stimulates the terminal differentiation of alveolar macrophages in the murine lung.

### GM-CSF 'therapy'

The observation that GM-CSF levels in SPC-GM-CSF+/+/GM-CSF−/− mice were 700-fold higher in the lungs than in blood suggested pulmonary GM-CSF may be compartmentalized by a 'lung–blood barrier.' These results further suggested that GM-CSF acts locally within the lung to preserve lung surfactant homeostasis and lung host defense. This was confirmed by correction of PAP in GM-CSF−/− mice by adenovirus-mediated GM-CSF gene transfer to the lung, i.e., 'pulmonary gene therapy.'[110] PAP in these mice was also corrected by aerosol administration of murine GM-CSF to the lungs.[111] Notably, systemic administration by peritoneal injection did not correct the lung disease in GM-CSF−/− mice. These studies demonstrate that PAP caused by the absence of GM-CSF can be corrected in mice by GM-CSF replacement 'therapy.'

Taken together, the serendipitous discovery and subsequent studies of PAP in mice lacking GM-CSF or GM-CSF signaling provided an important 'road map' for studying the pathogenesis and therapy of idiopathic PAP in humans.

## PATHOGENESIS

In their initial description in 1958, Rosen et al.[54] established the abnormal alveolar accumulations in PAP to consist primarily of phospholipids and proteins. While subsequent studies demonstrated this material to be surfactant, investigations over more than three decades failed to determine whether surfactant accumulation was due to increased production, decreased clearance, or the expression of abnormal surfactant lipid(s) or protein(s).[112] The most widely held theory during this time was that a presumed 'irritant,' e.g., silica dust or an infectious agent, for example, mycoplasma, stimulated increased surfactant production.[75,113] However, despite a prolonged search, no such 'irritant' could be consistently demonstrated in the alveolar material recovered from PAP patients. Ultrastructural,[70,114] biochemical,[115,116] and functional[117] analysis of the PAP material and data from murine PAP models, support a pathogenesis due to reduced clearance rather than overproduction or abnormal surfactant lipid or protein.[96]

In the 1970s and 1980s, a number of abnormalities of alveolar macrophages were identified in PAP patients. These included morphological defects such as giant secondary lysosomes filled with lipoproteinaceous material[118] and functional abnormalities, such as defects in chemotaxis,[118] adhesion,[118] phagocytosis,[119] microbicidal activity,[118] and phagolysosome fusion.[120] One theory held that these abnormalities were due to excessive ingestion of the lipoproteinaceous material, i.e., the 'overstuffed alveolar macrophage' theory.[121] Support for the theory was weakened by the finding that BAL fluid from PAP patients could recapitulate some of these abnormalities in normal alveolar macrophages.[122,123] Further, identification of an 'immuno-inhibitory' activity in the lungs and sera of these patients, that blocked mitogen-stimulated proliferation of normal allogeneic and autologous monocytes, suggested that a circulating factor might be involved in the pathogenesis of PAP.[124]

The identification of PAP in GM-CSF−/− and GM-CSF Rβc−/− mice prompted a re-evaluation of the pathogenesis of human idiopathic PAP with respect to GM-CSF. One early approach evaluating the systemic administration of recombinant human GM-CSF in one idiopathic PAP patient resulted in radiographic, physiologic, and symptomatic improvement.[125] However, treatment of additional patients had mixed results and failed to produce the expected peripheral neutrophilic response,[125] a curious finding confirmed in subsequent studies.[80,126] Paradoxically, GM-CSF was not absent in the BAL fluid and serum in idiopathic PAP, but rather, was increased in eight cases evaluated by several experimental techniques.[127] Further, attempts to identify mutations in the genes encoding either GM-CSF or its receptor in adult individuals with idiopathic PAP have been unsuccessful to date,[128] in contrast to findings in cases of congenital PAP (see below).[129]

This puzzle was solved by Nakata et al. who made a critical observation linking the pathogenesis of human acquired PAP to GM-CSF through a series of experiments that re-examined the 'immunoinhibitory' activity present in these patients. BAL fluid from PAP patients but not normal individuals inhibited the proliferation of GM-CSF-dependent TF-1 cells and competitively blocked GM-CSF binding to cellular receptors or an anti-GM-CSF monoclonal antibody.[86] Ultimately, the activity was shown to consist of polyclonal anti-GM-CSF autoantibodies primarily of the immunoglobulin G isotype class.[87] Importantly, these autoantibodies were present at high levels in all cases of idiopathic PAP, but not in any cases of congenital or secondary PAP, other lung disorders, or in normal individuals.[87] Further, they were present in both blood and lungs of PAP patients, bound GM-CSF with very high affinity, and were capable of neutralizing GM-CSF bioactivity.[90] Because anti-GM-CSF autoantibodies are present in PAP patients at levels exceeding normal circulating GM-CSF levels by up to 25 000 fold, GM-CSF bioactivity is absent in the blood and lungs. Thus, idiopathic PAP represents a 'functional GM-CSF knockout' equivalent to the GM-CSF$-/-$ or GM-CSF R$\beta$c$-/-$ mouse.

The absence of GM-CSF signaling results in a pattern of abnormalities of pulmonary cytokine expression that is similar in idiopathic PAP in humans and GM-CSF$-/-$ mice. For example, the macrophage growth and differentiation factor, macrophage colony-stimulating factor (M-CSF), is similarly elevated in both human and murine forms of PAP.[88,130] Similarly, monocyte chemotactic protein 1 is elevated in the lungs of both.[85,106] The mechanism of these cytokine abnormalities is currently unknown. However, the similar pattern of abnormalities in human and murine PAP where GM-CSF signaling is disrupted by very different mechanisms strongly suggests a common molecular pathophysiology.

Taken together, the observations on idiopathic PAP in humans and PAP in GM-CSF$-/-$ and GM-CSF R$\beta$c$-/-$ mice strongly suggest a common cellular and molecular pathophysiology wherein disruption of GM-CSF signaling impairs alveolar macrophage terminal differentiation and the ability to catabolize surfactant lipids and proteins, thus disrupting surfactant homeostasis.

### Monogenic disease components

There are no monogenic disease components that have been described in idiopathic PAP. In contrast, there are well-described monogenic components of congenital PAP arising from recessive mutations in the gene encoding the GM-CSF receptor (CSFR2B; see below). Previous reports have described the lung disease arising from mutations in SFTPB associated with SP-B deficiency as a congenital form of PAP. However, since the clinical features, pathophysiology, histopathology, and molecular pathogenesis of these two congenital lung diseases are quite distinct and now more clearly understood, disorders arising from SFTPB mutations should no longer be considered to be a congenital form of PAP.

### Complex disease components
#### Familial aggregation

No ethnic predominance has been reported in PAP. Notwithstanding, in one series of 15 patients diagnosed with PAP in Israel between 1976 and 1997, ethnic and familial clustering and the rarity of cases among Ashkenazi Jews was interpreted as suggesting a genetic predisposition.[56] Anti-GM-CSF autoantibody testing (see below) was not available at the time of this report, so the proportion of cases that were antibody positive in this report was not determined.

#### Linkage analysis
There are no linkage studies that have been reported in idiopathic PAP.

#### Association analysis
No data are available describing associations with human leukocyte antigen or other candidate genes. Seven of 410 published cases of PAP (two male, five female) were found to have had co-existing autoimmune disorders or positive autoimmune serology.[55] The autoimmune abnormalities included clinical rheumatoid arthritis in two cases, positive smooth-muscle antibodies in two cases (one with positive rheumatoid factor), immunoglobulin A nephropathy, multiple sclerosis, and possible celiac disease.[55]

### Environmental factors
#### Smoking
Smoking is associated with development of idiopathic PAP. Analysis of 410 published cases revealed that most PAP patients are men (male:female ratio, 2.65:1.0) and 72 percent had a history of smoking.[55] Interestingly, there was no gender difference among nonsmokers with PAP (male:female ratio, 0.69:1.0), suggesting that the male predominance may be linked to their more frequent use of tobacco.[55]

### TREATMENT

Early therapeutic approaches for PAP were empiric and included antibiotics, corticosteroids, digestive enzymes (streptokinase, trypsin), heparin, and mucolytics (acetylcysteine, potassium iodide, ambroxol).[55,75,114,131] The first effective therapy for PAP, performed in 1960 by Dr Jose Ramirez-Rivera, was an attempt to physically remove the accumulated alveolar material by 'segmental flooding' coupled with cough clearance.[132] The procedure employed a percutaneous transtracheal endobronchial catheter to blindly instill 100 mL of warmed saline drop-wise into an affected region of lung. This stimulated violent coughing typically productive of 30–40 mL of white viscid material. The procedure was repeated up to four times per day for 2–3 weeks with postural positioning to target different lung segments. Although impractical, radical, and not particularly well accepted at the time, with refinements this procedure ultimately led to the development of whole lung lavage.

### Whole lung lavage

Whole lung lavage is widely considered today to be the cornerstone of therapy for idiopathic PAP.[57,132–135] Despite wide acceptance, a standardized procedure for whole lung lavage has not been developed and no randomized trial or formal prospective trial has ever been conducted to evaluate its effects on the natural history of PAP. Specific criteria indicating the need for or timing of, or therapeutic response to whole lung lavage have not been developed. Commonly, the procedure is done under general anesthesia using a Carlens tube and mechanical ventilation. The patient is supine with the lung to be treated in a dependent position. The lung is filled to functional residual capacity with normal saline at 37°C with or without addition of acetylcysteine or heparin. Then, aliquots of 500–1000 mL of warmed saline are infused and then aspirated followed by vigorous endobronchial suctioning at the end of the procedure in order to remove as much of the accumulated material as possible. Chest percussion performed manually or mechanically, is used by some groups in an effort to maximize the removal of the accumulated material.[136]

Notwithstanding the lack of a uniform approach or prospective evaluation, a number of studies have shown that whole lung lavage improves the clinical, physiologic, and radiographic findings in idiopathic PAP patients.[83,134,137–142] In one meta-analysis involving 146 cases with adequate documentation, the 5-year survival in PAP patients undergoing whole lung lavage was higher (95 ± 2 percent) compared to individuals who did not have the procedure (85 ± 5 percent) ($P = 0.04$).[55] This study also showed that the interval between the diagnosis of PAP and the first treatment by whole lung lavage ranged from 0 (immediate) to 210 months with a median of 2 months. Fewer data are available from which to determine the length of the therapeutic effect. However, among 55 PAP patients for whom sufficient data were available, the median duration of benefit from lavage was 15 months.[55] Biochemical evidence also supports the therapeutic efficacy of whole lung lavage.[143,144] Lobar lavage by fiberoptic bronchoscopy has also been reported for the treatment of PAP, although the practical clinical utility of this approach is unclear.[140]

## GM–CSF

Prompted by the demonstration of PAP in GM-CSF−/− mice, Seymour first evaluated the therapeutic potential of GM-CSF in an individual with idiopathic PAP.[125] Daily subcutaneous injection of GM-CSF (up to 6 µg/kg/ day) was accompanied by significant improvement in exercise tolerance and reduction in the alveolar-arterial oxygen gradient ([A-a]DO$_2$) within 35 days after initiating therapy. Improvement deteriorated upon GM-CSF withdrawal and could be restored by reinstitution of GM-CSF administration. Seymour et al. then led a multinational trial conducted from 1995 to 1998 to test the effectiveness of subcutaneous GM-CSF administration (5 µg/kg/day for 6–12 weeks) in 14 PAP patients. Five patients responded to initial therapy with mean improvement in [A-a]DO$_2$ of 23.2 mmHg. The dose was escalated to 20 µg/kg/day in non-responders; the overall response rate was 43 percent.[80] An ongoing study, initiated in the USA in 1998, reported a response in three of four initial patients receiving daily subcutaneous GM-CSF injections in escalating doses over 12 weeks.[126] Responders had symptomatic, physiologic, and radiographic improvement and a reduction in [A-a]DO$_2$ from 48.3 mmHg at baseline to 18.3 mmHg after 16 weeks of treatment. Together, these reports[80,126] and an update of the American study reporting on their first 7 patients[145] indicate an overall response rate to daily subcutaneous GM-CSF therapy of 48 percent.[55] In Japan, a network of collaborating

investigators is evaluating aerosolized GM-CSF in acquired PAP. While early results from these trials are encouraging, no firm conclusions can yet be drawn regarding the effectiveness of GM-CSF therapy for acquired PAP. Interestingly, however, a decrease in pulmonary anti-GM-CSF antibody levels in association with clinical improvement has suggested that 'desensitization' to GM-CSF may be involved.[84,146]

### Other therapeutic approaches

Recognition of idiopathic PAP as an autoimmune disease mediated by the presence of high levels of neutralizing anti-GM-CSF autoantibodies suggests several alternative immunological therapeutic approaches. One potential approach is use of plasmapheresis to remove the antibody.[147] The potential beneficial effects of this approach include improvement in both surfactant clearance and host defense functions of macrophages due to improved GM-CSF signaling. Another immunological approach is the use of anti-B-lymphocyte antibodies to decrease the number of anti-GM-CSF antibody producing cells. Future studies will be needed to evaluate these potential therapeutic approaches.

## FUTURE DIRECTIONS

Great strides have been made over the last decade in our understanding of the pathogenesis of PAP, stimulated in large measure by the serendipitous finding that GM-CSF-deficient mice develop PAP. Still, the precise mechanism(s) by which GM-CSF regulates surfactant homeostasis have not been identified in mice or man. GM-CSF is clearly critical in the regulation of many immune and other functions of murine alveolar macrophages; however, the mechanisms by which these pathways operate have not been defined. An understanding of how GM-CSF regulates PU.1 levels in macrophages could provide important molecular targets of drug development eventually providing the means to regulate macrophage functions relevant to surfactant homeostasis and innate immunity in the lungs. Since the total anti-GM-CSF autoantibody level in idiopathic PAP does not appear to correlate with the disease severity, other correlates must be sought. It will be important to determine if the level of neutralizing anti-GM-CSF antibody correlates with disease. It will also be essential to understand if there is a genetic predisposition to PAP, as well as pharmacogenetic influences on responses to treatment. Finally, recognition of idiopathic PAP as an autoimmune disorder opens the door to a number of testable immunological therapies for treatment of PAP. Regarding this latter point, the National Institutes of Health has recently established the Rare Diseases Clinical Research Network, including the Rare Lung Diseases Consortium, the mission of which includes testing of novel therapeutic approaches for PAP.

## Congenital PAP

Cases of lung disease occurring in infants that resembled idiopathic PAP were reported in the 1950s and 1960s, but were not initially recognized as distinct from idiopathic PAP that occurred in adults. Congenital PAP was first recognized clearly as distinct from idiopathic PAP and likely genetic in origin in 1981, by the finding of four affected siblings in a consanguineous family.[148] Careful histopathological analysis and detailed molecular investigations have demonstrated that congenital PAP is actually a heterogeneous group of disorders with distinct histopathological features and a clinical course quite different from idiopathic PAP in adults. The disease arises from mutations in one of several genes including those encoding surfactant protein (SP)-B, SP-C, or the ABCA3 lipid transporter molecule (see above), or the GM-CSF receptor βc chain[149–152] (recently reviewed by deMello and Lin[153]). The treatment approach to PAP depends on the underlying etiology. Current therapy for congenital PAP is supportive,[153] although successful lung transplantation has been reported.[15]

## Secondary PAP

Secondary PAP occurs as a secondary consequence of clinical conditions associated with functional impairment or reduced numbers of alveolar macrophages. Such diseases include hematological malignancies, pharmacological immunosuppression, inhalation of inorganic dusts (e.g., silica) or toxic fumes, and certain infections.[129,154–160] Therapy for secondary PAP generally involves treatment of the underlying condition, for example, in PAP associated with hematological malignancies, successful chemotherapy or bone marrow transplantation corrects the associated pulmonary disorder.[158]

## Key learning points

### HEREDITARY SP-B DEFICIENCY

- Hereditary SP-B deficiency is a rare cause of neonatal respiratory insufficiency caused by mutations in the SFTPB gene.

- Infants with this disorder develop fulminant respiratory failure that is refractory to supplemental oxygen, mechanical ventilation, surfactant replacement, and extracorporeal membrane oxygenation.

- Pulmonary histopathology demonstrates copious amounts of proteinaceous material and desquamated epithelial cells within the alveolar space and ultrastructural studies show rare, aberrant lamellar bodies.

- SP-B protein is generally absent and SP-C is usually present as an incompletely processed, biologically inactive protein.

- Lung transplantation is the only therapy that has been demonstrated to prolong survival.

### ABCA3 DEFICIENCY

- The ABCA3 gene is highly expressed in lung; it encodes a 150 kDa protein that localizes to lamellar body membranes and is believed to mediate lipid transport.

- Mutations in the ABCA3 gene have been demonstrated in infants who developed respiratory insufficiency within the first 3 months of life.

- Abnormalities in lamellar body ultrastructure have been demonstrated in lung tissue from infants dying with mutations in the ABCA3 gene.

### PULMONARY ALVEOLAR PROTEINOSIS

- PAP occurs in three clinically distinct forms: idiopathic, congenital, and secondary, of which 90 percent of PAP cases are idiopathic.

- High levels of neutralizing anti-GM-CSF antibodies are present in all individuals with idiopathic PAP examined to date, but not in individuals with congenital or secondary PAP, other lung diseases or normal individuals.

- The levels of GM-CSF neutralizing capacity in individuals with idiopathic PAP are up to 50 000-fold higher than physiological GM-CSF concentrations.

- In mice, GM-CSF deficiency causes PAP due to impaired surfactant clearance by alveolar macrophages.

- GM-CSF, via the transcription factor PU.1, stimulates terminal differentiation of alveolar macrophages in the lungs in mice and likely also in humans.

- GM-CSF plays a critical role in pulmonary surfactant homeostasis and innate immunity in mice, and likely also in humans.

## REFERENCES

◆1  McCormack FX, Whitsett JA. The pulmonary collectins, SP-A and SP-D, orchestrate innate immunity in the lung. *J Clin Invest* 2002; **109**: 707–12.

2  Korfhagen TR, Bruno MD, Ross GF et al. Altered surfactant function and structure in SP-A gene targeted mice. *Proc Natl Acad Sci USA* 1996; **93**: 9594–9.

3  Botas C, Poulain F, Akiyama J et al. Altered surfactant homeostasis and alveolar type II cell morphology in mice lacking surfactant protein D. *Proc Natl Acad Sci USA* 1998; **95**: 11869–74.

4  Wert SE, Yoshida M, LeVine AM et al. Increased metalloproteinase activity, oxidant production, and emphysema in surfactant protein D gene-inactivated mice. *Proc Natl Acad Sci USA* 2000; **97**: 5972–7.

◆5  Whitsett JA, Weaver TE. Hydrophobic surfactant proteins in lung function and disease. *N Engl J Med* 2002; **347**: 2141–8.

◆6   Whitsett JA, Wert SE, Trapnell BC. Genetic disorders influencing lung formation and function at birth. *Hum Mol Genet* 2004; **13** (Spec No 2): R207–15.

◆7   Nogee LM. Alterations in SP-B and SP-C expression in neonatal lung disease. *Annu Rev Physiol* 2004; **66**: 601–23.

8   Nogee LM. Genetic mechanisms of surfactant deficiency. *Biol Neonate* 2004; **85**: 314–8.

9   Hamvas A. Inherited surfactant protein-B deficiency. *Adv Pediatr* 1997; **44**: 369–88.

10   Cole FS, Hamvas A, Rubinstein P et al. Population-based estimates of surfactant protein B deficiency. *Pediatrics* 2000; **105** (3 Pt 1): 538–41.

11   Lin Z, deMello DE, Wallot M, Floros J. An SP-B gene mutation responsible for SP-B deficiency in fatal congenital alveolar proteinosis: evidence for a mutation hotspot in exon 4. *Mol Genet Metab* 1998; **64**: 25–35.

12   Nogee LM, Wert SE, Proffit SA, Hull WM, Whitsett JA. Allelic heterogeneity in hereditary surfactant protein B (SP-B) deficiency. *Am J Respir Crit Care Med* 2000; **161** (3 Pt 1): 973–81.

13   Dunbar AE 3rd, Wert SE, Ikegami M et al. Prolonged survival in hereditary surfactant protein B (SP-B) deficiency associated with a novel splicing mutation. *Pediatr Res* 2000; **48**: 275–82.

14   Wallot M, Wagenvoort C, deMello D et al. Congenital alveolar proteinosis caused by a novel mutation of the surfactant protein B gene and misalignment of lung vessels in consanguineous kindred infants. *Eur J Pediatr* 1999; **158**: 513–8.

✳15   Hamvas A, Nogee LM, Mallory GB Jr et al. Lung transplantation for treatment of infants with surfactant protein B deficiency. *J Pediatr* 1997; **130**: 231–9.

16   Ballard PL, Nogee LM, Beers MF et al. Partial deficiency of surfactant protein B in an infant with chronic lung disease. *Pediatrics* 1995; **96**: 1046–52.

17   Klein JM, Thompson MW, Snyder JM et al. Transient surfactant protein B deficiency in a term infant with severe respiratory failure. *J Pediatr* 1998; **132**: 244–8.

18   Yusen RD, Cohen AH, Hamvas A. Normal lung function in subjects heterozygous for surfactant protein-B deficiency. *Am J Respir Crit Care Med* 1999; **159**: 411–4.

19   Quasney MW, Waterer GW, Dahmer MK et al. Association between surfactant protein B+ 1580 polymorphism and the risk of respiratory failure in adults with community-acquired pneumonia. *Crit Care Med* 2004; **32**: 1115–9.

20   Haataja R, Ramet M, Marttila R, Hallman M. Surfactant proteins A and B as interactive genetic determinants of neonatal respiratory distress syndrome. *Hum Mol Genet* 2000; **9**: 2751–60.

21   Marttila R, Haataja R, Guttentag S, Hallman M. Surfactant protein A and B genetic variants in respiratory distress syndrome in singletons and twins. *Am J Respir Crit Care Med* 2003; **168**: 1216–22.

22   Gong MN, Wei Z, Xu LL et al. Polymorphism in the surfactant protein-B gene, gender, and the risk of direct pulmonary injury and ARDS. *Chest* 2004; **125**: 203–11.

23   Lin Z, Pearson C, Chinchilli V et al. Polymorphisms of human SP-A, SP-B, and SP-D genes: association of SP-B Thr131Ile with ARDS. *Clin Genet* 2000; **58**: 181–91.

24   Max M, Pison U, Floros J. Frequency of SP-B and SP-A1 gene polymorphisms in the acute respiratory distress syndrome (ARDS). *Appl Cardiopulm Pathophysiol* 1996; **6**: 111–8.

24   Makri V, Hospes B, Stoll-Becker S, Borkhardt A, Gortner L. Polymorphisms of surfactant protein B encoding gene: modifiers of the course of neonatal respiratory distress syndrome? *Eur J Pediatr* 2002; **161**: 604–8.

26   Seifart C, Plagens A, Brodje D et al. Surfactant protein B intron 4 variation in German patients with COPD and acute respiratory failure. *Dis Markers* 2002; **18**: 129–36.

27   Selman M, Lin HM, Montano M et al. Surfactant protein A and B genetic variants predispose to idiopathic pulmonary fibrosis. *Hum Genet* 2003; **113**: 542–50.

28   deMello DE, Nogee LM, Heyman S et al. Molecular and phenotypic variability in the congenital alveolar proteinosis syndrome associated with inherited surfactant protein B deficiency. *J Pediatr* 1994; **125**: 43–50.

29   deMello DE, Heyman S, Phelps DS et al. Ultrastructure of lung in surfactant protein B deficiency. *Am J Respir Cell Mol Biol* 1994; **11**: 230–9.

30   Vorbroker DK, Profitt SA, Nogee LM, Whitsett JA. Aberrant processing of surfactant protein C in hereditary SP-B deficiency. *Am J Physiol* 1995; **268** (4 Pt 1): L647–56.

31   Beers MF, Hamvas A, Moxley MA et al. Pulmonary surfactant metabolism in infants lacking surfactant protein B. *Am J Respir Cell Mol Biol* 2000; **22**: 380–91.

32   Guttentag S, Robinson L, Zhang P et al. Cysteine protease activity is required for surfactant protein B processing and lamellar body genesis. *Am J Respir Cell Mol Biol* 2003; **28**: 69–79.

33   Ueno T, Linder S, Na CL et al. Processing of pulmonary surfactant protein B by napsin and cathepsin H. *J Biol Chem* 2004; **279**: 16178–84.

34   Li J, Ikegami M, Na CL et al. N-terminally extended surfactant protein (SP) C isolated from SP-B-deficient children has reduced surface activity and inhibited lipopolysaccharide binding. *Biochemistry* 2004; **43**: 3891–8.

35   Tredano M, van Elburg RM, Kaspers AG et al. Compound SFTPB 1549C–>GAA (121ins2) and 457delC heterozygosity in severe congenital lung disease and surfactant protein B (SP-B) deficiency. *Hum Mutat* 1999; **14**: 502–9.

36   Herman TE, Nogee LM, McAlister WH, Dehner LP. Surfactant protein B deficiency: radiographic manifestations. *Pediatr Radiol* 1993; **23**: 373–5.

37   Newman B, Kuhn JP, Kramer SS, Carcillo JA. Congenital surfactant protein B deficiency – emphasis on imaging. *Pediatr Radiol* 2001; **31**: 327–31.

38   Stuhrmann M, Bohnhorst B, Peters U et al. Prenatal diagnosis of congenital alveolar proteinosis (surfactant protein B deficiency). *Prenat Diagn* 1998; **18**: 953–5.

39   Hamvas A, Cole FS, deMello DE et al. Surfactant protein B deficiency: antenatal diagnosis and prospective treatment with surfactant replacement. *J Pediatr* 1994; **125**: 356–61.

40   Clark JC, Wert SE, Bachurski CJ et al. Targeted disruption of the surfactant protein B gene disrupts surfactant homeostasis, causing respiratory failure in newborn mice. *Proc Natl Acad Sci USA* 1995; **92**: 7794–8.

41   Tokieda K, Whitsett JA, Clark JC et al. Pulmonary dysfunction in neonatal SP-B-deficient mice. *Am J Physiol* 1997; **273** (4 Pt 1): L875–82.

42   Melton KR, Nesslein LL, Ikegami M et al. SP-B deficiency causes respiratory failure in adult mice. *Am J Physiol Lung Cell Mol Physiol* 2003; **285**: L543–9.

43 Foster CD, Zhang PX, Gonzales LW, Guttentag SH. In vitro surfactant protein B deficiency inhibits lamellar body formation. *Am J Respir Cell Mol Biol* 2003; **29**: 259–66.

44 Clark SC, Kamen R. The human hematopoietic colony-stimulating factors. *Science* 1987; **236**: 1229–37.

45 Tokieda K, Iwamoto HS, Bachurski C et al. Surfactant protein-B-deficient mice are susceptible to hyperoxic lung injury. *Am J Respir Cell Mol Biol* 1999; **21**: 463–72.

46 Lin S, Na CL, Akinbi HT et al. Surfactant protein B (SP-B)−/− mice are rescued by restoration of SP-B expression in alveolar type II cells but not Clara cells. *J Biol Chem* 1999; **274**: 19168–74.

47 Klein I, Sarkadi B, Varadi A. An inventory of the human ABC proteins. *Biochim Biophys Acta* 1999; **1461**: 237–62.

48 Lefevre C, Audebert S, Jobard F et al. Mutations in the transporter ABCA12 are associated with lamellar ichthyosis type 2. *Hum Mol Genet* 2003; **12**: 2369–78.

●49 Shulenin S, Nogee LM, Annilo T et al. ABCA3 gene mutations in newborns with fatal surfactant deficiency. *New Engl J Med* 2004; **350**: 1296–303.

50 Mulugeta S, Gray JM, Notarfrancesco KL et al. Identification of LBM180, a lamellar body limiting membrane protein of alveolar type II cells, as the ABC transporter protein ABCA3. *J Biol Chem* 2002; **277**: 22147–55.

51 Yamano G, Funahashi H, Kawanami O et al. ABCA3 is a lamellar body membrane protein in human lung alveolar type II cells. *FEBS Lett* 2001; **508**: 221–5.

52 Yoshida I, Ban N, Inagaki N. Expression of ABCA3, a causative gene for fatal surfactant deficiency, is up-regulated by glucocorticoids in lung alveolar type II cells. *Biochem Biophys Res Commun* 2004; **323**: 547–55.

53 Nagata K, Yamamoto A, Ban N et al. Human ABCA3, a product of a responsible gene for abca3 for fatal surfactant deficiency in newborns, exhibits unique ATP hydrolysis activity and generates intracellular multilamellar vesicles. *Biochem Biophys Res Commun* 2004; **324**: 262–8.

●54 Rosen SG, Castleman B, Liebow AA. Pulmonary alveolar proteinosis. *New Engl J Med* 1958; **258**: 1123–42.

◆55 Seymour JF, Presneill JJ. Pulmonary alveolar proteinosis: progress in the first 44 years. *Am J Respir Crit Care Med* 2002; **166**: 215–35.

56 Ben-Dov I, Kishinevski Y, Roznman J et al. Pulmonary alveolar proteinosis in Israel: ethnic clustering. *Isr Med Assoc J* 1999; **1**: 75–8.

57 Wasserman K, Masson GR. Pulmonary alveolar proteinosis. In: Murray JF, Nadel JA (eds). *Textbook of respiratory medicine*. Philadelphia: Saunders, 1994: 1933–46.

58 Presneill JJ, Nakata K, Inoue Y, Seymour JF. Pulmonary alveolar proteinosis. *Clin Chest Med* 2004; **25**: 593–613, viii.

59 Asamoto H, Kitaichi M, Nishimura K et al. [Primary pulmonary alveolar proteinosis – clinical observation of 68 patients in Japan]. *Nihon Kyobu Shikkan Gakkai Zasshi* 1995; **33**: 835–45.

60 Goldstein LS, Kavuru MS, Curtis-McCarthy P et al. Pulmonary alveolar proteinosis: clinical features and outcomes. *Chest* 1998; **114**: 1357–62.

◆61 Prakash UB, Barham SS, Carpenter HA et al. Pulmonary alveolar phospholipoproteinosis: experience with 34 cases and a review. *Mayo Clin Proc* 1987; **62**: 499–518.

62 Shah PL, Hansell D, Lawson PR et al. Pulmonary alveolar proteinosis: clinical aspects and current concepts on pathogenesis. *Thorax* 2000; **55**: 67–77.

63 Bedrossian CW, Luna MA, Conklin RH, Miller WC. Alveolar proteinosis as a consequence of immunosuppression. A hypothesis based on clinical and pathologic observations. *Hum Pathol* 1980; **11** (5 Suppl): 527–35.

64 Andriole MT, Ballas M, Wilson GL. The Association of Nocardiosis and Pulmonary Alveolar Proteinosis: a case study. *Ann Intern Med* 1963; **60**: 266–75.

65 Supena R, Karlin D, Strate R, Cramer PG. Pulmonary alveolar proteinosis and Nocardia brain abscess. Report of a case. *Arch Neurol* 1974; **30**: 266–8.

66 Oerlemans WG, Jansen EN, Prevo RL, Eijsvogel MM. Primary cerebellar nocardiosis and alveolar proteinosis. *Acta Neurol Scand* 1998; **97**: 138–41.

67 Walker DA, McMahon SM. Pulmonary alveolar proteinosis complicated by cerebral abscess: report of a case. *J Am Osteopath Assoc* 1986; **86**: 447–50.

68 Wang BM, Stern EJ, Schmidt RA, Pierson DJ. Diagnosing pulmonary alveolar proteinosis. A review and an update. *Chest* 1997; **111**: 460–6.

69 Fraser RS, Muller NL, Colman N, Pare PD. Pulmonary alveolar proteinosis. In: Fraser RS, Muller NL, Colman N, Pare PD (eds). *Diagnosis of diseases of the chest*. Philadelphia: Saunders, 1999: 2700–8.

70 Costello JF, Moriarty DC, Branthwaite MA, Turner-Warwick M, Corrin B. Diagnosis and management of alveolar proteinosis: the role of electron microscopy. *Thorax* 1975; **30**: 121–32.

●71 Kitamura T, Uchida K, Tanaka N et al. Serological diagnosis of idiopathic pulmonary alveolar proteinosis. *Am J Respir Crit Care Med* 2000; **162** (2 Pt 1): 658–62.

72 Preger L. Pulmonary alveolar proteinosis. *Radiology* 1969; **92**: 1291–5.

73 Lee KN, Levin DL, Webb WR et al. Pulmonary alveolar proteinosis: high-resolution CT, chest radiographic, and functional correlations. *Chest* 1997; **111**: 989–95.

74 Johkoh T, Itoh H, Muller NL et al. Crazy-paving appearance at thin-section CT: spectrum of disease and pathologic findings. *Radiology* 1999; **211**: 155–60.

75 De Sanctis PN. Pulmonary alveolar proteinosis: a review of the findings and theories to date with a digression on *Pneumocystis carinii* pneumonia. *Boston Med Q* 1962; **13**: 19–35.

76 Fountain FF Jr. Lactate dehydrogenase isoenzymes in alveolar proteinosis. *J Am Med Assoc* 1969; **210**: 1283.

77 Fujishima T, Honda Y, Shijubo N, Takahashi H, Abe S. Increased carcinoembryonic antigen concentrations in sera and bronchoalveolar lavage fluids of patients with pulmonary alveolar proteinosis. *Respiration* 1995; **62**: 317–21.

78 Minakata Y, Kida Y, Nakanishi H, Nishimoto T, Yukawa S. Change in cytokeratin 19 fragment level according to the severity of pulmonary alveolar proteinosis. *Intern Med* 2001; **40**: 1024–7.

79 Takahashi T, Munakata M, Suzuki I, Kawakami Y. Serum and bronchoalveolar fluid KL-6 levels in patients with pulmonary alveolar proteinosis. *Am J Respir Crit Care Med* 1998; **158**: 1294–8.

80 Seymour JF, Presneill JJ, Schoch OD et al. Therapeutic efficacy of granulocyte-macrophage colony-stimulating factor in patients with idiopathic acquired alveolar proteinosis. *Am J Respir Crit Care Med* 2001; **163**: 524–31.

81 Kuroki Y, Takahashi H, Chiba H, Akino T. Surfactant proteins A and D: disease markers. *Biochim Biophys Acta* 1998; **1408**: 334–45.

82    Fraimow W, Cathcart RT, Taylor RC. Physiologic and clinical aspects of pulmonary alveolar proteinosis. *Ann Intern Med* 1960; **52**: 1177.

83    Selecky PA, Wasserman K, Benfield JR, Lippmann M. The clinical and physiological effect of whole-lung lavage in pulmonary alveolar proteinosis: a ten-year experience. *Ann Thorac Surg* 1977; **24**: 451–61.

84    Schoch OD, Schanz U, Koller M et al. BAL findings in a patient with pulmonary alveolar proteinosis successfully treated with GM-CSF. *Thorax* 2002; **57**: 277–80.

85    Iyonaga K, Suga M, Yamamoto T et al. Elevated bronchoalveolar concentrations of MCP-1 in patients with pulmonary alveolar proteinosis. *Eur Respir J* 1999; **14**: 383–9.

86    Tanaka N, Watanabe J, Kitamura T et al. Lungs of patients with idiopathic pulmonary alveolar proteinosis express a factor which neutralizes granulocyte-macrophage colony stimulating factor. *FEBS Lett* 1999; **442**: 246–50.

●87    Kitamura T, Tanaka N, Watanabe J et al. Idiopathic pulmonary alveolar proteinosis as an autoimmune disease with neutralizing antibody against granulocyte/macrophage colony-stimulating factor. *J Exp Med* 1999; **190**: 875–80.

88    Bonfield TL, Russell D, Burgess S et al. Autoantibodies against granulocyte macrophage colony-stimulating factor are diagnostic for pulmonary alveolar proteinosis. *Am J Respir Cell Mol Biol* 2002; **27**: 481–6.

◆89    Trapnell BC, Whitsett JA, Nakata K. Pulmonary alveolar proteinosis. *New Engl J Med* 2003; **349**: 2527–39.

●90    Uchida K, Nakata K, Trapnell BC et al. High-affinity autoantibodies specifically eliminate granulocyte-macrophage colony-stimulating factor activity in the lungs of patients with idiopathic pulmonary alveolar proteinosis. *Blood* 2004; **103**: 1089–98.

91    Burgess AW, Camakaris J, Metcalf D. Purification and properties of colony-stimulating factor from mouse lung-conditioned medium. *J Biol Chem* 1977; **252**: 1998–2003.

92    Miyatake S, Otsuka T, Yokota T, Lee F, Arai K. Structure of the chromosomal gene for granulocyte–macrophage colony stimulating factor: comparison of the mouse and human genes. *EMBO J* 1985; **4**: 2561–8.

93    Rasko JE. Granulocyte–macrophage colony stimulating factor. In: Thomson AW (ed.) *The cytokine handbook*, 2nd edn. London: Academic Press, 1994: 343–69.

●94    Dranoff G, Crawford AD, Sadelain M et al. Involvement of granulocyte–macrophage colony-stimulating factor in pulmonary homeostasis. *Science* 1994; **264**: 713–6.

●95    Stanley E, Lieschke GJ, Grail D et al. Granulocyte/macrophage colony-stimulating factor-deficient mice show no major perturbation of hematopoiesis but develop a characteristic pulmonary pathology. *Proc Natl Acad Sci USA* 1994; **91**: 5592–6.

96    Ramirez J, Harlan WR Jr. Pulmonary alveolar proteinosis. Nature and origin of alveolar lipid. *Am J Med* 1968; **45**: 502–12.

97    Yoshida M, Ikegami M, Reed JA et al. GM-CSF regulates surfactant Protein-A and lipid catabolism by alveolar macrophages. *Am J Physiol Lung Cell Mol Physiol* 2001; **280**: L379–86.

98    Huffman JA, Hull WM, Dranoff G, Mulligan RC, Whitsett JA. Pulmonary epithelial cell expression of GM-CSF corrects the alveolar proteinosis in GM-CSF-deficient mice. *J Clin Invest* 1996; **97**: 649–55.

99    Hayashida K, Kitamura T, Gorman DM et al. Molecular cloning of a second subunit of the receptor for human granulocyte–macrophage colony-stimulating factor (GM-CSF): reconstitution of a high-affinity GM-CSF receptor. *Proc Natl Acad Sci USA* 1990; **87**: 9655–9.

●100    Robb L, Drinkwater CC, Metcalf D et al. Hematopoietic and lung abnormalities in mice with a null mutation of the common beta subunit of the receptors for granulocyte–macrophage colony-stimulating factor and interleukins 3 and 5. *Proc Natl Acad Sci USA* 1995; **92**: 9565–9.

●101    Nishinakamura R, Nakayama N, Hirabayashi Y et al. Mice deficient for the IL-3/GM-CSF/IL-5 beta c receptor exhibit lung pathology and impaired immune response, while beta IL3 receptor- deficient mice are normal. *Immunity* 1995; **2**: 211–22.

102    LeVine AM, Reed JA, Kurak KE, Cianciolo E, Whitsett JA. GM-CSF-deficient mice are susceptible to pulmonary group B streptococcal infection. *J Clin Invest* 1999; **103**: 563–9.

103    Paine R 3rd, Preston AM, Wilcoxen S et al. Granulocyte–macrophage colony-stimulating factor in the innate immune response to *Pneumocystis carinii* pneumonia in mice. *J Immunol* 2000; **164**: 2602–9.

104    Berclaz PY, Zsengeller Z, Shibata Y et al. Endocytic internalization of adenovirus, nonspecific phagocytosis, and cytoskeletal organization are coordinately regulated in alveolar macrophages by GM-CSF and PU.1. *J Immunol* 2002; **169**: 6332–42.

105    Berclaz PY, Shibata Y, Whitsett JA, Trapnell BC. GM-CSF, via PU.1, regulates alveolar macrophage Fcgamma R-mediated phagocytosis and the IL-18/IFN-gamma-mediated molecular connection between innate and adaptive immunity in the lung. *Blood* 2002; **100**: 4193–200.

106    Paine R 3rd, Morris SB, Jin H et al. Impaired functional activity of alveolar macrophages from GM-CSF- deficient mice. *Am J Physiol Lung Cell Mol Physiol* 2001; **281**: L1210–8.

●107    Shibata Y, Berclaz P-Y, Chroneos Z et al. GM-CSF regulates alveolar macrophage differentiation and innate immunity in the lung through PU.1. *Immunity* 2001; **15**: 557–67.

◆108    Lloberas J, Soler C, Celada A. The key role of PU.1/SPI-1 in B cells, myeloid cells and macrophages. *Immunol Today* 1999; **20**: 184–9.

◆109    Trapnell BC, Whitsett JA. GM-CSF regulates pulmonary surfactant homeostasis and alveolar macrophage-mediated innate host defense. *Annu Rev Physiol* 2002; **64**: 775–802.

●110    Zsengeller ZK, Reed JA, Bachurski CJ et al. Adenovirus-mediated granulocyte–macrophage colony-stimulating factor improves lung pathology of pulmonary alveolar proteinosis in granulocyte–macrophage colony-stimulating factor-deficient mice. *Hum Gene Ther* 1998; **9**: 2101–9.

111    Reed JA, Ikegami M, Cianciolo ER et al. Aerosolized GM-CSF ameliorates pulmonary alveolar proteinosis in GM-CSF-deficient mice. *Am J Physiol* 1999; **276** (4 Pt 1): L556–63.

112    Pattle RE, Thomas LC. Lipoprotein composition of the film lining the lung. *Nature* 1961; **189**: 844.

113    Larson RK, Gordinier R. Pulmonary alveolar proteinosis: report of six cases, review of the literature, and formulation of a new theory. *Ann Intern Med* 1965; **62**: 292–312.

114    Davidson JM, Macleod WM. Pulmonary alveolar proteinosis. *Br J Dis Chest* 1969; **63**: 13–28.

115    Singh G, Katyal SL, Bedrossian CW, Rogers RM. Pulmonary alveolar proteinosis. Staining for surfactant apoprotein in

alveolar proteinosis and in conditions simulating it. *Chest* 1983; **83**: 82–6.

116 Honda Y, Takahashi H, Shijubo N, Kuroki Y, Akino T. Surfactant protein-A concentration in bronchoalveolar lavage fluids of patients with pulmonary alveolar proteinosis. *Chest* 1993; **103**: 496–9.

117 McClenahan JB. Pulmonary alveolar proteinosis. *Arch Intern Med* 1974; **133**: 284–7.

118 Golde DW, Territo M, Finley TN, Cline MJ. Defective lung macrophages in pulmonary alveolar proteinosis. *Ann Intern Med* 1976; **85**: 304–9.

119 Harris JO. Pulmonary alveolar proteinosis: abnormal in vitro function of alveolar macrophages. *Chest* 1979; **76**: 156–9.

120 Gonzalez-Rothi RJ, Harris JO. Pulmonary alveolar proteinosis. Further evaluation of abnormal alveolar macrophages. *Chest* 1986; **90**: 656–61.

121 Golde DW. Alveolar proteinosis and the overfed macrophage (editorial). *Chest* 1979; **76**: 119–20.

122 Muller-Quernheim J, Schopf RE, Benes P, Schulz V, Ferlinz R. A macrophage-suppressing 40-kD protein in a case of pulmonary alveolar proteinosis. *Klin Wochenschr* 1987; **65**: 893–7.

123 Nugent KM, Pesanti EL. Macrophage function in pulmonary alveolar proteinosis. *Am Rev Respir Dis* 1983; **127**: 780–1.

124 Stratton JA, Sieger L, Wasserman K. The immunoinhibitory activities of the lung lavage materials and sera from patients with pulmonary alveolar proteinosis (PAP). *J Clin Lab Immunol* 1981; **5**: 81–6.

◆125 Seymour JF, Dunn AR, Vincent JM, Presneill JJ, Pain MC. Efficacy of granulocyte–macrophage colony-stimulating factor in acquired alveolar proteinosis. *New Engl J Med* 1996; **335**: 1924–5.

126 Kavuru MS, Sullivan EJ, Piccin R, Thomassen MJ, Stoller JK. Exogenous granulocyte–macrophage colony-stimulating factor administration for pulmonary alveolar proteinosis. *Am J Respir Crit Care Med* 2000; **161** (4 Pt 1): 1143–8.

127 Carraway MS, Ghio AJ, Carter JD, Piantadosi CA. Detection of granulocyte–macrophage colony-stimulating factor in patients with pulmonary alveolar proteinosis. *Am J Respir Crit Care Med* 2000; **161** (4 Pt 1): 1294–9.

128 Bewig B, Wang XD, Kirsten D, Dalhoff K, Schafer H. GM-CSF and GM-CSF beta c receptor in adult patients with pulmonary alveolar proteinosis. *Eur Respir J* 2000; **15**: 350–7.

129 Dirksen U, Hattenhorst U, Schneider P et al. Defective expression of granulocyte–macrophage colony-stimulating factor/interleukin-3/interleukin-5 receptor common beta chain in children with acute myeloid leukemia associated with respiratory failure. *Blood* 1998; **92**: 1097–103.

130 Shibata Y, Berclaz P-Y, Whitsett JA, Trapnell B. GM-CSF regulates innate immunity in the lung by coordinate, marked stimulation of phagocytosis, pathogen killing and toll receptor signaling in alveolar macrophages through the transcription factor PU.1. *Ped Pulmonol* 2001, Abstr. **22**: 279.

131 Diaz JP, Manresa Presas F, Benasco C et al. Response to surfactant activator (ambroxol) in alveolar proteinosis. *Lancet* 1984; **1**: 1023.

●132 Ramirez-Rivera J, Schultz RB, Dutton RE. Pulmonary alveolar proteinosis: a new technique and rational for treatment. *Arch Intern Med* 1963; **112**: 173–85.

◆133 Ramirez-Rivera J, Nyka W, McLaughlin J. Pulmonary alveolar proteinosis: diagnostic technics and observations. *New Engl J Med* 1963; **268**: 165–71.

134 Du Bois RM, McAllister WA, Branthwaite MA. Alveolar proteinosis: diagnosis and treatment over a 10-year period. *Thorax* 1983; **38**: 360–3.

135 Kariman K, Kylstra JA, Spock A. Pulmonary alveolar proteinosis: prospective clinical experience in 23 patients for 15 years. *Lung* 1984; **162**: 223–31.

136 Hammon WE, McCaffree DR, Cucchiara AJ. A comparison of manual to mechanical chest percussion for clearance of alveolar material in patients with pulmonary alveolar proteinosis (phospholipidosis). *Chest* 1993; **103**: 1409–12.

137 Wasserman K, Blank N, Fletcher G. Lung lavage (alveolar washing) in alveolar proteinosis. *Am J Med* 1968; **44**: 611–7.

138 Ramirez J. Pulmonary alveolar proteinosis. Treatment by massive bronchopulmonary lavage. *Arch Intern Med* 1967; **119**: 147–56.

139 Kavuru MS, Popovich M. Therapeutic whole lung lavage: a stop-gap therapy for alveolar proteinosis. *Chest* 2002; **122**: 1123–4.

140 Cheng SL, Chang HT, Lau HP, Lee LN, Yang PC. Pulmonary alveolar proteinosis: treatment by bronchofiberscopic lobar lavage. *Chest* 2002; **122**: 1480–5.

141 Beccaria M, Luisetti M, Rodi G et al. Long-term durable benefit after whole lung lavage in pulmonary alveolar proteinosis. *Eur Respir J* 2004; **23**: 526–31.

142 Ramirez J, Campbell GD. Pulmonary alveolar proteinosis. Endobronchial treatment. *Ann Intern Med* 1965; **63**: 429–41.

143 Hoffman RM, Dauber JH, Rogers RM. Improvement in alveolar macrophage migration after therapeutic whole lung lavage in pulmonary alveolar proteinosis. *Am Rev Respir Dis* 1989; **139**: 1030–2.

144 Bury T, Corhay JL, Saint-Remy P, Radermecker M. [Alveolar proteinosis: restoration of the function of the alveolar macrophages after therapeutic lavage]. *Rev Mal Respir* 1989; **6**: 373–5.

145 Mazzone PJ, Sullivan EJ, Piccin R et al. Granulocyte macrophage-colony stimulating factor therapy for pulmonary alveolar proteinosis. *Am Rev Respir Dis* 2000; **161**: A888.

146 Tazawa R, Ishimoto O, Ohta H et al. Granulocyte–macrophage colony stimulating factor and lung immunity in pulmonary alveolar proteinosis. *Am J Resp Crit Care* 2005; **171**: 1142–9.

147 Kavuru MS, Bonfield TL, Thomassen MJ. Plasmapheresis, GM-CSF, and alveolar proteinosis. *Am J Respir Crit Care Med* 2003; **167**: 1036.

148 Teja K, Cooper PH, Squires JE, Schnatterly PT. Pulmonary alveolar proteinosis in four siblings. *New Engl J Med* 1981; **305**: 1390–2.

149 Nogee LM, de Mello DE, Dehner LP, Colten HR. Brief report: deficiency of pulmonary surfactant protein B in congenital alveolar proteinosis. *New Engl J Med* 1993; **328**: 406–10.

150 Nogee LM, Dunbar AE 3rd, Wert SE et al. A mutation in the surfactant protein C gene associated with familial interstitial lung disease. *New Engl J Med* 2001; **344**: 573–9.

151 Nogee LM, Garnier G, Dietz HC et al. A mutation in the surfactant protein B gene responsible for fatal neonatal respiratory disease in multiple kindreds. *J Clin Invest* 1994; **93**: 1860–3.

152 Dirksen U, Nishinakamura R, Groneck P et al. Human pulmonary alveolar proteinosis associated with a defect in GM-CSF/IL-3/IL-5 receptor common beta chain expression. *J Clin Invest* 1997; **100**: 2211–7.

◆153 deMello DE, Lin Z. Pulmonary alveolar proteinosis: a review. *Pediatr Pathol Mol Med* 2001; **20**: 413–32.

154  Cordonnier C, Fleury-Feith J, Escudier E, Atassi K, Bernaudin JF. Secondary alveolar proteinosis is a reversible cause of respiratory failure in leukemic patients. *Am J Respir Crit Care Med* 1994; **149** (3 Pt 1): 788–94.

155  Keller CA, Frost A, Cagle PT, Abraham JL. Pulmonary alveolar proteinosis in a painter with elevated pulmonary concentrations of titanium. *Chest* 1995; **108**: 277–80.

156  Ruben FL, Talamo TS. Secondary pulmonary alveolar proteinosis occurring in two patients with acquired immune deficiency syndrome. *Am J Med* 1986; **80**: 1187–90.

157  Buechner HA, Ansari A. Acute silico-proteinosis. A new pathologic variant of acute silicosis in sandblasters, characterized by histologic features resembling alveolar proteinosis. *Dis Chest* 1969; **55**: 274–8.

158  Ladeb S, Fleury-Feith J, Escudier E et al. Secondary alveolar proteinosis in cancer patients. *Support Care Cancer* 1996; **4**: 420–6.

159  Doyle AP, Balcerzak SP, Wells CL, Crittenden JO. Pulmonary alveolar proteinosis with hematologic disorders. *Arch Intern Med* 1963; **112**: 178–84.

160  Garcia Rio F, Alvarez-Sala R, Caballero P et al. Six cases of pulmonary alveolar proteinosis: presentation of unusual associations. *Monaldi Arch Chest Dis* 1995; **50**: 12–5.

# Lymphangioleiomyomatosis

FRANCIS X. McCORMACK

## DEFINITION

Lymphangioleiomyomatosis (LAM) is an uncommon, progressive, cystic lung disease that predominantly affects young women. LAM presents with progressive dyspnea on exertion, chylothorax, and the highest rates of secondary spontaneous pneumothorax and recurrence of any chronic lung disease. The histopathological hallmarks of LAM are dilated, cystic distal airspaces and diffuse expansion of the pulmonary interstitium with spindle-shaped cells epitheloid smooth muscle cells. LAM lesions stain with smooth muscle markers and, curiously, with an antibody called HMB-45, which recognizes a protein epitope in the melanogenic pathway. Infiltration of tissues surrounding airways, vessels, and lymphatics results in airflow obstruction, hemoptysis and chylous reflux into the pleural, peritoneal, or pericardial spaces. In the most advanced presentations of LAM, the high resolution computed tomography (CT) scan of the chest reveals a dramatic and nearly pathognomonic appearance of reticular networks of thin-walled cysts. Airflow obstruction, gas trapping, hypoxemia, and a reduced diffusing capacity of carbon monoxide are the most common findings on pulmonary function testing. Many LAM patients have a benign, fatty renal tumor called an angiomyolipoma (AML), as well as axial lymphadenopathy. Lung function is lost at the rate of approximately 7–9 cc of $FEV_1$ per month, and respiratory insufficiency, including the need for chronic oxygen therapy, often develops. There are no known effective therapies, and lung transplantation is often performed as a last resort. Recent advances in our understanding of the genetic and cellular basis of cell growth dysregulation in LAM, many arising from the study of fruit flies, yeast, and worms, have led to the identification of well-defined molecular targets for clinical trials.

## EPIDEMIOLOGY

The LAM Foundation has registered 1028 LAM patients in 40 countries and on six continents. Case series of 30 or more patients have been reported from Asia, Europe, and North America.[1–6] Diligent efforts to identify all LAM patients in the UK, France, and the USA have revealed a minimum prevalence of approximately 1–5 per million and have suggested the existence of at least 6000–30 000 LAM patients on earth. LAM affects women almost exclusively, usually between menarche and menopause. However, rare presentations in prepubertal children and in postmenopausal women have been reported. All races and ethnicities are affected. In one LAM Foundation survey of 432 patients, however, Caucasians made up 91 percent, Asians 4 percent, African-Americans 3 percent, and Hispanics 1 percent of registrants. Access to healthcare, level of education, and use of the internet likely play important roles in the skewed ethnic and racial distribution for LAM reflected in the Foundation database.

## MONOGENIC DISORDERS

Cystic pulmonary changes consistent with LAM are present in up to one-third of postpubertal women with the neurocutaneous disease, tuberous sclerosis.[7–9] Tuberous sclerosis complex (TSC) is an autosomal dominant, tumor suppressor syndrome caused by biallelic mutations in either of two genes, *TSC1* or *TSC2*.[10] The classical manifestations of tuberous sclerosis are cognitive impairment, seizures, and skin lesions.[11] Although the disease is usually apparent in childhood, penetrance is variable and subtle adult presentations are not uncommon. In patients with TSC, germline mutations are found in the blood and 'second hit' somatic mutations, usually deletions, are found in the tumors and lesions of affected patients.[12] Only about one-third of TSC (and TSC-LAM) is inherited; the majority of cases arise from mutations that occur after conception. Rarely, TSC mutation-negative parents with multiple affected children are found to have germline mosaicism for TSC mutations (i.e., mutations are only present in the germ cells of one of the parents, not in their blood or somatic tissues).[13] TSC due to mutations in TSC1 is less common and results in slightly less severe disease manifestations than TSC2-associated disease.[14] Although it is clear that mutations in either locus can cause LAM, the number of genotyped TSC patients with LAM is small and it is not known how genotype affects the severity of pulmonary manifestations. In contrast to the profound gender restriction in LAM, there is no known gender or racial predilection for TSC. Biopsy-documented TSC-LAM has been reported in many women and in only three men,[15–18] but radiographically apparent cystic lung disease in males with TSC has been recognized in several series.[19] The estimated number of TSC patients worldwide is approximately 1.5 million, suggesting that there may be as many as 250 000 women with TSC-LAM on earth. TSC-LAM is heritable.[20] Although not carefully studied, there is a general impression that respiratory issues rise to the level of clinical priority in only about 5–10 percent of TSC-LAM patients.[21]

LAM also occurs in a noninheritable, sporadic form (S-LAM), in women who do not have TSC.[22] About 85 percent of 230 patients in the NHLBI LAM Registry[23] and LAM Foundation database, as well as most patients described in studies in the literature have S-LAM. Disease manifestations in S-LAM are usually limited to cystic disease in the lung, axial lymphadenopathy and renal, hepatic, or splenic angiomyolipomas.[22] In S-LAM, TSC mutations are detectable in the diseased lung and kidney tissue, but not in the normal lung, normal kidney, or blood, suggesting that two somatic mutations cause S-LAM.[24,25] To date, only TSC2 mutations have been described in S-LAM. S-LAM has been reported in postmenopausal females but never in males.

The observation that S-LAM is 10-fold more prevalent than TSC-LAM in pulmonary clinics, despite the prediction that TSC-LAM is 10-fold more prevalent on earth, has led to speculation that TSC-LAM is a milder disease than S-LAM.

## NATURAL HISTORY

LAM occurs predominantly in women, usually between menarche and menopause. The average age at diagnosis of S-LAM is about 35 years.[2,5,6] However, new diagnoses of LAM have been reported in patients ranging from age 12 to 75 years.[26]

LAM is usually recognized after a delay of 3–5 years from the onset of symptoms. Typically, patients are told that they have chronic obstructive pulmonary disease or asthma, and despite clues from the failure to manifest the exacerbations and remissions that are characteristic of those disorders, most will suffer at least one pneumothorax before the diagnosis is made. The clinical course is usually characterized by one of three patterns: chronic dyspnea, chronic dyspnea followed by pneumothorax, or pneumothorax without antecedent dyspnea. The most common presentation of LAM is slowly progressive dyspnea on exertion in the setting

of a normal or uninformative chest X-ray. The rate of loss of lung function is 90–110 cc of $FEV_1$ per year, or about 7–9 cc/month.[6,27,28] About 55 percent of LAM patients will reach MRC grade 3 dyspnea (shortness of breath after walking 100 yards on level ground) within 10 years of the onset of symptoms.[27] Over the same period, 23 percent will require supplemental oxygen.

Approximately 45–50 percent of women reported in clinical series complained of dyspnea on exertion at disease onset, but eventually 83–94 percent will experience exertional dyspnea.[3,6] Symptoms of cough, chest pain, hemoptysis, chyloptysis, and wheezing are each present in approximately 10 percent of patients at disease onset and 30–40 percent over the course of illness. Pneumothorax occurs in about 50 percent of patients at the time when symptoms develop, and eventually occurs in 65–80 percent of LAM patients.[29] Over 70 percent of patients with LAM who have a pneumothorax will have a recurrent event, either an ispilateral recurrence or a contralateral pneumothorax, and the average number of pneumothoraces per LAM patient that has had at least one pneumothorax is 3.5.[4,5]

Chylothorax occurs in about 10–39 percent of LAM patients at some point in their illness, and is the presenting manifestation in about 0–14 percent of patients.[30] Renal angiomyolipomas, unusual hamartomas containing fat, smooth muscle, and blood vessels,[31] are present in about 70–80 percent of patients with TSC-associated LAM and 50 percent of patients with sporadic LAM (S-LAM).[32] Spontaneous hemorrhage into angiomyolipomas may produce severe flank or abdominal pain, acute hypotension, and/or anemia, occasionally in association with circulatory collapse. Rarely, LAM presents as retroperitoneal masses or adenopathy which mimic lymphoma, ovarian or renal cancer, or other malignancy.[33] Large lymph filled abdominal lymphangiomyomas have also been described, and may vary in size with gravitational influences in supine and erect positions.[34]

The prognosis of LAM varies considerably. Johnson et al. recently reported a 91 percent 10-year survival from the onset of symptoms, considerably higher than the 20–80 percent 10-year survival reported in prior studies.[2,3,35,36] Although never proven, it is likely that patients who present with a sentinel pneumothorax without antecedent exercise limitation have a better prognosis than those who present with dyspnea. Similarly, screening of asymptomatic female TSC patients identifies a population with a more favorable prognosis and fewer and less severe pulmonary manifestations,[8] including lower incidence of associated manifestations of chylous pleural effusions, pneumothoraces, hemoptysis, and chest X-ray and lung function abnormalities.[37] Ascertainment biases related to screening and mode of presentation almost certainly play an important role in the differences in disease manifestations that have been described for TSC-LAM and S-LAM in the literature.

## PATHOGENESIS

Tumor suppressor proteins regulate orderly cell growth and differentiation by sensing the surrounding environment, transmitting signals to the nucleus, and directly affecting transcription, translation, or cell division. In the classic tumor suppressor 'two hit' paradigm,[38] a mutant copy of a growth control gene is inherited, and a tumor or dysplastic lesion develops when the second copy of the gene is inactivated through a random, somatic mutation. This second mutational event is often a large deletion, resulting in loss of whole segments of chromosomes. A polymerase chain reaction (PCR) technique can be used to detect the 'loss of heterozygosity (LOH)' for the region containing the genetic locus. When both copies of the TSC gene contain critical mutations, the protein produced by the gene is defective or deficient, function is lost, and cell growth, survival, or function becomes dysregulated.

Although TSC-LAM and S-LAM had identical histopathological presentations, the genetic relationship between these diseases was obscure until 1998, when loss of heterozygosity (LOH) for TSC2 was discovered in angiomyolipomas (AMLs) and lymph nodes from patients with S-LAM.[39] Missense and protein truncating TSC2 mutations associated with LOH were subsequently described in the lung and kidney lesions of patients with S-LAM.[25] Adjacent normal lung tissue and circulating blood cells were free from mutations, and within a given patient the mutations in the lung and kidney were identical, consistent with origin from a common precursor.[24,25] These data suggested that LAM may arise by benign metastasis of LAM cells from another site; perhaps a kidney tumor, axial lymph nodes, or a progenitor cell in the bone marrow.[40] Reports of recurrence of LAM in the donor lung of LAM patients who had undergone lung transplantation are also consistent with the metastatic theory,[41–44] including two in which the lesional cells were proven to

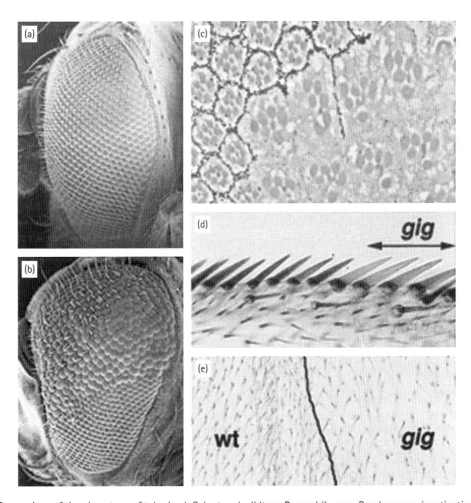

**Figure 18B.1**  *Comparison of the phenotype of tuberin-deficient and wildtype Drosophila eyes. Random gene inactivation was followed by characterization of eye phenotypes. Enlarged eyes cells in tuberin-deficient flies (b) compared to wildtype flies (a) were discovered. Phase microscopy revealed differences between normal pigmented wildtype eye cells (c, upper left), compared to enlarged, nonpigmented cells in tuberin-deficient flies (c, lower right). Bristles (d) arising from cells at the anterior edge of the wing were larger and less pigmented in those containing tuberin mutations (gig). Photomicrographs of cells in the wing revealed enlargement in those containing the tuberin (gig) mutant compared to wildtype (e) (From Ref. 48) (See Plate 5 for colour version.).*

originate from recipient tissues by molecular techniques.[44,45] Other rare diseases which result from metastases of benign smooth muscle cells in women include leiomyomatosis peritonealis disseminata, intravenous leiomyomatosis, and benign metastasizing leiomyomatosis.[40]

TSC is known to result from mutations in either of two tumor suppressor genes: the hamartin gene (*TSC1*) on chromosome 9 (9q34),[46] or the tuberin gene (*TSC2*) locus on chromosome 16 (16p13.3).[47] Hamartin has no informative homologies with other proteins in the NCBI database, while tuberin has a domain with GAP (GTPase activating protein) homology. Prior to 2000, all that was known was that tuberin and hamartin associate and restrain cell growth. Data from recent studies have shed light on the roles of tuberin and hamartin in altered cell function in TSC and LAM. Drosophila experiments have shown loss of tuberin results in a defect in cell cycle control, which causes cells to repeat S phase without entering M phase.[48] In these studies, tuberin and hamartin were found to be key members of the PI3K/PKB(Akt)/mTOR/S6K signaling pathway that regulates nutrient uptake, cell size, and cell proliferation (see Fig. 18B.1).[49–51]

Tuberin and hamartin associate into a complex that functions as a master regulator for the kinase mTOR (mammalian target of rapamycin, encoded by the FRAP1 gene in humans) in the Akt pathway, by modulating the activity of an intermediate G protein called Rheb (Fig. 18B.2).[52,53] The GAP activity of the tuberin/hamartin complex maintains Rheb in an inactivated, nonphosphorylated state (Rheb GDP). Phosphorylation of tuberin by Akt inactivates the GAP activity of tuberin/hamartin, and perhaps dissociates the complex. Tuberin can also be phosphorylated by a variety of mechanisms that are responsive to the energy and nutrient status of the cell. Tuberin GAP inactivation increases the abundance of Rheb-GTP, which phosphorylates the downstream target mTOR, which in turn phosphorylates S6 and the protein translation initiation factor 4E binding protein (4E-BP1). The end result is initiation of protein translation and stimulation of angiogenesis through production of vascular endothelial growth factor.[54] Thus genetic mutations that result in the absence or dysfunction of tuberin or hamartin, as occur in patients with tuberous sclerosis and LAM, result in constitutive activation of S6K and 4E-BP1, loss of growth control, stimulation of angiogenesis, and

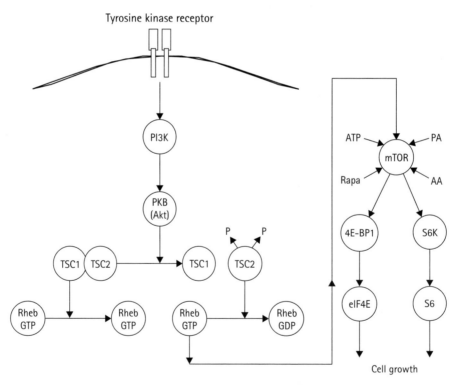

**Figure 18B.2** *Tuberous sclerosis proteins regulate signaling through the Akt growth and protein translation pathway. A phosphorylated growth factor receptor activates PI3K followed by Akt. Activated pAkt phosphorylates TSC2, which blocks its GAP (GTPase activating protein) activity. When not phosphorylated, TSC2 complexed with TSC1 functions as a GAP for Rheb, maintaining Rheb in an inactivated Rheb-GDP (guanosine diphosphate) state. Activated Rheb (Rheb-GTP) is therefore abundant when TSC1 or TSC2 is missing or when TSC2 is phosphorylated. Rheb-GTP activates mTOR in a manner that is potentiated by the availability of amino acids (AA), phosphatidic acid (PA), and ATP, and blocked by the absence of these substrates or the presence of rapamycin. Activated mTOR phosphorylates downstream targets S6K and 4E-BP1. pS6K phosphorylates S6 and 4E-BP1 releases eIF4E, which together activate the translational machinery and promote cell growth.*

inhibition of apoptosis.[55] Inappropriate cellular proliferation, survival, and/or infiltration can be blocked by inhibitors of Akt pathway signaling, such as sirolimus. Sirolimus binds to FK-506 binding protein 12 (FKBP-12, also known as FKBP1A) and irreversibly inactivates mTOR. Sirolimus has been shown to reverse the cell size defect in tuberous sclerosis flies and to shrink neoplastic growths in tuberous sclerosis rats[56] and mice. These studies form the basis for the trials of sirolimus in patients with tuberous sclerosis and LAM, currently underway in the USA and Europe.

## CLINICAL EVALUATION

### Presentation

LAM should be considered in any woman with an unexplained pneumothorax, particularly in the pregnant or young, nonsmoking patient. Chylothorax should also suggest the diagnosis in any female of childbearing age without a readily apparent alternative etiology. LAM can also present less frequently with hemoptysis (especially with exertion), chyloptysis, chyluria, chylous ascites, or chylopericardium. Rarely, abdominal complaints may predominate. Extensive lymphadenopathy may prompt an evaluation for malignancy, such as ovarian cancer or lymphoma.

A detailed history of dyspnea, exercise limitation, cough, expectoration, and pleurisy or atypical chest pain should be taken. Evidence for TSC, including a personal or family history of seizures or cognitive impairment, should be sought. Use of birth control pills or other estrogen-containing therapies should be noted.

### Physical examination

A careful skin examination by a physician who has expertise in the dermatologic and ocular manifestations of tuberous sclerosis should be performed. Typical findings include hamartomas of the retina, angiofibromas of the face, forehead patches, subungual fibromas and confetti lesions of the upper and lower extremities, ash leaf lesions and Shagreen patches of the trunk. Lung examination is usually unremarkable, but can reveal crackles in a minority of patients.

### Radiology

We recommend a high resolution CT scan of the chest in any young, nonsmoking female who presents with pneumothorax. Although large series report that the chest radiograph is retrospectively abnormal in most cases,[2,6] in our experience the chest X-ray can be deceptively unremarkable, even in the presence of moderately advanced disease.[4] Basilar reticulonodular changes are occasionally apparent, and lung volumes can be normal or increased. Cystic and bullous changes, pleural effusions (unilateral or bilateral), hilar and mediastinal adenopathy, and pneumothoraces may be apparent. High resolution CT scanning of the chest is the most helpful radiologic modality in LAM, and usually demonstrates profuse thin-walled (1–2 mm) cysts (2–40 mm in diameter) in all lung fields (Fig. 18B.3).[4] Diffuse nodular changes consistent with micronodular pneumocyte hyperplasia, a condition associated with innumerable adenomatous lesions composed of well-differentiated type II cells, may be present.[57] Mediastinal and hilar adenopathy are not uncommon.[4] Abdominal CT

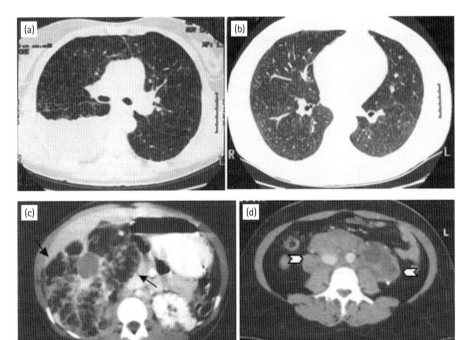

**Figure 18B.3** *Computed tomography of LAM. (a) High resolution CT of the chest showing diffuse cystic change and right pleural (chylous) effusion consistent with LAM. (b) High resolution CT of the chest showing diffuse nodular changes of multifocal micronodular pneumocyte hyperplasia. (c) CT scan of the abdomen showing large angiomyolipoma (arrows) containing abundant fat density. (d) CT scan of the abdomen showing solid and fluid-filled paraspinal masses consistent with LAM (chevrons).*

scanning is positive in over 50 percent of patients, and may reveal fat containing renal or extrarenal angiomyolipomas, axial lymphadenopathy, cystic or noncystic lymphangiomyomas, or chylous ascites (Figure 18B.3).[4] HRCT is recommended in all young women with tuberous sclerosis upon reaching maturity.[58] CT or MRI scanning of the brain is recommended at least once in the lifetime of all S-LAM patients to rule out findings of subclinical TSC such as cortical tubers, subependymal nodules, or subependymal giant cell astrocytomas.

## Pulmonary physiology

Lung function may be normal in LAM, especially in TSC-LAM patients identified through screening.[8] LAM most commonly presents with reductions in $FEV_1$ out of proportion to reduction in FVC, consistent with obstructive physiology.[59] Reversible airflow obstruction is present in up to 17–25 percent of patients.[4] Elevations in RV and the ratio of RV/TLC consistent with air trapping are frequently noted, and together with reductions in diffusing capacity, are often the earliest physiologic abnormalities to develop. Hyperinflation may also occur, which is unusual among the interstitial lung diseases. Mixed physiologic defects with superimposed restrictive changes are not uncommon, but it is unclear to what extent prior surgeries and pleural symphysis procedures may contribute to restrictive physiology. Impaired gas exchange and hypoxemia occur, but hypercapnea is rare even in end-stage disease. Diffusion capacity for carbon monoxide (DLCO) is frequently reduced, and in some cases may be reduced out of proportion to the obstructive defect.[60,61]

## Laboratory findings

There are no consistent laboratory findings or clinical markers that are helpful in the diagnosis or management of LAM. TSC1 and TSC2 genotype analysis on DNA from peripheral blood cells is commercially available, but mutations are not present in peripheral blood cells from S-LAM patients and the clinical utility of genotype analysis in TSC-LAM patients has not yet been established.

## Differential diagnosis

The differential diagnosis of pneumothorax in a young woman includes secondary pneumothorax related to asthma, emphysema, Langerhan's cell histiocytosis or other chronic lung disease, catamenial pneumothorax, and primary spontaneous pneumothorax.[22] The differential diagnosis of thin-walled cystic change on HRCT includes emphysema, Langerhan's cell histiocytosis, lymphocytic interstitial pneumonitis, bartotrauma associated with mechanical ventilation, Sjogren's syndrome, and Birt–Hogg–Dube syndrome.[62] Rare syndromes of benign or malignant smooth

muscle metastasis may also produce cystic change in the lung, including benign metastasizing leiomyoma and low-grade leiomyosarcomas.[63] Endometrial stromal sarcoma has been reported to mimic LAM.[64,65] Lymphatic malformations, such as pulmonary lymphangiectasis and diffuse pulmonary lymphangiomatosis, are usually diagnosed in childhood but can present in adults.[66]

## Diagnostic evaluation

The diagnosis of LAM can be made on clinical grounds without a biopsy in the presence of a compatible HRCT showing multiple thin-walled cysts and any one of the following: TSC, an angiomyolipoma, or a chylous effusion. Angiomyolipomas are occasionally visible on the abdominal cuts of the HRCT, but if not, an MRI or dedicated abdominal CT should be obtained to identify renal, hepatic, splenic, or paraaortic masses containing fat density that may obviate the need for biopsy. A CT or MRI of the head demonstrating subclinical subependymal nodules or cortical tubers can also establish the diagnosis of TSC noninvasively. In the absence of these corroborating features, thoracoscopic lung biopsy is usually prudent. Diagnostic transbronchial biopsy procedures are the exception in LAM, and we usually proceed directly to surgical approaches.

## Pathology

Grossly, the LAM lung is diffusely cystic and enlarged.[67] The pleural surface often reveals a remarkable profusion of blebs. Most cysts are 0.5–2.0 cm in diameter, but can measure over 10 cm. At the microscopic level, at low magnification, diffuse cystic change is apparent. LAM cell infiltration is typically found in small clusters or nests at the edges of cysts or along pulmonary lymphatics (Fig. 18B.4). LAM cells are identified by their round, ovoid, or spindle shape, haphazard arrangement, moderate eosinophilic cytoplasm, and fine or vesicular chromatin. In early stages, LAM cells may be inconspicuous but in more advanced lesions they may be so profuse that identification of normal structures becomes difficult. LAM cells stain positively with smooth muscle actin, desmin, vimentin, and HMB-45, an antibody which recognizes the epitope Pmel 17 in the melanin biosynthesis pathway.[68] It is unclear why the melanin pathway is perturbed in LAM.

## Treatment

### OVERVIEW

Patients with LAM should avoid exposure to tobacco smoke, discontinue estrogen-containing medications and supplements, and become informed regarding the potential risks of pregnancy. Current therapies for LAM are targeted at antagonizing the action of estrogen, especially

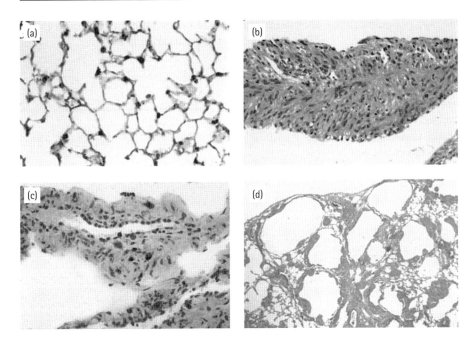

**Figure 18B.4**  *Pathology of LAM. (a) Normal lung histology; (b) Alveolar septum expanded by spindle-shaped smooth muscle; (c) HMB-45 staining of smooth muscle in LAM; (d) Smooth muscle infiltration, cyst formation, tissue destruction in LAM (See Plate 6 for colour version.).*

with progesterone- or gonadotropin-releasing hormone (GnRh) agonists, but there is no convincing evidence that these empiric strategies are effective. Pneumothorax should be managed aggressively with pleural symphysis procedures, because the likelihood of recurrence is >70 percent.[29] Large angiomyolipomas (>4 cm) should be evaluated for angiographic embolization.[31] Lung transplantation is an important option for patients with end-stage LAM and outcomes are similar to other diseases, but the perioperative bleeding rate appears to be somewhat higher.[69]

## PHARMACOLOGIC THERAPIES AND OTHER ISSUES

There are no properly designed trials to guide therapy in LAM. The retrospective studies that have analyzed the effectiveness of various treatments are inconclusive, flawed by unavoidable biases, and potentially misleading. Patients should be fully informed of the primitive state of therapeutic knowledge in the disease, the risks and benefits of therapy, and the option to be monitored without intervention. For asymptomatic patients, especially those with TSC identified through screening, observation is the most common recommendation in our clinic. In the face of worsening symptoms or objective evidence of disease progression, patients may be offered one of several empiric pharmacologic options including progestins (both oral and intramuscular) or gonadotropin-releasing hormone (GnRH) agonists. We generally recommend oral progestins at doses that are sufficient to suppress serum estrogen production (e.g., Agestyn 5–10 mg p.o. per day).[22] The suprapharmacologic intramuscular progesterone doses that have been propagated in the literature (e.g., intramuscular Depoprovera 400 mg every month) accumulate in fat, and may cause prolonged amenorrhea, fluid retention, and mood swings. Gonadotropin-releasing hormone agonists (e.g., Lupron)

have been used in patients with LAM, but benefits are unproven and induction of early menopause is often poorly tolerated in young women. There is no proven role for corticosteroids, immunomodulatory cytoxic agents, or ovarian irradiation in the treatment of LAM. Ovarectomy is rarely recommended by experts caring for LAM patients because the benefits are unknown and the risk of bone and heart disease is increased.

Patients should be advised that pregnancy has been reported to result in exacerbations of LAM, including decline in pulmonary function or pneumothorax in at least 10 percent of patients.[6,29] However, the risk of pregnancy in LAM has not been rigorously studied, and decisions regarding the advisability of pregnancy should be made on an individual basis.

A trial of bronchodilators should be considered in patients with LAM, since about 20 percent have been shown to exhibit reversible airflow obstruction.[4] Oxygen should be administered to maintain oxyhemoglobin saturations of greater than 90 percent with rest, exercise, and sleep. Bone densitometry should be considered in all patients who are immobilized and/or on antiestrogen therapies.[70] Calcium, vitamin D and bisphosphonate, or other therapies should be initiated in osteoporotic patients. Proper attention should be paid to cardiovascular health in patients who are rendered menopausal by therapy. Pulmonary rehabilitation should be considered for motivated patients.

The risk of pneumothorax in flight is small and we do not restrict air travel in LAM patients. Our recommendation is to obtain a chest X-ray prior to boarding a plane if pleuritic chest pain or new and unexplained shortness of breath is present.

Pleural disease should be aggressively managed.[29] We advocate the use of a pleural symphysis procedure on the first pneumothorax, given the >70 percent chance of recurrence.

Chemical pleurodesis (preferably with talc), mechanical abrasion, talc poudrage, and pleurectomy have all been effective in patients with LAM, but the failure rate of each approaches 30 percent, much higher than for other cystic lung diseases such as Langerhan's cell histiocytosis. Chyle does not cause pleural inflammation or fibrosis, and small chylous effusions do not always require intervention once the diagnosis is made. Shortness of breath may mandate drainage, however, and in some cases repeatedly. Pleural symphysis may be required to prevent nutritional and lymphocyte deficiencies that can result from repeated taps or persistent drainage.

As with other obstructive lung diseases, referral for lung transplantation should be considered as $FEV_1$ approaches 25–30 percent of predicted. Some patients who do not meet this criteria may qualify based on disabling dyspnea or problems maintaining oxygen saturation with lesser degrees of airflow obstruction. Although not studied in LAM, bilateral lung transplantation produces slightly better functional outcomes in other obstructive lung diseases, but is not always feasible due to the limited availability of organs and urgency of the need for transplant.[71]

Renal angiomyolipomas may require embolization or cauterization if bleeding occurs, which is thought to be more common when the diameter of the tumor exceeds 4 cm. Nephron-sparing partial resection is an alternative approach for large tumors. Resection of the kidney for AML may be required in special cases or for life-threatening hemorrhage, but too often is a regrettable and unnecessary consequence of unfamiliarity with the recognition and management of AML.[31]

## Disease models

There are no known animal models which exhibit pulmonary pathology that is characteristic of LAM. Epistatic analyses using readouts of larval, eye cell, and whole animal size have proven to be a spectacularly powerful tool in deciphering the complex circuitry of the mTOR pathway.[72] The Eker rat, which harbors a naturally occurring mutation in the TSC2 locus, develops renal cystadenomas, uterine leiomyomas, and extremity angiosarcomas.[73] Cell lines derived from the Eker uterine leiomyomas (called ELT3) exhibit LOH for TSC2 and estrogen-dependent growth, making them a useful cell model for LAM.[55] TSC1 and TSC2 heterozygous null mice also develop renal adenomas, as well as smooth muscle and endothelial cell-rich, HMB-45 positive hepatic hemangiomas. Sex-dependent hemorrhage into the liver lesions of TSC1+/− mice results in lethality in approximately 45 percent of the females and 10 percent of the males by 18 months of age.[74] This liver lesion is currently being studied as a model to test antiestrogen strategies in LAM. TSC1+/− and TSC2+/− mice have elevated VEGF levels.[75] TSC1 and TSC2 homozygous null mice die in utero at gestational day 9 of hepatic agenesis, but tissue-specific conditional knockout mice develop authentic TSC features, including seizures and cardiac rhabdomyomas.

## FUTURE DIRECTIONS

Trials of mTOR inhibitors in LAM are underway. The role of estrogen, metastasis, angiogenesis, and matrix degrading enzymes in the progression of LAM are important future therapeutic targets which are just beginning to be explored.

The gender restriction in LAM is the most striking of any human condition outside of diseases of the reproductive tract. Several investigators have postulated that estrogen plays a role in LAM cell migration, infiltration, proliferation, or secretion of destructive proteases.[76,77] Estrogen has been shown to modulate signaling through the Akt pathway that is known to be dysregulated in LAM,[77,78] and may contribute to the modulation of genes that play a causative or permissive role in a variety of pathological cellular processes. All of the advances in the genetics and signaling biology of LAM in the past 5 years notwithstanding, our understanding of the pathogenesis of LAM will remain woefully incomplete until the molecular basis of hormonal influences in LAM is revealed.

The evidence that LAM cells can metastasize is incontrovertible, at least in the two cases verified using genetic markers. It is unclear if all LAM is metastatic, however. Only 50 percent of sporadic LAM patients have angiomyolipomas, so AMLs cannot be the only source.[32] It is possible that a tuberin- or hamartin-deficient stem cell that originates in the bone marrow or the lymphatic system seeds the lung and the kidney. Identification of the source of LAM cells may suggest therapeutic strategies and prophylactic interventions.

Inhibition of matrix degrading enzymes may prevent cyst formation in LAM. LAM lesions have been shown to be associated with protease imbalances, including upregulation of MMP-2 and MMP-9,[79,80] and downregulation of TIMP-3.[81] Several metalloproteinase inhibitors are currently undergoing clinical testing in other diseases.

Loss of TSC2 results in accumulation of HIF1-α and increased expression of HIF-responsive genes including vascular endothelial growth factor (VEGF).[54,82,83] TSC1+/− mice have elevated levels of VEGF in hepatic lesions and in serum.[75] mTOR-independent pathways also clearly regulate VEGF production in TSC2 null cells, however, based on the observation that sirolimus only partially inhibits VEGF production. Angiogenesis inhibitors (which include rapamycin) are certainly attractive candidates for future LAM trials.

Other promising drug categories include farnesyl transferase inhibitors, which interfere with the action of Rheb, and cytokines such as interferon-γ, which has a beneficial effect on renal tumor size in TSC2+/− mice.[21,84] Combination therapies of mTOR inhibitors with metalloproteinase inhibitors, cytokines, farnesyl transferase inhibitors, estrogen blocking agents, and angiogenesis inhibitors may ultimately be the most promising approach to address the mTOR-dependent and mTOR-independent consequences of TSC1 and TSC2 deficiency.

## Key learning points

- LAM is a rare cystic lung disease that affects women almost exclusively.

- Both S-LAM and TSC-LAM are caused by mutations in tuberous sclerosis genes, which result in deficiency or defective function of the tuberin/hamartin complex that regulates activation of mTOR, a master switch that interprets the nutrient and energy status of the cell and governs cell growth and survival.

- Currently available approaches to management of LAM include observation and antagonism of estrogen action. A trial of symptomatic treatment with bronchodilators is recommended. Supplemental oxygen therapy may also be required.

- Recurrent pneumothorax is common in LAM, and we recommend that the initial event should be aggressively managed with pleurodesis.

- Rapamycin, an irreversible mTOR inhibitor, corrects the cell size defect in tuberous sclerosis Drosophila models and shrinks hepatic and renal tumors in tuberous sclerosis rodents. Rapamycin is currently being tested in clinical trials in patients with TSC and LAM.

- Support organizations available for LAM patients include The LAM Foundation (www.lam.uc.edu), LAM organizations in Japan (JLAM), France (FLAM), England (LAM Action), New Zealand (LAM Trust), Italy, and The Tuberous Sclerosis Alliance (www.tsa.org).

## REFERENCES

◆1  Oh YM, Mo EK, Jang SH et al. Pulmonary lymphangioleio-myomatosis in Korea. *Thorax* 1999; **54**: 618–21.

◆2  Kitaichi M, Nishimura K, Itoh H, Izumi T. Pulmonary lymphangioleiomyomatosis: a report of 46 patients including a clinicopathologic study of prognostic factors. *Am J Respir Crit Care Med* 1995; **151**: 527–33.

◆3  Taylor JR, Ryu J, Colby TV, Raffin TA. Lymphangioleiomyomatosis. Clinical course in 32 patients. *New Engl J Med* 1990; **323**: 1254–60.

◆4  Chu SC, Horiba K, Usuki J et al. Comprehensive evaluation of 35 patients with lymphangioleiomyomatosis. *Chest* 1999; **115**: 1041–52.

◆5  Johnson SR, Tattersfield AE. Treatment and outcome of lymphangioleiomyomatosis in the UK. *Am J Respir Crit Care Med* 1997; **155**: A327.

◆6  Urban T, Lazor R, Lacronique J et al. Pulmonary lymphangioleiomyomatosis. A study of 69 patients. Groupe d'Etudes et de Recherche sur les Maladies 'Orphelines' Pulmonaires (GERM'O'P). *Medicine* 1999; **78**: 321–37.

●7  Costello LC, Hartman TE, Ryu JH. High frequency of pulmonary lymphangioleiomyomatosis in women with tuberous sclerosis complex. *Mayo Clin Proc* 2000; **75**: 591–4.

8  Franz DN, Brody A, Meyer C et al. Mutational and radiographic analysis of pulmonary disease consistent with lymphangioleiomyomatosis and micronodular pneumocyte hyperplasia in women with tuberous sclerosis. *Am J Respir Crit Care Med* 2001; **164**: 661–8.

9  Moss J, Avila NA, Barnes PM et al. Prevalence and clinical characteristics of lymphangioleiomyomatosis (LAM) in patients with tuberous sclerosis complex. *Am J Respir Crit Care Med* 2001; **164**: 669–71.

10  Cheadle JP, Reeve MP, Sampson JR, Kwiatkowski DJ. Molecular genetic advances in tuberous sclerosis. *Hum Genet* 2000; **107**: 97–114.

11  Gomez M, Sampson J, Whittemore V. *The tuberous sclerosis complex*, 3rd edn. Oxford, UK: Oxford University Press, 1999.

12  Jones AC, Shyamsundar MM, Thomas MW et al. Comprehensive mutation analysis of TSC1 and TSC2 and phenotypic correlations in 150 families with tuberous sclerosis. *Am J Hum Genet* 1999; **64**: 1305–15.

13  Kwiatkowska J, Wigowska-Sowinska J, Napierala D et al. Mosaicism in tuberous sclerosis as a potential cause of the failure of molecular diagnosis. *New Engl J Med* 1999; **340**: 703–7.

14  Dabora SL, Jozwiak S, Franz DN et al. Mutational analysis in a cohort of 224 tuberous sclerosis patients indicates increased severity of TSC2, compared with TSC1, disease in multiple organs. *Am J Hum Genet* 2001; **68**: 64–80.

15  Aubry MC, Myers JL, Ryu JH et al. Pulmonary lymphangioleiomyomatosis in a man. *Am J Respir Crit Care Med* 2000; **162**(2 Pt 1): 749–52.

16  Korobowicz E, Sierocinska-Sawa J. Pulmonary lymphangioleiomyomatosis – a case report. *Pol J Pathol* 1996; **47**: 83–6.

17  Kaptanoglu M, Hatipoglu A, Kutluay L et al. Bilateral chylothorax caused by pleuropulmonary lymphangiomyomatosis: a challenging problem in thoracic surgery. *Scand Cardiovasc J* 2001; **35**: 151–4.

18  Kim NR, Chung MP, Park CK et al. Pulmonary lymphangioleiomyomatosis and multiple hepatic angiomyolipomas in a man. *Pathol Int* 2003; **53**: 231–5.

19  Dwyer JM, Hickie JB, Garvan J. Pulmonary tuberous sclerosis. Report of three patients and a review of the literature. *Q J Med* 1971; **40**: 115–25.

20  Slingerland JM, Grossman RF, Chamerlain D, Tremblay CE. Pulmonary manifestations of tuberous sclerosis in first degree realtives. *Thorax* 1989; **44**: 212–4.

◆21  Kwiatkowski DJ. Rhebbing up mTOR: new Insights on TSC1 and TSC2, and the pathogenesis of tuberous sclerosis. *Cancer Biol Ther* 2003; **2**: 471–6.

◆22  Sullivan EJ. Lymphangioleiomyomatosis: a review. *Chest* 1998; **114**: 1689–703.

23 Sullivan EJ, Beck GJ, Peavy HH, Fanburg BL. Lymphangioleiomyomatosis Registry. *Chest* 1999; **115**: 301.

24 Astrinidis A, Khare L, Carsillo T et al. Mutational analysis of the tuberous sclerosis gene TSC2 in patients with pulmonary lymphangioleiomyomatosis. *J Med Genet* 2000; **37**: 55–7.

●25 Carsillo T, Astrinidis A, Henske E. Mutations in the tuberous sclerosis complex gene TSC2 are a cause of sporadic pulmonary lymphangioleiomyomatosis. *Proc Natl Acad Sci USA* 2000; **97**: 6085–90.

26 Baldi S, Papotti M, Valente ML et al. Pulmonary lymphangioleiomyomatosis in postmenopausal women: report of two cases and review of the literature. *Eur Respir J* 1994; **7**: 1013–6.

27 Johnson SR, Whale CI, Hubbard RB et al. Survival and disease progression in UK patients with lymphangioleiomyomatosis. *Thorax* 2004; **59**: 800–3.

28 Johnson SR, Tattersfield AE. Clinical experience of lymphangioleiomyomatosis in the UK. *Thorax* 2000; **55**: 1052–7.

❉29 Almoosa KF et al. Clinical features and management of pneumothorax in lymphangioleiomyomatosis. Submitted.

◆30 Ryu JH, Doerr CH, Fisher SD et al. Chylothorax in lymphangioleiomyomatosis. *Chest* 2003; **123**: 623–7.

31 Bissler JJ, Kingswood JC. Renal angiomyolipomata. *Kid Intl* 2004; **66**: 924–34.

32 Bernstein SM, Newell JD Jr, Adamczyk D et al. How common are renal angiomyolipomas in patients with pulmonary lymphangiomyomatosis? *Am J Respir Crit Care Med* 1995; **152**: 2138–43.

33 Matsui K, Tatsuguchi A, Valencia J et al. Extrapulmonary lymphangioleiomyomatosis (LAM): clinicopathologic features in 22 cases. *Hum Pathol* 2000; **31**: 1242–8.

34 Avila NA, Bechtle J, Dwyer AJ et al. Lymphangioleiomyomatosis: CT of diurnal variation of lymphangioleiomyomas. *Radiology* 2001; **221**: 415–21.

35 Silverstein EF, Ellis K, Wolff M, Jaretzki A 3rd. Pulmonary lymphangiomyomatosis. *Am J Roentgenol Radium Ther Nucl Med* 1974; **120**: 832–50.

36 Corrin B, Leibow AA, Friedman PJ. Pulmonary lymphangiomyomatosis: a review. *Am J Pathol* 1975; **79**: 348–82.

37 Castro M, Shepherd CW, Gomez MR et al. Pulmonary tuberous sclerosis. *Chest* 1995; **107**: 189–95.

38 Knudson AG. Two genetic hits (more or less) to cancer. *Nat Rev Cancer* 2001; **1**: 157–62.

●39 Smolarek TA, Wessner LL, McCormack FX et al. Evidence that lymphangiomyomatosis is caused by TSC2 mutations: chromosome 16p13 loss of heterozygosity in angiomyolipomas and lymph nodes from women with lymphangiomyomatosis. *Am J Hum Genet* 1998; **62**: 810–5.

40 Henske EP. Metastasis of benign tumor cells in tuberous sclerosis complex. *Genes Chromosomes Cancer* 2003; **38**: 376–81.

41 Bittmann I, Dose TB, Miller C et al. Lymphangioleiomyomatosis: recurrence after single lung transplantations. *Hum Pathol* 1997; **28**: 1420–3.

42 Nine JS, Yousem SA, Paradis IL et al. Lymphangioleiomyomatosis: recurrence after lung transplantation. *J Heart Lung Transplant* 1994; **13**: 714–9.

43 O'Brien JD, Lium JH, Parosa JF et al. Lymphangioleiomyomatosis recurrence in the allograft after single lung transplantation. *Am J Respir Crit Care Med* 1995; **151**: 2033–6.

44 Bittmann I, Rolf B, Amann G, Lohrs U. Recurrence of lymphangioleiomyomatosis after single lung transplantation: new insights into pathogenesis. *Hum Pathol* 2003; **34**: 95–8.

●45 Karbowniczek M, Astrinidis A, Balsara BR et al. Recurrent lymphangiomyomatosis after transplantation: genetic analyses reveal a metastatic mechanism. *Am J Respir Crit Care Med* 2002; **31**: 31.

●46 van Slegtenhorst M, de Hoogt R, Hermans C et al. Identification of the tuberous sclerosis gene TSC1 on chromosome 9q34. *Science* 1997; **277**: 805–8.

●47 The European Chromosome 16 Tuberous Sclerosis Consortium. Identification and characterization of the tuberous sclerosis gene on chromosome 16. *Cell* 1993; **75**: 1305–15.

●48 Ito N, Rubin GM. Gigas, a Drosophila homolog of tuberous sclerosis gene product-2, regulates the cell cycle. *Cell* 1999; **96**: 529–39.

49 Potter CJ, Huang H, Xu T. Drosophila TSC1 functions with TSC2 to antagonize insulin signaling in regulating cell growth, cell proliferation, and organ size. *Cell* 2001; **105**: 357–68.

50 Tapon N, Ito N, Dickson BJ et al. The Drosophila tuberous sclerosis complex gene homologs restrict cell growth and cell proliferation. *Cell* 2001; **105**: 345–55.

51 Gao X, Pan D. TSC1 and TSC2 tumor suppressors antagonize insulin signaling in cell growth. *Genes Dev* 2001; **15**: 1383–92.

52 Stocker H, Radimerski T, Schindelholz B et al. Rheb is an essential regulator of S6K in controlling cell growth in Drosophila. *Nat Cell Biol* 2003; **5**: 559–65.

53 Zhang Y, Gao X, Saucedo LJ et al. Rheb is a direct target of the tuberous sclerosis tumour suppressor proteins. *Nat Cell Biol* 2003; **5**: 578–81.

●54 Brugarolas JB, Vazquez F, Reddy A et al. TSC2 regulates VEGF through mTOR-dependent and -independent pathways. *Cancer Cell* 2003; **4**: 147–58.

●55 Goncharova EA, Goncharov DA, Eszterhas A et al. Tuberin regulates p70 S6 kinase activation and ribosomal protein S6 phosphorylation. A role for the TSC2 tumor suppressor gene in pulmonary lymphangioleiomyomatosis (LAM). *J Biol Chem* 2002; **277**: 30958–67.

●56 Kenerson HL, Aicher LD, True LD, Yeung RS. Activated mammalian target of rapamycin pathway in the pathogenesis of tuberous sclerosis complex renal tumors. *Cancer Res* 2002; **62**: 5645–50.

57 Muir TE, Leslie KO, Popper H et al. Micronodular pneumocyte hyperplasia. *Am J Surg Pathol* 1998; **22**: 465–72.

58 Roach ES, Gomez MR, Northrup H. Tuberous sclerosis complex consensus conference: revised clinical diagnostic criteria. *J Child Neurol* 1998; **13**: 624–8.

59 Crausman RS, Lynch DA, Mortenson RL et al. Quantitative CT predicts the severity of physiologic dysfunction in patients with lymphangioleiomyomatosis. *Chest* 1996; **109**: 131–7.

60 Avila NA, Kelly JA, Dwyer AJ et al. Lymphangioleiomyomatosis: correlation of qualitative and quantitative thin-section CT with pulmonary function tests and assessment of dependence on pleurodesis. *Radiology* 2002; **223**: 189–97.

61 Taveira-DaSilva AM, Stylianou MP, Hedin CJ et al. Maximal oxygen uptake and severity of disease in lymphangioleiomyomatosis. *Am J Respir Crit Care Med* 2003; **168**: 1427–31.

62 Koyama M, Johkoh T, Honda O et al. Chronic cystic lung disease: diagnostic accuracy of high-resolution CT in 92 patients. *AJR Am J Roentgenol* 2003; **180**: 827–35.

63 Shin MS, Fulmer JD, Ho KJ. Unusual computed tomographic manifestations of benign metastasizing leiomyomas as cavitary nodular lesions or interstitial lung disease. *Clin Imaging* 1996; **20**: 45–9.

64 Yilmaz A, Rush DS, Soslow RA. Endometrial stromal sarcomas with unusual histologic features: a report of 24 primary and metastatic tumors emphasizing fibroblastic and smooth muscle differentiation. *Am J Surg Pathol* 2002; **26**: 1142–50.

65 Aubry MC, Myers JL, Colby TV et al. Endometrial stromal sarcoma metastatic to the lung: a detailed analysis of 16 patients. *Am J Surg Pathol* 2002; **26**: 440–9.

66 Faul JL, Berry GJ, Colby TV et al. Thoracic lymphangiomas, lymphangiectasis, lymphangiomatosis, and lymphatic dysplasia syndrome. *Am J Respir Crit Care Med* 2000; **161**(3 Pt 1): 1037–46.

67 Ferrans VJ, Yu ZX, Nelson WK et al. Lymphangioleiomyomatosis (LAM) (A review of clinical and morphological features). *J Nippon Med Sch* 2000; **67**: 311–29.

68 Zhe X, Schuger L. Combined smooth muscle and melanocytic differentiation in lymphangioleiomyomatosis. *J Histochem Cytochem* 2004; **52**: 1537–42.

69 Boehler A, Speich R, Russi EW, Weder W. Lung transplantation for lymphangioleiomyomatosis. *New Engl J Med* 1996; **335**: 1275–80.

70 Taveira-Dasilva AM, Stylianou MP, Hedin CJ et al. Bone mineral density in lymphangioleiomyomatosis. *Am J Respir Crit Care Med* 2005; **171**: 61–7.

71 Bando K, Paradis IL, Keenan RJ et al. Comparison of outcomes after single and bilateral lung transplantation for obstructive lung disease. *J Heart Lung Transplant* 1995; **14**: 692–8.

●72 Montagne J, Stewart MJ, Stocker H et al. Drosophila S6 kinase: a regulator of cell size. *Science* 1999; **285**: 2126–9.

73 Cook JD, Walker CL. The Eker rat: establishing a genetic paradigm linking renal cell carcinoma and uterine leiomyoma. *Curr Mol Med* 2004; **4**: 813–24.

●74 Kwiatkowski DJ, Zhang H, Bandura JL et al. A mouse model of TSC1 reveals sex-dependent lethality from liver hemangiomas, and up-regulation of p70S6 kinase activity in TSC1 null cells. *Hum Mol Genet* 2002; **11**: 525–34.

●75 El-Hashemite N, Walker V, Zhang H, Kwiatkowski DJ. Loss of TSC1 or TSC2 induces vascular endothelial growth factor production through mammalian target of rapamycin. *Cancer Res* 2003; **63**: 5173–7.

76 Astrinidis A, Cash TP, Hunter DS et al. Tuberin, the tuberous sclerosis complex 2 tumor suppressor gene product, regulates Rho activation, cell adhesion and migration. *Oncogene* 2002; **21**: 8470–6.

77 Razandi M, Pedram A, Park ST, Levin ER. Proximal events in signaling by plasma membrane estrogen receptors. *J Biol Chem* 2003; **278**: 2701–12.

78 Pedram A, Razandi M, Aitkenhead M et al. Integration of the non-genomic and genomic actions of estrogen. Membrane-initiated signaling by steroid to transcription and cell biology. *J Biol Chem* 2002; **277**: 50768–75.

79 Hayashi T, Fleming MV, Stetler-Stevenson WG, Liotta LA. Immunohistochemical study of matrix metalloproteinases (MMPs) and their tissue inhibitors (TIMPs) in pulmonary lymphangioleiomyomatosis. *Hum Pathol* 1997; **28**: 1071–8.

80 Hayashi T, Stetler-Stevenson WG, Fleming MV et al. Immunohistochemical study of metalloproteinases and their inhibitors in the lungs of patients with diffuse alveolar damage and idiopathic pulmonary fibrosis. *Am J Pathol* 1996; **149**: 1241–56.

81 Zhe X, Yang Y, Jakkaraju S, Schuger L. Tissue inhibitor of metalloproteinase-3 downregulation in lymphangioleiomyomatosis: potential consequence of abnormal serum response factor expression. *Am J Respir Cell Mol Biol* 2003; **28**: 504–11.

●82 Brugarolas J, Lei K, Hurley RL et al. Regulation of mTOR function in response to hypoxia by REDD1 and the TSC1/TSC2 tumor suppressor complex. *Genes Dev* 2004; **18**: 2893–904.

83 Brugarolas J, Kaelin WG Jr. Dysregulation of HIF and VEGF is a unifying feature of the familial hamartoma syndromes. *Cancer Cell* 2004; **6**: 7–10.

84 Lee L, Sudentas P, Donoghue B et al. Efficacy of a rapamycin analog (CCI-779) and IFN-gamma in tuberous sclerosis mouse models. *Genes Chromosomes Cancer* 2005; **42**: 213–27.

# Hermansky–Pudlak Syndrome

LISA R. YOUNG AND FRANCIS X. McCORMACK

## DEFINITION

Hermansky–Pudlak Syndrome (HPS) is a rare autosomal recessive disorder of organelle biogenesis, characterized by oculocutaneous albinism, platelet dysfunction, and lysosomal accumulation of ceroid lipofuscin in reticuloendothelial cells. The disorder was first described in 1959 by the Czechoslavakian physicians Hermansky and Pudlak.[1] Clinical manifestations include a variable deficiency of skin and hair pigmentation, reduced visual acuity, congenital nystagmus, and a platelet related bleeding diathesis. As introduced in Chapter 12, pulmonary disease, which is highly penetrant in HPS, manifests as a restrictive disorder with interstitial infiltrates, and can progress to respiratory insufficiency and death by the fourth or fifth decade.[2,3]

## EPIDEMIOLOGY

While rare, HPS may be the most common single gene disorder in Puerto Rico, where 1/20 people carry the gene and the disease is found in 1/1800.[4] Most HPS in Puerto Ricans is caused by mutations in the *HPS1* gene, which have been identified in about 450 patients in the northwest part of the country.[5–8] Mutations in *HPS3* have also been identified in Puerto Rico, but are much less common.[7,8]

Outside Puerto Rico, HPS-1 has been identified in approximately 40 additional patients. Nakatani et al.[9] identified 65 total cases of HPS reported in Japan, and HPS has now been reported in individuals of almost every nationality. The total number of individuals with HPS is unknown and is likely underestimated based on the low index of suspicion for the disorder, but HPS is thought to affect 1000 patients worldwide.[10] Approximately 400 patients are registered with the Hermansky–Pudlak Syndrome Network, a not-for-profit patient advocacy and support organization (Donna Appell, RN, personal communication).

## GENETIC ETIOLOGY

There are seven genetic loci known to be associated with HPS in humans. The existence of 14 genetically distinct mouse models of HPS suggest that there are several additional HPS loci to be discovered in humans.[11] Table 18C.1 summarizes the HPS subtypes and genetic etiologies, as well as prominent clinical features and mouse models. All of the known HPS genes are ubiquitously expressed.[11–13] All manifestations of HPS appear to arise from defects in genes involved in biogenesis of lysosomes or specialized intracellular organelles that are related to lysosomes, including melanosomes and platelet dense granules. However, only the HPS2 protein product, adaptor protein 3 (AP-3), has informative homologies to functionally characterized proteins. Sets of the other HPS gene products interact and form protein complexes termed BLOCs (biogenesis of lysosomal-related organelles complexes), numbered 1, 2, or 3. BLOC1 contains the HPS7 gene product, BLOC2 contains HPS3, HPS5, and HPS6 subunits, and HPS1 and HPS4 interact in BLOC3.[14] The corresponding mouse models are discussed later in this chapter.

### HPS-1

*HPS1* spans 20 exons on 10q23.1–23.2 and encodes a ubiquitously expressed, 700 amino acid, 79.3-kDa protein with no known function or informative homologies to other proteins. The most common mutation, which is responsible for the Puerto Rican founder effect, is a 16-bp duplication in exon 15 of *HPS1*; this mutation has also been identified in several families in the Swiss Alps.[15] Among non-Puerto Rican individuals, at least 18 other *HPS1* mutations have been described, with the most common being the insC974 mutation. The protein product of HPS1 is contained in two distinct high-molecular weight complexes distributed between uncoated vesicles, early stage melanosomes and the cytosol.

**Table 18C.1**   *Summary of HPS subtypes, genetic loci, and associated features*

| Type | Chr. locus | Locus name | Protein function/complex | Pulmonary disease | Other clinical features | Mouse model |
|------|-----------|-----------|------------------------|------------------|------------------------|-------------|
| HPS-1 | 10q23.1–23.3 | HPS1 | Unknown function/ BLOC-3 | Most common and severe pulmonary fibrosis | Granulomatous colitis | Pale ear |
| HPS-2 | 5q14.1 | HPS2/ AP3B1 | Adaptor protein 3 | Mild ILD reported | Neutropenia; frequent infections | Pearl |
| HPS-3 | 3q24 | HPS3 | Unknown function/ BLOC-2 | ? mild ILD | | Cocoa |
| HPS-4 | 22q11.2–12.2 | HPS4 | Unknown function/ BLOC-3 | + pulmonary fibrosis | Granulomatous colitis | Light ear |
| HPS-5 | 11p14 | HPS5 | Unknown function/ BLOC-2 | Unknown | | Ruby-eye 2 |
| HPS-6 | 10q24.32 | HPS6 | Unknown function/ BLOC-2 | Unknown | | Ruby-eye |
| HPS-7 | 6p22.3 | HPS7/ DTNBP1 | Unknown function/ BLOC-1 | Unknown | | Sandy |

## HPS-2

Of all the HPS subtypes, only HPS-2 results from mutations in an HPS gene that produces a product (AP3β1) of known function. The recognition of an HPS-like phenotype in Drosophila, including pigment granule defects, first led to the identification of the HSP2 locus on human chromosome 5.[16] The observation that the Drosophila pigmentation gene *garnet* encodes the β3A subunit of the AP-3 adaptor complex suggested an association between HPS and mutations in proteins which mediate trafficking of vesicular cargo proteins to cytoplasmic organelles. Dell'Angelica et al.[16] subsequently identified mutations in the gene for the β3A subunit of the heterotetrameric AP-3 complex in two patients with HPS. The cDNA for β3A predicted a protein composed of 1094 amino acids and a mass of 140 kDa. Fibroblasts from these subjects contained markedly reduced levels of AP-3 due to enhanced ubiquitin-mediated degradation of mutant β3A and the AP-3 complex. The AP-3 deficiency resulted in inappropriate cell surface expression of the lysosomal membrane proteins CD63, LAMP1, and LAMP2, but not of nonlysosomal proteins, suggesting that HPS2 is required at an early stage of melanosome biogenesis and maturation.[16]

## HPS-3

Aniskter and Oh identified a subset of 13 Puerto Rican HPS patients who did not have the 16-bp duplication characteristic of HPS-1, and used homozygosity mapping of pooled DNA from their six families to identify a new HPS susceptibility locus on 3q24, called HPS3.[7,8] The *HPS3* gene encodes a cytoplasmic 113.7-kDa protein and consists of 1004 amino acids, including a clathrin-binding motif

and signals for targeting to lysosomal vesicles. The exact function of the HPS3 protein is unknown.

## HPS-4

Naturally occurring mutations in mice that result in pigment dilution and platelet dysfunction have revealed an additional HPS gene, *HPS4*.[17] The gene responsible for the phenotype in the 'light ear' mouse was mapped to a region of the mouse chromosome that is syntenic with human chromosome 22q11.2–12.2. The human gene, termed *HPS4*, encodes a 708 amino acid protein with an apparent MW of 76.9 kDa. Of 21 unrelated Puerto Rican HPS patients lacking the HPS1 mutation who were screened, seven were found to have nonsense, frameshift, and in-frame insertion mutations in HPS4. The HPS1 and HPS4 proteins interact in BLOC-3.[17]

## HPS-5

HPS-5 was initially described in a young child, and has recently been further characterized in four additional patients.[18] HPS5 is located on chromosome 11p14, consists of 23 exons, and is expressed in at least three splice variants. Immunohistochemical studies in fibroblasts suggest that HPS5 functions in the movement of vesicles from the perinuclear region to the periphery of the cell.

## HPS-6

HPS-6 has been described in a single patient. The HPS5 and HPS6 proteins interact with HPS3 as components of BLOC-2.[14]

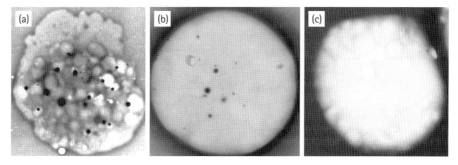

**Figure 18C.1**   *Electron micrograph of platelets from a normal subject (a) and from patients with Hermansky–Pudlak Syndrome (b and c). Note the reduction (b) and absence (c) of dense bodies in the HPS patients. (Images provided by James G. White MD and the Hermansky–Pudlak Syndrome Network.)*

## HPS-7

HPS-7 has been reported in a Portuguese woman and is caused by mutation in the human ortholog DTNBP1 of dysbindin, a component of BLOC-1 which interacts with the pallidin protein.[19]

## PATHOGENESIS

The manifestations of HPS highlight the importance of HPS genes in the genesis of lysosomal related organelles. Individuals with HPS have tyrosinase-positive oculocutaneous albinism.[20,21] Melanocytes are ultrastructurally normal, but contain predominantly early premelanosomes.[22] In HPS1, hypopigmentation is due to mistranslocation of tyrosinase and tyrosinase-related protein 1 to large granular complexes rather than melanosomes, thereby compromising melanin synthesis.[23]

The bleeding diathesis in HPS patients is due to an absence or reduction in the number of platelet dense granules, as demonstrated on wet mount electron microscopic analysis of platelets (Fig. 18C.1). HPS platelets appear unable to form the dense granules, or alternatively, cannot concentrate the products within them.[24,25] The absence of platelet-dense bodies results in a diminished secondary aggregation response of platelets.

Lysosomal accumulation of a poorly characterized lipoproteinaceous material, called ceroid lipofuscin, in macrophages has been associated with HPS pulmonary fibrosis and granulomatous colitis.[26–28] HPS patients have large foamy alveolar macrophages (Fig. 18C.2), though airspace accumulation of lipoproteinaceous material as occurs in pulmonary alveolar proteinosis has not been reported.[29,30] Although frequently implicated in the pathogenesis of lung disease in HPS, the role, if any, that these cellular accumulations play in pulmonary fibrosis is unclear. Elevated levels of inflammatory cytokines and mononuclear cells have also been identified in bronchoalveolar lavage of patients with mild lung function abnormalities (personal communication, Mark Brantly, MD). The mechanisms of

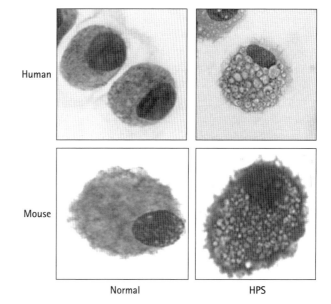

**Figure 18C.2**   *Abnormal appearance of alveolar macrophages from HPS patients and the Pearl mouse model. Macrophages containing lysosomal inclusions from a patient with HPS (left panel) are compared to a normal subject (right panel). (Human macrophage images provided by Mark Brantly MD). Similar abnormalities are observed in alveolar macrophages from Pearl mice.*

these cellular and inflammatory abnormalities and their potential role in pathogenesis of fibrosis in HPS have not been determined.

The pathogenesis of some of the clinical manifestations of HPS-2 is best understood in the context of known functions of the HPS2 product, the adaptor protein-3 complex (AP-3). The AP-3 complex has been implicated in several potential mechanisms of immune recognition which may explain the increased susceptibility to infections observed in HPS-2 patients. First, AP-3 regulates the trafficking of CD1b (humans) and CD1d (mice), which are transmembrane proteins required for the presentation of mycobacterial lipid antigens to T cells.[31] Additionally, the AP-3 complex is involved in the movement of lytic granules of cytotoxic T-lymphocytes (CTLs) to the immunological

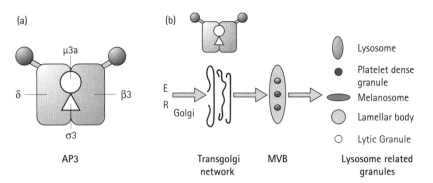

**Figure 18C.3** *Role of AP-3 in organelle biogenesis and protein trafficking. (a) Complex hetero-oligomeric structure of AP-3. HPS-2 is caused by mutations in the β3A subunit, which results in instability and degradation of the entire AP-3 complex. (b) The AP-3 complex escorts nascent proteins to lysosome-related organelles.*

synapse. In the absence of AP-3, loss of cytotoxicity by CTLs is observed.[32] Finally, AP-3 has also been demonstrated to be critical for directing neutrophil elastase to the azurophilic granule, another lysosomal-related organelle. Frameshift mutations in the Ap3b1 subunit of AP-3 in the gray collie lead to hypopigmentation, but also cyclic hematopoiesis with neutropenia, as neutrophil elastase is misdirected to the default destination at the plasma membrane.[33,34] These clues provide powerful insights into the role of AP-3 in intracellular protein trafficking (Fig. 18C.3), and may provide a foundation for understanding how abnormal intracellular protein trafficking impacts the type II cells and macrophages in the HPS lung.

No clinical features have been reported with the HPS carrier state, though a recent report of a Spanish family with HPS-1 found in vitro platelet dysfunction in two asymptomatic relatives carrying only one HPS1 mutation (insC974). Gonzalez-Conejero et al.[35] report that these carriers had a decreased content of platelet dense granules and showed significant reductions in platelet aggregation, expression of CD63 after platelet activation, and serotonin uptake.

## CLINICAL PRESENTATION AND EVALUATION

Albinism in HPS consists of highly variable hypopigmentation of the skin, hair, and ivides. Ocular albinism manifests with decreased visual acuity, transillumination of the iris, congenital horizontal nystagmus, and difficulty with dark adaptation.

The bleeding diathesis in patients with HPS varies from mild to severe and may include easy bruising, epistaxis, or prolonged or heavy bleeding with menses, dental procedures, and surgeries. Fatal hemorrhage is a common cause of early mortality in HPS patients,[26] and has been reported with dental extractions and parturition.[3] Individuals with HPS will have a history of prolonged bleeding, but normal platelet counts and general coagulation cascade parameters. While the diagnosis of HPS may be suspected in individuals with other features of HPS (albinism) and a prolonged bleeding

time, the sine qua non of the diagnosis of HPS is the absence of platelet dense granules on wet mount electron microscopic analysis of platelets (Fig. 18C.1).

Other clinical features of HPS may be directly related to the specific HPS subtype, as patients with HPS-2 have also been reported to have neutropenia and recurrent childhood infections.[36] In contrast, a study of 15 Puerto Rican HPS patients found no evidence of defects in peripheral blood lymphocyte or neutrophil function.[37] Some subjects with HPS-1 and HPS-4 develop a granulomatous colitis that is similar to Crohn's disease,[29] and renal or cardiac failure have also been reported.[7]

Interstitial lung disease (ILD) develops in most patients with HPS who survive into adulthood.[38–40] Nonproductive cough and progressive dyspnea on exertion are the most common presenting pulmonary symptoms, with a mean age of onset of pulmonary symptoms of about 35 years. There is no known gender predominance. Pulmonary function tests reveal a restrictive defect, although superimposed obstructive defects have been reported in smokers. Chest radiograph patterns vary from normal to fine reticular changes to end-stage honeycombing (Fig. 18C.4), and bulla and bronchiectasis have been reported.[41,42] Screening with high resolution computed tomography (HRCT) scans identifies ground-glass and fibrotic changes in a majority of HPS patients, though in early cases chest radiographs may be normal.[42,43]

Because of risk associated with lung biopsy in patients with a bleeding diathesis, only limited lung tissue is available for analysis. The available lung histology suggests that HPS shares some features of usual interstitial pneumonitis (UIP), but the key findings of fibroblastic foci and lower-lobe predominance have not been reported in HPS. As shown in Fig. 18C.5, large hyperplastic alveolar type II cells, with characteristic swelling and foamy degeneration, and lymphocytic and histiocytic infiltration of respiratory bronchioles are also present.[9,40] At the ultrastructural level, HPS type II cells also contain bizarre enlarged lamellar bodies.[9] Lamellar body abnormalities have also been reported in other forms of inherited pulmonary fibrosis, such as autosomal recessive ABCA-3 deficiency and autosomal dominant SP-C ILD.[44,45]

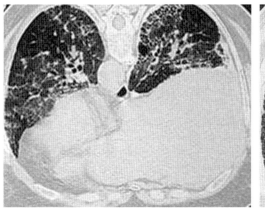
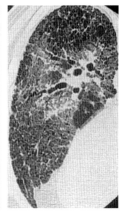

**Figure 18C.4**   *HRCT from a patient with HPS demonstrating reticulonodular infiltrates and honeycombing. (Images provided by Mark Brantly MD.)*

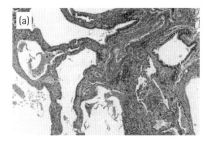
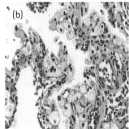
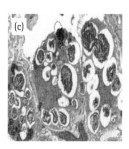

**Figure 18C.5**   *HPS lung histology. Note findings of end-stage fibrosis (a), lymphocytic infiltration and hyperplastic type II cells (b). At the ultrastructural level, type II cells from HPS patients contain abnormally large and irregular lamellar bodies with electron dense inclusions (c). (Extraction artifact is also present) Nakatani et al., with kind permission of Springer Science and Business Media. (Extraction artifact is also present.)*

There is significant interindividual variability in the severity of pulmonary disease which is not clearly related to age or specific mutations. In HPS1 patients followed at the NIH, some individuals had pulmonary fibrosis which progressed to death by approximately age 40, while others had a later onset of disease, but a subsequent rapid rate of decline in pulmonary function after disease onset. This variability may derive from environmental factors or may be due to epigenetic phenomena.[7,42]

## GENOTYPE–PHENOTYPE CORRELATIONS

The 16-bp duplication in HPS-1 that is prevalent in Puerto Rico is associated with an increased risk of interstitial lung disease.[7] Gahl et al.[27] reported that 9/16 HPS patients with the duplication, but none of the 10 HPS patients without it, had a DLCO less than 80 percent of predicted. HRCT analysis of the patients with the duplication showed a greater incidence and severity of pulmonary fibrosis than in patients with other HPS mutations. Patients with HPS-1 also have a significant incidence of granulomatous colitis (up to 15 percent),[27,46] and poor visual acuity has also been associated with HPS-1.[21] However, Swiss HPS-1 patients have been reported to have a normal life expectancy without pulmonary manifestations.[47] Although descriptions of HPS-4

patients are limited, HPS4 is reported to have a phenotype similar to Puerto Rican patients with HPS-1.[10] Mutations in HPS3 have been described to result in a milder overall disorder.[8] The rare HPS-2 subtype results in a distinct phenotype with neutropenia and increased infections, but two brothers with HPS-2 also had radiographic evidence of mild lung disease in their twenties.[48] While pulmonary fibrosis has not been reported in patients with HPS-5, the majority of HPS-5 patients described to date are younger than the age at which HPS pulmonary manifestations are typical.[18]

## TREATMENT

Limited therapy exists for individuals with HPS, but prevention and management of bleeding complications is a priority. Patients with HPS are counseled to wear medical alert bracelets, and medications such as aspirin, ibuprofen, and warfarin are generally avoided. Platelet transfusions may be required in the setting of trauma, bleeding episodes, or surgical procedures. Desmopressin (DDAVP) has been administered to many patients, but with inconsistent efficacy. Cordova et al.[49] reported that DDAVP had no effect on bleeding time in 19 pediatric Puerto Rican patients.

No definitive treatment exists for the pulmonary fibrosis associated with HPS and respiratory failure is the most common cause of death after bleeding complications. Steroids and other immunomodulating agents have been used, but there are no controlled studies to guide therapy and no definite benefits have been reported.[9] In a trial of pirfenidone in HPS patients, pirfenidone-treated patients lost lung function as assessed by forced vital capacity (FVC) at a rate of 5 percent of predicted (approximately 400 mL) per year slower than placebo-treated patients, with greater benefit to patients with an initial FVC of >50 percent of predicted. Dizziness was reported in three patients receiving Pirfenidone, but no significant adverse events occurred.[10] Pirfenidone is an anti-inflammatory drug which inhibits TGF-β expression. While the molecular targets of this therapy have not been fully elucidated, further investigations into the role of targeted anti-inflammatory therapy in HPS are clearly warranted.

Vigilance and early intervention for respiratory infections may be beneficial in patients with HPS, in addition to prophylaxis with influenza and pneumococcal vaccinations. Smoking cessation should be recommended for all patients with HPS. While bleeding complications are a significant consideration, lung transplantation may be an option for some HPS patients with advanced pulmonary fibrosis.

## DISEASE MODELS

Mice are the species of choice for the study of HPS. At least 14 different murine models of HPS exist, with genes identified by positional cloning.[13] The pale ear mouse is the murine analogue of HPS-1 in humans,[50,51] and the light ear mouse is the HPS-4 model.[17] The gene mutated in the cocoa (coa) mouse is homologous to the human HPS3 locus.[52] The HPS-5 and HPS-6 models are the ruby-eye 2 and ruby eye, respectively.[53]

Five HPS genes encode known vesicle trafficking proteins. Nine HPS genes are novel, found only in higher eukaryotes, and encode members of BLOCs 1, 2, or 3. Ten of the HPS models are maintained on the C57BL/6J inbred strain. A mutation in one subunit of a BLOC often results in secondary degradation of other components of the complex, and mutations affecting any component in a given BLOC tend to produce similar coat phenotypes in mice.[13] For example, the 'pallid,' 'cappuccino,' 'muted,' and 'sandy' mice all have mutations that affect BLOC1 proteins, and all four have very light gray coats and ears. In contrast, the 'pale ear' and 'light ear' mice have mutations that affect BLOC3 proteins, and both have relatively preserved and naturally dark tones in their coats but their ears and tails are hypopigmented.[13]

HPS mouse models share many of the physiological and cellular effects of HPS mutations seen in humans with HPS. Varying degrees of hypopigmentation are observed in all models, and all have a marked deficiency of platelet dense granules in comparison to wildtype mice.[13]

Lysosomal-related organelles occur in many cell types and abnormalities have been demonstrated in many HPS mouse models. These examples include: decreased secretion of cytotoxic T-lymphocyte lytic granules in ashen, gunmetal, and pearl mice[32,54] and abnormal secretion of mast cell granules in ruby-eye.[53]

The pulmonary phenotype of HPS mouse models described to date does not include prominent pulmonary fibrosis. Pale ear HPS1 mice exhibit relatively limited lung abnormalities. Pearl HPS2 mice have foamy alveolar macrophages (Fig. 18C.2) and a proliferation of foamy type II cells with abnormal lamellar bodies. To enhance the murine pulmonary phenotype, Swank and colleagues created an HPS1/HPS2 pale ear/pearl double-mutant mouse line. This model has markedly elevated whole lung lipid levels, foamy macrophages, and type II cell changes similar to those seen in patients with HPS. However, although the double mutant mice exhibit age-dependent airspace enlargement and subtle interstitial expansion at the ultrastructural level, histologic evidence of fibrosis does not occur to 1 year of age.[28,55] Late onset of emphysema also occurs in the pallid mouse.[56]

## SUMMARY

HPS is strongly associated with ILD, which is radiographically similar to idiopathic pulmonary fibrosis (IPF) and may share some, but not all, of the histologic features of UIP. The mechanism of lung fibrosis of HPS is unknown but aberrant lysosomal processing and ceroid accumulation resulting in macrophage and/or alveolar epithelial dysfunction are thought to play a role. The locus heterogeneity of HPS phenotypes in mice suggests that there may be several additional HPS gene loci to be discovered in humans. All patients with albinism and a bruising or bleeding diathesis should be screened for HPS. All patients with HPS should be monitored for pulmonary involvement with pulmonary function tests and chest radiographs. When indicated, bronchoscopy should be performed via the oral route and to avoid nasal bleeding. Furthermore, because of bleeding complications, lung biopsy is frequently contraindicated. There are currently no treatments available for the pulmonary manifestations of HPS, although pirfenidone may have some promise. Vigilance and early treatment for respiratory infections and avoidance of smoking should be encouraged. Mouse models of HPS share many of the phenotypic characteristics of HPS and may provide insight into mechanisms of vesicle trafficking and ultimately the pathogenesis of the pulmonary fibrosis associated with HPS. Monogenic disorders associated with highly penetrant pulmonary fibrosis, such as Hermansky–Pudlak syndrome, may shed light on disease mechanisms of other scarring lung diseases, such as IPF.

## Key learning points

- HPS is a rare disorder characterized by albinism, platelet dysfunction, and highly penetrant pulmonary fibrosis. Pigment deficiencies can be quite subtle; all patients with a bleeding diathesis and any degree of ocular or cutaneous albinism should be screened for HPS with electron microscopy of peripheral blood platelets. Patients with known HPS should be radiographically and physiologically monitored for restrictive lung disease.

- Pulmonary fibrosis in HPS has a histological appearance which is similar to usual interstitial pneumonia in several respects, but is also accompanied by hyperplastic, hypertrophic type II cells containing enlarged lamellar bodies, and lipid-filled, activated alveolar macrophages. The study of HPS associated pulmonary fibrosis provides an opportunity to approach fibrogenesis from the vantage point of a primary molecular defect.

- There are at least seven genetic loci associated with HPS in humans, which result in defects in the biogenesis of lysosomes and lysosome-related intracellular organelles including melanosomes and platelet dense granules, and lamellar bodies.

- None of the known naturally occurring mouse models of HPS develop histologically apparent pulmonary fibrosis spontaneously, but they may provide insight into mechanisms of abnormal vesicular trafficking and cellular dysfunction in HPS.

- Currently available approaches to treatment of HPS are limited but include smoking cessation and prevention and management of bleeding complications. Pirfenidone and other targeted anti-inflammatory agents warrant further study.

- The Hermansky–Pudlak Syndrome Network, Inc (www.hpsnetwork.org) is a support organization that serves for patients with HPS.

## REFERENCES

●1 Hermansky F, Pudlak P. Albinism associated with hemorrhagic diathesis and unusual pigmented reticular cells in the bone marrow: report of two cases with histochemical studies. *Blood* 1959; **14**: 162–9.

2 Davies BH, Tuddenham EG. Familial pulmonary fibrosis associated with oculocutaneous albinism and platelet function defect. A new syndrome. *Q J Med* 1976; **45**: 219–32.

3 DePinho RA, Kaplan KL. The Hermansky–Pudlak syndrome. Report of three cases and review of pathophysiology and management considerations. *Medicine* 1985; **64**: 192–202.

●4 Wildenberg SC, Oetting WS, Almodovar C et al. A gene causing Hermansky–Pudlak syndrome in a Puerto Rican population maps to chromosome 10q2. *Am J Hum Genet* 1995; **57**: 755–65.

5 Fukai K, Oh J, Frenk F et al. Linkage disequilibrium mapping of the gene for Hermansky–Pudlak syndrome to chromosome 10q23.1-q23.3. *Hum Mol Genet* 1995; **4**: 1665–9.

6 Hazelwood S, Shotelersuk V, Wildenberg SC et al. Evidence for locus heterogeneity in Puerto Ricans with Hermansky–Pudlak syndrome. *Am J Hum Genet* 1997; **61**: 1088–94.

7 Boissy RE, Zhao Y, Gahl WA. Altered protein localization in melanocytes from Hermansky–Pudlak syndrome: support for the role of the HPS gene product in intracellular trafficking. *Lab Invest* 1998; **78**: 1037–48.

●8 Anikster Y, Huizing M, White J et al. Mutation of a new gene causes a unique form of Hermansky–Pudlak syndrome in a genetic isolate of central Puerto Rico. *Nat Genet* 2001; **28**: 376–80.

9 Nakatani Y, Nakamura N, Sano J et al. Interstitial pneumonia in Hermansky–Pudlak syndrome: significance of florid foamy swelling/degeneration (giant lamellar body degeneration) of type-2 pneumocytes. *Virch Arch* 2000; **437**: 304–13.

●10 Gahl WA, Brantly M, Troendle J et al. Effect of pirfenidone on the pulmonary fibrosis of Hermansky–Pudlak syndrome. *Mol Genet Metab* 2002; **76**: 234–42.

◆11 Swank RT, Novak EK, McGarry MP et al. Mouse models of Hermansky–Pudlak syndrome: a review. *Pigment Cell Res* 1998; **11**: 60–80.

◆12 Huizing M, Boissy RE, Gahl WA. Hermansky–Pudlak syndrome: vesicle formation from yeast to man. *Pigment Cell Res* 2002; **15**: 405–19.

◆13 Li W, Rusiniak ME, Chintala S et al. Murine Hermansky– Pudlak syndrome genes: regulators of lysosome-related organelles. *Bioessays* 2004; **26**: 616–28.

◆14 Dell'Angelica EC. The building BLOC(k)s of lysosomes and related organelles. *Curr Opin Cell Biol* 2004; **16**: 458–64.

●15 Oh J, Ho L, Ala-Mello S et al. Mutation analysis of patients with Hermansky–Pudlak syndrome: a frameshift hot spot in the HPS gene and apparent locus heterogeneity. *Am J Hum Genet* 1998; **62**: 593–8.

16 Dell'Angelica EC, Shotelersuk V, Aguilar RC et al. Altered trafficking of lysosomal proteins in Hermansky–Pudlak syndrome due to mutations in the beta 3A subunit of the AP-3 adaptor. *Mol Cell* 1999; **3**: 11–21.

17 Suzuki T, Li W, Zhang Q et al. Hermansky–Pudlak syndrome is caused by mutations in HPS4, the human homolog of the mouse light-ear gene. *Nat Genet* 2002; **30**: 321–4.

18 Huizing M, Hess R, Dorward H et al. Cellular, molecular and clinical characterization of patients with Hermansky–Pudlak syndrome type 5. *Traffic* 2004; **5**: 711–22.

19 Li W, Zhang Q, Oiso N et al. Hermansky–Pudlak syndrome type 7 (HPS-7) results from mutant dysbindin, a member of the biogenesis of lysosome-related organelles complex 1 (BLOC-1). *Nat Genet* 2003; **35**: 84–9.

20 Izquierdo NJ, Townsend W, Hussels IE. Ocular findings in the Hermansky–Pudlak syndrome. *Trans Am Ophthalmol Soc* 1995; **93**: 191–200; discussion 200–2.

21 Iwata F, Reed GF, Caruso RC et al. Correlation of visual acuity and ocular pigmentation with the 16-bp duplication in the HPS-1 gene of Hermansky–Pudlak syndrome, a form of albinism. *Ophthalmology* 2000; **107**: 783–9.

22 Boissy RE, Nordlund JJ. Molecular basis of congenital hypopigmentary disorders in humans: a review. *Pigment Cell Res* 1997; **10**: 12–24.

23  Sarangarajan R, Budev A, Zhao Y et al. Abnormal translocation of tyrosinase and tyrosinase-related protein 1 in cutaneous melanocytes of Hermansky–Pudlak syndrome and in melanoma cells transfected with anti-sense HPS1 cDNA. *J Invest Dermatol* 2001; **117**: 641–6.

24  White JG. Membrane defects in inherited disorders of platelet function. *Am J Pediatr Hematol Oncol* 1982; **4**: 83–94.

25  Weiss HJ, Lages B, Viviv W et al. Heterogeneous abnormalities of platelet dense granule ultrastructure in 20 patients with congenital storage pool deficiency. *Br J Haematol* 1993; **83**: 282–95.

26  Witkop CJ, Townsend D, Bitterman PB, Harmon K. The role of ceroid in lung and gastrointestinal disease in Hermansky–Pudlak syndrome. *Adv Exp Med Biol* 1989; **266**: 283–96; discussion 297.

●27  Gahl WA, Brantly M, Kaiser-Kupfer MI et al. Genetic defects and clinical characteristics of patients with a form of oculocutaneous albinism (Hermansky–Pudlak syndrome). *New Engl J Med* 1998; **338**: 1258–64.

28  Feng L, Novak EK, Hartnell LM et al. The Hermansky–Pudlak syndrome 1 (HPS1) and HPS2 genes independently contribute to the production and function of platelet dense granules, melanosomes, and lysosomes. *Blood* 2002; **99**: 1651–8.

●29  Garay SM, Gardella JE, Fassini EP, Goldring RM. Hermansky–Pudlak syndrome. Pulmonary manifestations of a ceroid storage disorder. *Am J Med* 1979; **66**: 737–47.

30  Harmon KR, Witkop CJ, White JG et al. Pathogenesis of pulmonary fibrosis: platelet-derived growth factor precedes structural alterations in the Hermansky–Pudlak syndrome. *J Lab Clin Med* 1994; **123**: 617–27.

31  Sugita M, Cao X, Watts GF et al. Failure of trafficking and antigen presentation by CD1 in AP-3-deficient cells. *Immunity* 2002; **16**: 697–706.

32  Clark RH, Stinchcombe JC, Day A et al. Adaptor protein 3-dependent microtubule-mediated movement of lytic granules to the immunological synapse. *Nat Immunol* 2003; **4**: 1111–20.

33  Benson KF, Li FQ, Person RE et al. Mutations associated with neutropenia in dogs and humans disrupt intracellular transport of neutrophil elastase. *Nat Genet* 2003; **35**: 90–6.

34  Horwitz M, Benson KF, Duan Z et al. Hereditary neutropenia: dogs explain human neutrophil elastase mutations. *Trends Mol Med* 2004; **10**: 163–70.

35  Gonzalez-Conejero R, Rivera J, Escolar G et al. Molecular, ultrastructural and functional characterization of a Spanish family with Hermansky–Pudlak syndrome: role of insC974 in platelet function and clinical relevance. *Br J Haematol* 2003; **123**: 132–8.

●36  Shotelersuk V, Dell'Angelica EC, Hartnell L et al. A new variant of Hermansky–Pudlak syndrome due to mutations in a gene responsible for vesicle formation. *Am J Med* 2000; **108**: 423–7.

37  Shanahan F, Randolph L, King R et al. Hermansky–Pudlak syndrome: an immunologic assessment of 15 cases. *Am J Med* 1988; **85**: 823–8.

38  Shimizu K, Matsumoto T, Miura G et al. Hermansky–Pudlak syndrome with diffuse pulmonary fibrosis: radiologic-pathologic correlation. *J Comput Assist Tomogr* 1998; **22**: 249–51.

39  Reynolds SP, Davies BH, Gibbs AR. Diffuse pulmonary fibrosis and the Hermansky–Pudlak syndrome: clinical course and postmortem findings. *Thorax* 1994; **49**: 617–8.

40  White DA, Smith GJ, Cooper JA Jr et al. Hermansky–Pudlak syndrome and interstitial lung disease: report of a case with lavage findings. *Am Rev Respir Dis* 1984; **130**: 138–41.

41  Leitman BS, Balthazar EJ, Garay SM et al. The Hermansky–Pudlak syndrome: radiographic features. *Can Assoc Radiol J* 1986; **37**: 42–5.

42  Avila NA, Brantly M, Premkumar A et al. Hermansky–Pudlak syndrome: radiography and CT of the chest compared with pulmonary function tests and genetic studies. *AJR Am J Roentgenol* 2002; **179**: 887–92.

●43  Brantly M, Avila NA, Shotelersuk V et al. Pulmonary function and high-resolution CT findings in patients with an inherited form of pulmonary fibrosis, Hermansky–Pudlak syndrome, due to mutations in HPS-1. *Chest* 2000; **117**: 129–36.

44  Shulenin S, Nogee LM, Annilo T et al. ABCA3 gene mutations in newborns with fatal surfactant deficiency. *New Engl J Med* 2004; **350**: 1296–303.

45  Nogee LM, Dunbar AE 3rd, Wert SE et al. A mutation in the surfactant protein C gene associated with familial interstitial lung disease. *New Engl J Med* 2001; **344**: 573–9.

◆46  Hermos CR, Huizing M, Kaiser-Kupfer MI et al. Hermansky–Pudlak syndrome type 1: gene organization, novel mutations, and clinical-molecular review of non-Puerto Rican cases. *Hum Mutat* 2002; **20**: 482.

47  Schallreuter KU, Frenk E, Wolfe WS et al. Hermansky–Pudlak syndrome in a Swiss population. *Dermatology* 1993; **187**: 248–56.

48  Shotelersuk V, Hazelwood S, Larson D et al. Three new mutations in a gene causing Hermansky–Pudlak syndrome: clinical correlations. *Mol Genet Metab* 1998; **64**: 99–107.

49  Cordova A, Barrios NJ, Ortiz I et al. Poor response to desmopressin acetate (DDAVP) in children with Hermansky–Pudlak syndrome. *Pediatr Blood Cancer* 2005; **44**: 51–54.

50  Bailin T, Oh J, Feng GH et al. Organization and nucleotide sequence of the human Hermansky–Pudlak syndrome (HPS) gene. *J Invest Dermatol* 1997; **108**: 923–7.

51  Gardner JM, Wildenberg SC, Keiper NM et al. The mouse pale ear (ep) mutation is the homologue of human Hermansky–Pudlak syndrome. *Proc Natl Acad Sci USA* 1997; **94**: 9238–43.

52  Suzuki T, Li W, Zhang O et al. The gene mutated in cocoa mice, carrying a defect of organelle biogenesis, is a homologue of the human Hermansky–Pudlak syndrome-3 gene. *Genomics* 2001; **78**: 30–7.

53  Zhang Q, Zhao B, Li W et al. Ru2 and Ru encode mouse orthologs of the genes mutated in human Hermansky–Pudlak syndrome types 5 and 6. *Nat Genet* 2003; **33**: 145–53.

54  Clark R, Griffiths GM. Lytic granules, secretory lysosomes and disease. *Curr Opin Immunol* 2003; **15**: 516–21.

55  Lyerla TA, Rusiniak ME, Borchers M et al. Aberrant lung structure, composition, and function in a murine model of Hermansky–Pudlak syndrome. *Am J Physiol Lung Cell Mol Physiol*, 2003; **285**: L643–53.

56  McGarry MP et al. Pulmonary pathologies in pallid mice result from nonhematopoietic defects. Exp Mol Pathol, 2002; **72**(3): 213–20.

# Glossary

**Acquired genetic mutation** *See* somatic cell genetic mutation

**Additive genetic effects** When the combined effects of alleles at different loci are equal to the sum of their individual effects. *See also* anticipation, complex trait

**Adenine** (A) A nitrogenous base, one member of the base pair AT (adenine-thymine). *See also* base pair, nucleotide

**Affected relative pair** Individuals related by blood, each of whom is affected with the same trait. Examples are affected sibling, cousin, and avuncular pairs. *See also* avuncular relationship

**Aggregation technique** A technique used in model organism studies in which embryos at the 8-cell stage of development are pushed together to yield a single embryo (used as an alternative to microinjection). *See also* model organisms

**Allele** Alternative form of a genetic locus; a single allele for each locus is inherited from each parent (e.g., at a locus for eye color the allele might result in blue or brown eyes). *See also* locus, gene expression

**Allogeneic** Variation in alleles among members of the same species

**Alternative splicing** Different ways of combining a gene's exons to make variants of the complete protein

**Amino acid** Any of a class of 20 molecules that are combined to form proteins in living things. The sequence of amino acids in a protein and hence protein function are determined by the genetic code

**Amplification** An increase in the number of copies of a specific DNA fragment; can be in vivo or in vitro. *See also* cloning, polymerase chain reaction

**Animal model** *See* model organisms

**Annotation** Adding pertinent information such as gene coded for, amino acid sequence, or other commentary to the database entry of raw sequence of DNA bases. *See also* bioinformatics

**Anticipation** Each generation of offspring has increased severity of a genetic disorder; e.g., a grandchild may have earlier onset and more severe symptoms than the parent, who had earlier onset than the grandparent. *See also* additive genetic effects, complex trait

**Antisense** Nucleic acid that has a sequence exactly opposite to an mRNA molecule made by the body; binds to the mRNA molecule to prevent a protein from being made. *See also* transcription

**Apoptosis** Programmed cell death, the body's normal method of disposing of damaged, unwanted, or unneeded cells. *See also* cell

**Arrayed library** Individual primary recombinant clones (hosted in phage, cosmid, YAC, or other vector) that are placed in two-dimensional arrays in microtiter dishes. Each primary clone can be identified by the identity of the plate and the clone location (row and column) on that plate. Arrayed libraries of clones can be used for many applications, including screening for a specific gene or genomic region of interest. *See also* library, genomic library, gene chip technology

**Assembly** Putting sequenced fragments of DNA into their correct chromosomal positions

**Autoradiography** A technique that uses X-ray film to visualize radioactively labeled molecules or fragments of molecules; used in analyzing length and number of DNA fragments after they are separated by gel electrophoresis

**Autosomal dominant** A gene on one of the non-sex chromosomes that is always expressed, even if only one copy is present. The chance of passing the gene to offspring is 50 percent for each pregnancy. *See also* autosome, dominant, gene

**Autosome** A chromosome not involved in sex determination. The diploid human genome consists of a total of 46 chromosomes, 22 pairs of autosomes, and 1 pair of sex chromosomes (the X and Y chromosomes). *See also* sex chromosome

**Avuncular relationship** The genetic relationship between nieces and nephews and their aunts and uncles.

**Backcross** A cross between an animal that is heterozygous for alleles obtained from two parental strains and a second animal from one of those parental strains. Also used to describe the breeding protocol of an outcross followed by a backcross. *See also* model organisms

**Bacterial artificial chromosome** (BAC)   A vector used to clone DNA fragments (100- to 300-kb insert size; average, 150 kb) in *Escherichia coli* cells. Based on naturally occurring F-factor plasmid found in the bacterium *E. coli*. *See also* cloning vector

**Bacteriophage**   *See* phage

**Base**   One of the molecules that form DNA and RNA molecules. *See also* nucleotide, base pair, base sequence

**Base pair** (bp)   Two nitrogenous bases (adenine and thymine or guanine and cytosine) held together by weak bonds. Two strands of DNA are held together in the shape of a double helix by the bonds between base pairs

**Base sequence**   The order of nucleotide bases in a DNA molecule; determines structure of proteins encoded by that DNA

**Base sequence analysis**   A method, sometimes automated, for determining the base sequence

**Behavioral genetics**   The study of genes that may influence behavior

**Bioinformatics**   The science of managing and analyzing biological data using advanced computing techniques. Especially important in analyzing genomic research data. *See also* informatics

**Bioremediation**   The use of biological organisms such as plants or microbes to aid in removing hazardous substances from an area

**Biotechnology**   A set of biological techniques developed through basic research and now applied to research and product development. In particular, biotechnology refers to the use by industry of recombinant DNA, cell fusion, and new bioprocessing techniques

**Birth defect**   Any harmful trait, physical or biochemical, present at birth, whether a result of a genetic mutation or some other nongenetic factor. *See also* congenital, gene, mutation, syndrome

**BLAST**   A computer program that identifies homologous (similar) genes in different organisms, such as human, fruit fly, or nematode

**Cancer**   Diseases in which abnormal cells divide and grow unchecked. Cancer can spread from its original site to other parts of the body and can be fatal. *See also* hereditary cancer, sporadic cancer

**Candidate gene**   A gene located in a chromosome region suspected of being involved in a disease. *See also* positional cloning, protein

**Capillary array**   Gel-filled silica capillaries used to separate fragments for DNA sequencing. The small diameter of the capillaries permit the application of higher electric fields, providing high speed, high throughput separations that are significantly faster than traditional slab gels

**Carcinogen**   Something which causes cancer to occur by causing changes in a cell's DNA. *See also* mutagene

**Carrier**   An individual who possesses an unexpressed, recessive trait

**cDNA library**   A collection of DNA sequences that code for genes. The sequences are generated in the laboratory from mRNA sequences. *See also* messenger RNA

**Cell**   The basic unit of any living organism that carries on the biochemical processes of life. *See also* genome, nucleus

**Centimorgan** (cM)   A unit of measure of recombination frequency. One centimorgan is equal to a 1% chance that a marker at one genetic locus will be separated from a marker at a second locus due to crossing over in a single generation. In human beings, one centimorgan is equivalent, on average, to one million base pairs. *See also* megabase

**Centromere**   A specialized chromosome region to which spindle fibers attach during cell division

**Chimera (pl. chimaera)**   An organism that contains cells or tissues with a different genotype. These can be mutated cells of the host organism or cells from a different organism or species

**Chimeraplasty**   An experimental targeted repair process in which a desirable sequence of DNA is combined with RNA to form a chimeraplast. These molecules bind selectively to the target DNA. Once bound, the chimeraplast activates a naturally occurring gene-correcting mechanism. Does not use viral or other conventional gene-delivery vectors. *See also* gene therapy, cloning vector

**Chloroplast chromosome**   Circular DNA found in the photosynthesizing organelle (chloroplast) of plants instead of the cell nucleus where most genetic material is located

**Chromomere**   One of the serially aligned beads or granules of a eukaryotic chromosome, resulting from local coiling of a continuous DNA thread

**Chromosomal deletion**   The loss of part of a chromosome's DNA

**Chromosomal inversion**   Chromosome segments that have been turned 180 degrees. The gene sequence for the segment is reversed with respect to the rest of the chromosome

**Chromosome**   The self-replicating genetic structure of cells containing the cellular DNA that bears in its nucleotide sequence the linear array of genes. In prokaryotes, chromosomal DNA is circular, and the entire genome is carried on one chromosome. Eukaryotic genomes consist of a number of chromosomes whose DNA is associated with different kinds of proteins

**Chromosome painting** Attachment of certain fluorescent dyes to targeted parts of the chromosome. Used as a diagnositic for particular diseases, e.g. types of leukemia

**Chromosome region p** A designation for the short arm of a chromosome

**Chromosome region q** A designation for the long arm of a chromosome

**Clone** An exact copy made of biological material such as a DNA segment (e.g., a gene or other region), a whole cell, or a complete organism

**Clone bank** *See* genomic library

**Cloning** Using specialized DNA technology to produce multiple, exact copies of a single gene or other segment of DNA to obtain enough material for further study. This process, used by researchers in the Human Genome Project, is referred to as cloning DNA. The resulting cloned (copied) collections of DNA molecules are called clone libraries. A second type of cloning exploits the natural process of cell division to make many copies of an entire cell. The genetic makeup of these cloned cells, called a cell line, is identical to the original cell. A third type of cloning produces complete, genetically identical animals such as the famous Scottish sheep, Dolly. *See also* cloning vector

**Cloning vector** DNA molecule originating from a virus, a plasmid, or the cell of a higher organism into which another DNA fragment of appropriate size can be integrated without loss of the vector's capacity for self-replication; vectors introduce foreign DNA into host cells, where the DNA can be reproduced in large quantities. Examples are plasmids, cosmids, and yeast artificial chromosomes; vectors are often recombinant molecules containing DNA sequences from several sources

**Code** *See* genetic code

**Codominance** Situation in which two different alleles for a genetic trait are both expressed. *See also* autosomal dominant, recessive gene

**Codon** *See* genetic code

**Coisogenic or congenic** Nearly identical strains of an organism; they vary at only a single locus

**Comparative genomics** The study of human genetics by comparisons with model organisms such as mice, the fruit fly, and the bacterium *E. coli*

**Complementary DNA** (cDNA) DNA that is synthesized in the laboratory from a messenger RNA template

**Complementary sequence** Nucleic acid base sequence that can form a double-stranded structure with another DNA fragment by following base-pairing rules (A pairs with T and C with G). The complementary sequence to GTAC for example, is CATG

**Complex trait** Trait that has a genetic component that does not follow strict Mendelian inheritance. May involve the interaction of two or more genes or gene-environment interactions. *See also* Mendelian inheritance, additive genetic effects

**Computational biology** *See* bioinformatics

**Confidentiality** In genetics, the expectation that genetic material and the information gained from testing that material will not be available without the donor's consent

**Congenital** Any trait present at birth, whether the result of a genetic or nongenetic factor. *See also* birth defect

**Conserved sequence** A base sequence in a DNA molecule (or an amino acid sequence in a protein) that has remained essentially unchanged throughout evolution

**Constitutive ablation** Gene expression that results in cell death

**Contig** Group of cloned (copied) pieces of DNA representing overlapping regions of a particular chromosome

**Contig map** A map depicting the relative order of a linked library of overlapping clones representing a complete chromosomal segment

**Cosmid** Artificially constructed cloning vector containing the cos gene of phage lambda. Cosmids can be packaged in lambda phage particles for infection into *E. coli*; this permits cloning of larger DNA fragments (up to 45 kb) than can be introduced into bacterial hosts in plasmid vectors

**Crossing over** The breaking during meiosis of one maternal and one paternal chromosome, the exchange of corresponding sections of DNA, and the rejoining of the chromosomes. This process can result in an exchange of alleles between chromosomes. *See also* recombination

**Cytogenetics** The study of the physical appearance of chromosomes. *See also* karyotype

**Cytological band** An area of the chromosome that stains differently from areas around it. *See also* cytological map

**Cytological map** A type of chromosome map whereby genes are located on the basis of cytological findings obtained with the aid of chromosome mutations

**Cytoplasmic (uniparental) inheritance** *See* cytoplasmic trait

**Cytoplasmic trait** A genetic characteristic in which the genes are found outside the nucleus, in chloroplasts or mitochondria. Results in offspring inheriting genetic material from only one parent

**Cytosine** (C) A nitrogenous base, one member of the base pair GC (guanine and cytosine) in DNA. *See also* base pair, nucleotide

**Data warehouse** A collection of databases, data tables, and mechanisms to access the data on a single subject

**Deletion** A loss of part of the DNA from a chromosome; can lead to a disease or abnormality. *See also* chromosome, mutation

**Deletion map** A description of a specific chromosome that uses defined mutations – specific deleted areas in the genome – as 'biochemical signposts,' or markers for specific areas

**Deoxyribonucleotide** *See* nucleotide

**Deoxyribose** A type of sugar that is one component of DNA (deoxyribonucleic acid)

**Diploid** A full set of genetic material consisting of paired chromosomes, one from each parental set. Most animal cells except the gametes have a diploid set of chromosomes. The diploid human genome has 46 chromosomes. *See also* haploid

**Directed evolution** A laboratory process used on isolated molecules or microbes to cause mutations and identify subsequent adaptations to novel environments

**Directed mutagenesis** Alteration of DNA at a specific site and its reinsertion into an organism to study any effects of the change

**Directed sequencing** Successively sequencing DNA from adjacent stretches of chromosome

**Disease-associated genes** Alleles carrying particular DNA sequences associated with the presence of disease

**DNA** (deoxyribonucleic acid) The molecule that encodes genetic information. DNA is a double-stranded molecule held together by weak bonds between base pairs of nucleotides. The four nucleotides in DNA contain the bases adenine (A), guanine (G), cytosine (C), and thymine (T). In nature, base pairs form only between A and T and between G and C; thus the base sequence of each single strand can be deduced from that of its partner

**DNA bank** A service that stores DNA extracted from blood samples or other human tissue

**DNA probe** *See* probe

**DNA repair genes** Genes encoding proteins that correct errors in DNA sequencing

**DNA replication** The use of existing DNA as a template for the synthesis of new DNA strands. In humans and other eukaryotes, replication occurs in the cell nucleus

**DNA sequence** The relative order of base pairs, whether in a DNA fragment, gene, chromosome, or an entire genome. *See also* base sequence analysis

**Domain** A discrete portion of a protein with its own function. The combination of domains in a single protein determines its overall function

**Dominant** An allele that is almost always expressed, even if only one copy is present. *See also* gene, genome

**Double helix** The twisted-ladder shape that two linear strands of DNA assume when complementary nucleotides on opposing strands bond together

**Draft sequence** The sequence generated by the HGP as of June 2000 that, while incomplete, offers a virtual road map to an estimated 95 percent of all human genes. Draft sequence data are mostly in the form of 10 000 base pair-sized fragments whose approximate chromosomal locations are known. *See also* sequencing, finished DNA sequence, working draft DNA sequence

**Electrophoresis** A method of separating large molecules (such as DNA fragments or proteins) from a mixture of similar molecules. An electric current is passed through a medium containing the mixture, and each kind of molecule travels through the medium at a different rate, depending on its electrical charge and size. Agarose and acrylamide gels are the media commonly used for electrophoresis of proteins and nucleic acids

**Electroporation** A process using high-voltage current to make cell membranes permeable to allow the introduction of new DNA; commonly used in recombinant DNA technology. *See also* transfection

**Embryonic stem (ES) cells** An embryonic cell that can replicate indefinitely, transform into other types of cells, and serve as a continuous source of new cells

**Endonuclease** *See* restriction enzyme

**Enzyme** A protein that acts as a catalyst, speeding the rate at which a biochemical reaction proceeds but not altering the direction or nature of the reaction

**Epistasis** One gene interacts with or prevents the expression of another gene located at a different locus

**Escherichia coli** Common bacterium that has been studied intensively by geneticists because of its small genome size, normal lack of pathogenicity, and ease of growth in the laboratory

**Eugenics** The study of improving a species by artificial selection; usually refers to the selective breeding of humans

**Eukaryote** Cell or organism with membrane-bound, structurally discrete nucleus and other well-developed subcellular compartments. Eukaryotes include all organisms except viruses, bacteria, and bluegreen algae. *See also* prokaryote, chromosome

**Evolutionarily conserved** *See* conserved sequence

**Exogenous DNA** DNA originating outside an organism that has been introduced into the organism

**Exon** The protein-coding DNA sequence of a gene. *See also* intron

**Exonuclease** An enzyme that cleaves nucleotides sequentially from free ends of a linear nucleic acid substrate

**Expressed gene** *See* gene expression

**Expressed sequence tag** (EST) A short strand of DNA that is a part of a cDNA molecule and can act as identifier of a gene. Used in locating and mapping genes. *See also* cDNA, sequence tagged site

**Filial generation** (F1, F2) Each generation of offspring in a breeding program, designated F1, F2, etc.

**Fingerprinting** In genetics, the identification of multiple specific alleles on a person's DNA to produce a unique identifier for that person. *See also* forensics

**Finished DNA Sequence** High-quality, low error, gap-free DNA sequence of the human genome. Achieving this HGP goal required additional sequencing to close gaps, reduce ambiguities, and allow for only a single error every 10 000 bases, the agreed-upon standard for HGP finished sequence. *See also* sequencing, draft sequence

**Flow cytometry** Analysis of biological material by detection of the light-absorbing or fluorescing properties of cells or subcellular fractions (i.e., chromosomes) passing in a narrow stream through a laser beam. An absorbance or fluorescence profile of the sample is produced. Automated sorting devices, used to fractionate samples, sort successive droplets of the analyzed stream into different fractions depending on the fluorescence emitted by each droplet

**Flow karyotyping** Use of flow cytometry to analyze and separate chromosomes according to their DNA content

**Fluorescence in situ hybridization** (FISH) A physical mapping approach that uses fluorescein tags to detect hybridization of probes with metaphase chromosomes and with the less-condensed somatic interphase chromatin

**Forensics** The use of DNA for identification. Some examples of DNA use are to establish paternity in child support cases; establish the presence of a suspect at a crime scene, and identify accident victims

**Fraternal twin** Siblings born at the same time as the result of fertilization of two ova by two sperm. They share the same genetic relationship to each other as any other siblings. Also known as dizygotic twin. *See also* identical twin

**Full gene sequence** The complete order of bases in a gene. This order determines which protein a gene will produce

**Functional genomics** The study of genes, their resulting proteins, and the role played by the proteins the body's biochemical processes

**Gamete** Mature male or female reproductive cell (sperm or ovum) with a haploid set of chromosomes (23 for humans)

**GC-rich area** Many DNA sequences carry long stretches of repeated G and C which often indicate a gene-rich region

**Gel electrophoresis** *See* electrophoresis

**Gene** The fundamental physical and functional unit of heredity. A gene is an ordered sequence of nucleotides located in a particular position on a particular chromosome that encodes a specific functional product (i.e., a protein or RNA molecule). *See also* gene expression

**Gene amplification** Repeated copying of a piece of DNA; a characteristic of tumor cells. *See also* gene, oncogene

**Gene chip technology** Development of cDNA or oligonucleotide microarrays from a large number of genes. Used to monitor and measure changes in gene expression for each gene represented on the chip

**Gene expression** The process by which a gene's coded information is converted into the structures present and operating in the cell. Expressed genes include those that are transcribed into mRNA and then translated into protein and those that are transcribed into RNA but not translated into protein (e.g., transfer and ribosomal RNAs)

**Gene family** Group of closely related genes that make similar products

**Gene library** *See* genomic library

**Gene mapping** Determination of the relative positions of genes on a DNA molecule (chromosome or plasmid) and of the distance, in linkage units or physical units, between them

**Gene pool** All the variations of genes in a species. *See also* allele, gene, polymorphism

**Gene prediction** Predictions of possible genes made by a computer program based on how well a stretch of DNA sequence matches known gene sequences

**Gene product** The biochemical material, either RNA or protein, resulting from expression of a gene. The amount of gene product is used to measure how active a gene is; abnormal amounts can be correlated with disease-causing alleles

**Gene testing** *See* genetic testing, genetic screening

**Gene therapy** An experimental procedure aimed at replacing, manipulating, or supplementing nonfunctional or misfunctioning genes with healthy genes. *See also* gene, inherit, somatic cell gene therapy, germ line gene therapy

**Gene transfer** Incorporation of new DNA into an organism's cells, usually by a vector such as a modified virus. Used in gene therapy. *See also* mutation, gene therapy, vector

**Genetic code** The sequence of nucleotides, coded in triplets (codons) along the mRNA, that determines the sequence of amino acids in protein synthesis. A gene's DNA sequence can be used to predict the mRNA sequence, and the genetic code can in turn be used to predict the amino acid sequence

**Genetic counseling**    Provides patients and their families with education and information about genetic-related conditions and helps them make informed decisions

**Genetic discrimination**    Prejudice against those who have or are likely to develop an inherited disorder

**Genetic engineering**    Altering the genetic material of cells or organisms to enable them to make new substances or perform new functions

**Genetic engineering technology**    *See* recombinant DNA technology

**Genetic illness**    Sickness, physical disability, or other disorder resulting from the inheritance of one or more deleterious alleles

**Genetic informatics**    *See* bioinformatics

**Genetic map**    *See* linkage map

**Genetic marker**    A gene or other identifiable portion of DNA whose inheritance can be followed. *See also* chromosome, DNA, gene, inherit

**Genetic material**    *See* genome

**Genetic mosaic**    An organism in which different cells contain different genetic sequence. This can be the result of a mutation during development or fusion of embryos at an early developmental stage

**Genetic polymorphism**    Difference in DNA sequence among individuals, groups, or populations (e.g., genes for blue eyes versus brown eyes)

**Genetic predisposition**    Susceptibility to a genetic disease. May or may not result in actual development of the disease

**Genetic screening**    Testing a group of people to identify individuals at high risk of having or passing on a specific genetic disorder

**Genetic testing**    Analyzing an individual's genetic material to determine predisposition to a particular health condition or to confirm a diagnosis of genetic disease

**Genetics**    The study of inheritance patterns of specific traits

**Genome**    All the genetic material in the chromosomes of a particular organism; its size is generally given as its total number of base pairs

**Genome project**    Research and technology-development effort aimed at mapping and sequencing the genome of human beings and certain model organisms. *See also* Human Genome Initiative

**Genomic library**    A collection of clones made from a set of randomly generated overlapping DNA fragments that represent the entire genome of an organism. *See also* library, arrayed library

**Genomic sequence**    *See* DNA

**Genomics**    The study of genes and their function

**Genotype**    The genetic constitution of an organism, as distinguished from its physical appearance (its phenotype)

**Germ cell**    Sperm and egg cells and their precursors. Germ cells are haploid and have only one set of chromosomes (23 in all), while all other cells have two copies (46 in all)

**Germ line**    The continuation of a set of genetic information from one generation to the next. *See also* inherit

**Germ line gene therapy**    An experimental process of inserting genes into germ cells or fertilized eggs to cause a genetic change that can be passed on to offspring. May be used to alleviate effects associated with a genetic disease. *See also* genomics, somatic cell gene therapy

**Germ line genetic mutation**    *See* mutation

**Guanine** (G)    A nitrogenous base, one member of the base pair GC (guanine and cytosine) in DNA. *See also* base pair, nucleotide

**Gyandromorph**    Organisms that have both male and female cells and therefore express both male and female characteristics

**Haploid**    A single set of chromosomes (half the full set of genetic material) present in the egg and sperm cells of animals and in the egg and pollen cells of plants. Human beings have 23 chromosomes in their reproductive cells. *See also* diploid

**Haplotype**    A way of denoting the collective genotype of a number of closely linked loci on a chromosome

**Hemizygous**    Having only one copy of a particular gene. For example, in humans, males are hemizygous for genes found on the Y chromosome

**Hereditary cancer**    Cancer that occurs due to the inheritance of an altered gene within a family. *See also* sporadic cancer

**Heterozygosity**    The presence of different alleles at one or more loci on homologous chromosomes

**Heterozygote**    *See* heterozygosity

**Highly conserved sequence**    DNA sequence that is very similar across several different types of organisms. *See also* gene, mutation

**High-throughput sequencing**    A fast method of determining the order of bases in DNA. *See also* sequencing

**Homeobox**    A short stretch of nucleotides whose base sequence is virtually identical in all the genes that contain it. Homeoboxes have been found in many organisms from fruit flies to human beings. In the fruit fly, a homeobox appears to determine when particular groups of genes are expressed during development

**Homolog**    A member of a chromosome pair in diploid organisms or a gene that has the same origin and functions in two or more species

**Homologous chromosome**    Chromosome containing the same linear gene sequences as another, each derived from one parent

**Homologous recombination**    Swapping of DNA fragments between paired chromosomes

**Homology**    Similarity in DNA or protein sequences between individuals of the same species or among different species

**Homozygote**    An organism that has two identical alleles of a gene. *See also* heterozygote

**Homozygous**    *See* homozygote

**Human artificial chromosome** (HAC)    A vector used to hold large DNA fragments. *See also* chromosome, DNA

**Human gene therapy**    *See* gene therapy

**Human Genome Initiative**    Collective name for several projects begun in 1986 by DOE to create an ordered set of DNA segments from known chromosomal locations, develop new computational methods for analyzing genetic map and DNA sequence data, and develop new techniques and instruments for detecting and analyzing DNA. This DOE initiative is now known as the Human Genome Program. The joint national effort, led by DOE and NIH, is known as the Human Genome Project

**Human Genome Project** (HGP)    Formerly titled Human Genome Initiative. *See also* Human Genome Initiative

**Hybrid**    The offspring of genetically different parents. *See also* heterozygote

**Hybridization**    The process of joining two complementary strands of DNA or one each of DNA and RNA to form a double-stranded molecule

**Identical twin**    Twins produced by the division of a single zygote; both have identical genotypes. Also known as monozygotic twin. *See also* fraternal twin

**Immunotherapy**    Using the immune system to treat disease, for example, in the development of vaccines. May also refer to the therapy of diseases caused by the immune system. *See also* cancer

**Imprinting**    A phenomenon in which the disease phenotype depends on which parent passed on the disease gene. For instance, both Prader-Willi and Angelman syndromes are inherited when the same part of chromosome 15 is missing. When the father's complement of 15 is missing, the child has Prader-Willi, but when the mother's complement of 15 is missing, the child has Angelman syndrome

**In situ hybridization**    Use of a DNA or RNA probe to detect the presence of the complementary DNA sequence in cloned bacterial or cultured eukaryotic cells

**In vitro**    Studies performed outside a living organism such as in a laboratory

**In vivo**    Studies carried out in living organisms

**Independent assortment**    During meiosis each of the two copies of a gene is distributed to the germ cells independently of the distribution of other genes. *See also* linkage

**Informatics**    *See* bioinformatics

**Informed consent**    An individual willingly agrees to participate in an activity after first being advised of the risks and benefits. *See also* privacy

**Inherit**    In genetics, to receive genetic material from parents through biological processes

**Inherited**    *See* inherit

**Insertion**    A chromosome abnormality in which a piece of DNA is incorporated into a gene and thereby disrupts the gene's normal function. *See also* chromosome, DNA, gene, mutation

**Insertional mutation**    *See* insertion

**Intellectual property rights**    Patents, copyrights, and trademarks. *See also* patent

**Interference**    One crossover event inhibits the chances of another crossover event. Also known as positive interference. Negative interference increases the chance of a second crossover. *See also* crossing over

**Interphase**    The period in the cell cycle when DNA is replicated in the nucleus; followed by mitosis

**Intron**    DNA sequence that interrupts the protein-coding sequence of a gene; an intron is transcribed into RNA but is cut out of the message before it is translated into protein. *See also* exon

**Isoenzyme**    An enzyme performing the same function as another enzyme but having a different set of amino acids. The two enzymes may function at different speeds

**Junk DNA**    Stretches of DNA that do not code for genes; most of the genome consists of so-called junk DNA which may have regulatory and other functions. Also called non-coding DNA

**Karyotype**    A photomicrograph of an individual's chromosomes arranged in a standard format showing the number, size, and shape of each chromosome type; used in low-resolution physical mapping to correlate gross chromosomal abnormalities with the characteristics of specific diseases

**Kilobase** (kb)    Unit of length for DNA fragments equal to 1000 nucleotides

**Knockout**    Deactivation of specific genes; used in laboratory organisms to study gene function. *See also* gene, locus, model organisms

**Library**    An unordered collection of clones (i.e., cloned DNA from a particular organism) whose relationship to each other can be established by physical mapping. *See also* genomic library, arrayed library

**Linkage**    The proximity of two or more markers (e.g., genes, RFLP markers) on a chromosome; the closer the markers, the lower the probability that they will be separated during DNA repair or replication processes (binary fission in prokaryotes, mitosis or meiosis in eukaryotes), and hence the greater the probability that they will be inherited together

**Linkage disequilibrium**    Where alleles occur together more often than can be accounted for by chance. Indicates that the two alleles are physically close on the DNA strand. *See also* Mendelian inheritance

**Linkage map**    A map of the relative positions of genetic loci on a chromosome, determined on the basis of how often the loci are inherited together. Distance is measured in centimorgans (cM)

**Localize**    Determination of the original position (locus) of a gene or other marker on a chromosome

**Locus (pl. loci)**    The position on a chromosome of a gene or other chromosome marker; also, the DNA at that position. The use of locus is sometimes restricted to mean expressed DNA regions. *See also* gene expression

**Long-Range Restriction Mapping**    Restriction enzymes are proteins that cut DNA at precise locations. Restriction maps depict the chromosomal positions of restriction-enzyme cutting sites. These are used as biochemical 'signposts,' or markers of specific areas along the chromosomes. The map will detail the positions where the DNA molecule is cut by particular restriction enzymes

**Macrorestriction map**    Map depicting the order of and distance between sites at which restriction enzymes cleave chromosomes

**Mapping**    *See* gene mapping, linkage map, physical map

**Mapping population**    The group of related organisms used in constructing a genetic map

**Marker**    *See* genetic marker

**Mass spectrometry**    An instrument used to identify chemicals in a substance by their mass and charge

**Megabase** (Mb)    Unit of length for DNA fragments equal to 1 million nucleotides and roughly equal to 1 cM. *See also* centimorgan

**Meiosis**    The process of two consecutive cell divisions in the diploid progenitors of sex cells. Meiosis results in four rather than two daughter cells, each with a haploid set of chromosomes. *See also* mitosis

**Mendelian inheritance**    One method in which genetic traits are passed from parents to offspring. Named for Gregor Mendel, who first studied and recognized the existence of genes and this method of inheritance. *See also* autosomal dominant, recessive gene, sex-linked

**Messenger RNA** (mRNA)    RNA that serves as a template for protein synthesis. *See also* genetic code

**Metaphase**    A stage in mitosis or meiosis during which the chromosomes are aligned along the equatorial plane of the cell

**Microarray**    Sets of miniaturized chemical reaction areas that may also be used to test DNA fragments, antibodies, or proteins

**Microbial genetics**    The study of genes and gene function in bacteria, archaea, and other microorganisms. Often used in research in the fields of bioremediation, alternative energy, and disease prevention. *See also* model organisms, biotechnology, bioremediation

**Microinjection**    A technique for introducing a solution of DNA into a cell using a fine microcapillary pipet

**Micronuclei**    Chromosome fragments that are not incorporated into the nucleus at cell division

**Mitochondrial DNA**    The genetic material found in mitochondria, the organelles that generate energy for the cell. Not inherited in the same fashion as nucleic DNA. *See also* cell, DNA, genome, nucleus

**Mitosis**    The process of nuclear division in cells that produces daughter cells that are genetically identical to each other and to the parent cell. *See also* meiosis

**Model organisms**    A laboratory animal or other organism useful for research

**Modeling**    The use of statistical analysis, computer analysis, or model organisms to predict outcomes of research

**Molecular biology**    The study of the structure, function, and makeup of biologically important molecules

**Molecular farming**    The development of transgenic animals to produce human proteins for medical use

**Molecular genetics**    The study of macromolecules important in biological inheritance

**Molecular medicine**    The treatment of injury or disease at the molecular level. Examples include the use of DNA-based diagnostic tests or medicine derived from DNA sequence information

**Monogenic disorder** A disorder caused by mutation of a single gene. *See also* mutation, polygenic disorder

**Monogenic inheritance** *See* monogenic disorder

**Monosomy** Possessing only one copy of a particular chromosome instead of the normal two copies. *See also* cell, chromosome, gene expression, trisomy

**Morbid map** A diagram showing the chromosomal location of genes associated with disease

**Mouse model** *See* model organisms

**Multifactorial or multigenic disorder** *See* polygenic disorder

**Multiplexing** A laboratory approach that performs multiple sets of reactions in parallel (simultaneously); greatly increasing speed and throughput

**Murine** Organism in the genus Mus. A rat or mouse

**Mutagen** An agent that causes a permanent genetic change in a cell. Does not include changes occurring during normal genetic recombination

**Mutagenicity** The capacity of a chemical or physical agent to cause permanent genetic alterations. *See also* somatic cell genetic mutation

**Mutation** Any heritable change in DNA sequence. *See also* polymorphism

**Nitrogenous base** A nitrogen-containing molecule having the chemical properties of a base. DNA contains the nitrogenous bases adenine (A), guanine (G), cytosine (C), and thymine (T). *See also* DNA

**Northern blot** A gel-based laboratory procedure that locates mRNA sequences on a gel that are complementary to a piece of DNA used as a probe. *See also* DNA, library

**Nuclear transfer** A laboratory procedure in which a cell's nucleus is removed and placed into an oocyte with its own nucleus removed so the genetic information from the donor nucleus controls the resulting cell. Such cells can be induced to form embryos. This process was used to create the cloned sheep 'Dolly'. *See also* cloning

**Nucleic acid** A large molecule composed of nucleotide subunits. *See also* DNA

**Nucleolar organizing region** A part of the chromosome containing rRNA genes

**Nucleotide** A subunit of DNA or RNA consisting of a nitrogenous base (adenine, guanine, thymine, or cytosine in DNA; adenine, guanine, uracil, or cytosine in RNA), a phosphate molecule, and a sugar molecule (deoxyribose in DNA and ribose in RNA). Thousands of nucleotides are linked to form a DNA or RNA molecule. *See also* DNA, base pair, RNA

**Nucleus** The cellular organelle in eukaryotes that contains most of the genetic material

**Oligo** *See* oligonucleotide

**Oligogenic** A phenotypic trait produced by two or more genes working together. *See also* polygenic disorder

**Oligonucleotide** A molecule usually composed of 25 or fewer nucleotides; used as a DNA synthesis primer. *See also* nucleotide

**Oncogene** A gene, one or more forms of which is associated with cancer. Many oncogenes are involved, directly or indirectly, in controlling the rate of cell growth

**Open reading frame** (ORF) The sequence of DNA or RNA located between the start-code sequence (initiation codon) and the stop-code sequence (termination codon)

**Operon** A set of genes transcribed under the control of an operator gene

**Overlapping clones** *See* genomic library

**P1-derived artificial chromosome** (PAC) One type of vector used to clone DNA fragments (100- to 300-kb insert size; average, 150 kb) in *Escherichia coli* cells. Based on bacteriophage (a virus) P1 genome. *See also* cloning vector

**Patent** In genetics, conferring the right or title to genes, gene variations, or identifiable portions of sequenced genetic material to an individual or organization. *See also* gene

**Pedigree** A family tree diagram that shows how a particular genetic trait or disease has been inherited. *See also* inherit

**Penetrance** The probability of a gene or genetic trait being expressed. 'Complete' penetrance means the gene or genes for a trait are expressed in all the population who have the genes. 'Incomplete' penetrance means the genetic trait is expressed in only part of the population. The percent penetrance also may change with the age range of the population

**Peptide** Two or more amino acids joined by a bond called a 'peptide bond.' *See also* polypeptide

**Phage** A virus for which the natural host is a bacterial cell

**Pharmacogenomics** The study of the interaction of an individual's genetic makeup and response to a drug

**Phenocopy** A trait not caused by inheritance of a gene but appears to be identical to a genetic trait

**Phenotype** The physical characteristics of an organism or the presence of a disease that may or may not be genetic. *See also* genotype

**Physical map** A map of the locations of identifiable landmarks on DNA (e.g., restriction-enzyme cutting sites, genes), regardless of inheritance. Distance is measured in base pairs. For the human genome, the lowest-resolution physical map is the banding patterns on the 24 different chromosomes; the highest-resolution map is the complete nucleotide sequence of the chromosomes

**Plasmid**   Autonomously replicating extra-chromosomal circular DNA molecules, distinct from the normal bacterial genome and nonessential for cell survival under nonselective conditions. Some plasmids are capable of integrating into the host genome. A number of artificially constructed plasmids are used as cloning vectors

**Pleiotropy**   One gene that causes many different physical traits such as multiple disease symptoms

**Pluripotency**   The potential of a cell to develop into more than one type of mature cell, depending on environment

**Polygenic disorder**   Genetic disorder resulting from the combined action of alleles of more than one gene (e.g., heart disease, diabetes, and some cancers). Although such disorders are inherited, they depend on the simultaneous presence of several alleles; thus the hereditary patterns usually are more complex than those of single-gene disorders. *See also* single-gene disorder

**Polymerase chain reaction** (PCR)   A method for amplifying a DNA base sequence using a heat-stable polymerase and two oligonucleotide primers, one complementary to the (+) strand at one end of the sequence to be amplified and one complementary to the (−) strand at the other end. Because the newly synthesized DNA strands can subsequently serve as additional templates for the same primer sequences, successive rounds of primer annealing, strand elongation, and dissociation produce rapid and highly specific amplification of the desired sequence. PCR also can be used to detect the existence of the defined sequence in a DNA sample

**Polymerase, DNA or RNA**   Enzyme that catalyzes the synthesis of nucleic acids on preexisting nucleic acid templates, assembling RNA from ribonucleotides or DNA from deoxyribonucleotides

**Polymorphism**   Difference in DNA sequence among individuals that may underlie differences in health. Genetic variations occurring in more than 1 percent of a population would be considered useful polymorphisms for genetic linkage analysis. *See also* mutation

**Polypeptide**   A protein or part of a protein made of a chain of amino acids joined by a peptide bond

**Population genetics**   The study of variation in genes among a group of individuals

**Positional cloning**   A technique used to identify genes, usually those that are associated with diseases, based on their location on a chromosome

**Premature chromosome condensation** (PCC)   A method of studying chromosomes in the interphase stage of the cell cycle

**Primer**   Short preexisting polynucleotide chain to which new deoxyribonucleotides can be added by DNA polymerase

**Privacy**   In genetics, the right of people to restrict access to their genetic information

**Probe**   Single-stranded DNA or RNA molecules of specific base sequence, labeled either radioactively or immunologically, that are used to detect the complementary base sequence by hybridization

**Prokaryote**   Cell or organism lacking a membrane-bound, structurally discrete nucleus and other subcellular compartments. Bacteria are examples of prokaryotes. *See also* chromosome, eukaryote

**Promoter**   A DNA site to which RNA polymerase will bind and initiate transcription

**Pronucleus**   The nucleus of a sperm or egg prior to fertilization. *See also* nucleus, transgenic

**Protein**   A large molecule composed of one or more chains of amino acids in a specific order; the order is determined by the base sequence of nucleotides in the gene that codes for the protein. Proteins are required for the structure, function, and regulation of the body's cells, tissues, and organs; and each protein has unique functions. Examples are hormones, enzymes, and antibodies

**Proteome**   Proteins expressed by a cell or organ at a particular time and under specific conditions

**Proteomics**   The study of the full set of proteins encoded by a genome

**Pseudogene**   A sequence of DNA similar to a gene but nonfunctional; probably the remnant of a once-functional gene that accumulated mutations

**Purine**   A nitrogen-containing, double-ring, basic compound that occurs in nucleic acids. The purines in DNA and RNA are adenine and guanine. *See also* base pair

**Pyrimidine**   A nitrogen-containing, single-ring, basic compound that occurs in nucleic acids. The pyrimidines in DNA are cytosine and thymine; in RNA, cytosine and uracil. *See also* base pair

**Radiation hybrid**   A hybrid cell containing small fragments of irradiated human chromosomes. Maps of irradiation sites on chromosomes for the human, rat, mouse, and other genomes provide important markers, allowing the construction of very precise STS maps indispensable to studying multifactorial diseases. *See also* sequence tagged site

**Rare-cutter enzyme**   *See* restriction-enzyme cutting site

**Recessive gene**   A gene which will be expressed only if there are two identical copies or, for a male, if one copy is present on the X chromosome

**Reciprocal translocation**   When a pair of chromosomes exchange exactly the same length and area of DNA. Results in a shuffling of genes

**Recombinant clone**   Clone containing recombinant DNA molecules. *See also* recombinant DNA technology

**Recombinant DNA molecules**   A combination of DNA molecules of different origin that are joined using recombinant DNA technologies

**Recombinant DNA technology**   Procedure used to join together DNA segments in a cell-free system (an environment outside a cell or organism). Under appropriate conditions, a recombinant DNA molecule can enter a cell and replicate there, either autonomously or after it has become integrated into a cellular chromosome

**Recombination**   The process by which progeny derive a combination of genes different from that of either parent. In higher organisms, this can occur by crossing over. *See also* crossing over, mutation

**Regulatory region or sequence**   A DNA base sequence that controls gene expression

**Repetitive DNA**   Sequences of varying lengths that occur in multiple copies in the genome; it represents much of the human genome

**Reporter gene**   *See* marker

**Resolution**   Degree of molecular detail on a physical map of DNA, ranging from low to high

**Restriction enzyme, endonuclease**   A protein that recognizes specific, short nucleotide sequences and cuts DNA at those sites. Bacteria contain over 400 such enzymes that recognize and cut more than 100 different DNA sequences. *See also* restriction enzyme cutting site

**Restriction fragment length polymorphism**   (RFLP) Variation between individuals in DNA fragment sizes cut by specific restriction enzymes; polymorphic sequences that result in RFLPs are used as markers on both physical maps and genetic linkage maps. RFLPs usually are caused by mutation at a cutting site. *See also* marker, polymorphism

**Restriction-enzyme cutting site**   A specific nucleotide sequence of DNA at which a particular restriction enzyme cuts the DNA. Some sites occur frequently in DNA (e.g., every several hundred base pairs); others much less frequently (rare-cutter; e.g., every 10 000 base pairs)

**Retroviral infection**   The presence of retroviral vectors, such as some viruses, which use their recombinant DNA to insert their genetic material into the chromosomes of the host's cells. The virus is then propogated by the host cell

**Reverse transcriptase**   An enzyme used by retroviruses to form a complementary DNA sequence (cDNA) from their RNA. The resulting DNA is then inserted into the chromosome of the host cell

**Ribonucleotide**   *See* nucleotide

**Ribose**   The five-carbon sugar that serves as a component of RNA. *See also* ribonucleic acid, deoxyribose

**Ribosomal RNA** (rRNA)   A class of RNA found in the ribosomes of cells

**Ribosomes**   Small cellular components composed of specialized ribosomal RNA and protein; site of protein synthesis. *See also* RNA

**Risk communication**   In genetics, a process in which a genetic counselor or other medical professional interprets genetic test results and advises patients of the consequences for them and their offspring

**RNA** (Ribonucleic acid)   A chemical found in the nucleus and cytoplasm of cells; it plays an important role in protein synthesis and other chemical activities of the cell. The structure of RNA is similar to that of DNA. There are several classes of RNA molecules, including messenger RNA, transfer RNA, ribosomal RNA, and other small RNAs, each serving a different purpose

**Sanger sequencing**   A widely used method of determining the order of bases in DNA. *See also* sequencing, shotgun sequencing

**Satellite**   A chromosomal segment that branches off from the rest of the chromosome but is still connected by a thin filament or stalk

**Scaffold**   In genomic mapping, a series of contigs that are in the right order but not necessarily connected in one continuous stretch of sequence

**Segregation**   The normal biological process whereby the two pieces of a chromosome pair are separated during meiosis and randomly distributed to the germ cells

**Sequence**   *See* base sequence

**Sequence assembly**   A process whereby the order of multiple sequenced DNA fragments is determined

**Sequence tagged site** (STS)   Short (200 to 500 base pairs) DNA sequence that has a single occurrence in the human genome and whose location and base sequence are known. Detectable by polymerase chain reaction, STSs are useful for localizing and orienting the mapping and sequence data reported from many different laboratories and serve as landmarks on the developing physical map of the human genome. Expressed sequence tags (ESTs) are STSs derived from cDNAs

**Sequencing**   Determination of the order of nucleotides (base sequences) in a DNA or RNA molecule or the order of amino acids in a protein

**Sequencing technology**    The instrumentation and procedures used to determine the order of nucleotides in DNA

**Sex chromosome**    The X or Y chromosome in human beings that determines the sex of an individual. Females have two X chromosomes in diploid cells; males have an X and a Y chromosome. The sex chromosomes comprise the 23rd chromosome pair in a karyotype. *See also* autosome

**Sex-linked**    Traits or diseases associated with the X or Y chromosome; generally seen in males. *See also* gene, mutation, sex chromosome

**Shotgun method**    Sequencing method that involves randomly sequenced cloned pieces of the genome, with no foreknowledge of where the piece originally came from. This can be contrasted with 'directed' strategies, in which pieces of DNA from known chromosomal locations are sequenced. Because there are advantages to both strategies, researchers use both random (or shotgun) and directed strategies in combination to sequence the human genome. *See also* library, genomic library

**Single nucleotide polymorphism** (SNP)    DNA sequence variations that occur when a single nucleotide (A, T, C, or G) in the genome sequence is altered. *See also* mutation, polymorphism, single-gene disorder

**Single-gene disorder**    Hereditary disorder caused by a mutant allele of a single gene (e.g., Duchenne muscular dystrophy, retinoblastoma, sickle cell disease). *See also* polygenic disorders

**Somatic cell**    Any cell in the body except gametes and their precursors. *See also* gamete

**Somatic cell gene therapy**    Incorporating new genetic material into cells for therapeutic purposes. The new genetic material cannot be passed to offspring. *See also* gene therapy

**Somatic cell genetic mutation**    A change in the genetic structure that is neither inherited nor passed to offspring. Also called acquired mutations. *See also* germ line genetic mutation

**Southern blotting**    Transfer by absorption of DNA fragments separated in electrophoretic gels to membrane filters for detection of specific base sequences by radiolabeled complementary probes

**Spectral karyotype** (SKY)    A graphic of all an organism's chromosomes, each labeled with a different color. Useful for identifying chromosomal abnormalities. *See also* chromosome

**Splice site**    Location in the DNA sequence where RNA removes the noncoding areas to form a continuous gene transcript for translation into a protein

**Sporadic cancer**    Cancer that occurs randomly and is not inherited from parents. Caused by DNA changes in one cell that grows and divides, spreading throughout the body. *See also* hereditary cancer

**Stem cell**    Undifferentiated, primitive cells in the bone marrow that have the ability both to multiply and to differentiate into specific blood cells

**Structural genomics**    The effort to determine the 3D structures of large numbers of proteins using both experimental techniques and computer simulation

**Substitution**    In genetics, a type of mutation due to replacement of one nucleotide in a DNA sequence by another nucleotide or replacement of one amino acid in a protein by another amino acid. *See also* mutation

**Suppressor gene**    A gene that can suppress the action of another gene

**Syndrome**    The group or recognizable pattern of symptoms or abnormalities that indicate a particular trait or disease

**Syngeneic**    Genetically identical members of the same species

**Synteny**    Genes occurring in the same order on chromosomes of different species. *See also* linkage, conserved sequence

**Tandem repeat sequences**    Multiple copies of the same base sequence on a chromosome; used as markers in physical mapping. *See also* physical map

**Targeted mutagenesis**    Deliberate change in the genetic structure directed at a specific site on the chromosome. Used in research to determine the targeted region's function. *See also* mutation, polymorphism

**Technology transfer**    The process of transferring scientific findings from research laboratories to the commercial sector

**Telomerase**    The enzyme that directs the replication of telomeres

**Telomere**    The end of a chromosome. This specialized structure is involved in the replication and stability of linear DNA molecules. *See also* DNA replication

**Teratogenic**    Substances such as chemicals or radiation that cause abnormal development of a embryo. *See also* mutatgen

**Thymine** (T)    A nitrogenous base, one member of the base pair AT (adenine-thymine). *See also* base pair, nucleotide

**Toxicogenomics**    The study of how genomes respond to environmental stressors or toxicants. Combines genome-wide mRNA expression profiling with protein expression patterns using bioinformatics to understand the role of gene-environment interactions in disease and dysfunction

**Transcription**    The synthesis of an RNA copy from a sequence of DNA (a gene); the first step in gene expression. *See also* translation

**Transcription factor** A protein that binds to regulatory regions and helps control gene expression

**Transcriptome** The full complement of activated genes, mRNAs, or transcripts in a particular tissue at a particular time

**Transfection** The introduction of foreign DNA into a host cell. *See also* cloning vector, gene therapy

**Transfer RNA** (tRNA) A class of RNA having structures with triplet nucleotide sequences that are complementary to the triplet nucleotide coding sequences of mRNA. The role of tRNAs in protein synthesis is to bond with amino acids and transfer them to the ribosomes, where proteins are assembled according to the genetic code carried by mRNA

**Transformation** A process by which the genetic material carried by an individual cell is altered by incorporation of exogenous DNA into its genome

**Transgenic** An experimentally produced organism in which DNA has been artificially introduced and incorporated into the organism's germ line. *See also* cell, DNA, gene, nucleus, germ line

**Translation** The process in which the genetic code carried by mRNA directs the synthesis of proteins from amino acids. *See also* transcription

**Translocation** A mutation in which a large segment of one chromosome breaks off and attaches to another chromosome. *See also* mutation

**Transposable element** A class of DNA sequences that can move from one chromosomal site to another

**Trisomy** Possessing three copies of a particular chromosome instead of the normal two copies. *See also* cell, gene, gene expression, chromosome

**Uracil** A nitrogenous base normally found in RNA but not DNA; uracil is capable of forming a base pair with adenine. *See also* base pair, nucleotide

**Vector** *See* cloning vector

**Virus** A noncellular biological entity that can reproduce only within a host cell. Viruses consist of nucleic acid covered by protein; some animal viruses are also surrounded by membrane. Inside the infected cell, the virus uses the synthetic capability of the host to produce progeny virus. *See also* cloning vector

**Western blot** A technique used to identify and locate proteins based on their ability to bind to specific antibodies. *See also* DNA, Northern blot, protein, RNA, Southern blotting

**Wild type** The form of an organism that occurs most frequently in nature

**Working Draft DNA Sequence** *See* Draft DNA Sequence

**X chromosome** One of the two sex chromosomes, X and Y. *See also* Y chromosome, sex chromosome

**Xenograft** Tissue or organs from an individual of one species transplanted into or grafted onto an organism of another species, genus, or family. A common example is the use of pig heart valves in humans

**Y chromosome** One of the two sex chromosomes, X and Y. *See also* X chromosome, sex chromosome

**Yeast artificial chromosome** (YAC) Constructed from yeast DNA, it is a vector used to clone large DNA fragments. *See also* cloning vector, cosmid

**Zinc-finger protein** A secondary feature of some proteins containing a zinc atom; a DNA-binding protein

# Index

Abbreviations: BMP/BMPR, bone morphogenetic protein/bone morphogenetic protein receptor; CF, cystic fibrosis; COPD, chronic obstructive lung disease; incl., including; SP, surfactant protein. Page numbers in bold indicate glossary references.